COMPREHENSIVE GERIATRIC ONCOLOGY

COMPREHENSIVE GERIATRIC ONCOLOGY

Edited by

Lodovico Balducci

H. Lee Moffitt Cancer Center & Research Institute
Florida, USA

Gary H. Lyman

H. Lee Moffitt Cancer Center & Research Institute
Florida, USA

and

William B. Ershler

Gerontology Research Center, National Institute on Aging,
Baltimore, Maryland, USA

harwood academic publishers
Australia • Canada • China • France • Germany • India
Japan • Luxembourg • Malaysia • The Netherlands • Russia
Singapore • Switzerland • Thailand • United Kingdom

Amsteldijk 166
1st Floor
1079 LH Amsterdam
The Netherlands

British Library Cataloguing in Publication Data

A catalogue record for this book is available from the British Library.

ISBN 90-5702-225-7 (hard cover)

CONTENTS

PART VIII   REHABILITATION AND SUPPORTIVE CARE

INTRODUCTION

Management of cancer in the older-aged person is an increasingly common problem. The issues of geriatric oncology are as complicated and elusive as the definition of aging, a highly individualized process involving changes in physical, cognitive, emotional, social and economic domains. In epidemiological studies the changes of aging have been well recognized as restricted physiologic reserve, higher prevalence of comorbidity, diminished and delayed processing of new information, enhanced susceptibility to depression, limited social support, decreased financial resources, and confinement. However, the occurrence, the severity of the interactions, and the overall impact of these changes in the individual person are not predictable from one's chronologic age.

Despite the inability to establish certain chronologic boundaries of senescence, that has handicapped the study of the interactions of aging and disease, in 1992 we endeavored to publish the first treatise of geriatric oncology. Our effort was inspired and supported by the conviction that cancer in older persons may be considered a different disease from cancer in the younger persons, that the biology of the aged tumor host influenced the growth of cancer, that the management of cancer in the older person deserved an individualized approach in terms of prevention and treatment, and that medical decisions involving the older person with cancer involved the knowledge and the awareness of the multidimensional changes of age. This view, which was then a minority view, has been largely vindicated by recent molecular and epidemiologic discoveries, and by recent approaches to cancer treatment. Just to quote a few examples, age is today a well recognized negative prognostic factor for large cell lymphoma and for ovarian cancer, the prevalence of multidrug resistance in leukemic myeloblasts in persons aged 60 and over was found to be as high as 57% (versus 17% in younger patients), and a number of treatment protocols aimed at older persons with special forms of cancer, such as non-Hodgkin's lymphoma and breast cancer, have been developed. In the introduction to a previous publication we stated that the characteristics of aging are influenced by evolving cultural and environmental factors. Accordingly, we proposed to lay the foundation for a continuing discourse on aging and cancer. We believe the time is ripe for reframing and restating our original propositions in the light of the information accumulated during the last five years.

Unquestionably, the issues of cancer and aging have elicited more interest during the past five years than ever before: for example, all major cooperative oncology groups both in the USA and in Europe have included committees devoted to the issues of aging, three international conferences devoted to cancer and age, with multinational support, have been held at biennial intervals in Argentina, Italy and the USA; the National Institute on Aging has issued a RFA for the study of breast cancer in the older woman, and the number of scientific articles, communications, and reviews concerning management of cancer in the older person have increased dramatically. At the same time, the spectacular advances in molecular biology have shed unexpected light on the interactions of aging and cancer. The flourishing of these diverse activities has yielded a host of new information that will deeply affect the approach to the older person with cancer.

Our previous publication highlighted a number of areas where interactions of aging and cancer appeared likely. This book addresses the major areas of cancer biology, cancer prevention and cancer treatment in the light of newly acquired knowledge. Among the major additions to our new book we would like to underline an international epidemiological perspective, an analysis of age-related molecular and immunologic changes, a review of the physiology of aging, an 'in depth' analysis of chemoprevention, a guide to the assessment of life-expectancy, comorbidity, and quality of life, new advances in the use of anesthesia in the older person with cancer, and an examination of gastrointestinal and thoracic malignancies in older individuals. In addition, the issues of surgery, chemotherapy, radiotherapy and nutrition, as well as the chapters related to screening, decision analysis, supportive management, nursing issues, breast cancer, lymphomas and multiple myeloma, have been expanded to accommodate new knowledge and new problems.

The aim of this book is threefold. First and foremost, we wish to assist the practitioner in delivering the best possible cancer care to older patients. For this purpose, we provide an extensive review of current information on the effects of age on tolerance of antineoplastic treatments, such as surgery, radiation therapy, cytotoxic chemotherapy, hormonal and biologic therapy and we explore the role of novel interventions, such as bone marrow transplantation, administration of hemopoietic growth factors and endoscopic surgery. We also take a close look at the management of common malignancies in the elderly and we examine the influence of age on treatment choice. A painstaking analysis of major clinical trials is included, whenever possible, to identify data pertinent to older patients. Frequently, when cancer occurs in the very old, supportive care is the most appropriate form of management. Accordingly, we study supportive care of the older-aged person with cancer, focusing on symptom management, rehabilitation, quality of life assessment, and support structures. Information on patients, disease, and treatment has been prefaced by a chapter devoted to decision analysis. We feel that decision analysis represents a valuable clinical tool to plan the most favorable course of action in complex clinical situations, such as those involving elderly cancer patients. The clinical aspects of these situations present the practitioner with complex and often competing forces. Familiarity with decision analysis may guide the practitioner toward the management strategy associated with optimal outcome and may aid health policy decisions in the cost effective utilization of limited resources.

Second, we wish to promote cancer prevention in the older-aged person. The incidence of most malignancies increases with age and, therefore, the elderly represent an ideal target for both secondary and tertiary prevention of cancer. Secondary prevention involves reversal of late carcinogenic stages, while tertiary prevention is achievable through screening asymptomatic persons for early cancer. For this reason we will illustrate the biological basis of increased cancer risk with aging, we entertain pharmacologic interventions that may lessen the risk of cancer and we review the results of clinical trials exploring early detection of common cancers in older persons. The data on cervical cancer may represent the first direct demonstration of the life-saving effect of screening in older persons. As in the case of cancer management, decision analysis may direct the institution of the safest and most cost-effective preventative strategy in individual situations.

Third, we wish to highlight emerging issues of geriatric oncology and present a research agenda for geriatric cancer in the older person. We believe that care delivery to the older-aged person with cancer is an area of major controversy and that this issue should be studied directly in the community where the elderly patient receives care. For this purpose, practitioners of oncology and of geriatrics should be ready to participate in community-based clinical trials that will embrace the data provided in this or similar volumes in the future.

This book is directed primarily at the practicing oncologist. For this reason, the general principles of cancer treatment and the standard management of specific diseases were streamlined. We hope, however, that the book may also appeal to general surgeons, geriatricians and health professionals who provide primary care to elderly patients. It is possible that biologists may find in this book a rapid and exhaustive review of molecular and cellular interactions of aging and cancer, behavioral and social scientists may find a comprehensive outline of emotional and social problems of the older cancer patients, and clinical epidemiologists and health care planners may find important information related to the incidence of cancer in older patients and cancer care delivery to the older patients around the world. We hope to entice practitioners of various specialities and scientists of different disciplines to reflect on the multidimensional nature of aging and to work together to enhance our understanding of this important subject.

The future of this book depends upon the feedback we receive from our interested readership. We do not know of any other clinical area which depends on the contribution of different disciplines and on the input from clinical practice to a higher degree than geriatric oncology.

CONTRIBUTORS

Vladimir N. Anisimov, MD, DSc
Chief, Laboratory of Experimental Tumors
N.N. Petrov Research Institute of Oncology
St. Petersburg, Russia

Scott J. Antonia, MD
Assistant Professor
University of South Florida College of Medicine
Department of Medical Oncology/Hematology
H. Lee Moffitt Cancer Center & Research Institute
Tampa, Florida, USA

Paul Baekey, MD
Associate Professor of Pathology
Pathology Chair
Breast Program
H. Lee Moffitt Cancer Center
Tampa, Florida, USA

Marion R.S. Bain, MB, ChB
Consultant in Public Health Medicine
Scottish Cancer Registry
Scottish Health Service
Edinburgh, UK

Lodovico Balducci, MD
Professor of Medicine
University of South Florida College of Medicine
Program Leader, Senior Adult Oncology Program
H. Lee Moffitt Cancer Center & Research Institute
Tampa, Florida, USA

Oscar F. Ballester, MD
Assistant Professor of Medicine
Division of Bone Marrow Transplantation
University of South Florida College of Medicine
Tampa, Florida, USA

Joan A. Balmes
Assistant Director
Interdisciplinary Team Training in Geriatrics
James A. Haley Veterans' Hospital
Tampa, Florida, USA

Patricia P. Barry, MD
Associate Professor of Internal Medicine
Chief of Geriatrics Section
Boston University
Boston, Massachusetts, USA

Gianni Berretta, MD
Professor of Chemotherapy
Chief, Medical Oncology
Geriatric and Rehabilitation Department
Trivulzio Institute
Milan, Italy

Karen Smith Blesch, RN, PhD
Hoffman LaRoche, Inc.
Nutley, New Jersey, USA

Patrick G. Brady, MD
Professor of Medicine
Department of Internal Medicine
University of South Florida College of Medicine
Tampa, Florida, USA

Thomas Büchner, MD
Professor of Medicine and Hematology
Head, Leukemia Research Section
Department of Internal Medicine
University Hospital
Munster, Germany

Edith A. Burns, MD
Assistant Professor of Medicine
Section of Geriatrics
Sinai Samaritan Medical Center
Milwaukee, Wisconsin, USA

Antonino Carbone
Division of Medical Oncology
Centro di Riferimento Oncologico Istituto Nazionale
    Centroeuropeo
Aviano, Italy

J.F. Cleary, MD
University of Wisconsin Comprehensive Cancer
    Center
Madison, Wisconsin, USA

Mary E. Corcoran, RPh, CRPh
Clinical Pharmacist
H. Lee Moffitt Cancer Center and Research Institute
Tampa, Florida, USA

Claudia Corrado, MD
Attending Physician
National Academy of Medicine
Buenos Aires, Argentina

Mary E. Costanza, MD
Professor of Medicine
University of Massachusetts Medical School Cancer
    Center
Worcester, Massachusetts, USA

Dario Cova, MD
European Institute of Oncology
Milan, Italy

Charles E. Cox, MD
Professor
University of South Florida College of Medicine
Breast Program
H. Lee Moffitt Cancer Center and Research Institute
Tampa, Florida, USA

Maria Grazia Daidone, PhD
Experimental Oncology C
National Cancer Institute
Milan, Italy

Giovanni Di Fronzo, PhD
Centro di Studio della Patologia Cellulare
Consiglio Nazionale delle Ricerche
Milan, Italy

Dario Dini, MD
Head of the Division of Cancer Rehabilation
National Cancer Research Institute
Genoa, Italy

Edmund H. Duthie, Jr, MD
Professor of Medicine
Chief, Division of Geriatrics/Gerontology
Medical College of Wisconsin
VA Medical Center Milwaukee
Milwaukee, Wisconsin, USA

John R. Eckardt, MD
Director, Clinical Research Program
Division of Hematology/Oncology
St. John's Mercy Medical Center
St. Louis, Missouri, USA

Kathryn L. Edmiston, MD
Associate Professor of Medicine
University of Massachusetts Medical School Cancer
   Center
Worcester, Massachusetts, USA

Laurie A. Ehrbar, BA
Department of Psychology
University of South Florida
Tampa, Florida, USA

Albert B. Einstein, MD
Professor, Department of Internal Medicine
University of South Florida College of Medicine
Tampa, Florida, USA

Gerald J. Elfenbein, MD, FACP
Professor, Department of Internal Medicine
University of South Florida College of Medicine
Tampa, Florida, USA

James N. Endicott, MD
Professor of Surgery
Division of Otolaryngology
University of South Florida College of Medicine
Tampa, Florida, USA

William B. Ershler, MD
John Franklin Professor of Medicine
Glennan Center for Geriatrics and Gerontology
Norfolk, Virginia, USA

Martine Extermann, MD
Instructor
University of South Florida College of Medicine
H. Lee Moffitt Cancer Center & Research Institute
Tampa, Florida, USA

Peter J. Fabri, MD
Professor of Surgery and Associate Dean for
   Clinical Affairs
University of South Florida College of Medicine
Tampa, Florida, USA

J. Albert Fernandez-Pol, MD
Department of Medicine, Division of Nuclear
   Medicine
Laboratory of Molecular Oncology and Clinical
   Immunoassay
Veterans Affairs Medical Center
St. Louis, Missouri, USA

Karen K. Fields, MD
Associate Professor of Internal Medicine
Director, Bone Marrow Transplant Program
H. Lee Moffitt Cancer Center and Research Institute
Tampa, Florida, USA

David E. Fisher, MD, PhD
Assistant Professor, Harvard Medical School
Dana Farber Cancer Institute
Boston, Massachusetts, USA

Alexandra Flowers, MD
Coordinator Neuro-Oncology Program
Department of Neurology
Hartford Hospital
Hartford, Connecticut, USA

Sarah Fox, EdD, MPH
Associate Professor of Medicine
University of California, Los Angeles
Senior Behavioural Scientist
RAND Corporation
Santa Monica, California, USA

Jay Friedland, MD
Assistant Professor
Department of Radiology
University of South Florida College of Medicine
Tampa, Florida, USA

Patricia A. Ganz, MD
Professor, Schools of Medicine & Public Health
Director, Cancer Prevention & Control Research
Jonsson Comprehensive Cancer Center
UCLA Schools of Medicine & Public Health
Los Angeles, California, USA

Walter Gianni, MD
Institute of Geriatrics
University "La Sapienza"
Rome, Italy

James S. Goodwin, MD
George and Cynthia Mitchell Distinguished Professor
Director, Sealy Center on Aging
University of Texas Medical Branch
Galveston, Texas, USA

Alberto Gozza, MD
National Cancer Research Institute
Genoa, Italy

Cristina Granetto, MD
Department of Medical Oncology I
National Cancer Research Institute
Genoa, Italy

Harvey Greenberg, MD
Associate Professor
Director of Division of Radiation Oncology
H. Lee Moffitt Cancer Center
Tampa, Florida, USA

John N. Greene, MD
Associate Professor
Division of Infectious Diseases
Department of Internal Medicine
University of South Florida College of Medicine
Tampa, Florida, USA

William E. Haley, PhD
Professor and Chair, Department of Gerontology
Professor, Department of Psychology
University of South Florida
Consulting Psychologist
H. Lee Moffitt Cancer Center & Research Institute
    Tampa, Florida, USA

Jean C. Harvey
Scottish Cancer Registry
Scottish Health Service
Edinburgh, UK

Edward G. Helm, MD
Department of Surgery and LSU Center on Aging
Louisiana State University Medical Center
New Orleans, Louisiana, USA

David Heber, MD, PhD
UCLA Center for Human Nutrition
UCLA School of Medicine
Los Angeles, California, USA

Stephanie B. Hoffman, PhD
Director, Interdisciplinary Team Training in
    Geriatrics
James A. Haley Veterans' Hospital
Tampa, Florida, USA

Frederick F. Holmes, MD, FACP
Edward Hashinger Distinguished Professor
Department of Internal Medicine
The University of Kansas Medical Center
Kansas City, Kansas, USA

Mary M. Horowitz, MD
Professor of Medicine, Scientific Director
IBMTR/ABMTR
Medical College of Wisconsin
Milwaukee, Wisconsin, USA

Jeanne Hudson, RD, LD
Clinical Dietitian
H. Lee Moffitt Cancer Center and Research Institute
Tampa, Florida, USA

S. Michal Jazwinski, PhD
Department of Biochemistry and Molecular Biology
    and LSU Center on Aging
Louisiana State University Medical Center
New Orleans, Louisiana, USA

James C. Jiang, PhD
Department of Biochemistry and Molecular Biology
    and LSU Center on Aging
Louisiana State University Medical Center
New Orleans, Louisiana, USA

Paul Kaesberg, MD
Chairman
Department of Oncology and Hematology
Physicians Plus Medical Group
Madison, Wisconsin, USA

Richard Karl, MD
Chief of Surgery
Program Leader
Gastrointestinal Tumor Program
University of South Florida College of Medicine
H. Lee Moffitt Cancer Center & Research Institute
Tampa, Florida, USA

B.J. Kennedy, MD
Regents Professor of Medicine, Emeritus
Masonic Professor of Oncology, Emeritus
Division of Medical Oncology
University of Minnesota Medical School
Minneapolis, Minnesota, USA

Sangkyu Kim, PhD
Department of Biochemistry and Molecular Biology
    and LSU Center on Aging
Louisiana State University Medical Center
New Orleans, Louisiana, USA

Raynard S. Kingston, MD, PhD
Assistant Professor, Geriatrics
University of California, Los Angeles
Senior Natural Scientist, RAND
Santa Monica, California, USA

Paul A. Kirchman, PhD
Department of Biochemistry and Molecular Biology
    and LSU Center on Aging
Louisiana State University Medical Center
New Orleans, Louisiana, USA

Nicole M. Kuderer
Albert Ludwigs University
Freiburg, Germany

Carlo La Vecchia, MD
Institute of Medical Statistics and Biometrics
University of Milan
Milan, Italy

Fabio Levi, MD
University Institute of Social and Preventitive
    Medicine
Lausanne, Switzerland

Franca Lucchini, MD
University Institute of Social and Preventitive
    Medicine
Lausanne, Switzerland

Antonella Luisi, PhD
Experimental Oncology C
National Cancer Institute
Milan, Italy

Gary H. Lyman, MD, MPH
Professor of Medicine, Epidemiology & Biostatistics
Department of Medical Oncology & Hematology
University of South Florida College of Medicine
H. Lee Moffitt Cancer Center & Research Institute
Tampa, Florida, USA

Rafael Miguel, MD
Associate Professor of Anesthesiology
University of South Florida College of Medicine
Chief of Anesthesiology
H. Lee Moffitt Cancer Center and Research Institute
Tampa, Florida, USA

Susan E. Minton, DO
Division of Medical Oncology and Hematology
Department of Internal Medicine
University of South Florida College of Medicine
High Risk Breast Screening Program
H. Lee Moffitt Cancer Center and Research Institute
Tampa, Florida, USA

Silvio Monfardini, MD
Scientific Director
Istituto Nazionale per lo Studio e la Cura dei Tumori
Naples, Italy

Timothy D. Moon, MD
Department of Surgery, Division of Urology
University of Wisconsin – Madison Medical School
Madison, Wisconsin, USA

Lynn C. Moscinski, MD
Department of Pathology
H. Lee Moffitt Cancer Center and Research Institute
Tampa, Florida, USA

Calum S. Muir, MB, ChB
Scottish Cancer Registry
Scottish Health Service
Edinburgh, UK

Evan Negri, MD
Institute of Pharmacological Research "Mario Negri"
Milan, Italy

Barbara A. Neilan, MD
Associate Professor of Medicine
Allegheny University of the Health Sciences
Allegheny University Hospitals, MCP Division
Philadelphia, Pennsylvania, USA

Janine Overcash, MD
H. Lee Moffitt Cancer Center and Research Institute
Tampa, Florida, USA

Dobromir Pencev, MD
Assistant Professor of Medicine
Department of Internal Medicine
University of South Florida College of Medicine
Tampa, Florida, USA

Thierry Pignon, MD
Department of Radiotherapy
Hopital de la Timone
Marseille, France

Haim Pinkas, MD
Associate Professor of Medicine
Department of Internal Medicine
University of South Florida College of Medicine
Tampa, Florida, USA

Antonio Pinto, MD
Head, The Leukemia Unit
Division of Medical Oncology
Centro di Riferimento Oncologico
Istituto Nazionale di Ricovero e Cura a Carattere
    Scientifico (IRCCS)
Aviano, Italy

Julio Pow-Sang, MD
Associate Professor
Department of Surgery
University of South Florida College of Medicine
Tampa, Florida, USA

Lazzaro Repetto, MD
Department of Medical Oncology I
National Cancer Research Institute
Genoa, Italy

Lynn A. Ries, MS
Cancer Statistics Branch Surveillance Program
Division of Cancer Prevention and Control
National Cancer Institute
Bethesda, Maryland, USA

Cleora S. Roberts, PhD, ACSW
Research Social Worker
H. Lee Moffitt Cancer Center and Research Institute
Tampa, Florida, USA

Lary A. Robinson, MD
Associate Professor
Department of Surgery
H. Lee Moffitt Cancer Center and Research Institute
University of South Florida College of Medicine
Tampa, Florida, USA

Richard G. Roetzheim, MD, MPH
Associate Professor, Family Medicine
University of South Florida College of Medicine
Tampa, Florida, USA

Riccardo Rosso, MD
Department of Medical Oncology I
National Cancer Research Institute
Genoa, Italy

Philip A. Rowlings, MBBS, FRACD, FRCPA
Assistant Professor, Assistant Scientific Director
IBMTR/ABMTR
Medical College of Wisconsin
Milwaukee, Wisconsin, USA

Ivaca Rubelj, MD
Department of Biochemistry and Molecular Biology
Louisiana State University Medical Center
New Orleans, Louisiana, USA

John C. Ruckdeschel, MD
Professor and Center Director
H. Lee Moffitt Cancer Center and Research Institute
University of Florida College of Medicine
Tampa, Florida, USA

Leonardo Santi, MD
Scientific Director
National Cancer Research Institute
Genoa, Italy

Pierre Scalliet, MD, PhD
Professor of Clinical Oncology
University Hospital St Luc – Catholic University of
    Louvain
Brussels, Belgium

Ronald S. Schonwetter, MD
Associate Professor
Division of Geriatric Medicine
Department of Internal Medicine
University of South Florida College of Medicine
Medical Director, Hospice of Hillsborough Inc.
Tampa, Florida, USA

Gail L. Shaw, MD, FACP
Division of Medical Oncology and Hematology
Department of Internal Medicine
University of South Florida College of Medicine
Program Leader, Cancer Prevention and Lifetime
    Cancer Screening Programs
H. Lee Moffitt Cancer Center and Research Institute
Tampa, Florida, USA

Rebecca A. Silliman, MD, PhD
Associate Professor of Medicine and Public Health
Geriatrics Section
Boston University School of Medicine
Boston, Massachusetts, USA

Rosella Silvestrini, PhD
Experimental Oncology C
National Cancer Institute
Milan, Italy

Alexander S.D. Spiers, TD, MD, PhD, FRCPE
Professor of Medicine
University of South Florida College of Medicine
Director, Leukemia & Lymphoma Center
H. Lee Moffitt Cancer Center and Research Institute
Tampa, Florida, USA

Giorgio Stanta, MD
Department of Pathology
University of Trieste
Trieste, Italy

N. Simon Tchekmedyian, MD
Associate Clinical Professor of Medicine
UCLA School of Medicine
Medical Director
Pacific Shores Medical Group
Long Beach, California, USA

Tate Thigpen, MD
Professor of Medicine
Director of the Division of Oncology
Department of Medicine
University of Mississippi School of Medicine
Jackson, Mississippi, USA

Antonella Venturino, MD
Department of Medical Oncology I
National Cancer Research Institute
Genoa, Italy

David H. Vesole, MD, PhD, FACP
Associate Professor of Medicine
Division of Hematology/Oncology
University of Arkansas for Medical Sciences
Little Rock, Arkansas, USA

Daniel D. Von Hoff, MD, FACP
Chief Executive Officer and Director
Institute for Drug Development
Cancer Therapy and Research Center
Clinical Professor Medical Oncology
The University of Texas Health Science Center
San Antonio, Texas, USA

Henry Wagner, MD
Associate Professor
Department of Radiation Oncology
H. Lee Moffitt Cancer Center and Research Institute
University of South Florida College of Medicine
Tampa, Florida, USA

Rosemary Yancik, PhD
Chief, Cancer and Aging Section, Geriatrics
    Program
National Institutes of Health
National Institute on Aging
Bethesda, Maryland, USA

Vittorina Zagonel, MD
Associate Director
Division of Medical Oncology
Centro di Riferimento Oncologico
Istituto Nazionale di Ricovero e Cura a Carattere
    Scientifico (IRCCS)
Aviano, Italy

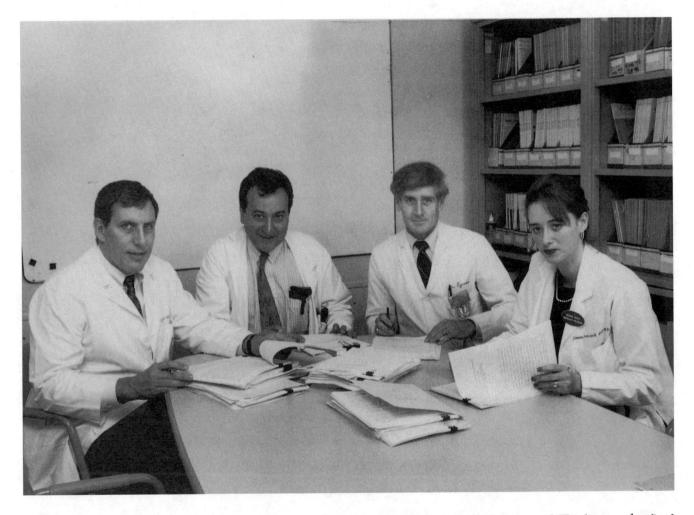

Editors (from left): William B. Ershler, MD, Lodovico Balducci, MD, and Gary H. Lyman, MD, discuss the final preparations of the book with Janine Overcash, ARNP, associate leader of the Senior Adult Oncology Program.

1. Aging and Cancer

B.J. Kennedy

Aging is a normal process of our life span, not a disease. In many countries, the population is aging and older persons are living longer. With aging, the incidence of cancer increases, and our expanding older population makes the prevalence of cancer more apparent. Recent reviews of geriatric oncology have characterized the problem in terms of the volume of patients and the diagnosis and treatment of the older person with cancer (1–6). To meet this challenge, there will be emphasis on physician education in geriatrics, increase in basic and clinical research of cancer in older persons, and adjustment in physician's methods of care of older persons.

Attitudes towards aging are undergoing a major change. Aging has been perceived as the end of life, with older persons having little potential for growth. As a result, efforts for maintenance of health of older persons have been impaired.

To reverse this negative perception, elimination of the terms "senior citizens," "golden age," "elderly," "frail old," "older-old" has been encouraged. The preferred term is "older persons" which specifies no numerical age limit to the aging process with more emphasis on the physiologic status of the patient.

America is growing older (7). The U.S. population over the age of 65 has increased ten-fold since 1900. Today, 31.1 million Americans, one in every eight are over 65 (12.5% of the total U.S. population) compared

Table 1.1 Year and age of baby boomers born between 1945 and 1965 (8).

Year	Age
1975	10–30
1990	25–45
2010	45–65
2030	65–85

Table 1.2 Projected number of persons over age 65 in the United States.

Year	Millions	% of Population
1990	31	12.5
2020	51	17.3
2030	65	21.1

Table 1.3 Average life expectancy.

Year	Length of life
100	22
Middle Ages	33
1900	49
1950	68
1990	75
2050	85

Table 1.4 Remaining years of white female life expectancy (8).

Current Age	Years Remaining
65	18.8
75	11.7
85	6.3

to only one of every fifteen persons in 1930. It is projected that in 2020 one in every five Americans will be over 65 (8).

In 2010 the first wave of "baby boomers" — the 76 million babies born between 1946 and 1965 — will reach 65 (Table 1.1). The predicted increased longevity and increased size of this group will trigger a dramatic growth in the number of persons over 65 (Table 1.2).

The average length of life continues to increase. Life expectancy in the United States has increased by 25 years since the turn of the century (Table 1.3). Life expectancy for white women born today is 85 years and for white men born today it is 77 years (9). More impressive is the number of years remaining for older persons (Table 1.4).

The maximum life span has been projected to be about 120 years. The number of older aged persons is increasing dramatically. Survival to the age of 80 and beyond has increased in many developed countries (10). There are 37,000 persons over age 100 and this is expected to double by 2000. Fifty percent of these live in nursing homes. Those aged 85 and over are the most rapidly growing group having represented 1% of the population in 1982, and projected to represent 2.4% in 2010 and 5% in 2050. Currently 21% of all deaths occur in people over 85 years.

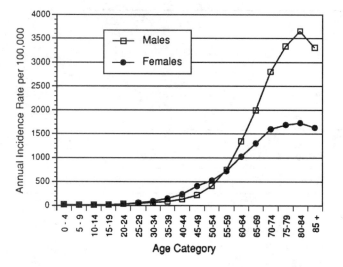

Figure 1.1 Annual age-specific cancer incidence rates.

Progress against infectious diseases during the past 50+ years has made it possible for people to live longer. Yet, because of fatty diets, cigarette smoking, and sedentary life style, coronary heart disease was the number one killer. In the past 20 years, however, the death rate from coronary heart disease has plunged 48% because of the adoption of healthier life styles. With new drugs and treatment strategies the coronary heart disease death rate is predicted to plummet still further this decade. With the decrease in coronary heart disease and vascular diseases, people are living longer, which resulted in a new era of degenerative diseases, including Alzheimer's disease and cancer.

Cancer is a disease primarily of older persons (Figure 1) (9). Over 60% of all cases of cancer are diagnosed after age 65, an age group that constitutes only 12.5% of our current U.S. population. By 2030, 70% of patients with cancer will be over 65. More than 67% of cancer deaths occur in this older group. The risk of persons over 65 years of age developing cancer is 10 times that of those under 65. Up to the age of 50, the incidence of cancer is higher in women. After age 60 there is a remarkable increase in cancer incidence among men.

There are multiple reasons for more cancer in older persons. They have less resistance to carcinogens, longer exposure to carcinogens, decline in immune competence, alteration of anti-tumor defenses, decrease DNA repair, defects in tumor suppressor genes and differences in biologic behavior including such factors as angiogenesis.

Because of the increased incidence and prevalence of cancer in older persons, as well as their higher mortality rate from cancer, it has been implied that no progress has been made in the fight against cancer. The data suggests otherwise (Table 1.5). The higher rate of cure of acute leukemia in children, testis cancer in men, and Hodgkin's disease is responsible for a 23% decrease in cancer mortality in persons under 55 years. However, there has been a 17% increase in cancer mortality in those over 55 years (11).

Table 1.5 U.S. cancer mortality per 100,000 (10).

Age	<55 years	>55 years
1968	43	775
1985	35	905
% change	–23%	+17%

Physiology of Aging

The normal process of aging is associated with a progressive age-related reduction in function of many organs including losses such as renal, pulmonary, immune, cardiac, hematologic, hepatic, muscle, sight, hearing, osseous, and brain functions. Physiologic functions of various organ systems at age 70 may be 50% of those observed at age 30. The volume of the liver decreases and blood flow to the liver decreases about 1% per year with age. A decrease of hepatic clearance and metabolism of drugs by the liver is also apparent.

The most consistent physiologic change of aging is a decline of renal function. With a concomitant decrease in muscle mass, the serum creatinine level remains normal, making the creatinine clearance a more reliable indicator of renal function. It has been clearly shown that nephrotoxicity of cisplatinum does not worsen with advancing age.

Advancing age is associated with a decline in immune competence as suggested by the higher incidence of cancer in older persons and their greater susceptibility to infections. The diminished immune functions reflected by lymphocyte response to stimulation, delayed-type sensitivity, and antibody responses. With the involution of the thymus, T-cell deficiency may be a factor. Furthermore, Interleukin-2 synthesis decreases with age. Mice with restricted caloric intake have a longer life span than those fed *ad libitum*. This prolonged life-span is credited to the preservation of immune function.

The consequences of these changes with age added to co-morbid diseases have profound effects on tolerance to treatments of cancer including those of surgery, radiation therapy and chemotherapy. Although such changes should be taken into consideration when treating older patients for cancer, the use of chronologic age alone should not be used as a guide to cancer prevention or therapy. It is the physiologic performance of the patient that is of prime importance.

Specific Neoplasms

The leading sites for the incidence of cancer for all ages (Table 1.6), differ from the leading sites for cancer mortality in the older persons (Table 1.7). Most elderly patients benefit from thoughtful consideration of specific, comprehensive management plans to cure, control or palliate a cancer. Advanced age is not a contraindication to major surgery providing comorbid

Table 1.6 Estimated leading sites for cancer incidence, 1997, all ages.

Female	Male
Breast	Prostate
Lung	
Colon and Rectum	
Uterus	Urinary bladder
Ovary	Lymphoma

Table 1.7 Leading sites for cancer mortality in persons over 75 years of age.

Female	Male
Lung	Lung
Colon and Rectum	Prostate
Breast	Colon and Rectum
Pancreas	Pancreas
Ovary	Bladder

diseases will not influence the potential mortality. Radiotherapy may be an excellent alternative. Chemotherapy is well tolerated when used with appropriate caution.

Breast

Breast cancer is the most common cancer in women. The incidence increases with age with approximately 48% of all cases occurring in women older than 65 years. Older women are less likely to perform self examination of the breast, have an annual breast examination, or have an annual mammogram. In fact, about two thirds of women over age 65 do not have regular mammograms despite payment by Medicare (12). A greater proportion of older persons has estrogen receptor positive tumors than the younger population, reflecting a biologic difference of this cancer with age. The tumors are more likely to be well differentiated, have lower proliferative rates, and have more favorable histologic types. The approach to definitive therapy in early stages of the disease is comparable to the younger population. In older persons, the chronologic and physiologic differences result in altered hormonal or chemotherapy approaches compared to younger patients in the use of adjuvant therapies or treatment of disseminated disease. The limited data on treatment efficacy in older women with breast cancer and selection bias in clinical trials has resulted in substantial variations in treatments (13). Treatment of the older patient is often influenced by factors other than the medical condition.

Lung

Lung cancer is the leading cause of death from cancer in both sexes over age 75. There is a three-fold greater risk for lung cancer in men over 65 years. Lung cancer is probably not a direct result of the aging process, but reflects the period of time necessary to induce lung cancer from long-term tobacco use. After age 70, the age-specific incidence of lung cancer decreases, which may reflect a decline in smoking habits as people approach age 50. Of course, those who developed lung cancer earlier have already died. There also is a biologic difference in lung cancer in older persons. There is more squamous cell cancer in patients over 70 years of age (71%) than those under 50 years (58%) which may reflect the less advanced stage of the disease in the elderly. Although older persons may have a greater risk of early death after thoracotomy, the likelihood of long-term survival following surgery is not diminished by age alone. Hence, the risk of surgery is well worth the benefit in selected patients. Older patients fare just as well as younger ones with palliative chemotherapy.

Colorectal

Colorectal cancer is the third most common malignancy in the United States, and age is a leading risk factor. Over 90% of cases occur in those over 50 years of age, and the survival rates decrease with age. Unfortunately, the diagnosis of colorectal cancer is made in the late phase of the disease because the elderly are less likely to receive routine health examinations. Stage for stage, surgery or chemotherapy should be employed as in younger persons.

Prostate

Prostate cancer is the most common cancer in American men, and a major cause of death from cancer, second only to lung cancer. After the age of 80 years, 50% of all men may have Stage A1 cancer (not clinically apparent). However, when initially diagnosed nearly 70% of patients will have advanced disease. The introduction of the PSA blood test has resulted in a greater number of patients diagnosed in the earlier phase of the disease. Introduction of free PSA may result in fewer ultrasounds and biopsies. Because prostate cancer is a relatively understudied disease among elderly men, data is lacking on the preferred method of management, especially in those over 75 years of age. The factors of tumor size and histologic grade influence the decision making process. Prostatectomy, radiation therapy, hormonal therapies, or watchful waiting are alternatives to be considered.

Pancreas

The incidence of pancreas cancer is increasing world wide. Because of the aggressiveness of this cancer and its low curability rate, the mortality figures are similar for both sexes. Palliative surgery, radiotherapy for localized disease, or chemotherapy are selectively employed.

Melanoma

The incidence and mortality rate of melanoma are increasing at a faster rate than any other cancer except

Table 1.8 Pap screening for cervical cancer.

Age	% Tested
18–39	81%
40–59	67%
>60	52%

Source: U.S. Center for Disease Control

for lung cancer in women, as is the mortality rate (14). With increasing age, there is an increasing incidence of melanoma. Prolonged sun exposure is a factor. Survival can be substantial for these older patients providing that constraints are not placed on providing curative treatment.

Cervix

Cervical cancer in women over 60 years of age accounts for 24% of new cases and 40% of deaths from this disease. Increasing age is associated with increased stage at time of presentation, yet in regions where the older women have been aggressively screened, their death rates have declined. Less than 50% of women over 65 years of age have been screened for cervical cancer (Table 1.8).

Leukemia

Chronic lymphatic leukemia is one of the principal hematologic neoplastic diseases of older persons, and its incidence may be greater than reported, since its indolent nature may result in its failure to be registered in tumor registries. Treatment is usually initiated when specific signs or symptoms occur. Chemotherapy in persons over 70 years of age is implied to be of benefit.

Nearly 60% of patients with acute myeloid leukemia are older than 60 years of age (14). Treatment in this age group has improved. As each decade passed, the complete remission rate for those surviving treatment has increased (6). The duration of remission and survival time of older responders to therapy are comparable to younger patients. Increasing age is associated with a lower CR rate, slower neutrophil recovery, and longer hospitalizations than younger adults (16).

Hodgkin's Disease

Hodgkin's disease has a bimodal age incidence curve, peaking in the late 20s then declining to age 45, after which the incident increases steadily with age. Age is a major prognostic factor influencing treatment response, duration of response, and survival. In advanced disease, the response rate to chemotherapies was lower in patients over 60 years of age compared with younger persons. In a national pattern of care study, as the age of the patient at diagnosis increased, the survival decreased (17). Analysis revealed that both age and stage, independent of each other, are significant prognostic factors for Hodgkin's disease. There may be biologic differences in patients at advancing age, resulting in a poorer prognosis.

Non-Hodgkin's Lymphoma

The incidence of lymphoma has dramatically increased over the past decade and is expected to continue to rise. The disease presentation is the same in younger and older persons. Stage lll and IV non-Hodgkin's lymphocytic lymphomas have an indolent course and are responsive to chemotherapy, yet do not attain complete remissions (18). Incomplete remission may not require maintenance chemotherapy. A few elderly patients may never require treatment (18). Patients older than 65 years of age have had greater treatment-related toxicity, lower complete response rates, and decreased survival when compared to younger patients. Overall survival is affected by co-morbid conditions (20).

Treatment Considerations

An age bias in the management of cancer has been recognized in a number of studies (6). Attitudes toward aging, rather than scientific facts have affected decisions by physicians. Chronologic age is associated with perceived negative characteristics including poor prognosis, cognitive impairment, decreased quality of life, limited life expectancy, and decreased social worth. Older patients are discriminated against based on chronologic age.

Older age has been associated with less screening for cancer, less staging of diagnosed cancer, less aggressive therapy, or no treatment at all. Fewer older women have had a Pap test for cancer (Table 1.6). Women over 80 have had fewer mammogram screenings for breast cancer, and staging was less vigorous. Because of older patients' impaired physiologic reserve and a fear of excessive operative mortality in older patients with cancer, some physicians have been reluctant to recommend curative major surgical procedures and to favor more conservative treatment, thereby losing the potential curability of cancer by surgery. Study of the outcomes of surgery in patients 90 years of age and older revealed that these extremely old patients fared quite well, and survival at 5 years was comparable to that expected. During the ten year period of study from 1975 through 1985, operative rates increased in this age group (21). Advanced age is not a contraindication to major surgery providing that the presence of co-morbid diseases will not influence the potential mortality. Radiotherapy or chemotherapy is often less aggressive as well, and for some patients, no treatment is administered.

The lack of progress against cancer in older patients may be due to failure to apply standard therapy as fully for them as for younger people. The decision for management of cancer in older persons should be based upon the individual needs of a patient and not based on chronologic age alone.

Clinical Trials

Patients over ages 65 to 70 generally are under represented in cancer treatment trials. Data on cooperative group phase III studies have shown a declining entry in the past five years of patients over 65 years. Age restriction is not a valid eligibility criterion for NCI trials. Possible explanations have been suggested (22). These include: 1) presence of comorbidity, 2) a research focus on aggressive therapy, the toxicity of which is unacceptable to the elderly, 3) fewer trials available aimed at older patients, 4) limited expectations for long term benefit by providers, relatives and patients, 5) lack of financial social, and logistic support for participation in trials. Because of the importance of research on the interaction between chronologic age and chemotherapy effectiveness, older patients should be allowed and encouraged to enroll in clinical trials (5, 21). The apparent discrimination in not treating older patients as aggressively as younger patients, and in excluding older patients from research trials is not justified.

Costs

The rapid growth in the older population and their increased medical care utilization is a major determinant of increasing health care costs in the United States. Medicare expenditures for health care services continue to expand, despite efforts to the contrary. Some of the expanding costs are due to the growing fraction of Medicare providers in specialty fields, the expansion of technologies that are useful to patients, services that became available for conditions that were untreatable 30 years ago and the ever enlarging older population. Currently, there are four working Americans supporting each retiree. In the future, there will be only two per retiree, and there will be fewer sons and daughters to support and care for the older persons. The government will not be able to meet the cost. Hence, plans need to be developed that allow people to save for their own retirement health care needs. As the demand for long-term care facilities increases, long-term care will become the most important health care issue. In the next several decades, geriatric and cancer care will become a significant medical, public health, economic, and social challenge.

Manpower

In the evolution of the subspecialty of Medical Oncology, the initial definition of the subjects of relevance of this subspecialty included gerontology (23). It was perceived that cancer in the aging population would be a major health problem. The number of certified medical oncologists has grown at an awesome rate since 1973, and now is over 6500. Yet a surplus of medical oncologists is not anticipated. By the year 2000, the need for oncology manpower will surpass that for cardiology. Because of the increased number of visits for their therapy, an expanded need for more oncologists must be anticipated to meet the requirements for care of patients with cancer in the early part of the 21st century (24). It is reasonable to assume that primary care physicians will be more responsible for

teaching cancer prevention, emphasizing early cancer detection, and administering some of the standard therapies. Moreover, since many cancers are now cured, the overall healthcare of the patient becomes increasingly important as that patient continues to grow older.

Conclusion

The United States population is growing older. Physicians need to be more familiar with the medical needs of older patients and their greater chance of developing cancer. The importance of geriatric oncology was recognized 25 years ago when the subjects of relevance in medical oncology training were specified. Primary care physicians and oncologists need to be prepared for the impending increase of cancer in older persons.

References

1. Multiple authors. National Conference on Cancer and the Older Person. *Cancer* 1994; **74**: No. 7.
2. Yancik R and Ries LA. Cancer in older persons. *Cancer* 1994; **74**: 1995–2003.
3. Cohen HJ, editor. Cancer l: General aspects, in *Clinics in Geriatric Medicine*. Philadelphia, PA: W.B. Saunders Co., 1987.
4. Holmes FF. Aging and Cancer. *Recent Results in Cancer Research*. Berlin: Springer Verlag, 1983.
5. Kennedy BJ. Specific considerations for the older patient with cancer. In *Medical Oncology*, edited by P Calabresi and PS Schein. New York: McGraw-Hill, Inc., pp. 1219–1230, 1993.
6. Kennedy BJ. Aging and cancer. *J Clin Oncol* 1988; **6**: 1903–1911.
7. Spencer G. Projections of the population of the United States, by age, sex, and race: 1988 to 2080. Washington (DC): U.S. Government Printing Office, 1989. Current Population Reports, Series P-25, no. 1018.
8. Taeuber CM. Sixty-five plus in America. Rev. ed. Washington (PC): U.S. Government Printing Office, 1993. Current Population Reports, Special Studies, pp. 23–178 RV.
9. Kennedy BJ, Bushhouse SA, Bender AP. Minnesota population cancer risk. *Cancer* 1994; **73**: 724–729.
10. Manton KG and Vaupel JW. Survival after the age of 80 in the United States, Sweden, France, England, and Japan. *New England Journal of Medicine* 1995; **333**: 1232–1235.
11. Division of Chronic Disease Control: Years of potential life lost due to cancer — United States, 1968–1985. *JAMA* 1989; **261**: 209.
12. Trontell AE, Franey EW. Use of mammography services by women aged ≥65 years enrolled in Medicare — United States, 1991–1993, *JAMA* 1995; **274**: 1420.
13. Silliman RA, Balducci L, Goodwin JS, Holmes FF, Leventhal EA. Breast cancer care in old age: what we know, don't know, and do. *J Natl Cancer Inst* 1993; **85**: 190–199.
14. Cohen HJ, Cox E, Manton K, and Woodbury M. Malignant melanoma in the elderly. *J Clin Oncol* 1987; **5**: 100–106.
15. Brincker H. Estimates of overall treatment results in acute non-lymphocytic leukemia based on age-specific rates of incidence and of complete remission. *Cancer Treat Rep* 1985; **69**: 5–11.
16. Schiffer CA, McIntyre OR. Age related changes in adults with acute leukemia. In *The Underlying Molecular, Cellular and Immunological Factors in Cancer and Aging*, edited by SS Yang and HR Warner. New York: Plenum Press, pp. 215–229, 1993.
17. Kennedy BJ, Loeb V Jr, Peterson V, Donegan WL, Natarajan N, and Mettlin C. National patterns of care for Hodgkin's disease. *Cancer* 1985; **56**: 2547–2556.
18. Vose JM, Armitage JO, Weisbenburger DD, Bierman PJ, Sorensen S, Hutchins M, Moravec DF, Howe D, Dowling MD, Mailliard J, Johnson PS, Pernick W, Packard WM, Okerbloom J, Thompson RF, Langdon Jr RM, Soori Y, and Peterson C. The importance of age in survival of patients treated with chemotherapy for aggressive non-Hodgkin's lymphoma. *J Clin Oncol* 1988; **6**: 1838–1844.

19. Rosenberg SA. Non-Hodgkin's lymphoma — selection of treatment on the basis of histologic type. *N Engl J Med* 1979; **301**: 924–928.

20. Lichtman SM. Lymphoma in the older patient. *Sem Onc* 1995; **22** (Suppl. 1): 25–28.

21. Hosking MP, Warner MA, Lobdell CM, Offord KP, and Melton III W. Outcomes of surgery in patients 90 years of age and older. *JAMA* 1989; **261**: 1909–1915.

22. Trimble EL, Carter CL, Cain D, Freidlin B, Ungerleider RS, Friedman MA. Representation of older patients in cancer treatment trials. *Cancer* 1994; **74**: 2209–2214.

23. Kennedy BJ, Calabresi P, Carbone P, *et al.* Training program in medial oncology. *Ann Intern Med* 1973; **78**: 127–130.

24. Kennedy BJ. Future Manpower needs in caring for an older cancer-patient population. *J Ca Ed* 1994; **9**:11–13.

2. Essentials of Clinical Decision Analysis: A New Way to Think about Cancer and Aging

Gary H. Lyman

Introduction

Clinical medicine is fundamentally an effort to make decisions in the setting of uncertainty based on a set of facts and a set of rules applied to these facts (1). The knowledge base represents an enormous collection of facts gathered over years of formal education, training and experience in both preclinical and clinical settings. On the other hand, our understanding of how to gather information and evaluate it in order to arrive at correct decisions is obtained in a much less direct manner largely through observation of experienced clinicians and trial and error. It is only in recent years that a discipline of decision analysis has been extended to clinical medicine from other disciplines (2,3).

The factual basis of our clinical knowledge will vary substantially over time and from one setting to another while the rules of reasoning that we use to make decisions based on this information is fundamentally the same regardless of the setting. However, clinical reasoning skills vary greatly from clinician to clinician and from subject to subject (4–6). This chapter discusses the application of these methods and the unique features of cancer in the elderly that should be considered in making clinical decisions.

Essentials of Clinical Decision Making

Decision making in any clinical or public health situation is based on a structuring of the problem, knowledge of the performance of diagnostic tests and therapeutic modalities, and a reasonable understanding of the likelihood and value of various outcomes based on experience or the literature (7,8). Decision making in the elderly patient with cancer requires a specific understanding of the epidemiology and natural history of the disease, as well as the diagnostic, therapeutic, and supportive care strategies available. The value of establishing the diagnosis and/or treating elderly patients with cancer may differ from that in younger patients because of such factors as the greater prevalence of cancer and the limited life expectancy. The value of early diagnosis and responsiveness to systemic therapy may also differ greatly among cancers afflicting the elderly.

Test Performance

As in any testing situation, the major objective of cancer screening and diagnostic testing is to separate those with disease from those without disease. Ideally, positive test results should be seen only in those with disease (true positive) and negative test results should be seen only in those without disease (true negative). However, clinical testing is almost always associated with a certain number of false positive results in those without disease and false negative results in those with disease. The performance of screening and diagnostic tests is assessed on the basis of several measures (see appendix 1) (9–13). The *sensitivity* of a test is the probability of a positive test result in those with the disease. The specificity of a test is the probability of a negative test result in those without the disease. Of greater interest to clinicians, perhaps, are the measures of predictive value. The positive predictive value is the probability of the disease in someone with a positive test. Alternatively, the negative predictive value is the probability of being without disease if the test is negative. The predictive value of a test depends not only on the sensitivity and specificity of the test but also on the prevalence of the disease in those being tested. Prevalence represents the probability of disease in the population at a given time the relationship between test performance, prevalence and the post test probability of disease is described by Bayes' theorem (Appendix 2). Since the incidence and prevalence of cancer increase dramatically with increasing age, the positive predictive value of a screening or diagnostic test increases with increasing age. With increasing disease prevalence, there is a decreasing proportion of false-positive results potentially increasing the diagnostic yield per unit cost (14–16). We have observed that physicians frequently overestimate posttest probabilities particularly when disease prevalence is low in the population (15,16) We have strongly urged that health care professionals should receive formal training in the proper evaluation of test information (16).

Outcome Measures

Patient outcome may be measured in a variety of ways. Outcome measures from clinical trials generally refer to treatment efficacy in terms of survival, time to recurrence, or disease-free survival. Outcome measures applied to the population of diseased individuals define treatment effectiveness. Outcomes may assess both clinical effectiveness and economic cost. Both direct and indirect measures are available. The most common direct measures of outcome effectiveness are survival or life expectancy. The most common direct measures of cost are the actual cost of resources utilized or the charges for services as an approximation of cost. Indirect measures of outcome effectiveness include treatment response, the duration of response or the time to disease recurrence. Measures of indirect cost include lost income from illness and other costs not directly related to the services provided.

A survival function represents the cumulative proportion alive or alive and free of disease (disease-free survival) over time. Survival is directly related to the risk of dying over each unit of time (mortality rate). The survival of a group of individuals may be summarized by various measures such as the median (50th percentile) or the proportion alive at certain time points such as one year or five years. Life expectancy represents the average number of years of life remaining at any given age. In seriously ill patients, including elderly cancer patients, life is relatively short and the mortality rate is approximately constant. When the mortality rate is constant, the relationship between survival and time is described by a declining exponential function. Such an approximation is sufficiently close for most decision making applications. Under the assumption of a declining exponential approximation for life expectancy (DEALE), life expectancy is the inverse of the mortality rate. In addition, the total mortality rate may be considered the sum of the age-specific mortality rate and the mortality rates for any disease(s) (see Appendix 3). In some clinical settings, the mortality rate may vary overtime. In this situation, other models are utilized to estimate life expectancy. When a patient is likely to experience several different health states over time, a Markov model may be utilized. If the transition probabilities of moving from one health state to another over time are known, life expectancy can be estimated. The Markov model assumes that the transition probability to a new health state is determined by the current health state and not previous states. Costs are generally measured in monetary units such as dollars. Marginal costs as well as marginal effectiveness refer to the differences in these measures between two strategies. In a cost benefit analysis, benefits must be converted into the common monetary unit. In a cost-effectiveness analysis, the cost for each unit of added effectiveness over time is calculated; this allows the comparison of different strategies with the same effectiveness measures.

A variety of methods are available to adjust these outcome measures for the impact on quality of life. Patient willingness to pay to achieve effectiveness or to avoid toxicity can be incorporated into a cost-benefit analysis. Utility analysis attempts to adjust the outcome value based on patient perception of quality of life in different outcome states. After ranking possible outcomes and assigning values of 0 and 1 to the outcomes with the lowest and highest quality of life, the intermediate outcomes can be assigned values by means of a standard reference gamble or a time trade off equating the amount of time in good health to a specified period of time in the disease state. Each of these methods of adjustment have limitations in implementation and interpretation. However they do begin to address a dimension of management outcome not adequately considered in the past.

Decision Analysis

A useful decision model requires three elements: a) a structure in the form of a decision tree leading forward from two or more choices at a decision node ($\square$), b) a set of probabilities for each branch in the model leading from a chance node (O) and c) a value for each possible pathway through the model leading up to a terminal node ($\blacksquare$). With each branch that follows a chance event, a probability or probability variable is assigned a baseline value. The baseline value may be derived from the literature or represent an individual best guess. Probabilities must be between 0 and 1 and must add up to 1 for the branches of an given chance node. Outcome measures can be formatted in a variety of ways and often involve either a negative value such as cost or a positive value or effectiveness.

The strategy utilized in decision analysis involves determining the decision choice associated with the greatest expected value (7–11). This can be expressed as the greatest expected effectiveness or the least expected cost or cost/effectiveness. Once baseline probabilities and outcome values have been assigned, each node can be evaluated by multiplying the ultimate outcome value by the probability of each branch and adding the products of the branches from each node together. The expected value, therefore, represents a weighted sum of the expected values of all possible paths where the weights are represented by the probabilities of the various chance events. The resulting expected value is then utilized as the outcome value for the immediately preceding branch. In this fashion, the model is 'folded back' achieving an expected outcome value for each decision choice. The choice associated with the greatest expected value should represent the desired choice for reasonable decision makers. There are times when decisions involve immediate versus delayed effects or costs where reasonable decision makers may differ as to the optimal choice. Confidence limits on the expected value can be estimated if the distribution of the individual probabilities and outcome values are known. Utilizing a Monte Carlo technique, the distribution of expected values can be estimated by sampling the known distributions in the model as the model is evaluated repeatedly.

One of the most powerful features of decision modeling is the ability to conduct a sensitivity analysis. In a simple (one-way) sensitivity analysis, the baseline value of a variable is varied over the range of possible values. As the value of a variable is varied, the expected outcome value of each choice varies forming a functional relationship or curve relating the variable and the expected outcome value from the model. The value of the variable at which the curves associated with two choices intersect represents the threshold were the outcome values for two strategies are equal. The threshold is the value of any variable for which the expected value of any two choices are equal. Above and below the threshold, one or the other choice is favored on the basis of having the greatest expected value. The values of two variables may be varied, simultaneously generating a threshold function. Obviously, any combination of values of the two variables that do not lie on the threshold curve will result in expected values favoring one strategy or the other. Likewise, the value of three variables may be varied simultaneously yielding a family of threshold curves. In theory, any number of variable may be varied simultaneously although such analysis is limited by the ability to conceptualize and graphically depict such relationships.

The application of decision analytic techniques to clinical medicine in general and the management of the elderly cancer patient in particular has many potential benefits. These strategies force the clinician to explicitly state the question being asked, the data and assumptions to be utilized and how these will be analyzed to formulate a decision. Different clinicians utilizing the same data and the same logic should arrive at the same conclusion. The ability to assess the effect of variation in the assumptions on the optimal choice in a sensitivity analysis is a major strength of this approach. These techniques should be most helpful clinically in the most complex cases with the greatest degree of uncertainty. Decision analysis should also be a useful aid to teaching students and resident physicians how to utilize clinical data even relatively early in their clinical experience. Decision analysis may also facilitate research into the process of clinical reasoning. And finally, these techniques may be applied to health outcomes and health policy research and facilitate the development of reasonable clinical practice guidelines for management of the elderly cancer patient.

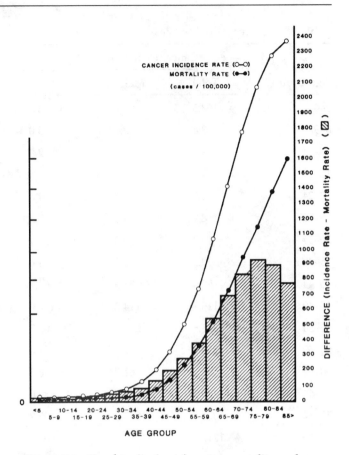

Figure 2.2 Graphic display of cancer mortality and cancer incidence rates for U.S. population by 5-year age group. Cancer mortality in deaths per 100,000 per year is displayed as solid circles. Cancer incidence rates in cases per 100,000 per year are displayed as open circles. The differences in cancer incidence rates and cancer mortality rates by 5-year age group are displayed as vertical bars.

Aging and Cancer

Increasing age represents the single most important risk factor for cancer. As shown in Figure 2.1, the number of cancer deaths in the United States peaks between the ages of 65 and 75 and then decreases due to competing risks for mortality in the declining population at risk. Cancer incidence and mortality rates, however, continue to increase throughout life (Figure 2.2). As shown in Table 2.1, cancer mortality rates increase with age more dramatically for males than for females, with a nearly twofold difference in those over the age of 85 (17).

Cancer incidence and mortality rates have increased considerably over the past several decades in the United States (18,19). Although age-adjusted cancer mortality rates have also increased, most of this increase is attributable to increasing cancer mortality in individuals over the age of 65. Age-specific cancer mortality rates have actually decreased substantially in younger age groups over the past two decades while they have increased in those 65 years of age and over (Table 2.2). Most of the increase in cancer mortality rates in those

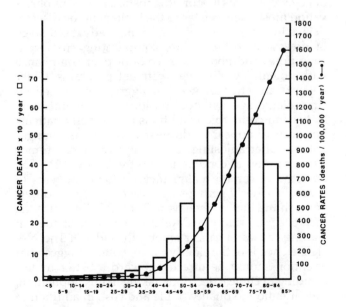

Figure 2.1 Graphic display of cancer mortality and cancer mortality rates for U.S. population by 5-year age group. Cancer mortality in deaths × 10³/year is displayed as vertical bars. Cancer mortality rates in deaths per 100,000 per year are displayed as solid circles.

Table 2.1 Cancer mortality tates.

Age Group	Cancer Deaths/100,000/year		
	Total	Males	Females
0–4	3.5	3.7	3.3
5–9	3.4	3.9	3.0
10–14	3.1	3.5	2.8
15–19	4.3	5.0	3.6
20–24	5.7	6.7	4.6
25–29	8.9	9.6	8.3
30–34	16.2	15.3	17.1
35–39	30.9	27.1	34.6
40–44	59.4	53.9	64.7
45–49	116.7	114.3	119.0
50–54	215.5	229.0	202.7
55–59	357.1	410.7	308.4
60–64	546.1	661.7	446.1
65–69	750.7	949.7	589.0
70–74	1001.4	1333.3	757.7
75–79	1217.9	1712.9	902.2
80–85	1454.1	2161.8	1080.8
85+	1682.7	2585.6	1329.5

National Center for Health Statistics, 1986–1990
SEER Cancer Statistics Review, 1973–1990

Table 2.2 Changes in cancer mortality rates (1950–1990).

Age Group	Mortality Rates/100,000/Year			Percent Change
	1950	1975	1990	1950–90
0–4	11.1	5.2	3.2	–71.2
5–14	6.6	4.7	3.1	–50.4
15–24	8.5	6.6	4.8	–44.1
25–34	19.8	14.6	12.2	–38.4
35–44	64.2	53.9	44.7	–29.9
45–54	175.2	179.2	161.5	–8.1
55–64	394.0	423.2	441.9	12.6
65–7	4700.0	769.8	871.2	24.5
75–79	1160.9	1156.0	1344.5	15.7
81+	1450.7	1437.9	1752.9	18.7
All Ages	158.1	162.3	174.0	10.0

National Center for Health Statistics
SEER Cancer Statistics Review, 1973–1990

Table 2.3 Cancer incidence, mortality, and survival rates*.

	Age 65 and over 1984–88 Ten Leading Causes of Cancer		
	Incidence	Mortality	5-year Survival (%)
All sites	2014	1044	55
Colon/Rectum	337	143	55
Lung	312	270	11
Prostate	304	81	73
Breast	251	75	78
Bladder	108	27	73
Lymphomas	68	38	40
Pancreas	62	57	2
Uterus	59	15	76
Stomach	52	33	16
Leukemia	50	37	29

*Rates are per 100,000 population per year and are age-adjusted to the 1970 US standard population
National Center for Health Statistics
SEER Cancer Statistics Review 1973–1990

age 65 and over has been due to lung cancer, with lesser contributions from genitourinary cancer and the hematologic malignancies.

The increase in cancer mortality rates among the elderly appears to be related, at least in part, to increasing cancer incidence rates. For some types of cancer, old age represents a poor prognostic factor. This observation most likely relates to the biology of the disease, delays in diagnosis resulting in more advanced stage of disease at presentation, complicating co-morbid conditions, and poor tolerance of or poor compliance with potentially effective treatment programs. Older patients are often treated less aggressively based on chronologic age without consideration of functional status and co-morbid conditions (20). Elderly patients with cancer appear to do nearly as well as younger patients after adjusting for the type of cancer, tumor stage, co-morbid conditions, and treatment (2,21). The outcome of certain malignancies actually appears to favor the elderly perhaps because of biological differences in the tumor's behavior. Table 2.3 illustrates the incidence, mortality and relative survival of the ten leading causes of cancer among the elderly. The specialized needs of the elderly cancer patient suggest that attention should be directed toward a better understanding of clinical decision making in this population. Full attention to quality of life and cost, in addition to measures of survival or longevity, is of paramount importance in the elderly cancer patient (3,23). In addition, a better understanding is needed of those factors which influence a clinicians's decisions when caring for elderly cancer patients.

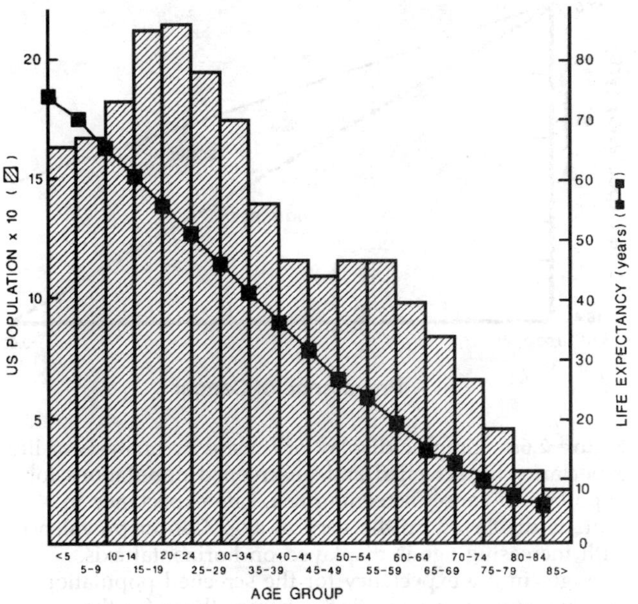

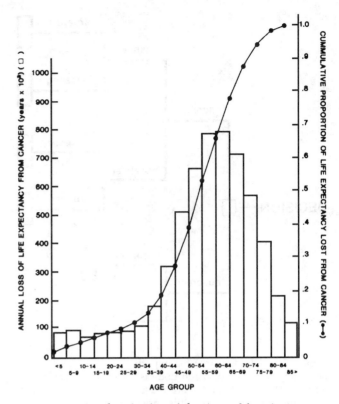

Figure 2.3 Graphic display of U.S. population and life expectancy by 5-year age group. Age-specific U.S. population × 10⁶ for 1980 is displayed as shaded vertical bars. Life expectancy in years for U.S. population from birth and for 5-year age-specific groups is displayed as solid squares.

Figure 2.4 Graphic display of the Annual loss in age-specific life expectancy from (years × 10³) for the US Population by five year age groups. Also illustrated is the cumulative proportion of life expectancy lost from cancer.

Optimal decision making in the elderly requires knowledge of the life expectancy associated with different age groups. Figure 2.3 reveals the relationship between increasing age and decreasing life expectancy (17). It is important to note that, although life expectancy from birth has increased dramatically since the

turn of the century, there has been little increase in the life expectancy of those age 65 and over or of the total life-span (Table 2.4) (24). Decision making in the elderly must consider both the increase in cancer mortality as well as the decrease in life expectancy with increasing age. Figure 2.4 illustrates this complex relationship by displaying the age specific loss in life expectancy due to cancer with age. Clearly, the greatest impact of cancer on years of productive life is in the range of 50 to 70 years of age.

The relative importance of prolonging survival and the acceptability of certain types of discomfort or costs vary among individuals. Physicians must be aware that such factors as age, race, sex, and socioeconomic status may influence treatment decisions in a subtle and often unrecognized manner. Where feasible, the patient's values should be incorporated into any decision analysis performed (25–27). Appropriate adjustment of survival by the anticipated impact on quality of life is particularly important in decision making in the elderly. This chapter illustrates the usefulness of decision analysis in improving our understanding of those factors important in medical and public health decisions in the elderly. The issues important for clinical decision making related to cancer and aging will be illustrated with regard to both cancer screening and treatment.

Table 2.4 Life expectancy (years).

Year	From Birth		From Age 65	
	Males	Females	Males	Females
1900	48	51	11	12
1910	50	53	11	12
1920	56	57	12	13
1930	58	61	12	13
1940	62	66	12	14
1950	65	71	13	15
1960	67	73	13	16
1970	67	75	13	17
1980	70	78	14	18
1990	72	79	15	19

Vital Statistics of the United States, 1990
Center for Disease Control and Prevention
National Center for Health Statistics

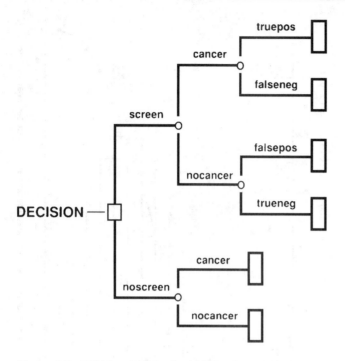

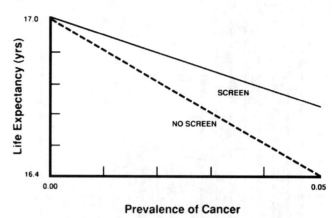

Figure 2.5 Decision tree for hypothetical cancer screening test. The decision node is illustrated as an open square. The chance nodes are illustrated as open circles. The outcome values or utilities are illustrated as open rectangles. The following abbreviations are utilized: truepos: true-positive test, falseneg: false-negative test, falsepos: false-positive test, trueneg: true-negative test.

Figure 2.6a Graphic display of sensitivity analysis of life expectancy for screened and unscreened populations for hypothetical cancer screening test. Life expectancy in years is displayed on the vertical axis. Cancer prevalence with increasing age is displayed on horizontal axis. Changes in life expectancy for the screened population are displayed as a solid line, whereas those for the unscreened population are shown as a dashed line.

Cancer Screening

The ideal test for screening for disease at any age would have perfect sensitivity and specificity and would detect disease early with no cost or toxicity. In addition, when considering screening tests, the disease being sought should be treatable when diagnosed early and yet cause morbidity or even mortality if not detected early. In reality, screening tests have less than perfect sensitivity and specificity. Such tests are often costly and may be associated with significant morbidity and mortality either due to the testing procedure or the evaluation of individuals with positive test results. A diagnostic test associated with only a modest probability of enhancing the beneficial outcome may be justified if it is associated with little or no harmful effect and minimal cost. In contrast, a test associated with frequent morbidity or considerable cost is only justified if it is associated with a high probability of improved patient survival.

The impact of any screening test or strategy must ultimately be evaluated in the population to be screened. To illustrate issues related to aging and cancer screening, a hypothetical screening test for cancer is presented (Figure 2.5). It is assumed that this test is capable of detecting a cancer earlier than in those not screened. It is also assumed that earlier detection for this cancer can improve survival. The impact of age on the value of this screening test will be assessed both with regards to cost and effectiveness.

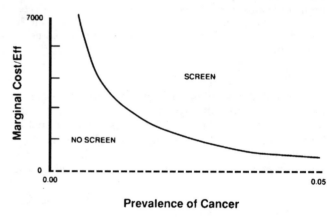

Figure 2.6b Graphic display of sensitivity analysis of cost effectiveness for screened and unscreened populations for hypothetical cancer screening test. Marginal cost effectiveness in cost in dollars per year of life expectancy extended is displayed on the vertical axis. Cancer prevalence with increasing age is displayed on the horizontal axis. Changes in cost effectiveness for the screened population are shown by the solid line, whereas those for the unscreened population is shown by the horizontal dashed line.

When considering a malignancy for which there is effective treatment when diagnosed early, screening is associated with the greatest expected value for most reasonable assumptions. However, since disease prevalence and thus the positive predictive value increase while life expectancy decreases with advancing age, the net effectiveness of screening in the elderly is a complex function.

As shown in Figure 2.6A, expected value based on life expectancy decreases with increasing age in both

Table 2.5 Age and screening test performance.

Age Group	Life Expectancy (yr)	Prevalence	Years Gained†	Cost per Year ($)
25–35	50	.004	540	36,919
35–45	41	.0014	1,670	11,978
45–55	32	.0053	5,240	3,783
55–65	24	.0132	10,290	1,899
65–75	16	.0248	13,010	1,471
75–85	10	.0372	11,350	1,647
85+	6	.0480	7,380	2,481

* Based on a preclinical duration of disease of 24 months
† Per 100,000 individuals screened.
‡ Based on a cost of screening ($100) and cost of diagnosis ($1000)

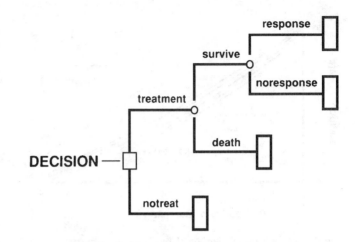

Figure 2.7 Decision tree for hypothetical cancer treatment program. The decision node is illustrated as an open square. The chance nodes are displayed as open circles, and the outcome values or utilities are illustrated as open rectangles.

screened and unscreened populations. The fall in life expectancy, however, is less rapid in the screened population than in the unscreened population. Therefore, the comparative effectiveness of such screening is greater with increasing age and increasing disease prevalence. Figure 2.6B demonstrates that the cost effectiveness of screening improves with increasing age and disease prevalence.

Table 2.5 illustrates the effect of age on the cost effectiveness of screening for a hypothetical malignancy. In this example, it is assumed that the 5-year survival of patients diagnosed routinely at the time of symptom onset is 50%, whereas the survival of those detected by screening while asymptomatic is 90%. Under these assumptions, the optimal effectiveness and cost effectiveness of screening is observed in individuals 65 to 75 years of age. This observation is the result of the increasing positive predictive value associated with increasing disease prevalence but a corresponding fall in life expectancy with increasing age.

The effectiveness and cost effectiveness of cancer screening increase as the magnitude of the absolute difference in survival between unscreened and screened individuals increases. Test sensitivity and specificity have noticeably less impact on the calculated expected value. Although cost estimates affect the measured cost effectiveness, they do not alter the basic relationships and conclusions of the model. Screening for a malignancy in which early intervention is beneficial can be effectively and cost effectively applied in the elderly.

Cancer Treatment

For cancer treatment decisions, the diagnosis must already be established. Therefore, disease prevalence is no longer an issue in cost-effectiveness analysis. Alternatively, issues related to cost and quality of life often take on even greater importance than with screening. A variety of factors must be considered, including the type, stage and grade of tumor, the patient's functional status, the presence of any complicating medical con-

ditions, and a number of psychological and socioeconomic factors. The clinician should consider the age-specific life expectancy of the individual before committing the patient to treatment associated with considerable morbidity. The types of malignancies which afflict the elderly are in general less responsive to systemic therapy than malignancies found in younger individuals. Alternatively, many malignancies found in elderly patients are most effectively treated by surgical resection when early diagnosis is possible. When palliation with little impact on longevity is the most likely outcome, the limited life expectancy of the elderly and quality of life issues may favor no treatment. When highly treatable and potentially curable disorders are involved, the greatest expected value will almost always favor the decision to treat regardless of age. However, since both treatment response and toxicity correlate directly with treatment intensity, the clinician is often faced with a very difficult clinician decision.

These points can be illustrated by reference to a hypothetical treatment program for advanced cancer shown in Figure 2.7. In this example, we assume that responding patients with a certain malignancy experience a doubling in median survival although with some risk of early mortality. Outcome is assessed in terms of both treatment cost and effectiveness. Effectiveness is measured in terms of life expectancy adjusted for the impact on quality of life. The average quality-adjusted life expectancy and cost effectiveness associated with treatment increase as treatment mortality decreases, the response rate increases, or the impact of treatment on median survival increases. Based on initial conditions for individuals over age 65, including a median survival of 1 year untreated, a 5% risk of treatment mortality, and a quality adjustment of treatment of 3 months, the threshold for response rate of 28% is estimated. Regimen response rates above this threshold

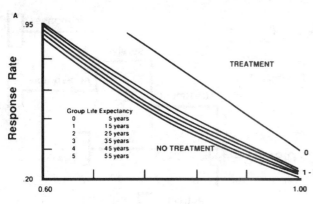

Probability of Surviving Treatment

Figure 2.8 Graphic display of two-way sensitivity analysis for hypothetical cancer treatment program. Response rate as the proportion responding is displayed on the vertical axis. The probability of early survival of the treatment program is displayed on the horizontal axis. The curved lines represent the decision thresholds where the expected value of treatment equals the expected value of no treatment. Any combination of response rate and probability of survival above the threshold line is associated with a greater expected value for treatment. Any combination of response rate and probability of survival below the threshold line is associated with a greater expected value for no treatment. A family of threshold curves for varying group life expectancies with age are illustrated. The decision threshold line moves upward with decreasing life expectancy or increasing age.

would favor treatment while those below the threshold would favor no treatment. The threshold for treatment increases with increasing age due to a decrease in life expectancy. Under the hypothetical conditions illus-

trated here, treatment of an individual age 85 and over is favored only when a response rate more than 44% is anticipated. The conditions under which treatment is favored in this treatment model become more restrictive with increasing age. The impact of life expectancy and, therefore, age on the decision to treat based on response rate and treatment mortality is illustrated in Figure 2.8. The treatment decision threshold increases with increasing age, but may still favor treatment in responsive malignancies under a wide variety of assumptions.

Discussion

Managing the elderly cancer patient involves decisions based on a wide variety of factors aimed at providing the patient with the optimal duration and quality of life. Careful attention to the entire patient situation, familiarity with advances in cancer diagnosis and treatment, and an understanding of the rational use of clinical data and measured outcomes should assist physicians in making the appropriate clinical decision for each patient.

The risk of most cancers increases progressively with increasing age. Based on the observed natural history of many cancers and the availability of effective treatment modalities when localized, early and accurate detection appears to offer the best opportunity for improving cancer survival in the elderly. Several available cancer screening strategies have been shown to be cost effective when applied to an elderly population. Current recommendations for cancer screening among those age 50 and older are presented in Table 2.6.

The value of available treatment strategies in treating elderly patients with malignancy is less clear and depends greatly upon the type of cancer involved and the treatment strategy utilized.

Table 2.6 Recommendations for cancer screening patients over the age 50.

Cancer	Procedure	Recommended Frequency
Cervix	Papanicolaou Test	Yearly until 3 consecutive negative tests then every 3 years
Breast	Self Examination	Monthly
	Physical Examination	Yearly
	Mammography	Yearly
Colon/Rectum	Digital Rectal Exam	Yearly
	Fecal Occult Blood Test	Yearly
	Sigmoidoscopy	Every 3–5 years
Prostate	Digital Rectal Exam	Yearly
	Prostate Specific Antigen	Yearly
Uterus	Endometrial Sample	Once at menopause
Ovary	Pelvic Exam	Yearly
Multiple	General Physical Exam	Yearly

American Cancer Society, 1995

Several studies have demonstrated that elderly patients selected on the basis of underlying risk factors tolerate definitive cancer treatment, including surgery, radiation therapy, and chemotherapy (21,22). The only potential for cure in most elderly patients with malignancy is provided by early and complete surgical removal. The clinician must recognize, however, that major surgery is associated with greater risk in the elderly than in younger patients, largely due to the increased frequency of comorbid medical disorders (28). The greater operative risk among the elderly is most problematic when palliation is the goal, rather than when curative resection is undertaken (29).

Several malignancies may be cured or controlled effectively by the application of radiation therapy. Radiation therapy is often effective in relieving tumor symptoms related to compression and obstruction in patients with advanced disease. The therapeutic ratio of normal tissue tolerance to tumor lethal dose falls with increasing age (30).

Systemic chemotherapy is capable of prolonging the survival of patients with a variety of advanced malignancies, with cure possible in such disorders as the malignant lymphomas, breast cancer, and small cell lung cancer. The magnitude and duration of treatment response often depends directly on treatment intensity. The greater the impact of treatment on prolonging patient survival, the more toxicity that is generally considered acceptable. On the other hand, the more that quality of life is compromised by treatment, the less important mere prolongation of survival becomes. When chemotherapy is administered with the intention of prolonging survival, dose reduction may significantly compromise disease control (31). The acute toxic effects of chemotherapy on proliferating normal elements, such as hematopoietic stem cells and intestinal mucosa, may be increased in patients exposed to previous treatment and in those with reduced functional and nutritional status that limits tolerable treatment intensity. The toxicity of chemotherapy in the elderly may be increased by the associated physiologic and pathologic changes that occur with aging. It should be remembered that hormonal manipulation may produce tumor regression with acceptable toxicity in a variety of malignancies, including breast cancer, prostate cancer, and uterine cancer.

Elderly cancer patients should be considered potential subjects for approved clinical trials with the exception of those with serious complicating medical conditions and those incapable of informed consent. Elderly patients eligible for prospective multi-institutional clinical trials have been found to experience no increase in the frequency or severity of chemotherapy toxicity (32). In addition, elderly patients in these studies did not differ in important risk factors or compliance with treatment dosage and had equivalent response rates to younger patients. Although the tumor response and toxicity associated with systemic treatment depend more on physiologic factors than on actual age, experimental drugs should generally be avoided in the very elderly. The malignancies afflicting the elderly are less likely to be those that respond to new treatment modalities. In addition, unusual and potentially life-threatening toxicities must be anticipated in this group. If experimental treatment is undertaken, it should be performed as a part of a well designed, controlled clinical trial with fully informed consent.

When aggressive treatment approaches are not a reasonable consideration, much may still be offered to the aged cancer patient, including the control of pain and other symptoms of the underlying malignancy. Aggressive psychosocial support is essential in managing the elderly cancer patient. Due to the limitations in life expectancy and frequent co-morbid conditions in the elderly, quality of life must be a primary concern of the treating clinician. Decisions to limit treatment in the elderly cancer patient with untreatable or refractory disease eventually must also be considered.

Decision analysis provides both a framework for thinking about health care in the elderly and a fertile area for methodologic and health care outcomes research. Decision analysis is particularly suited to assessing the usefulness of prevention and early detection strategies in complex settings with mixed outcomes, as exemplified in the elderly. Such an approach is particularly valuable in situations where a decision based on simple survival is incomplete or unsatisfactory. In health care planning for the elderly, any useful medical and public health strategy must consider performance outcome both in terms of benefits and risks including costs. Decision analysis is ideally suited for assessing the value of new therapeutic strategies, as well as technologies aimed at reducing disease and treatment related toxicity. Finally, it provides a useful framework for continuous objective evaluation of rapidly evolving clinical strategies in an era of increasing health awareness and cost containment. The application of decision analysis methods to health care in the elderly should not only improve our understanding of this rapidly expanding field but should also result in improved quality of care and quality of life for the elderly patient with cancer.

References

1. Kahneman D, Slovic P, Tversky A. *Judgement under uncertainty: Heuristics and biases.* Cambridge: Cambridge University Press, 1982.
2. Pauker SG, Kassirer JP. Decision analysis. *N Engl J Med* 1987; **316**: 250–258.
3. Kassirer JP, Moskowitz AJ, Lau J, Pauker SG. Decision analysis: A progress report. *Ann Int Med* 1987; **106**: 275–291.
4. Albert DA, Munson R, Resnik MD. *Reasoning in medicine: An introduction to clinical inference.* Baltimore: John Hopkins University Press, 1988.
5. Sox HC, Blatt MA, Higgins MC, Maston KI. *Medical Decision Making.* Boston: Butterworth, 1988.
6. Kassirer JP, Gorry GA. Clinical problem solving: A behavioral analysis. *Ann Int. Med* 1978; **89**: 245–255.
7. Weinstein MC, Fineberg HV. *Clinical Decision Analysis.* Philadelphia: WB Saunders, 1980.
8. Kong A, Barnett GO, Mosteller F, Youtz C. How medical professionals evaluate expressions of probability. *N Engl J Med* 1986; **315**: 740–744.

9. Wasson JH, Sox HC, Goldman L, Neff RK. Clinical prediction rules: Applications and methodological standards. *N Engl J Med* 1985; **313**: 793–799.

10. Schwartz S, Griffin T. *Medical thinking: The psychology of medical judgement and decision making.* New York: Springer-Verlag, 1986.

11. Schwartz WB, Gorry GA, Kassirer JP, Essig A. A decision analysis and clinical judgment. *Am J Med* 1973; **55**: 459–472.

12. Mushlin AI. Diagnostic tests in breast cancer: Clinical strategies based on diagnostic probabilities. *Ann Int Med* 1985; **103**: 79–85.

13. Rembold CM, Watson D. Posttest probability calculation by weights: A simple form of Bayes' theorem. *Ann Int Med* 1988; **108**: 115–120.

14. Sox HC. Probability theory in the use of diagnostic tests: An introduction to critical study of the literature. *Ann Int Med* 1986; **104**: 60–66.

15. Selection and interpretation of diagnostic tests and procedures. Principles and applications. *Ann Int Med* 1981; **94**: 553–600.

16. Health and Public Policy Committee. American College of Physicians: The use of diagnostic tests for screening and evaluating breast lesions. *Ann Int Med* 1985; **103**: 147–151.

17. *Vital Statistics of the United States, II, Mortality, Part A 1950–1983.* Washington, DC: US Government Printing Office, 1984.

18. *Cancer in Florida 1981–1983.* Health Program Office, Epidemiology Program, Department of Health and Rehabilitative Services, 1986.

19. *Third National Cancer Survey: Incidence Data.* National Cancer Institute Monograph 41, DHEW publication No. 75–787. Washington, DC, US Government Printing Office, 1975.

20. Greenfield S, Blanco DM, Elashoff RM, Gaaz PA. Patterns of care related to age of breast cancer patients. *JAMA* 1987; **251**: 2766–2770.

21. Peterson BA, Kennedy BJ. Aging and cancer management. Part 1: Clinical observations. *Cancer* 1979; **29**: 322–332.

22. Butler RN, Gastel B. Aging and cancer management: Research perspectives. *Cancer* 1979; **29**: 322–32.

23. Beghe C, Balducci L. Geriatric oncology: Perspectives from decision analysis. A review. *Arch Gerontol Geriatr* 1990; **10**: 141–162.

24. Miller BA, Ries LAG, Hankey BF, Kosary CL, Harras A, Devesa SS, Edwards BK (ed). *SEER Cancer Statistics Review 1973–1990,* National Cancer Institute, NIH Pub. No. 93–2789, 1993.

25. Brody DS. The patient's role in clinical decision making. *Ann Intern Med* 1980; **93**: 718–722.

26. Lo B, Jonsen AR. Clinical decisions to limit treatment. *Ann Intern Med* 1980; **93**: 764–768.

27. Beck Jr, Kassirer JP, Parker SG. A convenient approximation of life expectancy (the DEALE) 1. Validation of the method. *Am J Med* 1982; **72**: 883–888.

28. Sherman S, Suidot CE. The feasibility of thoracotomy for lung cancer in the elderly. *JAMA* 1987; **258**: 927–930.

29. Lewis AAM, Khoury GA. Resection for colorectal cancer in the very old: Are the risks too high? *Br Med J* 1988; **296**: 459–461.

30. Samet J, Hunt WC, Key C, *et al.* Choice of cancer therapy varies with age of patient. *JAMA* 1986; **225**: 3385–3390.

31. Frei E III, Canellos GP. Dose: A critical factor in cancer chemotherapy. *Am J Med* 1980; **69**: 585–594.

32. Begg CB, Cohen JL, Ellerton J. Are the elderly predisposed to toxicity from cancer chemotherapy? *Cancer Clin Trials* 1980; **3**: 369–374.

Glossary

Probability   A number between 0 and 1 representing the likelihood of an event.

Odds   The ratio of the probability that an event occurs divided by the probability that the event does not occur.

Conditional probability   The probability of an event given the occurrence of another event.

Prior probability   The pretest probability of an event or the prevalence.

Posterior probability   The conditional probability of an event given that another event of a specific test outcome has occurred.

True-positive rate   The probability of a positive test result in diseased individuals (sensitivity).

False-positive rate   The probability of a positive test result in those without disease.

True-negative rate   The probability of a negative test result in those without disease (specificity).

False-negative rate   The probability of a negative test result in those without disease.

Predictive value positive   The probability of disease in those with a positive test result.

Predictive value negative   The probability of no disease in those with negative test results.

Sensitivity analysis   A study of changes in outcome measures with changes in probabilities, value outcomes, or decision assumptions.

Life expectancy   The average life remaining for individuals of a given age.

Expected value   The average outcome value over possible outcome paths, with the value of each path weighted by the probability of the path.

Cost effectiveness   The cost for each unit of outcome value gained, such as years of additional life expectancy.

Appendix 2.1

Test Performance

The following summarizes test performance characteristics useful in decision analysis based on probability theory when $P(X)$ is defined as the probability of an event X. $P(X|Y)$ represents the conditional probability of event X given that event Y has occurred. The odds of X is defined as $P(X)/1-P(X)$:

Sensitivity = P(Positive test | Disease)
Specificity = P(Negative test | No Disease)
Predictive value positive = P(Disease | Positive Test)
Predictive value negative = P(Disease | Negative Test)

Appendix 2.2

Expressions for Bayes' Theorem

$$\text{predictive value positive} = \frac{\text{sensitivity} \cdot \text{prevalence}}{\text{sensitivity} \cdot \text{prevalence} + (1 - \text{specificity}) \cdot (1 - \text{prevalence})}$$

$$\text{predictive value negative} = \frac{(1 - \text{sensitivity}) \cdot \text{prevalence}}{\text{sensitivity} \cdot \text{prevalence} + (1 - \text{specificity}) \cdot (1 - \text{prevalence})}$$

2. Posttest odds = pretest odds • likelihood ratio

$$\text{probability} = \frac{\text{odds}}{1 + \text{odds}}$$

$$\text{likelihood ratio (LR)} = \frac{\text{probability of result} \in \text{a person without disease}}{\text{probability of result} \in \text{a person without disease}}$$

$$LR_+ = \frac{\text{true positive rate}}{\text{false positive rate}} = \frac{\text{sensitivity}}{1 - \text{specificity}}$$

$$LR_- = \frac{\text{false negative rate}}{\text{true negative rate}} = \frac{1 - \text{sensitivity}}{\text{specificity}}$$

3. ln (posttest odds) = (ln (pretest odds) + ln (LR)
   Where ln = natural logarithm

Appendix 2.3

Declining Exponential Approximation of Life Expectancy (DEALE)

$S = S_0 \, e^{-mt}$
Where S_0 = number of patients alive at time 0,
S = number of patients alive at time t
e = base of the natural logarithm, and
m = mortality rate
$m_{\text{total}} = m_{\text{age-specific}} + m_{\text{disease-specific}}$

$$\frac{S}{S_0} = e^{-mt} \quad m = -\frac{1}{t} \ln\left(\frac{S}{S_0}\right)$$

3. International Perspectives of Cancer and Aging

Carlo La Vecchia, Fabio Levi, Franca Lucchini and Eva Negri

Introduction

Incidence and mortality in most common cancer sites, and in particular in non hormone-related epithelial carcinomas, increase with age (1). Consequently, cancer cases and deaths in the elderly represent a significant proportion of the cancer burden on a population level.

However, analysis and interpretation of international trends in cancer and aging are hampered by major difficulties and greater changes in diagnosis and certification of several cancer sites in the elderly when compared to younger and middle age subjects. Thus, cancer rates and trends are largely different when considering population of the young and middle aged as opposed to populations from middle age onwards (2-4).

For instance, Doll (3) concluded on the basis of cancer death certification data at age 20-44, that patterns in trends were favorable for most cancer sites in developed countries, with the major exception of eastern Europe. In contrast, Hoel et al. (4) concluded that upward trends in mortality from several common cancers were increasing in most developed countries, on the basis of inspection of rates at ages 45 to 84, and that these trends could not be explained only by changes in cigarette smoking and aging.

It is more difficult to infer the causes and the consequences of cancer in older than in younger persons. This is because collection of data is hampered by the difficulties of the interview, in the elderly, and because death certificates and data from the tumor registry are less reliable.

With this public health focus, we present in this chapter in graphical form, trends in mortality from major cancer sites over the period 1950-1992 for the population aged 65 to 84 years in 33 countries from 4 continents. A summary review of these data, beginning in 1955, in tabular form has been presented elsewhere (5).

Material and Methods

Official death certification numbers for 23 European countries, excluding the former Soviet Union, Albania and a few countries with a population of <1 million (Andorra, Iceland, Liechtenstein, Luxembourg and Malta), the United States and Canada, 4 South American countries (Argentina, Costa Rica, Uruguay and Venezuela), 2 Asian countries (Hong Kong and Japan), Australia and New Zealand, were derived from the World Health Organization (WHO) database. During the calendar period considered (1950-1992), four different Revisions of the International Classification of Diseases (ICD) were used (6-9). Classification of cancer deaths were thus re-coded, for all the calendar periods, according to the Ninth Revision (ICD-9) (9). To improve comparability of data throughout different countries and calendar periods, we pooled together all intestinal sites including rectum, all uterine cancers (cervix and endometrium), all skin neoplasms (melanoma and non-melanomatous), and all non-Hodgkin's lymphomas. Neoplasms whose classification changed substantially in the examined period, e.g. liver, pleural and bone cancer, and those which pose major diagnosis and classification problems, particularly in the elderly, such as brain cancer (2,10) are not considered in the present report. Table 3.1 gives the cancers or groups of cancers considered, together with the corresponding ICD codes under subsequent Revisions.

Estimates of the resident population, generally based on official censuses, were obtained from the same WHO data bank. From the matrices of certified deaths and resident populations, age-specific rates for each 5-year age group considered and calendar period were computed. Age-standardized rates were based on the world standard population (11).

In a few countries, data were missing for part of one or more calendar periods (Table 3.2). When a single year was missing within a quinquennium, numerators and denominators were interpolated linearly from the previous and subsequent calendar year. No extrapolation was made for missing data at the beginning or the end of the calendar period considered, or when data on one or more quinquennia were not available.

Results

Trends in world-standardized rates at age 65-84 for each 5-year calendar period by sex in each country are given in Figure 3.1. A large number of scales has been adopted to optimize the description of trends for each country. For any comparison between countries, careful inspection of the absolute value of rates is required. Although this is essentially a descriptive report, a short comment is enclosed in order to recall major patterns of trends for each cancer site. This, however, cannot substitute for careful inspection of trends for each country and sex.

Table 3.1 Cancers or groups of cancers considered.

Type of cancer	6 I.C.D.	7 I.C.D.	8 I.C.D.	9 I.C.D.
Oral cavity and pharynx	140–148	140–148	140–149	140–149
Esophagus	150	150	150	150
Stomach	151	151	151	151
Intestines, mainly colon and rectum	152–154	152–154	152–154	152–154 + 159.0
Gallbladder and bile ducts	–	155.1	156	156
Pancreas	157	157	157	157
Larynx	161	161	161	161
Trachea, bronchus and lung	162	(162 + 163) – 162.2	162	162
Skin, including melanoma	190 + 191	190 + 191	172 + 173	172 + 173
Breast	170	170	174	174(M)/175(F)
Uterus (cervix and corpus)	171–174	171–174	180–182	179–182
Ovary	175	175	183	183
Prostate	177	177	185	185
Testis	178	178	186	186
Bladder	181*	181*	188	188
Kidney	180	180	189*	189*
Thyroid	194	194	193	193
Hodgkin's disease	201	201	201	201
Non-Hodgkin's lymphomas	200 + 202 + 205	200 + 202 + 205	200 + 202 + 208 + 209	200 + 202
Multiple myeloma	203	203	203	203
Leukemias	204	204	204–207	204–208
All neoplasms, benign and malignant	140–239	140–239	140–239	140–239

*And other urinary sites
I.C.D. = International Classification of Diseases

Cancer of the Oral Cavity and Pharynx

Within Europe, a major excess of cancer of the oral cavity and pharynx was observed in France, whose rates were 72/100,000 males in the late 1970s, but declined thereafter to reach 60/100,000 in the early 1990s. Thus, in the most recent calendar period death rates from cancers of the oral cavity for elderly males were similar in Hungary (55/100,000) and in France. The upward trends in Hungary were reflected, to a lesser degree, in most other central and eastern European countries, including Germany. Oral cancer death rates in elderly males were between 28 and 32/100,000 in Portugal, Spain and Italy, with a recent upward trend in Spain. In contrast, most northern European countries showed recent declines in oral cancer rates not only in males, but (particularly in Sweden and Norway) in elderly females, too, over the most recent calendar period reaching values around or below 20/100,000 males and 10/100,000 females.

Oral cancer death rates in elderly males were moderately declining in North America and Venezuela, in females, too, and also in Australia and New Zealand. Japan had rather low oral cancer rates in males in the 1950s (below 10/100,000), but a steady upward trend was observed over the last three decades.

Cancer of the Esophagus

As for oral cavity and pharynx, some of the highest esophageal cancer death rates in elderly males were in France in the mid 1960s, with a peak around 100/100,000. Swiss rates in the early 1950s were over 120/100,000 and Finnish rates over 80. In these countries, as well as in Austria, Germany and Italy, esophageal cancer rates have been declining over the last few decades in elderly males. In contrast, a recent upward trend was registered in Denmark, the Netherlands, Czechoslovakia and the United Kingdom. Rates for females were much lower and often unremarkable, except in Nordic countries, where esophageal cancer rates were relatively high in females in the 1950s and 1960s, and declines in elderly females paralleled those in males. In these countries, besides

Table 3.2 Calendar years for which data were missing for each country and cancer site.

Country	Oral cavity & pharynx	Esophagus	Stomach	Intestines	Gallbladder	Pancreas	Larynx	Lung	Skin
Austria	50-54	50-54	50-54	50-54	50-68	50-54	50-54	50-54	50-54
Belgium	50-53,85,90-92	50-53,85,90-92	50-53,85,90-92	50-53,85,80-92	50-67,85	50-54,77-78,85,90-92	50-54,85,90-92	50-54,85,90-92	50-53,83,85,87-89,90-92
Bulgaria	50-63	50-63	50-63	50-63	50-67,83	50-65	50-63	50-63	50-63
Czechoslovakia	50-52,92	50-52,92	50-52,92	50-52,92	50-67,83-84,92	50-54,92	50-52,92	50-52,92	50-52,92
Denmark	50	50	50	50	50-66,68	50-54	50	50	50
Finland	50-51	50-51	50-51	50-51	50-57,88	50-54	50-51	50-51	50-51
France	92	92	92	92	50-57,92	50-54,92	92	92	50-54,92
Germany	50-51,92	50-51,92	50-51,92	50-51,92	50-67,92	50-54,92	50-51,92	50-51,92	50-51,92
Greece	50-60,92	50-60,92	50-60,92	50-60,92	50-65,92	50-65,92	50-60,92	50-60,92	50-60,92
Hungary	50-54	50-54	50-54	50-54	50-69	50-69	50-54	50-54	50-54
Ireland	92	92	92	92	50-67,92	50-54,92	92	92	92
Italy	50,91-92	50,91-92	50,91-92	50,91-92	50-57,91-92	50-54,91-92	50,91-92	50,91-92	50,91-92
Netherlands	92	92	92	92	50-68,92	50-54,92	92	92	92
Norway	50,92	50,92	50,92	50,92	50-68,92	50-54,92	50,92	50,92	50,92
Poland	50-58	50-58	50-58	50-58	50-69,72-92	50-60,69,72-79	50-58	50-58	50-58
Portugal	50-54	50-54	50-54	50-54	50-83	50-79	50-54	50-54	50-54
Romania	50-58,79	50-58,79	50-58,79	50-58,79	50-92	50-79	50-58,79	50-58,79	50-58,79
Spain	50,92	50,92	50,92	50,92	50-67,92	50,92	50,92	50,92	50,92
Sweden	50,91-92	50,91-92	50,91-92	50,91-92	50-67,91-92	50,91-92	50,91-92	50,91-92	50,91-92
Switzerland	50	50	50	50	50-68	50-54	50	50	50
UK, England & Wales	91-92	91-92	91-92	91-92	50-67,91-92	50-54,91-92	91-92	91-92	91-92
UK, Scotland	92	92	92	92	50-57,91-92	50-54,91-92	92	92	92
Yugoslavia, former	50-60,91-92	50-60,91-92	50-60,91-92	50-60,91-92	50-57,91-92	50-59,91-92	50-60,91-92	50-60,91-92	50-60,91-92
Canada	92	92	92	92	50-57,92	92	92	92	92
USA	91-92	91-92	91-92	91-92	50-61,78,91-92	50-54,78,91-92	91-92	91-92	91-92
Argentina	50-65,71-76,91-92	50-65,71-76,91-92	50-65,71-76,91-92	50-65,71-76,91-92	50-92	50-92	50-65,71-76,91-92	50-65,71-76,91-92	50-65,71-76,91-92
Costa Rica	50-60,92	50-60,92	50-60,92	50-60,92	50-92	50-65,68-92	50-60,92	50-60,92	50-60,92
Uruguay	50-54,61-62,78,91-92	50-54,61-62,79,91-92	50-54,61-62,79,91-92	50-54,61-62,79,91-92	50-65,68-92	50-65,68-92	50-54,61-62,79,91-92	50-54,61-62,79,91-92	50-54,61-62,79,91-92
Venezuela	50-54,84,90-92	50-54,84,90-92	50-54,84,90-92	50-54,84,90-92	50-57,68-69,79,81-92	50-54,68-69,79,81-92	50-54,84,90-92	50-54,84,90-92	50-54,84,90-92
Hong Kong	50-59,90-92	50-59,90-92	50-59,90-92	50-59,90-92	50-68,82,88-92	50-69,90-92	50-59,90-92	50-59,90-92	50-59,90-92
Japan	-	-	-	-	50-57	-	-	-	-
Australia	-	-	-	-	50-67	-	-	-	50-57
New Zealand	92	92	92	92	50-65,92	50-54,92	92	92	50-57,92

Table 3.2   Calendar years for which data were missing for each country and cancer site.

Country	Breast	Uterus	Ovary	Prostate	Testis	Bladder	Kidney	Thyroid	Hodgkin's disease
Austria	50–54	50–54	50–68	–	–	50–68	50–68	50–58	68
Belgium	50–53,85,90–92	50–53,85,90–92	50–53,80–83,85,90–92	50–53,85,90–92	50–53,85,90–92	50–53,85,90–92	50–53,85,90–92	50–53,85,90–92	50–53,85,90–92
Bulgaria	50–63	50–63	50–65	50–63	50–65	50–65	50–65,83	50–65,83	50–64
Czechoslovakia	50–52,92	50–52,92	50–54,79,81,84–86,92	50–52,92	50–54,92	50–54,92	50–54,92	50–54,92	50–54,92
Denmark	50	50	50–54	50–54	50–54	50–54	50–54	50–54	50–54
Finland	50–51	50–51	50–54,87–92	50–51	50–54	50–54	50–54,88	50–54,88	50–54
France	92	92	50–54,92	92	50–54,92	50–54,92	50–54,92	50–54,92	50–54,92
Germany	50–51,92	50–51,92	50–67,92	50–51,92	50–54,92	50–67,92	50–67,92	50–54,92	50–54,92
Greece	50–60,92	50–60,92	50–65,92	50–60,92	50–65,92	50–65,92	50–65,92	50–65,92	50–63,92
Hungary	50–54	50–54	50–69	50–54	50–69	50–69	50–69	50–69	50–69
Ireland	92	92	50–54,92	92	50–54,92	50–54,92	50–54,92	50–54,92	50–54,92
Italy	50,91–92	50,91–92	50–54,91–92	50,91–92	50–54,91–92	50–54,91–92	50–54,91–92	50–55,68,91–92	50–54,91–92
Netherlands	92	92	50–54,92	92	50–54,92	50–54,92	50–54,92	50–54,92	50–54,92
Norway	50,92	50,92	50–54,92	50,92	50–54,92	50–54,92	50–54,92	50–54,92	50–54,92
Poland	50–58	50–58	50–60,69	50–58	50–60,69,72–79	50–60,69	50–60,69,72–79	50–60,72–92	50–60,69,72–92
Portugal	50–54	50–54	50–83	–	50–79	50–79	50–83	50–83	50–79
Romania	50–58,79	50–58,79	50–92	50–68,79	50–69,70	50–68,79	50–92	50–92	50–68,79
Spain	50–92	50,92	50–54,92	50,92	50–92	50–54,92	50–54,92	50–54,92	50–54,92
Sweden	50,91–92	50,91–92	50–54,91–92	50,91–92	50–54,91–92	50–54,91–92	50–54,91–92	50–54,91–92	50–54,91–92
Switzerland	50	50	50–54	50	50–54	50–54	50–54	50–54	50–54
UK, England & Wales	91–92	91–92	50–54,91–92	91–92	50–54,91–92	50–54,91–92	50–54,91–92	50–54,91–92	50–54,91–92
UK, Scotland	92	92	50–54,91–92	91–92	50–54,91–92	50–54,91–92	50–54,91–92	50–54,91–92	50–54,91–92
Yugoslavia, former	50–60,91–92	50–60,91–92	50–59,79–92	50–60,91–92	50–59,91–92	50–59,91–92	50–59,91–92	50–59,89,91–92	50–59,91–92
Canada	92	92	92	92	92	92	92	92	92
USA	91–92	91–92	76,91–92	91–92	91–92	78,91–92	78,91–92	78,91–92	74,78,91–92
Argentina	50–65,71–76,91–92	50–65,71–76,91–92	55–92	50–65,71–76,80–81,91–92	50–92	50–78,80–81,91–92	50–92	50–92	50–92
Costa Rica	50–60,92	50–60,92	50–65,68–92	50–60,92	50–65,68–92	50–65,68–79,92	50–65,68–92	50–65,68–92	50–60,63–66,68–92
Uruguay	50–54,61–62,79,91–92	50–54,61–62,79,91–92	50–65,68–92	50–54,61–62,79,91–92	50–65,68–92	50–68,79,91–92	50–65,68–92	50–65,68–92	50–65,68–92
Venezuela	50–54,84,90–92	50–54,84,90–92	50–54,68–69,79–92	50–54,84,90–92	50–54,68–69,79,81–92	50–54,84,90–92	50–54,68–69,79,81–92	50–54,68–69,79,81–92	68–69,79,81–92
Hong Kong	50–59,90–92	50–59,90–92	50–65,79–92	50–59,90–92	50–65,90–92	50–65,90–92	50–65,82,88–92	50–65,82,88–92	50–63,90–92
Japan	–	–	–	–	–	–	–	–	50–57
Australia	–	–	81–84	–	–	–	–	50–57	50–57
New Zealand	92	92	92	92	92	92	92	50–57,92	50–57,92

Table 3.2 Calendar years for which data were missing for each country and cancer site.

Country	Non-Hodgkin's lymphomas	Multiple myeloma	Leukemias	Total, all sites
Austria	50–54	50–68	50–54	50–54
Belgium	50–53	50–53,85,90–92	50–53,85,90–92	50–53,85,90–92
Bulgaria	50–65,83	50–64,83	50–63	50–63
Czechoslovakia	50–54,92	50–54,92	50–52,92	50–52,92
Denmark	50–54	50–54	50	50
Finland	50–54,88	50–54,88	50–54	50–54
France	50–54,92	50–54,92	50–54,92	50–54,92
Germany	50–54,92	50–67	50–51,92	50–51,92
Greece	50–65,92	50–63,92	50–63,92	50–60,92
Hungary	50–69	50–69	50–54	50–54
Ireland	50–54,92	50–54,92	92	92
Italy	50–54,91–92	50,55,91–92	50,91–92	50,91–92
Netherlands	50–54,92	50–54,92	92	92
Norway	50–54,92	50–54,92	50,92	50,92
Poland	50–60,69,72–92	50–60,69,72–92	50–58	50–58
Portugal	50–83	50–83	50–54	50–54
Romania	50–92	50–92	50–58	50–58,79
Spain	50–54,92	50–54,92	50,92	50,92
Sweden	50–54,91–92	50–54,91–92	50,91–92	50,91–92
Switzerland	50–54	50–54	50	50
UK, England & Wales	50–54,91–92	50–54,91–92	91–92	91–92
UK, Scotland	50–54,91–92	50–54,91–92	91–92	91–92
Yugoslavia, former	50–59,91–92	50–59,91–92	50–60,91–92	50–59,91–92
Canada	50–68,92	50–68,92	92	92
USA	55–67,78,91–92	55–67,74–78,91–92	91–92	91–92
Argentina	50–92	50–92	50–65,71–76,91–92	50–65,71–76,91–92
Costa Rica	50–92	50–92	50–60,92	50–60,92
Uruguay	50–92	50–92	50–54,61–62,79,91–92	50–54,61–62,79,91–92
Venezuela	50–69,79,81–92	55–68,79, 90–92	84,90–92	84,90–92
Hong Kong	50–68,82,88–92	50–68,82,88–92	50–59,90–92	50–59,90–92
Japan	50–67	50–67	50–57	–
Australia	50–67	50–67	50–57	–
New Zealand	50–67,92	50–67,92	50–57,92	92

alcohol and tobacco, dietary deficiencies were probably important causes of esophageal cancer in the past (12).

In North America, esophageal cancer rates in the elderly were stable or slightly upwards over more recent calendar periods, as were the rates in Australia and New Zealand. A substantial decline was reported in Argentina and Uruguay, starting from rates over 100/100,000 in males and over 60/100,000 in females in Uruguay, where hot mate drinking is a major cause of esophageal cancer (13). Rates were also high in Japan and Hong Kong (around 70/100,000 males), with a moderately upward trend between 1950 and 1970, and some decline thereafter.

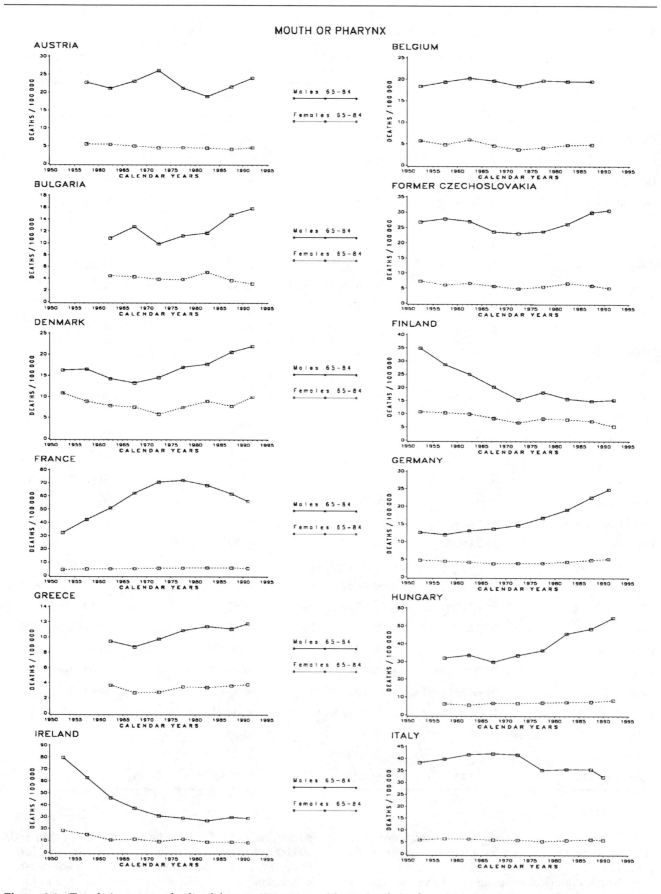

Figure 3.1 Trends in age-standardized (at age 65 to 84, world standard) death certification rates per 100,000 population from selected cancers or groups of cancers in various areas of the world, 1950–1992.

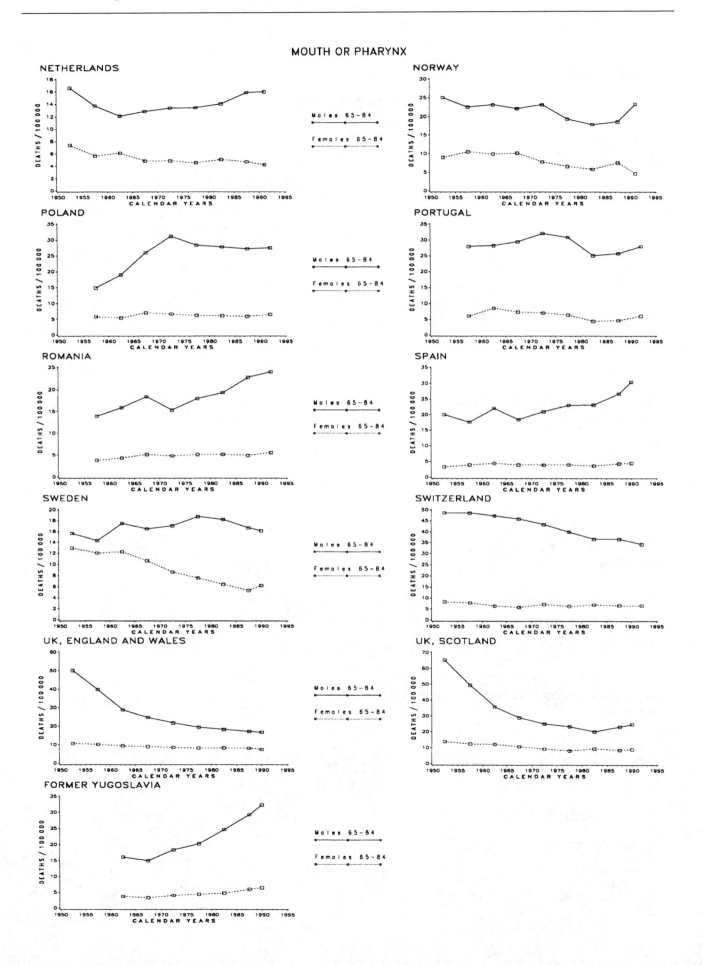

MOUTH OR PHARYNX

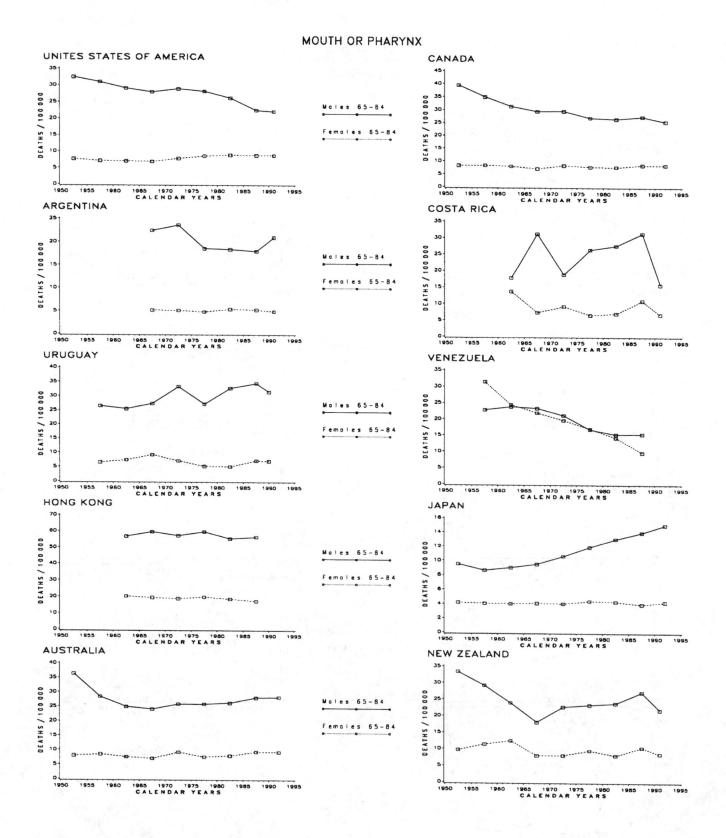

MOUTH OR PHARYNX

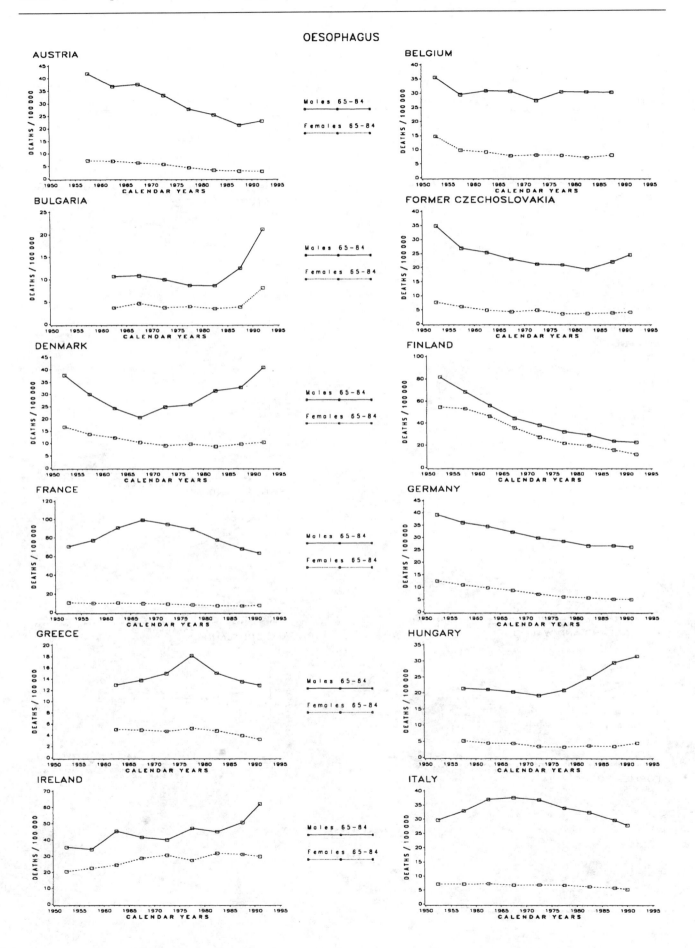

OESOPHAGUS

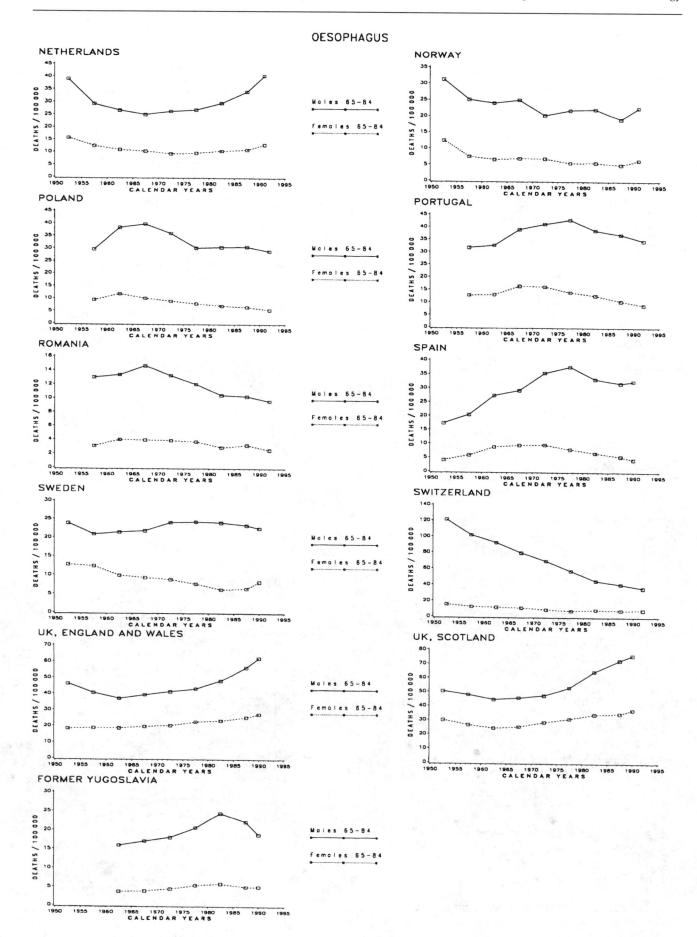

OESOPHAGUS

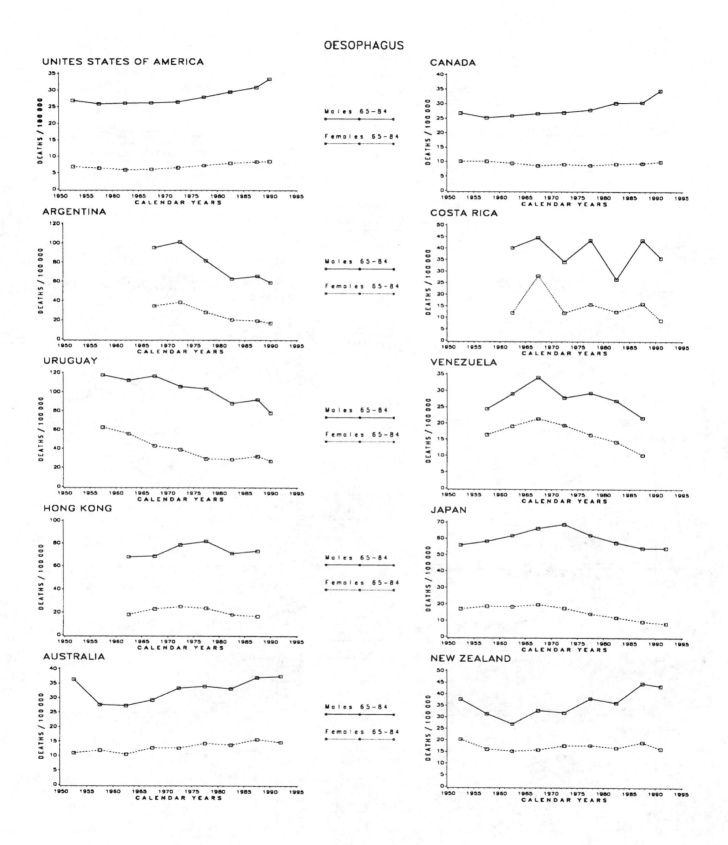

OESOPHAGUS

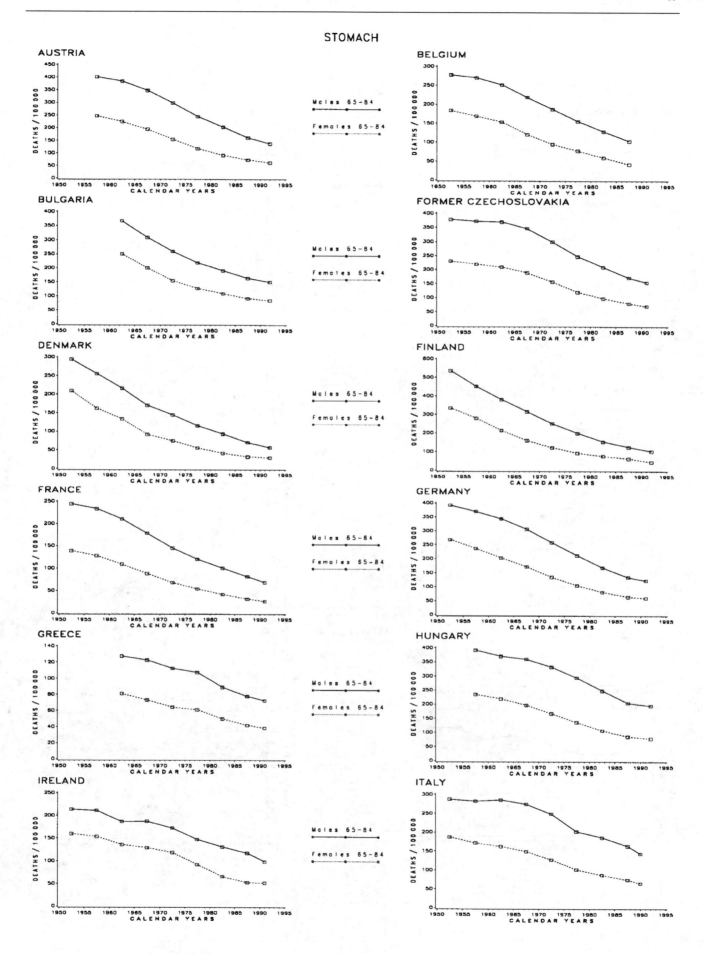

STOMACH

STOMACH

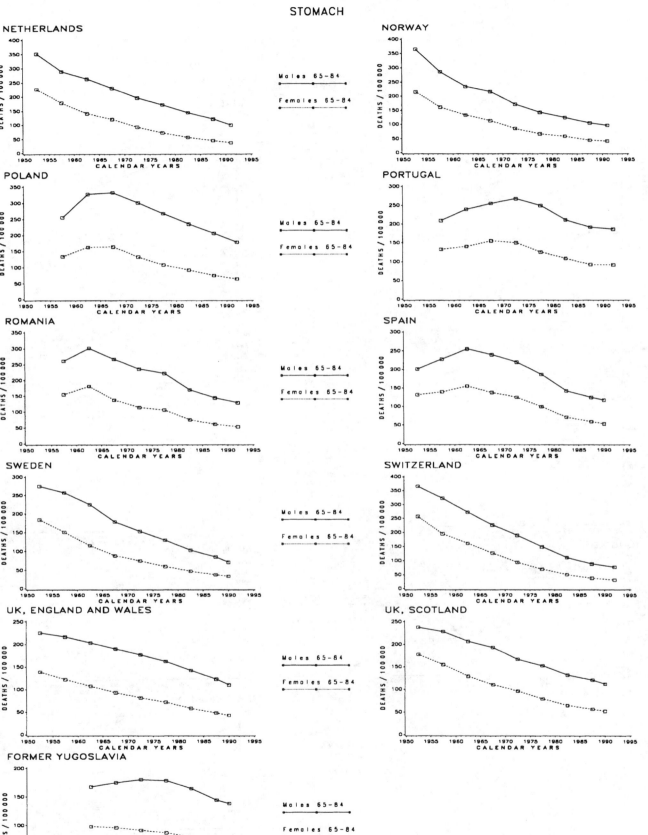

NETHERLANDS

NORWAY

POLAND

PORTUGAL

ROMANIA

SPAIN

SWEDEN

SWITZERLAND

UK, ENGLAND AND WALES

UK, SCOTLAND

FORMER YUGOSLAVIA

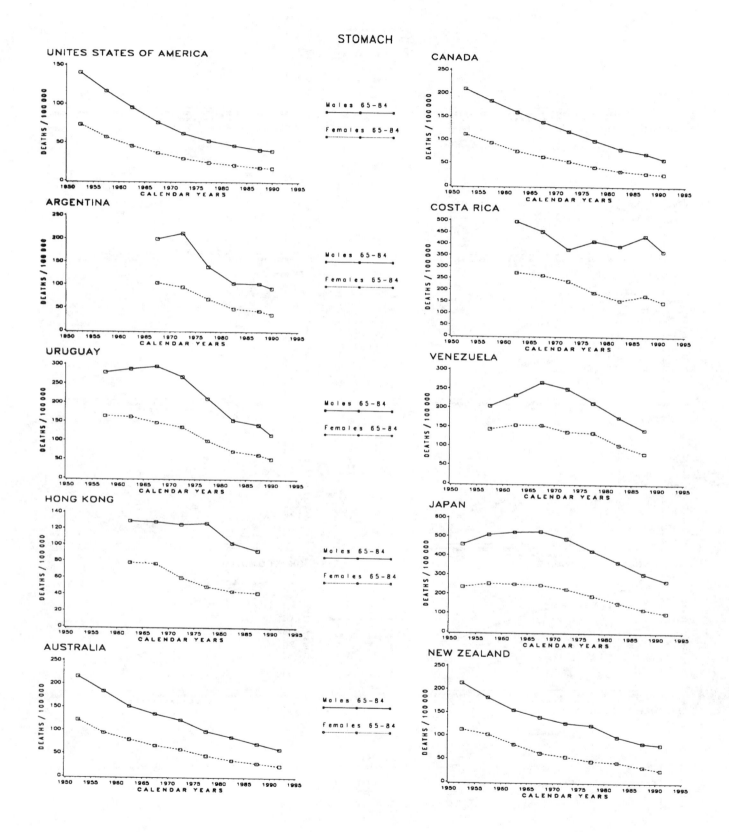

STOMACH

UNITES STATES OF AMERICA

ARGENTINA

URUGUAY

HONG KONG

AUSTRALIA

CANADA

COSTA RICA

VENEZUELA

JAPAN

NEW ZEALAND

Males 65-84

Females 65-84

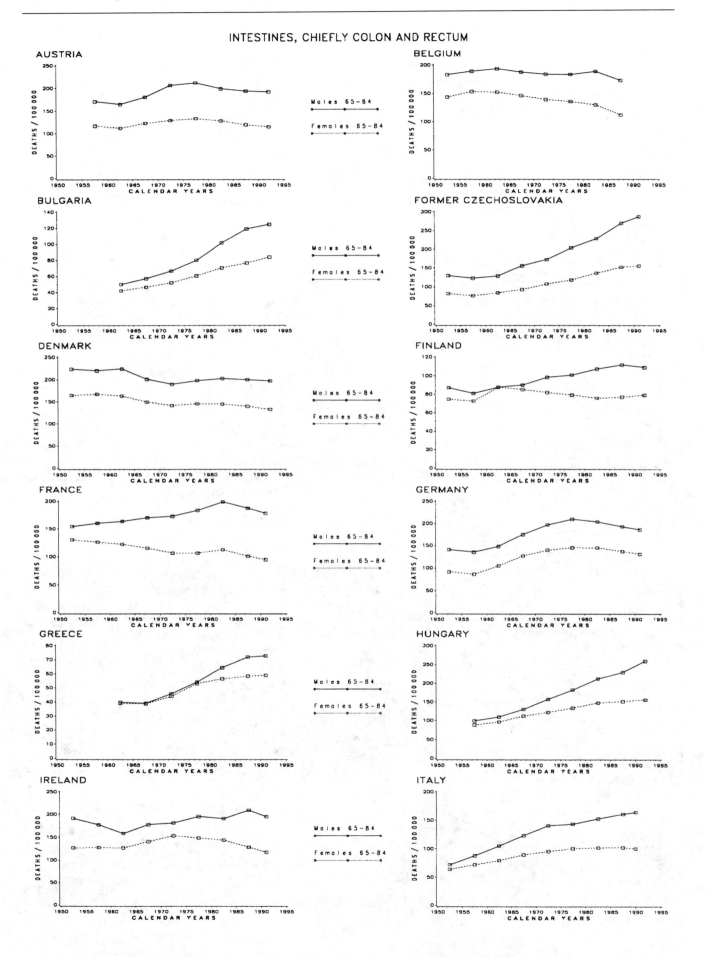

INTESTINES, CHIEFLY COLON AND RECTUM

INTESTINES, CHIEFLY COLON AND RECTUM

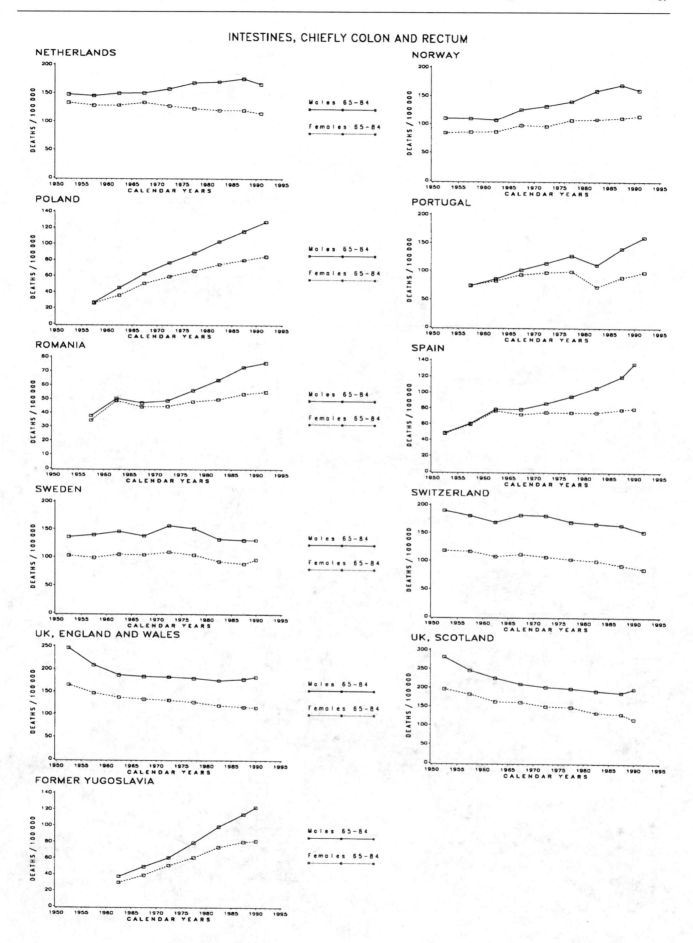

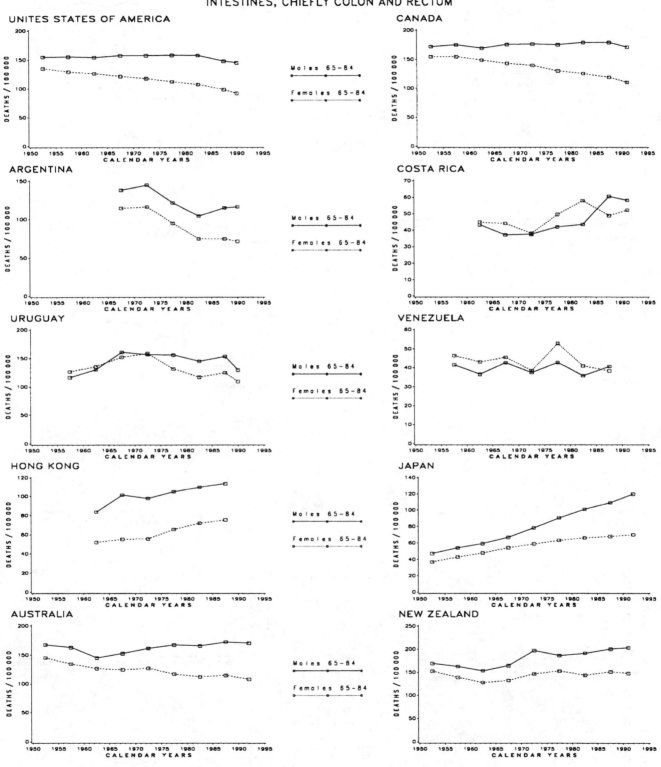

INTESTINES, CHIEFLY COLON AND RECTUM

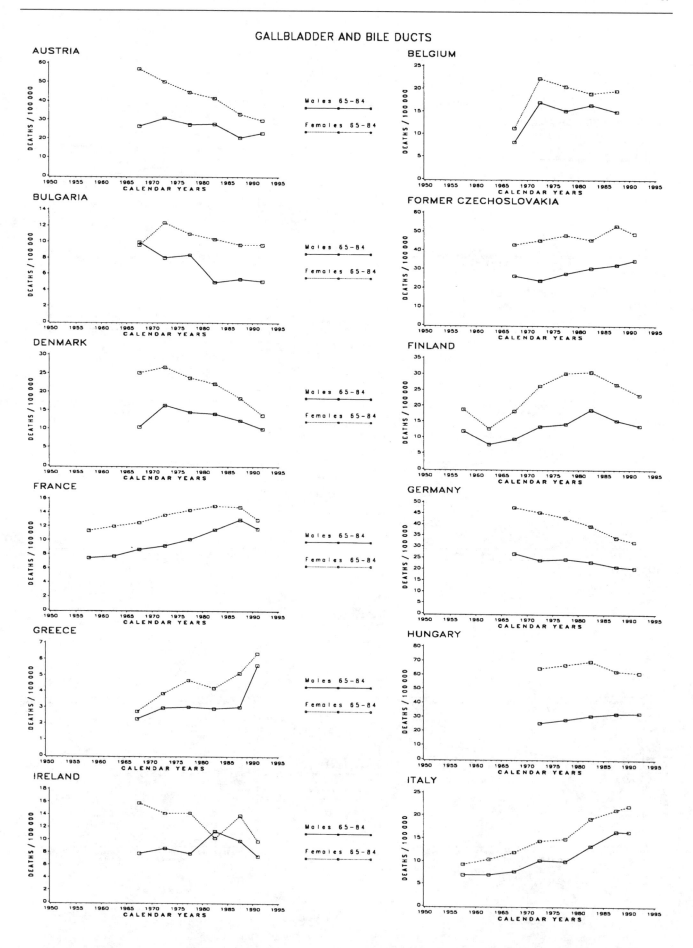

GALLBLADDER AND BILE DUCTS

GALLBLADDER AND BILE DUCTS

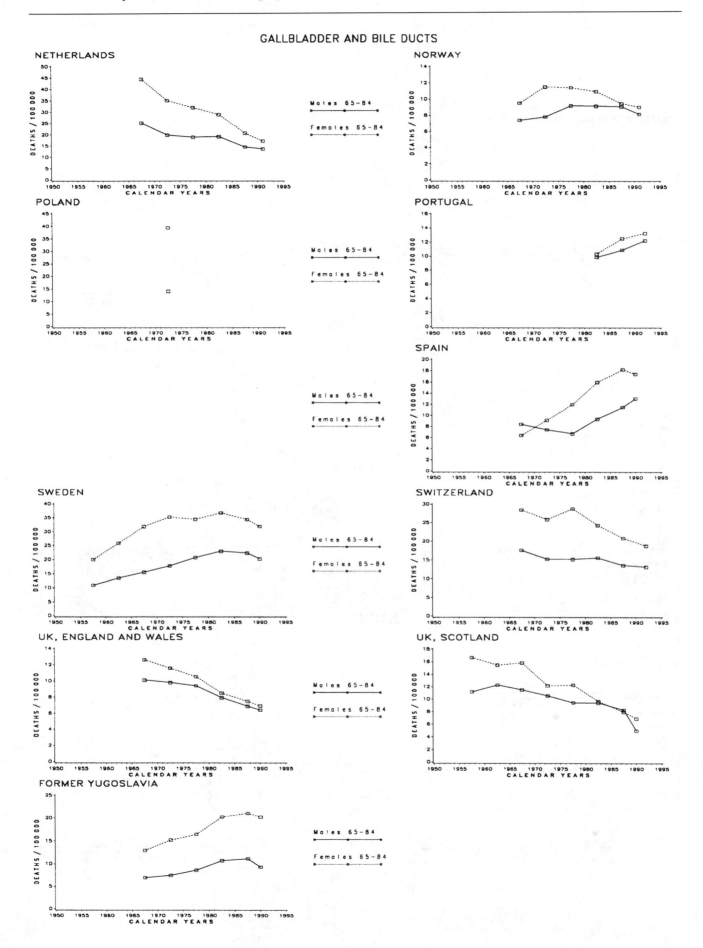

GALLBLADDER AND BILE DUCTS

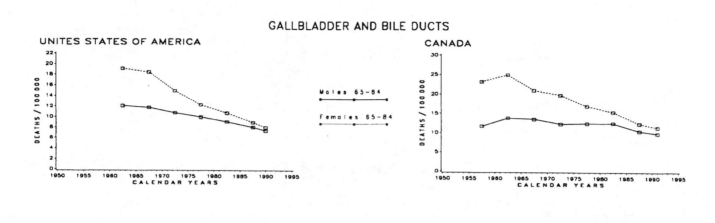

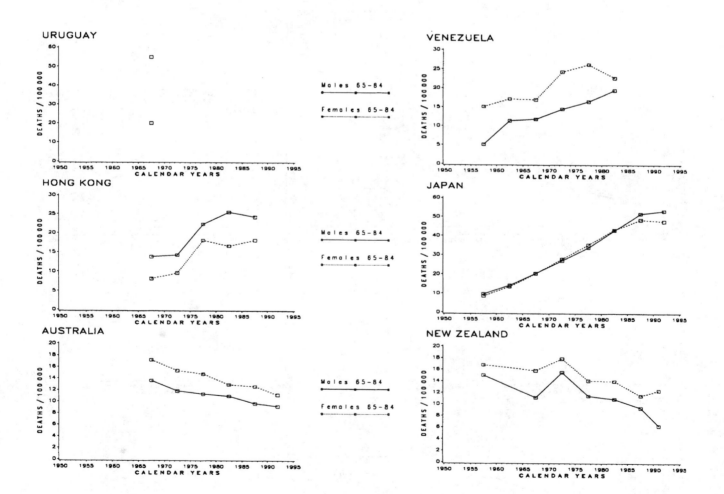

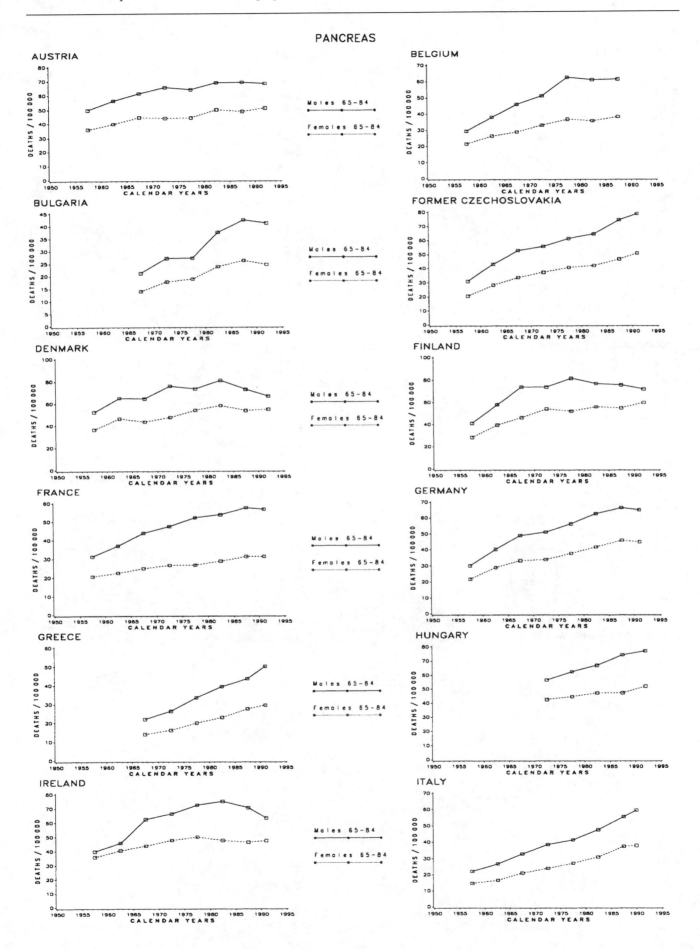

PANCREAS

PANCREAS

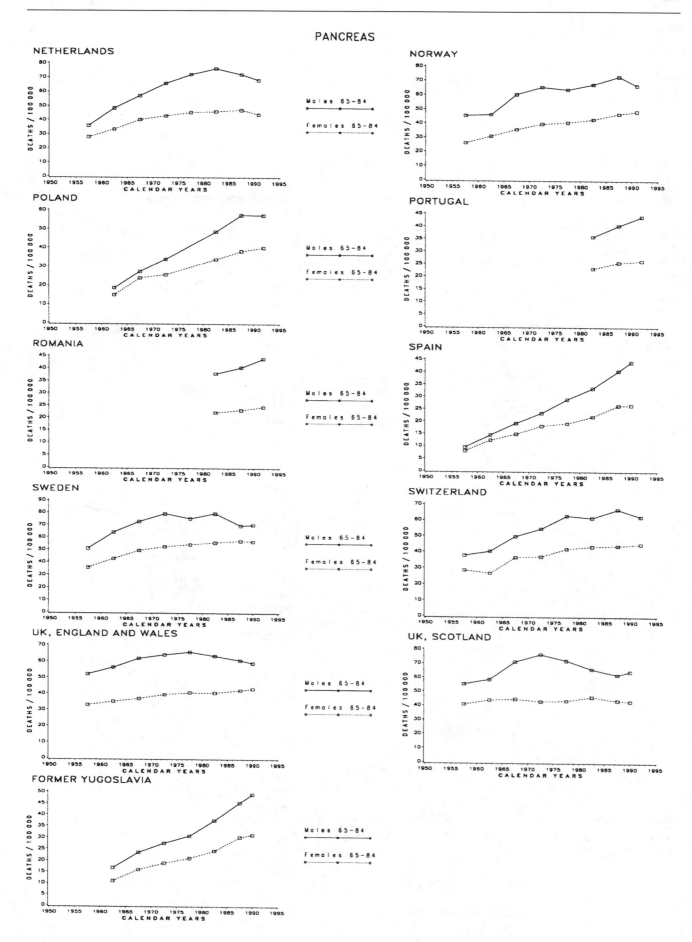

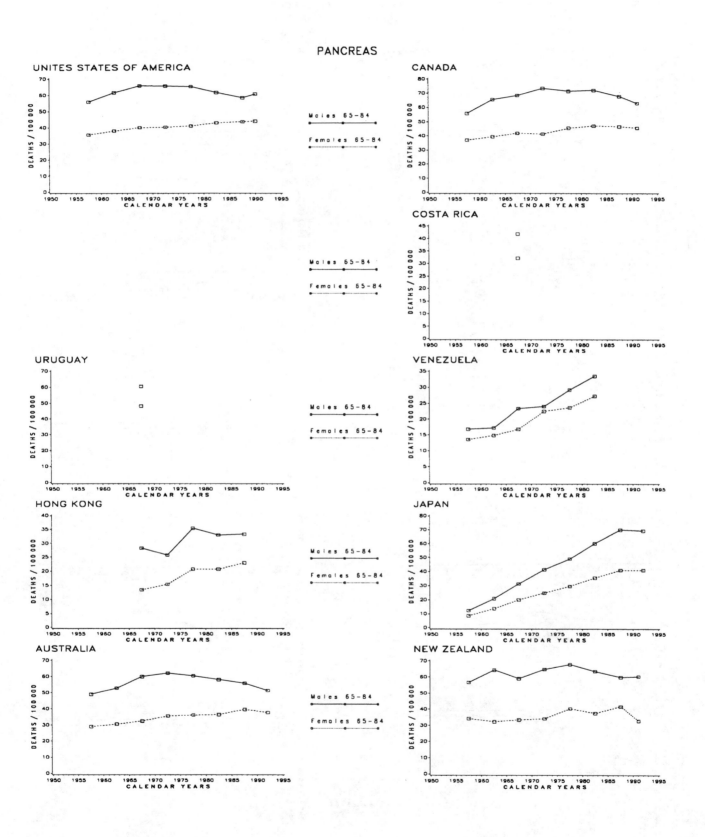

PANCREAS

LARYNX

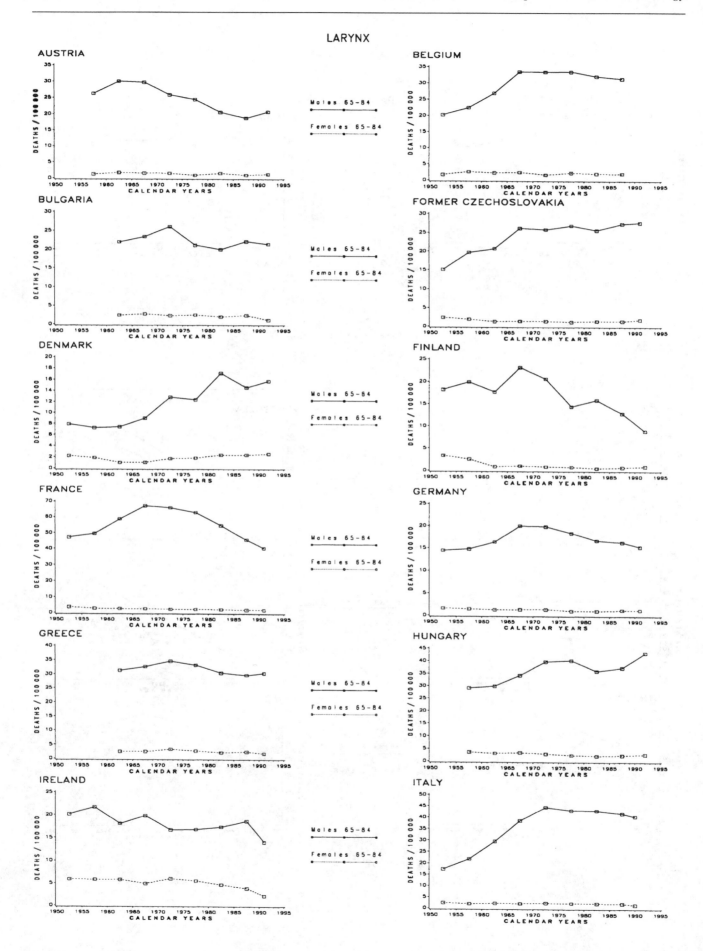

LARYNX

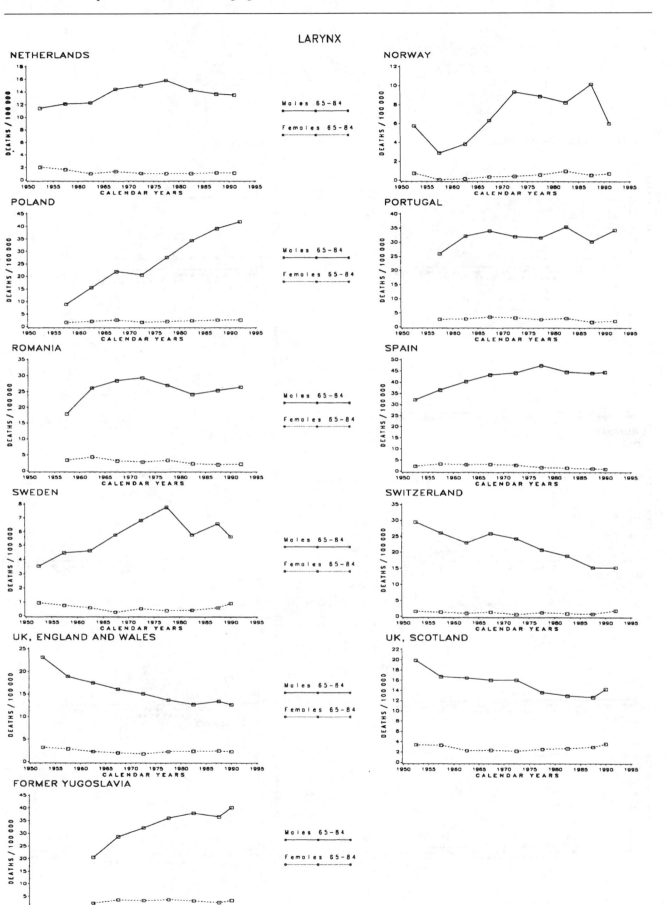

LARYNX

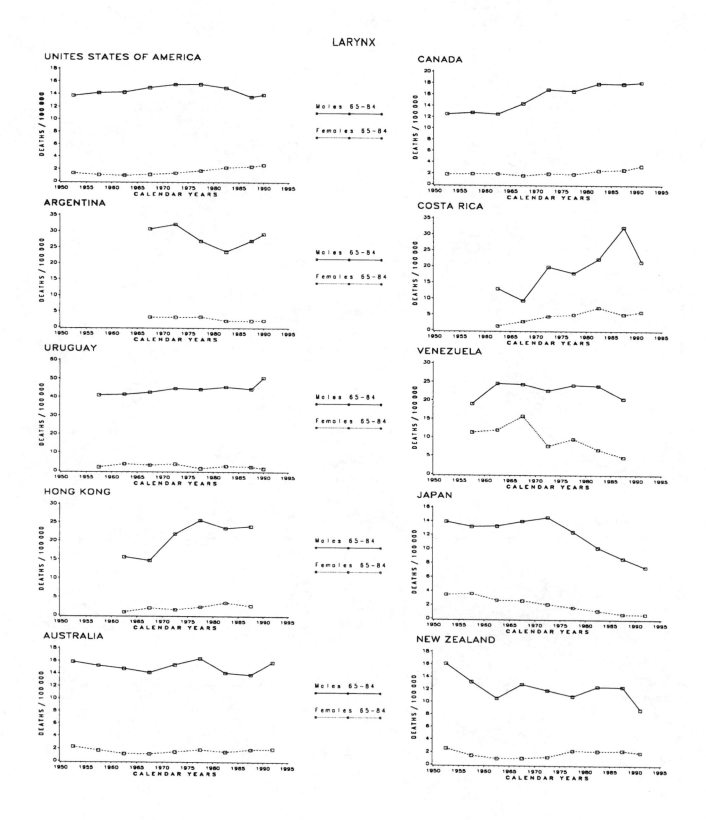

TRACHEA, BRONCHUS AND LUNG

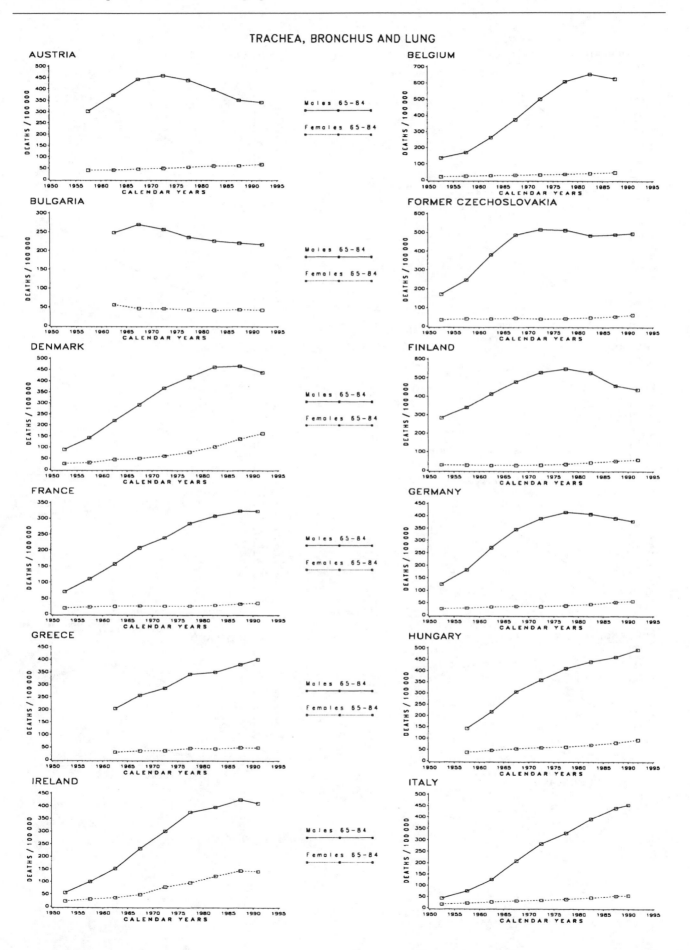

TRACHEA, BRONCHUS AND LUNG

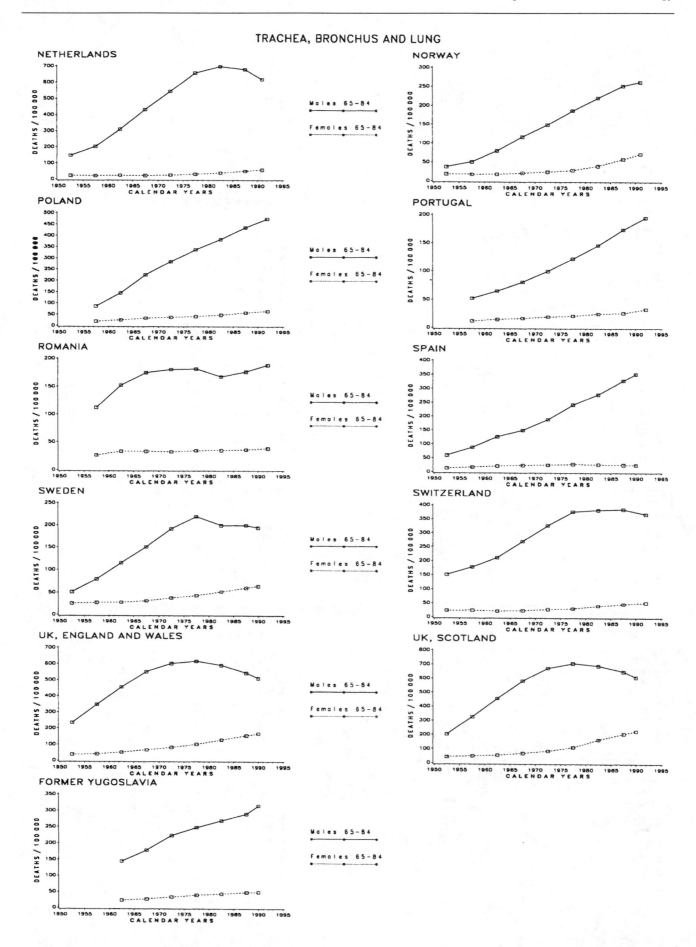

TRACHEA, BRONCHUS AND LUNG

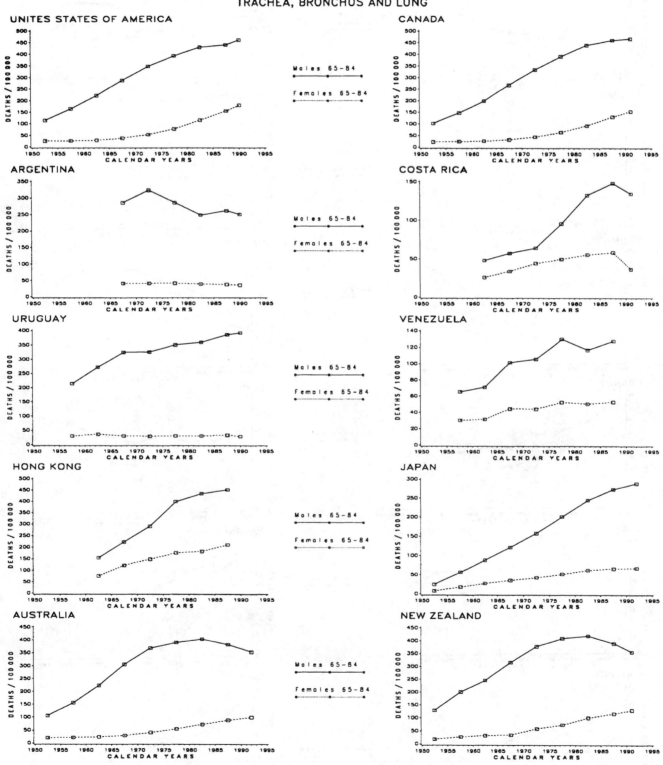

SKIN INCLUDING MELANOMA

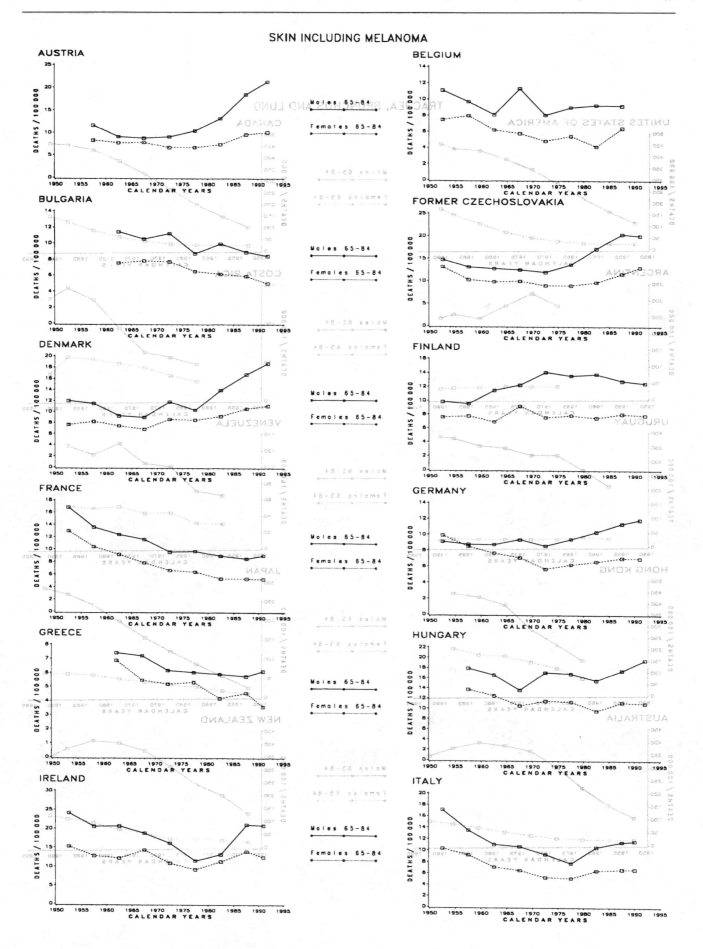

SKIN INCLUDING MELANOMA

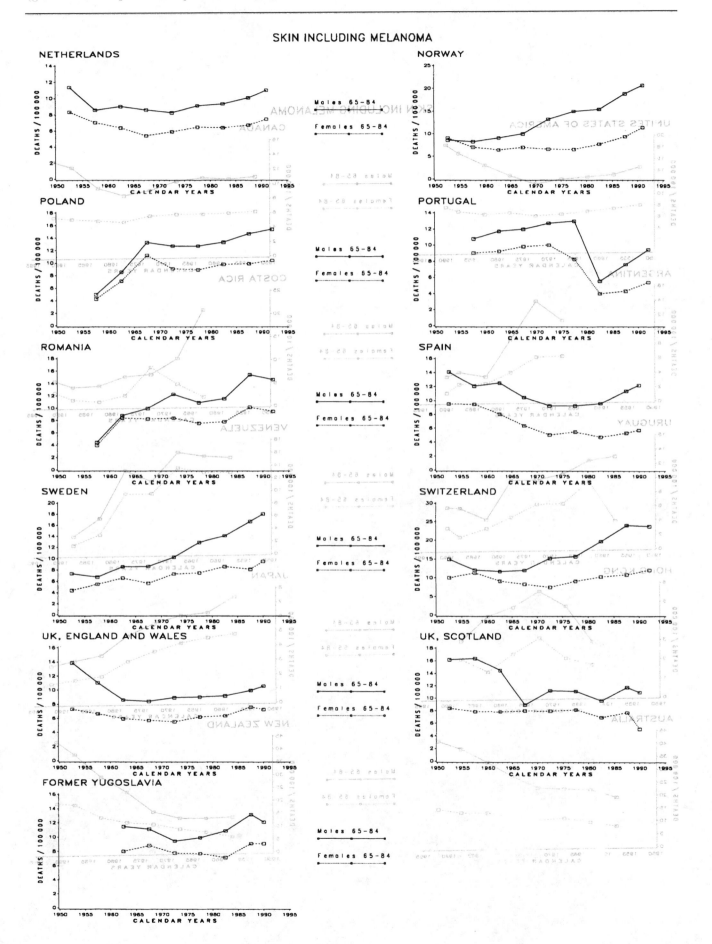

SKIN INCLUDING MELANOMA

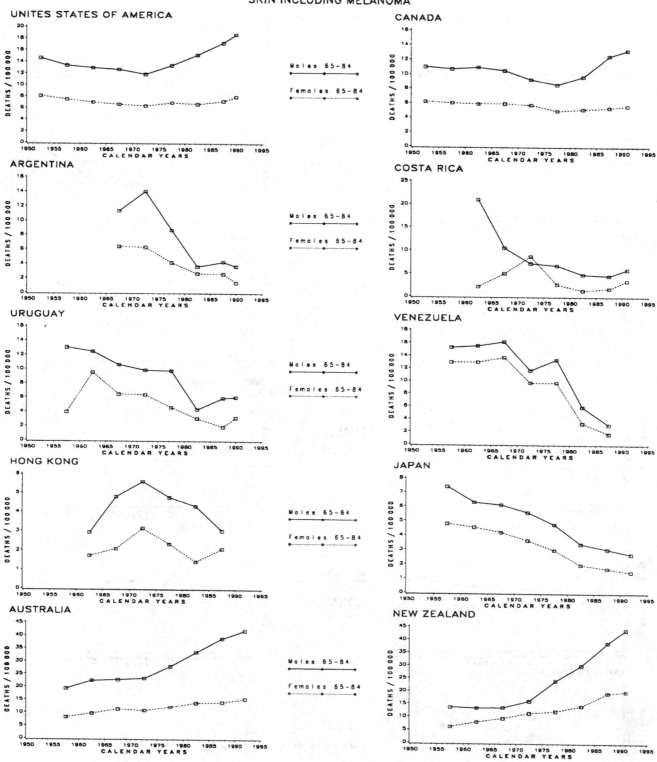

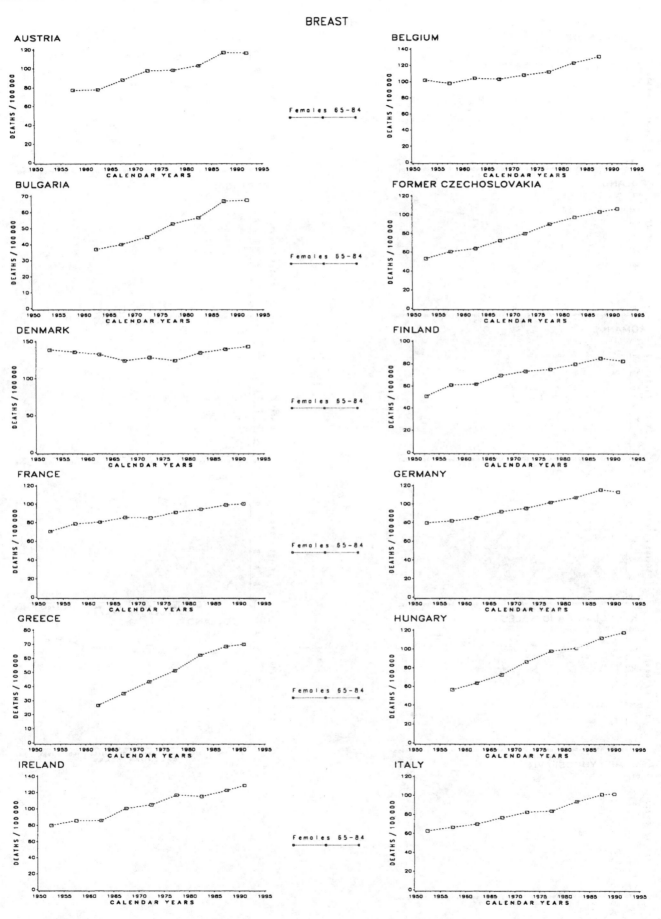

BREAST

BREAST

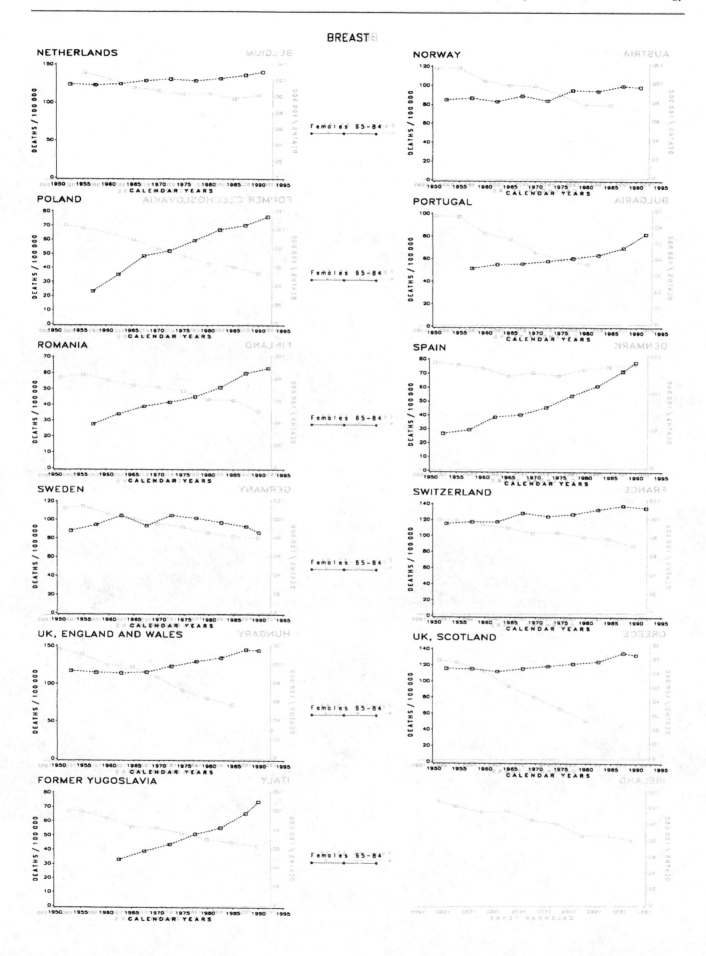

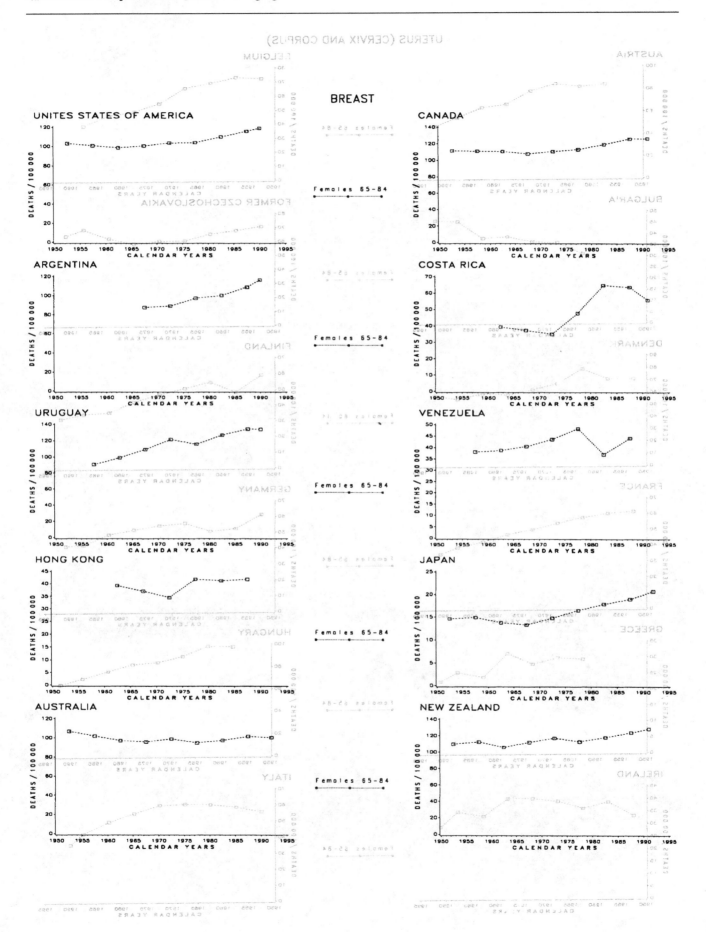

BREAST

UTERUS (CERVIX AND CORPUS)

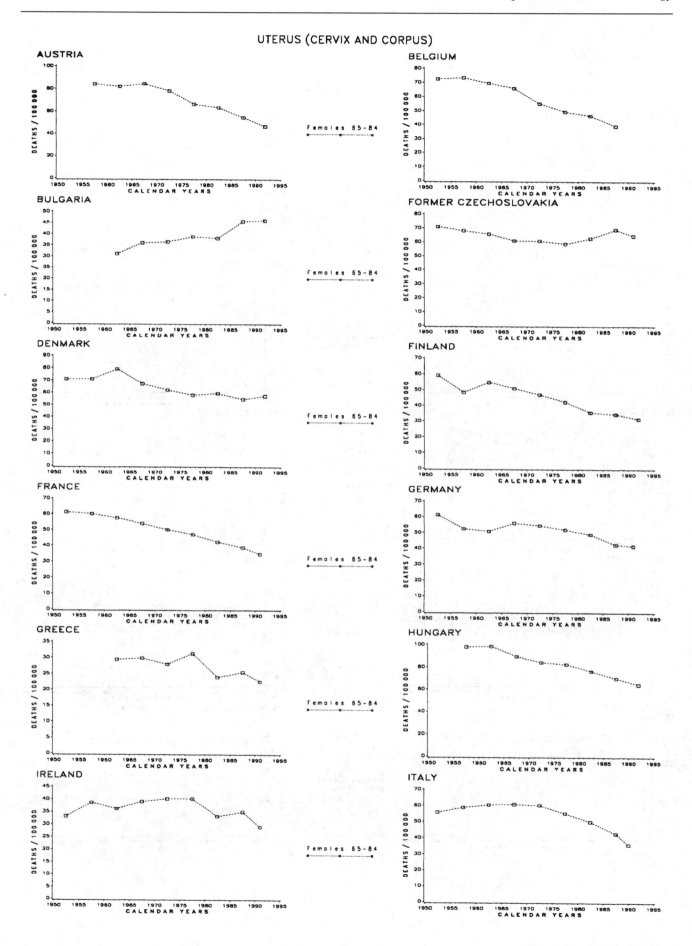

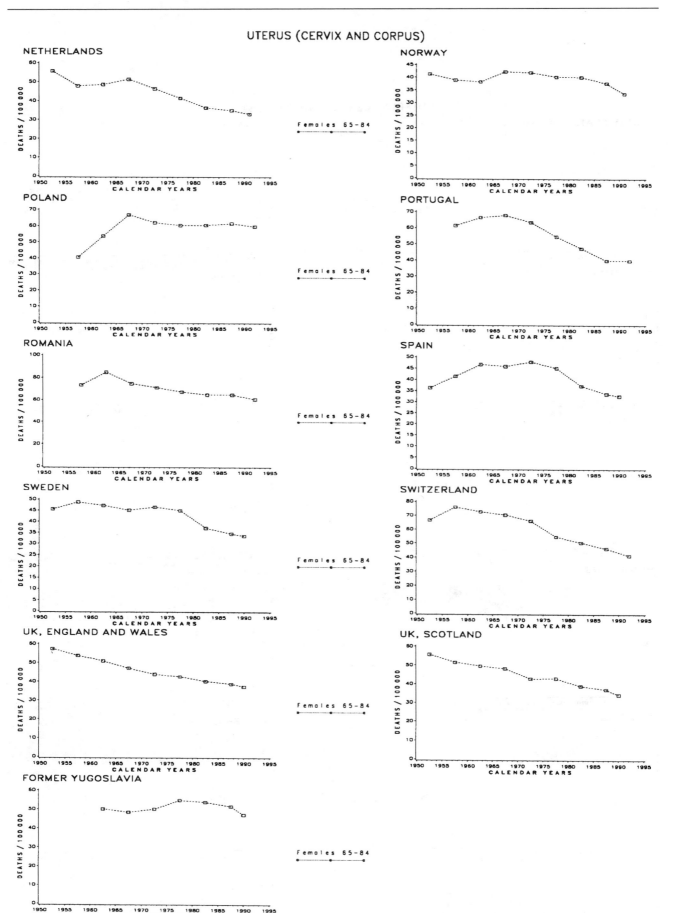

UTERUS (CERVIX AND CORPUS)

UTERUS (CERVIX AND CORPUS)

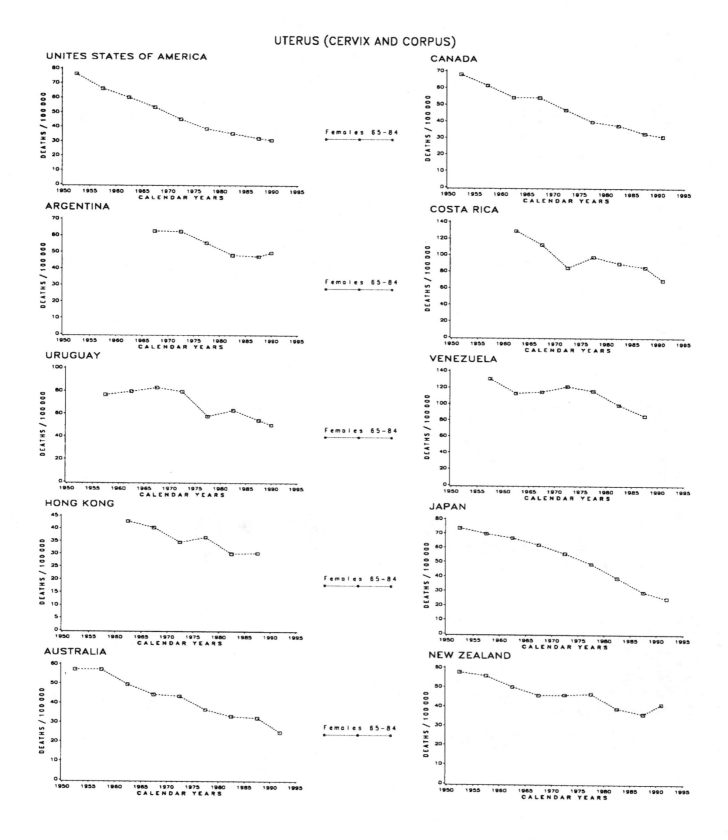

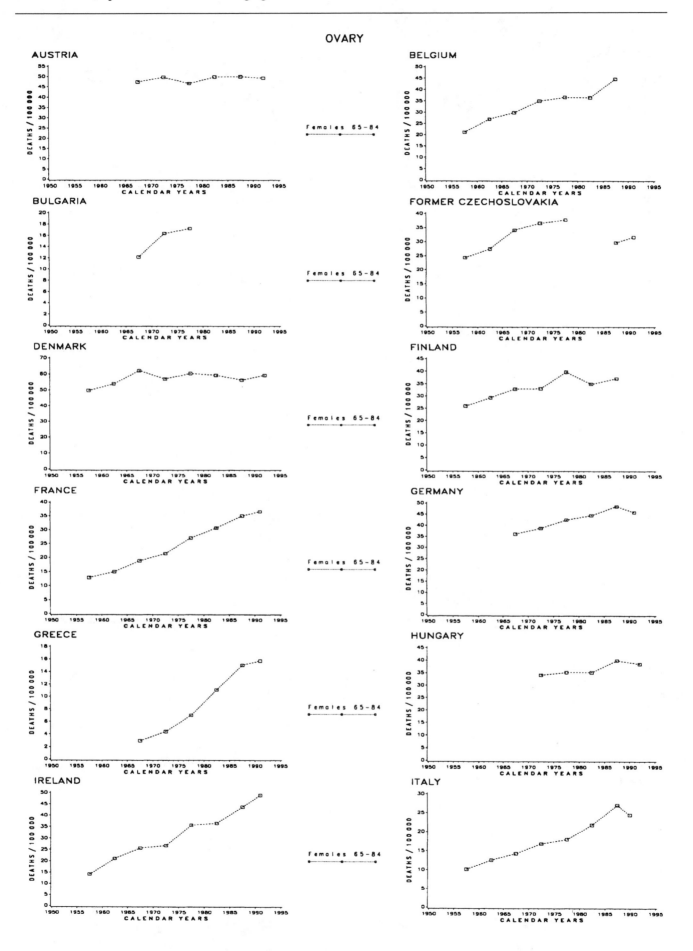

OVARY

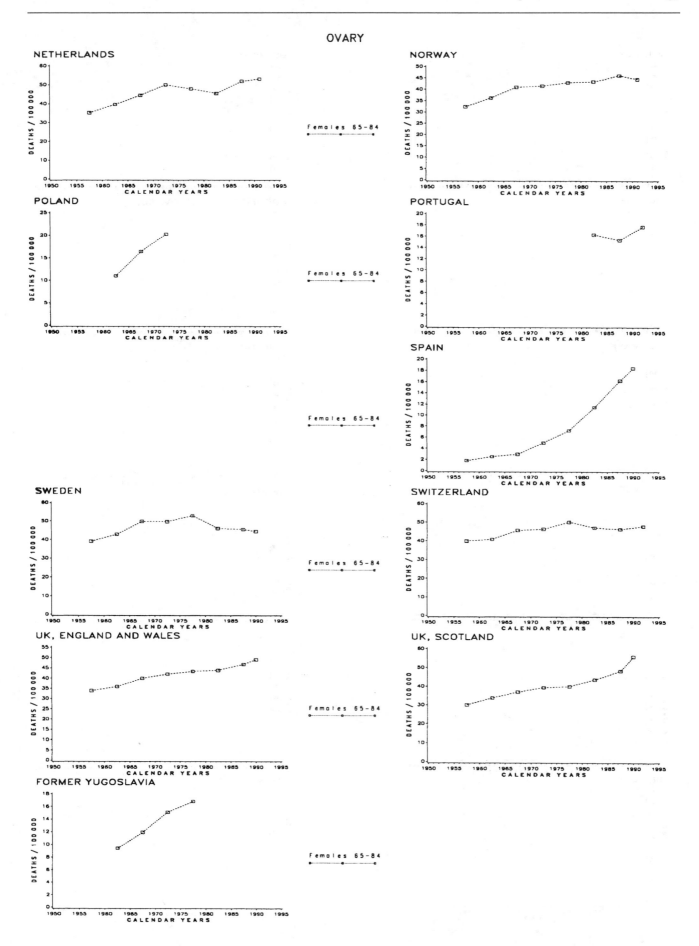

OVARY

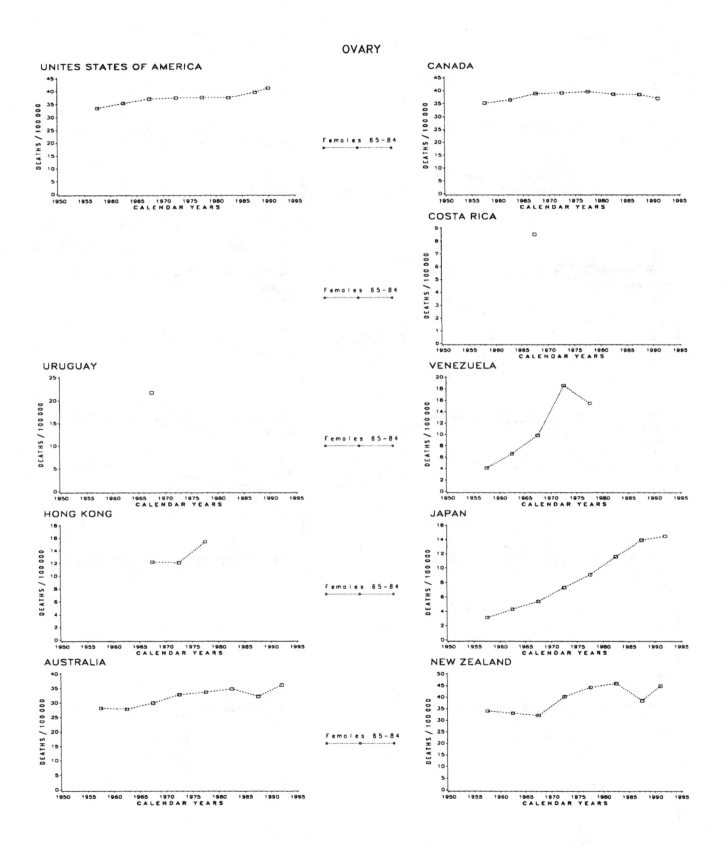

OVARY

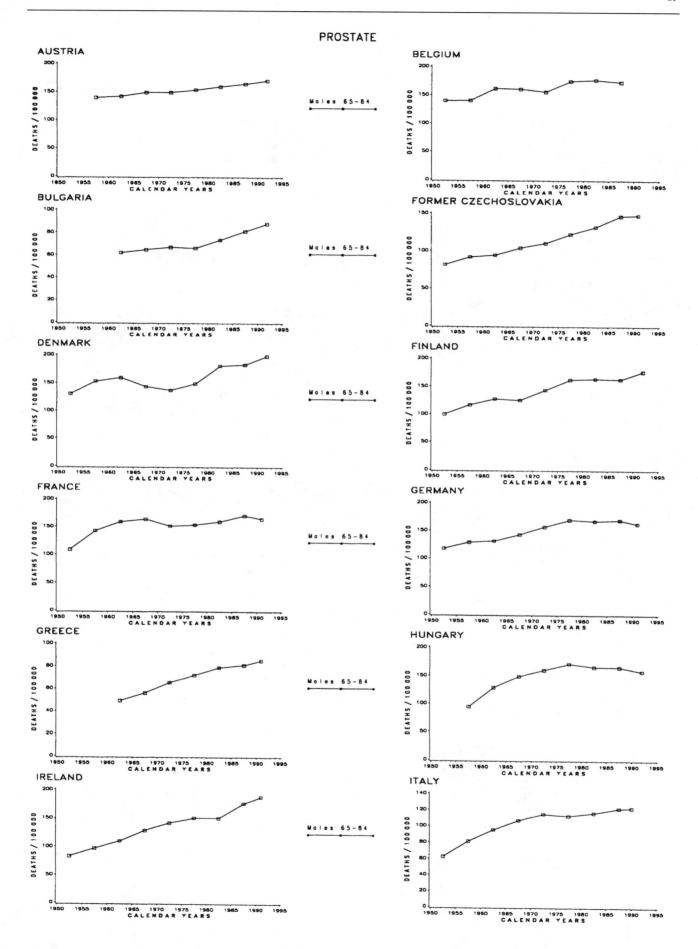

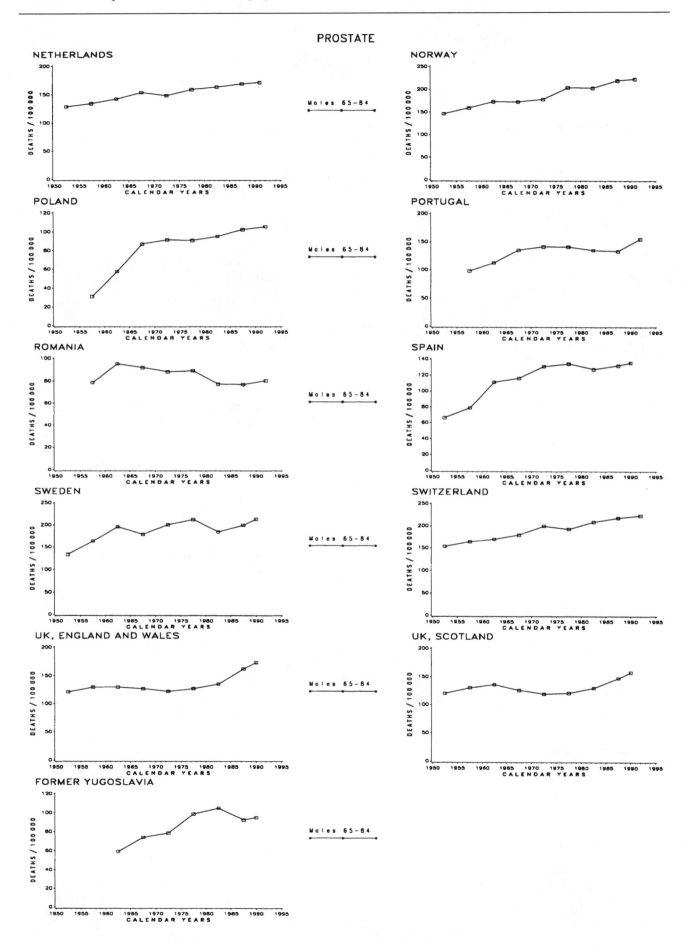

PROSTATE

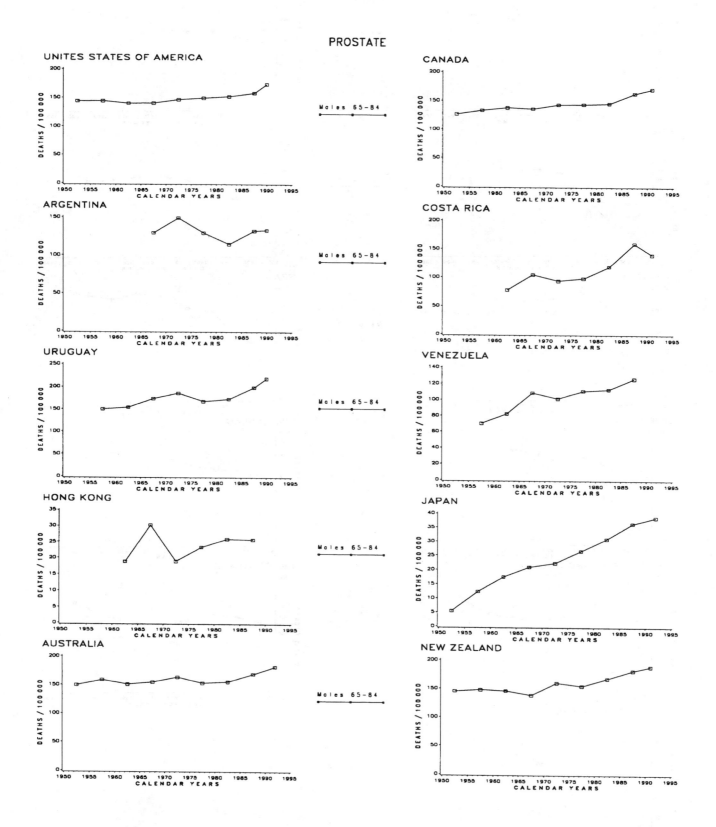

TESTIS

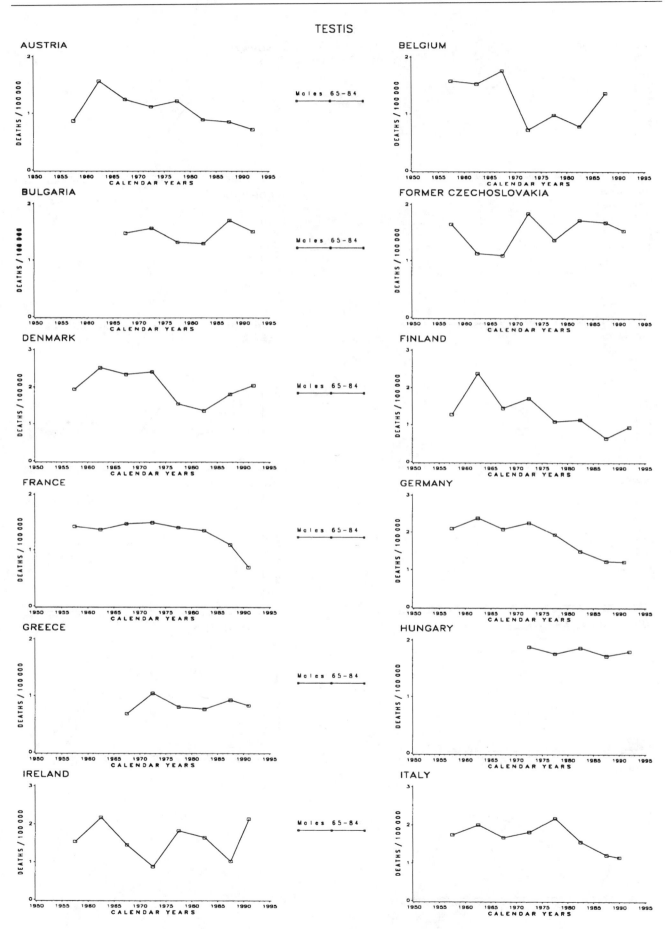

Males 65-84

TESTIS

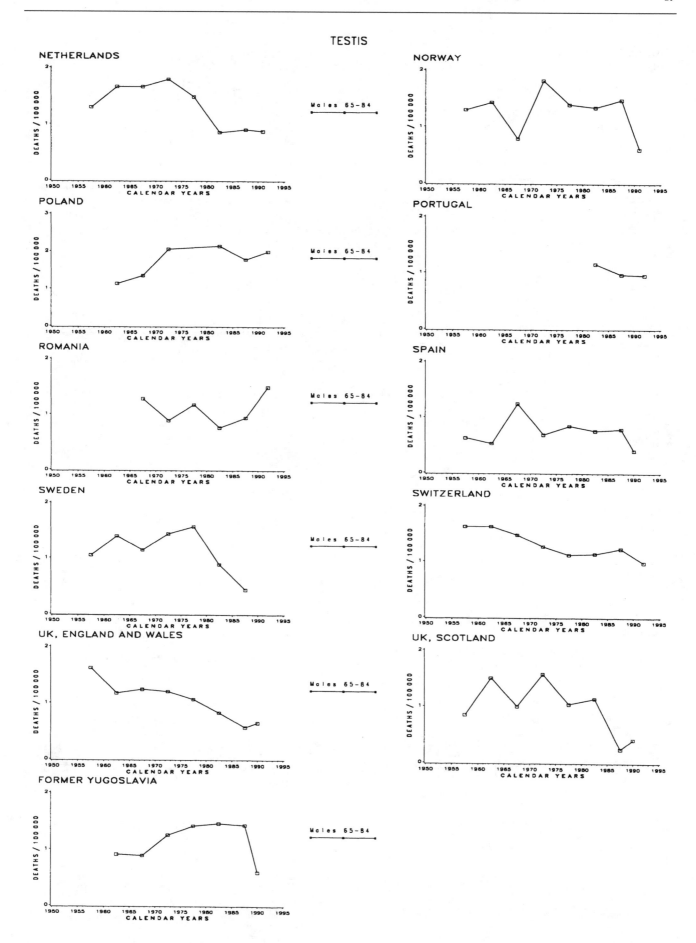

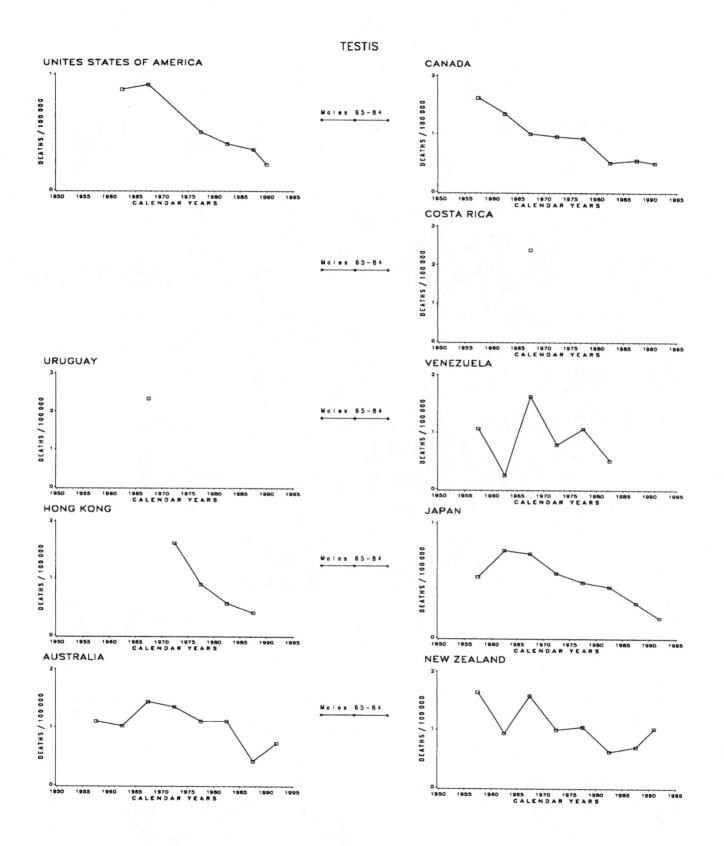

TESTIS

BLADDER

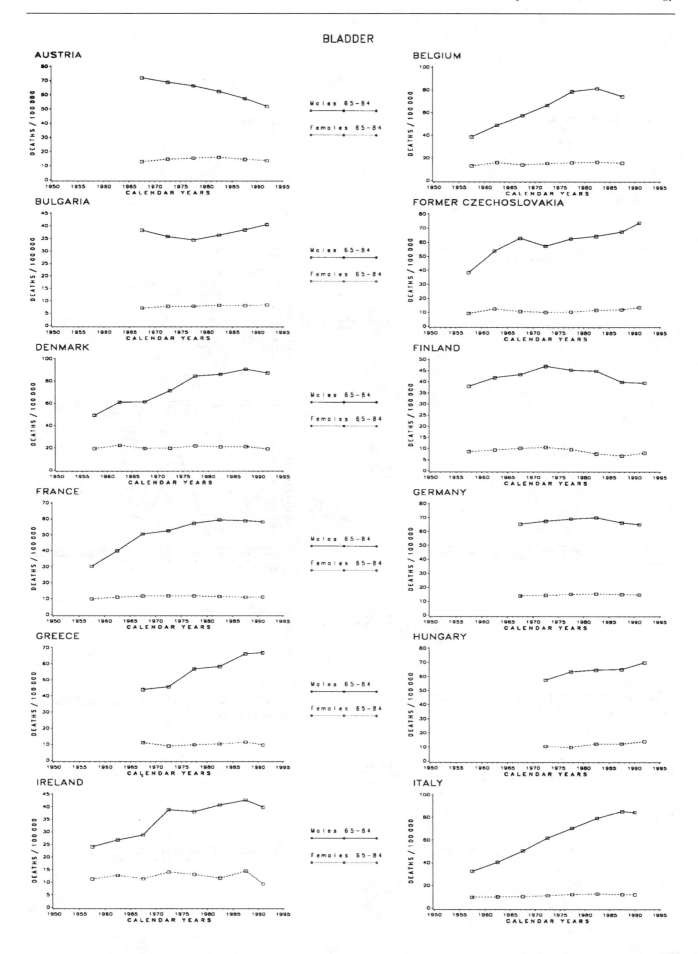

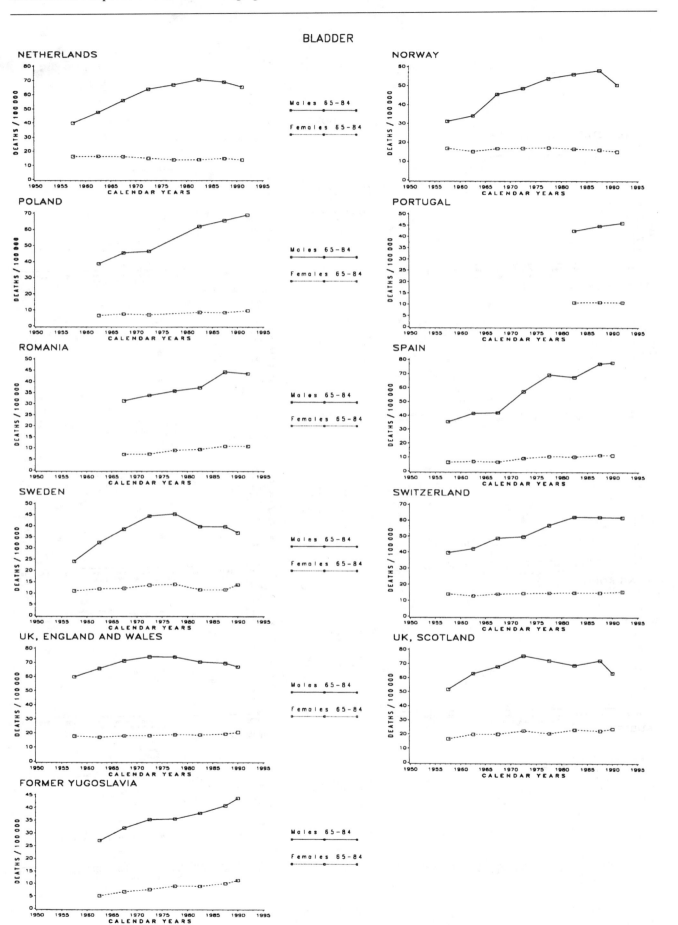

BLADDER

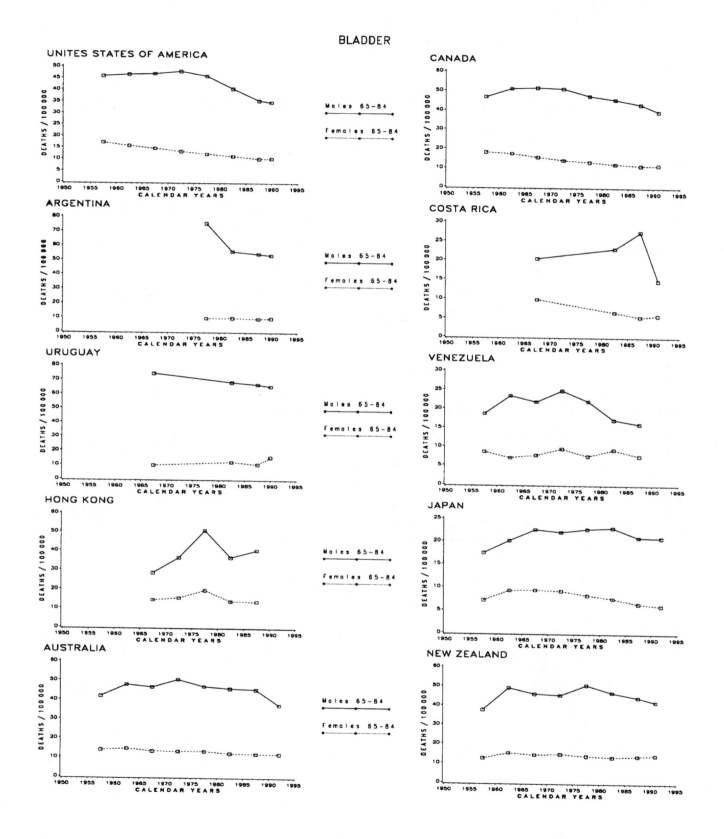

BLADDER

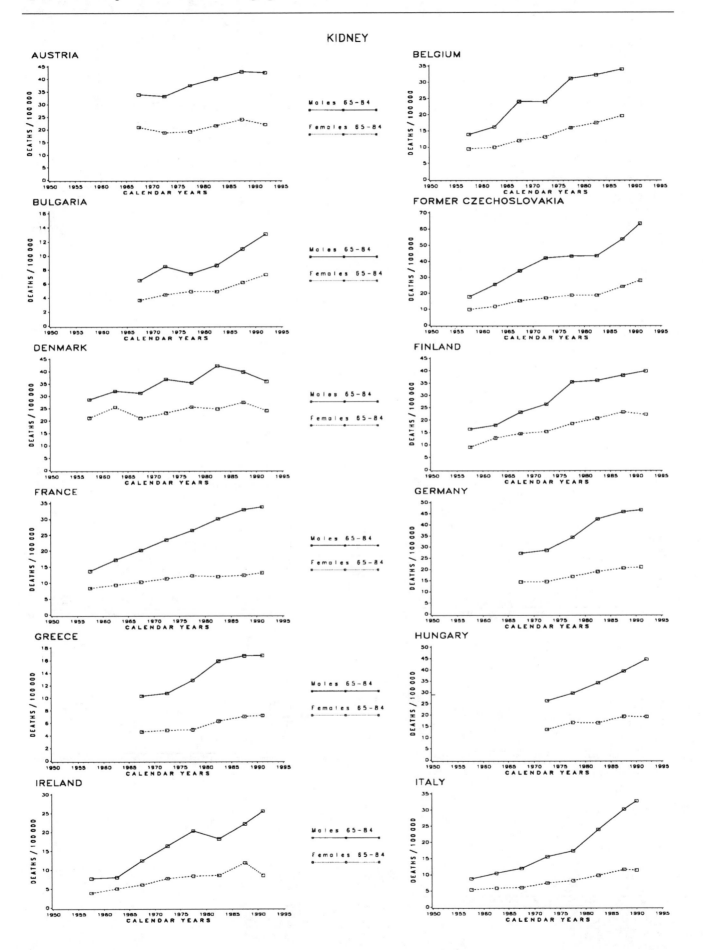

KIDNEY

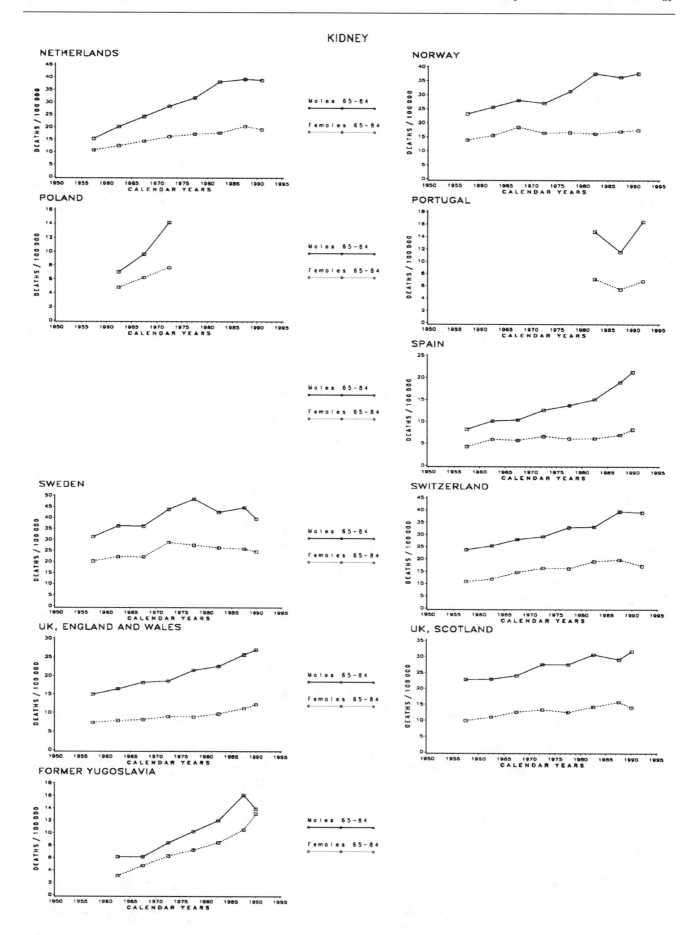

KIDNEY

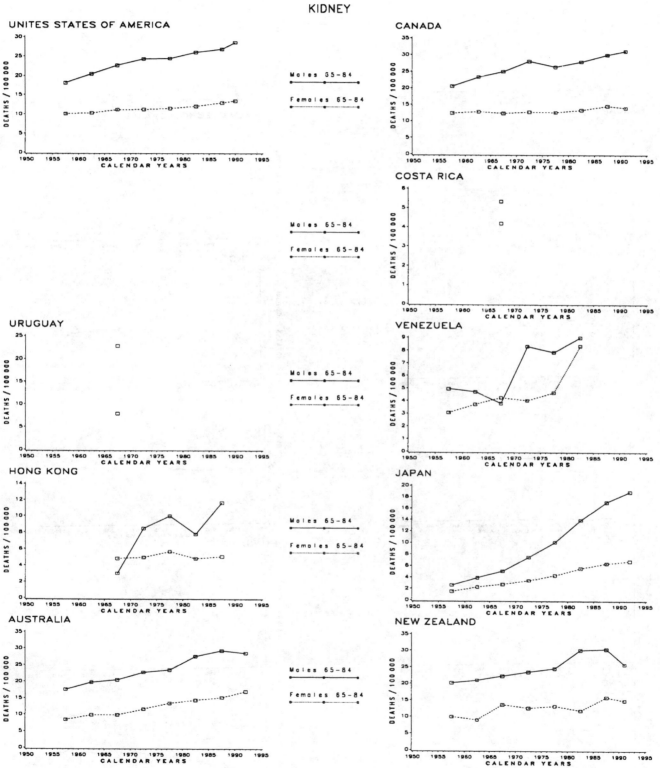

KIDNEY

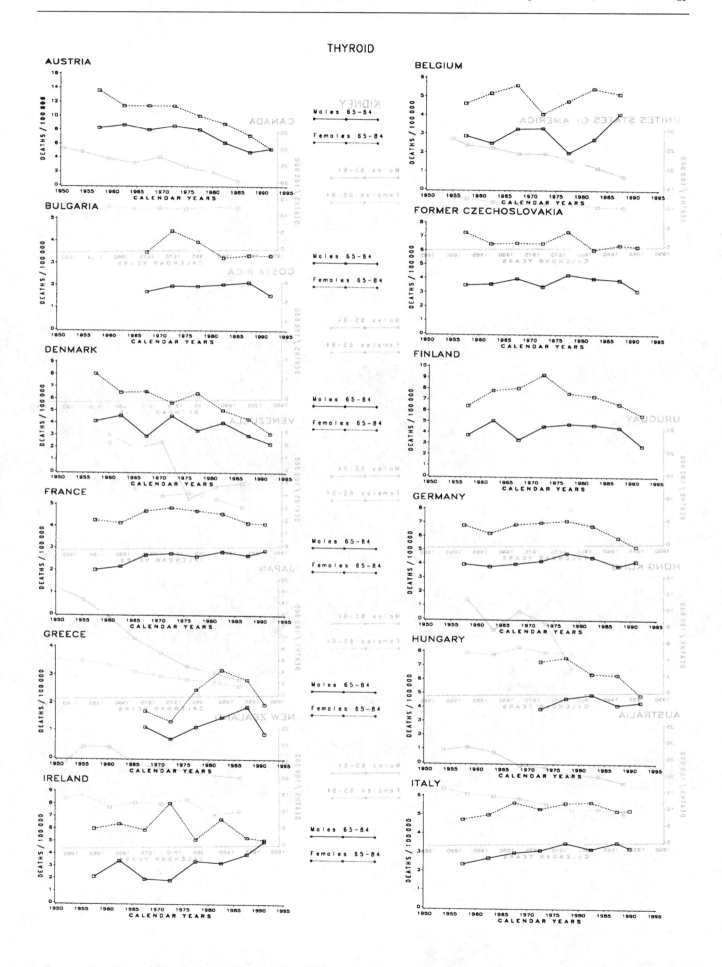

THYROID

THYROID

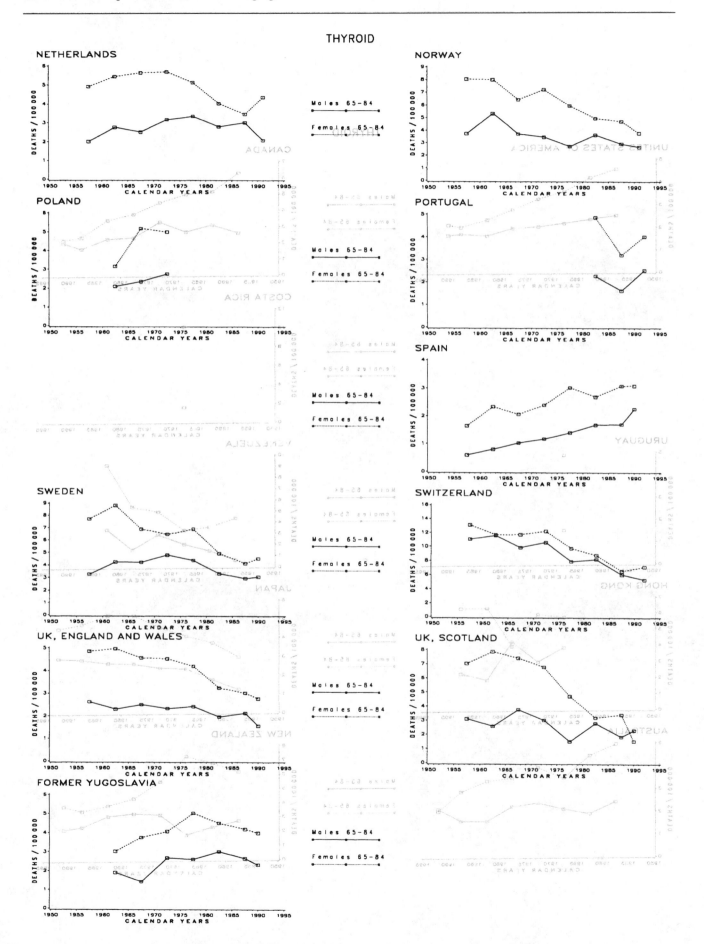

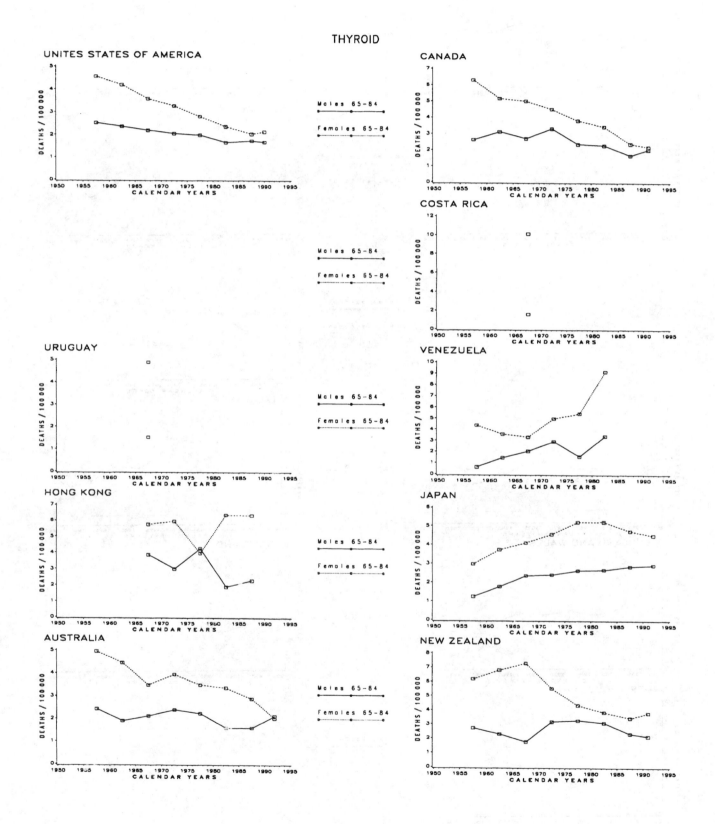

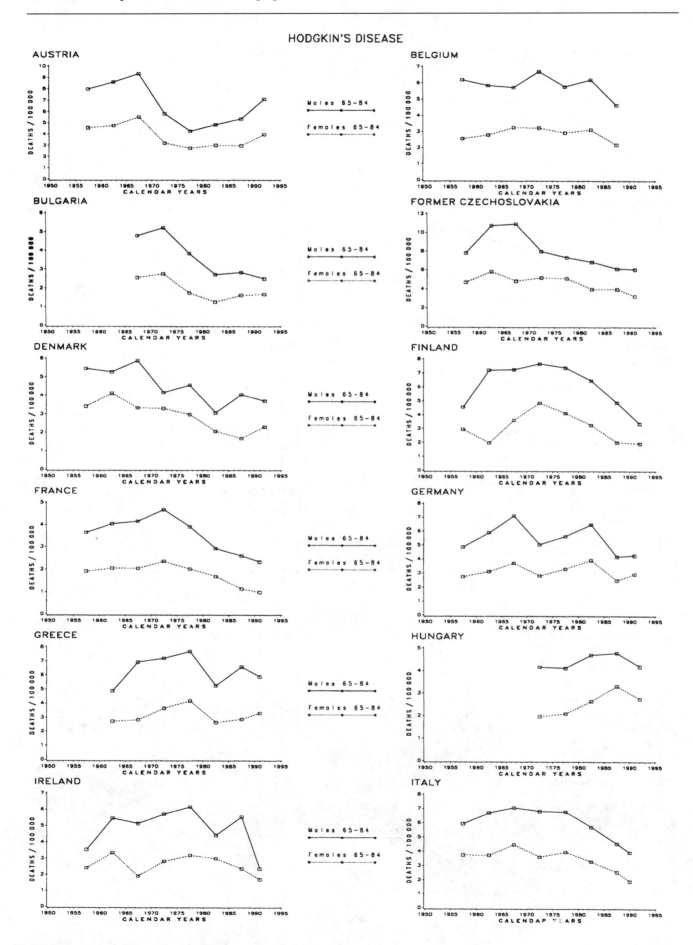

HODGKIN'S DISEASE

HODGKIN'S DISEASE

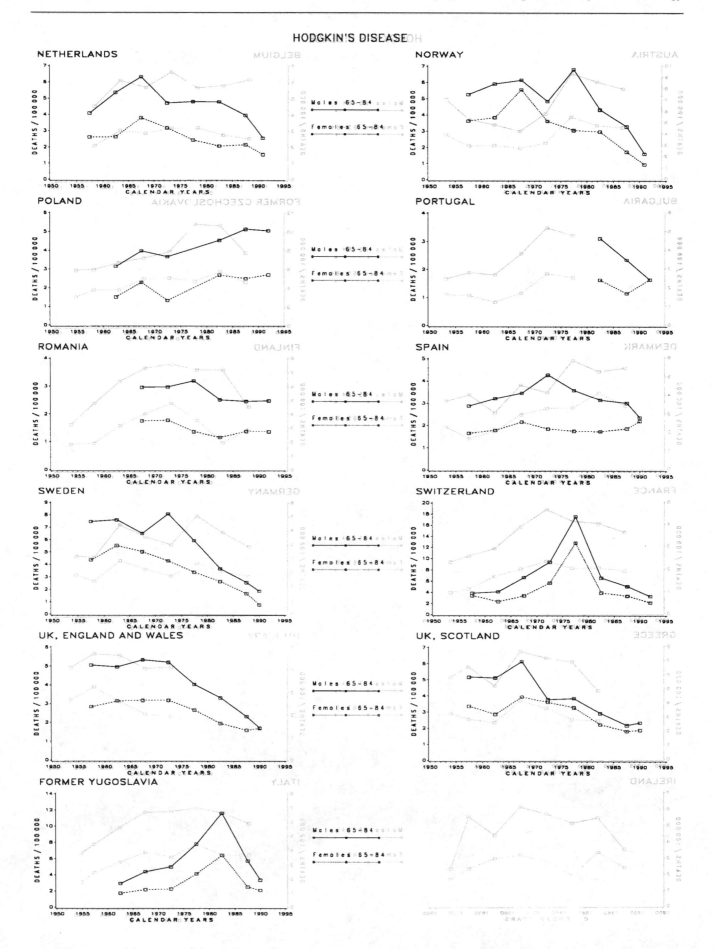

HODGKIN'S DISEASE

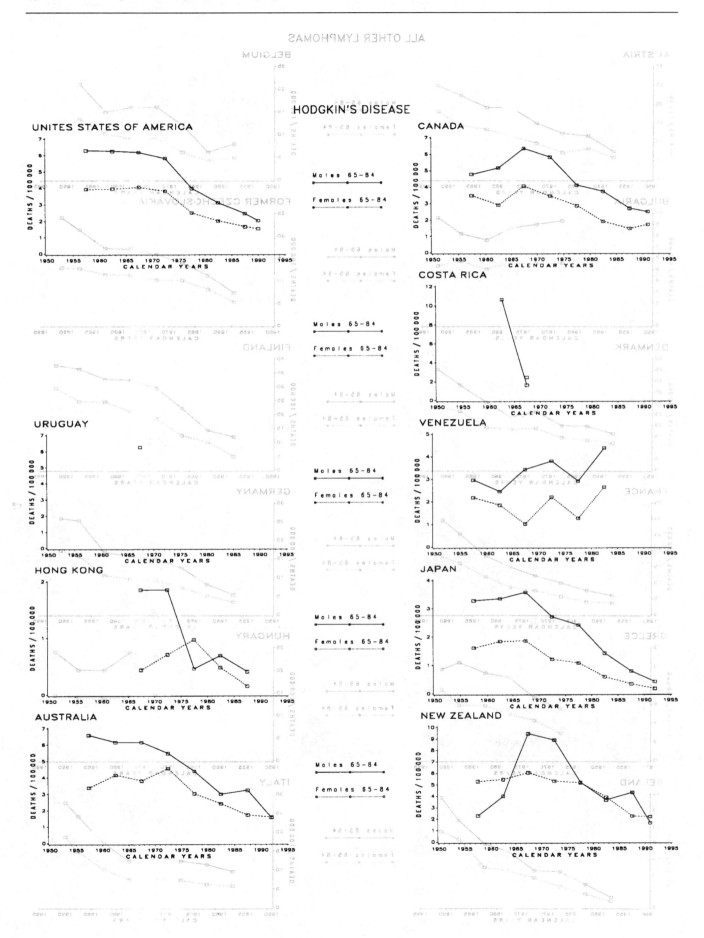

ALL OTHER LYMPHOMAS

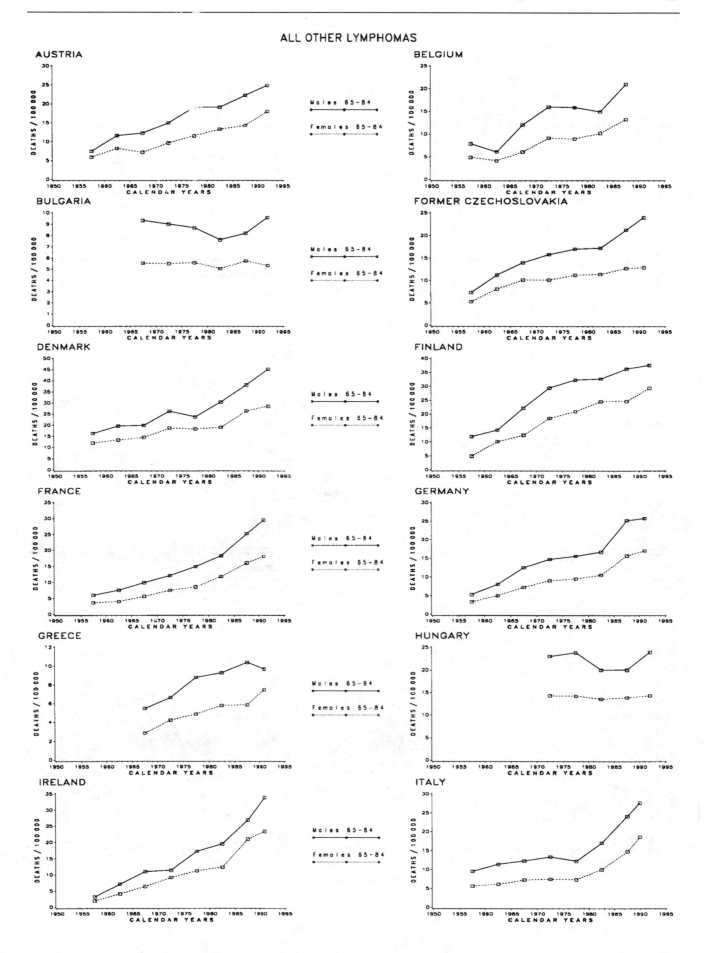

ALL OTHER LYMPHOMAS

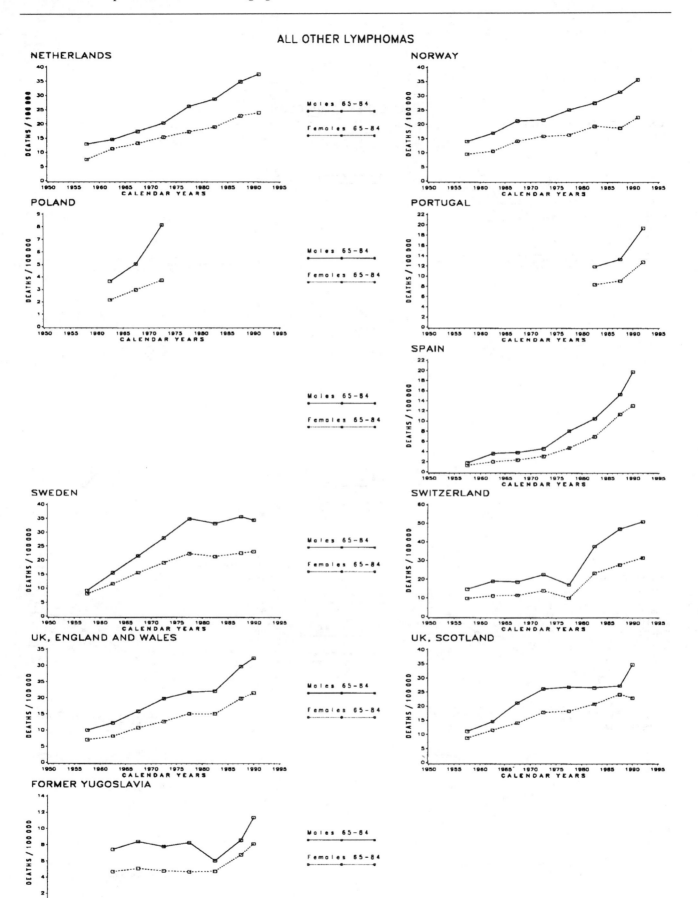

ALL OTHER LYMPHOMAS

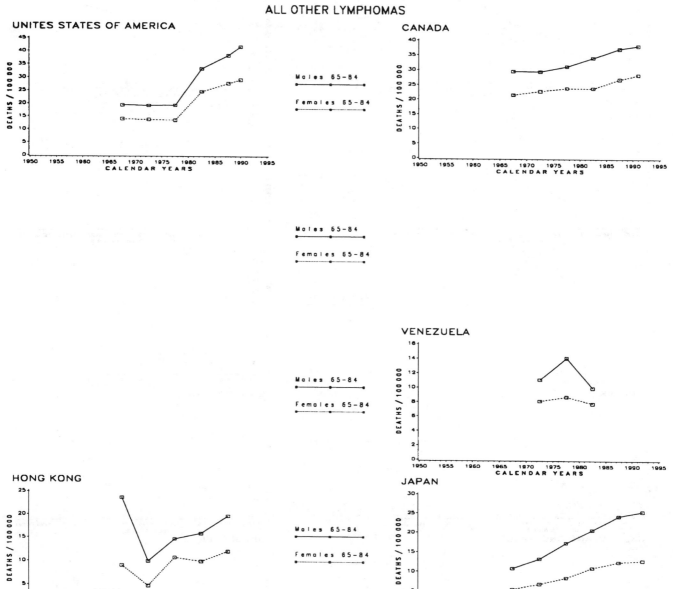

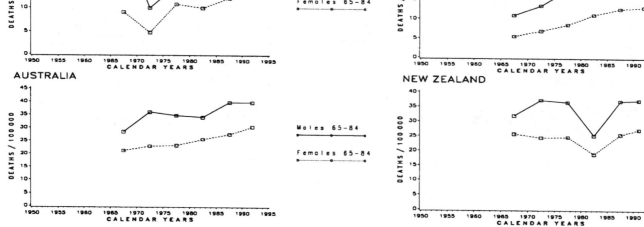

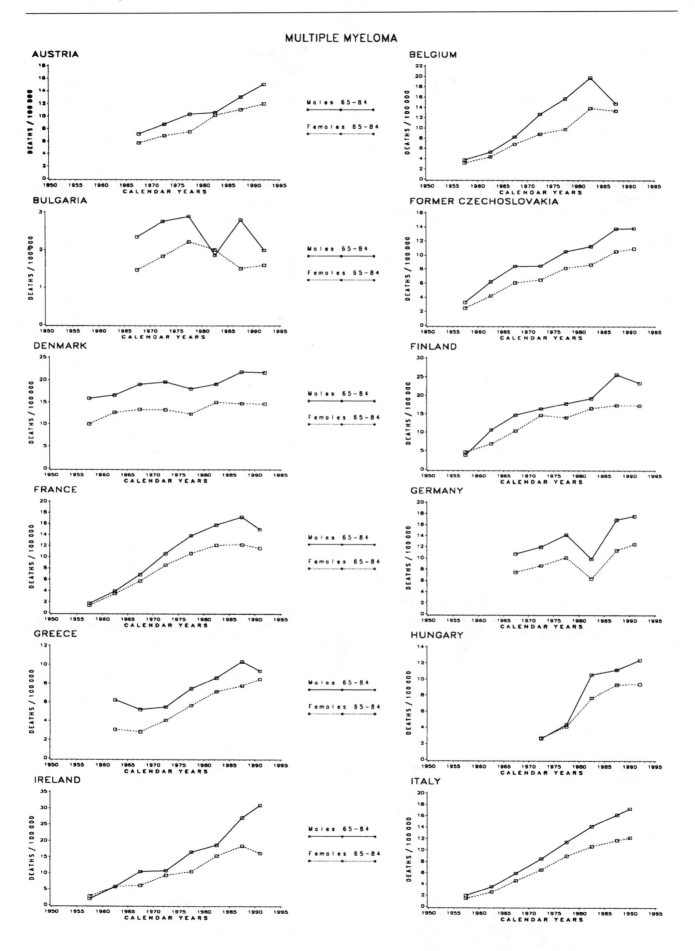

MULTIPLE MYELOMA

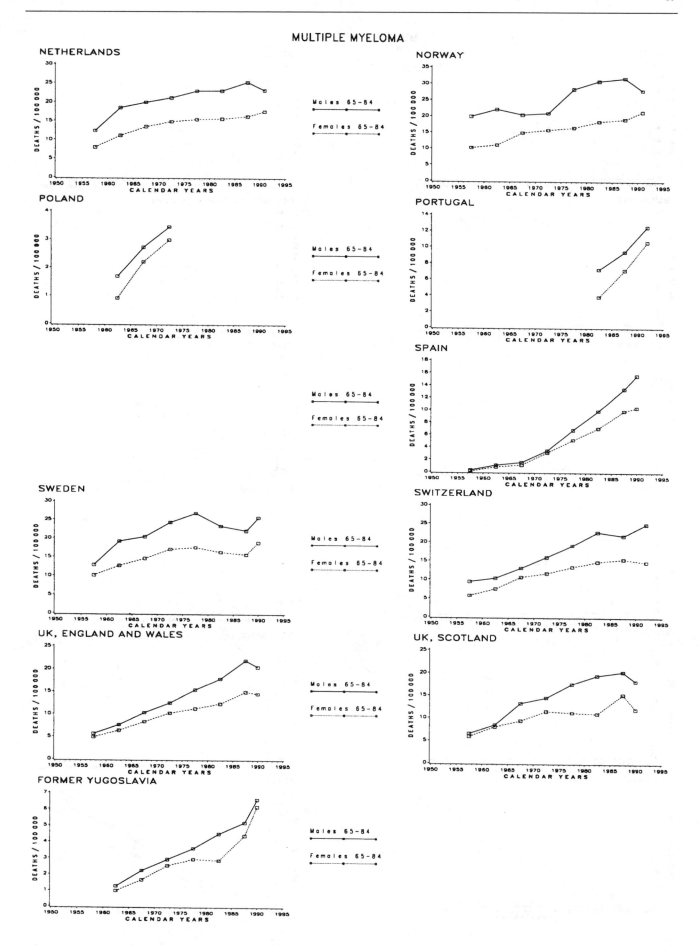

MULTIPLE MYELOMA

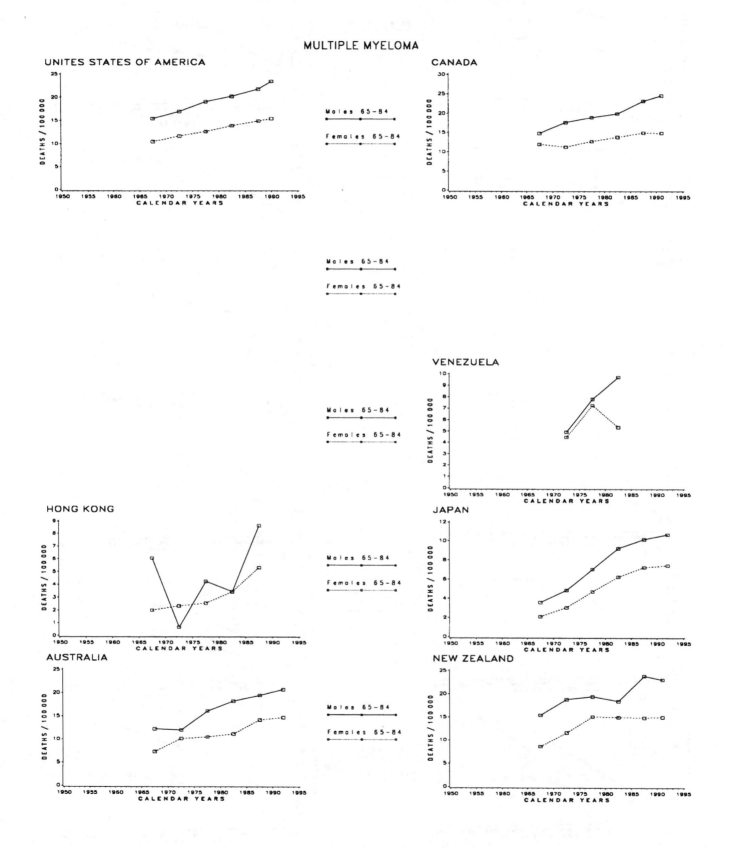

MULTIPLE MYELOMA

UNITES STATES OF AMERICA

CANADA

VENEZUELA

HONG KONG

JAPAN

AUSTRALIA

NEW ZEALAND

Males 65-84

Females 65-84

LEUKAEMIAS

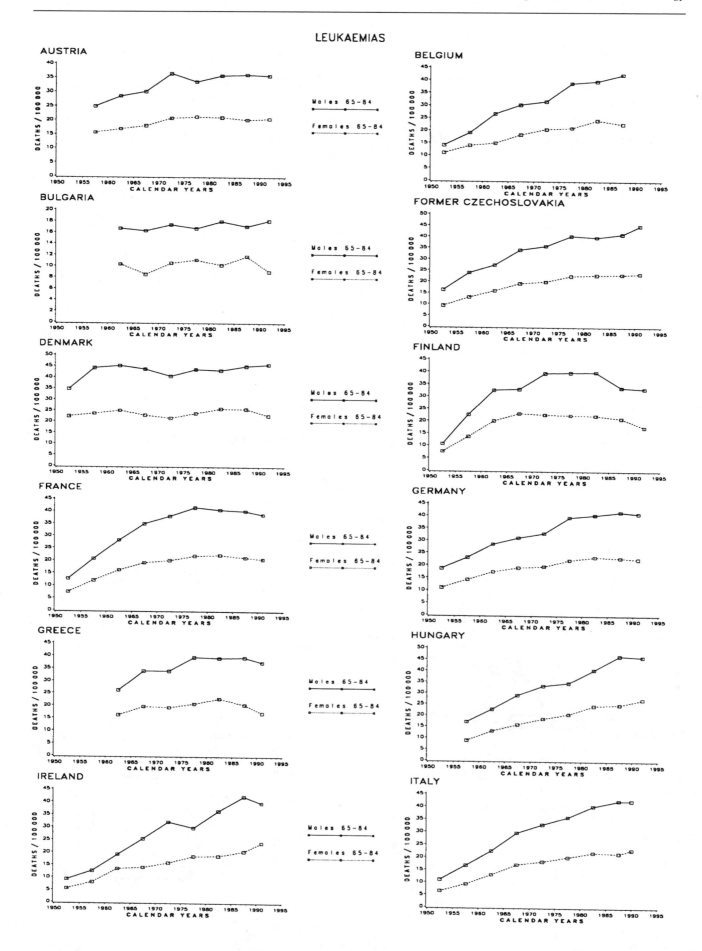

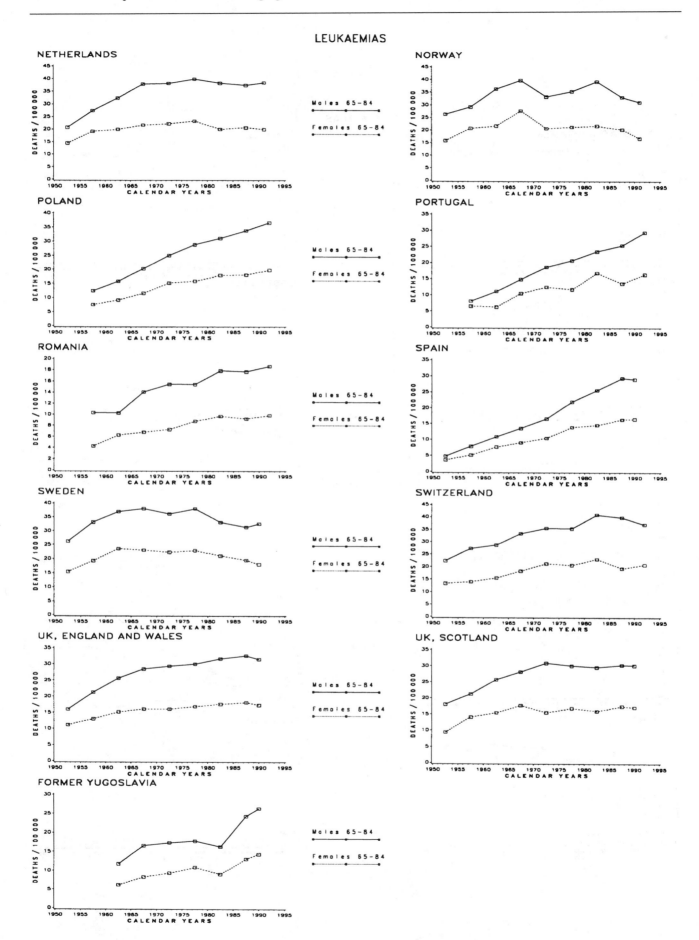

LEUKAEMIAS

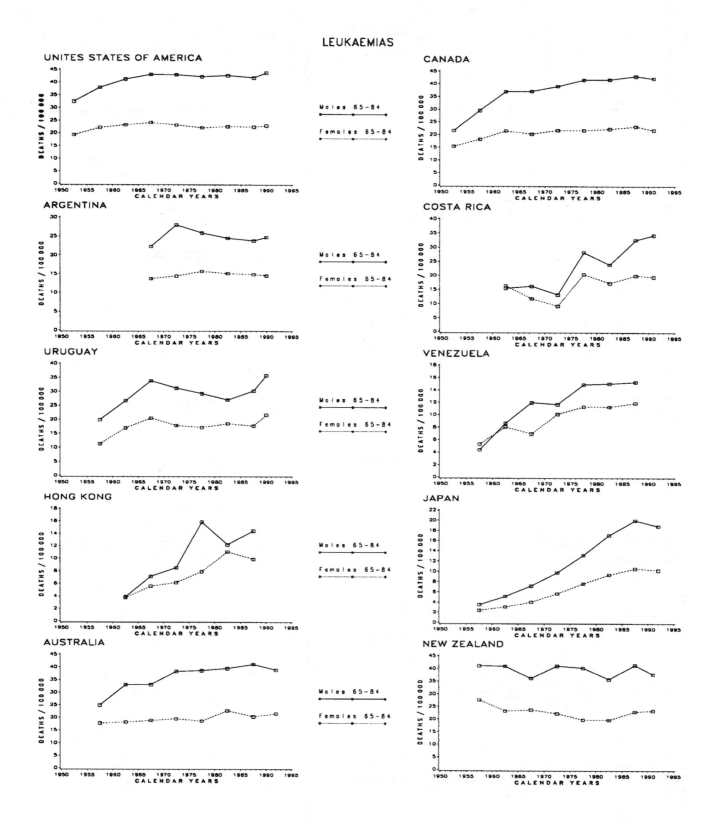

LEUKAEMIAS

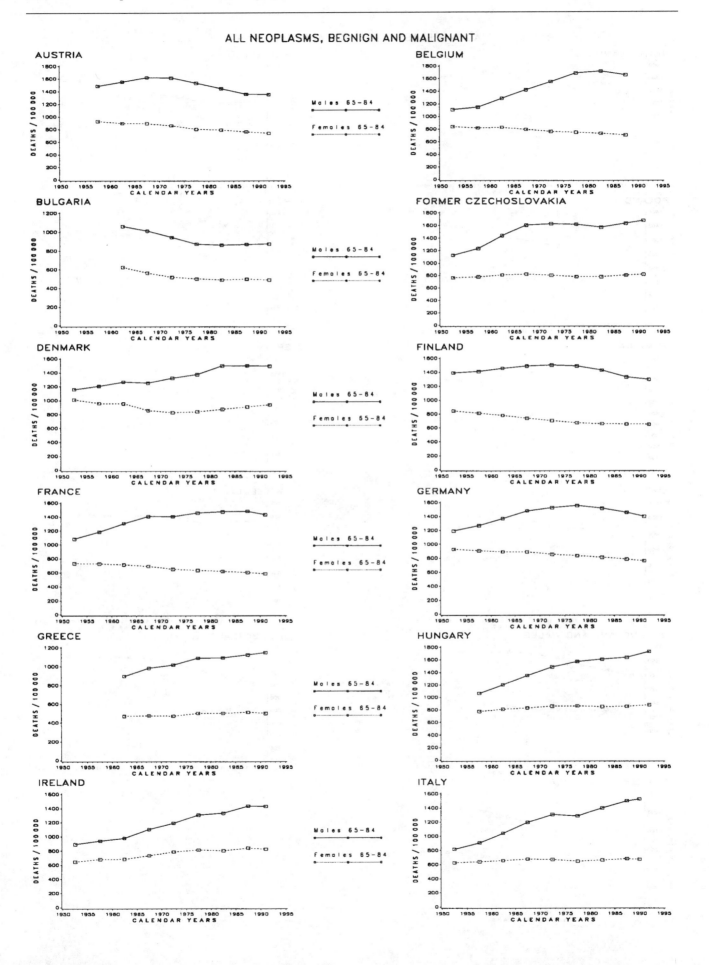

ALL NEOPLASMS, BEGNIGN AND MALIGNANT

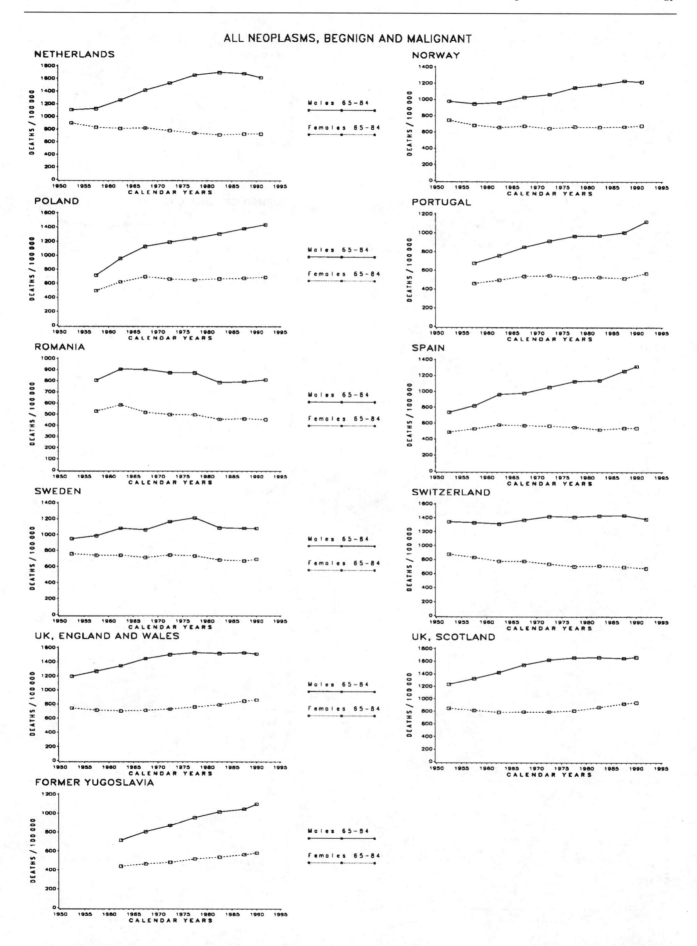

ALL NEOPLASMS, BEGNIGN AND MALIGNANT

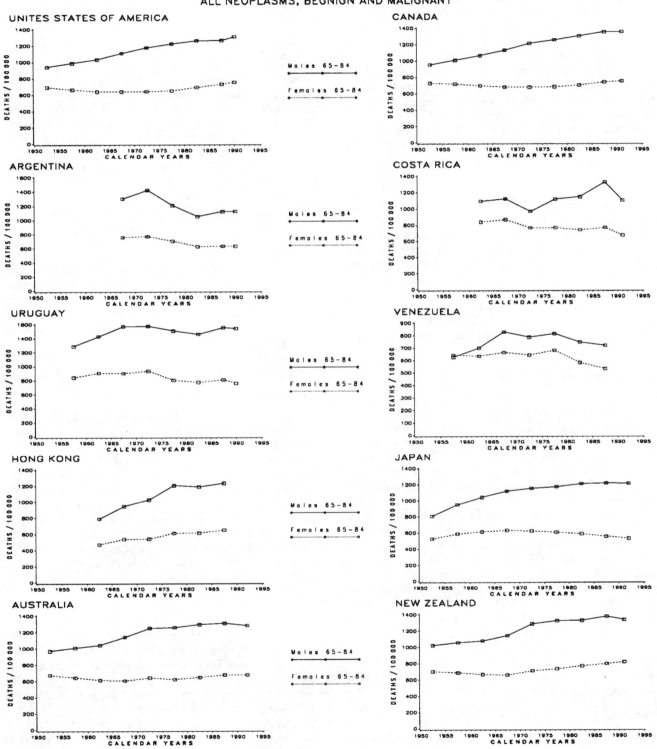

ALL NEOPLASMS, BEGNIGN AND MALIGNANT

Stomach

The decline in stomach cancer rates has been the most favorable pattern in mortality for any common cancer site over the last several decades (14). In the 1950s, gastric cancer was still by far the most common cause of cancer death in the elderly of both sexes. In most western and northern European countries, the decline was steady from the 1950s onward and reached 50% to 70%. In Italy, the decline started in the late 1960s for males, whereas in Spain, Portugal and most eastern European countries early rises, mostly in males, were followed by declines from the 1970s onward. Steady declines in both sexes were observed in North America, Australia and New Zealand, too, while in South America and Japan the decline was evident only from the 1970s onward.

Colorectum

Colorectal cancer rates in the elderly were stable, or even moderately downward, in several countries in Northern Europe, America and Australia. In contrast, death rates have tended to increase, often substantially, in most countries of southern and eastern Europe, and in Japan as well, where rates were exceedingly low in the 1950s. Thus, differences in colorectal cancer mortality in the elderly of both sexes across various countries and areas of the world have tended to level off during the last four decades, although an appreciable variation still remains.

Gallbladder and Bile Ducts

Besides the observation that death rates from gallbladder cancer were systematically higher in elderly females than males (except in Hong Kong and Japan), the pattern of gallbladder cancer rates in various countries is substantially heterogeneous. Thus, rates were upward in France, Italy, Spain, Greece, Finland and Sweden (at least in the late 1980s), and downward in Austria, Germany, the Netherlands, Britain, North America, Australia and New Zealand. Japan showed both a steady and substantial upward trend, and had the highest gallbladder cancer rates in the elderly for both sexes in the 1990s (53/100,000 males, 48/100,000 females). These patterns of trends are partly attributable to difficulties in diagnosis and certification of gallbladder cancer, particularly in the elderly, partly due to a leveling of rates in various countries around similar values (with the major exception of the excess in Japan), and partly due to the different patterns of cholecystectomy in various countries and calendar years, since gallstones are the major recognized risk factor for gallbladder cancer (15,16).

Pancreas

Pancreatic cancer mortality increased appreciably and systematically to reach rates around 70/100,000 males aged 65 to 84 and 40/100,000 females aged 65–84 in most countries of the world, including Japan. However it is unclear how much of this systematic increase is due to improved diagnosis and certification, and how much is due to tobacco smoking and other potential risk factors for pancreatic cancer (17).

In some Nordic countries, Britain, Ireland, Germany and Switzerland, the Netherlands, North America, Australia and New Zealand pancreatic cancers in the elderly have tended to level off over the last two decades.

Larynx

In the elderly, as in other age groups, laryngeal cancer is extremely rare in females, and therefore its trends are unremarkable in women, with the sole exception of a downward trend in Ireland (whose rates were around 5/100,000 women in the 1950s), and steady rates around 4/100,000 in Scotland. In the mid 1960s, France had the highest laryngeal cancer rates in elderly males (67/100,000), but the rates have declined thereafter to approach 40/100,000. A similar pattern of trends (i.e., earlier rises followed by a leveling of rates) was observed in Austria, Germany, the Netherlands, most Nordic countries, and Italy, although the absolute values were appreciably lower. In contrast, substantial rises have been observed in Poland, Hungary (which now have the highest rates of laryngeal cancer in elderly males worldwide, 43.2/100,000), and most other eastern European countries. Laryngeal cancer rates in elderly males were approximately stable in the United States, Canada, the few Latin American countries providing data and Australia, but appreciably declining in Japan over the last few years, although absolute values were relatively low in this country.

Trachea, Bronchus and Lung

The rise of lung cancer was the single major pandemic registered in cancer mortality among elderly males over the last few decades (18). Lung cancer death rates in males aged 65 to 84 reached 700/100,000 in the late 1970s in Scotland, as well as in the early 1980s in the Netherlands and Belgium. Death rates reached 600/100,000 in the late 1970s in England and Wales. In most of these countries, lung cancer rates in elderly males have now started to level off or decline, but the epidemic is still expanding in most eastern Europe, approaching 500/100,000 in Poland and Hungary, and in southern Europe, approaching 400 to 450/100,000 in Italy and Greece, as well as in the United States and Canada. In North America, the start of an important epidemic of lung cancer in elderly females has also become evident, with rates over 100/100,000 women aged 65 to 84 in the early 1990s, and appreciable rises in females have been observed in Denmark, Australia and New Zealand as well as in Hong Kong, which started from higher rates in the 1960's. A steady and substantial rise in lung cancer in the elderly has also been registered in Japan, although absolute values are still lower than in other areas of the world (around 300/100,000 males and 70/100,000 females).

Skin, Including Melanoma

Trends in skin cancer mortality in the elderly are very difficult to interpret, since 1) skin cancer mortality includes various histotypes (mainly melanoma and squamous cell carcinoma), and 2) only a fraction of all skin cancers is the underlying and direct cause of death, thus leaving ample scope for variable completeness and validity of death certification in various countries. These cautions notwithstanding, it is nonetheless clear at inspection of skin cancer death rates in the elderly that no major and systematic epidemic has been observed over the last few decades, when substantial rises were evident in middle age in both sexes, largely or totally attributable to increased mortality from melanoma of the skin (19). Major exceptions were Australia and New Zealand, where an over 2-fold rise in skin cancer rates has been registered, and skin cancer death rates were over 40/100,000 males and 10/100,000 females aged 65 to 84 in recent years, together with some rise in North America from the mid 1970s onward, particularly for males.

Breast

There were at least two different patterns in breast cancer mortality among elderly women. One was typical of several northern European countries, North America, Australia and New Zealand, with rates around 120–140/100,000, which remained approximately stable during the four decades considered. A second one was observed in most southern and eastern European countries, Argentina and Uruguay, and was characterized by appreciably lower rates in earlier calendar periods, but substantial rises thereafter to reach values around or over 100/100,000 in the late 1980s and early 1990s. Norway and Sweden had relatively low rates (around 80/100,000) and have remained constant over time, but the most peculiar and remarkable pattern was in Japan, whose rates started around 15/100,000 women aged 65 to 84 in the early 1950s to reach only 20 in 1990–92 (20).

Uterus (cervix and corpus)

Mortality from uterine cancer has declined in most countries of the world, particularly since the late 1960s or early 1970s onward. This is most likely attributable to reduced incidence and/or early detection and diagnosis of cervical cancer, due to changed sexual habits, improved personal hygiene and more widespread adoption of cervical screening (21). The only area of the world where uterine cancer death rates were not consistently downward was in eastern European countries, thus indicating a delay in the adoption of adequate prevention measures.

Ovary

Certified mortality from ovarian cancer in women aged 65 to 84 was between 30 and 45/100,000 in most northern European and American countries, Australia and New Zealand, with some inconsistent rise, but in the absence of systematic trends in rates. In the 1950s and 1960s, rates were much lower in most southern and eastern European countries, Latin America and Japan. Apparent rises over time were registered in these countries, although the rates in the late 1980s or early 1990s

remain generally lower than those of North America or Europe.

Prostate

Prostatic cancer mortality in elderly males has risen in most countries of the world, although substantial differences remain between the rates. There were around 150–200/100,000 males aged 65 to 84 in North America, most northern European countries and Oceania, around 100/100,000 in eastern and southern Europe, and only 35–40/100,000 in Hong Kong or Singapore. Certified mortality from prostatic cancer, particularly in the elderly, is strongly influenced by diagnostic and certification accuracy; however, it is difficult to assess how much of the apparent increase is real, and how much is attributable to improved knowledge and diagnosis of the disease (22,23).

Testis

An appreciable decline in testicular cancer rates over the last two decades was observed for elderly males in most countries of Western Europe, North America, Japan and Oceania. Little evidence of decline was evident in Eastern Europe or South America. As in younger males, this probably reflects the impact of newer platinum-based chemotherapies in reducing testicular cancer mortality, and the delay of adequate adoption of these therapies in several areas of the world (24).

Bladder

This is another neoplasm that, besides occupational exposure to chemical carcinogens, is related to tobacco smoking (25,26). Not surprisingly, therefore, the trends in elderly males largely reflect those of lung cancer, with a peak in the 1970s in most northern European and American countries (as well as in Japan), and the presence of persistent and steady rises in southern and eastern Europe.

Kidney

Kidney cancer rates increased steadily and substantially in most countries considered, except in a few Nordic countries whose rates were particularly high and had reached a peak in the late 1970s or early 1980s. This steady and substantial rise is in part attributable to the delayed effects of cigarette smoking — the single best recognized risk factor in kidney cancer (26) and, partly, to improved diagnosis and certification mostly in the elderly, but remains, at least at present, open to interpretation.

Thyroid

Thyroid cancer mortality in the 1950s was elevated, particularly in elderly females living in central Europe, including the Alpine areas of Austria and Switzerland (27). Over the last four decades, steady and substantial declines in thyroid cancer rates were observed for both sexes in these areas, as well as in most western European countries (except Spain), North America and Oceania. These favorable trends are most likely attributable to the reduction of iodine deficiency, and hence of the related benign thyroid conditions which are risk factors for thyroid cancer (27). In Japan, thyroid cancer rates were low in the 1950s, increased up to the mid 1970s, and leveled off thereafter.

Hodgkin's Disease

In most (developed) countries of the world Hodgkin's disease mortality in population aged 65 to 84 declined appreciably from the mid 1970s onwards. These generalized downward trends are likely attributable to improved treatment of the disease, following newer chemo- and radiotherapy schemes (24). Exceptions to this favorable pattern are a few countries in southern and eastern Europe and South America, where treatment of the disease has not been optimal (24).

All Other Lymphomas

Mortality from non-Hodgkin's lymphomas in the elderly increased several-fold in most countries considered, to reach values around 30–40/100,000 males aged 65 to 84 and 15–20/100,000 females. The pattern of trends, however, was dichotomous, with sharp rises since the late 1960s in North America and a few western European countries. This indicates that the upward trend is, at least in part, attributable to changed criteria of diagnosis or classification (with Hodgkin's disease and other causes of death) (28). Whether improved diagnosis and certification largely explains the extent of the upward trends, or whether there are other causes for the systematic increase in non-Hodgkin's lymphomas observed in most countries over the world, remains an open issue (28,29).

Multiple Myeloma

This is another lymphohaemopoietic neoplasm showing substantial and systematic upward trends in certified mortality in the elderly in most areas of the world. However, since diagnosis and hence certification of multiple myeloma substantially improved after the introduction of serum electrophoresis and other diagnostic techniques, it is unclear how much of the increase is real and how much is due to changed criteria of classification (2,30). Indeed, countries like Sweden and Norway, where a diagnostic attention for the disease has been present longer, showed a tendency toward the leveling of death certification rates from myeloma in the elderly over the last two decades.

Leukaemias

Certified mortality from leukaemias in elderly males and females increased appreciably in most countries, particularly in the earlier calendar period. However, a leveling off, or a decline in rates, was observed in several Nordic countries, France and Britain, suggesting that the generalized rise registered for elderly males and females in most other areas of the world were largely or totally attributable to improved diagnosis and certification. It is possible that some of the recent declines observed in Norway, Sweden and Finland, are due to improved treatment of the disease, but the interpretation of this pattern, too, remains open to discussion (31).

All Neoplasms, Benign and Malignant

Certified mortality for all neoplasms for the population aged 65 to 84 showed a rather heterogeneous pattern in the two sexes and various geographical areas. In general, trends were systematically more favorable for females than for males, reflecting the earlier and more prevalent appearance of lung cancer (and other tobacco-related neoplasm) epidemic in elderly males, and the widespread decline of cervical cancer in females. In several countries, particularly in western Europe (but also Japan), the trends in both sexes were more favorable over the last two decades than in earlier calendar periods. Furthermore some areas of central Europe, including Austria and Switzerland, as well as Argentina, showed stable or even favorable trends over time for total cancer mortality in both sexes. This reflects a different pattern from the tobacco-related (lung) cancer epidemic in various countries, as well as the role of a few other major neoplasms, including the systematic downward trends in stomach cancer rates. In contrast, rates were moderately upward for males in North America. Several countries in southern and eastern Europe, where rates in the 1950s and 1960s were relatively low, showed appreciable upward trends, mostly in males. There was a general tendency towards a leveling of the differences in overall registered cancer mortality in elderly populations in various areas of the world.

Conclusion

It is important, particularly for the elderly, to stress the limits and uncertainties of cancer death certification and trends over time. Although the exact influence of changing certification accuracy of trends in cancer rates is uncertain, almost certainly this data implies some systematic upward trends over time, following generalized improvement of diagnosis and certification of selected cancer sites including, in particular, prostate and multiple myeloma (2).

Brain cancer was not included as a separate entity in this overview because 1) the major difficulties in classifying and distinguishing malignant, benign and undefined malignancy brain cancers at death, particularly in the elderly (10), 2) the impact of newer diagnostic technology and changed attitudes toward the elderly in the medical environment (32,33), and 3) the relatively modest impact in absolute terms of even substantial proportional rises in brain cancer rates in overall cancer mortality in the elderly (34).

These cautions notwithstanding, it is clear that there is no single and simple pattern of cancer mortality in the elderly in various areas of the world, aside from the major impact of the various phases of the widespread tobacco-related epidemic of lung cancer and other tobacco-related neoplasms (35).

A second pattern emerging from this overview is a systematic tendency towards increasing certified cancer mortality in the elderly, particularly in elderly males — in areas where rates were lower in the 1950s and 1960s, thus leading to a leveling of differences in cancer mortality values in various areas of the world.

Finally, there is the presence of a widespread favorable pattern in females, whose lung cancer epidemic in the elderly is still in its early phases in most countries, and for whom the earlier downward trends in stomach and cervical cancer mortality were particularly relevant.

In conclusion, in the elderly, after expressing due caution concerning death certification reliability in this age group, there is no widespread and generalized upward trend in cancer mortality, with the major exceptions of lung and other tobacco-related neoplasms. However, age-standardized cancer rates in the elderly, have an essential epidemiologic interest. On a public health scale, the aging of the population and, hence, the increased proportion and number of elderly people in all (developed) countries and areas of the world, implies *per se* an increased number of cases in the elderly, and thus a substantially increased health care and socio-economic burden.

Acknowledgments

This study has been made possible by a core grant of the Swiss (Aargau and St-Gall) League against Cancer (Contract FOR No. 305.93). Supports were also received by the Italian Association for Cancer Research and the Italian League against Cancer. This study was conducted within the framework of the CNR (Italian National Research Council) Applied Project "Clinical Application of Oncological Research" (Contract No. 94.01321.PF39) and of the "Europe Against Cancer" Programme of the Commission of the European Communities.

References

1. Cook PJ, Doll R, Fellingham SA. A mathematical model for the age distribution of cancer in man. *Int J Cancer* 1969; **4**: 93–112.

2. Doll R, Peto R. The causes of cancer: quantitative estimates of avoidable risks of cancer in the United States today. *JNCI* 1981; **66**: 1191–1308.

3. Doll R. Are we winning the fight against cancer? An epidemiological assessment. *Eur J Cancer* 1990; **26**: 500–508.

4. Hoel DG, Davis DL, Miller AB, Sondik EJ, Swerdlow AJ. Trends in cancer mortality in 15 industrialized countries, 1969–1986. *JNCI* 1992; **84**: 313–320.

5. Levi F, La Vecchia C, Lucchini F, Negri E. Worldwide trends in cancer mortality in the elderly, 1955–1992. *Europ J Cancer* 1996; 32A: 652–672.

6. World Health Organization. International Classification of Diseases: 6th Revision. Geneva: *World Health Organization*, 1950.

7. World Health Organization. International Classification of Diseases: 7th Revision. Geneva: *World Health Organization*, 1957.

8. World Health Organization. International Classification of Diseases: 8th Revision. Geneva: *World Health Organization*, 1967.

9. World Health Organization. International Classification of Diseases: 9th Revision. Geneva: *World Health Organization*, 1977.

10. Boyle P, Maisonneuve P, Saracci R, Muir CS. Is the increased incidence of primary malignant brain tumors in the elderly real? *JNCI* 1990; **82**: 1594–1596.

11. Doll R, Smith PG. Comparison between registries: age-standardized rates. In *Cancer Incidence in Five Continents, Vol IV*, edited by JAH Waterhouse, CS Muir, K Shanmugaratnam, J Powell, D Peachan, S Whelan. *IARC Scientific Publication No 42, Lyon: International Agency for Research on Cancer*, 671–675, 1982.

12. Graham S, Marshall J, Haughey B, *et al*. Nutritional epidemiology of cancer of the esophagus. *Am J Epidemiol* 1990; **131**: 454–457

13. Victora CG, Munoz N, Day NE, Barcelos LB, Peccin DA, Braga NM. Hot beverages and esophageal cancer in Southern Brazil: a case-control study. *Int J Cancer* 1987; **39**: 710–716.

14. Howson CP, Hiyama T, Wynder EL. The decline of gastric cancer: epidemiology of an unplanned triumph. *Epidemiol Rev* 1986; **8**: 1–27.

15. Diehl AK. Epidemiology of gallbladder cancer: a synthesis of recent data. *JNCI* 1980; **65**: 1209–1213.

16. Zatonski W, La Vecchia C, Levi F, Negri E, Lucchini F. Descriptive epidemiology of gall-bladder cancer in Europe. *J Cancer Res Clin Oncol* 1993; **119**: 165–171.

17. Boyle P, Hsieh CC, Maisonneuve P, *et al*. Epidemiology of pancreas cancer. *Int J Pancreatol* 1989; **5**: 327–346.

18. Doll R. Major epidemics of the 20th century: from coronary thrombosis to AIDS. *J R Statist Soc* A 1987; **150**: 373–395.

19. Glass AG, Hoover RN. The emerging epidemic of melanoma and squamous cell skin cancer. *JAMA* 1989; **262**: 1097–2100.

20. Boyle P, Levi F, Lucchini F, La Vecchia C. Trends in diet-related cancers in Japan. A conundrum? *Lancet* 1993; **342**: 752.

21. La Vecchia C. The epidemiology of cervical neoplasia. *Biomed Pharmacother* 1985; **39**: 426–433.

22. Zaridze DG, Boyle P. Cancer of the prostate: epidemiology and aetiology. *Brit J Urol* 1987; **59**: 493–502.

23. Potoski AL, Kessler L, Gridley G. *et al*: Rise in prostatic cancer incidence associated with increased use of transurethral resection. *J. Natl Cancer Inst* 1990; **82**: 1624–1628.

24. La Vecchia C, Levi F, Lucchini F, Garattini S: Progress from anticancer drugs in reducing mortality from selected cancers in Europe: an assessment. *Anti-cancer Drugs* 1991; **2**: 215–221.

25. Matanoski GM, Elliott FA. Bladder cancer epidemiology. *Epidemiol Rev* 1981; **3**: 203–229.

26. US Department of Health and Human Services: *Reducing the Health Consequences of Smoking: 25 Years of Progress*. A Report of the Surgeon General, US Department of Health and Human Services, Public Health Service, Centers for Disease Control, Center for Chronic Disease Prevention and Health Promotion, Office on Smoking and Health, Washington DC, USA. GPO DHHS Publication No (CDC) 89-8411: 1989.

27. Franceschi S, Boyle P, Maisonneuve P, *et al*. The epidemiology of thyroid carcinoma. *Crit Rev Oncogen* 1993; **4**: 25–52.

28. Devesa SS, Fears T. Non-Hodgkin's lymphoma time trends: United States and international data. *Cancer Res.* 1992; **52**(suppl): 5432- 5440.

29. Hartge P, Devesa S. Quantification of the impact of known risk factors on time trends in non-Hodgkin's lymphoma incidence. *Cancer Res* 1992; **52**(suppl): 5566–5569.

30. Cuzick J. Multiple myeloma. *Cancer Surveys.* 1994; **19–20**: 455–474.

31. Linet MS. *The Leukemia: Epidemiological aspects*. In *Monographs in Epidemiology and Biostatistics, Vol 6*, edited by AM Lilienfeld. New York: Oxford University Press, 20–65, 1985.

32. Modan B, Wagener DK, Feldman JJ, Rosenberg HM, Feinleib M. Increased mortality from brain tumors: a combined diagnostic technology and change in attitude toward the elderly. *Am J Epidemiol* 1992; **135**: 1349–1357.

33. Desmeules M, Mikkelson T, Mao Y. Increasing incidence of primary brain tumors: influence of diagnostic methods. *JNCI* 1992; **84**: 442–445.

34. Levi F, Lucchini F, La Vecchia C. Worldwide patterns of cancer mortality, 1985–89. *Eur J Cancer Prev* 1994; **3**: 109–143.

35. Peto R, Lopez AD, Boreham J, Thun M, Heath Jr C. Mortality from tobacco in developed countries: indirect estimation from national vital statistics. *Lancet* 1992; **339**: 1268–1278.

4. Cancer in Older Persons Magnitude of the Problem — How Do We Apply What We Know?

Rosemary Yancik and Lynn A. Ries

Acknowledgement

"Originally published in *Cancer* 1994; **74**: 1995–2003, ©1994 American Cancer Society. Reprinted with permission of J.B. Lippincott Company, Philadelphia, Pennsylvania."

Introduction

Persons 65 years and older bear the brunt of the cancer burden. Incidence data from the National Cancer Institute Surveillance, Epidemiology, and End Results (SEER) program, clearly indicate that aging is a high risk factor for cancer (1). The incidence rate for those 65 years or older is 2085.3 per 100,000 persons, as compared with 193.9 per 100,000 for those younger than 65 years, a dramatic tenfold difference in overall cancer incidence rates (i.e., the number of newly diagnoses cases occurring per 100,000 persons during a given time).

Incidence of Selected Tumors

More than 58% of all cancers occur in the elderly subgroup of the population. The impact of aging is made even more clear and apparent when specific tumors are considered.

Table 4.1 lists the American Cancer Society's (ACS) estimate of the number of new cancer cases for 1994 and the SEER estimates for individuals 65 years of age and older to illustrate the scope of the problem of cancer in the elderly by individual tumors. Proportions for the elderly are derived from calculations using the SEER incidence rates (2,3).

Two-thirds to three-quarters of the major sites of malignancies common to both men and women — colon, rectum, stomach, pancreas, urinary bladder — occur in the elderly. The percentages of lung and bronchus cancers that occur in the elderly are 63% and 61% for men and women, respectively. These percentages are expected to increase in the older age group as the smoking exposure time effects on birth cohorts becomes more apparent. Lung and bronchus cancers will increase for older persons within the next decade, reflecting the high rates of smoking behavior of persons currently in their 50s and early 60s.

As to the gender-specific malignancies, prostate cancer is particularly severe for men 65 years and older, with a high proportion of cases (84%) occurring in this age group. Breast and ovarian cancers are special prob-

Table 4.1 1994 estimates of cancer patients: men women, all ages and proportion 65 years of age and older.

Cancer site	Men			Women		
	All Ages (no.)	≥65 yr (no.)	>65 yr (%)	All ages (no.)	≥65 yr (no.)	>65 yr (%)
Lung	100,000	63,000	63	72,000	43,920	61
Colon	52,000	37,960	73	55,000	42,900	78
Rectum	3,000	14,950	65	19,000	13,490	71
Urinary bladder	38,000	26,600	70	13,200	9768	74
Stomach	15,000	10,200	68	9000	675	75
Pancreas	13,000	8840	68	14,000	10,780	77
Breast (female)	–	–	–	182,000	91,000	50
Ovary	–	–	–	24,000	11,760	49
Prostate	200,000	168,000	84	–	–	–

Data from American Cancer Society. *Cancer facts and figures — 1994*. American Cancer Society, 1994. Number of 65+ estimated from National Cancer Institute Seer Program Data, 1985–1989 and applied to American Cancer Society estimates.

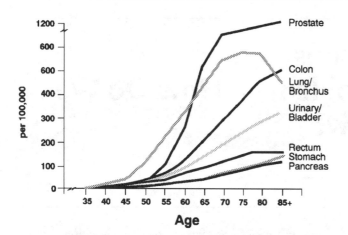

Figure 4.1 Cancer incidence rates in men.

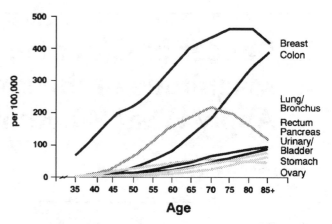

Figure 4.2 Cancer incidence rates in women.

lems for older women. These two malignancies generally have been considered early postmenopausal diseases rather than late postmenopausal tumors. In most discussions and research reports on prevention and treatment, a perimenopausal age-break of 50 years generally is used, with no reference to the actuality that 50% of breast cancers and 49% of ovarian cancers occur in women 65 years and older.

Unfortunately, as the population-based tumor registry data reveal, old age is the "normal time" at which cancer develops. The numbers shown in Table 4.1 alone persuasively suggest the urgent need to address the problems unique to persons aged 65 years and older. Compared with the rest of the population, these individuals suffer disproportionately from the morbidity, adversity, and hardship brought on by these malignancies. This age group, however, has been under-represented historically in clinical studies that generate knowledge about cancer treatment.

Incidence curves emphasize the escalation of increased cancer rates with advancing age and show contrasts by 5-year age groups beginning at 35 years of age. It is important to illustrate the increase in cancer incidence rates with advancing age. Incidence differentials are delineated by age for the selected tumors for men and women, respectively, as seen in Figures 4.1 and 4.2.

The curves, based on incidence rates per 100,000 persons (shown on the vertical axis), portray the gradients for selected tumors as they rise with advancing age (shown on the horizontal axis). The highest incidences and greatest number of cancer for men are associated with three tumors types: prostate cancer, lung cancer, and colon cancer. The scale shown for men reaches to a high of 1200.0 per 100,000 to accommodate the incidence rates for prostate cancer in the age-specific groups for men after the age of 65. Two other malignancies also have extremely high incidence rates in men: Colon cancer rates range from 188.7 per 100,000 for the 65–69-year-old age group to almost 493.6 for those aged 85 and older. Lung cancer rates escalate to more than 500.0 for those aged 70–84 years. The peak rate of 567.0 per 100,000 is in the 80–84-year-old group.

Urinary bladder cancer rates crest at 317.2 for men aged 85 and older. Incidence rates for tumors of the rectum, stomach, and pancreas do not reach the elevated levels of the preceding three cancers, but all rates increase with advancing age to more than 100 per 100,000.

Eight malignancies that are most common in women are shown in Figure 4.2. The vertical axis scale extends to 500 per 100,000 persons. Breast cancer has the highest incidence rates of all tumors affecting women. All age groups older than 65 years of age have rates exceeding 400.0 per 100,000 persons. Two specific age groups, 75–79 and 80–84, show the highest rate: 465 per 100,000. It should be noted here (and it is discussed in detail in other papers in the conference proceedings), that there is less emphasis placed on knowledge of the need for regular mammograms in older age groups even though cancer incidence is extremely high for older women. There has been a continuing debate within the past year regarding the effectiveness of breast cancer screening for women aged 40–49 years (4). Incidence rates of 126.6 and 188.4 per 100,000 for women aged 40–44 and 45–49, respectively, are one-third to less than one-half the rates shown for women aged 65 years and older. Even though rates are highest in the older age groups, especially those 70 years and older, there has been no emphasis on early detection for elderly women.

Lung cancer incidence rates peak in the 70–79 year-old age group with more than 200.0 per 100,000 persons. Colon cancer rates are highest for women 65 years of age and older and increase dramatically for women in their 80s, with rates of 339 and 391 per 100,000 persons, respectively. Incidence rates for ovarian cancer are close to those for rectal cancer, pancreatic cancer, urinary bladder cancer, and stomach cancer. These five tumors have rates that peak under 100.0 per 100,000 persons in the older age groups.

The unique National Cancer Institute (NCI) SEER population-based data furnishes the initial framework to describe the magnitude of the cancer problem for older persons (1,2). The SEER program covers approximately 10% of the U.S. Population. Incidence, mortality, and stage of disease at initial diagnosis and age

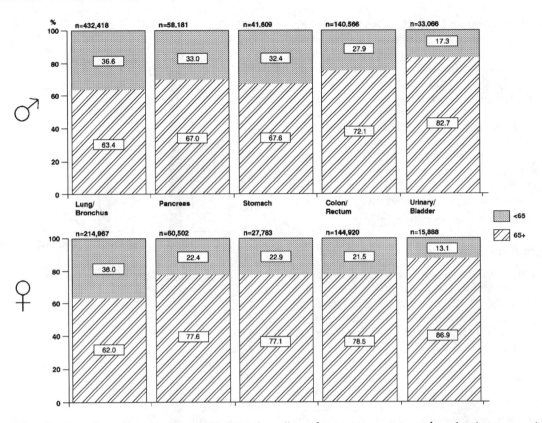

Figure 4.3 Mortality for selected cancer sites, 1985–1989 (lung/bronchus, pancreas, stomach, colon/rectum, urinary tract/bladder).

contrasts are made with SEER data for 1985–89 from the tumor registries of Connecticut, Iowa, New Mexico, Utah, and Hawaii, and the reporting regions of Detroit, Atlanta, San Francisco, and Seattle (2). A comprehensive description of the SEER program and its procedures are available in several publications (1,5,6). Mortality data from the National Center for Health Statistics and demographic data from the U.S. Bureau of the Census complete the picture (7,8).

Mortality

Two-thirds (67%) of all cancer mortalities in the United States occur in individuals in the 65-years-and-older age group (1,8). Mortality rates have increased significantly for the elderly in recent years in numbers and proportion. Less than 10 years ago, the percentage of cancer deaths for persons aged 65 and older was close to 60% (9).

The nine malignancies addressed in particular for this paper represent 45% of the cancer mortality in the United States during 1985–1989 (2). This is a high proportion of the approximately 66 different categories of tumor registration on which SEER reports routinely (1,5,6). Figures 4.3 and 4.4 show the number of cancer deaths and the percentages of those that occurred in

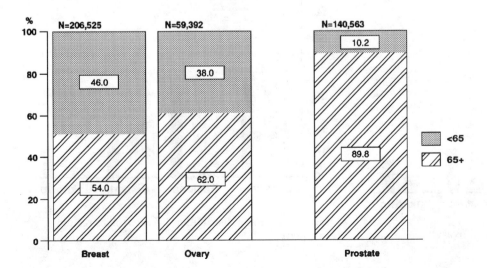

Figure 4.4 Mortality for selected cancer sites, 1985–1989 (breast, ovary, prostate).

individuals younger than 65 and those 65 years of age and older for the nine tumors discussed in this paper.

First distinguishing the tumors common to men and women, colon and rectum, urinary bladder, stomach, and pancreas, the percentages of those aged 65 years and older range from 67% (for pancreatic cancer deaths in men) to 87% (for urinary bladder deaths in women). For lung and bronchial cancer, 62% of cancer mortality is in older women; 63% is in older men.

For the gender specific malignancies, 90% of mortalities from prostate cancer occur in men ages 65 and older. The mortality rates for breast cancer and ovarian cancer for women are greater in women aged 65 years and older — 54% and 62%, respectively.

Stage Distribution by Age

As with most tumors, anatomic staging of the extent of tumor progression at initial diagnosis is extremely important. Staging governs prognosis and treatment. Early diagnosis of cancer is more likely to have positive consequences for the length and quality of survival and cure potential. The NCI SEER data on the extent of disease at initial diagnosis — localized, regional, distant (metastatic), or stage unknown or not recorded — is stratified by age groups for selected tumors to illustrate the relationships between stage and age. The question for each age group is: What is the stage distribution? The progression of stage severity and stage-unknown categories for ovary, breast, and prostate cancer are shown in Figures 4.5–4.7. Rates for colon and rectal cancers for both men and women are shown in Figures 4.8 and 4.9.

Ovary

Differences in stage distribution are striking by age. The younger than 55 age group has the highest proportion of localized disease, whereas the older age groups have more distant disease. In addition, the oldest age group has the highest proportion of unstaged disease. The stage/age distribution for this cohort is consistent

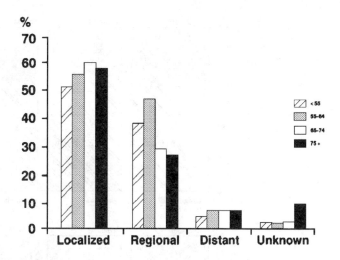

Figure 4.6 Stage distribution by age: prostate.

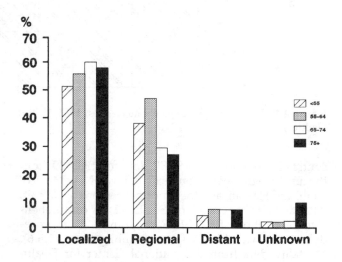

Figure 4.7 Stage distribution by age: breast.

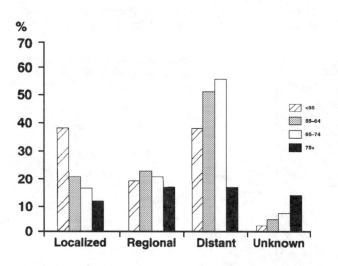

Figure 4.5 Stage distribution by age: ovary.

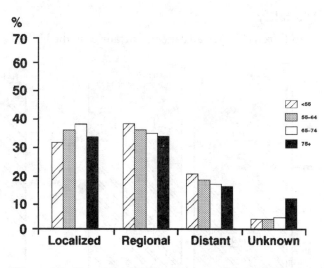

Figure 4.8 Stage distribution by age: colon/rectum (women).

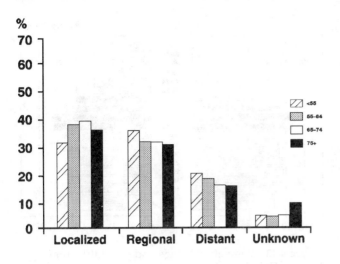

Figure 4.9 Stage distribution by age: colon/rectum (men).

with a previous report on ovarian cancer in the elderly using the SEER data for an earlier time period (10).

Prostate

Prostate cancer is diagnosed in the localized stage for 50–59% of each age category for the patient cohort illustrated in Figure 4.6. Regional disease diagnosis shows a descending profile of percentages from the younger to older age groups. There are high proportions in the distant-stage and stage-unknown categories for patients 75 years of age and older. It has been surmised that increases in prostatectomy procedures for younger men have led to a shift in diagnosis from localized to more advanced disease stages in recent years.

Breast

More than half of the breast cancer patients in all age groups are diagnosed with localized stage disease. A difference in regional disease stage is observed in age groups. The percentage of distant disease is similar across age groups. More women 75 years of age and older have a higher percentage of stage-unknown disease.

Colorectal — Men and Women

Distribution of colorectal cancer cases by disease stage, including those for which the stage was unknown, are shown for both genders. Once again, we see that the percentage in the stage-unknown category for the 75 and older age group is quite large. For both sexes, there is a consistency in the disease stage distribution across age groups. There is little variation in stage distribution by age for these malignancies.

In summary, there does not appear to be an age/stage relationship in prostate, breast, and colorectal cancers. Only in the case of cancer are older patients more likely to be diagnosed initially with a more severe disease stage. Without classifying information on the patients in the stage-unknown category, this con-

clusion is not certain. Because of the preponderance of percentages in the stage-unknown category for the older age group, one analytic interpretation derived from these data is that cancer in the older person cannot be labeled as "less often metastatic" or "less aggressive." Another interpretation is an interference that older cancer patients are receiving less than full workups (i.e., the greater proportion of older persons in the stage-unknown categories) resulting in less than complete staging procedures.

Our Aging Nation

The elderly population (i.e., persons aged 65 years and older) of the United states currently is 31.1 million, constituting 12.5% of the total U.S. population; the cancer control need of this group should receive prompt and systematic attention (7). In preparation for the forthcoming dramatic expansion of this age group in the next 40 years, we should be anticipating the greater need for health care resources. If the overall cancer rates remain the same, the aged population prevalence (the number of persons living at a specific point in time with a history of cancer or with a newly diagnosed malignancy) would increase from 8 million individuals, the current figure reported recently by the American Cancer Society, to 12 million (3). The later figure is based on projections derived from calculations made by the NCI using data from the SEER Connecticut Tumor Registry and established modeling procedures (NCI, unpublished data, 1993) (9). Of the cancer patients in 2030, 70% will be 65 years of age or older.

Figure 4.10 describes the recent past and near future in a 10-decade comparison of population estimates and projections with data from the U.S. Bureau of the Census (11). The total U.S. population has doubled from 122.8 million in 1930 to 248.7 million persons in the past 60 years. The proportion of the population aged 65 years and older also has almost doubled, from one in fifteen of the population in the 1930s to one in eight in the 1990s. Looking forward 40 years, one in five persons will be 65 years of age or older in 2030.

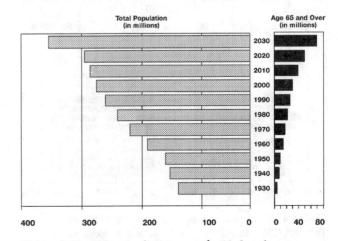

Figure 4.10 U.S. population growth: 10-decade comparison — total population/age –65 segment.

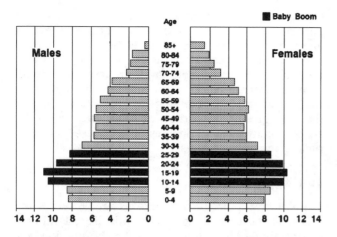

Figure 4.11 Population by age and sex: 1975. From Taeuber CM. Sixty-five plus in America. Rev. ed. Washington (DC): U.S. Govt Printing Office, 1993. U.S. Bureau of the Census, Current Population Reports, Special Studies, P23-178RV.

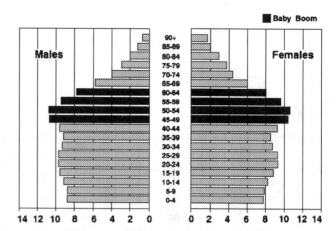

Figure 4.13 Population by age and sex: 2010. From Taeuber CM. Sixty-five plus in America. Rev. ed. Washington (DC): U.S. Govt Printing Office, 1993. U.S. Bureau of the Census, Current Population Reports, Special Studies, P23-178RV.

Not only is the U.S. population aging; the age structure is changing over time. More older people are living longer. There are and will continue to be more older-old persons (i.e., 75–84 and 85 and older) in the older-age segment of the population. (11). Low fertility, elimination of certain infectious diseases, and longer life expectancies are contributing to the U.S. demographic imperative (12).

Age pyramids, depicting age structure, often are featured in the U.S. Bureau of the Census publications. They portray the changes that have occurred and will occur. Figures 4.11–4.14, from C.M. Taeuber's recent publication, "Sixty-Five Plus in America," describe age-specific changes for selected years (11).

The first age pyramid depicts the post-World War II "baby boom" as it was in 1975 when the cohort was between 10 and 30 years of age. Changes over time in

the United States for selected decades show the shifting age structure in the United States. The configurations seen in Figures 4.12, 4.13, and 4.14 reflect the changes that will occur as we advance toward 2030. The age structure pyramid will become rectangular in shape.

Figure 4.12 represents this cohort (the cohort now aged between 25 and 45 years) as it was in 1990. The first wave of the "baby boomers" will become 65 years old in 2010, as indicated in Figure 4.13. By 2030, the entire cohort will be 65 years or older (Figure 4.14).

As the post war baby-boom cohorts reach age 65, the numbers of older persons will not only rapidly increase, there will be significant age shifts in the population, resulting in even more persons in the oldest-age category (i.e., 85 years and older) as shown in Figure 4.14. The old will get older between now and the peak year of population growth, 2030.

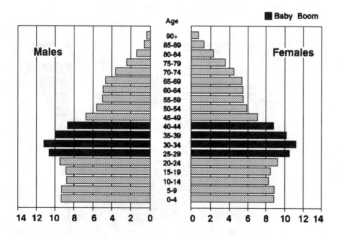

Figure 4.12 Population by age and sex: 1990. From Taeuber CM. Sixty-Five plus in America. Rev. ed. Washington (DC): U.S. Govt Printing Office, 1993. U.S. Bureau of the Census, Current Population Reports. Special Studies, P23-178RV.

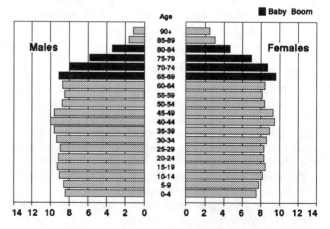

Figure 4.14 Population by age and sex: 2030. From Taeuber CM. Sixty-five plus in America. Rev. ed. Washington(DC): U.S. Govt Printing Office, 1993. U.S. Bureau of the Census, Current Population Reports, Special Studies, P23-178RV.

Table 4.2 Life expectancy: average number of years of life remaining.

Age (yr)	Male		Female	
	White	Black	White	Black
0–1	72.3	64.9	78.9	73.4
65–70	14.9	13.4	18.7	16.9
70–75	11.8	10.9	15.0	13.8
75–80	9.1	8.6	11.7	10.9
80–85	6.8	6.8	8.7	8.4
≥ 85	5.1	5.5	6.3	6.6

Data from Taeuber CM. *Sixty-five plus in America.* Washington, DC: U.S. Govt Printing Office, 1993. U.S. Bureau of the Census, Current Population Reports, Special Studies, P23-178RV.

Life Expectancy

There have been vast improvements in life expectancy at birth (i.e., the average number of years a person will live given the age-specific mortality rates of a particular year) has increased from 47 years in 1900 to 75.7 in 1992. Table 4.2 shows the average number of years of life remaining under the mortality conditions of 1988 at the selected ages according to gender and race. Life expectancy at age 65 ranges from 13 years (for black males) to 19 years (for white females). For the 80–85 year average group, the range is 7–9 years. Black women who survive to age 85 have the highest average number of years of life remaining (12).

The Aged and How They Differ from Younger Persons

We have been referring to the aged (or the elderly) as a group, using the traditional cut-off age of 65 years. As we have emphasized elsewhere (and shall do so here), however, definitions of old age for clinical purposes should be flexible and dependent on criteria other than calendar age (13,14). Persons 65 years of age and older include the young old (i.e., 65–74 years), the older-old (i.e., 75–84 years of age), and the oldest-old (i.e., 85 years of age and older) — a subdivision of age cohorts that reflect the heterogeneity of age within the older population. To sharpen the focus on the unique problems that may be present in older persons in need of information on cancer prevention or those who have been newly-diagnosed with cancer, we first must acknowledge the greater variability in health and age-related declines in functioning. We know that the pace of aging varies from individual to individual. It has been suggested that no two individuals accumulate identical environmental or other types of insults alike. It is preferable to ask which patients would benefit from which treatments. The use of chronologic age as a guide for cancer on prevention and therapy is not a good strategy for the elderly (13).

With respect to cancer detection, there may be a nonspecific presentation of a malignancy, sometimes unique to the aged, that requires clinicians to be alert to masked symptomatology or to look for subtle signs of additional adverse conditions in the presence of the presenting complaint (15). For many older cancer patients, there may be competing concurrent chronic conditions (i.e., comorbidity) and decreased physical and physiologic functioning. When cancer is linked with the chronic disabling conditions acquired over the course of a lifetime, there is a high probability that the residual consequences of previous illnesses and the effects of the normal and pathologic processes of aging, including frailty, will be present. There are differences in drug metabolism and changing levels of absorption, distribution, metabolism, and excretion that predominate in older persons (16). Cancer treatment strategies are challenged also by the potential for secondary complications of disease and treatment and the development of unrelated conditions during the course of cancer therapy. Other relevant concerns are comprehension deficits, diminished social support, and limited financial resources (17). These are several examples of the multiplicity of age-related conditions that may exist concurrently with cancer management for the elderly.

Why are Aging and Cancer Linked?

What accounts for this phenomenon? How does aging influence the incidence of most major malignancies? Incidence data, providing details from the epidemiologic perspective, powerfully describe the age-dependency contribution to most of the major tumors, but do not explain it.

Perhaps older people are less resistant to carcinogens, having had a longer exposure time to such substances. Over the courses of one's lifetime, there are successive insults from different carcinogenic substances. Possibly the cells go through all the multistep processes over time (18). Perhaps aging alters the body's antitumor defenses (19). Whatever is occurring, fortunately, cancer is not inevitable for all older persons. Not all older persons are afflicted with cancer, but perhaps persons in the older age group are more vulnerable to malignancies as our population-based data show.

Implications for Research and Practice

Cancer in the elderly is a major health care concern that has failed largely to generate much enthusiasm. The stark and concise summary statistics on cancer and aging indicate that the older segment of the United States population is an important target group for cancer research and control activities. Studies using the SEER information base, with documentation presented by descriptive analyses such those presented in this chapter, are capable of stratifying large amounts of patient data to raise issues for targeting clinical trials, cancer control, and biologic and epidemiologic investigations. They tell us where we should concentrate our efforts.

The scientific approach to cancer treatment has not permitted the complexities of older patients with cancer to be addresses, given the presence of the normal process of aging and multiple pathology of other chronic diseases and disabilities that the old are likely to have. Furthermore, the quality of life issues for care of the elderly have not been linked with the psychologic and social support that older persons must have to cope with cancer and its treatment (20).

How Do We Apply What We Know?

At a minimum, there should be special efforts to accomplish the following: (1) focus on screening and early detection for malignancies that could be prevented or diagnosed in the early stages (e.g., breast cancer in older women); (2) increase the awareness of oncologists, primary care physicians, and geriatricians about masked signs of malignancies and/or altered presentation of signs and symptoms of cancer in the elderly; (3) assess how concomitant diseases, illnesses, and the normal processes of aging affect the management of cancers in older persons; and (4) document systematically the differences and sensitivities of older cancer patients to conventional forms of treatment.

Persistent efforts regarding the effects of cancer have been made on behalf of older persons by some individuals in geriatric medicine, oncology, social science, and the health care professions in the last 10 years or so. Stimulating conferences, workshops and their proceedings, several review articles, and some research have been published more recently. The NCI, in collaboration with the National Institute on Aging, has issued research initiatives on breast and ovarian cancer in older women. Ovarian cancer in older women was the special theme of a conference initiated by the National Institute on Aging, and jointly sponsored by the NCI and ACS in 1991 (21). Several research recommendations from this particular workshop have been implemented. The NCI Office of Cancer Communications has had a focus on older Americans for cancer prevention. The National Institute on Aging is joining the NCI Cancer Centers Branch in a request for research applications on breast cancer in the NCI-designated cancer centers that includes a component that would address this malignancy in women aged 65 and older. A National Institute on Aging/NCI collaborative study on the comorbidity burden of cancer in the elderly is underway, using six geographic SEER areas as a base for the field study.

We believe that many more individuals and organizations are sensitive to the problems of cancer in the older person. We have been applying the demographic and epidemiologic data on aging to a wide scope of activities.

What Don't We Know?

Fundamental knowledge on cancer detection, treatment, and prevention for older persons, major aspects of cancer control activities, and cancer research has not been developed to any great extent. There is a paucity of data available for inclusion in the professional mainstream of information in gerontology, geriatric medicine, medical oncology, and oncology nursing.

Information on the magnitude of the cancer burden for the elderly has not been persuasive or has failed to reach leaders in medical research and practice. While great progress has been made in gerontology, geriatric medicine, and oncology as separate fields, we need to develop stronger ties between aging and cancer research. We need to pursue vigorously the answers to what we do not know in parallel to applying what we do know.

The National Conference on Cancer and the Older Person, sponsored by the ACS and the Centers for Disease Control and Prevention, provided an excellent review of the extent of the problem of cancer in the elderly. Many issues were addressed about cancer in the elderly as we attempted to provide objective insights, formulated hypotheses for research, and identified research and knowledge gaps. Indeed, it is a setting like the ACS/Centers for Disease Control and Prevention national conference, and the proceedings generated from those presentations, that reinforces the need for information on cancer in the elderly.

The issues noted below relate to the spectrum of cancer control research and application that are in urgent need of being addressed.

Early Detection and Screening

Does mammography screening in older asymptomatic women reduce the mortality of breast cancer in this age group? It was indicated earlier in this paper that SEER data show that peak rates of 434–465 per 100,000 persons occur in those in the 75–84-years age group. By contrast, incidence rates for the 40–49-years age group are 126.6–188.4 per 100,000. Currently primary and secondary preventive technology for the major tumors must be applied to the older age groups (22).

Treatment and Comorbidity in the Aged

Cancer is diagnosed in bodies already rife with comorbid conditions. Therefore, there are competing diseases for treatment. There may be poor physical functioning due to age-associated disabilities. It is not known to what extent concurrent health problems complicate cancer management in the older person or if nonspecific signs and symptoms are masked by multiple pathology or frailty in the older person.

Are the research treatment questions under examination in the clinical trials and research efforts beneficial and pertinent to the majority of persons afflicted with the common tumors? Prospective clinical trials do not enroll older persons. If they do, the individuals are most likely comorbidity-free and, therefore, a select group.

Do answers to key questions on cancer therapy for older persons factor in the concurrent chronic disease problems that are prominent in the elderly? We know very little about how older cancer patients are treated or the health and illness experience of these individuals.

A specially designed clinical trial research effort that focuses on older cancer patients is needed for those whose tumors are concurrent with the multiple pathology often associated with advanced age. One leading suggestion for this type of research calls for forming an international working group to develop guidelines for organizing prospective studies on the major tumors that occur in persons aged 65 years and older (20).

Final Comments

Oncology practice includes older cancer patients. Cancer prevention and early detection apply to older persons. The strong epidemiologic and demographic data are more than sufficient to urge us to go beyond mere description of cancer to the older population — we must apply the insights gained from this information. The collection of papers from the national conference furnish the occasion not only for looking back, but for looking forward to what we can do for our ever-increasing elderly population.

References

1. Miller BA, Ries LAG, Hankey BF, Kor CL, Harras A, Devesa SS, et al. *SEER Cancer statistics review: 1973–1989.* Bethesda (MD): National Cancer Institute, 1992. NIH Report No. 92-2789.

2. Miller BA, Ries LAG, Hankey BF, Kor CL, Edwards BK. *Cancer Statistics Review: 1973–1989.* Bethesda (MD): National Cancer Institute, 1992. NIH Report No. 92-2789.

3. American Cancer Society. *Cancer facts and figures — 1994.* Atlanta (GA): The Society, 1994.

4. Fletcher W, Black W, Harris R, Rimer BK, Shapiro S. Report of the International Workshop on Screening for Breast Cancer. *J Natl Cancer Inst* 1993; **85**: 1644–56.

5. Ries LAG, Hankey BF, Edwards BK. *Cancer Statistics Review: 1973–1987.* Bethesda (MD): National Cancer Institute, 1990. NIH Report No. 90-2789.

6. Young JL, Percy CL, Asire AJ. *Incidence and Mortality Data: 1973–77.* Washington (DC): U.S. Government Printing Office, 1981. National Cancer Institute monograph 57. DHHS Report No NIH-81-2330.

7. Spencer G. *Projections of the population of the United States, by age sex, and race: 1988 to 2080.* Washington (DC): U.S. Government Printing Office, 1989. Current Population Reports, series P-25, no. 1018.

8. National Center for Health Statistics. *Vital Statistics of the United States 1989.* Vol. 2 Mortality, part B. Hyattsville (MD): National Center for Health Statistics, 1991.

9. Yancik R, Kessler L, Yates JW. The elderly population opportunities for cancer prevention and detection. *Cancer* 1988; **62** (Suppl): 1823–8.

10. Yancik R, Ries LG, Yates JW. Ovarian cancer in the elderly: an analysis of Surveillance, epidemiology, and End Results program data. *Am J Obstet Gynecol* 1986; **154**: 639–47.

11. Taeuber CM. *Sixty-five plus in America.* Rev. ed. Washington (DC): U.S. Government Printing Office, 1993. Current Population Reports, Special Studies, P23-178RV.

12. Mansourian BP, Davies AM. Research strategies for health based on the technical discussions at the 43rd World Health Assembly on the Role of Health Research in the Strategy for Health for All by the Year 2000. New York: Hogrefe and Huber, **1**, 1992.

13. Yancik R, Carbone PP, Patterson WB, Steel K, Terry WD. *Perspective on Prevention and Treatment of Cancer in the Elderly.* New York: Raven Press, 1983.

14. Yancik R, Ries LAG. Cancer in the aged: an epidemiologic perspective on treatment issues. *Cancer* 1991; **68**(11 Suppl): 2502–10.

15. Adams G. *Essentials of Geriatric Medicine.* Oxford (UK): Oxford University Press, 1977.

16. Bressler R. Drug use in the geriatric patient. In *Handbook of Clinical Gerontology*, edited by LL Carstensen, BA Edelstein. New York: Pergamon Press, 1987.

17. Patterson WB, Yancik R, Carbone PP. Malignant Diseases. In *Practice of Geriatrics*, edited by E Calkins, AB Ford, PR Katz. Philadelphia (PA): Saunders, 1992.

18. Cairns J. Aging and the national history of cancer. In *Perspectives on and Treatment of Cancer in the Elderly*, edited by R Yancik, PP Carbone, WB Patterson, K Steel, WD Terry. New York: Raven Press, 19–23, 1983.

19. Miller R. Gerontology as oncology: research on aging as the key to the understanding of cancer. *Cancer* 1991; **68**: 2496–501.

20. Monfardini S, Yancik R. Cancer in the elderly: Meeting the challenge of an aging population. *J Natl Cancer Inst* 1993; **85**: 532–8.

21. National Institute on Aging. National Cancer Institute, American Cancer Society. Perspectives on ovarian cancer in older-aged women: current knowledge and recommendations for research. *Cancer* 1993; **71**(Suppl): 513–660.

22. American Cancer Society. National workshop on cancer control and the older person. *Cancer* 1991; **68**(11): 2493–5.

5. Epidemiology Research in Aging: Perspectives and Limitations

Marion R.S. Bain, Jean C. Harvey and Callum S. Muir

Introduction

Improved standards of living, improved nutrition, better prevention and health care have led to increased life expectancy in many parts of the world. The birth rate has also declined substantially in many countries. The consequence of these changes is an increasing average age in many populations. As the risk of most epithelial cancers increases with age, numbers of people with cancers can also be expected to grow.

The United Nations (1) calculated that in Southern Europe the total population would increase by 15% between 1975 and 2000. The proportion of the population over 60 would increase by 24% in males and 27% in females. In Northern Europe, the population size and age structure were considered to be virtually stable. Assuming these projections occur and taking into account probable secular trends in cancer risk, the effect on cancer burden has been assessed (2). The numbers of cases in Northern Europe (including the United Kingdom and the Scandinavian countries) would change little. However, increases of between 60 and 80% in Eastern Europe (countries such as Poland, Romania, Hungary and the former Czechoslovakia) and Southern Europe (Greece, Italy, Spain, Portugal and the former Yugoslavia) and between 10 and 30% in Western Europe (for example, France, Germany, Switzerland and the Netherlands) would be expected.

Sources of Information on Cancer in a Population

The two main sources of information on cancer in a population are mortality (derived from death certificates) and incidence (collected by cancer registries). Population based survival data can be calculated when these two sources are available for the population as a whole.

Mortality Data

The accuracy of mortality data has generally been assessed in studies by one of two methods:

1. Comparison of the clinical diagnosis with autopsy findings
2. Comparison between the clinical diagnosis recorded in case notes and the death certificate diagnosis

Studies from several countries have compared clinical diagnoses with autopsy findings (including 3, 4, 5,

Table 5.1 Percentage of clinical diagnoses of cancer confirmed by autopsy in different age groups.

Age	% Confirmed
<55	100
55–64	88
65–74	90
>75	75

Adapted from Cameron et al., 1980 (9)

6, 7, 8). These studies vary in the source of cases and the percentage of deaths autopsied. However, in general, cancer uncovered at autopsy had been diagnosed clinically in 80 to 90 % of cases. Within this group, in 10 to 25% the cancer site was either not known or attributed to the wrong site. The cancers which were most often missed or wrongly assigned clinically were lung, liver and pancreatic cancers. Missed clinical diagnoses of cancer were commonly attributed to vascular or respiratory causes.

A high percentage of clinical diagnoses of cancer were confirmed by autopsy (80 to 90%), although again up to one quarter had an incorrect or unknown site. Clinically over-diagnosed cancers were commonly large bowel cancers and pancreatic cancers. Vascular causes were the most common autopsy detected cause of death in incorrect clinical diagnoses of cancer.

Incorrect diagnoses occur more frequently with increasing age. In one study looking at routine autopsies (25% of all deaths) in Royal Infirmary of Edinburgh, less than 50% of all clinical diagnoses were confirmed in those over 74 years (5). This low confirmation rate probably reflects greater diagnostic uncertainty in cases undergoing routine autopsy. A further study (9), with a higher percentage of deaths being subjected to autopsy (65%) showed higher confirmation rates, but a similar pattern of increasing diagnostic inaccuracy with increasing age (Table 5.1).

Therefore, death certificates completed before or without autopsy are frequently incorrect. The presence of cancer may be missed or wrongly diagnosed or the wrong primary site identified. Diagnostic inaccuracy is more common in the elderly. This presumably reflects the complicating effects of co-existing diseases in the elderly and, in many countries, perhaps fewer diagnostic investigations in the older age groups. The

Table 5.2 Comparison of detection and confirmation rates for selected cancer sites.

High detection rates and high confirmation rates (>80%)	Low detection rates and low confirmation rates (<80%)	Detection rate higher than confirmation rate (over-reporting on death certificates)	Confirmation rate higher than detection rate (under-reporting on death certificates)
Stomach	Mouth NOS	Colon	Buccal cavity
Pancreas	Small Intestine	Larynx	Rectum
Bronchus/Lung	Connective Tissue	Bone	Cervix
Melanoma of Skin		Uterus NOS	Corpus
Breast		Pharynx NOS	Eye
Ovary		Ill defined and	Myeloid Leukemia
Prostate		unknown sites	Transverse Colon
Bladder			Sigmoid Colon
Thyroid			
Multiple Myelomas			

Notes:

Detection rate: the proportion of hospital diagnoses with cancer of a certain site in which the cause of death reflects the same hospital diagnosis.

Confirmation rate: the proportion of cancer deaths in which the specified underlying cause is confirmed by the hospital diagnosis.

Adapted from Percy et al., 1981 (12)

frequency of autopsy in different areas will have an effect on the accuracy of death certificate data. Autopsies are carried out less frequently in the elderly in all countries (10). The overall frequency of autopsy is also generally falling (11).

Inaccurate recording of the clinical diagnosis on the death certificate has also been shown to occur. A large study (12) compared cause of death on the death certificate with the hospital diagnosis. For most of the leading causes of cancer mortality, the death certificate was a fairly reliable indicator of the hospital diagnosis (Table 5.2). However cancer of the colon was often over-reported and cancer of the rectum under-reported on death certificates. Rarer cancers showed considerable disagreement between the hospital diagnosis and the death certificate cause of death. Bone tumors were over reported on death certificates, presumably because metastatic bone tumors from other primary sites were misclassified. For many sites, a non-specific site was stated on the death certificate despite a specific diagnosis having been made in hospital. For example, over 60% of the death certificate cases of cancer of the uterus, not otherwise specified, had actually been diagnosed as cervical cancer or corpus cancer in hospital. There were no significant differences in accuracy of death certification with age.

Coding rules for large intestine neoplasms may also lead to inaccuracies. The International Classification of Diseases (ICD) requires neoplasms of the rectosigmoid junction to be allocated to the rectum. It may be dif-

ficult to decide whether a neoplasm is in the sigmoid colon or the rectosigmoid junction. In addition, the terms "sigmoid colon" and "rectosigmoid junction" may be used interchangeably by surgeons and pathologists (13). The same coding rules assign cancer of the large bowel to the colon.

Incidence Data

Incidence data is collected by cancer registries throughout the world. Information from registries has been collected by the International Association of Cancer Registries (IACR) and the International Agency for Research on Cancer (IARC) and published in successive volumes of *Cancer Incidence in Five Continents* (14). Several indices of data reliability are requested from contributing registries including:

1. The proportion of diagnoses reported to the registry with histological verification (HV%). For some sites other reliable methods of diagnosis exist (e.g. serum fetoprotein levels for primary liver cancer, radiology for cancer of the esophagus, exfoliative cytology of the cervix uteri). HV% may therefore vary between sites. Some registries include cytological diagnoses with histology, others do not. Registry practice should therefore be considered before making comparisons.

2. The proportion of all notifications for which the existence of a cancer was only identified from a statement on a death certificate. This is usually less

Table 5.3 Indicators of data quality: Stomach cancer in selected cancer registries, 1983–1987.

	0–34	35–64	65–74	75+	All Ages
Canada – Males					
HV%	84	91	87	77	85
DCO%	1	1	1	4	2
Switzerland – Basel – Males					
HV%	99	99	99	98	99
DCO%	–	–	–	–	–
Denmark – Males					
HV%	99	96	95	94	91
DCO%	0	1	2	4	3
US SEER – White males					
HV%	99	99	98	92	97
DCO%	0	0	1	2	1
Scotland – Males					
HV%	99	87	79	68	78
DCO%	0	4	5	7	5

Source: Parkin *et al.*, 1992 (14)

than 1 in 20 notifications. Higher values indicate incomplete registration or poor quality death certification.

3. The proportion of notifications with age unknown. This should be very low (with the exception of non-melanoma skin cancer).

4. The ratio of mortality to incidence for a given cancer in the registration area at a particular time (M/I%). This varies substantially from site to site. Rapidly fatal forms of malignancy give values close to unity while non-melanoma skin cancer gives very low ratios. For a given cancer site, this ratio will depend on the results of treatment (and possibly the definition of what constitutes a cancer). It will therefore vary between medical centers.

Selected results from several areas are presented in Tables 5.3 and 5.4.

Table 5.3 compares HV% and DCO% for stomach cancer in males in Canada, Basel in Switzerland, Denmark, Scotland and the US SEER (Surveillance, Epidemiology and End Results) Registries (white population). The commonly held belief that diagnosis is less reliable in the elderly is supported by the findings in Canada, Denmark, Scotland and the US. The HV% decreased and the DCO% increased with age. However, this was not invariably the case in all countries. In Basel the HV% was very high across the age bands. (In Switzerland it is not possible to identify DCO cases because

Table 5.4 SEER registries 1983–1986: Indices of data reliability.

Age Group		65–69				70–74				75–79				80–84				85+			
Mode of Diagnosis	HV	A	C	DCO	HV	A	C	DCO	HV	A	C	DCO	HV	A	C	DCO	HV	A	C	DCO
Esophagus	M 97.5	0.2	1.6	0.2	93.9	0.5	4.3	0.5	92.5	1.6	4.0	2.0	91.8	0.8	5.2	1.5	80.6	1.0	15.3	3.1
	F 98.8	–	–	0.6	95.6	0.6	1.9	1.2	92.7	0.7	2.9	3.7	93.0	–	7.5	3.5	79.1	–	16.3	4.7
Stomach	M 97.6	0.4	0.9	0.9	96.5	1.0	1.0	1.0	94.5	0.6	3.9	0.5	92.8	1.2	4.0	1.4	84.6	1.3	11.2	2.4
	F 98.5	–	–	0.5	94.4	0.4	3.3	2.0	92.8	0.6	4.2	2.0	90.0	1.6	7.5	0.7	70.9	1.8	20.4	5.7
Liver	M 73.9	5.1	17.1	2.3	72.5	8.2	13.0	4.8	71.5	7.8	16.8	3.4	69.0	6.0	18.1	6.9	58.6	8.6	20.7	10.3
	F 81.1	2.1	12.6	4.2	76.7	1.9	13.6	4.9	71.1	4.4	18.9	5.6	72.6	5.5	19.2	2.7	52.9	2.9	25.7	11.4
Pancreas	M 80.5	1.7	14.3	2.2	77.8	1.7	17.7	1.8	69.9	2.0	23.6	3.3	54.6	1.2	39.8	3.6	43.1	1.5	45.2	7.5
	F 83.4	1.1	13.8	1.1	77.3	0.9	19.2	1.9	69.7	1.0	24.5	4.1	57.7	1.1	36.7	3.9	34.7	1.7	55.5	6.8
Lung	M 93.8	0.9	3.8	1.0	91.3	1.0	6.2	1.1	96.8	1.4	9.4	1.9	77.1	1.0	18.1	3.1	58.5	2.0	31.8	6.8
	F 93.3	0.7	4.3	1.1	90.8	0.8	6.2	1.7	85.6	1.1	10.6	2.0	70.3	2.0	23.7	3.5	54.8	1.3	32.9	4.1
Breast	F 99.3	–	0.4	0.2	98.3	0.1	1.0	0.5	97.5	0.1	1.5	0.7	94.7	0.2	3.6	1.5	85.8	0.1	9.4	8.9
Prostate	M 97.5	1.4	0.9	0.2	97.1	1.4	1.2	0.2	95.2	1.4	2.5	0.5	92.2	1.8	4.6	0.9	83.6	2.6	10.6	2.4
Brain	M 90.2	0.3	8.3	0.9	82.1	–	14.9	3.1	69.9	2.9	28.3	1.7	56.1	–	36.6	6.1	42.9	–	47.6	7.1
	F 83.3	–	15.7	0.4	80.5	–	17.5	1.6	71.4	0.5	22.9	3.7	44.1	2.5	46.9	5.9	35.3	–	52.9	5.9
All Sites	M 95.5	0.9	2.6	0.9	94.0	1.0	1.9	0.8	91.6	1.2	5.6	1.1	87.4	1.3	8.8	1.9	79.2	1.7	14.5	3.7
	F 96.6	0.3	2.2	0.6	94.6	0.4	3.7	1.0	92.3	0.6	5.3	1.4	87.2	0.7	9.4	2.2	76.6	0.7	16.7	4.9

* Basic data were kindly provided by Ms V. Van Hoten and Mrs C. Percy of the US National Cancer Institute. Totals are less than 100% due to small number of cases diagnosed in hospital for which the record did not indicate one way or another whether diagnosis was histologically confirmed or not.

HV = histological verification; A = diagnosed at autopsy; DCO = death certificate only; C = clinical diagnosis only.

the problem of medical confidentiality prevents matching of pathology records with death certification data.) Large differences in the indices are seen in different parts of the world.

More detailed data concerning the elderly population from the SEER registries of the United States are given in Table 5.4. Indices of data quality are given by age and sex for selected sites of cancer. The percentage with histological verification is generally the same for the sites listed at ages 65–69 and 70–74, but after the age of 75 the HV% gradually falls, along with an increase in those diagnosed clinically and an increase in DCO%.

The indices are useful guides to data quality. However, they must be interpreted with an awareness of

Table 5.5 Percentage relative survival from lung, large bowel, prostate and breast cancer, Scotland 1983–1987, by broad age-group, both sexes combined.

Age-Group	Lung	Large Bowel	Prostate	Breast
35–44	10.9	47.3	–	70.5
45–54	9.0	43.7	32.3	67.1
55–64	8.3	38.8	50.9	63.4
65–74	5.6	39.7	48.3	63.1
75–84	2.7	36.2	43.1	56.0
All Ages	6.6	39.6	46.7	64.3

Source: Black *et al.*, 1993 (15)

Table 5.6 Comparison of five-year relative survival for selected cancer sites: Scotland (1983–1987)[a], Denmark (1983–1987)[b], Geneva (1982–1986)[c], Quebec (1984–1986)[d], and US Whites (1981–1987)[e].

	Scotland M+F	Denmark M	Denmark F	Geneva M	Geneva F	Quebec M	Quebec F	US M	US F
Esophagus	7.1	2.9	6.8	*	*	11	10	7.7	11.5
Stomach	10.6	11.9	12.8	18	18	22	26	14.7	18.0
Large bowel	39.6	38.2	40.5	50	45	52	52	57.0	57.0
Pancreas	4.0	2.1	1.9	*	*	6	7	2.4	3.2
Larynx	65.9	60.6	62.3	57	59	62	65	68.4	65.6
Lung	6.6	5.6	6.0	13	16	15	20	11.8	16.3
Melanoma skin	78.5	77.7	84.6	80	87	57	77	76.8	86.7
Breast	64.3	58.2	69.4	*	80	83	73	74.4	78.2
Cervix uteri	58.7	–	63.9	–	66	–	74	–	67.5
Corpus uteri	71.2	–	77.2	–	74	–	81	–	84.4
Ovary	29.4	–	30.4	–	38	–	42	–	38.7
Prostate	46.7	39.0	–	57	–	68	–	75.6	–
Testis	89.1	91.1	–	*	–	83	–	92.8	–
Bladder	63.5	63.1	56.4	57	55	78	78	80.2	75.4
Kidney	35.3	34.9	36.3	58	44	53	57	54.1	51.6
Brain etc.	18.4	35.9	47.6	*	*	24	27	23.0	25.8
Thyroid	73.5	57.9	68.1	*	90	72	83	92.2	94.2
Hodgkins disease	67.0	69.5	74.5	76	71	75	76	75.7	78.2
Non-Hodgkins Lymphoma	43.3	40.9	45.0	34	34	*	*	50.2	52.7
Leukemia	29.4	27.7	27.7	*	*	29	34	36.0	36.7
All sites	34.6	*	*	*	*	40	54	52.0	57.4

* Data not provided or not comparable
– not applicable

[a] Population based survival data for all Scotland (15). In general there is little difference in survival between the sexes, malignant melanoma of skin excepted, a form of cancer with a 20% advantage for females.
[b] Population based survival data for Denmark (22).
[c] Population based survival data of Canton of Geneva (23).
[d] Population based survival data for the Province of Quebec (24).
[e] Population based survival data providing information of the 10% of the US population covered by the SEER (Surveillance, Epidemiology and End Results) Program of the US NCI (25).

Table adapted from reference (26).

local circumstances. A high HV% may be due to complete reporting by pathologists and lesser degrees of reporting by other sources. A low HV% may reflect an inadequate number of pathologists, a high proportion of cancer that can be diagnosed by other means, failure to notify the registry that biopsy or autopsy was performed, or an unwillingness to investigate older persons exhaustively. A high proportion of DCO (for example in Japan) may be due to the inability to link hospital records with death certificates. The M/I ratio may be distorted by poor or imprecise death certification. For example there are usually more deaths attributed to unspecified leukemia than there are incident cases, as the more precise data on cell type available to the clinician and cancer registry do not appear on the death certificate.

Generally the results support the commonly held view that diagnosis is less accurate in the elderly. This may reflect the reluctance to investigate patients in whom treatment is not contemplated. Concomitant disease may rule out cancer therapy. However, large differences are seen in different parts of the world. The enthusiasm of physicians to investigate and treat elderly people undoubtedly varies in different cultures.

Survival Data

Estimating cancer survival for the population as a whole requires knowledge of all persons with newly diagnosed cancer, their date of diagnosis, and their date of death. Obtaining this information requires either national cancer registration, or, if registration covers only part of a country, the ability to determine whether registered cancer patients have died. In many countries this is not possible. In several western European countries considerations of patient confidentiality prevent such matches being made. Population figures are required. Results from controlled clinical trials are not representative of the cancer survival of a given population, as patients entered in these trials are highly selected so that valid comparisons of comparable patient groups can be made between treatment regimes. Such trials frequently exclude patients over 65 years of age.

Relative survival in Scotland has been analyzed (15). As, with the exception of malignant melanoma, survival was similar for both sexes the data were published for both sexes combined for the non sex-specific cancers. Survival is not provided for those aged 85 years and over as the quality and completeness of the cancer registration data is poorer for this age group than for younger cases.

For the sites shown in Table 5.5, and for all sites combined, relative survival is poorer with advancing age (with the exception of prostatic cancer where mortality is highest in those aged 45 to 54). For all sites combined, the rate for the 65–74 age group is nearly half that of those in the 35–44 age group. For those aged 75–84, the chance of survival is further reduced. This pattern is found for one, three and five year follow-up periods. Nearly 60% of 35–44 year olds survived five years after diagnosis. Only 28% of the 65–74 age group

Table 5.7 Five year relative survival in colon cancer by stage and sex in Norway, 1968–75.

Stage		<55	55–74	75+
Localized	M	.77	.69	.60
	F	.79	.71	.56
Regional Spread	M	.48	.42	.35
	F	.45	.42	.36
Distant Spread	M	.05	.04	.08
	F	.08	.06	.05

Source: Cancer Registry of Norway, 1980 (16)

Table 5.8 Five year relative survival in breast cancer by stage and age in Norway, 1968–79.

Age	Stage 1	Stage II	Stage III	Stage IV	All cases
<45	.90	.60	.48	.14	.72
45–55	.89	.62	.47	.16	.71
55–74	.86	.56	.48	.12	.65
75+	.76	.48	.40	.09	.58
All ages	.86	.58	.46	.12	.67
No of Cases	4,743	3,305	772	912	10,591

Source: Cancer registry of Norway, 1980 (16)

survived and only 24.5% of those aged 75–84 remained alive.

A decline in survival with advancing age is seen in all population based series. Comparative figures of five year relative survival for selected cancer sites in five countries is given in Table 5.6.

Survival differences need to be interpreted in the light of stage distribution of the presenting cancer. Staging data is rarely available, however the Norwegian Cancer Registry has published such data (16). Five year relative survival for colon cancer and breast cancer by stage are given in Tables 5.7 and 5.8. At any stage, survival is poorer in those over 74. However, at any age, stage is a more important prognostic factor than age *per se*. Staging data is required for analyzing survival data. Brewster *et al.* (17) examined a probability sample of 2,200 records of Scottish cancer patients. The proportion of cancers for which stage was explicitly given varied by site. However, sufficient information was given in the records for staging to be carried out in 80 to 90%. The proportion which were staged or stageable decreased with age but remained over 75% up to the age of 84 (Table 5.9).

Size of the Cancer Burden in the Elderly

Incidence data can be used to estimate the size of the cancer burden in the elderly. The average annual

Table 5.9 Proportion of a sample of 420 cases of colorectal, breast and cervix uteri cancer diagnosed in Scotland in 1990 with information permitting staging by broad age-group.

Age Group	Staged (a) %	Stageable* (b) %	(a+b)	Not Staged %	Total %
<50	29	29	58–(92%)	5	63
50–64	63	72	135–(94%)	8	143
65–74	41	42	83–(81%)	20	103
75–84	33	37	70–(79%)	19	89
85+	4	7	11–(55%)	11	20
All ages	170	187	357–(85%)	63	420

*Stageable from information contained within medical records

(Data kindly provided by Dr. D. Brewster of the Scottish Cancer Registry)

number of cancers registered for all ages and for those over 75 years in the five years from 1983 to 1987 in selected countries is shown in Table 5.10. Between one quarter and one third of the overall cancer burden in these countries is found in those aged 75 and over.

Future Burden

The effect of demographic changes on the future size of the cancer burden can be estimated on the assumption that current age specific rates for the common cancers in those aged 75 years and over would still apply. An estimate of the number of cancers occurring in this same age span in 2029 in Scotland is given in Figure 5.1. This estimate is bound to be incorrect as it does not take into account the likely continued fall in lung cancer in males or possible increases for other sites. However the estimates of cancer incidence for all sites seem likely to be of the correct magnitude.

Predicting age specific rates beyond the year 2000 is difficult as they depend on the cumulated effect of carcinogenic exposures. For older persons born at a particular time, much of this exposure has already taken place, cellular damage has occurred and the resulting cancer risk is largely determined. However it is believed that prolonged exposure to promoting agents is required for initiated cells to be transformed. If exposure to promoters can be reduced or avoided or anti-promoters given, malignant transformation may be postponed or may not take place at all. Therefore, changes such as consuming more fresh fruit and vegetables or ceasing to smoke may reduce risk even in older persons. Only recently has extensive work begun in this area, including search for short term tests of promoting activity.

Younger birth cohorts may experience new carcinogenic risks and/or avoid exposure to known causes and hence their risk is much less easy to forecast. Sharp *et al.* (18) predicted cancer burden in Scotland up to the year 2000 using age-period-cohort mathematical models. However even these cannot take account of future risk in those who are presently relatively young.

Cancer Treatment in the Elderly

Place of Treatment

Many factors including the stage of the tumor, presence and extent of other diseases and the distance from treatment centers are likely to influence the place of treatment of older persons. In Scotland, fifteen Health Boards are responsible for providing all health services in their own area (Figure 5.2). The proportion of cancer patients in Scotland less than 75 years of age and aged 75 and over treated in their Health Board of residence has been examined by the Scottish Cancer Registry. The majority of patients, both under 75 and 75 and older, are treated within their Health Board of residence (Figure 5.3). However, in all areas except Orkney and Shetland persons aged 75 years and over seem less likely to be transferred to a different Health Board area compared with those under 75 years. This effect is

Table 5.10 Size of cancer burden in selected countries.

	Average number of cancers/year (excludes non-melanoma skin cancer (ICD–9 173))**			
Country	Total Population*	All ages	75+ Age-group	% of total cancers/year In 75+ age-group
Canada	25,037,770	90,397	23,950	26
Scotland	5,133,138	21,802	6,705	31
England and Wales	49,925,500	183,140	59,933	33
Denmark	5,117,434	23,843	7,405	31
USA SEER whites	18,318,686	74,858	21,246	28

* Average annual population 1983–87

** Average over period 1983–87

Source: Parkin *et al.*, 1992 (14)

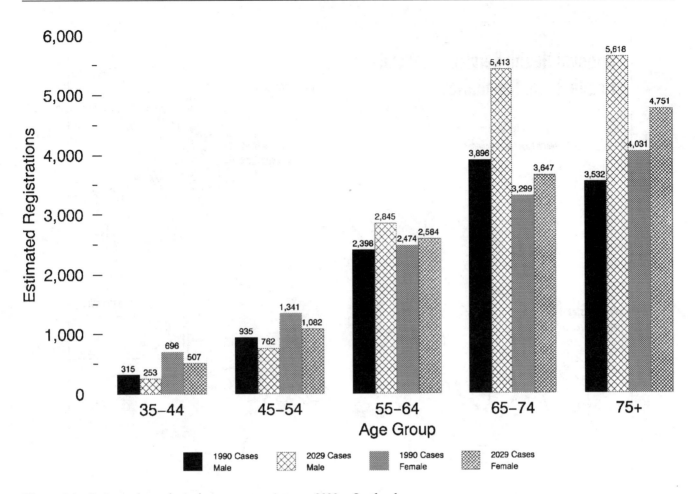

Figure 5.1   Estimated number of cancer cases in year 2029 – Scotland.

especially marked in rural Health Boards. For Health Boards containing cities, such as Lothian and Greater Glasgow, very few patients of any age are treated elsewhere. Those treated outside their own area would be most likely to have their treatment in Health Boards within cities as the medical facilities are concentrated there. A small proportion of cancer patients in Scotland are admitted to institutions which notify 10 or less patients with cancer a year to the cancer registry. The spectrum of cancers notified from these institutions is very similar to that for all cancers in Scotland. However the age distribution is quite different, a large majority of the patients being 75 years or older (Table 5.11).

Therefore, older patients in Scotland appear less likely to be referred outside their area of residence (especially in rural areas), and are more likely to be admitted to institutions which admit small numbers of cancer patients. These findings may be due to more advanced disease or co-morbid conditions in the elderly, which makes treatment less likely. There is no reason why elderly persons with cancer should not be treated as energetically as those who are younger (and, as the neoplasms often grow more slowly, with success). However, physicians may be reluctant to subject elderly patients to the discomfort of investiga-

tion and aggressive therapy. In addition, a proportion of elderly patients will be unsuitable for treatment because of co-existing cardiovascular, respiratory or other diseases. Patient preference may also influence treatment decisions.

Future Research

A significant proportion of the overall cancer burden occurs in the elderly. Cancer in the elderly is likely to be complicated by the presence of co-existing disease. More work needs to be done attempting to quantify co-morbidity, assessing its effects on cancer and its influence on decisions to treat elderly cancer patients.

Clinically, decisions have to be made considering the risks and discomfort of investigation and treatment and the effects on survival and quality of life. The balance tends to result in less investigation of elderly patients. This leads to poorer characterization of cancer in this age group which in turn affects the information available for planning of services.

Treatment also appears to be less likely in the elderly. The conspicuous lack of clinical trials involving the elderly means that information on which to base treatment decisions in this age group is often not available. More trials involving the elderly are required. Surveys of attitudes of general practitioners

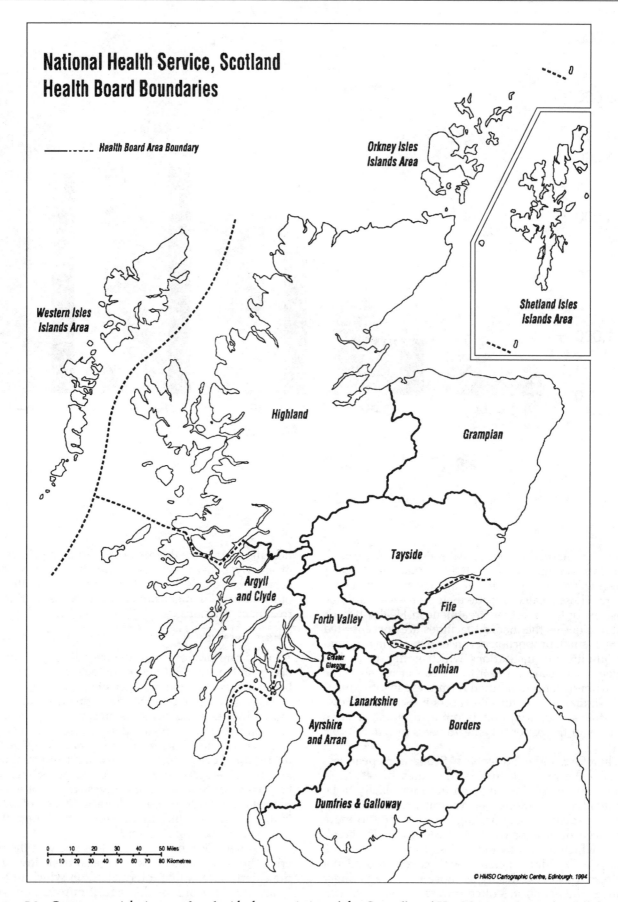

Figure 5.2 Crown copyright is reproduced with the permission of the Controller of Her Majesty's Stationery Office.

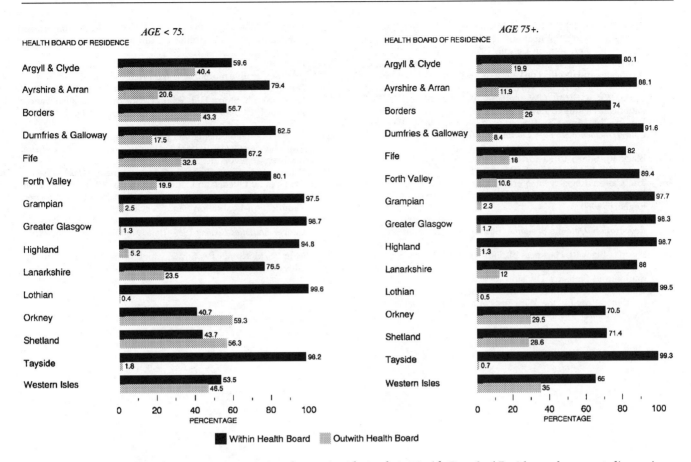

Figure 5.3 Percentage of cancer cases treated within and without their Health Board of Residence, by age at diagnosis, Scotland 1981–1990.

and hospital consultants to treatment of the elderly are also required. Whether funding for treatment has any effect may also be important in countries with private health care systems. In addition, the needs, expectations and wishes of older people with cancer need to be studied. The failure to refer older patients to cancer centers may be especially important if recent studies on the effect of type of hospital and treating physician on survival for ovarian cancer (19, 20) and large bowel cancer (21) are confirmed.

Table 5.11 Percentage age distribution of cancer notified for Scotland as a whole in 1990; compared with age distribution of cancer notified for Scottish hospitals treating fewer than 10 cases in 1990.

Age group	Scotland (%)	Hospitals treating <10 cases/year (%)
<55	24.2	7.6
55–64	18.4	7.6
65–74	27.3	16.4
>75	30.0	68.4

Source: Scottish Cancer Registry

References

1. United Nations Organization. *Demographic Indicators of Countries. Estimates and Projections as Assessed in 1984.* New York: UNO, 1986.
2. Muir CS. Changing international patterns of cancer incidence. In *Accomplishments in Cancer Research 1988*, edited by JG Fortner, JE Rhoads. Philadelphia: Lippincott Co, 1989.
3. Heasman MA, Lipworth L. *Accuracy of Certification of Cause of Death* HMSO, 1966.
4. Engel LW, Stauchen JA, Chiazze L, Jr, Heid M. Accuracy of death certification in an autopsied population with specific attention to malignant neoplasms and vascular diseases. *American Journal of Epidemiology* 1980; **111**: 99–112.
5. Cameron HM, McGoogan E. A prospective study of 1152 autopsies: 1. Inaccuracies in death certification. *The Journal of Pathology* 1981; **133**: 273–283.
6. Goldman L, Sayson R, Robbins S, Cohn LH, Bettman M, Weisberg M. The value of the autopsy in three medical eras. *The New England Journal of Medicine* 1983; **308**: 1000–1005.
7. Holzner JH. The role of autopsy in the control of mortality in Austria. In *Autopsy in Epidemiology and Medical Research.* Lyon: IARC, 25–35, 1991.
8. Modelmog D, Rahlenbeck S, Trichopoulos D. Accuracy of death certificates: A population based, complete-coverage, one-year autopsy study in East Germany. *Cancer Causes and Control* 1992; **3**: 541–546.
9. Cameron HM, McGoogan E, Watson H. Necropsy A yardstick for clinical diagnoses. *British Medical Journal* 1980; **281**: 985–988.
10. World Health Organization. *World Health Statistics 1990*, Table 5.2, Background information on mortality statistics. Geneva: WHO, 15–21, 1991.

11. Riboli E, Delendi M. *Autopsy in Epidemiology and Medical Research* (IARC Scientific Publications No.112). Lyon: International Agency for Research on Cancer, 1991.

12. Percy C, Stanek E, Gloeckler L. Accuracy of cancer death certificates and its effect on cancer mortality statistics. *American Journal of Public Health* 1981; **71**: 242–250.

13. Puffer RR, Griffith GW. *Patterns of Urban Mortality*. Pan American Health Organization, 1967.

14. Parkin DM, Muir CS, Whelan SL, Gao Y, Ferlay J, Powell J. *Cancer Incidence in Five Continents: Volume VI*. Lyon: IARC, 1992.

15. Black RJ, Sharp L, Kendrick S. *Trends in Cancer Survival in Scotland*. Edinburgh: Information and Statistics Division, 1993.

16. The Cancer Registry of Norway. *Survival of Cancer Patients: Cases Diagnosed in Norway 1968–1975*. Oslo: Norwegian Cancer Registry, 1980.

17. Brewster D, Crichton J, Muir CS. *Accuracy of 1990 Cancer Registration Data in Scotland*. Edinburgh: Information and Statistics Division, 1993.

18. Sharp L, Black RJ, Harkness EL, Finlayson AR, Muir CS. *Cancer Registration Statistics in Scotland 1981–1990*. Edinburgh: Information and Statistics Division, 1993.

19. Gillis CR. Medical audit, cancer registration and survival in ovarian cancer for the West of Scotland. In *Newsletter of the Scottish Cancer Therapy Network* 1993; **no. 1**: 2–4.

20. Junor EJ, Hole DJ, Gillis CR. Management of ovarian cancer referral to a multidisciplinary team matters. *British Journal of Cancer* 1994; **70**: 363–370.

21. McArdle CS, Hole DJ. Impact of variability among surgeons on postoperative morbidity and mortality and ultimate survival. *British Medical Journal* 1991; **302**: 1501–1505.

22. Carstensen B, Storm HH, Schou G. Survival in Danish Cancer Patients 1943–1987. *APMIS* 1993; (Supplement no 33) **101**: 1–213.

23. Register Genevois des Tumeurs: Le cancer a Geneve. Incidence, Mortalite, Survie: 1970–1990. *Les Cahiers de la sante No 2*. Geneva: Register Genevois des Tumeurs, 1993.

24. Pelletier G. La Survie Reliee au Cancer. Etude des Cas Nouveaux Declares au Quebec au Cours des Annees 1984, 1985 et 1986. *Collection Donnees Statistiques et Indicateurs No. 21*. Quebec, Planification-Evaluation Sante Services Sociaux, 1993.

25. Ries LAG, Hankey BF, Miller BA, Hartman AM, Edwards BK. Cancer *Statistics Review 1987–1988*. National Cancer Institute. NIH pub. No. 91-2789, 1991.

26. Muir CS, McKinney PA. Strategy for Cancer Control in Scotland. Glasgow: Scottish Forum for Public Health Medicine, 1994.

6. Factors Affecting the Diagnosis and Treatment of Older Persons with Cancer

James S. Goodwin

Introduction

Men and women over age 75 are different than men and women in their 50's. A recurring theme of geriatrics is that one cannot take rules generated from the study of the medical treatment of 50 year olds and unquestioningly apply them to the medical treatment of 80 year olds. Yet, most of the "rules" of oncology and the rest of internal medicine are generated from information obtained from studies of those under the age of 65 (1). There are no compelling *a priori* reasons to think that these rules will work very well in older patients. Similarly, the fact that older cancer patients are treated differently from younger cancer patients does not prove that older patients are being treated incorrectly.

In this chapter we will begin with an overview of the current status of how older patients with cancer are diagnosed and treated. The evidence shows that older people are less likely to be diagnosed at an early stage for those cancers for which there are accepted screening procedures. In addition, older patients are less likely to receive treatments that are considered definitive or potentially curative.

Because of the concepts raised in the first paragraph, we will then turn to a discussion of the evidence that the decrease in definitive treatment for older cancer patients is indeed inappropriate; that is, that it is associated with poor outcomes. We will discuss the specific characteristics of older cancer patients that put them at risk for delays in diagnosis and inadequate treatment. Finally, based on our understanding of the barriers to adequate medical care experienced by some older cancer patients, we will discuss ways to improve the diagnosis, treatment and outcomes of the older men or women with cancer.

Older Patients are Less Likely to be Diagnosed with Early Stage Cancer

One relatively recent breakthrough in the examination of medical practices is in the use of large scale disease registries, such as cancer registries, to examine issues such as patterns of diagnosis and treatment. It is important to realize that this was not the purpose for which these registries were created. Cancer registries were created to produce reliable data on the incidence of various cancers and how the incidence might vary with gender, race, age or geographic area. However,

Table 6.1 Effectiveness Versus Efficacy

- Efficacy
  - Demonstration of beneficial effect of a treatment in prospective controlled clinical trial.

- Effectiveness
  - Demonstration of beneficial effect of a treatment when used in a community.

the growth of effectiveness research has led to a greater appreciation that results of clinical trials were not always indicative of whether a particular treatment was effective in the "real world." Thus, the need arose for mechanisms to look at diagnosis and treatment of the entire population — so called "population-based" data. This is precisely what cancer registries provide. However, because these registries were not constructed to help us analyze appropriateness of diagnosis and treatment, one should be sensitive to the limitations of these data.

Holmes and Hearne (2) used data on 31,000 cancers between 1944 and 1979 in a regional cancer registry for Kansas and western Missouri to examine the relationship between stage at diagnosis and age of the patient. They found significant positive trends between age and stage for cancers of the bladder, breast, cervix, kidney, ovary, stomach, and uterus; that is, the older the patient, the more likely he or she was diagnosed at an advanced stage. Breslow (3) reported an increase in stage at diagnosis of cervical cancer in elderly patients in data from the California tumor Registry, which receives information on cancer patients treated at 40 California hospitals.

New Mexico Tumor Registry data were utilized to examine the relationships between stage of cancer at diagnosis and age, ethnic group, marital status, and place of residence (urban or rural) of men and women diagnosed with cancer in New Mexico (4,5,6). Cancers of the bladder, breast, cervix, ovary, thyroid, and uterus and malignant melanoma, were more likely to be diagnosed at more advanced stages in older patients (Table 6.2). The most striking relationship between stage at diagnosis and age was found for cervical cancer. More than 20% of cervical cancers were diagnosed at a remote stage in women older than 75 years of age compared with 3% for women 55 years of age and younger. With breast cancer there was an increase in

Table 6.2   Cancers more likely to be diagnosed at an advanced stage in older patients.

| Cancer site | Stage | Percentage of patients diagnosed at advanced stage Age group (years) | | | | |
		≤55	55–65	65–74	75–84	≥85
Bladder	Regional, remote*	5	12	13	13	15
Breast	Regional**	41	39	35	29	31
	Remote**	5	8	8	8	15
Cervix	Regional, remote**	3	20	23	26	34
Melanoma	Regional, remote*	13	18	21	21	29
Ovary	Regional, remote**	62	78	80	86	79
Thyroid	Regional, remote*	34	40	39	63	67
Uterus	Regional, remote*	13	10	15	24	19

Adapted from data presented in reference 4.

* p < 0.01 by Chi square for linear trend.
**p < 0.0001 by Chi square for linear trend.

the percentage of remote-stage cancers balanced by a decrease in the percentage of regional-stage cancers with age. Other population-based studies have reported no increase in advanced stage breast cancer with age, possibly because the regional and remote stages were combined and together considered as "advanced disease" (7,8).

There was an opposite pattern of stage at diagnosis versus age for cancers of the stomach, pancreas, rectum, and lung, with older patients diagnosed at less advanced stages of cancer (4). Stage of cancer at diagnosis is influenced by the extent of the diagnostic evaluation; a less extensive evaluation would tend to misclassify advanced cancers as local. Although 99% of cancers in those under 55 years of age are diagnosed by histopathology or cytopathology, more than 20% of cancers in those older than 85 years of age are diagnosed on a clinical or radiologic basis without pathological confirmation. Thus, less extensive evaluation may partially explain the finding that some cancers are diagnosed more frequently at local stages in elderly subjects.

Older Patients are less Likely to Receive Definitive Therapy for Cancer

The New Mexico Tumor Registry data base was used to assess the relationship between patient age and the use of potentially curative therapy, termed definitive treatment (9). Table 6.3 gives the percentage of patients in different age categories receiving definitive treatment after the diagnosis of a local cancer. For most sites there was a significant decline with age in the percentage of patients receiving definitive therapy. The pattern was generally similar for regional stage cases. To confirm the relationship between definitive treatment and age, the proportion of patients in each age group

Table 6.3   Percentage of patients in different age groups receiving definitive treatment for local stage cancers.

| Site | Age Group (years) | | | | |
	< 54	55–64	65–74	75–84	> 85
Bladder[†]	96	96	95	91	84
Breast[†]	96	96	95	84	69
Cervix[†]	96	92	87	87	61
Colon	89	94	86	87	65
Esophagus**	89	68	71	43	42
Gallbladder*	71	69	71	54	44
Kidney[†]	98	89	78	66	50
Lip	85	88	84	85	80
Lung[†]	55	51	32	13	0
Melanoma	98	100	96	97	91
Ovary	95	89	94	100	80
Pancreas[†]	19	30	13	0	0
Prostate[†]	82	89	88	81	75
Rectum[†]	92	92	90	75	54
Stomach[†]	84	71	75	29	30
Uterus[†]	94	96	88	68	23
All sites[†]	92	87	80	72	62

Adapted from data presented in reference 9.

* < P < 0.05, by X^2 for linear trend.
** P < 0.01, by X^2 for linear trend.
[†] < P < 0.001, by X^2 for linear trend.

that received no treatment recorded by the New Mexico Tumor Registry was also examined. The trends were the inverse of those found for definitive treatment. For all sites combined, the proportion of patients with no treatment increased progressively from 3% in those younger than 55 years to 29% in those 85 years and older.

Tumor registry data also allow the analysis of changes over time in the provision of treatments (10). For cancer patients over age 75, there was a clear increase in the percentage over time (from 1969 through 1982) of those receiving definitive therapy (9).

Older cancer patients are also less likely to receive chemotherapy after the diagnosis of local or advanced cancer. For example, Mor et al. (11) analyzed 1891 cancer cases from the National Hospice Survey and found decreasing chemotherapy use with age in patients with breast, lung and colorectal cancer.

Much of the attention to possible under treatment of older patients has focussed on breast cancer (12–25). Several studies conducted in a variety of health care settings and geographic regions have shown that many older women diagnosed with breast cancer receive less extensive diagnostic evaluations and initial treatments than are generally thought to be appropriate. For example, 56% of women aged 65 or older who received breast conserving surgery (BCS) between 1981–85 in New Mexico received no adjuvant radiotherapy (14). Older women are also less likely to receive axillary dissection (18,19), oncology referrals (17), and chemotherapy (11,15,17,19), in addition to being less likely to receive radiation (14,15,17,19,22,26,27).

Might Cancer Therapy Considered "Less than Definitive" Actually be Appropriate for Some Older Patients?

The answer to the question posed in the title to this section is yes. This is made obvious by considering the extreme case. Does one recommend definitive surgery for local rectal cancer in a 114 year old man? Does one perform either modified radical mastectomy or breast conserving surgery with subsequent radiation in a 95 year old woman? Would it not be more appropriate to remove the lump and prescribe Tamoxifen? It is not ageist to recognize the medical realities of extreme old age; indeed, not doing so involves sacrificing common sense and humane care to a false standard of ideological purity: the concept that differences in care are de facto evidence of inadequacies of care (28). Thus, the decrease in receipt of definitive treatment in older cancer patients that was documented in the preceding section is potentially justifiable; it may represent appropriate clinical decision making by patients and their physicians faced with the complex task of balancing several potentially conflicting values. Some patients may appropriately be judged to be unable to tolerate the rigors of diagnostic testing and treatment (e.g., those with serious comorbidities).

Furthermore, the patient with dementia poses a special problem. If the treating physician cannot obtain

informed consent, if the patient cannot understand the necessity of the treatment and give permission to the treating physician, any treatment, no matter how necessary to preserve health, can be seen as a form of assault. This takes an emotional toll on the physician, the other members of the health care team, and the patient's family, in addition to the patient.

The above comments notwithstanding, there is a clear consensus among those investigating the issue that the decrease in definitive treatment for older cancer patients is indeed inappropriate, or at least frequently inappropriate. The arguments supporting this opinion can be presented in four parts:

First, the observed less aggressive approach does not appear to be largely explained by comorbidity (18,19,23). For example, in a study of breast cancer care at seven southern California hospitals, 17% of women with local or regional diseased aged 70 or older and with low comorbidity did not receive definitive therapy, compared with 4.4% of women under 70.

Second, there are substantial geographic variations in the cancer care received by women that would be difficult to explain on the basis of distributional differences in comorbidity and physical frailty. This is best documented for breast cancer. For example, the percentage of women aged 65 or older with local breast cancer who underwent breast conserving surgery in 1986 varied from 3.5% in Kentucky to greater than 20% in New York, Pennsylvania, Massachusetts, and Vermont (29). The percentage of non-Hispanic white women aged 65–74 with local breast cancer who did not receive breast irradiation following breast-conserving surgery varied from 14% in Seattle, Washington to 46% in Connecticut (27). Other studies have demonstrated considerable variation in the types of care received by breast cancer patients among hospitals within a given state (26,30).

Third, several investigators have found that characteristics of patients other than their medical status or comorbidity are more important determinants of treatment received. These include ethnicity (27,31,32,33), advanced age (17–23,26,27) educational level (23), marital status (6,26,34), place of residence (26,30,35), cognitive status (23), access to transportation (23) and social support (23). Definitive therapy often involves several modalities. As shown in Table 6.4, advanced age, impaired access to transportation, functional dependence and impaired cognition all had a significant effect on receipt of radiation therapy but not on receipt of surgery (23). This reinforces the concept that the decrease in definitive treatments has more to do with issues of access to care than to medical considerations per se.

Fourth, choice of treatment has a strong influence on outcomes in older cancer patients. For example, breast conserving surgery without radiation is associated with a high rate of local recurrence in older women (36,37). Receipt of BCS without irradiation was associated with a two fold higher death rate compared to BCS plus radiation in a population-based study of women of all ages with breast cancer in Orange County, California

Table 6.4 Odds ratios for not receiving any surgery or any radiation therapy after the diagnosis of cancer in older subjects.

Factor	Categories compared	Odds ratio (95% confidence intervals)	
		No surgery	No radiation
Age	Increase of 10 years	0.96 (0.66–1.40)	2.14 (1.47–3.12)
Drives or lives with driver	No vs. Yes	0.72 (0.26–1.99)	3.35 (1.28–8.76)
Activities of daily living	Some problems vs none	0.80 (0.40–1.60)	2.49 (1.34–4.62)
Physical activity	Bottom 20% vs others	0.70 (0.37–1.31)	2.46 (1.31–4.64)
Mental status	Incompetent vs. No errors	0.29 (0.64–1.32)	13.5 (1.78–101.6)
	≥2 errors vs. No errors	1.18 (0.55–2.56)	1.60 (0.78–3.28)
	1 error vs. No errors	0.99 (0.54–1.80)	1.44 (0.86–2.40)

Adapted from data in reference 23. The cases include in situ, local, and regional stages of colorectal, breast, and prostate cancer. Odds ratios computed from separate logistic regressions with terms for site and stage.

(25). In a longitudinal study of older women diagnosed with breast cancer in New Mexico, women who did not receive definitive treatment for stage I or II breast cancer had twice the death rate (hazard ratio = 2.2; 95% CI = 1.4,3.4) during eight years post diagnosis as those receiving definitive treatment, after controlling for age, race, income, comorbidity, and such indicators of physical frailty as functional status, cognitive function and activity level (38). A similar pattern of results were reported for older men and women with local colorectal cancer (38).

In summary, the evidence for inappropriate undertreatment of some older cancer patients is substantial. However, it cannot be considered definitive, for several reasons. First, increased mortality associated with certain treatments in population-based studies does not prove those treatments are inappropriate. One can always posit that the same forces that influenced choice of therapy also influenced mortality. It is virtually impossible in large population-based studies to completely control for comorbidity or other factors that might simultaneously decrease survival and increase the choice of a "non-definitive" treatment. Second, geographic variation in use of treatments is not necessarily inappropriate; for example, if two treatments were roughly comparable. Similarly, if treatments are roughly comparable in outcome, variation in treatment by any patient characteristic — age, ethnicity, marital status, etc. — is not necessarily inappropriate. Personal goals and values may vary across these groups, and those values could appropriately influence choice of therapy.

The above arguments are dependent on therapies being "roughly comparable," which brings us to the third reason why we cannot conclude with absolute certainty that older patients receiving "less than definitive" treatments are being inappropriately treated: the lack of comprehensive information on outcomes of various cancer treatments in the elderly. While it is fairly well recognized that there are insufficient numbers of older people, particularly those over age 70, enrolled in clinical trials of cancer treatments, we should also consider the possibility that this may always be the case (1). The heterogeneity of the aging population, as well as the volunteer nature of prospective trials, may render unrealistic the goal of obtaining information on outcomes of cancer treatments on all the definable subpopulations of older men and women. Nevertheless, the recent attention given to enrolling older subjects in clinical trials, as well as the growing sophistication of population-based comparisons of treatment and outcomes in large populations, ensures that our level of knowledge about appropriate cancer treatments for older men and women will increase dramatically over the next decade.

Are Older Cancer Patients Also at Risk for Over Treatment?

The same underlying factors that put the older patient at risk for under-treatment can also contribute to over-treatment. These factors are the great heterogeneity among the elderly and the relative lack of information about effectiveness. Lack of sound data invariably leads to variation in practice patterns, and within that variation will exist both too much and too little treatment. There is better documentation for under-treatment, reviewed in the previous section, than for over-treatment. Every primary care physician has at least one "horror story" of a frail elderly patient spending the last weeks of life being shuttled from doctor to doctor, from treatment to treatment, with little time for reflection, for leave-taking. Ever since we declared the "war on cancer" in the late 1970's, there has been a tendency, particularly at academic medical centers, to see all patients as potential recruits, potential soldiers in that war. In that metaphorical structure, choosing no additional cancer-specific therapy can be viewed as a form of surrender. In addition, cancer therapists can become overly identified with their therapy, be it drugs or radiation, so that the patient may feel obligated to choose the proffered therapy so as not to reject the physician.

Over-treatment has always been difficult to define with sufficient rigor to study using population-based methods (39), but the recent growth of interest and expertise in measuring quality of life as an outcome of cancer therapy should change that (40). The greatest concerns about over-treatment have been raised for cancer of the prostate, where improvements in screening tests have led to a dramatic increase in diagnoses (41). This in turn has led to a four fold increase in the use of radical prostatectomy, a procedure of unproven benefit in this disease (42). This issue will be discussed in the chapters dealing with screening for and treatment of prostate cancer.

Perhaps easier to document than over-treatment of cancer is over-utilization of cancer screening tests in the elderly. The forces promoting over-utilization are complex, but include the high emotional content attached to cancer and a lack of understanding among most health professionals and the general public that over-utilization of screening tests can actually cause real harm. The arguments against screening are generally framed in economic terms, whether a given test is "cost effective" in a given population. In actuality, the strongest argument against over-utilization of screening tests is not economic; it is that they cause more harm than good. The emotional content of discussions of cancer has contributed to two strong but rarely enunciated belief systems. The first is that more is better: if Pap smears every two years are good, then yearly Paps are better; if routine mammograms in 50 to 70 year olds reduces breast cancer deaths, then mammograms in 40 year olds and 80 year olds must reduce cancer deaths, no matter what the data show. The second belief system is that any cancer screening system is efficacious until proven otherwise. The typical approach to a potential therapy is that it should be shown in rigorous prospective controlled trials to be efficacious, to reduce morbidity and/or mortality compared to no treatment or another treatment. However, with screening tests that standard is often put on its head, and the skeptic is asked to prove the test is not efficacious. This can lead to fairly absurd practices in the community. For example, a recent publication for health professionals put out by the American Association of Retired People (AARP) contained a long article describing the under utilization of mammography in nursing home patients, and several programs were proposed to overcome this deficiency (43). There was no realization that comorbidity and shortened life expectancies often undermine the theoretical underpinnings of screening for cancer (44). A recent small study of primary care physicians found that some physicians felt that all nursing home residents should undergo routine yearly testing for occult blood in the stool as a screen for colon cancer; these physicians used no upper age cutoff and felt testing should proceed in the face of essentially any comorbidity (45).

Table 6.5 The Seven Danger Signals of Cancer: Go to your doctor to learn if your signal means cancer.

- unusual bleeding or discharge
- a lump or thickening in the breast or elsewhere
- a sore that does not heal
- change in bowel or bladder habit
- hoarseness or cough
- indigestion or difficulty in swallowing
- change in a wart or mole

These "danger signals" were developed by the American Cancer Society to increase public awareness of cancer in the 1940's and 1960's. Several would have very poor specificity in the elderly.

No screening test is benign. The test itself may be painful. False positive results lead to undue concern as well as to follow-up testing of increasing invasiveness and morbidity (46–49). Thus, the concept that "it may help and certainly does not hurt" cannot be applied to cancer screening tests, as it often seems to be. There must be convincing evidence that use of the test improves health outcomes. A more general recognition of this reality may serve to balance the forces that now advocate for an unquestioning acceptance of screening for cancer in the elderly.

Why are Old People at Risk for Delays in Diagnosis and Inappropriate Treatment?

When the medical care system is performing some task less than well, one can assume that the task is difficult. This is an obvious but important conclusion to draw from the evidence reviewed in the previous two sections of this chapter. It is very very difficult to recognize the symptoms of cancer in an 80 year old. As an example of the difficulties in recognizing cancer, let us consider the "seven danger signals of cancer," a list of cancer symptoms that were widely publicized by the American Cancer Society from the 1940's through the 1960's. The problem is, there is a high prevalence of some of these symptoms in the elderly without cancer. There is a background of symptomatology in the elderly population — sleep disturbance, aches and pains, constipation, lumps and bumps, cognitive changes. A cancer-specific symptom appearing against that background is not as noticeable as it would be in a younger population. It is also difficult to make treatment decisions. Both patient and physician-related factors influence the decision to be treated and the selection of a particular treatment after the diagnosis of cancer. Patient and physician decisions concerning treatment may be influenced by numerous age dependent factors (50). These have been mentioned previously, and are summarized in Table 6.6.

Table 6.6 Difficulties in treating cancer in the elderly.

- Few controlled trials containing sufficient numbers of elderly to allow for conclusions about efficacy.

- Decrease in bone marrow reserve with age leads to increase in complications from chemotherapy.

- Increased perioperative mortality from cancer surgery in the elderly.

- Limited normal life expectancy in very elderly can make information on five and ten year survivals in younger patients irrelevant.

- Older patients may have difficulty getting to multiple appointments for radiation or chemotherapy because they do not drive and they have difficulty using public transportation.

- Oral prescription cancer drugs (e.g. tamoxifen, methotrexate) are expensive and not covered by Medicare.

- Cognitive dysfunction can lead to errors in medication and non-compliance with physician appointments and instructions.

Adding to the difficulty is the fact that the primary treatment of most cancer is performed by general surgeons practicing in community hospitals. For example, most women with breast cancer are operated on in hospitals that perform fewer than 15 such cases yearly (12). The great majority of older cancer patients do not experience the multidisciplinary approach available in a typical cancer center.

Improving the Outcomes of Older Cancer Patients

Those interested in improving the lives of older cancer patients are in a bind. On the one hand, to impose standard protocols or practice guidelines on this highly heterogeneous population would be inappropriate. On the other hand, it does not seem enough to simply state that the clinicians must use good judgement in tailoring the therapeutic plan depending on the specific physiologic, psychological and social state of the individual elderly patient. How does one form good judgements in the absence of information?

The best approach available to the older person today is seek care at a cancer center with special programs for the elderly (51). Clearly, several of the difficulties in cancer treatment for the elderly, as outlined in Table 6.6, are most amenable to a multidisciplinary approach, with participation by social work and nursing, supplemented by ongoing case-management. Other difficulties in Table 6.6 are purely medical in nature, but presumably would also be dealt with best in a multidisciplinary facility with a sufficient volume of elderly patients to generate good clinical experience in making difficult decisions (51). Increased volume is associated with decreased complications and mortality for tech-

nically difficult procedures such as coronary angioplasty (52). One might expect a similar relationship between volume and quality for the cognitively difficult procedure of caring for the older cancer patient.

References

1. Goodwin JS, Hunt WC, Key CR, *et al*. Cancer treatment protocols. Who gets chosen? *Arch Intern Med* 1988; **148**: 2258–2262.
2. Holmes FF, Hearne E. Cancer stage-to-age relationship: Implications for cancer screening in the elderly. *J Am Geriatr Soc* 1981; **29**: 55.
3. Breslow L. Early case finding, treatment, and mortality from cervix and breast cancer. *Prevent Med* 1971; **1**: 141.
4. Goodwin JS, Samet JM, Key CR. Stage at diagnosis of cancer varies with the age of the patient. *J Am Geriatr Soc* 1986; **34**: 20–26.
5. Goodwin JS, Hunt C, Key C, Samet J. Relationship of marital status to stage at diagnosis, choice of treatment, and survival in individuals with cancer. *JAMA* 1987; **258**: 3125–3130.
6. Samet JM, Hunt WC, Goodwin JS. Determinants of stage and size of cancer in elderly New Mexicans: A population-based study. *Cancer* 1990; **66**: 1302–1307.
7. Moritz DJ, Satariano WA. Factors predicting stage of breast cancer at diagnosis in middle-aged and elderly women: the role of living arrangements. *J Clin Epidemiol* 1993; **46**: 443–454.
8. Richardson JL, Langholz B, Bernstein L, Burciaga C, Dailey K, Ross R. Stage and delay in breast cancer diagnosis by race, socioeconomic status, age and year. *Br J Cancer* 1992; **65**: 922–926.
9. Samet J, Key C, Hunt C, Key C, Goodwin JS. Choice of cancer therapy varies with the age of the patient. *JAMA* 1986; **255**: 3385–3390.
10. Goodwin JS, Hunt WC, Key CR, Samet JM. Changes in surgical treatments: The example of hysterectomy versus conization for cervical carcinoma in situ. *J Clin Epidemiol* 1990; **43**: 977–982.
11. Mor V, Guadagnoli E, Silliman RA, *et al*. Relationship between age at diagnosis and treatments received by cancer patients. *J Am Geriatr Soc* 1985; **33**: 585–589.
12. Nattinger A, Gottlieb M, Hoffman RG, Walker AD and Goodwin JS. Lack of increase in use of breast-conserving surgery from 1986 to 1990. *Medical Care* 1996; **34**: 479–489.
13. Yancik R, Ries LB, Yates JW. Breast cancer in aging women: a population-based study of contrasts in stage, surgery, and survival. *Cancer* 1989; **63**: 164–169.
14. Mann B, Samet J, Key C, Goodwin, JM and Goodwin JS. Changing treatment of breast cancer in New Mexico from 1969 through 1985, *JAMA* 1988; **259**: 3413–3417.
15. Allen C, Cox EB, Manton KG, *et al*. Breast cancer in the elderly. Current patterns of care. *J Am Geriatr Soc* 1986; **34**: 637–642.
16. Samet J, Hunt WC, Key C, Goodwin JS. Choice of cancer therapy varies with age of patient. *JAMA* 1986; **255**: 3385–3390.
17. Chu J, Diehr P, Feigl P, *et al*. The effect of age on the care of women with breast cancer in community hospitals. *J Gerontol* 1987; **42**: 185–190.
18. Greenfield S, Blanco D, Elashof RM, Ganz PA. Patterns of care related to age of breast cancer patients. *JAMA* 1987; **257**: 2700–2760.
19. Silliman RA, Guadagnoli E, Weitberg AB, *et al*. Age as a predictor of diagnostic and initial treatment intensity in newly diagnosed breast cancer patients. *J Gerontol* 1989; **44**: M46–50.
20. Bergman L, Dekker G, VanLeeuwen FE, *et al*. The effect of age on treatment choice and survival in elderly breast cancer patients. *Cancer* 1991; **67**: 2227–2234.
21. Satariano ER, Swanson GM, Moll PP. Nonclinical factors associated with surgery received for treatment of early-stage breast cancer. *Am J Public Health* 1992; **82**: 195-198.
22. Bergman L, Kluck HM, VanLeeuwen FE, Crommelin MA, Dekker G, Hart AA, Coebergh JW. The influence of age on treatment choice and survival of elderly breast cancer patients in south-eastern Netherlands. *Eur J Cancer* 1992; **28**: 1475–1480.
23. Goodwin JS, Hunt WC, Samet JM. Determinants of cancer therapy in elderly patients. *Cancer* 1993; **72**: 594–601.

24. Hand R, Sener S, Imperato J, Chmiel JS, Sylvester J, Fremgen A. Hospital variables associated with quality of care for cancer patients. *JAMA* 1991; **266**: 3429–3432.

25. Lee-Feldstein A, Anton-Culver H, Feldstein PJ. Treatment differences and other prognostic factors related to breast cancer survival. *JAMA* 1994; **271**; 1163–68.

26. Lazovich D, White E, Thomas D, *et al*. Underutilization of breast conserving surgery and radiation therapy among women with stage I or II breast cancer. *JAMA* 1991; **266**: 3433–3438.

27. Farrow DC, Hunt WC, Samet JM. Geographic variation in the treatment of localized breast cancer. *N Engl J Med* 1992; **326**: 1097–1101.

28. Goodwin JS. Geriatric ideology: The myth of the myth of senility. *J Am Geriatr Soc* 1991; **39**: 627–631.

29. Nattinger AB, Gottlieb MS, Veum J, Yahnke D and Goodwin JS. Geographic variation in the use of breast-conserving treatment for breast cancer. *N Engl J Med* 1992; **326**: 1102–1107.

30. Hand R, Sener S, Imperato J, *et al*. Hospital variables associated with quality of care for breast cancer patients. *JAMA* 1991; **266**: 3429–3432.

31. Samet JM, Key CR, Hunt WC, Goodwin JS. Survival of American Indian and Hispanic Cancer patients in New Mexico and Arizona, 1969–82. *J Nat Cancer Instit* 1987; **79**: 457–463.

32. Bain RP, Greenberg RS, Whitaker JP. Racial differences in survival of women with breast cancer. *J Chronic Dis* 1986; **39**: 631–642.

33. Eloy JW, Hill H, Chun VW, *et al*. Racial differences in survival from breast cancer. *JAMA* 1994; **272**: 947–954.

34. Goodwin JS, Hunt C, Key C, Samet JM. The effect of marital status on stage, treatment, and survival of cancer patients. *JAMA* 1987; **258**: 3125–3130.

35. Samet J, Goodwin JS. Patterns of cancer care for non-Hispanic whites, Hispanics, and American Indians in New Mexico. In *Cancer in the Elderly*, edited by R Yancik, J Yates. New York: Springer Publishing Company, 1989.

36. Cantharis DA, Pouleter CA, Sischy B, Paterson E, Sobel S, Rubin P, Dvoretsky P, Mishalak W, Doane KL. Treatment of breast cancer among elderly women with segmental mastectomy or segmental mastectomy plus postoperative radiotherapy. *Int J Rad Oncol Biol Phys* 1988; **15**: 263–270.

37. Clark RM, McCulloch PB, Levine MN. Randomized clinical trial to assess the effectiveness of breast irradiation following lumpectomy and axillary dissection for node-negative breast cancer. *J Natl Cancer Inst* 1992; **84**: 683–689.

38. Goodwin JS, Hunt WC, Samet JS. Determinants of survival in older cancer patients. *J Natl Cancer Instit* 1996; **88**: 1031–1038.

39. Roos NP, Black C, Roos LL, Tate RB, Carriere KC. A population-based approach to monitoring adverse outcomes of medical care. *Medical Care* 1995; **33**: 127–138.

40. Litwin MS, Hays RD, Fink A, Ganz P, Leake B, Leach G, Brook RH. Quality of life outcomes in men treated for localized prostate cancer. *JAMA* 1995; **273**: 129 135.

41. Potosky A, Miller BA, Albertsen PC, Kramer BS. The role of increasing detection in the rising incidence of prostate cancer. *JAMA* 1995; **273**: 548–552

42. Albertsen PC, Fryback DG, Storer BE, Kolon TF, Fine J. Long term survival among men with conservatively treated localized prostate cancer. *JAMA* 1995; **274**: 626–631.

43. Anon. Breast screening for frail and disabled older women — an overlooked population. *Perspectives in Health Promotion and Aging* 1995; **10**: 10–12.

44. Satariano WA, Ragland DR. The effect of comorbidity on 3-year survival of women with primary breast cancer. *Ann Internal Med* 1994; **120**: 104–110.

45. Klos SE, Drink P, Goodwin JS. The utilization of fecal occult blood testing in the institutionalized elderly. *J Am Geriatr Soc* 1991; **39**: 1169–1173.

46. Lieberman DA. Colon cancer screening, the dilemma of positive screening tests. *Arch Intern Med* 1990; **150**: 740.

47. Allison JE, Feldman R, Tekawa IS. Hemoccult screening in detecting colorectal neoplasm: Sensitivity, and predictive value. *Ann Inter Med* 1990; **112**: 328.

48. Skegg DCG. Cervical screening blues. *Lancet* 1995; **345**: 1451–1452.

49. Lang CA, Ransohoff DF. Fecal occult blood screening for colorectal cancer. *JAMA* 1994; **271**: 1011–1013.

50. Levy SM. The aging cancer patient: Behavioral research issues. In *Perspectives on Prevention and Treatment of Cancer in the Elderly*, edited by R Yancik. New York: Raven Press, 1983, pp. 83–96.

51. Schipper H, Dick J. Herodotus and the multi disciplinary clinic. *Lancet* 1995; **346**: 1312–1313.

52. Jollis JG, Peterson ED, DeLong ER, Mark DB, Collins SR, Muhlbaier LH, Pryor DB. The relation between the volume of coronary angioplasty procedures at hospitals treating Medicare beneficiaries and short term mortality. *N Engl J Med* 1994; **331**: 1625–29.

7. Cellular and Molecular Aging

Sangkyu Kim, James C. Jiang, Paul A. Kirchman, Ivica Rubelj,
Edward G. Helm and S. Michal Jazwinski

Introduction

A rational approach to the treatment of diseases of
the elderly, including geriatric oncology, requires a
firm knowledge of the aging process. A comprehensive understanding of the aging process, in turn, is
predicated on a multifaceted approach that encompasses the description of molecular, cellular, and systemic changes during the life span of the organism.
Such a description has been assembled over the past
few decades, but it is only recently that causal associations have been the subject of concerted experimental
attack. This change in emphasis has coincided with the
introduction of molecular and genetic tools to aging
research. Thus, we have before us the perspective of
ultimately achieving a grasp of "how" we age, with the
attendant benefits of being able to assess the age-associated predispositions to a variety of disease states.
This suggests that in the longer term we will be able
to intervene in the development of these diseases and,
perhaps, even in the aging process itself. We accept
here the view that aging is not a disease, although
it may predispose to disease. The question that is of
prime medical relevance in this context concerns the
nature of the predisposition.

Another important development of the past decade
in aging research is the realization of "why" we age.
This is important because it circumscribes the plausible
physiological parameters of the aging process. It is not
our purpose here to review the literature dealing with
the evolutionary biology of aging. However, it is con-
sequential to note that it is difficult to refute that we
age not because of a deliberate design or program, but
because organisms have not been "engineered" to be
immortal. Indeed, there appears to be a balance between life maintenance and the expenditure of energy
and effort into reproduction. The latter, in fact, guarantees that the species, unlike the individual, is immortal. Thus given a particular "genetic constitution",
there comes a time in life when we become more and
more vulnerable to the predations of our environment.
The focus then of modern aging research is on the
physiological functions that provide for maintenance
of the organism, its efficient marshaling of energy
resources, and significantly its capacity to resist environmental stresses and insults. With these considerations in mind, it is difficult to escape the conclusion
that there is no one aging process, but that aging is
composed of several component processes. This diversity plays itself out in many ways in genetically outbred
species such as the human, because these component
aging processes are superimposed on a broad array of
genetic backgrounds. The comparative biology of aging lends support to the views enunciated above. Different species age differently, showing a wide variety
of overlapping manifestations of aging. Some of these
manifestations are major aspects of aging in one species and minor aspects in others. The point is that
different species have evolved to optimize their reproductive strategies under environmental conditions that
typify the ecological circumstances they encounter.

The purpose of this chapter is to review the molecular and cellular aspects of aging. Human biology is the
focus, but relevant information from other species is
included when it illuminates certain points. Physiological aging at the organismal level is not at the center of
this discussion. However, it is the vantage from which
the treatment begins and to which it tends, if not overtly.
Molecular and cellular aging is a vast topic. It encompasses the gamut of biological processes in both mitotic
and post-mitotic cells. In order to provide a meaningful
exposition for the geriatric oncologist, a broad, but not
all-inclusive, picture is painted. In the interest of clarity, the organizing theme of the cell during aging of the
organism has been selected. We discuss how aging
affects the cell and the functional consequences this has
for the organism. We have limited the discussion in
ways to improve the clarity. We must therefore apolo-
gize to authors for not citing all the important work in
biological research on aging.

This chapter begins with a discussion of proliferative homeostasis. Most of the research in this area is
based on the cellular senescence paradigm developed
using normal human diploid fibroblasts in tissue culture. The molecular events associated with cellular
immortalization are discussed on this backdrop. The
aging of endothelial cells is singled out for further
analysis, because of the importance of vascularization
in oncogenesis. This section ends with a discussion of
wound healing from a somewhat more clinical perspective. Proliferative homeostasis in normal tissue is
well illustrated by the wound healing phenomenon.
Immunosenescence is targeted for discussion given
the significance of the immune system in the destruction of abnormal cells. The problem of programmed
cell death is of obvious importance for the function
of the immune system, and it is dealt with briefly here.
The responses of cells and tissues to a variety of stresses,
and the age-associated deficits in this function, are
then presented. This leads to the final section which
touches on the importance of endocrine factors during
aging.

Proliferative Homeostasis

Cellular Senescence

Senescent phenotype

In 1961 Hayflick and Moorehead (1) reported that serially cultured human diploid fibroblasts could divide *in vitro* only a finite number of times. Since then this phenomenon of limited replicative life span has been investigated extensively and established well in human and other mammalian fibroblast strains (reviewed in 2 and 3). In early-passage cultures, most of the cells multiply actively with shorter generation times. This mitotic period of rapid growth is gradually followed by a static post-mitotic period, during which individual cells' replicative capacity declines, and the cells display an increased generation time (4). The major factor that determines the replicative life span of cultured populations is not the chronological time but the number of population doublings (5, 6). The finite number of population doublings for a given fibroblast strain is reproducible with some fluctuation in the range (4, 6, 7). The limited replicative life span *in vitro* appears to parallel cellular senescence *in vivo*. The replicative potential of cultured fibroblasts is inversely correlated with the donor age; *e.g.*, the replicative capacity *in vitro* decreases with increasing donor age, and vice versa (8–10). Differences in the *in vitro* replicative life span among different species are well correlated with the differences in their organismal life span (11). Thus, as Hayflick suggested, the limited life span of fibroblasts *in vitro* can be regarded as "an expression of aging or senescence at the cellular level" (12).

The phenotype associated with cellular senescence is similar to that of terminally differentiated cells. It was found in cultured populations of human skin fibroblast cells that rapidly growing mitotic populations consisted of three major cell types and stationary post-mitotic populations consisted of four major cell types (13). The latter cell types include the final degenerating type. These seven morphological types were distinct from each other in polypeptide synthesis patterns. It appeared that each of these cell types represents a differentiation stage in a sequential cell differentiation lineage. Another observation supporting the idea that senescence resembles cell differentiation can be found in mouse embryonic stem cells. Unlike human fibroblast cells, undifferentiated mouse embryonic stem cells have an unlimited life span (14). Once differentiated, however, these cells give rise to mortal somatic cells, suggesting that differentiation may initiate senescence (15).

It should be noted that cellular senescence is not a process of "programmed cell death." Programmed cell death is an active physiological process involving *de novo* gene expression in which individual cells die at a specific time during development (reviewed in 16 and 17). The process of programmed cell death in most mammalian cells involves a stereotypic set of events, and it is termed apoptosis. Apoptosis involves membrane blebbing, chromatin condensation, and DNA fragmentation. The idea that cellular senescence is not

apoptosis is strongly supported by a recent finding that senescent human fibroblasts are resistant to induced apoptosis and this resistance is correlated with the abundance of the *bcl2* gene product (18). The *bcl2* gene product is known to inhibit apoptosis (19).

One of the prominent phenotypic changes shown by senescent cells is their heterogeneous cell size increase as they approach the end of their replicative life span (20–24). The human skin fibroblast cells undergoing the seven major morphological changes, discussed above, also became larger and larger in size before they degenerated (13). The cell size increase is accompanied by or probably results from increase in the cellular content of macromolecules such as protein, RNA, and lipids (25, 26). Another interesting phenotypic change of senescent cells is that late-passage cultures, which predominantly contain senescent cells, display a reduced harvest density and a decreased saturation density upon subcultivation (27–29). Apparently senescent cells cannot tolerate cell-to-cell contact resulting from a high density.

The senescence phenotype is dominant over the normal proliferation phenotype. Evidence supporting this conclusion comes from heterokaryon and cell hybrid studies in which nonproliferating senescent cells were fused to actively dividing young cells (30–33). In each case, initiation of DNA synthesis in the next cell cycle was inhibited in young cells. This inhibition was abolished by pretreatment of the senescent cells with the protein synthesis inhibitor, cycloheximide, indicating that one or more protein factors from the senescent cells are involved in the inhibition of DNA synthesis initiation (30, 31, 34). Indeed, one study showed that injection of poly(A$^+$) RNA from senescent cells to young cells resulted in inhibition of DNA synthesis in young cells (35).

Another feature of senescent human fibroblast cells is that they are delayed or arrested in the late G1 phase, at the G1/S boundary of the cell cycle. The incorporation rate of [^{3}H]thymidine into DNA exponentially decreases in a human diploid fibroblast population (36). A majority of senescent diploid fibroblasts have a 2C DNA content (37). The nuclear fluorescence pattern of senescent cells stained with quinacrine dihydrochloride indicates their primary block in late G1 (38). Flow cytometric comparison of young and old cells indicated that late-passage cultures accumulate senescent cells with G1 DNA content (39). Senescent cells were comparable to young cells in expression level of the cell cycle regulated genes whose expression peaks at the G1/S boundary (40, 41). All these observations demonstrate that senescent cells are blocked in the late G1 phase. Progressive decline in replicative capacity and increasing population doubling time in late passage cultures are primarily due to increase in the fraction of G1-arrested cells (26, 28, 42, 43). It is interesting to note that, since the macromolecular content of senescent cells arrested in G1 increases as if they were preparing for initiation of the S phase, it appears that cell cycle progression is uncoupled from cell growth in senescent cells (20, 25).

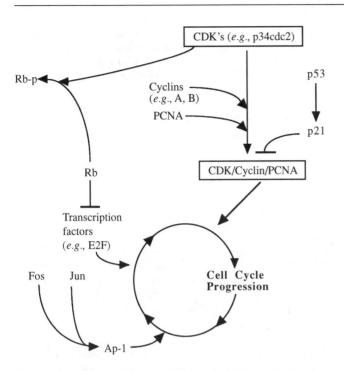

Figure 7.1 Key components in the regulation of cell cycle progression are the cyclin-dependent protein kinases (CDK's). CDK activation requires cyclins, and CDK/cyclin complexes are regulated by phosphorylation of both components. In addition to CDK's and cyclins, another protein factor, called PCNA (proliferating cell nuclear antigen), is required for DNA synthesis. p21, whose transcription is controlled by p53, is one of the CDK inhibitors (also called CDI's). p21 also inhibits PCNA. Thus, p53-dependent checkpoint control is mediated through p21. In normal human fibroblast cells, CDK's exist as quaternary complexes with a cyclin, PCNA, and p21. CDK's also regulate Rb function by phosphorylation. Unphosphorylated Rb inhibits cell cycle progression by binding to some transcription factors (E2F) necessary for cell cycle progression. c-fos together with c-jun form the transcription factor AP-1 which is necessary for transcription of AP-1 dependent genes.

In senescent human fibroblast cells, the number of receptors for growth factors and the receptor affinity for their ligands appear to be essentially intact (44, 45). Nevertheless, senescent cells are unresponsive to mitogen stimulation and show cell cycle arrest in G1. There is accumulating evidence indicating that the cell cycle arrest of senescent cells results from repression or inactivation of genes involved in cell cycle progression. These genes include *cdc2*, *cycA*, *cycB*, *Rb*, and *c-fos* (see Figure 7.1). In young fibroblast cells, the early induction of *c-fos* in the G1 phase is essential for continued cell proliferation (46–48). Fos forms a heterodimer with Jun and this Fos-Jun heterodimer binds to the AP-1 site as a transcription factor (48). In senescent cells, however, *c-fos* is repressed transcriptionally (49), resulting in a deficiency in the AP-1 activity (48). The retinoblastoma (*Rb*) tumor-suppressor gene is regarded as an anti-proliferative gene because it has the ability to suppress proliferation of tumor cells, and inactiva-

tion of the wild type gene leads to tumorigenesis (reviewed in 50; see below). The phosphorylation state of Rb oscillates in a cell-cycle dependent manner. Unphosphorylated Rb becomes phosphorylated at the G1/S boundary, indicating that phosphorylation may be necessary for entry into the S phase. Further evidence for the involvement of Rb in cell cycle progression comes from the finding that injection of purified unphosphorylated Rb protein blocked progress through the cell cycle in G1 (51). There is evidence that unphosphorylated Rb inhibits cell cycle progression by binding transcription factors necessary for cell cycle progression (reviewed in 50). One of the cellular targets of the Rb protein is E2F, which acts as a transcription factor for several cellular and viral genes (52, 53). Interestingly, senescent cells fail to phosphorylate the Rb gene product (54). Senescent cells also fail to express one of the cyclin-dependent protein kinase (cdk) genes, cdc2, and its cofactors cyclins A and B (55). p34cdc2 is a key component of maturation promoting factor (MPF), which is a complex of p34cdc2 and associated cyclins (reviewed in 56). The MPF activity is important in cell cycle progression from G1 to S and from G2 to M transitions (57, 58).

In summary, following a characteristic, limited number of population doublings, human diploid fibroblasts undergo cellular senescence. Cellular senescence is distinct from apoptosis. It resembles terminal differentiation. Human diploid fibroblast senescence is an important model for aging at the cellular level, although some controversy exists as to the nature of the *in vivo* processes that are modeled *in vitro*. Senescent human cells predominantly arrest in the late G1 phase, but remain viable and metabolically active. One major loss of function of senescent cells is the ability to synthesize DNA and divide, in part due to repressed expression of some components of the cell cycle machinery. However, the senescent state appears to have dominant features relative to the proliferative state.

Senescence and immortalization

Normally cultured human diploid fibroblasts cannot escape from cellular senescence; they degenerate gradually following cessation of proliferation (59–62). On the other hand, cultured rodent cells can easily escape from cellular senescence and achieve immortalization spontaneously (63–66). The frequency of immortalization varies greatly depending on animal species (65).

Interestingly, human diploid fibroblasts transformed with DNA tumor viruses such as simian virus 40 (SV40) and polyomavirus not only show extended replicative life span but also can give rise to immortal cell lines. Human fetal lung fibroblasts transformed with SV40 show typical, though not uniform among different cultures, transformation properties such as expression of T antigen, altered morphology, mitotic activity in confluent cultures (loss of contact inhibition), and ability to grow in low serum concentrations (67, 68). These SV40 transformed cells proliferate beyond the point at which normal uninfected cells undergo senescence. The extended life span of human diploid fibroblasts following SV40 transformation is about 20–40 population doublings longer than the life span of uninfected controls (69–71). At the end of the extended life span, the transformed cells enter a period of cellular deterioration, known as crisis. During crisis the number of cells in the population decreases, and usually most cultures are lost. On rare occasions, however, some cells survive crisis and these postcrisis cells can proliferate indefinitely (one to three in 10^7 transformed cells) (67, 68).

The SV40 large T antigen plays a key role in cellular transformation, life span expansion, and immortalization. This has been demonstrated by using mutant versions of the viral early region including temperature-sensitive mutants of T antigen (72–74). However, not much is known about the detailed molecular mechanisms of T antigen action in these processes. Since one of the major roles of T antigen is induction of cellular enzymes needed for viral and cellular DNA replication and the major functional loss of senescent cells is the inability to enter the S phase, the large T antigen can certainly play a key role in overcoming the DNA synthesis inhibitory activity of senescent cells (75). In fact, when T antigen expression was suppressed, both precrisis cells and postcrisis immortal cells arrested in the G1 phase (76). This implies that continued expression of T antigen is required for both the extended life span and the maintenance of immortality, and that the role of T antigen is to enable the cells to traverse the G1 cell cycle block and progress into the S phase. However, the T antigen's DNA synthesis induction alone cannot explain a number of cellular changes occurring in transformed cells. There is increasing evidence indicating that the large T antigen exerts its pleiotropic effect by interacting with other cellular proteins involved in cell proliferation and cell cycle control, such as the protein products of the p53 and retinoblastoma (Rb) genes (77, 78; see Figure 7.1 and below).

It is yet to be established why, unlike normal human diploid fibroblast cells, SV40-transformed cells enter crisis instead of senescence at the end of their extended life span, and what, if any, the relationship between crisis and senescence is. Stein (71) has shown that SV40-transformed precrisis cells, like normal senescent cells, show progressively decreasing ability to respond to mitogens in an age-dependent manner. Unlike normal senescent cells, however, SV40-transformed precrisis cells are refractory to the G1 cell cycle block in response to mitogen deprivation. This continued cell cycling of SV40 transformed cells results in life span extension and subsequent crisis rather than the normal G1 arrested senescent state (71). Wright et al. (76) proposed that cellular senescence and crisis are two distinct, independent events leading to immortalization.

Although the detailed molecular mechanisms of SV40-induced immortalization are unknown, several lines of evidence suggest that immortalization results from recessive mutational changes in the genes involved in cellular senescence. In a set of studies involving hybrids between normal human cells and immortal SV40-transformed cells, the majority of hybrids expressing the SV40 T antigen showed extremely limited division potential. This observation led to the conclusion that cellular senescence is dominant over immortality (79). Based on this finding, four distinct complementation groups were identified among various immortal human cell lines (80). This finding has also been successfully expanded to assignment of senescence-inducing genes to human chromosomes 1, 4, and 6 (81–83). Interestingly, in the immortality complementation study mentioned above, most immortal SV40-transformed cell lines examined were assigned to the same complementation group. This finding suggests that there is one major mutational pathway to immortalization of human cells by SV40. In fact, various mutational changes occur in the genome of the SV40-transformed cells just before or during crisis (67, 68, 74). Taken together, all these observations strongly suggest that immortality results from recessive mutational changes in the genes that are directly or indirectly involved in cell proliferation.

Telomeres and senescence

Telomere shortening. The termini of all linear eukaryotic chromosomes have unique structures called telomeres. Telomeres consist of characteristic repetitive DNA sequences, and form telosomes when associated with protein factors (reviewed in 84; see Figure 7.2). Telomeres are necessary for stable maintenance of linear chromosomes (reviewed in 85). For example, chromosomes without telomeres are unstable and bound for loss (86). A broken chromosome can fuse end to end with its sister chromatid to form a dicentric chromosome, which can lead to loss of genetic material during cell division (87, 88).

DNA replication is initiated from an RNA primer which is elongated only in a 5' to 3' direction by DNA polymerases. Therefore, successive rounds of replication would result in progressive loss of chromosomal ends without a special mechanism to compensate for the loss. Telomerase is an enzyme that adds new telomeric repeats *de novo* to chromosomal ends (89–92; see Figure 7.3). Its activity was first detected in *Tetrahymena* (93) and then in yeast (94), *Xenopus* (95), and immortalized human cells (96). Telomerase activity from cell extracts is inhibited *in vitro* by RNase or phenol treatment, suggesting that it is composed of RNA and protein components. The RNA or protein components of telomerase have been cloned and sequenced in ciliates such as *Tetrahymena* (97, 98), yeast (99), and human cells (100). The RNA moiety contains telomere-complementary sequence and serves as the template for addition of telomeric repeats. In bakers' yeast, *S. cerevisiae*, telomerase-mediated acquisition of new single-stranded telomeric repeats (5'-TG_{1-3}-3' or 5'-$C_{1-3}A$-3') occurs in the late S phase, probably immediately following the replication of terminal sequences (101, 102).

A number of studies in human cells suggest that telomeres may play a role in cellular senescence. The proposal is that the limited replicative life span of mammalian cells is due to the gradual loss of telomere sequences (103, 104). Specifically, it is hypothesized

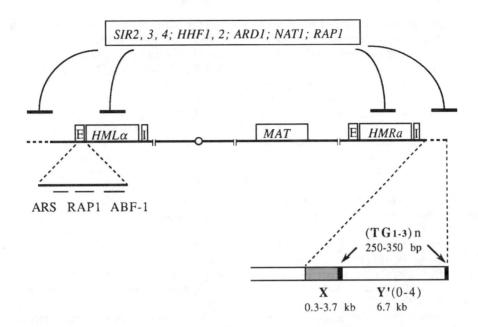

Figure 7.2 Chromosome III of the yeast *S. cerevisiae* is diagrammatically illustrated. The open circle on the line represents the centromere, and the dotted lines at both ends of the line represent telomeric regions. Note that although the silent copies of the *MAT* locus, *HML* and *HMR*, are located near the end of the left and right arm, respectively, they are not in the telomeric region. *HML* and *HMR* are each flanked by silencers denoted "E" and "I" and display a position effect. The E silencer is composed of smaller DNA binding sites including ARS, and Rap1 and Abf-1 binding sites. There are a number of gene products known to participate in *HM* silencing, as shown at the top of the figure. Also shown, at the bottom right, is an illustration of the yeast telomere structure. The tip of a chromosome ends in about 250–350 bp of $C_{1-3}A$ (or TG_{1-3}) repeats. Individual telomeres also contain zero to several copies of X and Y' subtelomeric sequences. The function of these subtelomeric sequences is largely unknown. There are 50–130 bp of the $C_{1-3}A$ repeats at the X-Y' junction. Most of the gene products involved in *HM* silencing also participate in telomeric silencing.

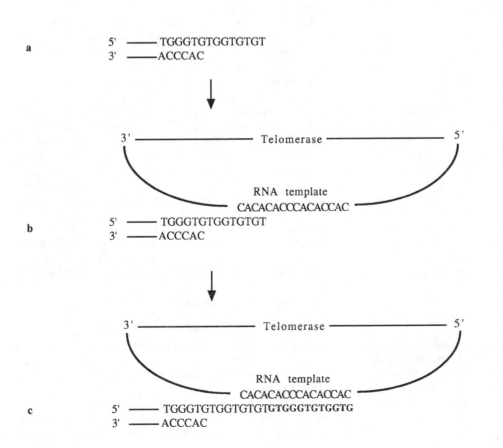

Figure 7.3 Role of telomeres and telomerase in preserving the information at chromosomal ends. a) The 3' end of eukaryotic linear chromosomes is incompletely replicated because DNA synthesis by DNA polymerases requires an RNA primer and proceeds only in the 5' to 3' direction. b) The RNA component of telomerase (shown in this diagram as an example is the *TLC1*-encoded template RNA in *S. cerevisiae*) anneals to the complementary single-stranded G-rich overhanging strand at the end of the chromosome. c) Telomeric DNA synthesis is elongated *de novo* according to the RNA template of telomerase. A second round of synthesis may be initiated by translocation of the newly-elongated strand to the 3' end of the template RNA.

that telomere shortening beyond a certain point will not only lead to chromosome instability but also to gradual erosion of essential genes, which will lead to cellular senescence and death.

There are three major observations that support the proposed role of telomere shortening in cellular senescence. First, both telomere length and replicative capacity appear to be dependant on the level of telomerease activity. Human somatic cells show low telomerase activity and progressively lose their telomeric sequences with replicative age (103–110). On the other hand, in germline cells, tumor cells, and immortal cells, telomerase activity is relatively abundant and there is no telomere shortening (108, 111–114). The RNA component level of human telomerase was also high in germline tissues and tumor cell lines but low in normal somatic cells and tissues (100). Second, there is a good correlation between the telomere length of initial fibroblast cultures and their replicative capacity. Human fibroblast strains with longer telomeres showed longer replicative life span than those with shorter telomeres (104). Third, when transfected with an antisense RNA of the RNA component gene of human telomerase, immortal HeLa cells, which express telomerase and maintain normal telomere length, lose telomeric DNA and replicative capacity (100). In S. cerevisiae, est1 mutant cells show telomere shortening, longer generation time, and gradual loss of viability (115). The tlc1 mutant, which is defective in the RNA component of yeast telomerase, displays a similar mutant phenotype (99). All these observations support the essential role of human telomerase in unlimited replicative life span.

However, the telomere shortening hypothesis in cellular senescence has some drawbacks. First of all, in human diploid fibroblasts, it is not easy to explain the dominance of senescence over immortality in cell-to-cell fusion experiments between senescent and immortalized cell lines. Second, it is unclear whether SV40-immortalized cells have acquired the ability to maintain normal telomere length. Moreover, if there is a causal link between telomere shortening and senescence, it is puzzling to observe the rapid cell cycle arrest (after one or two cell divisions) of SV40-immortalized human fibroblast cells upon deinduction of T antigen expression (76). Third, in some species, telomere length cannot be a biomarker for senescence. In Mus musculus, which is a short lived species, there is no perceptible decrease in telomere length over the life cycle and there is no difference in the length between somatic and germ line cells (116). S. cerevisiae and Paramecium tetraurelia show no detectable telomere shortening but undergo cellular senescence and cell death (117, 118).

Telomere position effect. Another interesting hypothesis for the role of telomeres in aging is that there might be essential genes involved in regulation of cellular senescence located near telomeres and these "senescence-regulatory genes" could be in turn regulated by telomere sequences (119). This hypothesis appears to be attractive in that it can explain those observations

that the telomere shortening hypothesis cannot explain.

In fact, a gene's function is affected by its chromosomal location. This phenomenon, chromosomal position effect, has been studied extensively in *Drosophila melanogaster* and in many other eukaryotes (reviewed in 120). In *Drosophila*, when a gene originally located in euchromatic regions is translocated to heterochromatic regions, its expression pattern is altered due to position effect (121). In a population of cells, the gene is expressed in some cells and not in others, resulting in a mosaic or variegated phenotype pattern. In *S. cerevisiae*, the two silent mating type loci, *HML* and *HMR*, also show a position effect. The mating type genes, which are expressed when located at the *MAT* locus, are transcriptionally silent when present at *HML* and *HMR* (see Figure 7.2). Other genes located adjacent to the *HML* and *HMR* loci are also subjected to transcriptional silencing (reviewed in 122). Thus the yeast *HM* loci resemble other eukaryotic heterochromatic regions.

Protein products of more than a dozen genes are known to participate in *HM* silencing. These include *SIR1*, *SIR2* (*MAR1*), *SIR3* (*MAR2,CMT*), *SIR4*, *ARD1*, *NAT1*, two genes encoding histone H4 (*HHF1* and *HHF2*), *RAP1*, *ORC2*, and *CDC7* (reviewed in 122). Mutations in any of these genes result in derepression of the normally silent mating genes at the *HM* loci. These gene products interact directly or indirectly with DNA sequences known as "silencers" flanking both *HML* and *HMR*. The *HM* silencers are composed of smaller functional units including *ARS*, and *RAP1* and *ABF-1* binding sites.

In addition to transcriptional silencing at the *HM* loci, there is also a position effect of telomeres on the transcription of nearby genes. When several genes were inserted individually near telomeres, there was a significant reduction in mRNA level compared with the mRNA level from the original locus (123). In a population of cells examined, some yeast cells expressed individual genes while others did not. A number of genes involved in the HM silencing are also involved in telomeric silencing; these include *SIR2*, *SIR3*, *SIR4*, *RAP1*, *HHF2*, *ARD1*, and *NAT1* (124–127). Other gene products, such as Sir1 are not recruited to telomeres, though *SIR1* has silencing potential at telomeres (128). It appears, therefore, that there are both common and specific protein factors involved in heterochromatization of individual chromosomal regions. The Rap1 protein plays a major structural role in telosome formation (129, 130). Loss of function mutations in *SIR2*, *SIR3*, and *SIR4* have been shown to relieve telomeric silencing and also result in telomere shortening (125, 126). Sir3, Sir4, and Rap1 proteins are found in the nuclear periphery of yeast spheroplasts and interact with one another, implying that they participate in telosome formation (125, 131). Especially the C-terminal domain of Rap1 is essential for telomeric silencing (132, 133).

Some properties of telomeric silencing give insight into the mechanism. The transcriptional repression is reversible; the expression pattern switches between on and off in approximately 15–20 generations (123, 126, 134). It was suggested that this reversible transcriptional repression may result from competition between the stable transcription complex and the normal telosome formation effective for transcriptional repression (123). In support of this suggestion, the major telosome structural protein, Rap1, is also involved in transcriptional regulation (reviewed in 135), and induced transcription of a telomere sequence has been shown to weaken transcriptional repression of a gene inserted near the telomere (136). The other interesting property of telomeric silencing is that silencing telomere domains spread continuously from the telomere such that the probability of a gene to be transcriptionally silenced decreases with increasing distance of the gene's promoter from the telomere (124). Based on this property, it could be imagined that the telosome structure might be cone-shaped, tapered toward the centromere.

Recently, an observation has been reported implying that there may exist senescence-regulating genes whose expression could be altered by position effect (137). The major finding is that a specific mutation in *SIR4* called *sir4-42*, which abolishes silencing in both *HM* loci and telomeres, extends yeast replicative life span. The *sir4-42* mutation is a deletion mutation of 121 amino acid residues from the C-terminal wild-type Sir4 protein, according to DNA sequencing analysis. Life span expansion by *sir4-42* requires *SIR2* and *SIR3*.

A complete deletion of the wild-type *SIR4* shortened life span, though its other mutant phenotypes are similar to those of *sir4-42*. Since both *sir4-42* and *sir4Δ* result in telomere shortening and alleviation of telomeric silencing, but only *sir4-42* extends life span, it follows that life span extension by *sir4-42* is not related to telomere length or telomeric silencing. It was envisioned that senescence-promoting genes are located not near telomeres nor *HM* loci but at other chromosomal regions with which the Sir proteins can interact. Thus, it was speculated that the Sir4-42-Sir2-Sir3 protein complex is able to bind to other chromosomal regions containing senescence-promoting genes and repress their expression, resulting in life span extension. The observation that overexpression of a C-terminal fragment extended life span in a wild-type strain-but not in a *sir4Δ* strain-seems to support the model.

Theoretically, senescence-regulating genes, if any, could be located anywhere in the genome. Nevertheless, the hypothesis of telomere position effect of senescence-regulating genes appears to be more attractive and amenable to further tests. The reason for this is that there is a significant link between telomere shortening and cellular senescence at least in human cells. Furthermore, telomere shortening and telomere position effect can influence each other. In other words, telomere shortening could be a consequence of altered telosome assembly and telomere position effect could change as a consequence of change in telomere length. One good example for this argument is that mutations in *SIR2*, *SIR3*, and *SIR4* result in both loss of silencing and telomere shortening. One important test for the telomere position effect hypothesis of cellular senescence is to see if there is any age-dependent change in expression level of genes located close to telomeres.

Genomic instability

Nuclear DNA. Genomic instability is another feature of senescent cells. As human diploid fibroblast cells reach the end of the replicative life span, the frequencies of cells with increased ploidy and with aberrant metaphase chromosomes increase progressively (39). The frequencies of aneuploid or multi-nucleated cells also increase over the life span (29, 138).

Not only does genomic instability lead to tumorigenesis (or carcinogenesis) but it accelerates its progression. Most cancer cells show aneuploidy and chromosomal abnormalities, and these gross chromosomal rearrangements become more severe as tumor development progresses. For example, chronic myeloid leukemia is characterized by the presence of the Philadelphia chromosome (139). As the disease eventually becomes more aggressive one or more chromosome abnormalities emerge (140). Moreover, rates of gene amplification are higher in tumor cells than in normal cells, though rates of point mutation are not significantly different (141, 142).

One of the key gene products involved in tumor suppression is p53. Cells homozygous for mutant p53 amplify the gene encoding *CAD* (a protein containing three functions: carbamoyl phosphate synthetase, aspartate transcarbamoylase, and dihydroorotase) at a high frequency, indicating that loss of p53 function leads to genomic instability (143, 144). In fact, mutations in p53 are the most common cause of genomic instability and cancers in humans (reviewed in 145; 146, 147). In the Li-Fraumeni syndrome (LFS), for example, patients are at a higher risk to develop various types of tumors with an early age of onset (148, 149). Patients with LFS have germline mutations in the p53 gene (150, 151). Another gene known to be involved in tumor suppression is the retinoblastoma (Rb) tumor-suppressor gene, which was initially found in the developing ocular lens (reviewed in 50; 51). Inactivation of both copies of Rb gives rise to eye tumors, as well as other tumor types. The human Ha-*ras* oncogene, when induced, also results in markedly increased genomic instability in p53-defective murine fibroblasts (152).

The ability of p53 to maintain genomic stability, thus suppressing tumorigenesis, comes from its involvement in checkpoint control. Especially, p53 is necessary for the G1-S checkpoint. A high level of expression of p53 inhibits cell cycle progression at the G1-S boundary (153–156) and p53 binds to and inhibits SV40 T antigen (156). When genomic DNA is damaged or cells are limited for nucleotide precursors of DNA synthesis, cell cycle progression is blocked or delayed in the G1 phase in wild-type cells. On the other hand, mutant cells defective in p53 function fail to arrest (143, 144, 157, 158).

The function of p53 appears to be pleiotropic because in addition to its checkpoint control, it is a transcription factor (reviewed in 159; 160) and also involved in regulation of apoptosis upon DNA damage (161–163). However, recent studies show that the cell cycle control by p53 is in part mediated through its transcriptional regulation of p21 (see Figure 7.1). p21 is an inhibitor of the cyclin-dependent kinases (CDKs) (164, 165). CDKs, in association with regulatory subunits called cyclins, regulate mammalian cell cycle progression (166). The activity of these multiple binary cyclin/CDK complexes is primarily controlled by activation (dephosphorylation) and inactivation (phosphorylation) of the CDK subunits (reviewed in 167). In addition to p21 in cyclin/CDK complexes, there is another protein factor called PCNA (proliferating-cell nuclear antigen). PCNA is involved in DNA synthesis during DNA repair (168) or during DNA replication (169–172). In normal human fibroblasts, each of the CDKs exists in quaternary complexes consisting of a cyclin, a CDK, PCNA, and p21 (164, 173). However, in many transformed fibroblasts (e.g., by SV40 T antigen), the quaternary complexes are found without PCNA and p21 (164). Moreover, dissociation of p21 from the CDK complexes is also found in p53-deficient cells from Li-Fraumeni patients that carry no known DNA tumor virus (164). Further studies showed that transcription of the p21 gene product is controlled by p53 (164, 174–177), and that p21 is an inhibitor of both the activities of cyclin/CDK complexes and PCNA-activated DNA replication (164, 165). p53-dependent cell cycle arrest upon DNA damage is mediated through p21 induction (178). Indeed, p21-/- mice are defective in the G1 checkpoint (179).

As mentioned above, the cell cycle block in G1 is one of the major features of senescent cells. Therefore, it will be very interesting to examine the function and expression profile of p53 and p21, among others, in cellular senescence. Evidence accumulated so far indicates that the mRNA levels of p53 and p21 increase with age in human fibroblasts and the cell cycle block in senescent cells is effected by p21 (180, 181). In fact, p21 was first cloned as a senescent cell-derived inhibitor (sdi1) of DNA synthesis in senescent human fibroblasts (181).

Mitochondrial DNA. In filamentous fungi, such as *Podospora anserina, Neurospora crassa,* and *Neurospora intermedia,* the mitochrondrial genome plays an important role in cellular senescence (for review, see 182). The primary cause of senescence in these obligate aerobes is respiratory failure due to increasing instability of the mitochondrial genome.

A number of studies with human cells indicate that mitochrondrial DNA instability also contributes to senescence. The primary cause of the mitochondrial dysfunction is abnormalities in mitochondrial DNA (183–186). In humans, the frequency of aberrant mtDNA with various deletions increases and the respiratory activity declines with age in muscle cells (187) and in liver cells (188). Flow cytometric analysis also indicates that mitochondria of human epidermal cells deteriorate in an age-dependent manner (189).

More attention has been drawn to the role of the F1 subunit of the F0F1–ATP synthetase, also called F1-ATPase (190). The F1-ATP synthetase, located in the inner mitochondrial membrane, is the main ATP producer (191). Activity of the F1-ATP synthetase has been shown to decrease during aging (192, 193). It is very likely that instability of the mitochondrial genome may lead to loss of key metabolic enzymes, and the loss of key metabolic enzymes may precipitate cellular aging. It will be interesting to know whether the same gene products (*e.g.*, p53) involved in maintaining nuclear genome stability are also involved in mitochondrial genome stability.

Aging of Endothelial Cells

The endothelium maintains functional integrity of the vascular wall. It occupies a histologically unique and strategic location forming the luminal surface of the entire cardiovascular and lymphatic systems, and as such it is of crucial importance in many normal functions and pathological conditions. As a major histological cell type (2kg/70kg human) (194), it contributes significantly to high morbidity and mortality rate (50%) in the elderly (195). Since age is associated with changes in the cardiovascular system, mainly in the structure and function of arteries, and diseases such as atherosclerosis and neoplasia, it is of particular interest to study changes that endothelial cells undergo during senescence.

Several normal human diploid cell types have been studied *in vitro*, and they all show a limited replicative lifespan (12, 196). Isolation and *in vitro* growth of endothelial cells has been achieved (194, 197), and their proliferative characteristics are well described (198). It has also been indicated that this *in vitro* system is suitable for investigating *in vivo* aging of vascular endothelial cells (199).

Cultures of human umbilical vein endothelial cells (HUVEC) achieve cellular senescence near 30 cumulative population doublings. Senescence is characterized by growth arrest and increase in cell size (199). Changes of many other properties of vascular endothelial cells have been observed during *in vitro* senescence, such as decrease in cell density (200), a change in the production of vasoactive factors (195), an increase in number of multinucleated cells, as well as a decrease in negative charge of the cell surface (201). This line of research also enabled isolation and examination of differentially expressed genes from selective cDNA libraries and monoclonal antibody pools. Dozens of such genes were identified and many of them have yet to be characterized (3). In addition, the expression of many known genes is altered during senescence of HUVEC (Table 7.1).

Alterations in gene expression and signal transduction

Prostacyclin (PGI$_2$) is an arachidonic acid metabolite, and it is mainly produced by endothelial cells and has various important functions. As the most potent inhibitor of platelet aggregation, it is responsible for maintenance of nonthrombogenicity (202). PGI$_2$ production by endothelial cells decreases during senescence *in vitro* (203) as well as *in vivo* (204). Because of its role as a

Table 7.1 Changes in gene expression during senescence of endothelial cells.

Gene	Change	Reference
Prostacyclin	decrease	199
Opioid peptide	increase	206
Endothelin	increase	209
IL 1-α	increase	213
Cyclooxygenase	increase	214
Plasminogen activator inhibitor 1	increase	214

potent antithrombic agent, the age-related reduction of prostacyclin production can lead to various vascular diseases such as myocardial infarction.

Opioid peptide production in the heart is known to modify cardiovascular function and can negatively modulate several characteristics of cardiac myocyte contraction. It was found that cardiac proenkephalin (PENK), methionine enkephalin (ME) and leucine enkephalin (LE) mRNA increase with advancing age in the rat (205). Another study showed that both enkephalins and the mRNA coding for them are increased in older versus younger rats (206). These age-related alterations in opioid production could contribute to increase in cardiovascular disease in the elderly.

Another important protein, endothelin-1 (ET-1), a 21 amino-acid peptide, is a very potent vasoconstrictor and was first identified in endothelial cell culture medium (207, 208). ET-1 is one of three endothelins identified, and the only one produced in endothelial cells. It is also produced in vascular smooth-muscle cells. Levels of ET-1 mRNA in aorta from young donors are undetectable, in contrast to the levels in older donors. ET-1 mRNA and peptide are also elevated in cultured endothelial cells (209). The age-related increase of ET-1 in endothelial cells may contribute to the higher level of ET-1 concentration in blood observed in the elderly (210), which then might cause high blood pressure by constricting capillaries and other blood vessels.

The interleukin-1 (IL-1) polypeptides are multifunctional cytokines that are involved in inflammatory responses and regulation of function in diverse cell types of the immune and vascular systems. The IL-1 gene family consists of IL-1α and IL-1β prototypes, and IL-1 receptor antagonist. IL-1α is an inhibitor of human endothelial cell growth (211) and also regulates human endothelial cell differentiation *in vitro*. It shows a nuclear localization in the cell (212). It has been demonstrated that senescent human endothelial cells express high steady state levels of IL-1α mRNA in comparison to populations of young endothelial cells (213). The level of the IL-1α polypeptide was also elevated in senescent cell populations relative to young populations. Subsequently, an age-related increase in the steady-state expression of the IL-1α response genes such as plasminogen activator inhibitor 1 (PAI-1) and cyclooxygenase

2 has been observed (214). Since transformed human endothelial cells did not contain detectable IL-1α mRNA, intracellular IL-1α may contribute to the formation of the senescent phenotype of HUVECs *in vitro* and possibly *in vivo*. Recently, it has been shown that treatment of human endothelial cells with an IL-1α antisense oligomer can delay onset of cellular senescence *in vitro* while removal of the IL-1α antisense oligomer resulted in the generation of the senescent phenotype and loss of proliferative potential (213). Since IL-1α can induce cyclooxygenase, a gene involved in prostaglandin production, it is directly involved in various physiological responses and pathological processes, such as inflammation (215). A more complete description of age-related changes in vascular responses can be found in Marin (195).

Proliferative response

Another important function of endothelial cells is their involvement in the proliferative response during some pathological processes such as inflammation, injury, and tumor growth. Probably the most studied role of endothelial cells in such processes is angiogenesis or neovascularisation.

Angiogenesis is the formation of new capillary blood vessels which happens through the process of sprouting from pre-existing vessels. It is very important during development, female reproductive function, and collateral blood vessel formation in ischemia and wound healing. It also occurs in pathological situations such as proliferative retinopathy, and it is necessary for the continued growth of solid tumors (216). After breakdown of the basement membrane of the parent vessel, endothelial cells migrate into the surrounding matrix. There, they form a capillary sprout, and as a result of further migration and endothelial cell proliferation, the sprout elongates proximal to the migrating front. A capillary loop is formed after fusion with another maturing sprout. Functional capillary is completed after reconstruction of basement membrane and formation of lumen (217). To execute such a complex series of events, endothelial cells have to alter their interactions with the surrounding extracellular matrix. This requires production of matrix degrading proteolytic enzymes. Also, the cells need to reach the angiogenic location by initiation of locomotion, which allows them to migrate towards the angiogenic stimulus, and they have to start proliferation which provides new cells for the newly-forming vessel.

Matrix degrading proteolytic enzymes play a central role in endothelial cell invasion. They are directly involved in overcoming the mechanical barriers imposed by the surrounding extracellular matrix. They also regulate cytokine activity by proteolytic activation of latent cytokines such as transforming growth factor-β (TGF-β) and by releasing matrix bound cytokines such as fibroblast growth factor-2 (FGF-2).

Plasminogen activator (PA)-plasmin is an extracellular proteolytic system involved in both matrix degradation and modulation of cytokine activity, and plasmin plays a central role in these processes. Plasmin is a protease which degrades laminin and proteoglycans, components of extracellular matrix. It also activates metalloprotease zymogens which degrade collagens and other glycoproteins. Although extracellular proteolytic activity is necessary for endothelial cell migration and invasion, it has to be localized and strictly controlled so that matrix integrity can be preserved. Thus, the role of protease inhibitors is of equal importance during angiogenesis. Precise protease-antiprotease equilibrium is necessary for angiogenesis (217). It has been demonstrated that angiogenesis associated with some processes, such as wound healing, is impaired in aged animals (218). Surprisingly, the proliferative capacity of wound derived capillary endothelial cells from aged rats was significantly higher than that from young animals after serum stimulation in spite of diminished vascular response in the aged (219).

Endothelial cells, through angiogenesis, contribute not only to wound healing and inflammation but also to solid tumor growth and metastasis (220). The growth of solid tumors depends on the establishment of a new vascular system (221), which occurs only in response to the secretion of a tumor angiogenesis factor (TAF) by the tumor cells. Without neovascularisation, solid tumors reach a maximum diameter of 1–2 mm, fail to invade tissue, and often die (222). The incidence of some cancers increases with age, but tumor growth is often slow and prolonged in the elderly (223). Since some poorly immunogenic tumors grow slowly in old hosts but very aggressively in young ones, it might be that impaired vascular response in the elderly underlies this effect. As it was recently reported, alteration of growth and morphology of some tumors with age is at least partially due to a reduced capacity to vascularize the tumors because of a lack of angiogenic factors (220).

Wound Healing

The features of proliferative homeostasis discussed above circumscribe medically-relevant processes such as wound healing. Knowledge of wound healing continues to play a critical role in all aspects of human life. The body's ability to repair itself is a complex process dependent on the extent of the injury, the environment in which the injury occurred and the competency of the body's defense mechanisms. A healthy, immunologically competent individual will handle a clean puncture wound differently than a contaminated puncture. Lacerations occurring in a sterile environment will be processed and handled differently than a laceration occurring in a dirty contaminated environment. Avulsion and crush injuries continue to present major challenges to patient and physician. Elderly, dehydrated, nutritionally depleted diabetic patients with an associated collagen-vascular disease and arterial occlusive disease will require hospitalization with hydration, appropriate antibiotics, surgical debridement and aggressive daily wound care for optimal treatment of significant wounds. Simple clean wounds in this setting demand prompt attention, appropriate treatment and close observation in an outpatient setting.

The past decade has witnessed major advances in the molecular biologic aspects of wound repair. Distinct but overlapping phases of wound repair are now well recognized. These processes unfold in a predictable and somewhat orderly fashion. Although these processes are intertwined and many occur simultaneously, they can be divided for the sake of discussion into inflammation, proliferation, connective tissue formation, and wound remodeling.

Inflammation

Injury to immunologically-competent living human tissue is always followed by inflammation. The inflammatory process defends the body against invading microorganisms and foreign substances and effects the removal of dead and dying tissue. The inflammatory process can be characterized as a complex interaction between vascular, cellular, and numerous extracellular components directed at minimizing the insult, destroying and removing cellular and unwanted debris, while preparing the injured area for repair to subsequently occur. The extent of the inflammatory process is directly related to the severity of trauma, the virulence of the microorganisms gaining access to devitalized tissue and the body's ability to defend itself.

The vascular response to injury is one of the most significant components of the inflammatory process. The initial response of injured blood vessels and that of surrounding small vessels is vasoconstriction in an attempt to limit intravascular volume losses. Vasoconstriction is mediated by local tissue factors, catecholamines and other vasoactive modulators such as thromboxane A2 which promotes vasoconstriction as well as platelet aggregation. Control of hemorrhage by vasoconstriction is short-lived and vasodilatation ensues within several minutes. Many vasoactive mediators such as nitric oxide, histamine, the kinins, the interleukins and the prostaglandins promote vasodilatation.

Disruption of blood vessels and lymphatics causes a leakage of intravascular fluid, lymph, blood components, and cells into the traumatized wound. Polymorphonuclear leukocytes are the predominant cell type during the early phase of inflammation. Mononuclear cells arrive later and become the predominant cell type during ongoing or chronic inflammatory processes. Exposure of disrupted blood vessels, subendothelial collagen and other elements stimulate the binding and aggregation of platelets (224–227).

Activated platelets release a number of inflammatory mediators which include: von Willebrand factor, fibronectin, serotonin, platelet derived growth factor, adenosine diphosphate (ADP), platelet activating factor, thromboxane A2 and 12-hydroxyeicosatetraenoic acid (228, 229). During the elaboration of these and other mediators, the platelet surface becomes "sticky" to facilitate surface bindings to other platelets. Exposed blood vessel wall components and activated platelets continue to attract and bind other platelets. ADP, platelet activating factor and thromboxane A2 play a significant role in augmenting platelet aggregation. Activation of clotting factors V and X stimulates the production of thrombin which regulates the formation of fibrin by catalyzing fibrinogen breakdown. It is the fibrin which forms a strand-like structure that fills or plugs the interstices between aggregating platelets. This aggregated platelet-fibrin structure traps red blood cells and clinically appears as a clot.

While the body is attempting to achieve hemostasis by vasoconstriction and clot formation in vascular and lymphatic vessels, many other inflammatory processes are occurring simultaneously. Pathogens are localized and the immediate area is walled off. Destruction and removal of invading microorganisms are conducted by polymorphonuclear leukocytes, macrophages, monocytes and lymphocytes. This process which includes phagocytosis is aided and augmented by complement, cytokines, antibody, coagulation factors, fibrinolytic factors, vitamins, minerals, electrolytes and the body's ability to localize or wall off the injured area. Clinically, the involved area appears warm, red and swollen and the patient complains of pain. These clear and established signs of inflammation are due to vasodilation, leakage of fluid into the extravascular space, toxins, and cell to cell interactions focused on destruction and removal of pathogens and devitalized tissue (228–231).

Cellular proliferation and epithelization

The inflammatory process prepares an appropriate environment in which cellular proliferation can occur. Inflammatory cells including macrophages and platelets communicate with fibroblasts to migrate into the wound area. Additional signals for cell proliferation are processed by the fibroblast. The intercellular signals which stimulate migration and initiate proliferation of the fibroblast are poorly understood. Biologic mediators produced by inflammatory cells appear to have both chemotactic and proliferative activity. Platelet derived growth factor (PDGF) and transforming growth factor-β play a significant role in this communication process (232–234).

The incoming fibroblasts migrate into a framework of fibrin and fibronectin and proliferate. Glycoprotein and other protein — carbohydrate substrates destined to become ground substances are produced at this time. The appearance of fibroblasts is accompanied by endothelial cells and capillary budding. This process of fibroblast and endothelial proliferation is inhibited by invading microorganisms and devitalized tissue. Simple wounds are usually ready for the proliferation phase by the third to the fifth post injury day. By this time the wound contains minimum inflammatory debris and is loaded with fibroblasts and capillaries. Clinically, this granulating tissue (fibroblasts and capillaries) appears as a pink, bumpy, friable surface which is a marked change from the scab or eschar noted during the inflammatory phase (235–238).

The proliferation phase also witnesses a great deal of activity at the surface where epithelial cells attempt to close the wound area. Two days after the injury, the basal cells of the epidermis detach themselves from the basement membrane and migrate toward the open, injured area. Proliferation and differentiation continue until the wound is closed. The leading edge of epithelial cells advances across the wound in a single layer. The zone following the advancing edge contains actively proliferating cells. This zone is followed by a zone of stratification where multiple layers of cells exist. This is the area of differentiation. Regeneration of epithelial appendages occurs in the stratified zone. Clinically, this zone appears as a prominent, slightly raised, smooth, edge-like area with a bluish hue that surrounds the entire granulating base. Various biologically active molecules that influence wound healing are listed in Table 7.2.

Contraction

Contraction is the process in which the overall dimensions of the wound decrease. Contraction is characterized by the outer boundary of the wound moving in a steady and progressive manner toward the center of the wound. Contraction begins approximately four days after injury. The mechanisms involved in the initiation, termination, or control of the contraction process are poorly understood. The ability of a contracting wound to achieve complete closure appears to be dependent on the mobility or stretchability of the skin and tissue surrounding the defect and the amount of skin available in a given area. Wound contraction plays an important role in closing defects of the skin in the neck region of elderly patients where redundant skin exists. Contraction also plays an important role in the healing of wounds that extend across joints where redundant skin is not available. The cosmetic effects will differ depending on the amount of excess and mobile skin. The elderly patient with a cervical wound should heal without a cosmetic or functional defect. Patients with wounds across a joint may end up with a functional deformity as wound contraction pulls and fixes the joint in a position of reduced tension (231).

Connective tissue formation and remodeling

The fibroblast becomes visible in the wound by the third post-injury day. The number of fibroblasts markedly increases over the next seven days. Following activation, the fibroblast becomes involved in synthesizing collagen. Osteoblasts and chrondrocytes perform a similar function in bone and cartilage. Collagen synthesis is an intracellular process which is associated with activation of cytoplasmic organelles. Ribosomes and the Golgi apparatus become prominent. The rough endoplasmic reticulum begins to form columns in parallel to facilitate the secretion of collagen macromolecules. The basic unit synthesized by the fibroblast is often called tropocollagen. Tropocollagen has a molecular weight of 300,000, a width of 15 Å and a length of 2,800 Å (231). Once the tropocollagen is secreted into the extracellular environment it is processed into collagen by crosslinks of various types and by polymerization. The collagen fibers form a triple helix that contains hydroxyproline and hydroxylysine. Arginine is essential for collagen synthesis. Arginine is suspected to perform its role not only in nitrogen metabolism in wound healing but also by augmenting

Table 7.2 Molecules of the wound environment that may influence epidermal wound closure.

Molecule	Molecular mass	Source	Action
Basic fibroblast growth factor	18 kDa	Keratinocytes, fibroblasts	Stimulates epidermal cell growth (246, 247)
Calcium	111 daltons (CaC1_2)	Milieux	Stimulates differentiation in high concentration, stimulates proliferation in low concentration (248)
Epidermal growth factor (EGF)	6 kDa (single chain)	Salivary gland	Stimulates epidermal cell proliferation (249–252)
Hypothalamic keratinocyte growth factor	~1.7 kDa	Hypothalamus	Stimulates epidermal cell growth (253)
Interleukin-1	31 kDa	Macrophages, epidermal cells	Stimulates epidermal growth and motility (254–255)
Platelet-derived growth factor (PDGF)	Dimer of 30–32 kDa and 14–18 kDa	Platelets, endothelium	Stimulates epidermal hyperplasia in combination with EGF (256)
Placental growth factor	Nondialyzable, heat sensitive	Placenta	Enhances keratinocyte growth (257)
Scatter factor	50 kDa	Fibroblasts	Stimulates epidermal cell motility (258)
Transforming growth factor-α	5.6 kDa	Transformed cells, placenta, embryonic tissue	Stimulates epidermal growth (259, 260)
Transforming growth factor-β	23–25 kDa (two subunits that may combine as TGF-β_1, TGF-β_2, or TGF-$\beta_{1,2}$)	Fibroblasts, platelets	All forms inhibit epidermal cell proliferation but stimulate motility (261–265)

the release of growth hormone, insulin, glucagon, prolactin and somatostatin (239, 240). Vitamin C appears to play a significant role in the secretion and crosslinking of collagen. This process also requires copper and zinc (232, 241, 242).

Post-injury days four through six witness a dramatic increase in collagen synthesis. This increase in collagen synthesis is associated with a rapid gain in the tensile strength of the wound. The collagen content of the wound continues to increase rapidly for an additional two weeks. Little increase in collagen deposition is noted after 45 days.

The terminal process of wound healing is the production of a scar. The disorderly orientation of the collagen fibers within the scar undergoes remodeling. Some of these fibers will be broken down and removed, while new collagen fibers will be deposited in an orderly arrangement along the lines of tension. The wound will remodel itself for up to two years. Any gain in tensile strength after the 15th to 20th day is primarily due to the remodeling of collagen.

Aging and wound repair

Little is known how aging affects the wound healing process. Human cells do age and ultimately die. Al-

though there appears to be a high correlation between patient age and a wide variety of disorders such as arteriosclerosis, nephrosclerosis, diabetes, anemia, and thromboembolic phenomena, there is no major biochemical difference in the hemostatic process between young and elderly patients (243). In one of the best animal studies, it was found that *in vitro* proliferative capacity and *in vivo* wound healing capacity of dermal fibroblasts was correlated. There was a continuous decline in both parameters with age in this longitudinal study. However, these changes were not progressive beyond the mean life span of the species, and they were not a predictor of the ultimate life span of any individual animal (244).

Clinically, it is difficult to evaluate aging and its effects on wound healing in the elderly patient. Elderly patients who seek medical attention have multiple associated disorders. It is rare to find an elderly patient who presents to an office or hospital with an open wound (lacerations, decubitus ulcers, significant trauma or ischemic injury) that is not impacted upon by various other pathologic processes. Elderly patients who present with malignancies or severe infections necessitating surgical intervention also have multiple associated disorders. One of the most common disorders

Table 7.3 Similarities between changes in immune and hematopoietic function caused by aging or protein energy malnutrition (Reproduced from ref. 245 with permission from Williams & Wilkins).

	Aging	Protein energy malnutrition
Cell-mediated immunity		
Delayed cutaneous hypersensitivity	decreased	decreased
T cell number	decreased	decreased
Percent T suppressor cells	increased	increased
Blastogenic response to mitogen	decreased	decreased
Humoral immunity		
B cell number	unchanged	unchanged
Antibody production	moderately decreased	moderately decreased
Erythropoiesis		
Hemoglobin	decreased	decreased
Marrow erythroid cells	decreased	decreased
CFU-E[1] number	decreased	decreased
BFU-E[2] number	normal	normal
Myelopoiesis		
Granulocyte number	reduced	reduced
Granulocytosis after endotoxin administration	decreased	decreased
CFU-C[3] number	decreased	decreased

[1] colony forming unit-erythroid

[2] burst forming unit-erythroid

[3] colony forming unit-culture

affecting the elderly are nutritional deficiencies. Nutritional deficiencies can exert profound effects on the wound healing process and actually mimic changes associated with aging. Similarities between changes in immunologic and hematopoietic function that occur with aging and those which occur with malnutrition can be seen in Table 7.3 (245). This suggests the possibility that malnutrition may contribute to some of the cellular changes that have been previously attributed to aging.

Clearly, our knowledge of exactly how aging affects the wound healing process is limited. Elderly patients appear to have a reduced cellular reserve capacity. The prolongation of the gain in tensile strength of the wound may be the result of a combination of factors including nutrition rather than simply an age related phenomenon. The wound healing process of the elderly may at times be slower due to a reduced cellular reserve capacity; however, the effectiveness remains intact.

Immunosenescence

Aging results in increased susceptibility to infectious diseases and increased incidence of cancer (266, 267). It is generally accepted that these increased incidences of disease are due to a decline with age in immune function (268). In humans, decline in cell mediated immunity is demonstrated in tests of delayed type hypersensitivity reactions to recall antigens (269). In animal model systems, cell mediated responses such as rejection of tumors and graft versus host reactions also decline with increasing age (270, 271). A deficit in humoral immunity with increasing age in humans is demonstrated by diminished antibody response to immunization and by the appearance of autoantibodies (266, 272). We will examine the molecular and cellular basis for this decline in immune function with age.

T Cells

In vitro models of T cell activity use polyclonal activators such as concanavalin A (ConA), phytohemagglutinin (PHA), or antibodies to the T cell receptor (TCR) to induce proliferation and lymphokine production. In these systems, the proliferative ability of T cells from mice and humans declines with increasing donor age (271, 273). Production of the lymphokine IL-2 by T cells from elderly humans and mice also declines relative to production by T cells from young donors (274). It appears that this lowered production of IL-2 is due to a decline, with age, in the proportion of T cells able to express this lymphokine (275). IL-2 provides a signal necessary to induce proliferation of T cells in

Table 7.4 T cell surface antigens.

Antigen (CD = Cluster of Differentiation)	Expression pattern
CD4	T helper subset
CD8	T cytotoxic subset
CD44^{hi}; CD44^{low}	High levels in memory T cells; low in naive
CD45RA	Naive T cells
CD45RO	Memory T cells

response to antigen or mitogen stimulation. In addition to the lowered ability of T cells from older mice and humans to express IL-2, there is also a decrease in the ability to express the high affinity receptor for IL-2 (IL-2R). The lowered expression of IL-2R in activated T cell cultures from old donors is also due to a decrease, with age, in the number of cells responding to stimulation (276). This apparent shift in proliferative ability is not due to changes in the ratio of helper (CD4) to cytotoxic (CD8) T cell subsets. Although age associated changes in the ratio of CD4 to CD8 cells can sometimes be found in individuals, they are not consistent enough or large enough to account for the large changes in proliferative capacity (268). These age related declines in proliferation and the production of components necessary for proliferation correlate with the loss of T cell mediated immunity with increasing age.

The most striking age related change in the anatomy of the immune system is involution of the thymus. The thymus reaches its maximum size prior to puberty and steadily declines in mass through adult life (277). Involution of the thymus results in decreased levels of serum thymic hormone activity and a loss of the thymic microenvironment necessary for differentiation of T lymphocyte precursors into mature T cells (278). A predictable result of thymic involution would be a decrease in the number of mature naive (as opposed to memory) T lymphocytes in peripheral blood. Identification of cell surface antigens (Table 7.4) that allow researchers to distinguish between naive and memory T cells made it possible to examine this prediction directly. Experimental evidence confirms that the number of naive T cells decreases dramatically in old age (279). However, thymic involution may not be the only mechanism responsible for the decrease in naive T cells. Globerson *et al.* (280) have shown that lymphopoietic precursors from the bone marrow of old mice are reduced in their capacity to colonize a lymphoid fetal thymus compared to precursors from young mice. Together, thymic involution and a reduced ability of T cell precursors to colonize the thymus account for a decline in the number of naive T cells entering the immune system.

While export of naive T cells from the thymus declines with age, conversion of naive T cells to memory

T cells due to stimulation by environmental antigens continues. This constant conversion to the longer-lived memory T cells and the slowed influx of naive T cells results in an increase in the ratio of memory to naive T cells in old age. In old mice, a 2.5-fold increase in the ratio of memory (CD44^{hi}) T cells to naive (CD44^{low}) T cells was found (281). This shift in the ratio of memory to naive T cells occurs in blood, spleen and lymph nodes, in both the CD8 and the CD4 T cell subsets. A decline in the ratio of naive CD4 cells to memory CD4 cells has also been detected in humans (279, 282).

This shift in the ratio of naive to memory T cells accounts for many of the age-related changes in T cell activation patterns. Not only have memory CD4 T cells been shown to proliferate less well than naive CD4 T cells, but high ratios of memory CD4 T cells can actually inhibit the proliferation of naive CD4 T cells (283). This inhibition may occur due to increased levels of IL-10, which is produced by memory T cells (284). Preliminary results have shown that antibodies to IL-10 block the inhibitory effects of memory CD4 T cells on the proliferative ability of naive CD4 T cells (283).

In addition to the possible production of inhibitory molecules, memory T cells may also proliferate less well due to defects in signal transduction. In response to stimulation with antigen- MHC complex or polyclonal mitogens, T cells rapidly activate one or more tyrosine kinases and phospholipase C (PLC). Phospholipase C cleaves phosphatidylinositol 4,5-bisphosphate (PIP$_2$) into 1,2-sn-diacylglycerol (DAG) and inositol 1,4,5-triphosphate (IP$_3$). IP$_3$ activates calcium channels, increasing the intracellular free calcium, while DAG activates the serine/threonine kinase, protein kinase C (PKC) (Figure 7.4) (285). Decreases in calcium mobilization and tyrosine phosphorylation of proteins, including PLC, have been found in T cells from old mice (286). Decreased phosphorylation of several proteins is also seen in memory T cells (287). Implication of a deficit in an early step of the signal transduction pathway is supported by the fact that T cells from old mice and humans can be stimulated to proliferate by bypassing early steps in signal transduction. Stimulation of old T cells with phorbol ester (which activates PKC) and calcium ionophore (which raises intracellular calcium) produces vigorous proliferation of T cells from young or old mice (288, 289).

The decrease in tyrosine phosphorylation may be due to an altered red-ox state of the cells. Thiol oxidation results in a phosphorylation pattern similar to the changes seen in T cells from old mice (290, 291). Increased oxidation in T cells from old mice or in the memory T-cell subtype might affect the interaction between CD4 and p56lck. Coupling is dependent on two cysteines in the amino terminus of p56^{lck} (292). Oxidation of the cysteines may affect the interaction of p56lck and its receptor on CD4 or CD8, resulting in a decrease of its activity and subsequently decreased phosphorylation of PLC (286). Interestingly, oxidation may be a means by which T cell activity is regulated. Response to mitogen stimulation is inhibited in T cells exposed to activated neutrophils due to H$_2$O$_2$ (293).

The accumulation of high proportions of memory T cells may be due to a defect in apoptosis. Apoptosis, or programed cell death, is a process by which cells activate a genetically regulated suicide program (294). Deletion of T cells by apoptosis is important in regulating autoreactive T cells in the thymus and in down regulating immune reactions (295, 296). Apoptosis can be induced by stimulation of Fas, a cell surface signaling molecule (297). T cells from old mice show decreased expression of Fas, and reduced Fas-induced apoptosis. Expression of transgenic Fas restores Fas-induced apoptosis in old mice. In addition, T cell proliferation and production of IL-2, IL-4 and IL-10 were comparable to levels from young mice (298). These results suggest that age-related T cell defects are a result of defective apoptosis.

B Cells

Age-related defects in B cell function are more difficult to interpret than defects in T cells. Whether the decline in humoral immune response is due to defects in B cells or the T helper cells on which they are dependent for development and activation is a difficult question to address. The data indicates that a combination of B and T cell defects may be responsible for age-related decline in humoral immunity.

The number of B cells secreting antibody is lower in old age as is the amount of antibody produced (potency) of individual cells (299). The reduction in the number of B cells secreting antibody may be due to the formation of fewer germinal centers (300). This low-ered frequency of germinal center formation with age may be due to reductions in costimulatory molecules on the surface of B cells. The molecules B7-1 and B7-2 are ligands for T helper surface molecules (301). B7-2 is not expressed in germinal centers of aged mice (302). Further, antibody to B7-2 inhibits germinal center formation in young mice (302). In addition to the lowered affinity of B cells for T cells in germinal centers, the T cells may be reduced in their ability to stimulate B cells. Many studies have shown that production of IL-4 , a lymphokine necessary for activation and proliferation of B cells, is increased with age. However, Li and Miller (303), have shown that under proliferative conditions IL-4 production by T cells from old donors is decreased 4-fold.

Pre B-lymphocytes that haven't expressed surface Ig do not show any age-specific defect, suggesting that diminished responsiveness of mature B cells may be due to defective T cell help (304). Aged mice also show an altered B cell repertoire. The frequency of B cells responsive to most antigenic determinants decreases, although the frequency of response to some determinants actually increases (305, 306). However, age-dependent decline in B cell frequencies is not found in athymic nude mice, indicating that these changes are due to T cell influences (307).

In addition to defective interactions with T cells, there is some evidence that signals from interaction with antigen may also show age-related impairment. Cross-linkage of surface Ig on B cells with antigen or antibody transmits a signal similar to the signal gen-

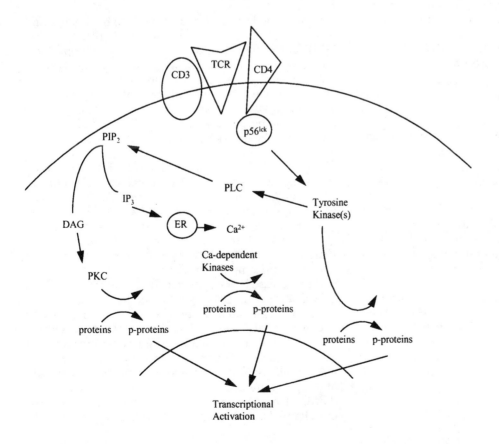

Figure 7.4 Signal transduction through the T cell receptor. Stimulation of the T cell receptor complex results in activation of tyrosine kinases and phospholipase C (PLC). Activated PLC cleaves phosphatidylinositol 4,5-bisphosphate (PIP$_2$) to diacylglycerol (DAG) and inositol 1,4,5-triphosphate (IP$_3$). DAG activates protein kinase C (PKC) while IP$_3$ stimulates the release of calcium, resulting in activation of Ca$^+$-dependent kinases. A similar pathway operates in cytotoxic T cells with CD8 in place of CD4.

erated during T cell activation (Figure 7.4). B cells from old donors did not proliferate as well in response to anti-IgM stimulation (308). Further characterization revealed that tyrosine phosphorylation and PKC activity are often lower in B cells from elderly subjects. However, some subjects with decreased PKC activity showed normal tyrosine phosphorylation (309).

Neutrophils and Macrophages

Few studies have been conducted on the age-related changes in immune cells other than B and T lymphocytes. The studies conducted have found defects in both neutrophils and macrophages. While the number of neutrophils from healthy elderly individuals is normal, there are defects found in their function. Neutrophils from elderly humans have been found to possess decreased plasma membrane viscosity, which may be responsible for reduced generation of oxygen free radicals (310). No defect in chemotaxis was found. While healthy elderly show normal numbers of neutrophils, there is a delayed recovery of neutrophil numbers after severe infection or chemotherapy. This slow recovery may be due to a defect in hematopoietic cells. Hematopoietic progenitors were found to be less responsive to G-CSF (granulocyte colony stimulating factor), which is necessary for development of neutrophils (311). While development of macrophages and antigen presentation by mature macrophages from aged mice seems unaffected, macrophages from old mice have been shown to produce less hydrogen peroxide and reactive nitrogen intermediates in response to stimulation (312, 313). However the production of INF-γ (interferon-γ) and the INF-γ receptor necessary to activate macrophages was not impaired. In a result similar to that seen in lymphocytes, early tyrosine phosphorylation events in response to INF-γ are severely reduced in macrophages from old mice (313).

Stress Responses

Stress has adverse effects on many physiological systems. The response to stress is an adaptation to the ever-changing environment, and it is found in all living organisms. The capacity to respond to stress usually declines with increasing age. Differential gene expression can be induced by a variety of acute stresses which include hypoxia, ischemia, reperfusion, hyperthermia, immobilization and oxidation. Signal transduction pathways translate stress signals into the expression of related genes, resulting in the synthesis of proteins which function in recovery or repair of injuries from stress.

Genes immediately induced by stresses are frequently proto-oncongenes that belong to several groups. The transcription of these genes occurs rapidly, transiently and precedes the other stress-induced genes. Some of them are transcription factors of these other induced genes. For example, the increase in AP-1 binding protein activity is mediated both by induction of two oncogenes, c-jun and c-fos, and post-translational modification of c-Jun. AP-1 can be activated by UV through the Ras pathway and is involved in protection against UV damage to cell components other than DNA (314). Hibi et al. (315) found that UV light can induce phosphorylation of serine 63 and threonine 73 in the activation domain of c-Jun. This occurs through the action of a serine/threonine protein kinase called JNK. Another investigation (316) showed that osmotic shock induced the phosphorylation of threonine and tyrosine of the mammalian protein kinase, JNK. The expression of the human Jnk gene in the yeast S. cerevisiae rescued a defect in growth on hyperosmotic media, which suggested that like the Hog 1 protein kinase in yeast, JNK may mediate osmosensing signal transduction in mammalian cells. Han et al. (317) found that endotoxin lipopolysaccharide or LPS induced the phosphorylation of tyrosine in mammalian protein kinase p38. Osmotic stress can also induce tyrosine phosphorylation in both mammalian p38 and yeast Hog1 which are members of mitogen-activated protein (MAP) kinase family. Beauchamp et al. (318) injected E. coli LPS into two to four-month-old Balb/c mice to determine whether acute systemic inflammation induces hepatic immediate-early gene expression. The analysis of extracts of total liver RNA, nuclear protein or total liver protein lysates showed that c-jun, jun-B, c-fos, zif 268 and nup475 mRNA in liver were induced by 5- to 13-fold. DNA binding activities of AP-1 and zif 268 increased, and the proteins, c-jun and jun-B, were detected in the AP-1 complex. This induction is similar to that following partial hepatectomy. These inducible transcription factors likely have important roles in the reprogramming of gene expression that leads to the acute-phase response.

C-myc is a transcription factor which has been found to control both cell proliferation and differentiation (319), and it is able to induce a variety of stress proteins including heat shock proteins (320). Heat shock genes are regulated at the transcriptional level by heat shock factor (HSF), which is quickly activated by heat shock or other stresses to form a trimer which is capable of binding the heat shock element (HSE) to induce transcription of heat shock genes. Before stress, HSF exists in the cell in the form of an inactive monomer.

Lowy et al. (321) reported that acute immobilization stress can increase the extracellular concentration of the endogenous excitatory amino acid (EAA), glutamate in the hippocampus. Further study (321) showed that during two periods of restraint a modest increase in glutamate level in the hippocampus of young rats (3–4 months) was observed. After the termination of the stress, hippocampal glutamate concentration continued to increase in the aged rat (22–24 months) reaching a level about 5-times higher than in the young rats, and it remained elevated for two hours. A similar pattern was observed in the medial prefrontal cortex with an augmented post-stress-induced glutamate response in the aged rats. Glutamate is a primary excitatory transmitter in the central nervous system, it binds to a variety of receptor families, it binds to the N-methyl-D-asparate (NMDA) receptor and opens relatively large membrane ion channels, and sodium and calcium flow directly into neurons. The enhanced post-stress glutamate response in aged rats may contribute to the increased sensitivity of aged rats to other neurotoxic insults.

Glucocorticoid secretion is also induced by stress. This induction appears to contribute to stress-induction of glutamate. Chronic administration of glucocorticoids can produce hippocampal damage in both rat and primate (322). Elevation of corticosterone, the major glucocorticoid in rats, also endangers hippocampal neurons after a variety of neurotoxic insults. The regulation of the hypothalamic — pituitary — adrenal (HPA) axis is influenced by the aging process. Aged rats have elevated basal corticosterone levels (323) and hypersecrete corticosterone after acute stress (324). Handling of neonatal rats prevents the later age-related increase in glucocorticoid secretion and attenuates the age-related loss of hippocampal neurons (325). It appears that the aging process makes the brain more susceptible to the deleterious effects of glucocorticoids and stress in general.

Heat Shock Response

The mechanism of induction of heat shock proteins has been intensively studied in the last decade, and it is the best characterized cellular response to stress. In all eukaryotes and prokaryotes a group of proteins known as heat shock proteins (HSPs) can be induced by hyperthermia. According to sequence homology and functional relatedness, the major HSPs can be grouped into four protein families: HSPs 90 (83–90 kDa), Hsps 70 (66–78 kDa), HSPs 60 (58–65 kDa) and small HSPs (15–30 kDa) (326). Despite the name, many other stresses (e.g. ethanol, amino acid analogs, heavy metals, free radicals, and a variety of acute stresses) induce HSPs. The number of HSPs varies from organism to organism and even among cell type in an organism, but HSP 70 family proteins are expressed in all organisms. Recent research shows Hsp 70 consists of three groups of proteins: Hsp 70 which is expressed in very low levels in unstressed cells and is dramatically induced by hyperthermia or other stresses, is the most conserved Hsp. Hsc 70 is expressed constitutively and only is slightly induced by heat. Finally, grp 78 is induced by glucose starvation but not by hyperthermia.

Hsp 70s are believed to function in a variety of cellular processes, including protein folding, translocation of proteins across membranes, and in stress responses (327). Hsp70 expression is regulated at the transcriptional level (328). In eukaryotic cells, a transcriptional factor known as heat shock factor (HSF) exists in the form of a monomer or dimer which has no DNA binding activity. When hyperthermia or other stresses are applied to cells, HSF is rapidly activated to assemble into a trimer which accumulates in the nucleus and binds to a specific DNA recognition sequence (5' nGAAnnTTCnnGAAn 3'), the heat shock element (HSE), located in the 5' flanking sequence of heat shock-response genes. It was also reported (329) that in yeast the Ras-cAMP pathway affected the induction of heat shock genes without changing the expression and biological activity of yeast HSF, but the exact mechanism of this regulation is unclear.

Hsp 70 appears to play a critical role in protecting cells against the adverse effects of hyperthermia. Evidence for this was provided by several studies. The thermotolerance of cells is altered if the expression of hsp 70 is enhanced or reduced. Microinjection of monoclonal antibody against hsp 70 rendered fibroblasts thermosensitive (330), and the inhibition of hsp 70 transcription had a similar effect (331). Cells transfected with vectors expressing hsp 70 protein had an increased thermotolerance (332). In the central nervous system pretreatment of animals with a submaximal thermal or ischemic stress, which induces HSP expression, confers protection from a subsequent ischemic insult (333). Interestingly, *in vitro* glutamate-neurotransmitter induced excitotoxicity is attenuated by the prior induction of the heat shock response.

One of the important adaptive abilities that is reduced in senescent organisms is the ability to respond to internal or external stress, such as the decline in hsp induction. From cultured cell to intact animal, more and more data on the alteration of hsp expression related to aging has accumulated (Table 7.5). The induction of hsp 70 mRNA and protein by heat shock was 40–50% lower in hepatocytes isolated from old rats than that from young rats. The age-related decrease arose from a decrease in the induction of HSF binding to the HSE (334). Fawcett et al. (335) showed that the activation of HSF by immobilization stress and adrenocorticotropic hormone decreased with age. Blake et al. (336) found that immobilization stress, known to activate the hypothalamic-pituitary-adrenal axis, induced the expression of hsp 70 mRNA selectively in the adrenal cortex of rats, and the magnitude of induction declined with increasing age. The induction decreased by 80% in 24-month-old rats compared to 2–4-month-old rats. Also, Udelsman et al. (337) found that the induction of restraint-induced hsp70 in the vasculature of the rat was dramatically reduced with age. In aging human IMR-90 diploid fibroblast cells, Liu et al. (338, 339) found a dramatic decrease in HSP induction at the protein, mRNA and transcriptional levels. In addition to the dramatic decline in HSP induction at the protein, mRNA and transcriptional levels in lymphocytes from old rats (Table 7.5), Pahlavani et al. (340) also found that the viability of the cells isolated from old rats was 30% lower than the viability of the cells isolated from young rats after the cell had been exposed to 45°C. It is possible that an age-related decline in the ability of cells to express heat shock protein might be a contributing factor in the increase in death from heat stroke observed in the elderly: the rate of heat stroke was more than 10-fold higher for persons of 65 years and older as compared to young persons (341).

The age-related decrease in the induction of hsp70 expression has been observed in many investigations (Table 7.5). This decrease is not due to the presence of a subpopulation of cells in the old animals that cannot respond to heat shock or to a shorter half life of hsp70 mRNA in old animals or old cells. The decrease occurs at the level of transcription. The decline in transcrip-

Table 7.5 The age-related decline of hps 70 induction in animal tissue and cultured cells (Adapted in part from ref. 381 with permission from Birkhauser Verlag).

Organism/tissue	Assay for hsp70	Age studied	Change with age	References
Animals				
Male Wistar rat/ lung, skin	protein mRNA	5 & 24 mo.	decrease 55% decrease	382
Male Wistar rat/ brain, lung, skin	mRNA	5–6 & 24–25 mo.	50–70% decrease	336
F344 rat/ adrenal aorta	protein protein	6 & 12 mo.	65% decrease 75% decrease	337
Male F344 rat/ hippocampus	mRNA	4 & 30 mo.	85% decrease	383
Male F344 rat/ hepatocytes	protein	5–7 & 25–27 mo.	37% decrease	384
Male F344 rat/ hepatocytes	protein mRNA transcription	4–6 & 26–28 mo.	45% decrease 40% decrease 31% decrease	334
Male F344 rat/ adrenal	transcription	5–6 & 24–25 mo.	90% decrease	335
Male F344 rat/ lymphocytes	protein mRNA transcription	4–6 & 24–26 mo.	37–75% decrease 52% decrease 56% decrease	340
Rhesus monkey/ lymphocytes	protein	5 & 21 yr.	75% decrease	340
Cultured cells (cellular senescence)				
Human/(IMR90) lung diploid fibroblasts	protein mRNA transcription	17–51 PDL[1]	65% decrease 80% decrease 50% decrease	339
Human/(IMR90) lung diploid firoblasts	mRNA	21 & 45 PDL	70% decrease	338
Human/(WI38) diploid fibroblasts	protein mRNA	50 & 90% of *in vitro* life span	decrease decrease	385
Human/T lymphocytes	protein mRNA	11 to 80% of *in vitro* life span	50% decrease 50% decrease	386

[1] population doubling level

tion of hsp70 with age was observed in several tissues, including: lung, skin, brain, and hippocampus from old rat, peripheral mononuclear cells and fibroblasts from human, and lung, skin and lymphocytes from both human and monkey. In cultured human fibroblasts and T-lymphocytes, the induction of hsp70 showed a decline at the end of the replicative life span. At both the organismal and cellular levels, the decline in induction of hsp70 with age is associated with a decreased activity of HSF. A plausible explanation for the decline in HSF activity is the accumulation of defective HSF in old cells. Defective HSF arises from conformational changes, the conformational changes in protein in old organisms occurs through post-synthetic modification, e.g. protein oxidation, amino acid racemization, deamination, glycation, and conformational drift (342, 343).

Oxidative Stress Response

At present, the most widely tested damage theory of aging is the free radical theory which was first proposed by Harman (344). Oxidative stress exists in all living organisms. Reactive oxygen species (ROS) are products of normal metabolism or radiation. They include superoxide radical, hydrogen peroxide, hydroxyl radical and singlet oxygen. They damage virtually all cellular constituents. The accumulation of irreversible oxidative damage, according to theory, not only causes aging, but also degenerative disorders, including cancer, atherosclerosis, cataracts and neurodegeneration. Although cells possess an elaborate network of antioxidative defenses, they are not totally effective. A small fraction of pro-oxidants escapes elimination and inflicts molecular damage (345). The level of oxidative stress seems to depend fundamentally on the intracellular preponderance of pro-oxidants over antioxidants. When human WI38 fibroblast cells were cultured under mild hyperoxia (40% oxygen) for one or two population doublings, their proliferation was blocked irreversibly. They were similar to senescent cells in general morphology and lipofuscin accumulation. The rate of telomere shortening, was much higher for cells cultured under hyperoxia (500 bp per population doubling) than that under normoxia (90 bp per population doubling) (346). This observation argues strongly against the telomere hypothesis of aging in its simplest form.

Ames et al. (347) estimated the number of oxidative hits to DNA per cell per day is about 100,000 in rats and about 10,000 in human. Such serious damage is repaired by a series of glycosylases, which are specific for a particular oxidized base, as well as by nonspecific excision repair enzymes. The DNA lesions are removed from DNA effectively, but not all of them. Oxidized DNA lesions accumulate with age. In a two-year-old rat, the number of DNA lesions could reach two million per cell which is about twice that in a young rat. The accumulation of DNA lesions with age leads to the accumulation of DNA mutations. The somatic mutation frequency in human lymphocytes is about nine times greater in elderly than in neonates. Two of the important DNA lesions, 8-hydroxyguanine and formamido-pyrimidine, are formed by hydroxyl or superoxide radical attack. 8-hydroxyguanine is highly mutagenic, since it base pairs with adenine instead of cytosine. Its content is often used as a measurement for the oxidative damage in DNA. Chen et al. (348) measured the oxidative DNA damage in cultured human diploid fibroblast cells. Senescent IMR90 cells excise from DNA four times more 8-hydroxyguanine per day than do early passage young cells. The steady-state level of 8-hydroxy-2'-deoxyguanosine in DNA is about 35% higher in senescent cells than in young cells. In contrast, the contents of protein carbonyls did not show a difference between senescent and young cells. Also, they found that when cells were cultured under 3% oxygen concentration, they achieved 50% more population doublings during their life span than those cultured under 20% oxygen concentration. An antioxidant α-phenyl-t-butyl nitrone, stimulated cell growth at late stages of the replicative life span. This antioxidant delayed senescence and rejuvenated near senescent cells in a dose-dependent manner (348). Oxidized nucleotides can be removed by DNA glycosylase, AP endonuclease and the excision repair system, and then excreted in the urine. Poly ADP ribosyltransferase is involved in DNA repair. Its activity was found to decline with age (349). This finding supports the hypothesis that the capacity for DNA repair declines with age.

Recently, the study of oxidative damage in DNA and its relationship to aging has focused on mitochondrial DNA (mtDNA). Mitochondria consume 90% of oxygen intake (respiration), and they are the most important source of intracellular reactive oxygen species. About 1–2% of the total oxygen consumed by mitochondria is converted to superoxide and hydrogen peroxide. These are converted by enzymatic and nonenzymatic antioxidants. The cell defends itself against the high rate of damage by a constant turnover of mitochondria and removal of damaged mitochondria which produce increased oxidants. Apparently, mtDNA is subject to much more severe oxidative damage than nuclear DNA (nDNA). mt DNA can be fragmented by ROS. The insertion of mtDNA fragments into the nucleus is continuously occurring, and it has been estimated that between 10–130 copies of various mtDNA sequence are in the human genome (350). Richter (351) suggested that mtDNA fragments escape from mitochondria and accumulate in a time-dependent manner in nDNA, which would progressively change the nuclear information content and therefore cause aging. Accumulation of chronic injury to mt DNA caused by free radicals generated in mitochondria results in respiratory-defective cells which limits the life span of individuals. This is especially the case in mtDNA of human heart (352).

The level of mt DNA modification in old organisms has been investigated. The content of 8-hydroxyguanine, the most widely used measurement of mtDNA modification, in liver of three-month-old rat is about 16-times more abundant in mtDNA than in nDNA (351). The 8-hydroxy-deoxyguanine in mtDNA is 3-times higher in 24-month-old rat than that in four-month-old rat, and it is twice as that of nDNA in old rat (347). Hayakawa *et al.* (353) reported an age-related accumulation of 8-hydroxy-deoxyguanine in mtDNA of human diaphragmatic and heart muscle, and mtDNA deletion was also found highly correlated with the 8-hydroxy-deoxyguanine. Corral-Debrinski *et al.* (354) found an increase in mtDNA modification in human brain with advancing age. 8-hydroxy-deoxyguanine content increased markedly with age in three regions of human cerebral cortex and cerebellum. It increased progressively with age from 42 to 97 in both mtDNA and nDNA, with the rate of increase being much greater in mtDNA. A 10-fold increase was observed in mtDNA as compared to nDNA in the entire age range, and a 15-fold increase was observed in subjects over 70 years. The increase of 8-hydroxy-deoxyguanine was also observed in nDNA in human liver, kidney and intestine (355). The first clear experimental evidence for a causal relationship between ROS production in mitochondria and mtDNA modification was provided by Adachi *et al.* (356). They reported that doxorubicin treatment of mice leads to a dose- and time-dependent formation of deletions in cardiac mtDNA. Doxorubicin stimulated ROS production in mitochondria and when used with ubiquinol-10 (an antioxidant), the extent of mtDNA modification was dramatically reduced (357).

More than a dozen diseases are found to be associated with mtDNA modifications at certain locations (358). Some of them are expressed in an age-related manner, such as Alzheimer's disease, Parkinson's disease, type II diabetes, deafness, and blindness. If the mutation occurred in a germ cell, it is maternally inherited, but time of expression depends on the extent of deleterious effects of this mutation. Persons who inherit mildly deleterious mtDNA mutations manifest late-onset degenerative diseases; those who inherit moderately severe mutations have adult-onset diseases; and persons who inherit severe mutations get childhood diseases. However, mtDNA mutations accumulate with age in somatic cells. Somatic mutations accumulate in post-mitotic tissues and exacerbate the oxidative phosphorylation defects that are inherited through the germ line (359). The characteristics of cells from patients with some diseases support the involvement of oxidative DNA lesions in human aging. In Cockayne syndrome (CS), cells exhibit a dramatic impairment of DNA repair. Cultured skin fibroblasts from young CS patients may exhibit accelerated replicative decline. Somatic cells from Werner's syndrome patients are prone to develop intragenic deletions (360) and multiple chromosome mutations (361). In addition, their cultured cells and those from Hutchinson-Gilford syndrome exhibit accelerated rate of accumulation of protein carbonyls (362).

Endogenous oxidants also damage protein and lipid, which leads to formation of protein carbonyls, glycoxidation and advanced glycosylation-end-products (AGEs). All amino acid residues of a protein are subject to attack by hydroxyl radicals which results in protein carbonyls. Tyrosine, phenylalanine, histidine, methionine, and cysteine residues are the preferred targets (363). Hydroxyl radicals are reactive oxygen species formed by ionizing radiation or the reaction of Fe (II) with H_2O_2 produced in metal catalyzed oxidation (MCO). ROS formed in MCO is not released into surrounding media, but preferentially reacts with functional groups of amino acid residues at the metal binding site.

Carbonyl derivatives of proteins can also form by interaction of lysine, cysteine, and histidine residues of protein with 4-hydroxy-2-nonenal (HNE), which is a product of peroxidation of polyunsaturated fatty acid, or interaction of another lipid peroxidation product, malondialdehyde, with lysine residues of protein (364). Collected evidence for a relationship between protein oxidation and protein damage is as follows: Many oxidized proteins are more susceptible than their native counterparts to degradation by most proteases, and especially by the 19S-multicatalytic cytosolic proteases (365). Nearly all animal tissues contain a neutral alkaline protease (the multicatalytic proteinase) that degrades oxidized enzymes but has no ability to degrade their unoxidized form (366, 367). Exposure of a cell to an oxygen radical-generating system or H_2O_2 greatly stimulates the degradation of endogenous protein in liver, red blood cell and heart mitochondria (368). The exposure of pure enzymes or protein to oxygen free radicals *in vitro* increases their susceptibility to degradation by adenosine 5'-triphosphate-independent proteases in extracts of *E. coli*, liver, red blood cell and heart mitochondria (363, 369). Reaction of protein with carbohydrates under oxidative conditions leads to cumulative irreversible chemical modification of proteins including formation of brown and fluorescent pigment and cross-links in protein which are termed glycoxidation proteins (GOPs). They are formed by sequential glycation and oxidation reactions. Only limited number of GOPs have been identified: N-ε (carboxymethyl) lysine (CML) and N-ε (carboxymethyl)-hydroxy lysine and the fluorescent arginine-lysine cross-link, pentosidine (370). GOPs accumulate linearly with age in extracellular protein, but the glycoxidation rate is not inversely related to the life span of the species.

Another group of products formed on prolonged incubation of sugar with protein are termed AGEs. The formation of AGEs from glucose is catalyzed by auto-oxidative cleavage of glucose. AGEs can be detected immunologically. Antibody formed against proteins browned by reaction with glucose *in vitro* detect an age-dependent increase in AGEs in human lens and erythrocyte proteins. The role of AGEs in aging, like that of GOPs, is uncertain. However they both may contribute to the pool of intracellular protein carbonyls and to the formation of lipofuscin pigments.

Lipoxidation products (LOPs) are formed by reaction of protein with products of lipid peroxidation. Reactive intermedials, such as HNE, are formed on oxidation of polyunsaturated lipid in membranes and lipoproteins, and they produce chemical modification and cross-links in proteins. There is no evidence for the accumulation of LOPs with age. Post-translational modifications of protein by LOPs and GOPs may also contribute to the pool of protein carbonyls in tissue. Therefore protein carbonyls may be formed not only by oxidation of amino acid, but also by adduction of oxidized carbohydrates and lipids to protein. In addition to modification of protein by oxygen radicals and oxidized sugar and lipid, there is peroxynitrite-mediated nitration of tyrosyl residues in protein. Nitration of a specific tyrosine residue in Cu-Zn superoxide dismutase has been reported (371). Nitration of tyrosine residues which are normally substrates for a protein kinase, prevents this enzyme from acting. This would leave the protein in a permanent "on" or "off" condition. It has been shown that membranes undergo substantial age-related lipid peroxidation, which can result in significant changes in fatty acid composition and in the membrane fluidity. The ratio of unsaturated/saturated fatty acid tends to decrease with age (372), and the membrane fluidity shows age-related loss (373). Lipid peroxidation of the membrane phospholipids is mainly responsible for the loss.

If the widely accepted hypothesis that more ROS are produced in old organisms and the capacity of these organism's antioxidation systems declines is true, oxidative damage may play an important role within aging organisms in the pathogenesis of major age-related diseases. An experiment underscoring the role of oxidative damage (374) showed that overexpression of the antioxidative genes for both superoxide dismutase and catalase in transgenic *D. melanogaster* increased the life span by one-third.

The increase in oxidative damage with age could be due to at least three factors: (1) the rate of oxidant generation increases with age, (2) antioxidative defenses decline during aging, (3) repair ability declines with age. Studies in houseflies (375, 376) reveal supporting data. They found susceptibility of tissues to undergo damage in response to exogenous oxidative stress increases with age. After various doses of x-ray radiation the concentration of carbonyl protein is significantly higher in the homogenates from 14-day-old houseflies than that from 5-day-old houseflies. The concentration of the molecular products of free radical reaction increased in houseflies with age. The comparison of carbonyl protein concentration in homogenates from aged male houseflies showed an increase with age from 5 days to 16 days. The concentration of carbonyl protein and the rate of mitochondrial H_2O_2 generation in 16-day-old houseflies is twice that of 5-day-old. Consistent with the above data, the O^{2-} generation by submitochondrial particles from liver, heart, and brain in 18-month-old rat is significantly higher than that in 3-month-old rat (377). Similarly, in cultured human fibroblasts the protein carbonyl content increases exponentially as a function of the age of the fibroblast donor (362). The same is true for human brain (378), human eye lens cortex (379), and rat heptocytes (380). Based on reasonable assumptions, it is estimated that oxidized protein in an old animal may represent 30–50% of the total cellular protein (343, 380).

This is consistent with the finding that in animals the catalytic activity of many enzymes is only 25–50% as high as that in young animals.

Longevity-determining Genes and Stress Responses

Stress responses, which encompass induced responses to heat, heavy metals and other toxic agents, oxidants, ultraviolet light (UV), and osmotic extremes, are physiological processes. Some of these can be rather complex, such as the inflammatory and acute phase response. The molecular mechanisms underlying these stress responses is the collection of cellular events known as signal transduction. Aging is frequently defined as a progressive decline in the ability to withstand environmental stress. This ability to respond to stress involves an interplay between the organism and the environment. Cellular signal transduction processes provide, par excellence, the interface between the cell and its milieu. It might, therefore, be expected that genes that determine longevity may be important in the signal transduction processes that govern the response to stress. This expectation has been richly fulfilled recently, in the genetic analyses of aging in yeasts, roundworms, and fruit flies.

Several longevity-assurance genes have been described in baker's yeast, *S. cerevisiae*. One of these is *RAS2* (387). In yeast, *RAS2* stimulates adenyl cyclase, much in the same way as the heterotrimeric G-proteins of higher organisms do (388). However, the extension of life span that this gene specifies involves some other pathway. This latter pathway may constitute a MAP kinase pathway, more akin to the function of c-*ras* in higher eukaryotes. *RAS1* has an effect opposite to that of *RAS2* in yeast longevity (387). This may not be surprising given the structural differences between the two, as well as the differences in expression between them (388).

RAS2, unlike *RAS1*, is essential for yeasts to mount a response to UV (314). This resistance to UV does not involve repair of damage to DNA. Rather, it appears that damage to lipids and proteins may be key. In this way, *RAS2* functions much like mammalian c-*ras*, which activates a protein kinase cascade that has as its final component JNK (314). The resistance of yeasts to UV during the life span shows a bimodal profile (389). UV resistance increases with age, peaks in mid-life, and then declines. The *RAS2* expression pattern during the life span corresponds closely to this UV resistance profile. This raises the possibility that one of the factors that determines yeast longevity is their capacity to withstand UV stress.

Another yeast gene that determines longevity is *LAG1* (390). This is a 'gene of youth' because it is preferentially expressed in young yeasts. The role of *LAG1* in yeast aging is complex. It appears to function as a homeostatic switch that sets both upper and lower limits to longevity. *LAG1* and *RAS2* do not interact genetically (Kirchman and Jazwinski, unpublished). Thus, the Ras2 and Lag1 proteins reside in separate signal transduction pathways.

The mutational analysis of aging in the roundworm *Caenorhabditis elegans* has ferreted out the involvement of several genes that determine longevity. The first such gene identified was *age-1* (391). *age-1* mutants are more resistant than wild-type to oxidative stress. This was demonstrated in experiments using paraquat, an oxygen free radical generator, and hydrogen peroxide (392, 393). Furthermore, *age-1⁻* mutant worms possess higher levels of superoxide dismutase and catalase activities starting at mid-life (392, 393). Lithgow *et al.* (394) have also found that *age1⁻* mutant worms have a higher intrinsic thermotolerance than wild-type. A variety of stresses lead to the induction of heat shock proteins, including oxidative stress (395). Thus, we may be observing a pleiotropic up-regulation of stress responses in the *age-1⁻* mutant.

An entire signal transduction pathway has been implicated in *C. elegans* longevity recently. The first genes identified were *daf-2* and *daf-16* (396). This gene is involved in dauer larva formation. The dauer is a developmental form that arises in response to stress, including overcrowding, starvation, and heat. Subsequently, *daf-12*, *daf-18*, and *daf-23* have been added to the list, forming one, more or less, coherent pathway (397). Lithgow *et al.* (398) have found that *daf-2⁻* mutants display an enhanced thermotolerance.

Apart from the relevance of oxidant defenses in the form of superoxide dismutase in combination with catalase demonstrated by Orr and Sohal (374), no other discrete genes have been implicated in aging in *Drosophila*. Genetic selection has, however, been used to develop strains of fruit flies that display extended longevity (399–401). In all three derivations, the flies were selected for delayed reproduction, yielding longer-lived flies. The principle behind the selection approach is that the alleles favoring longer life are ultimately brought together from among those present in the outbred population over many generations. As might be expected, the outcome in all three cited experiments was different in detail. This suggests that there are alternate routes to postponed senescence. The flies selected by Luckinbill *et al.* (399) display an enhanced resistance to oxygen free radicals (402). However, they show no accentuation in resistance to other stresses. On the other hand, Rose's (400) flies are more resistant to starvation, deccication, and ethanol vapors than the control (403). Interestingly, they also possess a more active electrophoretic allele of superoxide dismutase (404). Unfortunately, these important selection experiments were not designed in a way that would facilitate the identification of the individual genes involved in extended longevity. Nevertheless, the studies clearly implicate stress responses in aging.

Endocrine Effects

The foregoing discussion was designed to review the molecular and cellular aspects of aging. Although a thorough discussion of endocrine changes during the aging process is not an integral part of this topic, it is important to realize that many of the features associated with aging at the molecular and cellular levels are impacted by the neuroendocrine system. This is not surprising in a multicellular organism such as the human. The purpose of this section is to review a selected subset of the endocrine factors that are known to be important in aging. These will include those that impinge on the immune system and on glucose metabolism, because they are closely related to the cellular and molecular processes discussed earlier and because they are of some significance for geriatric oncology. Although issues such as those related to estrogen or growth hormone therapy are of obvious importance in oncology, they do not fulfill the former criterion, and therefore they will not be treated here. This is not to say that estrogen and growth hormone do not impinge on the immune system, for example. It is just that an understanding of their roles in this capacity is in its infancy.

Endocrine Status and the Immune System

The previous section sketched out the involvement of the hypothalamic-pituitary-adrenal axis in the response to stress. This response ultimately results in the secretion of glucocorticoids, which have profound systemic effects. These include the well-known stress adaptation response that includes a variety of metabolic effects such as the stimulation of gluconeogenesis. However, chronic glucocorticoid secretion has adverse influences. The involvement of such chronic stress in neuronal death has been highlighted earlier. It is also worth noting the role of glucocorticoids in T cell demise. Glucocorticoids appear to exert this effect through the induction of IκB synthesis, which inhibits the activity of the transcription factor NF-κB (405, 406). This transcription factor is important in a variety of immune responses, including the acute phase response.

The steroid, dehydroepiandrosterone (DHEA), has been touted in many quarters as an "anti-aging drug" (see editorial in 407). This effect of DHEA has been adduced from studies in mice (reviewed in 408). Among the consequences of DHEA administration, there have been reports of a decline in the incidence of certain tumors. Many of the effects of the drug may be mediated through its influence on the immune system. The age-related increase in serum amyloid P substance and tissue specific autoantibodies was correlated with a decline in the regulation of IL-6 production by lymphoid cells (409). These changes occurred concomitantly with the known decline in DHEA levels. Administration of the hormone reversed these age-related changes.

The rise in IL-6 levels seen during aging in mice and in humans is particularly portentous. This cytokine is an important effector of the acute phase inflammatory response, participating in signal transduction via a JAK-Stat pathway. Its rise with age again underlines the fact that older organisms are subject to chronic stress. The increase in IL-6 is largely obviated by dietary restriction in mice (410), a regimen that will be discussed more fully below. These studies have been extended demonstrating that dietary restriction not only

Table 7.6 Effect of dietary restriction on circulating hormone levels in aging rats.

Hormone	Age change	Dietary effect	Reference
Insulin	increase	decrease	418
Glucagon	increase	no effect	418
Calcitonin	increase	decrease	426
Parathyroid	increase	increase suppressed	427
FSH	no change in adult	decrease	428
LH	slight change	decrease in ovulatory peak	428
Progesterone	increase	decrease	428
Prolactin	increase	increase suppressed	429
Testosterone	decrease	decrease reversed	429
Glucocorticoids	increase	increase	424, 430

attenuates IL-6 dysregulation, but also the correlated increase in lymphoma production (411). It is still unclear whether the observations on mice can be extended to humans. Indeed, mice normally produce comparatively lower levels of DHEA than humans. The decline in DHEA levels in both human males and females is, however, one of the more striking hormonal deficits of aging (412). Certain negative aspects to DHEA administration may pertain (407).

Glucose Metabolism

A large literature relating to blood glucose and insulin levels during aging exists. This body of data includes studies in both humans and rodents (413, 414). The overall conclusion from these studies is that with age there is an increased resistance to insulin, which leads to hyperinsulinemia followed by hyperglycemia (415). This can result in a pathological state that includes hypertension and accelerated vascular aging. This general view is complicated by disparate results obtained in some of the studies. Some of the inconsistency is undoubtedly due to methodological factors. More recently, the view is emerging that the observed disturbances in glucose metabolism are likely due to underlying pathological changes rather than to aging *per se* (*e.g.*, 416). Regardless of the precise origin, the elevated insulin and glucose levels that are frequently encountered in older individuals exert detrimental effects. One of these is clearly the potential for elevated non- enzymatic glycation, which was discussed earlier in this chapter.

Dietary Restriction

The reduction of caloric intake is the only reliable method to extend life span and postpone aging in mammals. Dietary restriction induces a wide array of physiological and molecular changes (reviewed in 417). Importantly, it lowers blood glucose and insulin levels, ameliorating the age-related deficits in glucose metabolism (418). Perhaps not surprisingly in this context, dietary restriction decreases the accumulation of glycoxidation products during aging (419). In addition to this effect, this regimen up-regulates antioxidant defenses (417). Of great interest to the oncologist, dietary restriction reduces the incidence of tumors (420). The mechanism by which this occurs is of considerable interest. A clue to this may reside in the demonstration that dietary restriction delays spontaneous tumorigenesis in p53-knockout mice (421). Unfortunately however, we do not as yet know whether dietary restriction would be effective in humans.

The many physiologic, cellular, and molecular effects of dietary restriction cannot be random, because they result in the extension of life span. They must somehow be coordinated. The mechanism for this coordination is not known. However, the many changes in hormone levels that the dietary restriction response entails (417) suggest a neuroendocrine basis (Table 7.6). An analysis of the pattern of the many changes induced by dietary restriction has led Richardson and McCarter (422) to propose that dietary restriction involves a broad resetting of physiological thresholds rather than a change in rates. In any case, it would appear that dietary restriction ultimately results in a broad array of gene regulatory changes at many loci throughout the organism (417), and these may represent the ultimate effectors of the response to dietary restriction (423).

The sole surprise in terms of the hormonal alterations effected by dietary restriction is an increase in glucocorticoid levels (424). This elevation is necessary for dietary restriction to have its antitumorigenic effect (425). The elevation of glucocorticoids by dietary restriction seems paradoxical, given the deleterious effects these hormones have on both the nervous and immune systems. The question, of course, is whether the elevation in glucocorticoids is causal or coincidental, in the dietary restriction response. Perhaps the presence of chronic stress, in the form of glucocorticoids, can mobilize the stress adaptation responses to acute bouts of stress, in the hospitable background of the dietarily modified animal.

Conclusions and Perspectives

The organism struggles to maintain homeostatic balance by investing resources in maintenance and repair, and in the processes that collectively span resistance to environmental stress, damage, and disease. This struggle becomes more and more difficult with age. This campaign is ultimately waged at the level of individual cells. However, these cells do not exist in a vacuum. Instead, they influence each other, frequently at a distance. It is becoming clear that the aging organism is subjected to chronic stress with a concomitant decline in the ability to respond to acute stress. Both mitotic and post-mitotic cell populations are subject to this waning vitality. In post-mitotic cells, the result is frequently degenerative, leading to cell death.

Mitotic cells, at least those from the committed compartment, suffer a decline in proliferative capacity with replicative age. We are not certain whether this also pertains to human stem cells. This decline is coupled to other functional deficits, such as the diminished capacity for wound repair. Cellular senescence is not tantamount to cell death, however. Indeed, the genetic instabilities these cells suffer may predispose them to immortalization. In the immune system, the age-dependent loss of signal processing functions may not only result in proliferative deficits but in loss of the capacity of the system to respond to neo-antigens coupled to the development of autoimmune disease. All of these age-related changes can have profound influences on the oncogenic process in geriatric patients.

Biological aging research is clearly approaching the point at which we will have a rather well-developed understanding of the role of age-related functional decline in the appearance and progress of neoplastic lesions. The future will bring an exploitation of this knowledge in the form of practical interventions. Furthermore, we believe that a better comprehension of the genetics of aging will result in a deeper perception of the genetics of cancer.

References

1. Hayflick L, Moorhead PS. The serial cultivation of human diploid cell strains. *Exp. Cell Res.* 1961; **25**: 585–621.
2. Goldstein S. Replicative senescence: the human fibroblast comes of age. *Science* 1990; **249**: 1129–1133.
3. Cristofalo VJ, Pignolo RJ. Replicative senescence of human fibroblast-like cells in culture. *Physiol. Rev.* 1993; **73**: 617–638.
4. Harley CB, Goldstein S. Cultured human fibroblasts: distribution of cell generations and a critical limit. *J. Cell. Physiol.* 1978; **97**: 509–516.
5. Dell'Orco RT, Mertens JG, Kruse PF, Jr. Doubling potential, calender time, and donor age of human diploid cells in culture. *Exp. Cell Res.* 1974; **84**: 363–366.
6. Goldstein S, Singal DP. Senescence of cultured human fibroblasts: mitotic vs. metabolic time. *Exp. Cell Res.* 1974; **88**: 359–364.
7. Dell'Orco RT, Mertens JG, Kruse PF, Jr. Doubling potential, calendar time, and senescence of human diploid cells in culture. *Exp. Cell Res.* 1973; **77**: 356–360.
8. Martin GM, Sprague CA, Epstein CJ. Replicative lifespan of cultivated human cells-effects of donor age, tissue and genotype. *Lab. Invest.* 1970; **23**: 86–92.
9. Schneider EL, Mitsui Y. The relationship between *in vitro* cellular aging and *in vivo* human age. *Proc. Natl. Acad. Sci. USA* 1976; **73**: 3584–3588.
10. Goldstein S, Moerman EJ, Soeldner JS, Gleason RE, Barnett DM. Chronologic and physiologic age affect replicative lifespan of fibroblasts from diabetic, prediabetic, and normal donors. *Science* 1978; **199**: 781–782.
11. Rohme D. Evidence for a relationship between longevity of mammalian species and life-spans of normal fibroblasts *in vitro* and erythrocytes *in vivo*. *Proc. Natl. Acad. Sci. USA* 1981; **78**: 5009–5013.
12. Hayflick L. The limited *in vitro* lifetime of human diploid cell strains. *Exp. Cell Res.* 1965; **37**: 614–636.
13. Bayreuther K, Rodemann HP, Hommel R, Dittmann K, Albiez M, Francz PI. Human skin fibroblasts *in vitro* differentiate along a terminal cell lineage. *Proc. Natl. Acad. Sci. USA* 1988; **85**: 5112–5116.
14. Suda Y, Suzuki M, Ikawa Y, Aizawa S. Mouse embryonic stem cells exhibit indefinite proliferative potential. *J. Cell. Physiol.* 1987; **33**: 197–201.
15. Rosenberger RF. The initiation of senescence and its relationship to embryonic cell differentiation. *Bioessays* 1995; **17**: 257–260.
16. Ellis RE, Yuan J, Horvitz HR. Mechanisms and functions of cell death. *Annu. Rev. Cell Biol.* 1991; **7**: 663–698.
17. Cohen JJ, Duke RC, Fadok VA, Sellins KS. Apoptosis and programmed cell death in immunity. *Annu. Rev. Immunol.* 1992; **10**: 267–293.
18. Wang E. Senescent human fibroblasts resist programmed cell death, and failure to suppress bcl2 is involved. *Cancer Res.* 1995; **55**: 2284–2292.
19. Korsmeyer SJ. Bcl-2 initiates a new category of oncogenes: regulators of cell death. *Blood* 1992; **80**: 879–886.
20. Cristofalo VJ, Kritchevsky D. Cell size and nucleic acid content in the human diploid cell line WI-38 during aging. *Med. Exp.* 1969; **19**: 313–320.
21. Greenberg SB, Grove GL, Cristofalo VJ. Cell size in aging monolayer cultures. *In vitro Cell Dev. Biol.* 1977; **13**: 297–300.
22. Bowman PD, Meek RL, Daniels CW. Aging of human fibroblasts *in vitro*. Correlation between DNA synthesis ability and cell size. *Exp. Cell Res.* 1975; **93**: 184–190.
23. Mitsui Y, Schneider EL. Increased nuclear sizes in senescent human diploid fibroblast cultures. *Exp. Cell Res.* 1976; **100**: 147–152.
24. Schneider EL, Fowlkes BJ. Measurement of DNA content and cell volume in senescent human fibroblasts utilizing flow multiparameter single cell analysis. *Exp. Cell Res.* 1976; **98**: 298–302.
25. Schneider EL, Shorr SS. Alteration in cellular RNAs during the *in vitro* lifespan of cultured human diploid fibroblasts. *Cell* 1975; **6**: 179–184.
26. Cristofalo VJ, Doggett DL, Brooks-Frederich KM, Phillips PD. Growth factors as probes of cell aging. *Exp. Gerontol.* 1989; **24**: 367–374.
27. Cristofalo, VJ. Cellular biomarkers of aging. *Exp. Gerontol.* 1988; **23**: 297–305.
28. Macieira-Coelho A, Ponten J, Phillipson L. The division cycle and RNA synthesis in diploid human cells at different passage levels *in vitro*. *Exp. Cell Res.* 1966; **42**: 673–684.
29. Matsumura T, Zerrudo Z, Hayflick L. Senescent human diploid cells in culture: survival, DNA synthesis and morphology. *J. Gerontol.* 1979; **34**: 328–334.
30. Norwood TH, Pendergrass WR, Sprague CA, Martin, GM. Dominance of the senescent phenotype in heterokaryons between replicative and post-replicative human fibroblast-like cells. *Proc. Natl. Acad. Sci. USA* 1974; **71**: 2231–2235.
31. Burmer GC, Zeigler CJ, Norwood TH. Evidence for endogenous polypeptide-mediated inhibition of cell-cycle transit in human diploid cells. *J. Cell Biol.* 1982; **94**: 187–192.
32. Pereira-Smith OM, Smith JR. Phenotype of low proliferative potential is dominant in hybrids of normal human fibroblasts. *Somatic Cell Genet.* 1982; **8**: 731–742.
33. Yanishevsky RM, Stein GH. Ongoing DNA synthesis continues in young human diploid cells (HDC) fused to senescent HDC, but entry into S phase is inhibited. *Exp. Cell Res.* 1980; **126**: 469–472.

34. Drescher-Lincoln CK, Smith JR. Inhibition of DNA synthesis in senescent-proliferating human cybrids is mediated by endogenous proteins. *Exp. Cell Res.* 1984; **153**: 208–217.

35. Lumpkin CKJ, McClung JK, Pereira-Smith OM, Smith JR. Existence of high abundance antiproliferative mRNAs in senescent human diploid fibroblasts. *Science.* 1986; **232**: 393–395.

36. Cristofalo VJ, Sharf BB. Cellular senescence and DNA synthesis: thymidine incorporation as a measure of population age in human diploid cells. *Exp. Cell Res.* 1973; **76**: 419–429.

37. Yanishevsky, R, Mendelsohn ML, Mayall BH, Cristofalo VJ. Proliferative capacity and DNA content of aging human dipoid cells in culture: a cytophotometric and autoradiographic analysis. *J. Cell. Physiol.* 1974; **84**: 1265–1270.

38. Gorman SD, Cristofalo VJ. Analysis of the G1 arrest position of senescent WI-38 cells by quinacrine dihydrochloride nuclear fluorescence-evidence for a late G1 arrest. *Exp. Cell Res.* 1986; **167**: 87–94.

39. Sherwood SW, Rush D, Ellsworth JL, Schimke RT. Defining cellular senescence in IMR-90 cells: A flow cytometric analysis. *Proc. Natl. Acad. Sci. USA.* 1988; **85**: 9086–9090.

40. Olashaw NE, Kress ED, Cristofalo VJ. Thymidine triphosphate synthesis in senescent WI-38 cells. Relationship to loss of replicative capacity. *Exp. Cell Res.* 1983; **149**: 547–554.

41. Rittling SR, Brooks KM, Cristofalo VJ, Baserga R. Expression of cell cycle-dependent genes in young and senescent WI-38 fibroblasts. *Proc. Natl. Acad. Sci. USA* 1986; **83**: 3316–3320.

42. Macieira-Coelho A, Berumen L. The cell cycle during growth inhibition of human embryonic fibroblasts *in vitro. Proc. Soc. Exp. Biol. Med.* 1973; **144**: 43–47.

43. Macieira-Coelho A, Ponten J. Analogy in growth between late passage human embryonic and early passage human adult fibroblasts. *J. Cell Biol.* 1969; **43**: 374–377.

44. Phillips PD, Kuhnle E, Cristofalo VJ. [^{125}I]EGF binding ability is stable throughout the replicative life span of WI-38 cells. *J. Cell. Physiol.* 1983; **114**: 311–316.

45. Phillips PD, Pignolo RJ, Cristofalo VJ. Insulin-like growth factor-I: specific binding to high and low affinity sites and mitogen action throughout the life span of WI-38 cells. *J. Cell. Physiol.* 1987; **133**: 135–143.

46. Holt JT, Gopal TV, Moulton AD, Nienhuis AW. Inducible production of c-fos antisense RNA inhibits 3T3 cell proliferation. *Proc. Natl. Acad. Sci. USA* 1986; **83**: 4794–4798.

47. Nishikura K, Murray JM. Antisense RNA of proto-oncogene c-fos blocks renewed growth of quiescent 3T3 cell. *Mol. Cell. Biol.* 1987; **7**: 639–649.

48. Riabowol K, Schiff J, Gilman MZ. Transcription factor AP-1 activity is required for initiation of DNA synthesis and is lost during cellular aging. *Proc. Natl. Acad. Sci. USA* 1992; **89**: 157–161.

49. Seshadri T, Campisi J. Repression of c-fos transcription and an altered genetic program in senescent human fibroblasts. *Science.* 1990; **247**: 205–209.

50. Hollingsworth Jr. RE, Chen P-L, Lee W-H. Integration of cell cycle control with transcriptional regulation by the retinoblastoma protein. *Current Opin. Cell Biol.* 1993; **5**: 194–200.

51. Goodrich DW, Wang NP, Qian Y-W, Lee EY H-P, Lee WH. The retinoblastoma gene product regulates progression through the G1 phase of the cell cycle. *Cell* 1991; **67**: 293–302.

52. Nevins JR. Mechanism of viral-mediated trans-activation of transcription. *Adv. Virus Res.* 1989; **37**: 35–83.

53. Srikumar PC, Hiebert S, Mudryj M, Horowitz JM, Nevins JR. The E2F transcription factor is a cellular target for the RB protein. *Cell* 1991; **65**: 1053–1061.

54. Stein GH, Beeson M, Gordon L. Failure to phosphorylate the retinoblastoma gene product in senescent human fibroblasts. *Science* 1990; **249**: 666–669.

55. Stein GH, Drullinger LF, Robetorye RS, Pereira-Smith OM. Senescent cells fail to express cdc2, cycA, and cycB in response to mitogen stimulation. *Proc. Natl. Acad. Sci. USA* 1991; **88**: 11012–11016.

56. Murray AW. Creative blocks: cell-cycle checkpoints and feedback control. *Nature* 1992; **359**: 599–604.

57. Rosenblatt J, Gu Y, Morgan DO. Human cyclin-dependent kinase 2 is activated during the S and G2 phase of the cell cycle and associates with cyclin A. *Proc. Natl. Acad. Sci. USA* 1992; **89**: 2824–2828.

58. Welch PJ, Wang JJ. Coordinated synthesis and degradation of cdc2 in the mammalina cell cycle. *Proc. Natl. Acad. Sci. USA* 1992; **89**: 3093–3097.

59. Fry DG, Hurlin PJ, Maher VM, McCormick JJ. Transformation of diploid human fibroblasts by transfection with V-SIS, PDGF2/C-SIS or T24H-ras genes. *Mutat. Res.* 1988; **199**: 341–351.

60. Sager R, Tanaka K, Lau CC, Ebina Y, Anisowicz A. Resistance of human cells to tumorigenesis induced by cloned transforming genes. *Proc. Natl. Acad. Sci. USA* 1983; **80**: 7601–7605.

61. McCormick JJ, Maher VM. Towards an understanding of the malignant transformation of diploid human fibroblasts. *Mutat. Res.* 1988; **199**: 273–291.

62. Sager R. Resistance of human cells to oncogenic transformation. *Cancer Cells* 1984; **2**; 487–493.

63. Curatolo L, Erba E, Morasca L. Culture conditions induce the appearance of immortalized C3H mouse cell lines. *In Vitro* 1984; **20**: 597–601.

64. Kraemer PM, Ray FA, Brothman AR, Bartholdi MF, Cram LC. Spontaneous immortalization rate of cultured Chinese hamster cells. *J. Natl. Cancer Inst.* 1986; **76**: 703–709.

65. Macieira-Coelho A. Implications of the reorganization of the cell genome for aging or immortalization of dividing cells *in vitro. Gerontology* 1980; **26**: 276–282.

66. Meek RL, Bowman, PD, Daniel CW. Establishment of mouse embryo cells *in vitro*: relationship of DNA synthesis, senescence and malignant transformation. *Exp. Cell Res.* 1977; **107**: 277–284.

67. Huschtscha LI, Holliday R. Limited and unlimited growth of SV40-transformed cells from human diploid MRC-5 fibroblasts. *J. Cell Sci.* 1983; **63**: 77–99.

68. Imai S-I, Saito F, Ikeuchi T, Segawa K, Takano T. Escape from *in vitro* aging in SV40 large T antigen-transformed human diploid cells: a key event responsible for immortalization occurs during crisis. *Mech. Ageing Dev.* 1993; **69**: 149–158.

69. Ide T, Tsuji Y, Nakashima T, Ishibashi S. Progress of aging in human diploid cells transformed with a tsA mutant of simian virus 40. *Exp. Cell Res.* 1984; **150**: 321–328.

70. Lomax CA, Bradley E, Weber J, Bourgaux P. Transformation of human cells by temperature-sensitive mutants of simian virus 40. *Intervirology* 1978; **9**: 28–38

71. Stein GH. SV40-transformed human fibroblasts: evidence for cellular aging in precrisis cells. *J. Cell. Physiol.* 1985; **125**: 36–44.

72. Rinehart CA, Haskill JS, Morris JS, Butler TD, Kaufman DG. Extended life span of human endometrial stromal cells transfected with cloned origin-defective temperature-sensitive Simian Virus 40. *J. Virol.* 1991; **65**: 1458–1465.

73. Radna RL, Caton Y, Jha KK, Kaplan P, Li G, Tragamps F, Ozer HL. Growth of immortal Simian Virus 40 tsA-transformed human fibroblasts is temperature dependent. *Mol. Cell. Biol.* 1989; **9**: 3093–3096.

74. Stewart N, Bacchetti S. Expression of SV40 large T antigen, but not small t antigen, is required for the induction of chromosomal aberrations in transformed human cells. *Virology* 1991; **180**: 49–57.

75. Gorman SD, Cristofalo VJ. Reinitiation of cellular DNA synthesis in BrdU-selected nondividing senescent WI-38 cells by Simian Virus 40 infection. *J. Cell. Physiol.* 1985; **125**: 122–126.

76. Wright WE, Pereira-Smith OM, Shay JW. Reversible cellular senescence: implications for immortalization of normal human diploid fibroblasts. *Mol. Cell. Biol.* 1989; **9**: 3088–3092.

77. Kuhar SG, Lehman JM. T antigen and p53 in pre- and post-crisis simian virus 40-transformed human cell lines. *Oncogene* 1991; **6**: 1499–1506.

78. Bryan TM, Reddel RR. SV40-induced immortalization of human cells. *Crit. Rev. Oncog.* 1994; **5**: 331–357.

79. Pereira-Smith OM, Smith JR. Evidence for the recessive nature of cellular immortality. *Science* 1983; **221**: 964–966.

80. Pereira-Smith OM, Smith JR. Genetic analysis of indefinite division in human cells: identification of four complementation groups. *Proc. Natl. Acad. Sci. USA* 1988; **85**: 6042–6046.

81. Sandhu AK, Hubbard K, Kaur GP, Jha KK, Ozer HL, Athwal RS. Senescence of immortal human fibroblasts by the introduction of normal human chromosome 6. *Proc. Natl. Acad. Sci. USA* 1994; **91**: 5498–5502.

82. Sugawara O, Oshimura M, Koi M, Annab LA, Barrett C. Induction of cellular senescence in immortalized cells by human chromosome 1. *Science* 1990; **247**: 707–710.

83. Ning Y, Weber JL, Killary AM, Ledbetter DH, Smith JR, Pereira-Smith OM. Genetic analysis of indefinite division in human cells: evidence for a cell senescence-related gene(s) on human chromosome 4. *Proc. Natl. Acad. Sci. USA* 1991; **88**: 5635–5639.

84. Zakian VA. Structure and function of telomeres. *Ann. Rev. Genet.* 1989; **23**: 579–604.

85. Blackburn EH. Telomeres: No end in sight. *Cell* 1994; **77**: 621–623.

86. Sandell L, Zakian VA. Loss of a yeast telomere: arrest, recovery, and chromosome loss. *Cell* 1993; **75**: 729–739.

87. McClintock B. The behavior in successive nuclear divisions of a chromosome broken at meiosis. *Proc. Natl. Acad. Sci. USA* 1939; **25**: 405–416.

88. McClintock B. The stability of broken ends of chromosomes in Zea mays. *Genetics* 1941; **26**: 234–282.

89. Blackburn EH. RNA-dependent polymerase motifs in EST1: tentative identification of a protein component of an essential yeast telomerase. *Cell* 1990; **60**: 529–530.

90. Greider CW. Telomerase and telomere-length regulation: lessons from small eukaryotes to mammals. *Cold Spring Harbor Symp. Quant. Biol.* 1993; **58**: 719–723

91. Harley CB. Telomerases. *Pathol. Biol.* 1994; **42**: 342–345.

92. Cohen M, Blackburn EH. Telomerase in yeast. *Science* 1995; **269**: 396–400.

93. Greider CW, Blackburn EH. Identification of a specific telomere terminal transferase activity in Tetrahymena extracts. *Cell* 1985; **43**: 405–413.

94. Lin JJ, Zakian VA. An *in vitro* assay for Saccharomyces telomerase requires EST1. *Cell* 1995; **81**: 1127–1135.

95. Mantell LL, Greider CW. Telomerase activity in germline and embryonic cells of Xenopus. *EMBO J.* 1994; **13**: 3211–3217.

96. Morin GB. The human telomere terminal transferase enzyme is a ribonucleoprotein that synthesizes TTAGGG repeats. *Cell* 1989; **59**: 521–529.

97. Lundblad V, Blackburn EH. An alternate pathway for yeast telomere maintenance rescues est[1] senescence. *Cell* 1993; **73**: 347–360.

98. Collins K, Kobayashi R, Greider CW. Purification of Tetrahymena telomerase and cloning of genes encoding the two protein components of the enzyme. *Cell* 1995; **81**: 677–686.

99. Singer MS, Gottschling DE. TLC1: template RNA component of Saccharomyces cerevisiae telomerase. *Science* 1994; **266**: 404–409.

100. Feng J, Funk WD, Wang S-S, Weinrich SL, Avilion AA, Chiu C-P, Adams RR, Chang E, Allsopp RC, Yu J, Le S, West MD, Harley CB, Andrews WH, Greider CW, Villeponteau B. The RNA component of human telomerase. *Science* 1996; **269**: 1236–1241.

101. Wellinger RJ, Wolf AJ, Zakian VA. Saccharomyces telomeres acquire single-strand TG1-3 tails late in S phase. *Cell* 1993; **72**: 51–60.

102. Wellinger RJ, Wolf AJ, Zakian VA. Origin activation and formation of single-strand TG1-3 tails occur sequentially in late S phase on a yeast linear plasmid. *Mol. Cell. Biol.* 1993; **13**: 4057–4065.

103. Harley CB. Telomere loss: mitotic clock or genetic time bomb? *Mutat. Res.* 1991; **256**: 271–282.

104. Allsopp R, Vaziri H, Patterson C, Goldstein S, Younglai EV, Futcher AB, Greider CW, Harley CB. Telomere length predicts replicative capacity of human fibroblasts. *Proc. Natl. Acad. Sci. USA* 1992; **89**: 10114–10118.

105. Harley CB, Futcher AB, Greider CW. Telomeres shorten during ageing of human fibroblasts. *Nature* 1990; **345**: 458–460.

106. Hastie ND, Dempster M, Dunlop MG, Thompson AM, Green DK, Allshire RC. Telomere reduction in human colorectal carcinoma and with ageing. *Nature* 1990; **346**: 866–868.

107. Lindsey J, McGill NI, Lindsey LA, Green DK, Cooke HJ. *In vivo* loss of telomeric repeats with age in humans. *Mutat. Res.* 1991; **256**: 45–48.

108. Counter CM, Avilion AA, LeFeuvre CE, Stewart NG, Greider CW, Harley CB, Bacchetti S. Telomere shortening associated with chromosome instability is arrested in immortal cells which express telomerase activity. *EMBO J.* 1992; **11**: 1921–1929.

109. Vaziri H, Schachter F, Uchida I, Wei L, Zhu X, Effros R, Cohen D, Harley CB. Loss of telomeric DNA during aging of normal and trisomy 21 human lymphocytes. *Am. J. Human Genet.* 1993; **52**: 661–667.

110. Vaziri H, Dragowska W, Allsopp RC, Thoman TE, Harley CB, Lansdorp PM. Evidence for a mitotic clock in human hematopoietic stem cells: Loss of telomeric DNA with age. *Proc. Natl. Acad. Sci. USA* 1994; **91**: 9857–9860.

111. Counter CM, Botelho FM, Wang P, Harley CB, Bacchetti S. Stabilization of short telomeres and telomerase activity accompany immortalization of Epstein-Barr virus-transformed human B lymphocytes. *J. Virol.* 1994; **68**: 3410–3414.

112. Counter CM, Hirte HW, Bacchetti S, Harley CB. Telomerase activity in human ovarian carcinoma. *Proc. Natl. Acad. Sci. USA* 1994; **91**; 2900–2904.

113. Nilsson P, Mehle C, Remes K, Roos G. Telomerase activity *in vivo* in human malignant hematopoietic cells. *Oncogene* 1994; **9**: 3043–3048.

114. Kim NW, Piatyszek MA, Prowse KR, Harley CB, West, MD, Ho PL, Coviello GM, Wright WE, Weinrich SL, Shay JW. Specific association of human telomerase activity with immortal cells and cancer. *Science* 1994; **266**: 2011–2015.

115. Lundblad V, Szostak JW. A mutant with a defect in telomere elongation leads to senescence in yeast. *Cell* 1989; **57**: 633–643.

116. Kipling D, Cooke HJ. Hypervariable ultra-long telomeres in mice. *Nature* 1990; **347**: 400–402.

117. D'mello NP, Jazwinski SM. Telomere length constancy during aging of Saccharomyces cerevisiae. *J. Bacteriol.* 1991; **173**: 6709–6713.

118. Gilley D, Blackburn EH. Lack of telomere shortening during senescence in Paramecium. *Proc. Natl. Acad. Sci. USA* 1994; **91**: 1955–1958.

119. Wright WE, Shay JW. Telomere positional effects and the regulation of cellular senescence. *Trends in Genet.* 1992; **8**: 193–197.

120. Lima-de-Faria A. Organization and function of telomeres. In *Molecular Evolution and Organization of the Chromosome* (Amsterdam: Elsevier Science Publishers B.V.), pp. 701–721, 1983.

121. Spofford JB. Position effect variegation in Drosophila. *Genet. Biol. Dros. 1c*, 1976; 955–1018.

122. Laurenson P, Rine J. Silencers, Silencing, and heritable transcriptional states. *Microbiol. Rev.* 1992; **56**: 543–560.

123. Gottschling DE, Aparicio OM, Billington BL, Zakian VA. Position effect at S. cerevisiae telomeres: reversible repression of Pol II transcription. *Cell* 1990; **63**: 751–762.

124. Renauld H, Aparicio OM, Zierath PD, Billington BL, Chablani SK, Gottschling DE. Silent domains are assembled continuously from the telomere and are defined by promoter distance and strength, and by SIR3 dosage. *Genes Dev.* 1993; **7**: 1133–1145.

125. Palladino F, Laroche T, Gilson E, Axelrod A, Pillus L, Gasser SM. SIR3 and SIR4 proteins are required for the positioning and integrity of yeast telomeres. *Cell* 1993; **75**: 543–555.

126. Aparicio OM, Billington BL, Gottschling DE. Modifiers of position effect are shared between telomeric and silent mating-type loci in S. cerevisiae. *Cell* 1991; **66**: 1279–1287.

127. Hardy CF, Sussel L, Shore D. A RAP1-interacting protein involved in transcriptional silencing and telomere length regulation. *Genes Dev.* 1992; **6**: 801–814.

128. Chien CT, Buck S, Sternglanz R, Shore D. Targeting of SIR1 protein establishes transcriptional silencing at HM loci and telomeres in yeast. *Cell* 1993; **75**: 531–541.

129. Wright JH, Gottschling DE, Zakian VA. Saccharomyces telomeres assume a nonnucleosomal chromatin structure. *Genes Dev.* 1992; **6**: 197–210.

130. Wright JH, Zakian VA. Protein-DNA interactions in soluble telosomes from Saccharomyces cerevisiae. *Nucleic Acids Res.* 1995; **23**: 1454–1460.

131. Cockell M, Palladino F, Laroche T, Kyrion G, Liu C, Lustig AJ, Gasser SM. The carboxy termini of Sir4 and Rap1 affect Sir3 localization: evidence for a multicomponent complex required for yeast telomeric silencing, *J. Cell Biol.* 1995; **129**: 909–924.

132. Buck SW, Shore D. Action of a RAP1 carboxy-terminal silencing domain reveals an underlying competition between HMR and telomeres in yeast. *Genes Dev.* 1995; **9**: 370–384.

133. Liu C, Mao X, Lustig AJ. Mutational analysis defines a C-terminal tail domain of RAP1 essential for telomeric silencing in Saccharomyces cerevisiae. *Genetics* 1994; **138**: 1025–1040.

134. Pillus L, Rine J. Epigenetic inheritance of transcriptional states in S. cerevisiae. *Cell* 1989; **59**: 637–647.

135. Shore D. RAP1: a protein regulator in yeast. *Trends in Genet.* 1994; **10**: 408–411.

136. Sandell LL, Gottschling DE, Zakian VA. Transcription of a yeast telomere alleviates telomere position effect without affecting chromosome stability. *Proc. Natl. Acad. Sci. USA* 1994; **91**: 12061–12065.

137. Kennedy BK, Austriaco NR, Jr, Zhang J, Guarente L. Mutation in the silencing gene SIR4 can delay aging in S. cerevisiae. *Cell* 1995; **80**: 485–496.

138. Smith JR, Hayflick L. Variation in the lifespan of clones derived from human diploid cell strains. *J. Cell. Biol.* 1974; **62**; 48–53.

139. Yunis JJ. The chromosomal basis of human neoplasia. *Science* 1983; **221**: 227–236.

140. Nowell PC. Genetic instability and tumor development. In *Basic Life Sciences*, vol. 57, pp. 221–231. Boundaries between Promotion and Progression during Carcinogenesis, edited by O Sudilovsky, HC Pitot and LA Liotta. New York: Plenum Press, 1988.

141. Tlsty TD, Margolin BH, Lum KL. Difference in the rates of gene amplification in nontumorigenic and tumorigenic cell lines as measured by Luria-Delbruck fluctuation analysis. *Proc. Natl. Acad. Sci. USA* 1989; **86**: 9441–9445.

142. Wright JA, Smith HS, Watt FM, Hancock MC, Hudson DL, Stark GR. DNA amplification is rare in normal human cells. *Proc. Natl. Acad. Sci. USA* 1990; **87**: 1791–1795.

143. Livingstone LR, White A, Sprouse J, Livanos E, Jacks T, Tlsty TD. Altered cell cycle arrest and gene amplification potential accompany loss of wild-type p53. *Cell* 1992; **70**: 923–935.

144. Yin Y, Tainsky MA, Bischoff FZ, Strong LC, Wahl GM. Wild-type p53 restores cell cycle control and inhibits gene amplification in cells with mutant p53 alleles. *Cell* 1992; **70**: 937–948.

145. Lane DP, Benchimol S. p53: oncogene or antioncogene? *Genes Dev.* 1990; **4**: 1–8.

146. Levine AJ, Momand J, Finlay CA. The p53 tumor suppressor gene. *Nature* 1991; **351**: 453–456.

147. Smith ML, Fornace AJ, Jr. Genomic instability and the role of p53 mutations in cancer cells. *Curr. Opin. Oncol.* 1995; **7**: 69–75.

148. Li FP, Fraumeni, JF Jr. Rhabdomyosarcoma in children: epidemiology study and identification of a familial cancer syndrome. *J. Natl. Cancer Inst.* 1969; **43**: 1365–1373.

149. Li FP, Fraumeni JF, Jr., Mulvihill JJ, Blattner WA, Dreyfus MG, Tucker MA, Miller RW. A cancer family syndrome in twenty-four kindreds. *Cancer Res.* 1988; **48**: 5358–5362.

150. Malkin D, Li F, Strong LC, Fraumeni JF, Nelson CE, Kim DH, Gryka G, Bischoff FZ, Tainsky MA, Friend SH. Germ line p53 mutations in a familial syndrome of sarcoma breast cancer and other neoplasms. *Science* 1990; **250**: 1233–1238.

151. Srivastava S, Zou S, Pirollo K, Blattner W, Chang EH. Germ-line transmission of a mutated p53 gene in a cancer-prone family with Li-Fraumeni syndrome. *Nature* 1990; **348**: 747–749.

152. Denko NC, Giaccia AJ, Stringer JR, Stambrook PJ. The human Ha-*ras* oncogene induces genomic instability in murine fibroblasts within one cell cycle. *Proc. Natl. Acad. Sci. USA* 1994; **91**: 5124–5128.

153. Diller L, Kassel J, Nelson CE, Gryka MA, Litwak G. Gebhardt M, Bressac B, Ozturk M, Baker SJ, Vogelstein B, Friend SH. p53 functions as a cell cycle control protein in osteosarcomas. *Mol. Cell. Biol.* 1990; **10**: 5772–5781.

154. Martinez J, Georgoff I, Martinez J, Levine AJ. Cellular localization and cell cycle regulation by a temperature-sensitive p53 protein. *Genes Dev.* 1991; **5**: 151–159.

155. Mercer WE, Shields MT, Amin M, Sauve GJ, Appella E, Romano JW, Ullrich SJ. Negative growth regulation in a glioblastoma tumor cell line that conditionally expresses human wild-type p53. *Proc. Natl. Acad. Sci. USA* 1990; **87**: 6166–6170.

156. Kastan MB, Zhan Q, El-Deiry WS, Carrier F, Jacks T, Walsh WV, Plunkett BS, Vogelstein, B, Fornace AJ Jr. A mammalian cell cycle checkpoint pathway utilizing p53 and GADD45 is defective in Ataxia-Telangiectasia. *Cell* 1992; **71**: 587–597.

157. Kastan MB, Onyeskwere O, Sidransky D, Vogelstein B, Craig RW. Participation of p53 protein in the cellular response to DNA damage. *Cancer Res.* 1991; **51**: 6304–6311.

158. Kuerbitz SJ, Plunkett BS, Walsh WV, Kastan MB. Wild-type p53 is a cell cycle checkpoint determinant following irradiation. *Proc. Natl. Acad. Sci. USA* 1992; **89**: 7491–7495.

159. Hinds PW, Weinberg RA. Tumor suppressor genes. *Curr. Opin. Genet. Dev.* 1994; **4**: 135–141.

160. Cox LS, Lane DP. Tumor suppressors, kinases and clamps: how p53 regulates the cell cycle in response to DNA damage. *Bioessays.* 1995; **17**: 501–508.

161. Clarke AR, Purdie CA, Harrison DJ, Morris RG, Bird CC, Hooper ML, Wylie AH. Thymocyte apoptosis induced by p53-dependent and independent pathways. *Nature* 1993; **362**: 849–852.

162. Lotem J, Sachs L. Hematopoietic cells from mice deficient in wild-type p53 are more resistant to induction of apoptosis by some agents. *Blood.* 1993; **82**: 1092–1096.

163. Lowe SW, Schmitt SW, Smith BA, Osborne BA, Jacks T. p53 is required for radiation-induced apoptosis in mouse thymocytes. *Nature* 1993; **362**: 847–849.

164. Xiong Y, Hannon GJ, Zhang H, Casso D, Kobayashi R, Beach D. p21 is a universal inhibitor of cyclin kinases. *Nature* 1993; **366**: 701–704.

165. Waga S, Hannon GJ, Beach D, Stillman B. The p21 inhibitor of cyclin-dependent kinases controls DNA replication by interaction with PCNA. *Nature* 1994; **369**: 574–578.

166. Sherr CJ, Roberts JM. Inhibitors of mammalian G1 cyclin-dependent kinases. *Genes Dev.* 1995: **9**: 1149–1163.

167. Draetta G. Cell cycle control in eukaryotes: molecular mechanisms of *cdc2* activation. *Trends Biol. Sci.* 1990; **15**: 378–383.

168. Shivji MK, Kenny MK, Wood RD. Proliferating cell nuclear antigen is required for DNA excision repair. *Cell* 1992; **69**: 367–374.

169. Prelich G, Kostura M, Marshak DR, Mathews MB, Stillman B. The cell-cycle regulated proliferating cell nuclear antigen is required for SV40 DNA replication *in vitro*. *Nature* 1987; **326**: 471–475.

170. Prelich G, Stillman B. Coordinated leading and lagging strand synthesis during SV40 DNA replication *in vitro* requires PCNA. *Cell* 1988; **53**: 117–126.

171. Tsurimoto T, Melendy T, Stillman B. Sequential initiation of lagging and leading strand synthesis by two different polymerase complexes at the SV40 DNA replication origin. *Nature* 1990; **346**: 534–539.

172. Waga S, Stillman B. Anatomy of a DNA replication fork revealed by reconstitution of SV40 DNA replication *in vitro*. *Nature* 1994; **369**: 207–212.

173. Xiong Y, Zhang H, Beach, D. D type cyclins associate with multiple protein kinases and the DNA replication and repair factor PCNA. *Cell* 1992; **71**: 505–514.

174. El-Deiry WS, Tokino T, Velculescu VE, Levy DB, Parsons R, Trent JM, Lin D, Mercer WE, Kinzler KW, Vogelstein B. WAF1, a potential mediator of p53 tumor suppression. *Cell* 1993; **75**: 817–825.

175. Gu Y, Turck CW, Morgan DO. Inhibition of Cdk2 activity *in vivo* by an associated 20K regulatory subunits. *Nature* 1993; **366**: 707–710.

176. Harper JW, Adami GR, Wei N, Keyomarsi K, Elledge SJ. The p21Cdk-interacting protein Cip1 is a potent inhibitor of G1 cyclin-dependent kinases. *Cell* 1993; **75**: 805–816.

177. Dulic V, Kaufmann WK, Wilson SJ, Tlsty TD, Lees E, Harper JW, Elledge SJ, Reed SI. p53-dependent inhibition of cyclin-dependent kinase activities in human fibroblasts during radiation-induced G1 arrest. *Cell* 1994; **76**: 1013–1023.

178. Di Leonardo A, Linke SP, Clarkin K, Wahl GM. DNA damage triggers a prolonged p53-dependent G1 arrest and long-term induction of Cip1 in normal human fibroblasts. *Genes Dev.* 1994; **8**: 2540–2551.

179. Deng C, Zhang P, Harper JW, Elledge SJ, and Leder P. Mice lacking p21CIP1/WAF1 undergo normal development, but are defective in G1 checkpoint control. *Cell* 1995; **82**: 675–684.

180. Kulju KS, Lehman JM. Increased p53 protein associated with aging in human diploid fibroblasts. *Exp. Cell Res.* 1995; **217**: 336–345.

181. Noda A, Ning Y, Venable SF, Pereira-Smith OM, Smith JR. Cloning of senescent cell-derived inhibitors of DNA synthesis using an expression screen. *Exp. Cell Res.* 1994; **211**: 90–98.

182. Jazwinski SM. Lower eukaryotic models: fungi and invertebrates. In *Encyclopedia of Gerontology*, edited by JE Birren. San Diego: Academic Press, pp. 151–161, 1996.

183. Arnheim N, Cortopassi GA. Deleterious mitochondrial mutations accumulate in aging human tissues. *Mutat. Res.* 1992; **275**: 157–167.

184. Wallace DC. Mitochondrial genetics: a paradigm for aging and degenerative diseases? *Science* 1992; **256**: 628–632.

185. Linnane AW, Zhang C, Baumer A, Nagley P. Mitochondrial DNA mutation and the aging process: bioenergy and pharmacological intervention. *Mut. Res.* 1992; **66**: 1289–1293.

186. Miquel J. An integrated theory of aging as the result of mitochondrial DNA mutation in differentiated cells. *Arch Gerontol. Geriatr.* 1991; **12**: 99–117.

187. Hsieh RH, Hou JH, Hsu HS, Wei YH. Age-dependent respiratory function decline and DNA deletions in human muscle mitochondria. *Biochem. Mol. Biol. Int.* 1994; **32**: 1009–1022.

188. Yen TC, King KL, Lee HC, Yeh SH, Wei YH. Age-dependent increase of mitochondrial DNA deletions together with lipid peroxides and superoxide dismutase in human liver mitochondria. *Free Radic. Biol. Med.* 1994; **16**: 207–214.

189. Dumas M, Maftah A, Bonte F, Ratinaud MH, Meybeck A, Julien R. Flow cytometric analysis of human epidermal cell ageing using two fluorescent mitochondrial probes. *C. R. Acad. Sci. III.* 1995; **318**: 191–197.

190. Kroll J. The mitochondrial F1-ATPase and the aging process. *Med. Hypothesis.* 1994; **42**: 356–396.

191. Pedersen PL, Carafolie E. Ion motive ATPase. I. ubiquity, properties and significance. *Trends Biochem. Sci.* 1987; **12**: 146–150.

192. Tummino PJ, Gafni A. A comparative study of succinate-supported respiration and ATP/ADP translocation in liver mitochondria from adult and old rats. *Mech. Ageing Dev.* 1991; **59**: 177–188.

193. Guerrieri F, Capozza G, Kalous M, Zanotti F, Drahota Z, Papa S. Age-dependent changes in the mitochondrial F0F1 ATP syntase. *Arch Gerontol. Geriat.* 1992; **14**: 299–308.

194. Levine ME, Mueller SN. Cultured vascular endothelial cells as a model system for the study of cellular senescence. *Intern. Rev. Cytol. Suppl.* 1979; **10**: 67–76.

195. Marin J. Age-related changes in vascular responses: a review. *Mech. Ageing Dev.* 1995; **79**: 71–114.

196. Norwood TH, Smith JR. The cultured fibroblast-like cell as a model for the study of aging. In *The Handbook of Biology of Aging*, edited by EL Schneider and C Finch. New York: Van Nostrand Reinhold, pp. 291–311, 1985.

197. Mueller SN, Rosen EM, Levine EM. Cellular senescence in a cloned strain of bovine fetal aortic endothelial cells. *Science* 1980; **207**: 889–891.

198. Rosen EM, Mueller SN, Noveral JP, Levine EM. Proliferative characteristics of clonal endothelial cell strains. *J. Cell. Physiol.* 1981; **107**: 123–137.

199. Hasegawa N, Yamamoto M, Imamura T, Mitsui Y, Yamamoto K. Evaluation of long-term cultured endothelial cells as a model system for studying vascular ageing. *Mech. Ageing Dev.* 1988; **46**: 111–123.

200. Repin VS, Dolgov VV, Zaikina OE, Novikov ID, Antonov AS, Nikolaeva MA,. Smirnov VN. Heterogeneity of endothelium in human aorta. A quantitative analysis by scanning electron-microscopy. *Atherosclerosis.* 1984; **50**: 35–52.

201. Danon D, Laver-Rudich Z, Skutelsky E. Surface charge properties of endothelium of the aorta in young and old animals. In *State of prevention and therapy in human arteriosclerosis and in animal models*, edited by WH Hauss, RW Wissler and R Lehmann. International Symposium: Opladen, Westdeutscher Verlag, pp. 541–552, 1978.

202. Moncada S, Gryglewski RJ, Bunting S, Vane JR. An enzyme isolated from arteries transforms prostaglandin endoperoxides to an unstable substance that inhibits platelet aggregation. *Nature* 1976; **263**: 663–665.

203. Hasegawa N, Yamamoto K, Kusumoto S, Watanabe T, Osawa T. Elevated promotion of prostacyclin production by synthetic lipid A analogs in aged human endothelial cells in culture. *Mech. Ageing Dev.* 1995; **78**: 155–162.

204. Tokunaga O, Yamada T, Fan J, Watanabe T. Age-related decline in prostacyclin synthesis by human aortic endothelial cells. *Am. J. Pathol.* 1991; **138**: 941–949.

205. Caffrey J L, Boluyt MO, Younes A, Barron BA, O'Neill L, Crow MT, Lakatta EG. Aging, cardiac proenkephalin mRNA and enkephalin peptides in the Fisher 344 rat. *J. Mol. Cell Cardiol.* 1994; **26**: 701–711.

206. Boluyt M O, Younes A, Caffrey JL, O'Neill L, Barron BA, Crow MT, Lakatta EG. Age- associated increase in rat cardiac opioid production. *Am. J. Physiol.* 1993; **265**, (Heart Circ. Physiol. 34): H212–H218.

207. Levin E R. Endothelins. *N. Engl. J. Med.* 1995; **333**: 356–363.

208. Yanagisawa M., Kurihara H, Kimura S, Tomobe Y, Kobayashi M, Mitsui Y, Yazaki Y, Goto K, Masaki T. A novel potent vasoconstrictor peptide produced by vascular endothelial cells. *Nature* 1988: **332**: 411–415.

209. Kumazaki T, Fujii T, Kobayashi M, Mitsui Y. Aging- and growth-dependent modulation of endothelin-1 gene expression in human vascular endothelial cells. *Exp. Cell Res.* 1994; **211**: 6–11.

210. Tokunaga O, Fan J, Watanabe T, Kobayashi M, Kumazaki T, Mitsui Y. Endothelin. Immunohistologic localization in aorta and biosynthesis by cultured human aortic endothelial cells. *Lab. Invest.* 1992; **67**: 210–217.

211. Garfinkel S, Haines DS, Brown S, Wessendorf J, Gillespie DH, Maciag T. Interleukin 1-alpha mediates an alternative pathway for the antiproliferative action of poly (I. C) on human endothelial cells. *J. Biol. Chem.* 1992; **267**: 24375–24378.

212. Wessendorf JHM, Garfinkel S, Zhan X, Brown S, Maciag T. Identification of a nuclear localization sequence within the structure of the human interleukin-1α precursor. *J. Biol. Chem.* 1993; **268**: 22100–22104.

213. Maier JAM, Voulalas P, Roeder D, Maciag T. Extension of the life-span of human endothelial cells by an interleukin-1α antisense oligomer. *Science* 1990; **249**: 1570–1574.

214. Garfinkel S, Brown S, Wessendorf JHM, Maciag T. Post-transcriptional regulation of interleukin-1α in various strains of young and senescent human umbilical vein endothelial cells. *Proc. Natl. Acad. Sci. USA* 1994; **91**: 1559–1563.

215. Ristimaki A, Garfinkel S, Wessendorf J, Maciag T, Hla T. Induction of cyclooxygenase-2 by interleukin-1α. *J. Biol. Chem.* 1994: **269**: 11769–11775.

216. Folkman J, Klagsbrun M. Angiogenic factors. *Science* 1987; **235**: 442–447.

217. Pepper MS, Vassalli J-D, Wilks JW, Schweigerer L, Orci L, Montesano R. Modulation of bovine microvascular endothelial cell proteolytic properties by inhibitors of angiogenesis. *J. Cell. Biochem.* 1994; **55**: 419–434.

218. Holm-Pedersen P, Nilsson K, Branemark PI. The microvascular system of healing wounds in young and old rats. *Adv. Microcirc.* 1973; **5**: 80–106.

219. Phillips GD, Stone AM, Schultz JC, Jones BD, Knighton DR. Proliferation of wound derived capillary endothelial cells: young versus aged. *Mech. Ageing Dev.* 1994; **77**: 141–148.

220. Pili R, Guo Y, Chang J, Nakanishi H, Martin GR, Passaniti A. Altered angiogenesis underlying age-dependent changes in tumor growth. *J. Natl. Cancer Inst.* 1994; **86**: 1303–1314.

221. Folkman J. Anti-angiogenesis: new concept of therapy of solid tumors. *Ann. Surg.* 1972; **175**: 409–416.

222. Brem S, Brem H, Folkman J, Finkelstein D, Patz A. Prolonged tumor dormancy by prevention of neovascularisation in the vitreous. *Cancer. Res.* 1976; **36**: 2807–2812.

223. Armitage P, Doll R. A two stage theory of carcinogenesis in relation to the age distribution of human cancer. *Br. J. Cancer* 1957; **11**: 161–169.

224. Barnes MJ, Bailey AJ, Gordon JL, MacIntyre DE. Platelet aggregation by basement membrane-associated collagens. *Thromb. Res.* 1980; **18**: 375–388.

225. Chiang TM, Mainardi CL, Seyer JM, Kang AH. Platelet interaction. Type V (A-B) collagen induces platelet aggregation. *J. Lab. Clin. Med.* 1980; **95**: 99–107.

226. Legrand YJ, Fauvel F, Arbeille B, Leger D, Mouhli H, Gutman N, Muh JP. Activation of platelets by microfibrils and collagen. a comparative study. *Lab. Invest.* 1986; **54**: 566–573.

227. Tryggvason K, Oikarinen J, Viinikka L, Ylikorkala O. Effects of laminin, proteoglycan and type IV collagen, components of basement membranes, on platelet aggregation. *Biochem. Biophys. Res. Commun.* 1981; **100**: 233–239.

228. Cohen I, Diegelmann RF, Lindblad WJ. *Wound Healing: Biochemical and Clinical Aspects.* Philadelphia: W.B. Saunders, 1992.

229. Weksler BB. Platelets. In *Inflammation: Basic Principles and Clinical Correlates*, edited by JI Gallin, IM Goldstein, R Snyderman. New York: Raven Press, pp. 543–557, 1988.

230. Peacock E. *Wound Repair*, 3rd ed. Philadelphia: W.B. Saunders, 1984.

231. Peacock E. Wound Healing and Wound Care. In *Principles of Surgery*, edited by S Schwartz, G Shires, F Spencer, 5th ed. New York: McGraw-Hill, pp. 307–330, 1989.

232. Brown GL, Nanney, LB, Griffen J, Cramer AB, Yancey JM, Curtsinger LJ, Holtzin L, Schultz GS, Jurkiewicz MJ, Lynch JB. Enhancement of wound healing by topical treatment with epidermal growth factor. *N. Engl. J. Med.* 1989; **321**: 76–79.

233. Daynes RA, Dowell T, Aranco BA. Platelet-derived growth factor is a potent biologic response modifier of T cells. *J. Exp. Med.* 1991; **174**: 1323–1333.

234. Sporn MB, Roberts AB. Transforming growth factor-beta — multiple actions and potential clinical applications. *JAMA* 1989; **262**: 938–941.

235. Clark RAF. Cutaneous tissue repair: Basic biologic considerations. *J. Am. Acad. Dermatol.* 1985; **13**: 701–725.

236. Hunt TK. *Wound Healing and Wound Infection: Theory and Surgical Practice.* New York: Appleton-Century-Crofts, 1980.

237. Hunt TK, Van Winkle W Jr. Fundamentals of wound management in surgery. In *Surgery: Wound Healing: Normal Repair.* South Plainfield, NJ: Chirogecom, 1976.

238. Madden JW, Arem AJ. Wound Healing: Biological and Clinical Features. In *Textbook of Surgery*, edited by DC Sabiston, 12th ed. Philadelphia: W.B. Saunders, pp. 265–286, 1981.

239. Bower RH. Nutrition and immune function. *Nutrition Clin. Prac.* 1990; **5**: 189–195.

240. Daly JM, Reynolds J, Thom A, Kinsley L, Dietrick-Gallagher M, Shou J, Ruggieri B. Immune and metabolic effects of arginine in the surgical patient. *Ann. Surg.* 1988; **208**: 512–523.

241. Orgill D, Demling RH. Current concepts and approaches to wound healing. *Crit. Care Med.* 1988; **16**: 899–908.

242. Pessa ME, Bland KI, Copeland EM III. Growth factors and determinants of wound repair. *J. Surg. Res.* 1987; **42**: 207–217.

243. Mansouri A, Hutchins LF. Coagulation in the Elderly. In *Geriatric Surgery: Comprehensive Care of the Elderly Patient*, edited by M Katlic. Baltimore, MD: Urban and Schwarzenberg, pp. 139–152, 1990.

244. Bruce SA, Deamond SF. Longitudinal study of *in vivo* wound repair and *in vitro* cellular senescence of dermal fibroblasts. *Exp. Gerontol.* 1991; **26**: 17–27.

245. Lipschitz D. Hematologic Changes in the Elderly. In *Geriatric Surgery: Comprehensive Care of the Elderly Patient*, edited by M Katlic. Baltimore, MD: Urban and Schwarzenberg, pp. 129–137, 1990.

246. O'Keefe EJ, Chui ML, Payne RE. Stimulation of growth of keratinocytes by basic fibroblast growth factor. *J. Invest. Dermatol.* 1988; **90**: 767–769.

247. Halaban R, Langdon R, Birchall N, Cuono C, Baird A, Scott G, Moellmann G, McGuire J. Basic fibroblast growth factor from human keratinocytes is a natural mitogen for melanocytes. *J. Cell. Biol.* 1988; **67**: 1611–1619.

248. Hennings H, Michael D, Cheng C, Steinert P, Holbrook K, Yuspa SH. Calcium regulation of growth and differentiation in mouse epidermal cells in culture. *Cell* 1980; **19**: 245–254.

249. Cohen S. The stimulation of epidermal proliferation by a specific protein (EGF). *Develop. Biol.* 1965; **12**: 394–407.

250. Brown GL, Curtsinger L, Brightwell JR, Ackerman DM, Tobin CR, Polk HC, George-Nascimento C, Valenzuela P, Schultz GS. Enhancement of epidermal regeneration by biosynthetic epidermal growth factor. *J. Exp. Med.* 1986; **163**: 1319–1324.

251. Franklin JD, Lynch JB. Effects of topical applications of epidermal growth factor on wound healing. *Plast. Reconstr. Surg.* 1979; **64**: 766–770.

252. Mertz PM, Davis SC, Arakawa Y, Cohen A. Pulsed rhEGF treatment increased epithelialization of partial thickness wounds. *J. Invest. Dermatol.* 1988; **90**: 588a.

253. Gilchrest BA, Marshall WL, Karassik RL, Weinstein R, Maciag T. Characterization and partial purification of keratinocyte growth factor from the hypothalamus. *J. Cell. Physiol.* 1984; **120**: 377–383.

254. Martinet N, Harne LA, Grotendorst GR. Identification and characterization of chemoattractants for epidermal cells. *J. Invest. Dermatol.* 1988; **90**: 122–126.

255. Mertz PM, Davis SC, Kilian P, Saunder DN. The effect of topical interleukin-1 on the epidermal healing rate of partial thickness wound. *Clin. Res.* 1988; **36**: 378a.

256. Lynch SE, Nixon JC, Colvin RB, Antoniades HN. Role of platelet-derived growth factor in wound healing: synergistic effects with other growth factors. *Proc. Natl. Acad. Sci. USA* 1987; **84**: 7696–7700.

257. O'Keefe EJ, Payne RE, Russell N. Keratinocyte growth-promoting activity from human placenta. *J. Cell. Physiol.* 1985; **124**: 439–445.

258. Stoker M, Gherardi E, Perryman M, Gray J. Scatter factor is a fibroblast-derived modulator of epithelial cell mobility. *Nature* 1987; **327**: 239–242.

259. Schultz GS, White N, Mitchell R, Brown G, Lynch JT, Wardzik DR, Todaro GL. Epithelial wound healing enhanced by transforming growth factor alpha and vaccinia growth factor. *Science* 1987; **235**: 350–352.

260. Barrandoh Y, Green H. Cell migration is essential for sustained growth of keratinocyte colonies: The role of transforming growth factor-alpha and epidermal growth factor. *Cell* 1987; **50**: 1131–1137.

261. Varni J, Nickoloff B, Riser B, Mitra R, Dixit V. Regulation of keratinocyte motility and proliferation by extracellular matrix components and cytokines. *FASEB J.* 1988; **2**: 1821A.

262. Tucker RF, Shipley GD, Moses HL, Holley RW. Growth inhibition from BSC-1 cells closely related to platelet type beta transforming growth factor. *Science* 1984; **226**: 705–707.

263. Knabbe C, Lippman E, Wakefield LM, Flanders KC, Kasid A, Derynck R, Dickson RB. Evidence that transforming growth factor beta is a hormonally regulated negative growth factor in human breast cancer cells. *Cell* 1987; **48**: 417–428.

264. Mansbridge JN, Hanawalt PC. Role of transforming growth factor beta in the maturation of human epidermal keratinocytes. *J. Invest. Dermatol.* 1988; **90**: 336–341.

265. Moses HL, Coffey RJ, Leof EB, Lyons RM, Keski-Oja J. Transforming growth factor beta in the maturation of human epidermal keratinocytes. *J. Invest. Dermatol.* 1988; **90**: 336–341.

266. Schwab R, Walters CA, Weksler ME. Host defense mechanisms and aging. *Sem. Oncol.* 1989; **16**: 20–27.

267. Newell GR, Spitz MR, Sider JG. Cancer and age. *Sem. Oncol.* 1989; **16**: 3–9.

268. Miller RA. Aging and Immune function. *Int. Rev. Cytol.* 1991; **124**: 187–215.

269. Roberts-Thomson IC, Whittingham S, Youngchaiyud S, Mackay IR. Ageing, immune response, and mortality. *Lancet.* 1974; **2:** 368–370.

270. Flood PM, Urban JL, Kripke ML, Schreiber H. Loss of tumor-specific and idiotype-specific immunity with age. *J. Exp. Med.* 1981; **154:** 275–290.

271. Walters CS, Claman HN. Age-related changes in cell-mediated immunity in BALB/C mice. *J. Immunol.* 1975; **115:** 1438–1443.

272. Kishimoto S, Tomino S, Mitsuya H, Fujiwara H, Tsuda H. Age-related decline in the *in vitro* and *in vivo* syntheses of anti-tetanus toxoid antibody in humans. *J. Immunol.* 1980; **125:** 2347–2352.

273. Kay MMB, Mendoza J, Divan J, Denton T, Union N, Lajiness M. Age-related changes in the immune system of mice of eight medium and long lived strains and hybrids. 1. organ, cellular, and activity changes. *Mech. Ageing Dev.* 1979; **11:** 295–346.

274. Nagel JE, Chopra RK, Chrest FJ, McCoy MT, Schneider EL, Holbrook NJ, Adler WH. Decreased proliferation, interleukin 2 synthesis, and interlukin 2 receptor expression are accompanied by decreased mRNA expression in phytohemagglutinin-stimulated cells from elderly donors. *J. Clin. Invest.* 1988; **81:** 1096–1102.

275. Miller RA. Age-associated decline in precursor frequency for different T cell-mediated reactions, with preservation of helper or cytotoxic effect per precursor cell. *J. Immunol.* 1984; **132:** 63–68.

276. Vie H, Miller RA. Decline, with age, in the proportion of mouse T cells that express IL-2 receptors after mitogen stimulation. *Mech. Ageing Dev.* 1986; **33:** 313–322.

277. Hadden JW, Malec PH, Coto J, Hadden EM. Thymic involution in aging: Prospects for correction. *Ann. N. Y. Acad. Sci.* 1992; **673:** 231–239.

278. Lewis VM, Twomey JJ, Bealmear P, Goldstein G, Good RA. Age, thymic involution and circulating thymic hormone activity. *J. Clin. Endocrinol. Metab.* 1978; **47:** 145–150.

279. De Paoli P, Battistin S, Santini GF. Age-related changes in human lymphocyte subsets: Progressive reduction of the CD4 CD45R (suppressor inducer) population. *Clin. Immunol. Immunopath.* 1988; **48:** 290–296.

280. Globerson A, Sharp A, Fridkis-Hareli M, Kukulansky T, Abel L, Knyszynski A, Eren R. Aging in the T lymphocyte compartment: a developmental view. *Ann. N. Y. Acad. Sci.* 1992; **673:** 240–251.

281. Lerner A, Yamada T, Miller RA. Pgp-1^{hi} T lymphocytes accumulate with age in mice and respond poorly to concanavalin A. *Eur. J. Immunol.* 1989; **19:** 977–982.

282. Song, L, Kim YH, Chopra RK, Proust JJ, Nagel JE, Nordin AA, Adler WH. Age-related effects in T cell activation and proliferation. *Exp. Gerontol.* 1993; **28:** 313–321.

283. Dozmorov IM, Kalinichenko VV, Sidorov IA, Miller RA. Antagonistic interactions among T cell subsets of old mice revealed by limiting dilution analysis. *J. Immunol.* 1995; **154:** 4283–4293.

284. Hobbs MV, Weigle WO, Ernst DN. Interleukin-10 production by splenic CD4$^+$ cells and cell subsets from young and old mice. *Cell Immunol.* 1994; **154:** 264–272.

285. Berridge MJ. Inositol triphosphate and diacylglycerol: two interacting second messengers. *Annu. Rev. Biochem.* 1987; **56:** 159–193.

286. Grossman A, Rabinovitch PS, Kavanagh TJ, Jinneman JC, Gilliland LK, Ledbetter JA, Kanner SB. Activation of murine T-cells via phospholipase-Cγ1–associated protein tyrosine phosphorylation is reduced with aging. *J. Gerontol.* 1995; **50A:** B205–B212.

287. Shi J, Miller RA. Tyrosine-specific protein phosphorylation in response to anti-CD3 antibody is diminished in old mice. *J. Gerontol.* 1992; **47:** B147–B153.

288. Whisler RL, Beijing L, Wu L, Chen M. Reduced activation of transcriptional factor AP-1 among peripheral blood T cells from elderly humans after PHA stimulation: restorative effect of phorbol diesters. *Cell. Immunol.* 1993; **152:** 96–109.

289. Miller RA. Immunodeficiency of aging: Restorative effects of phorbol ester combined with calcium ionophore. *J. Immunol.* 1986; **137:** 805–808.

290. Kanner SB, Kavanagh TJ, Grossmann A, Hu S, Bolen JB, Rabinovitch PS, Ledbetter JA. Sulfhydryl oxidation down-regulates T-cell signaling and inhibits tyrosine phosphorylation of phospholipase Cγ1. *Proc. Natl. Acad. Sci. USA* 1992; **89:** 300–304.

291. Kavanagh TJ, Grossmann A, Jinneman JC, Kanner SB, White CC, Eaton DL, Ledbetter JA, Rabinovitch PS. The effect of 1-chloro-2,4-dinitrobenzene exposure on antigen receptor (CD3)-stimulated transmembrane signal transduction in purified subsets of human peripheral blood lymphocytes. *Toxicol. Appl. Pharmacol.* 1993; **119:** 91–99.

292. Shaw A, Thomas ML. Coordinate interactions of protein tyrosine kinases and protein tyrosine phosphatases in T-cell receptor-mediated signaling. *Curr. Opin. Cell Biol.* 1991; **3:** 862–868.

293. El-Hag A, Lipsky PE, Bennett M, Clark RA. Immunomodulation by neutrophil myeloperoxidase and hydrogen peroxide: Differential susceptibility of human lymphocyte functions. *J. Immunol.* 1986; **136:** 3420–3426.

294. Steller H. Mechanisms and genes of cellular suicide. *Science* 1995; **267:** 1445–1449.

295. D'Adamio L, Awad KM, Reinherz EL. Thymic and peripheral apoptosis of antigen-specific T cells might cooperate in establishing self tolerance. *Eur. J. Immunol.* 1993; **23:** 747–753.

296. Kabelitz D, Pohl T, Pechhold K. Activation-induced cell death (apoptosis) of mature peripheral T lymphocytes. *Immunol. Today.* 1993; **14:** 338–339.

297. Nagata S, Golstein P. The Fas death factor. *Science* 1995; **267:** 1449–1456.

298. Zhou T, Edwards CK III, Mountz JD. Prevention of age-related T cell apoptosis defect in CD2-*fas*-transgenic mice. *J. Exp. Med.* 1995; **182:** 129–137.

299. Burns EA, Lum LG, Hommedieu GL, Goodwin JS. Specific humoral immunity in the elderly: *in vivo* and *in vitro* response to vaccination. *J. Gerontol.* 1993; **48:** B231–B236.

300. Szakal AK, Taylor JK, Smith JP, Kosco MH, Burton GF, Tew JG. Kinetics of germinal center development in lymph nodes of young and aging immune mice. *Anat. Rec.* 1990; **227:** 475–482.

301. Hathcock KS, Laszlo G, Dickler HB, Bradshaw J, Linsley P, Hodes RJ. Identification of an alternative CTLA4 ligand co-stimulatory for T cell activation. *Science* 1993; **262:** 905–908.

302. Miller C, Kelsoe G, Han S. Lack of B7-2 expression in the germinal centers of aged mice. *Aging Immunol. Infect. Dis.* 1994; **5:** 249–257.

303. Li, SP, Miller RA. Age-associated decline in IL-4 production by murine T lymphocytes in extended culture. *Cell. Immunol.* 1993; **151:** 187–195.

304. Zharhary D, Klinman NR. Antigen responsiveness of the mature and generative B cell population of aged mice. *J. Exp. Med.* 1983; **157:** 1300–1308.

305. Zharhary D, Klinman NR. A selective increase in the generation of phosphorylcholine-specific B cells associated with aging. *J. Immunol.* 1986; **136:** 368–370.

306. Riley SC, Froscher BG, Linton PJ, Zharhary D, Marcu K, Klinman NR. Altered V$_H$ gene segment utilization in the response to phosphorylcholine by aged mice. *J. Immunol.* 1989; **143:** 3798–3805.

307. Zharhary D. T cell involvement in the decrease of antigen-responsive B cells in aged mice. *Eur. J. Immunol.* 1986; **16:** 1175–1178.

308. Whisler RL, Williams JW Jr, Newhouse YG. Human B cell proliferative responses during aging. Reduced RNA synthesis and DNA replication after signal transduction by surface immunoglobulins compared to B cell antigenic determinants CD20 and CD40. *Mech. Ageing Dev.* 1991; **61:** 209–222.

309. Whisler RL, Grants IS. Age-related alterations in the activation and expression of phosphotyrosine kinases and protein kinase C (PKC) among human B cells. *Mech. Ageing Dev.* 1993; **71:** 31–46.

310. Perskin MH, Cronstein BN. Age-related changes in neutrophil structure and function. *Mech. Ageing Dev.* 1992; **64:** 303–313.

311. Chatta GS, Andrews RG, Rodger E, Schrag M, Hammond WP, Dale DC. Hematopoietic progenitors and aging: alterations in granulocytic precursors and responsiveness to recombinant human G-CSF, GM-CSF, and IL-3. *J. Gerontol.* 1993; **48**: M207–M212.

312. Higashimoto Y, Fukuchi Y, Shimada Y, Ishida K, Ohata M, Furuse T, Shu C, Teramoto S, Matsuse T, Sudo E, Orimo H. The effects of aging on the function of aveolar macrophages in mice. *Mech. Ageing Dev.* 1993; **69**: 207–217.

313. Ding A, Hwang S, Schwab R. Effect of aging on murine macrophages: Diminished response to INF-γ for enhanced oxidative metabolism. *J. Immunol.* 1994; **153**: 2146–2152.

314. Engelberg D, Klein C, Martinetto H, Struhl K, Karin M. The UV response involving the Ras signaling pathway and AP-1 transcription factors is conserved between yeast and mammals. *Cell* 1994; **77**: 381–390.

315. Hibi M, Lin A, Smeal T, Minden A, Karin M. Identification of an oncoprotein and UV-responsive protein kinase that binds and potentiates the c-Jun activation domain. *Genes Dev.* 1993; **7**: 2135–2148.

316. Galcheva-Gargova Z, Derijard B, Wu I, Davis R. An osmo-sensing signal transduction pathway in mammalian cells. *Science* 1994; **265**: 806–808.

317. Han J, Lee JD, Bibbs L, Ulevitch RJ. A MAP kinase targeted by endotoxin and hyperosmolarity in mammalian cells. *Science* 1994; **265**: 808–811.

318. Beauchamp RD, Papaconstantinou J, Henderson AM, Shen HM, Townsend CM Jr, Thompson JC. Activation of hepatic proliferation-associated transcription factors by lipopolysaccharide. *Surgery*. 1994; **116**(2): 367–376.

319. Coppola JA, Coleb MD. Constitutive c-myc oncogene expression blocks mouse erythroleukemia cell differentiation but not commitment. *Nature* 1986; **320**: 760–763.

320. Kingston RE, Baldwin AS, Sharp PA. Regulation of heat shock protein 70 gene expression by c-myc. *Nature* 1984; **312**: 280–282.

321. Lowy MT, Wittenberg L, Yamamoto BK. Effect of acute stress on hippocampal glutamate levels and spectrin proteolysis in young and aged rats. *J. Neurochem.* 1995; **65**: 268–274.

322. Sapolsky RM. Glucocorticoids, hippocampal damage and glutamatergic synapse. In *Progress in Brain Research*, edited by E Coleman, G Higgin and C Phelps, No. 86. Amsterdam: Elsevier Science Publishers B.V., pp. 13–23, 1990.

323. Sapolsky, RM. Do glucocorticoid concentrations rise with age in the rat? *Neurobiol. Aging* 1991; **13**: 171–174.

324. Erisman S, Carnes M, Takahashi LK, Lent SJ. The effects of stress on plasma ACTH and corticosterone in young and aging pregnant rats and their fetuses. *Life Sci.* 1990; **47**: 1527–1533.

325. Meaney MJ, Aitken DH, van Berkel C, Bhatnagar S, Sapolsky RM. Effect of neonatal handling on age-related impairments associated with the hippocampus. *Science* 1988; **239**: 766–768.

326. Lindquist S, Craig EA. The heat shock proteins. *Ann. Rev. Genet.* 1988; **22**: 631–677.

327. Halladay JT, Craig EA. A heat shock transcription factor with reduced activity suppresses a yeast HSP 70 mutant. *Mol. Cell. Biol.* 1995; **15**: 4890–4897.

328. Morimoto R I. Cell in stress: transcriptional activation of heat shock genes. *Science* 1993; **259**: 1409–1410.

329. Engelberg D, Zandi E, Parker CS, Karin M. The yeast and mammalian Ras pathways control transcription of heat shock genes independently of heat shock transcription factor. *Mol. Cell Biol.* 1994; **14**: 4929–37.

330. Riabowol KT, Mizzen LA, Welch WJ. Heat shock is lethal to fibroblasts microinjected with antibodies against hsp 70. *Science* 1988; **242**: 433–436.

331. Johnston RN, Kucey BL. Competitive inhibition of hsp 70 gene expression causes thermosensitivity. *Science* 1988; **242**: 1551–1554.

332. Li GC, Li L, Liu YK, Mak JY, Chen L, Lee WM. Thermal response of rat fibroblasts stably transfected with the human 70-kDa heat shock protein-encoding gene. *Proc. Natl. Acad. Sci. USA* 1991; **88**: 1681–1685.

333. Koroshetz WJ, Bonventre JV. Heat shock response in the central nervous system. *Experientia* 1994; **50**: 1085–1091.

334. Heydari AR, Wu B, Takahashi R, Strong R, Richardson A. Expression of heat shock protein 70 is altered by age and diet at the level of transcription. *Mol. Cell. Biol.* 1993; **13**: 2909–2918.

335. Fawcett TW, Sylvester SL, Sarge KD, Morimoto RI, Holbrook NJ. Effects on neurohormonal stress and aging on the activation of mammalian heat shock factor 1. *J. Biol. Chem.* 1994; **269**: 32272–32278.

336. Blake MJ, Fargnoli J, Gershon D, Holbrook NJ. Concomitant decline in heat-induced hyperthermia and HSP70 mRNA expression in aged rat. *Am. J. Physiol.* 1991; **260**: 663–667.

337. Udelsman R, Blake MJ, Stage CA, Li D, Putney DJ, Holbrook NJ. Vascular heat shock protein expression in response to stress. Endocrine and autonomic regulation of this age-dependent response. *J. Clin. Invest.* 1993; **91**: 465–473.

338. Liu AY, Lin Z, Choi H, Sorhage F, Li. B Attenuated induction of heat shock gene expression in aging diploid fibroblasts. *J. Biol. Chem.* 1989; **264**: 12037–12045.

339. Liu AY, Choi H, Lee Y, Chen K. Molecular events involved in transcriptional activation of heat shock genes become progressively refractory to heat stimulation during aging of human diploid fibroblasts. *J. Cell. Physiol.* 1991; **149**: 560–566.

340. Pahlavani MA, Harris MD, Moore SA, Weindruch R, Richardson A. The expression of heat shock protein 70 decreases with age in lymphocytes from rats and rhesus monkeys. *Exp. Cell Res.* 1995; **218**: 310–318.

341. Jones TS, Liang AP, Kilbourne EM, Griffin MR, Patriarca PA, Wassilak SGF, Mullan RJ, Herrick RF, Donnell HD, Choi K, Thacker SB. Morbidity and mortality associated with the July 1980 heat wave in St. Louis and Kansas City, Mo. *J. Am. Med. Assoc.* 1982; **247**: 3327–3355.

342. Rothstein M. Enzymes, enzyme alteration, and protein turnover. In *Review of Biological Research in Aging*, edited by M Rothstein, vol. 1. New York: Alan R. Liss. Inc., pp. 305–314, 1983.

343. Stadtman ER. Protein oxidation and aging. *Science* 1992; **257**: 1220–1224.

344. Harman D. Role of free radical and radiation chemistry. *J. Gerontol.* 1956; **11**: 298–300.

345. Sohal RS, Orr WC. Is oxidative stress a causal factor in aging? In *Molecular Aspects of Aging*, edited by K Esser and GM Martin. Chichester: John Wiley & Sons Ltd., pp. 109–127, 1995.

346. Zglinicki T, Saretzki G, Docke W, Lotze C. Mild hyperoxia shortens telomeres and inhibits proliferation of fibroblasts: a model for senescence? *Exp. Cell Res.* 1995; **220**: 186–193.

347. Ames BN, Shigenaga MK, Hagen TM. Oxidants, antioxidants, and the degenerative diseases of aging. *Proc. Natl. Acad. Sci. USA* 1993; **90**: 7915–7922.

348. Chen Q, Fischer A, Reagan JR, Yan LJ, Ames BN. Oxidative DNA damage and senescence of human diploid fibroblast cell. *Proc. Natl. Acad. Sci. USA* 1995; **92**: 4337–4341.

349. Hirsch-Kauffmann M, Schwaiger H, Auer B, Schneider R, Herzog H, Klocker H, Schweiger M. Aging and DNA repair. In *Molecular Mechanism of Aging*, edited by K Beyreuther and G Schettler, pp. 51–59. Berlin: Springer, 1990.

350. Shay JW, Werbin H, Piatyszek MA. Does aging favor translocation of mitochondial DNA fragments to the nuclear genome? In *Molecular Aspects of Aging*, edited by K Esser and GM Martin. Chichester: John Wiley & Sons Ltd., pp. 179–189, 1995.

351. Richter C. Do mitochondial DNA fragments promote cancer and aging? *FEBS Lett.* 1988; **241**: 1–5.

352. Muller-Hocker J. Cytochrom c oxidase deficient fibers in the limb muscle and diaphragm of man without muscular disease: an age-related alteration. *J. Neurol. Sci.* 1990; **100**: 14–21.

353. Hayakawa M, Hattori H, Sugiyama S, Ozawa T. Age-associated oxygen damage and mutations in mitochondrial DNA in human heart. *Biochim. Biophys. Res. Comm.* 1992; **189**: 979–985.

354. Corral-Debrinski M, Horton T, Lott MT, Shoffner JM, Beal MF, Wallace DC. Mitochondrial DNA deletion in human brain: regional variability and increase with advanced age. *Nature Genet.* 1992; **2**: 324–329.

355. Fraga CG, Shigenaga MK, Park WJ, Degan P, Ames BN. Oxidative damage to DNA during aging: 8-hydroxy-2'-deoxyguanosine in rat organ DNA and urine. *Proc. Natl. Acad. Sci. USA* 1990; **87**: 4533–4537.

356. Adachi K, Fujiura Y, Mayumi F, Nozuhara A, Sugiu Y, Sakanashi T, Hidaka T, Toshima H. A deletion of mitochondrial DNA in murine doxorubicin-induced cardiotoxicity. *Biochem, Biophys. Res. Comm.* 1983; **195**: 945–951.

357. Asano K, Amagase S, Matsuura ET, Yamagishi H. Changes in the rat liver mitochondrial DNA upon aging. *Mech. Ageing Dev.* 1991; **60**: 275–284.

358. Wallace DC. Mitochondrial DNA mutations in human diseases and aging. In *Molecular Aspects of Aging*, edited by K Esser and GM Martin. Chichester: John Wiley & Sons Ltd., pp. 163–177, 1995.

359. Wallace DC. Diseases of the mitochondrial DNA. *Annu. Rev. Biochem.* 1992; **61**: 1175–1212.

360. Fukuchi K, Martin GM, Monnat RJ Jr. Mutator phenotype of Werner syndrome is charicterized by extensive deletions. *Proc. Natl. Acad. Sci. USA* 1989; **86**: 5893–5897.

361. Salk D, Au D, Hoehn H, Martin GM. Cytogenetics of Werner's syndrome cultured skin fibroblasts: variegated translocation mosaicism. *Cytogenet. Cell Genet.* 1981; **30**: 92–107.

362. Oliver CN, Ahn BW, Moerman EJ, Goldstein S. Age-related changes in oxidized protein. *J. Biol. Chem.* 1987; **262**: 5488–5491.

363. Davies KJA. Protein damage and degradation by oxygen radicals. I. general aspects. *J. Biol. Chem.* 1987; **262**: 9895–9901.

364. Stadtman ER. The status of oxidatively modified protein as a mark of aging. In *Molecular Aspects of Aging*, edited by K Esser and GM Martin. Chichester: John Wiley & Sons Ltd., pp. 129–143, 1995.

365. Dean RT, Gieseg S, Davies MJ. Reactive species and their accumulation on radical-damaged proteins. *Trends Biochem. Sci.* 1993; **18**: 437–441.

366. Rivett AJ. Preferential degradation of the oxidatively modified form of glutamine synthetase by intracellular mammalian proteases. *J. Biol. Chem.* 1985; **260**: 300–305.

367. Rivett AJ. The multicatalytic protease of mammalian cells. *Arch. Biochem. Biophys.* 1989; **268**: 1–8.

368. Davies KJA, Lin SW, Pacifici RE. Protein damage and degradation by oxygen radicals. IV. Degradation of denatured protein. *J. Biol. Chem.* 1987; **262**: 9914–9920

369. Davies KJA. The red cell as a model. In *Cellular and Molecular Aspects of Aging*, edited by JW Eaton, DK Konzen and JG White. New York: Liss, pp. 15–24, 1984.

370. Baynes JW. Role of oxidative stress in development of complications in diabetes. *Diabetes* 1991; **40**: 405–412.

371. Ischiropoulos H, Zhu L, Chen J, Tsai M, Martin JC, Smith CD, Beckman JS. Peroxynitrite-mediated tyrosine nitration catalyzed by superoxide dismutase. *Arch. Biochem. Biophys.* 1992; **298**: 431–437.

372. Laganiere S, Yu BP. Modulation of membrane phospholipid fatty acid composition by age and food restriction. *Gerontology* 1993; **39**: 7–18.

373. Yu BP, Suescun EA, Yang SY. Effect of age-related lipid peroxidation on membrane fluidity and phospholipase A_2: modulation by dietary restriction. *Mech. Ageing. Dev.* 1992; **65**: 17–33.

374. Orr WC, Sohal RS. Extension of life span by overexpression of superoxide dismutase and catalase in Drosophila melanogaster. *Science* 1994; **263**: 1128–1130.

375. Sohal RS, Allen RG. Relationship between oxygen metabolism, aging and development. *Adv. Free Rad. Biol. Med.* 1986; **2**: 117–160.

376. Agarwal S, Sohal RS. Relationship between aging and susceptibility to protein oxidative damage. *Biochem. Biophys. Res. Comm.* 1993; **194**: 1203–1206.

377. Sohal RS, Orr WC. Relationship between antioxidants, prooxidants, and the aging process. *Ann. N. Y. Acad. Sci.* 1992; **663**: 74–84.

378. Smith CD, Carney JM, Starke-Reed PE, Oliver CN, Stadtman ER, Floyd RA. Excess brain protein oxidation and enzyme dysfunction in normal and aging and Alzheimer's disease. *Proc. Natl. Acad. Sci. USA* 1991; **88**: 10540–10543.

379. Garland D, Russle P, Zigler JS. Oxidative modification of lens proteins. In *Oxygen Radicals in Biology and Medicine*, edited by MG Simic, KS Taylor, JF Ward, and C Sontag. New York: Plenum, pp. 347–353, 1988.

380. Starke-Reed PE, Oliver CN. Protein oxidation and proteolysis during aging and oxidative stress. *Arch. Biochem. Biophys.* 1989; **275**: 559–567.

381. Heydari AR, Takahashi R, Gutsmann A, You S, Richardson A. Hsp70 and aging. *Experientia* 1994; **50**: 1092–1098.

382. Fargnoli J, Kunisada T, Fornace AJ, Schneider EL, Holbrook NJ. Decreased expression of heat shock protein 70 mRNA and protein after heat treatment in cells of aged rats. *Proc. Natl. Acad. Sci. USA* 1990; **85**: 846–850.

383. Pardue S, Groshan JD Raese, Morrison-Bogorad M. Hsp 70 mRNA induction is reduced in neurons of aged rat hippocampus after thermal stress. *Neurobiol. Aging* 1992; **13**: 661–672.

384. Wu B, Gu MJ, Heydari AR, Richardson A. The effect of age on the synthesis of two heat shock proteins in the HSP 70 family. *J. Gerontol.* 1993; **48**: B50–B56.

385. Luce MC, Cristofalo VJ. Reduction in heat shock gene expression correlates with increased thermosensitivity in senescent human fibroblasts. *Exp. Cell Res.* 1992; **202**: 9–16.

386. Effros RB, Zhu X, Walford RL. Stress response of senescent T lymphocytes: Reduced hsp 70 is independent of the proliferative block. *J. Gerontol.* 1994; **49**: B65–B70.

387. Sun J, Kale SP, Childress AM, Pinswasdi C, Jazwinski SM. Divergent roles of *RAS1* and *RAS2* in yeast longevity. *J. Biol. Chem.* 1994; **269**: 18638–18645.

388. Broach, JR, Deschenes RJ. The function of *RAS* genes in *Saccharomyces cerevisiae*. *Adv. Cancer Res.* 1990; **54**: 79–139.

389. Kale SP, Jazwinski SM. Differential response to UV stress and DNA damage during the yeast replicative life span. *Dev. Genet.* 1996; **18**: 154–160.

390. D'mello NP, Childress AM, Franklin DS, Kale SP, Pinswasdi C, Jazwinski SM. Cloning and characterization of *LAG1*, a longevity-assurance gene in yeast. *J. Biol. Chem.* 1994; **269**: 15451–15459.

391. Friedman DB, Johnson TE. A mutation in the *age-1* gene in *Caenorhabditis elegans* lengthens life and reduces hermaphrodite fertility. *Genetics* 1988; **118**: 75–86.

392. Vanfleteren JR. Oxidative stress and ageing in *Caenorhabditis elegans*. *Biochem. J.* 1993; **292**: 605–608.

393. Larsen PL. Aging and resistance to oxidative damage in *Caenorhabditis elegans*. *Proc. Natl. Acad. Sci. USA* 1993; **90**: 8905–8909.

394. Lithgow GJ, White TM, Hinerfeld DA, Johnson TE. Thermotolerance of a long-lived mutant of *Caenorhabditis elegans*. *J. Gerontol. Biol. Sci.* 1994; **49**: B270–276.

395. Sanchez Y, Taulien J, Borkovich KA, Lindquist SL. Hsp104 is required for tolerance to many forms of stress. *EMBO J.* 1992; **11**: 2357–2364.

396. Kenyon C, Chang J, Gensch E, Rudner A, Tabtlang R. A *C. elegans* mutant that lives twice as long as wild type. *Nature* 1993; **366**: 461–464.

397. Larsen PL, Albert PS, Riddle DL. Genes that regulate both development and longevity in *Caenorhabditis elegans*. *Genetics* 1995; **139**: 1567–1583.

398. Lithgow GJ, White TM, Melov S, Johnson TE. Longevity mutants of *Caenorhabditis elegans* exhibit increased intrinsic thermotolerance. *Proc. Natl. Acad. Sci. USA* 1995; **92**: 7540–7544.

399. Luckinbill LS, Arking R, Clare MJ, Cirocco WC, Buck SA. Selection for delayed senescence in *Drosophila melanogaster*. *Evolution.* 1984; **38**: 996–1003.

400. Rose MR. Laboratory evolution of postponed senescence in *Drosophila melanogaster*. *Evolution* 1984; **38**: 1004–1010.

401. Partridge L, Fowler K. Direct and correlated responses to selection on age at reproduction in *Drosophila melanogaster*. *Evolution* 1992; **46**: 76–91.

402. Arking R, Dudas SP, Baker GT. Genetic and environmental factors regulating the expression of an extended longevity phenotype in a long lived strain of *Drosophila*. *Genetica*. 1993; **91**: 127–142.

403. Service PM, Hutchinson EW, Mackinley MD, Rose MR. Resistance to environmental stress in Drosophila melanogaster selected for postponed senescence. *Physiol. Zool.* 1985; **58**: 380–389.

404. Tyler RH, Brar H, Singh M, Latorre A, Graves JL, Mueller LD, Rose MR, Ayala FJ. The effect of superoxide dismutase alleles on aging in *Drosophila*. *Genetica* 1993; **91**: 143–149.

405. Scheinman RI, Cogswell PC, Lofquist AK, Baldwin AS. Role of transcriptional activation of IκBα in mediation of immunosuppression by glucocorticoids. *Science* 1995; **270**: 283–286.

406. Auphan N, DiDonato JA, Rosette C, Helmberg A, Karin M. Immunosuppression by glucocorticoids: inhibition of NF-kB activity through induction of IκB synthesis. *Science* 1995; **270**: 286–290.

407. Bilger B. Forever young. *The Sciences* 1995; **35**: 26–31.

408. Finch CE. *Longevity, Senescence, and the Genome*. Chicago, IL: University of Chicago Press, 1990.

409. Daynes RA, Araneo BA, Ershler WB, Maloney C, Li GZ, Ryu SY. Altered regulation of IL-6 production with normal aging. Possible linkage to the age-associated decline in dehydroepiandrosterone and its sulfated derivative. *J. Immunol*. 1993; **150**: 5219–5230.

410. Ershler WB, Sun WH, Binkley N, Gravenstein S, Volk MJ, Kamoske G, Klopp RG, Roecker EB, Daynes RA, Weindruch R. Interleukin-6 and aging: blood levels and mononuclear cell production increase with advancing age and *in vitro* production is modifiable by dietary restriction. *Lymphokine Cytokine Res.* 1993; **12**: 225–230.

411. Volk MJ, Pugh TD, Kim M, Frith CH, Daynes RA, Ershler WB, Weindruch R. Dietary restriction from middle age attenuates age-associated lymphoma development and interleukin 6 dysregulation in C57BL/6 mice. *Cancer Res.* 1994; **54**: 3054–3061.

412. Orentreich N, Brind JL, Rizer RL, Vogelman JH. Age changes and sex differences in serum dehydroepiandrosterone sulfate concentration throughout adulthood. *J. Clin. Endocrinol. Metab.* 1984; **59**: 551–555.

413. Harris MI, Hadden WC, Knowler WC, Bennett PH. Prevalence of diabetes and impaired glucose tolerance and plasma glucose levels in U. S. population aged 20–74. *Diabetes* 1987; **36**: 523–524.

414. Hayashi K. Insulin insensitivity and hyposuppressibility of glucagon by hyperglycemia in aged Wistar rats. *Gerontology* 1982; **28**: 10–18.

415. Mobbs CV. Neurotoxic effects of estrogen, glucose, and glucocorticoids: Neurohumoral hysteresis and its pathological consequences during aging. In *Review of Biological Research in Aging*, edited by M Rothstein, Vol. 4. New York, NY: Wiley-Liss, pp. 201–228, 1990.

416. Coordt MC, Ruhe RC, McDonald RB. Aging and insulin secretion. *Proc. Soc. Exp. Biol. Med.* 1995; **209**: 213–222.

417. Yu BP. Food restriction research: Past and present status. In *Review of Biological Research in Aging*, edited by M Rothstein. New York, NY: Wiley-Liss, 1990; **4**: 349–371.

418. Masoro EJ, Katz MS, McMahan CA. Evidence for the glycation hypothesis of aging from the food-restricted rodent model. *J. Gerontol.* 1989; **44**: B20–B22.

419. Cefalu WT, Bell-Farrow AD, Wang ZQ, Sonntag WE, Fu M-X, Baynes JW, Thorpe SR. Caloric restriction decreases age-dependent accumulation of the glycoxidation products, Nᵉ-(carboxymethyl)lysine and pentosidine, in rat skin collagen. *J. Gerontol. Biol. Sci.* 1995; **50A**: B337–B341.

420. Weindruch R, Walford RL. Dietary restriction in mice beginning at 1 year of age: effect on life-span and spontaneous cancer incidence. *Science* 1982; **215**: 1415–1418.

421. Hursting SD, Perkins SN, Phang JM. Calorie restriction delays spontaneous tumorigenesis in p53-knockout transgenic mice. *Proc. Natl. Acad. Sci. USA* 1994; **91**: 7036–7040.

422. Richardson A, McCarter R. Mechanism of food restriction: Change of rate or change of set point? In *The Potential for Nutritional Modulation of the Aging Processes*, edited by DK Ingram, GT Baker and NW Shock. Trumbull, CT: Food & Nutrition Press, pp. 177–192, 1991.

423. Heydari AR, Richardson A. Does gene expression play any role in the mechanism of the antiaging effect of dietary restriction? *Ann. N. Y. Acad. Sci.* 1992; **663**: 384–395.

424. Stewart J, Meaney MJ, Aitken D, Jensen L, Kalant N. The effects of acute and life-long food restriction on basal and stress-induced serum corticosterone levels in young and aged rats. *Endocrinology* 1988; **123**: 1934–1941.

425. Pashko LL, Schwartz AG. Reversal of food restriction-induced inhibition of mouse skin tumor promotion by adrenalectomy. *Carcinogenesis* 1992; **13**: 1925–1928.

426. Kalu DK, Cockerham R, Yu BP, Roos BA. Lifelong dietary modulation of calcitonin levels in rats. *Endocrinology* 1983; **113**: 2010–2016.

427. Kalu DK, Hardin RR, Cockerham R, Yu BP, Norling BK, Egan JW. Lifelong food restriction prevents senile osteopenia and hyperparathyroidism in F344 rats. *Mech. Ageing Dev.* 1984; **26**: 103–112.

428. Holehan AM, Merry BJ. The control of puberty in the dietary restricted female rat. *Mech. Ageing Dev.* 1985; **32**: 179–191.

429. Snyder DL, Towne B. The effect of dietary restriction on serum hormone and blood chemistry changes in aging Lobund-Wistar rats. In *Dietary Restriction and Aging*, edited by DL Snyder. New York: Alan R. Liss, pp. 135–146, 1989.

430. Sapolsky RM, Krey L, McEwen BS. The adrenocortical stress-response in the aged male rat: impairment of recovery from stress. *Exp. Gerontol.* 1983; **18**: 55–63.

8. Age as a Risk Factor in Multistage Carcinogenesis

Vladimir N. Anisimov

Introduction

Cancer is a common cause of disability and death in the elderly: over 50% of malignant neoplasms occur in persons over 70 (1–3). The relationship between aging and cancer is not clear: considerable controversy surrounds the mechanisms that lead to increased incidence of cancer in the aged. Two major hypotheses have been proposed to explain the association of cancer and age. The first hypothesis holds this association is a consequence of the duration of carcinogenesis. In other words, the sequential carcinogenic steps that are required for the neoplastic transformation of normal tissues develop over several years and cancer is more likely to become manifest in older individuals by a process of natural selection (4,5). In an article entitled, "There is no such thing as aging, and cancer is not related to it," Peto *et al.* (5) have proposed that the high prevalence of cancer in older individuals simply reflects a more prolonged exposure to carcinogens. In the estimate of these authors, the incidence of cancer is a power function of the duration of carcinogen exposure, rather than a power function of the tumor-host age.

The second hypothesis proposes that age-related progressive changes in the internal milieu of the organism may provide an increasingly favorable environment for the induction of new neoplasms and for the growth of already existent, but latent malignant cells (6,7). The internal milieu includes cells and tissue microenvironment. Predisposing factors to carcinogenesis include age-related disturbances in metabolism and DNA repair, immunesenescence, decreased ability of the tissue microenvironment to inhibit cell proliferation and to favor cell differentiation (6,8–10). These hypotheses have been reviewed elsewhere (6–8). The elucidation of causes of an age-related increase in cancer incidence may be the key to a strategy for primary cancer prevention.

Age and Spontaneous Tumor Development

It is well documented that the incidence of malignant tumors increases progressively with age, both in animals and humans (1–3,6,11). The term "spontaneous tumors" may be misleading, as the majority of these neoplasms are caused by environmental factors, including tobacco smoking, diet, alcohol consumption, sexual promiscuity, industrial byproducts, ultraviolet radiations, drugs, and oncogenic viruses (12).

The overall incidence of cancer increases with age, but this increment is not uniform for all types of cancer. In animals, genetic influences seem to control the occurrence of age-related cancers, which are to a large extent species and strain specific (6). For example, 80 to 90% of AKR mice develop fatal leukemia between the ages of 7 and 10 months, whereas 90% of 18-month-old strain A mice develop pulmonary adenomas. A similar incidence of spontaneous hepatoma is seen in 14-month-old male C3H mice, whereas mammary adenocarcinoma affects 90% of 18-month-old females of the same strain. Endocrine tumors arise in 80 to 85% of older rats from some specific strains. To examine whether a cooperative role exists between inherited p53 and Rb deficiency in tumorigenesis, crosses were made between p-53- and Rb-deficient mice and these animals were monitored for subsequent tumor incidence (13). It was shown that mice containing Rb or p53 mutant alleles developed pituitary adenomas or lymphomas and sarcomas, respectively, whereas mice deficient for both Rb and p53 showed a faster rate of tumorigenesis and a wider array of tumors than animals deficient only in Rb or p53. These are only a few examples of the well-known interactions of genetics, age, and cancer in laboratory animals.

In humans, more than 80% of malignancies are diagnosed after age 50. In older humans, the influences of inheritable genetic abnormalities on carcinogenesis are unknown. A well known site-specific variation in the age-related incidence of cancer (Figure 8.1) suggests a different susceptibility of different tissues to carcinogenesis. Die *et al.* (1) subdivided all human tumors (except for chorionepithelioma) into two classes. The first class included all tumors whose incidence presents a single peak after age 50. The majority of tumors belongs to this class. The second class is composed of tumors having two peaks of incidence: the first before age 35 and the second after age 50. This class includes acute lymphocytic leukemia, osteosarcoma, and Hodgkin's Disease.

For completeness, the relationship of age with the incidence of benign tumors has not been satisfactorily studied, though benign neoplasms are more common than the malignant ones. Also, there is scarce data on the age-related distribution of tumors of different histogenesis found in the same organ. For example, epithelial carcinomas account for only a minority of ovarian cancers in women under 15 and germ cell neoplasms are most common in this group of women.

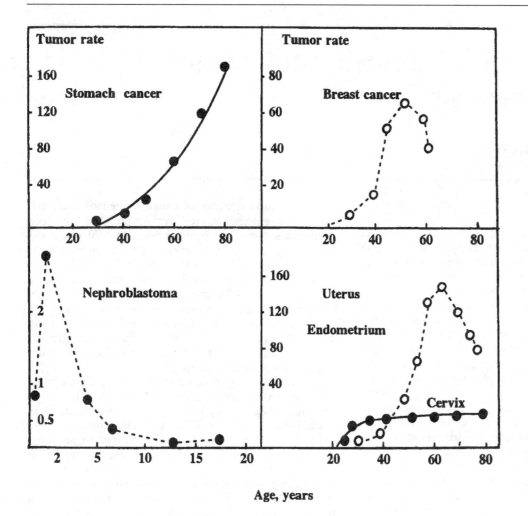

Figure 8.1 Incidence of cancer of various sites at different ages. Ordinate = tumor rate in 100,000 humans; abscissa = age, years.

The opposite is the case in women over 40. The example of ovarian cancer supports a variation in age-related incidence of tumors from different tissues and suggests two questions:

1. Do different tissues age at a different rate?
2. Does the susceptibility of different tissues to carcinogens vary with the person's age?

Susceptibility to Carcinogenesis at Different Age

Age-related variations in carcinogenesis from different agents (chemical, radioactive, hormonal, and viral) were explored in experimental studies with inconclusive results (Table 8.1). Overall, these experiments seem to confirm the hypothesis that there are age-related differences of carcinogen sensitivity in some tissues (6,7). Our own experiments and data from the literature show that, with age, susceptibility to carcinogens of some murine tissues decreases (mammary gland, small intestine and colon, thyroid, ovarian follicular epithelium), in other tissues it increases (subcutaneous tissue, cervix uteri, vagina) and in others it remains stable (lung, hemopoietic tissues) (6).

There are several possible reasons for this wide variation in experimental results. These include factors related to the experimental model and factors related to the tumor-host. Model-related factors involve the characteristics of different carcinogens (direct or indirect action, chemical structure, mechanism of action), route of administration, exposure duration, presence of local and systemic activity, and time of observation. Host-related factors involve animal species, strain, sex, and age. The effective dose of an indirect carcinogen, requiring metabolic activation, may vary significantly in old and young animals, because the activity of the enzymes necessary for carcinogen activation in the liver and/or target tissue(s) may change with age. Age-related changes in the activity of enzymes responsible for activation and inactivation of carcinogens are summarized in the Table 8.2 (6, 14–16). Due to age-related body weight gain, older animals may receive a greater relative amount of a carcinogen when dose is calculated per animal body weight. When these weight-related differences are eliminated by giving a dose of carcinogen sufficient to induce tumors in the majority of animals, it becomes difficult to detect differences in age-related sensitivity to that carcinogen.

Table 8.1 Effect of aging on susceptibility to carcinogenesis.

Target Tissue	Species	Carcinogenic Agent	Age groups (months)	Effect of aging
Skin	mouse	BP, DMBA, MCA,TC	2–4 and 12–13	no effect or decrease
		DMBA	14–20 and 22–24	increase
		NMU	2 and 13	no effect
		TPA	4 and 14	increase
		Ultra violet	2–3 and 10-l2	decrease or no effect
			12 and 24	increase
		beta-rays	2; 10 and 20	increase
	rat	fast neutrones,	1–3 and 21	decrease
		electrones	1; 8 and 13–15	decrease
	hamster	vinyl chloride	1 and 7,13,19	decrease
Zymbal gland	rat	DMAB	1 and 8	decrease
			1 and 15	increase
		NMU	1 and 12	increase
			12 and 23	decrease
Prepucial gland	rat	DMAB	1 and 8	increase
			1 and 15	decrease
Soft tissues	mouse	BP, DMBA	1–4 and 6–13	increase
		MCA	3–4 and 12	decrease
		MCA	6 and 20	increase
		DMBA	2–6 and 13	increase
		DMBA	1–2; 18 and 36	decrease
		polyurethane sponge	1 and 15, 5	increase
		Moloney virus	3 and 30	increase
	rat	BP, NMU	3–4 and 9–14	increase
		DMAB	2 and 15	no effect
Bone	mouse	224-Ra, 227-Th	1 and 5–6	no effect
		90-Sr; 137-Cs 144-Ce	0.5–1 and 4–12	decrease
	rat	239-Pu	1; 6 and 12	increase
		radio nuclides	2–3 and 8–10	no effect
	dog	239-Pu, Ra–226	3; 17 and 60	increase
		226-RA	17 and 60	decrease
Vessel wall	mouse	DENA	2.5 and 17	increase
		DMH	3 and 12–13	no effect
	rat	DENA	1;4; 6 and 12	decrease
		vinyl chloride	1.5–4 and 7–19	increase or decrease
Hemopoietic system	mouse	X-rays, -rays	1–4 and 12	decrease
		friend virus	2 and 24–25	decrease
		D-RadL virus	1; 3 and 12	no effect
		NMU	3 and 12	no effect
		NMU	12 and 24	increase
		Pristan	2–12 and 17–19	increase
		estrogens	1; 4 and 7	decrease
		PMS	6 and 10	no effect
	rat	X-rays	3–4 and 12–14	no effect or decrease
		radio nuclides	3 and 8–10	no effect
		NMU	3 and 14–15	no effect
		NMu	1; 12 and 23	decrease
	frog	DMNA, DMNO	1.5–2 and 12–18	decrease
Mammary gland	mouse	estrogens	1; 4 and 7	decrease
		vinyl chloride	1.5 and 13.5	decrease
	rat	DMBA, MCA, NMU	maximum susceptibility at the age of 50–75 days	

Table 8.1　Continued.

Target Tissue	Species	Carcinogenic Agent	Age groups (months)	Effect of aging
		DMBA, NMU, FBAA	1–6 and 12–16	decrease
		X-rays		
		beta-rays	1 and 12	no effect
		137-Cs	2 and 4	decrease
		60-Co	1–1.5 and 4	increase
		75-Se-selenomethionine	3; 12 and 24	increase
		estrogens	1 and 20	increase
Uterus	mouse	DMH	2 and 12	increase
		NMU	3 and 12	no effect
	rat	NMU, MAMNA	3 and 14 and 14–15	no effect
Cervix and vagina	mouse	DMBA	3 and 18	no effect
		MCA	2 and 15	no effect
Ovary	mouse	X-rays	2 and 12	decrease
		Biskinds' surgery	2–3 and 7–10	decrease
	rats	Biskinds' surgery	3 and 14	increase
		X-rays	3 and 14	decrease
		NMU	3 and 15	decrease
		DEH	3 and 14	increase
Testis	rat	fast neutrones	3 and 21	increase
		DMAB	1, 8 and 15	increase
Prostate	rat	DMNA	1; 8 and 15	no effect
Thyroid gland	rat	fast neutrones	1 and 21	decrease
		X-rays, BHOPA	2–3 and 14–15	decrease
	dog	131-I	2 and 15	decrease
Lung	mouse	DENA	1.5–2 and 12	increase
		NMU	3; 12 and 24	increase
		DBA, urethane	2–4 and 11–12	decrease
		vinyl chloride	1.5 and 13.5	decrease
		X-rays	1–2 and 6	increase
		X-rays	1–1.5 and 18–24	increase
	rat	MAMNA	3 and 14	no effect
		NBOPA	2 and 15	decrease
		fast neutrones	3 and 21	increase
Pleura	rat	Asbestos	2 and 10	increase
Liver	mouse	PB	1.5 and 12	increase
		DMTAA	1 and 4	decrease
	rat	FBAA, DENA, Aflatoxin B1	1–6 and 12	decrease
		DMNA, DENA	1 and 5–18	decrease
		Nitrosomorpholine	2 and 8	no effect
		NBOPA	2 and 8	increase
		CC14	1–6 and 12	increase
		PB	1.5 and 29	increase
		Nafenopin	3–8 and 13–24	increase
		Cyproteron, Cyclochloro-cyclohexane	8 and 24	increase
		WY–14, 643	2 and 15	increase
Pancreas	mouse	NMU	3; 12 and 24	increase
	rat	NMU	1 and 12	no effect
			12 and 23	decrease
		DMAB	1, 8 and 15	decrease
		Azaserine	0, 5 and 4–5	decrease
Tongue	rat	NMU	1 and 12	increase
		NMU	12 and 23	decrease

Table 8.1 Continued.

Target Tissue	Species	Carcinogenic Agent	Age groups (months)	Effect of aging
Esophagus	rat	DENA	1–6 and 12	decrease
		DENA	1–1, 5 and 5	no effect
		Nitrosomorpholine	2 and 12	no effect
Forestomach	mouse	DENA, NMU	2–3 and 12–17	decrease
	rat	NMU	1 and 12	no effect
		NMU	12 and 23	decrease
Stomach	rat	MNNG	1. 5–6 and 9–12	decrease
	hamster	vinyl chloride	1.5 and 7–19	decrease
Small bowels	rat	DMAB, MAMNA	1.3 and 14–15	decrease
		NMU	1 and 12	increase
		NMU	12 and 23	decrease
Colon	mouse	DMH	3 and 12	increase
		NMU	3; 12 and 24	increase
	rat	DMH	2 and 7	decrease
		DMH	8–10 and 18	decrease
		MAMNA, NMU	3 and 14–15	decrease
		NMU	1 and 12	increase
		NMU	12 and 23	decrease
Peritoneum	rat	DMAB	1; 8 and 15	decrease
Kidney	mouse	NMU	3 and 12	decrease
	rat	FBAA, DMNA, NMU	1–6 and 12–18	decrease
Kidney pelvis	mouse	BHBNA	1. 5–3 and 10	increase
	rat	NBOPA	2 and 15	increase
		NMU	1; 12 and 23	no effect
Bladder	mouse	BHBNA	1, 5–3 and 10	increase
		DMBA (in vitro)	1.5–2 and 28–30	increase
	rat	BHBNA	2 and 5	increase
		BHBNA	1.5; 12 and 23	increase
		NMU	1; 12 and 23	no effect

Abbreviations:
BHBNA — N-butyl-N-(4-hydroxybutyl)nitrosamine;
BP — benzo(a)pyrene;
CCl_4 — carbon tetrachloride;
DBA — 1, 2, 5, 6-dibenzanthracene;
DEH — 1, 2- diethylhydrazine;
DENA — N-nitrosodiethylamine;
DMAB — 3,2'-dimethyl-4-aminobiphenyl;
DMBA — 7, 12- dimethylbenz(a)anthracene;
DMH — 1, 2-dimethylhydrazine;
DMNA — N-nitrosodimethylamine;
DMNO — dimethylnitramine;
DMTAA — N, N-dimethyl-p(m-tolyazo)aniline;
FBAA — N-4- (fluorobipheny)acetamide;
MAMNA — methyl(acetoxymethyl)nitrosamine;
MCA — 20-methylcholanthrene;
MNNG — N-methyl-N'-nitro-N-nitrosoguanidine;
NBOPA — N-nitrosobis(2-oxopropyl)amine;
NMU — N-nitrosomethylurea;
PB — phenobarbital;
PMS — pregnant mare serum;
TC — tobacco condensate;
TPA — 12-0-tetradecanoylphorbol-13-acetate;
X-rays — whole-body X-ray irradiation

Table 8.2 Age-related changes of carcinogen-metabolizing enzymes in rat liver.

Enzyme	Age groups (months)	Effect of aging
Cytochrome p-450	3; 12 and 27 3–12 and 27 4–12; 18 and 27	no effect decrease decrease
Cytochrome b_5	3–5 and 14 3–6 and 24–30 7 and 24	decrease no effect decrease
NADPH-cytochrome c reductase	3–5 and 14 3, 4, 12, 24 and 36 3, 12 and 27	decrease decrease no effect
Aminopyrine-N-demethylase	6 and 25 1; 3; 10; 20 3; 6; 12; 24 and 28	no effect decrease decrease
Benzphetamine-N-demethylase	3; 12 and 27	decrease
Nitroanizole-N-demethylase	3–5 and 14 3; 6; 12; 24 and 28	increase decrease
Ethylmorphine-N-demethylase	3; 12 and 27 16 and 27	decrease decrease
Epoxide hydrase	3; 12 and 27	increase
Benzo(a)pyrene hydroxylase	3; 6; 12; 24; 27; 30	decrease
Aniline hydroxylase	1–6 and 18 3; 6; 12; 24; 28	decrease decrease
7-Ethoxycumarine-0-deethylase	3; 6; 12; 24 and 28	decrease
p-Dimethylaminoazo-benzene-reductase	1, 3, 10, 20	decrease
Nitroreductase	2 and 9	increase
Glutathione-reductase	1; 3 and 6 6; 12 and 24	increase decrease
Glutathione-S-transferase	3–4; 12 and 26–27 3 and 12 12 and 24	no effect or decrease increase decrease
o-Glucuronyl-transferase	4.5 and 24	decrease
p-Glucuronyl-transferase	4.5 and 24	increase
UDP-glucuronyl-transferase	2 and 9 3; 6; 12 and 24–26	no effect no effect
Beta-glucoronidase	2 and 9 6 and 28	increase increase
Aryl-sulphatase A and B	3 and 24	decrease
Glutathione peroxidase	3; 6; 12 and 24 12 and 24	increase no effect
UDP-glycodehydrogenase	3; 6; 12 and 24	increase

Table 8.3 Age-related changes in DNA repair in tissues exposed to carcinogens.

Type of DNA Damage	Carcinogen	Tissue	Species	Age groups	Effect of aging
Pyrimidine Dimers	UV	lymphocytes	human	13–94 years	decrease
				22 and 54 yrs	decrease
				17–69 yrs	no effect
		epidermis	human	0–70 yrs	no effect
				17–77 yrs	decrease
		skin	mouse	2 and 18 mo.	decrease
		kidney	human	30–82 yrs	no effect
		liver	rat	6 and 14 mo.	increase
				14 and 32 mo.	decrease
				2–3 and 28–30 mo.	no effect
		lens, epithelium	rat	14 and 40 mo.	no effect
		ganglium, opticum	rat	1–6 and 23 mo.	no effect
		kidney, lung brain, liver	hamster	1–2 and 17–18 mo.	no effect
		fibroblasts	mouse	2 and 30 mo.	decrease
			rat	6–10 and 32–44 mo.	decrease
		chondrocyte	rabbit	3 and 36 mo.	decrease
		thymocytes	mouse	2 and 22 mo.	no effect
DNA Strand Breaks	X-rays	lymphocytes	human	0–70 yrs	decrease
				17–60 and 60–78 yrs.	decrease
		cerebellum	dog	1, 5 mo. and 13 yrs.	no effect
			mouse	2 and 22 mo.	no effect
	Gamma rays	lymphocytes	human	0–70 yrs.	decrease
		liver	mouse	1, 5–2 and 18–22 mo.	decrease
		thymus	mouse	1 and 18 mo.	no effect
	electrons	skin	rat	1–6 and 13 mo.	decrease
Apurinic Sites	N-OH–2AAF	lymphocytes	human	0–10 and 51–60 yrs.	decrease
				51–60 and 71–80 yrs.	no effect
	4-NQO, DENA	ganglion opticum	rat	1–6 and 23 mo.	no effect
	4-HQO	skin	mouse	2 and 18 mo.	no effect
	DENA	fibroblasts	rat	13 wks and 24 mo.	decrease
	NMU	skin, lung, brain, heart, spleen, gonads	rat	6 and 24–26 mo.	decrease
	NMU	liver, kidney, duodenum, muscle	rat	6 and 24–26 mos.	no effect
	NMU	bone marrow	mouse	2 and 17 mo	decrease
	DMNA	kidney, duodenum, lung, liver, spleen, gonads	rat	6 and 24–26 mo.	decrease
	DMNA	skin, brain heart muscle	rat	6 and 24–26 mo.	no effect
	DMH	colon	rat	3–4 and 13–15 mo.	decrease
	MAMNA	colon, liver, ileum, lung, uterus	rat	3 and 14 mo.	decrease
	DMBA	mammary epithelium		1, 5 and 5 mo.	increase
Alkylation of Guanine at 0⁶ Position	DENA	liver	rat	3 and 14 mo.	decrease
		kidney	rat	3 and 14 mo.	increase
	MAMNA	liver	rat	3 and 14 mo.	increase
		colon, ileum	rat	3 and 14 mo.	decrease
		lung	rat	3 and 14 mo.	no effect

Abbreviations:
DENA — N-nitrosodiethylamine;
DMBA — 7, 12-dimethylbenz(a)anthracene;
DMNA — N-nitrodocimethylamine;
DMH — 1, 2-dimethylhydrazine;
MAMNA -methyl(acetoxymethyl)nitrosamine;
NMU — N-nitrosomethylurea;
N-OH-2AAF — N-OH-2-acetylaminofluorene;
4-HQO — 4-hydroxyaminoquinoline-1-oxide;
4-NQO — 4-nitroquinoline oxide.

Table 8.4 Age-related changes of DNA synthesis in various tissues.

Organ, tissue	Species	Age groups, months	Effect of aging
Esophagus basal layer of epithelium	mouse	1–2 and 19–21	decrease
Kidney cells of tubules	mouse	2 and 13	decrease
	rat	6 and 24	decrease
		17 and 24	increase
Liver	rat	2 and 24–36	decrease
	mouse	6 and 32	decrease
Tongue basal layer of epithelium	rat	2 and 19	decrease
		19 and 27	increase
Lung epithelium of alveolar wall	mouse	3 and 12	decrease
		12 and 24	no effect
Spleen	rat	6 and 22–24	increase
Mammary epithelium	rat	maximum at the 50 day of life	
Duodenum crypt epithelium	mouse	1–2 and 19–21	decrease
Colon crypt epithelium	mouse	1–2 and 19–21	decrease
Vessel wall endothelium	mouse	6; 12; 18 and 25	decrease

Critical factors that determine the susceptibility of a tissue to carcinogenesis include DNA synthesis and proliferative activity of that tissue at the time of carcinogen exposure, and the efficacy of repair of damaged DNA (17–21). The available data concerning age-related changes of these parameters have been discussed elsewhere (6,8) and are briefly summarized in Tables 8.3, 8.4 and 8.5. Obviously, there are no common patterns of age-related changes in DNA synthesis and repair or in proliferative activity of different tissues with age.

The homeostatic regulation of cell numbers in normal tissues reflect a precise balance between cell proliferation and cell death. Programmed cell death (apoptosis) provides a protective mechanism from cancer, by removing senescent, DNA-damaged, or diseased cells that could potentially interfere with normal function or lead to neoplastic transformation (22,23). With some reservations (24), apoptosis plays a substantial role in many other aspects of aging and cancer, including control of the life-span of most members of the immune complex, and the rate of growth of tumors (25). Recently it was suggested that p53 mediates apoptosis as a safeguard mechanism to prevent cell proliferation induced by oncogene activation (26).

When female rats older than 15–17 months are used in the experiment as the "old" group the majority of animals have a persistent estrus or anestrus that may strongly modify the susceptibility to some carcinogens (6).

Comparison of the carcinogenic effect in groups of animals with different life-expectancy presents an additional obstacle to the experimental study of carcinogenesis and age. The number of induced tumors may be underestimated in the animal with shorter life-expectancy, because competitive causes of death may prevent the clinical manifestations of cancer. Autoptic search for occult cancer should be performed in all animals, and tumors should be classified as "fatal" or "incidental" (27,28). This approach permits a more reliable comparison of incidence and lethality of tumors in young and old animals. Survival-related biases may be lessened when tumors discovered in an incidental context are analyzed by prevalence methods, while tumors discovered in a fatal context are analyzed by death-rate methods (27).

Age-related factors limiting the susceptibility to carcinogens are tissue-specific. This conclusion may explain, at least in part, both age-related changes in susceptibility to carcinogenesis in target tissues, and organ and tissue variability in age distribution of spontaneous tumor incidence. This conclusion generates a critical question: Is normal aging associated with an accumulation in cells that have undergone advanced carcinogenesis and are susceptible to the effects of late-stage carcinogens?

Table 8.5 Age-related changes of mitotic index in various tissues.

Organ, tissue	Species	Age groups, months/years	Effect of aging
Skin			
epidermis of abdominal wall	human	21–40 and 71–77	increase
ear epithelium	mouse	3–6 and 30–33	decrease
Epithelium			
oral cavity	human	25–34 and 50–78	increase
lacrimal gland	rat	1–3 and 30–33	decrease
forestomach	mouse	3 and 12	no effect
lung alveolar wall	mouse	3 and 12	no effect
Liver	rat	1–5 and 6–38	decrease
	mouse	3 and 12	decrease
Kidney			
proximal tubules	rat	4 and 38	decrease
Pituitary	rat	1–2 and 9–12	decrease
Thyroid gland	guinea pig	1–4 and 12–36	decrease
	rat	1–2 and 9	decrease
Parathyroid gland	guinea pig	1–4 and 12–36	decrease
	rat	1–2 and 9	decrease
Adrenal cortex	guinea pig	1–4 and 12–36	decrease
Endometrium	mouse	3 and 12	no effect
Duodenum crypts	mouse	1–2 and 19–21	decrease
Small intestine mucosa	rat	1–2 and 9	decrease
Descending colon	rat	4 and 18	decrease
Mammary epithelium	rat	maximum at 50th day of life	

Molecular Biology of Aging: Potential Relationship to Carcinogenesis

Both carcinogenesis and aging are associated with genomic alterations, which may act synergistically in causing cancer (29–32). In particular, three recently described age-related changes in DNA metabolism may favor cell transformation and cancer growth. These changes are genetic instability, DNA hypomethylation, and formation of DNA adducts (20,31,33).

Genetic instability involves activation of genes that are normally suppressed, such as the cellular proto-oncogenes, and/or inactivation of some tumor suppression genes (p53, Rb, etc.) (20,31,33–37). The role of genetic instability in linking aging and cancer may be clarified in the near future by new and promising laboratory techniques (38).

DNA hypomethylation is characteristic of aging, as well as of transformed cells (39–41). Hypomethylation, a potential mechanism of oncogene activation, may result in spontaneous deamination of cytosine and consequent base transition, i.e., substitution of the pair thymine:adenine. Accumulation of inappropriate base pairs may cause cell transformation by activation of cellular proto-oncogenes (35,37,42). Age-related abnormalities of DNA metabolism may be, to some extent, tissue- and gene-specific. For example, hypomethylation of the c-myc proto-oncogene has been found in the hepatocytes, but not in the neurons of old mice (43–45). Within the same cell, different DNA segments express different degrees of age-related hypomethylation. The uneven distribution of hypomethylation may underlie selective overexpression of proto-oncogenes by senescent cells (46–49). For example, the transcription of c-myc is progressively increased in the liver but not in the brain of rats between the ages of 4 and 22 months, whereas the transcription of c-sis and c-src does not appear to be age-related in any tissues (45,47). The different extent of DNA abnormalities among aging tissues may account in part for the different susceptibility of these tissues to carcinogens (32,41).

The formation of DNA adducts in target tissues is one of the key events in the process of chemical carcinogenesis (50,51). The majority of known carcinogens react with DNA through one of only three general types of chemical reaction. These involve the transfer to DNA of either alkyl, arylamine or aralkyl residues (51). The sites of alkylation and polycyclic aralkylation on DNA do not overlap, but monocyclic aralkylating agents (and possibly arylaminating agents) attack some sites that are targets for polycyclic aralkylating agents and some that are targets for simple alkylating agents. Accumulation of these substances, particularly of 7-methylguanine adducts in nuclear and mitochondrial DNA, may represent the linkage of aging and carcinogenesis (52).

It was shown that the DNA of various tissues of intact rodents contains adduct-like compounds (I-compounds) which accumulate with age (53). The production of I-compounds is not mediated by specific DNA-modifying enzymes, such as cytosine-5-methyltransferase, but it may involve microsomal oxydases and other xenobiotic metabolizing enzymes. Important characteristics of I-compounds are their capability to cause mutations, DNA chainbreaks, and gene rearrangements (53).

The damage caused by endogenous oxygen radicals has been proposed as a major contributor to both aging and cancer (54–57). Oxygen radicals are mainly produced *in vivo* as by-products of natural metabolism, from lipid peroxidation and from phagocytes (55–57). A variety of cellular defense systems are involved in protecting cellular macromolecules against devastating action of oxygen-based radicals. These systems include antioxidant enzymes (Cu- and Zn-containing superoxide dismutase (SOD), manganese-containing SOD, catalase, glutathione peroxidase, glutathione reductase, glucose-6-phosphate dehydrogenase), some vitamins (alpha-tocopherol, ascorbic acid), uric acid and pineal hormone melatonin (54–58).

There is evidence that an increased production of reactive oxygen species and/or a decreased efficiency of antioxidant defense systems is associated with aging (54–58). Endogenous oxidative damage to lipids and proteins increases with age (56). It was recently shown that oxygen free radicals may induce active mutations of the human c-Ha-ras proto-oncogene (59). The level of one oxidized nucleoside, 8-hydroxy-2'-deoxyguanosine (oh8dG) in the DNA increased with age in liver, kidney, and intestine but remained unchanged within brain and testes of rats, whereas the urinary excretion of the nucleoside decreased with age of rats (60). As it was recently discovered, oh8dG may hamper the function of human DNA methyltransferase (61). Some oxidized mutagenic nucleosides, such as 1,N6-ethenodeoxyadenosine and 3,N4-ethenodeoxycytidine, derived from spontaneous peroxidation of lipids and proteins, also have been detected in rodent tissues after treatment with chemical carcinogens (62).

In recent years, the importance of telomeres in aging has been highlighted. Telomeres are DNA sequences found at the end of eukaryotic chromosomes in somatic cells. During cell replication, telomeres are preserved by the enzyme telomerase, a ribonucleoprotein enzyme that adds the telomere sequences TTAGGG to chromosome ends (63–65). In the absence of telomerase, telomeres are shortened with each cell division. Loss of the distal region of telomeres correlates with the decline of the proliferative life-span of cells both *in vitro* and *in vivo* (63,65). There are serious arguments suggesting that telomere shortening and reactivation of telomerase are an important components of aging and carcinogenesis, respectively (63–65). It was suggested that a major function of wild-type p53 may be to signal growth arrest in response to telomere loss in senescent cells (66). This hypothesis is consistent with the behavior of most tumors that exhibit p53 mutation and also explain the existence and characteristics of rarer tumor types in which p53 function appear to be retained (66).

There is evidence of an age-related accumulation of spontaneous mutations in somatic and germ cells (67–70). Accumulation with age of some spontaneous mutations or mutations evoked by endogenous mutagens can induce genome instability and, hence, increase the sensitivity to carcinogens and/or tumor promoters. The progeny of 25-month-old male rats mated with 3-month-old females to chemical carcinogen, NMU, was significantly increased in comparison to the progeny of young males (71).

Thus, the data available show that some changes in structure and function of DNA are evolving with natural aging. The character of these changes could vary in different tissues and might cause uneven tissue aging. In turn, this may lead to both age-related increases in spontaneous tumor incidence and age-related changes in susceptibility to carcinogens in various organs.

Multistage Model of Carcinogenesis and Aging

Carcinogenesis is a multistage process: neoplastic transformation implies the engagement of a cell through sequential stages, and different agents may affect the transition between contiguous stages (11,72,73). Several lines of evidence support this conclusion (20):

1. Histopathology of tumors reveals multiple stages of tumor progression, such as dysplasia and carcinoma in situ.
2. The two-stage model of chemical carcinogenesis in mouse skin shows that different chemicals affect qualitatively different stages in the carcinogenic process.
3. The existence of individuals with genetic traits manifested by an early occurrence of cancer (e.g., familial retinoblastoma, colon and rectum adenomatosis) suggests that one of the carcinogenic steps is a germ-line mutation, but additional somatic effects are required for neoplastic development.
4. Mathematical models based on age-specific tumor incidence curves are consistent with the hypothesis that three to seven independent hits (effects of independent carcinogens) are required for tumor development.
5. Studies with chemical carcinogens in cell cultures reveal that different phenotypic properties of a tumor cell are required for tumor development.

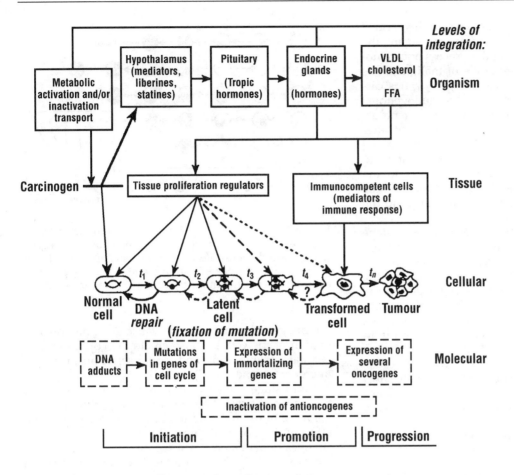

Figure 8.2 Integral scheme of carcinogeneses.

$t_1 \ldots t_{ii}$ = time of passage of cells from stage k_1 to stage $k_1 \ldots k_\eta$

6. Studies with viral and tumor-derived oncogenes in cell cultures show that neoplastic conversion of normal cells generally requires multiple cooperating oncogenes.

7. Transgenic mice that carry activated proto-oncogenes in their germ-line develop focal tumors, which are apparently monoclonal in origin, suggesting that additional somatic events are required for full malignant progression.

The process of neoplastic development is often divided into three operationally defined stages — initiation, promotion and progression. Initiation involves induction of permanent and irreversible alterations in the genome of the target cell by a carcinogen called an initiator. Promotion completes the neoplastic transformation of the initiated cells through the intervention of agent(s) called promoter(s) (73).

Unlike initiation, promotion requires prolonged exposure to the carcinogen and may be reversible to a large extent. A carcinogen that is able to act as both initiator and promoter is referred to as a full carcinogen. The dissection of carcinogenesis into initiation, promotion, and progression is useful as frame of reference. It should not be assumed, however, that only three carcinogenic stages exist: each stage can be subdivided into multiple substages. Promotion may involve the activation of several enzymes, such as protein kinase C and ornithine decarboxylase; enhanced hexose transport; increased polyamine production, prevention

of cell differentiation; and inhibition of cell-to-cell communication (19,74). It was found that 12-O-tetradecanoylforbol-13-acetate (TPA), a well-known skin tumor promoter, causes free-radical-mediated DNA alterations, such as sister chromatid exchanges and expression of proviruses and retroviruses (75).

Discovery of oncogenes and of their function has provided new insight into the carcinogenic process (33–35). One may view carcinogenesis as a "cascade" phenomenon, resulting in serial activation of multiple cellular oncogenes and/or inactivation of tumor-suppressing genes (e.g, p53) (33–36).

To overcome the obvious limitations of two (three)-stage model, a multistage model of carcinogenesis has been conceived, in which the number of stages is not limited, the stages are envisioned as a continuum, and the influence of factors other than specific carcinogens may be properly accounted for Figure 8.2 (11). The principles of this model are as follows. First, neoplastic transformation involves the transition of target cells through multiple stages, the number of which varies for different neoplasms (with minimum of one intermediate stage). Secondly, passage from one stage to another is a stochastic event, the rate of which depends on the dose of a carcinogen which affect the cell. Finally, all cells at any stage of carcinogenesis may enter the next stage independently of each other.

According to this model, the tumor develops only if at least one cell goes through all the necessary stages, and the clonal growth of this cell causes clinical cancer, as a critical tumor volume is achieved. In this model, the exact origin of the various stages is ignored and the changes in cell function during the process of carcinogenesis are not assessed. The grade of malignancy is considered to increase with every stage. Various carcinogenic agents (exogenous as well as endogenous) may modulate the process. In addition, some agents act at early stages of carcinogenesis and others at later stages (11). Epidemiological data, analyzed within the framework of a multi-stage model, have helped to estimate the contribution of various factors to the development of cancer. These factors include the time from the beginning of carcinogenic exposure, and the age of onset of exposure.

Important differences between early and late-stage carcinogens should be highlighted, to illustrate potential interactions of aging and carcinogenesis. Exposure to early stage carcinogens requires a *latent period* for the development of cancer. During the latent period the transformed cell goes through the subsequent carcinogenic stages. Clearly, elimination of early-stage carcinogens from the environment will not result in immediate cessation in the incidence of cancer. Carcinogens acting at late stages of carcinogenesis cause the tumor incidence rate to rise after a relatively short period of time. The increased rate of tumor incidence will be reversed immediately on cessation of exposure (Table 8.6) (11).

This risk of cancer after exposure to a carcinogen may be calculated as:

$$I = (age)^{k-1} - (t)^{k-1} \qquad (Eq.1)$$

Where I is the risk of cancer, t is the time from initial exposure to the carcinogen, and k is the number of stages that the target cells have undergone before the exposure to the carcinogen. This formula is based on the assumption that with aging there is a progressive accumulation of partially transformed cells primed to the effect of late-stage carcinogens (Figure 8.3).

Both experimental and epidemiologic studies illustrate the interaction of aging and carcinogenesis. The malignant transformation of normal cells involves both quantitative and qualitative changes. Figure 8.2 shows an integrated scheme of multi-stage carcinogenesis.

Table 8.6 Characteristics of early- and late-stage carcinogens.

Early-stage carcinogens
Prolonged latency
Persistence of the effect after withdrawal of the carcinogen

Late-stage carcinogens
Short latency
Rapid disappearance of the effect after withdrawal of the carcinogen

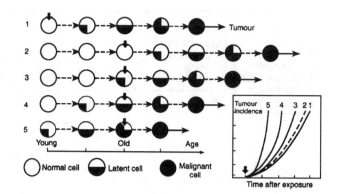

Figure 8.3 The multistage carcinogenesis inducted by single exposure to a carcinogenic agent at different ages. Groups 3–5 demonstrate the carcinogenic effect produced on a cell that has passed through one or more stages in accordance with the multistage model of carcinogenesis.

Carcinogenic agents not only cause genomic transformation of the cell, but also create the conditions that facilitate proliferation and clonal selection in the cell microenvironment (6,7).

Multi-stage carcinogenesis is accompanied by disturbances in tissue homeostasis and perturbations in nervous, hormonal, and metabolic factors which may affect antitumor resistance. The development of these changes depends on the susceptibility of various systems to a carcinogen and on the dose of the carcinogen. Changes in the microenvironment may condition key carcinogenic events and determine the duration of each carcinogenic stage, and sometimes they may even reverse the process of carcinogenesis. These microenvironmental changes influence the proliferation rate of transformed cells together, the total duration of carcinogenesis and, consequently, the latent period of tumor development.

Numerous experiments support this model. Thus, single skin application with DMBA in mice aged 8 and 48 weeks at doses ranging from 10 to 300 μg caused increased skin papilloma incidence in older mice (Table 8.7) (76). Also, the average diameter of the tumors was larger in the older animals. Likewise, the incidence of skin papillomas after TPA application was sixfold higher in 14-month-old mice than in 4-month-old. Of particular interest are the experiments using skin transplants. TPA failed to induce tumors in the skin of 2-month-old mice grafted to animals of different ages,

Table 8.7 Incidence of skin tumors in young and adult mice exposed to a single DMBA application.

	Dose, μg				
Age, weeks	300	100	%	30	10
8	30	21		0	0
48	47	18		6.3	1.3

but caused the same tumor incidence in the skin of 1-year-old donors irrespective of the recipient's age (77). These results indicate that the age of the target tissue, more than the age of the host, determines susceptibility to late-stage agents. Exposure of mice or F344 rats of various ages to phenobarbital resulted in hepatocarcinogenesis only in old animals (78,79). The incidence of proliferative foci and hepatic tumors induced by carbon tetrachloride or peroxisome proliferators in rodents is also a function of age (Table 8.1) (80–83).

Single intravenous injection of NMU at doses of 10, 20 and 50 mg/kg was administered to female rats aged 3 and 15 months (84). The NMU carcinogenic dose dependence in different age groups was considered in the context of a multi-stage model. It was calculated that the number of events necessary for complete malignant transformation in 15-month-old rats under the influence of NMU was lower than in 3-month-old. In this experiment as well as in another sets of experiments in rats and in mice it was shown that tumors developed earlier in older than in younger animals after exposure to the same doses of NMU(85,86).

Age-related accumulation of cells in advanced carcinogenic stages may also be inferred by other types of experiments. The mice model of hepatocarcinogenesis is very convenient for this purpose because of the availability of strains of animals with different susceptibility to hepatic carcinogenesis. In the liver of highly susceptible mice, the concentration of hepatocytes in advanced stages of carcinogenesis was increased early in life before the exposure to experimental carcinogens (87). In the liver of F344 rats the number of spontaneous proliferative foci is proportional to the animal age (79,83,88). Another pertinent model involves induction of lymphomas in mice receiving transplants of splenic, thymic and lymphoid cells from syngeneic donors (89). The incidence of neoplasms was related to the age of the donor, but not to the age of the recipient. Thus, transplants from 1-month-old donors to 14-month-old host failed to produce tumors, whereas transplants from 14-month-old donors into 1-month-old mice caused lymphomas in 59 to 65% of the recipients.

It is important to stress that in every tissue the number of events occurring in the stem cell before its complete transformation is variable and depends on many factors, in particular the rate of aging of the target tissue and its regulatory system(s) (6,90). This model is consistent with the analysis of age-related distribution of tumor incidence in different sites in humans and laboratory animals (1,6). It must be emphasized also that old animals can be used as an adequate model for long-term assay for carcinogenicity of suggested weak carcinogens and/or tumor promoters.

The multistage model of carcinogenesis and the distinction of early-and late-stage carcinogens are supported by epidemiologic studies in humans. Time from beginning of the exposure, duration of exposure, time since exposure was stopped, and age at first exposure are particularly important parameters. If an agent affected an early stage of cancer development, then the number of cells that pass through that stage will increase. These cells will have to pass through a series of further stages before expression of malignancy. Both the increase in tumor incidence after the start of exposure and the relative decrease after exposure is ceased will be considerably delayed. If a late stage is affected, the response to both the beginning and the end of the carcinogenic exposure will be much more rapid (11). As examples, the results of observations on patients treated with ionizing radiation or subjected to an organ transplantation would be considered. Thus, following a comparatively short exposure to ionizing radiation an excess risk of cancer tends to rise only after approximately 10 years and continues to rise fairly rapidly for at least several decades thereafter. This is typical example of an early-stage effect. In contrast, a marked excess of non-Hodgkin's lymphoma following organ transplantation becomes evident within six months, which suggest a late-stage effect (11).

As an example of "late stage" effect, the incidence rate of lung cancer from arsenic increases with the age at which the first exposure to arsenic occurs: persons exposed to arsenic at more advanced age are more likely to develop lung cancer. As an example of "early stage" effect, the risk of mesothelioma for a given duration of exposure to asbestos is independent from age at first exposure. The analysis of lung cancer mortality among smokers and ex-smokers suggests that tobacco smoke contains both early- and late-stage agents (11,73,91).

The terms "early" and "late" carcinogens do not necessarily imply specific events in experimental carcinogenesis. In addition to "mutagens," early stage carcinogens include substances that enhance the delivery of mutagens to the target tissue, substances that antagonize extracellular inhibition of mutagen effects, and substances that antagonize DNA repair mechanisms and stimulate cell proliferation and/or inhibit apoptosis. Late-stage agents may include, in addition to promoters, agents that antagonize several homeostatic mechanisms, such as immunosurveillance, agents which cause irreversibility of the tumor phenotype, and other agents whose effect is poorly understood. It is suggested that any of the carcinogens might in some circumstances act either early, late, or both, and a given agent might act early for one type of cancer and late for another (11,73). Research into the identification of tissue markers of early stages of carcinogenesis may yield insights into cancer prevention.

An important question related to the integrated carcinogenic model (6) concerns age-related changes in tissue microenvironment as these changes may both favor or oppose carcinogenesis in different circumstances. Should aging tissues alter the environment in which tumor develops, the growth rate of transplantable tumors may vary with the age of the tumor recipient (4). These experiments bypass the effect of age on carcinogenesis itself and explore the role of age-related changes in the organism on the growth and progression of transformed cells. Evaluation criteria for such experiments should include: (1) tumor transplantability, (2) rate of tumor growth, and (3) survival time of tumor bearing animals. The natural history of spontaneous tumors in humans (the rate of tumor doubling, metastazing potential) and on the survival of cancer patients newly diagnosed at different ages provide information on the effects of age on tumor growth in humans. Available data both in experimental animals and in humans are contradictory and support different effects of age on tumor development (6,91–96). In general, an "age effect" may be recognized both in experimental and in human malignancies.

Tissue origin (histogenesis) and immunogenicity of tumor are the principal factors determining age-related differences in tumor growth. There is increasing evidence that age-related changes in tumor microenvironment might play also a significant role. In our experiments, lung-affine cells of rat rhabdomyosarcoma RA-2 were intravenously inoculated into rats of different ages (97). It was observed that the number of lung tumor colonies was highest in 1-month-old and 15-month-old animals and lowest in 3- and 12-month-old animals. A positive correlation was found between the number of tumor lung colonies and somatomedine activity in the lung. In another experiment, RA-2 cells from a 3-month-old donor were inoculated into 2–3 or 21–23-month-old recipients and 3 weeks later were separately taken from "young" and "old" hosts and transplanted into 3-month-old recipients. The number of lung colonies was significantly decreased in 3-month-old recipients injected with RA-2 cell passed via "old" host (98). The results obtained suggest the critical role of host and donor microenvironment in lung colony forming potential of RA-2 cells.

McCullough et al. (99) have observed that transformed rat hepatocytic cells lines were only weakly tumorigenic following transplantation into the livers of young adult rats. The tumorigenicity of these cell lines increased progressively with the age of the tumor recipients. These results suggest strongly that the tissue microenvironment represents an important determinant in the age-related tumorigenic potential of transformed cells.

Carcinogens as Accelerators of Aging

Given the similarity of molecular changes of aging and carcinogenesis it is reasonable to ask whether and how carcinogens may affect aging. The ability of carcinogens to influence aging has been discussed for many years. Larionov (100) reports that the exposure of rodents to polycyclic hydrocarbons was followed by premature aging. Neonatal exposure to DMBA decreased the life-span of mice and has been accompanied by premature cessation of estral function, hair discoloration, and loss of body weight (101). In our own experiments, female rats treated with MCA manifested a number of endocrine changes typical of aging animals. These included cessation of estrus function (102). Chronic inhalation of tobacco smoke caused enhanced production of free radicals and signs of aging in rats (103). Acceleration of aging by ionizing radiation has been well documented and epitomizes dose-dependent effects of carcinogens on aging (104–107). Exposure to extremely low-frequency electromagnetic fields which has weak tumor-promoting effects in some experimental systems (108–112), was followed by the aging of endocrine and immune systems (113).

The effects of carcinogens on the neural, endocrine and immune systems, and on carbohydrate and lipid metabolism which may lead to acceleration of aging (6) are summarized in Table 8.8. Radioactive and chemical carcinogens appear to cause disturbances in the internal tissue milieu, similar to those of normal aging, but at an earlier age. Carcinogenic factors (including irradiation) cause a sharp transition to an "older" level of function in metabolic processes, hormonal and immune status. This transition is asynchronous and has different latent periods in various structures and systems of the exposed organism.

Some "in vitro" and "in vivo" effects of the thymidine analogue, bromodeoxyuridine (BrdUrd), suggest that BrdUrd may be used to investigate the role of selective DNA damage both in carcinogenesis and in aging. BrdUrd is incorporated into replicating DNA in place of thymidine, and this effect is mutagenic (114). In addition to the usual keto form, BrdUrd may assume an enoltautomeric form, which forms hydrogen bonds with guanine instead of adenine, the normal pair for thymidine and 5-bromouracil. In the absence of 5-bromouracil repair in rat DNA (115), if BrdUrd is incorporated into DNA as the enol tautomer, base pair substitution mutations are expected to occur (GC→AT and AT→GC transitions) during subsequent DNA replication (114,116).

Experiments with D.melanogaster (117) have shown that supplements of BrdUrd in the diet caused reduction of insect life-span. Craddock (118) observed a dose-dependent shortening in life-span of rats exposed to BrdUrd in early life, in uncontrolled experiments, without data on tumor incidence or on biomarkers of aging.

Assuming a fairly even level of BrdUrd incorporation into the DNA of various tissues of neonatal rats and long-term persistence in them (119,120), cells with highest proliferative activity would be more likely to undergo malignant transformation. Exposure to BrdUrd had dramatic effects on cellular functions including cell differentiation, inactivation of regulatory genes or master switch (121), and proliferation (122). These changes in cellular function may favor tumor development.

In a series of our experiments (86,120,123–127) rats received s.c. injections of BrdUrd at 1, 3, 7 and 21 days of postnatal life at the single dose of 3.2 mg per rat. BrdUrd persisted for up to 49 weeks in all tissues studied immunohistochemically, especially in tissues with normal low cell turnover. For cells with high turnover few or no BrdUrd labeled cells remained at 49 weeks (120). The exposure to BrdUrd was followed by the decrease in the mean life-span of the animals of 38% in males and 27% in females and by the increase in the rate of aging (calculated according to Gompertz equation) in comparison to controls. The monitoring

Table 8.8 Similarity of changes developing in organism during natural aging and carcinogenesis [6, with modifications].

Parameter	Aging	Chemical carcinogens	Ionizing radiation	Persistent estrus syndrome
Pineal melatonin secretion	decreases	decreases	decreases	
Catecholamine level and turnover in hypothalamus	decreases	decreases	decreases	decreases
Estradiol uptake by receptors	decreases	decreases	decreases	decreases
Threshold of sensitivity of hypothalamus to steroid feedback	increases	increases	increases	increases
Serum estradiol level before switching-off of reproductive function	increases			noncyclic secretion
Excretion of nonclassic phenol steroids	increases	increases	increases	increases
Incidence of persistent estrus	increases	increases	increases	increases
Adrenal cortex function	Hypercorticism	disfunction	disfunction	Hypercorticism
Tolerance to glucose	decreases	decreases	decreases	decreases
Sensitivity to insulin	decreases	decreases	decreases	decreases
Serum insulin level	increases	increases	decreases	
Serum cholesterol level	increases	increases	Hyperlipidemia	increases
Amount of fat in the body	increases		increases	increases
T-cell-mediated immunity	decreases	decreases	decreases	decreases
DNA repair efficacy	decreases	decreases	decreases	decreases
DNA adduct formation	increases	increases	increases	
Free radical production	increases	increases	increases	
"Errors" in DNA synthesis	increases	increases	increases	
Incidence of chromosome aberrations	increases	increases	increases	
Enzyme regulation	changes	changes	changes	
Cell bioenergetic	changes	changes	changes	changes
Clonal proliferation of stem cells	increases	increases	increases	increases
Derepression or activation of endogenous oncogenes and oncobiruses	increases	increases	increases	
Tumor incidence	increases	increases	increases	increases

of estrus showed acceleration of natural age-related switching-off of reproductive function in female rats, due to disturbances in central regulation of gonadotropic function in the pituitary. The exposure of rats to BrdUrd was followed by signs of immunodepression, by increase in the incidence of chromosome aberrations and spontaneous tumors. The latency of these tumors was decreased. In offspring of rats neonatally treated with BrdUrd the increased incidence of congenital malformation and of spontaneous tumors, and accelerated aging were both observed. Neonatal exposure of rats or mice to BrdUrd was followed by the initiation of the neoplastic process and, consequently, by increased tissue susceptibility to "early and late stage" carcinogens such as NMU; X-irradiation; urethan, estradiol-benzoate; persistent estrus syndrome; TPA.

This effect was tissue-specific and increased the susceptibility of the animals to a wider array of tumors (126).

We also evaluated the effect of DNA damages induced by neonatal exposure to BrdUrd on susceptibility of target tissues to carcinogenic effect of NMU injected at various ages (86). Rats exposed to BrdUrd in the neonatal period received single injections of NMU at doses of 10 or 50 ug/kg at the age of 3 or 15 months. In the absence of BrdUrd pretreatment, the carcinogenic effect of NMU was dose-dependent in the 3 month old rats, but not in the 15 year old. The susceptibility to NMU-induced tumor was decreased, but the tumor-related survival was also decreased in the older animals. These data suggest age-related decrement in the effect of NMU and, at the same time, age-related decrease in the number of events which are necessary for tumor development. The exposure to BrdUrd was followed by increased susceptibility to the carcinogenic effect of NMU both in 3- and 15-month-old rats. These effects were largely confined to NMU-target tissues. The incidence of tumors in rats exposed to BrdUrd plus NMU at the dose of 10 mg/kg was equal to that in the rats to whom the carcinogen was injected at the age of 3 or 15 months, however the survival of fatal tumor-bearing rats was significantly decreased for the older animals. When NMU was injected at the dose of 50 mg/kg in BrdUrd-pretreated rats, both the relative risk of tumors and the tumor-specific survival were decreased in the older animals. Thus, our data have shown the long-term persistence of initiating effect of neonatal treatment with BrdUrd and provided the evidence that a sole perturbation of DNA induced by BrdUrd contributed substantially to the initiation of tumorigenesis and to the acceleration of aging.

Premature Aging and Carcinogenesis

It is well known that some syndromes of untimely aging (progeria) are associated with an increased incidence of cancer (128,129). Alongside with the classical progeria syndromes, some diseases are accompanied by disturbances which might be regarded as signs of the intensified aging. For example, the syndrome of Stein-Leventhal (sclerocystic ovaries syndrome) occurs during puberty and is characterized by a bilateral sclerocystic enlargement of the ovaries, associated with a pronounced thickness of the capsule of the ovaries which forms a mechanical obstacle for the ovulatory rupture of a mature follicle. Follicular cysts and hyperplasia of theca tissue are found in such ovaries. Patients have anovulation, sterility, hirsutism, hyperlipidemia, lowered glucose tolerance, hyperinsulinemia, obesity, hypertension, and increased incidence of breast and endometrial cancer (130). In rodents, the syndrome of persistent estrus, which normally completes the reproductive period of life, can be induced by several methods, including neonatal administration of sex steroids, exposure to some chemical carcinogens or to ionizing irradiation, housing at the constant light regime, subtotal ovariectomy, orthotopic transplantation of an ovary into castrated animals, electrolytic lesion of anterior and/or mediobasal hypothalamus, etc. (6). Regardless of the method of the induction, premature aging and increase in tumor incidence have been observed in rats with persistent estrus (Table 8.8) (6).

The induction of persistent estrus in rats with chemical carcinogens (DMBA, NMU) was associated with increased tumor incidence when compared to animals without persistent estrus exposed to a carcinogen alone (6,111,131). These observations suggested promoting effect of the persistent estrus syndrome-associated intensified aging on carcinogenesis.

In mice genetically predisposed to premature immunodeficiency, increased incidence of spontaneous lymphoma has been observed (132). It must be emphasized that some agents leading to reduced life-spans can result from genetic defects unrelated directly to mechanisms of normal aging (133).

Life-Span Prolongation and Carcinogenesis

The effects of factors or drugs that increase life-span (geroprotectors) on spontaneous tumor development may provide important clues to the interactions of aging

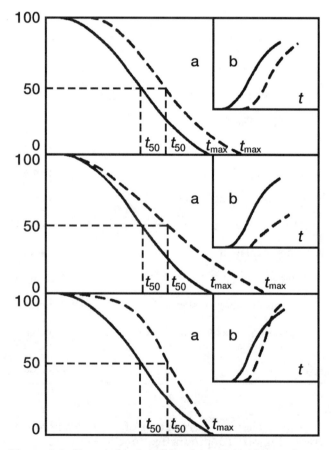

Figure 8.4 Types of aging delay (a) and incidence of spontaneous tumors (b) under influence of geroprotectors. Ordinate = (a) – number of survival animals, %;
(b) – tumor rate, %;
Abscissa = age; solid line = control; broken line = administration of geroprotector.

and carcinogenesis.

Life-span prolonging drugs and factors could be divided into three groups: a) geroprotectors that prolong the life-span equally in all members of the population: these substances postpone the beginning of population aging; b) geroprotectors that decrease the mortality of long-living subpopulation leading to a rise in maximal life-span: these substances slow down the population aging rate; c) geroprotectors that increase the survival in short-living subpopulation without change of the maximal life-span: in this case aging rate increases (Figure 8.4).

Available data from the literature and our own studies show a good correlation between the type of geroprotectors and the pattern of tumor development in the same population of animals (Table 8.9). As can be seen in Table 8.9 and Figure 8.4, geroprotectors of the first type do not influence the incidence of tumors but do prolong tumor latency. Geroprotectors of the second type are effective in inhibiting spontaneous carcinogenesis, prolonging tumor latency, and decreasing tumor incidence. Drugs of the third type can

sometimes increase the incidence of cancer (6–8).

Thus, the use of growth hormone for elimination of wrinkles and prolongation of life-expectancy (134–136) may be associated with increased incidence of cancer, as suggested by old observations (137). In the multi-stage model of carcinogenesis, growth hormone promotes initiated and partially transformed cells and acts like a late-stage agent or tumor promoter.

It should be noted that the mean life-span of animals increased equally with each type of geroprotectors (Figure 8.4), revealing no correlation between prolongation of survival and tumor incidence. At the same time, the correlation between the aging rate (aging rate could be estimated as α in Gompertz equation: $R = R_0 e^{\alpha t}$, where R – mortality, $R_0 = R$ at t (time) $= 0$; – constant) and malignant tumor incidence in the populations appeared to be high (6).

In the framework of multi-stage carcinogenesis, geroprotectors may both inhibit and enhance the passage of transformed cells through sequential carcinogenic stages. In general, the efficacy of geroprotectors in preventing cancer development decreases inversely

Table 8.9 Effects of geroprotectors on spontaneous tumor development in rodents.

Type of geroprotector Delay	Effect on aging	
	Tumor latency	Tumor incidence
1.　2-mercaptoethylamin	increases	no effect
2-ethyl-6-methyl-3-oxipyridine	increases	no effect
Procaine (gerovital)	no effect	no effect
2.　caloric restriction	increases	decreases
Tryptophan-deficient diet	no data	decreases
Antidiabetic biguanides	increases	decreases
L-DOPA	no effect	decreases
Phenytoin	no effect	decreases
Dehydroepiandrosterone	increases	decreases
Succinic acid	no effect	decreases
Epithalamin	increases	decreases
Melatonin	increases	decreases
Thymalin	increases	decreases
Levamisole	increases	decreases
3.　Selenium	no data	increases
Ethylenediaminetetra-acetate-Na$_2$	no data	increases
Deprenyl	no effect	no effect
Tritium oxide	no data	increases
Tocopherol (Vit.E):		
benign tumors	increases	increases
malignant tumors	increases	decreases

with the age of exposure to the carcinogen. It is important to emphasize that geroprotectors of the second type delay aging by influencing the "main" regulatory systems of the organism (nervous, endocrine, immune). These effects delay the development of age-related changes in the microenvironment of cells exposed to carcinogens.

Geroprotectors may also be classified into two main groups according to their mechanism of action. The first group includes drugs that prevent stochastic lesions of macromolecules. The theoretical basis for using these drugs is provided for by variants of the "catastrophe error" theory, which regards aging as a result of the accumulation of stochastic damages. The second group includes substances that appear to delay intrinsic aging, i.e. programmed cellular aging.

Antioxidants are the most typical representatives of the first class of geroprotectors. Age of initial administration and doses of environmental carcinogens influence the geroprotective and tumor-preventing effects of antioxidants. The effectiveness of these substances increases when the initial administration occurs early in life and decreases with the dose of environmental carcinogen(s) to which the organism was exposed.

The second class of geroprotectors includes antidiabetic biguanides (phenformin and buformin), the pineal peptide Epithalamin, melatonin and caloric-restricted diet. These factors influence the hormonal, metabolic and immunological functions of the body,

delaying age-related changes in these functions (6). It was suggested that caloric restriction retards cancer and aging by altering free radical metabolism (138) and by lessening the incidence of age-related spontaneous mutations (139). Recently it was shown that melatonin is a most potent endogenous scavenger of free radicals in vitro (58,140) and in vivo (141). Melatonin inhibits production of DNA adducts in carcinogen-exposed animals (140), protects chromosomes of human lymphocytes from radiation damages (142) and enhances gap junctional intercellular communications in vitro (143). The pineal peptide epithalamin stimulates synthesis and secretion of melatonin (144) and has antioxidant and lipid peroxidation inhibitory effects (141).

The data presented could provide an explanation for currently observed age-related increased incidence of cancer. Human survival is becoming more and more "rectangular" (145). This effect is due to a decline in early mortality, related mainly to infections. As a result, a significant increase in the mean life expectancy in human populations occurred (146). The changes in the shapes of the survival curves of human populations respond to the third type of aging delay presented in Figure 8.4. The changes of this type were shown experimentally and epidemiologically to be associated with an increase in tumor rate. In other words, for the increased mean life achieved by the reduction in mortality at an young age, mankind pays with an increased

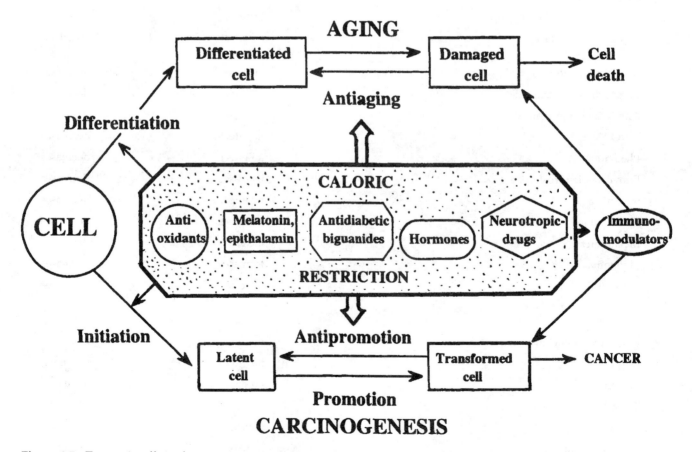

Figure 8.5 Targets in effect of geroprotectors on aging and carcinogenesis.

incidence of cancer and some other diseases of civilization, such as atherosclerosis or diabetes mellitus, at an older age.

Ongoing progress in preventive medicine may further prolong the average life-expectancy of the general population and mandate attention to the effects of a more prolonged life expectancy. Environmental protection represents one effective intervention in preventing some diseases of aging. However this intervention may have only limited success because irreversible processes such as industrialization and urbanization are associated with environmental pollution. New approaches to environmental protection involve substantial costs.

Changes in life style (tobacco smoking, alcohol drinking, diet, sexual mores and other dangerous habits) have already decreased the incidence of cancer and of other diseases of civilization with favorable effects on human longevity. It is becoming clearer and clearer that measures aimed at reversing age-related changes in internal milieu are the most effective prevention of premature aging and carcinogenesis. The substances which protect against the initiating action of harmful agents (antioxidants, antimutagens) may be important additional means of cancer prevention, especially under conditions of intensified risk of exposure to environmental factors (Figure 8.5).

The U.S. program for cancer prevention started in 1985, the goal for 15 years has been to diminish cancer mortality by 50% by the year 2000 and to promote healthy lifestyles (147). These include a fat-restricted diet (from 37–38% to <30% of all calories) and increased consumption of fruits and vegetables (by 50%). An increased intake of vitamins A, C, E, and of vegetable fiber may cause a decline in the incidence of cancers of the gastro-intestinal tract, breast, endometrium, prostate, lungs, and urinary bladder.

Conclusions

The incidence of cancer increases with age in humans and in laboratory animals alike, but patterns of age-related distribution of tumors is different for different tissues and different tumors. Aging may increase or decrease the susceptibility of individual tissues to early carcinogens and usually facilitates promotion and progression of carcinogenesis. Aging may predispose to cancer by two mechanisms: tissue accumulation of cells in late stages of carcinogenesis and alterations in internal homeostasis, in particular, alterations in immune and endocrine system. Increased susceptibility to the effects of late-stage carcinogens is found both in aged animals and aged humans, as predicted by the multistage model of carcinogenesis. Old animals should be included in standard protocol for the long-term assay for carcinogenicity, in particular, of compounds with suggested tumor-promoting activity. Strategies for cancer prevention must include not only measures to minimize exposure to exogenous carcinogenic agents, but also measures to normalize the age-

related alterations in internal milieu. Life-span prolonging drugs (geroprotectors) may either postpone population aging and prolong tumor latency or decrease the mortality in long-living individuals in populations and inhibit carcinogenesis. At least some geroprotectors may increase the survival of a short-living individuals in populations but increase the incidence of malignancy.

It is pertinent to remember E.S. Bauer (148) who wrote six decades ago that, "the problem of cancer apparently coincides with the problem of senility. The aim of science is to slow down the process of aging and to really decrease the probability of cancer development at the same time."

References

1. Dix D, Cohen P, Flannery J. On the role of aging in cancer incidence. *J Theor Biol* 1980; **83**: 163–173.
2. Napalkov P. The relation of human cancer incidence to age. General patterns and exceptions in the USSR. In *Age-Related Factors in Carcinogenesis*, edited by A Likhachev, V Anisimov, R Montesano. Lyon, France: IARC, 1985; **58**: 9–20.
3. Parkin DM, Muir CS, Whelan SL, Gao Y-T, Ferlay, Powell J. *Cancer Incidence in Five Continents*. Vol. VI. IARC Scientific Publication No. 120. Lyon, France: IARC, 1992.
4. Peto R, Roe FJC, Lee PN, et al. Cancer and ageing in mice and men. *Br J Cancer* 1975; **32**: 411–426.
5. Peto R, Parish SE, Gray RG. There is no such thing as ageing, and cancer is not related to it. In *Age-Related Factors in Carcinogenesis*, edited by A Likhachev, V Anisimov, R Montesano. Lyon, France: IARC, 1985; **58**: 43–53.
6. Anisimov VN. *Carcinogenesis and Aging*. Vols. 1 and 2. Boca Raton, FL: CRC Press, 1987.
7. Anisimov VN. Age-related mechanisms of susceptibility to carcinogenesis. *Seminars in Oncology* 1989; **16**: 10-19.
8. Anisimov VN. Age as a factor of risk in multistage carcinogenesis. In *Geriatric Oncology*, edited by L Balducci, GH Lyman, WB Ershler. Philadelphia: Lippincott, 53–59, 1992.
9. Dilman VH. Development, Aging, and Disease. *A New Rationale for and Intervention Strategy*. Switzerland: Harwood Acad Publ. Chur, 1994.
10. Miller RA. Gerontology as oncology. *Cancer* 1991; **68**: 2496–2501.
11. Kaldor JM, Day NE. *Interpretation of epidemiological studies in the context of the multistage model of carcinogenesis*. In *Mechanisms of Environmental carcinogenesis*, edited by JC Barrett. Boca Raton, FL: CRC Press, 1987; **2**: 21–57.
12. Tomatis L (ed). *Cancer. Causes, Occurrence and Control*. IARC Scientific Publication No.100. Lyon, France: IARC, 1990.
13. Harvey M, Voges H, Lee EYHP, et al. Mice deficient in both p53 and Rb develop tumors Primarily of endocrine origin. *Cancer Res* 1995; **55**: 1146–1151.
14. Birnbaum LS. Pharmacokinetic basis of age-related changes in sensitivity to toxicants. *Annu Rev Pharmacol Toxicol* 1991; **31**: 101–128.
15. Anisimov VN, Birnbaum LS, Butenko GM, et al. *Principles for Evaluating Chemical Effects on the Aged Population*. Environmental Health Criteria 144, Geneva: WHO 1993.
16. Mayersohn M, *Pharmacokinetics in the elderly*. Environmental Health Perspectives Supplement 11, 1994; **102**: 119–124.
17. Preston-Martin S, Pike MC, Ross RK, Jones PA, Henderson BE. Increased cell division as a cause of human cancer. *Cancer Res* 1990; **50**: 7415–7421.
18. Cohen SH, Ellwein LB. Genetic errors, cell proliferation, and carcinogenesis. *Cancer Res* 1991; **51**: 6493–6505.
19. Harris CC. Chemical and Physical carcinogenesis: advances and perspectives for the 1990s. *Cancer Res* 1991; **51**: 5023s–5044s.

20. Barrett JC. Mechanisms of action of known human carcinogens. In *Mechanisms of Carcinogenesis in Risk Identification*, edited by H Vainio, PN Magee, DB McGregor and AJ McMichael. Lyon, France: IARC, 1992; **116**: 115–134.

21. Likhachev AJ. Effects of age on DNA repair in relation to carcinogenesis. In *Cancer and Aging*, edited by A Macieira-Coelho and B Nordenskjold. Boca Raton, FL: CRC Press, Inc., 97–108, 1990.

22. McDonnell TJ. Cell division versus cell death: a functional model of multistep neoplasia. *Mol Carcinogenesis* 1993; **8**: 209–213.

23. James SJ, Muskhelishvili L. Rates of apoptosis and proliferation vary with caloric intake and may influence incidence of spontaneous hepatoma in C57BL/6 x C3H F1 mice. *Cancer Res* 1994; **54**: 5508–5510.

24. Farber E. Programmed cell death: necrosis versus apoptosis. *Modern Pathology* 1994; **7**: 605–609.

25. Zakeri Z, Lockshin RA. Physiological cell death during development and its relationship to aging. *Ann NY Acad Sci* 1994; **719**: 212–229.

26. Hermeking H, Eick E. Meditation of C-myc-induced apoptosis by p53. *Science* 1994; **265**: 2091–2096.

27. Peto R, Pike HC, Day NE, *et al.* Guidelines for simple, sensitive significance tests for carcinogenic effects in long-term animal experiments. In *Long-Term and Short-Term Screening Assays for Carcinogens. A Critical Appraisal*, (IARC Monographs Supplement 2). Lyon, France: IARC, 311–426, 1980.

28. Gart JJ, Krewski D, Lee PN, Tarone RE, Wahrendorf J (eds). *Statistical Methods in Cancer Research*. Volume III — The Design and Analysis of Long-Term Animal Experiments. (IARC Scientific Publication No. 79). Lyon, France: IARC, 1986.

29. Strehler BL. Genetic instability as the Primary cause of human aging. *Exp Gerontol* 1986; **21**: 283–319.

30. Kirkwood TBL. DNA, mutation and aging. *Mutat Res* 1989; **219**: 1–7.

31. Cheng KC, Loeb LA. Genomic instability and tumor progression. mechanistic considerations. *Adv Cancer Res* 1993; **60**: 121–156.

32. Lindahl T. Instability and decay of the primary structure of DNA. *Nature* 1993; **362**: 709–715.

33. Pitot HC. The molecular biology of carcinogenesis. *Cancer* 1993; **72**: 962–970.

34. Bishop JM. Molecular themes in oncogenesis. *Cell* 1991l; **64**: 235–248.

35. Harris CC. Tumor suppressor genes, multistage carcinogenesis and molecular epidemiology. In *Mechanisms of Carcinogenesis in Risk Identification*, edited by H Vainio, PN Magee, DB McGregor and AJ McMichael. Lyon, France: IARC, 1992; **116**: 67–86.

36. Knudson AG. Antioncogenes and human cancer. *Proc Natl Acad Sci USA* 1993; **9**: 10914–11113.

37. Lehman TA, Harris CC. Mutational spectra of Protooncogenes and tumor suppressor genes: clues in predicting cancer etiology. In *DNA Adducts: Identification and Biological Significance*, edited by A Dipple Hemminki, DEG Shuker, *et al.* Lyon, France: IARC, 1994; **125**: 399–414.

38. Wallace SS, Van Houten B, Wah Kow Y (eds). DNA Damage. Effects on DNA Structure and Protein Recognition. *Ann NY Acad Sci* 1994; 726.

39. Holliday R. Mechanisms for the control of gene activity during development. *Biol Res* 1990; **65**: 431–471.

40. Jones PA, Buckley JD. The role of DNA methylation in cancer. *Adv Cancer Res* 1990; **54**: 1–23.

41. Catania J, Fairweather DS. DNA methylation and cellular aging. *Mutat Res* 1991; **256**: 283–293.

42. Counts JL, Goodman JI. Hypomethylation of DNA, an epigenetic mechanism involved in tumor promotion. *Mol Carcinogenesis* 1994; **11**: 185–188.

43. Ono T, Uehara Y, Kurishita A, Tawa R, Sakurai H. Biological significance of DNA methylation in the aging Process. *Age & Aging* 1993; **22**: 534–543.

44. Ono T, Takahashi N, Okada S. Age-associated changes in DNA methylation and mRNA level of the c-myc gene in spleen and liver of mice. *Mutat Res* 1989; **219**: 39–50.

45. Matoha HF, Cosgrove JW, Atak JR, Rapoport SI. Selective elevation of c-myc transcript levels in the liver of the aging Fischer-344 rat. *Biochem Biophys Res Commun* 1987; **147**: 1–7.

46. Olafsson B, Chardin P, Touchot N, *et al.* Expression of the ras-related ralA, rhol2 and rab genes in adult mouse-tissues. *Oncogene* 1988; **3**: 231–234.

47. Ono T, Tawa R, Shinya K, *et al.* Methylation of the c-myc gene changes during aging process of mice. *Biochem Biophys Res Commun* 1986; **139**: 1299–1303.

48. Novikov LB, Tlevlesov NJ, Timoshenko MG, *et al.* Expression of proto-oncogenes in organs of adult intact rats. *Exp Oncol* 1989; **11**: 14–17.

49. Semsei I, Ma S, Culter RG. Tissue and age specific expression of the myc proto-oncogene family throughout the life span of the C57BL/6J mouse strain. *Oncogene* 1989; **4**: 465–470.

50. Hemminki K, Dipple A, Shuker DEG, *et al.* DNA Adducts: Identification and Biological Significance, (IARC Scientific Publication No. 125). Lyon, France: IARC, 1994.

51. Dipple A. DNA adducts of chemical carcinogens. *Carcinogenesis* 1995; **16**: 437–441.

52. Park JW, Ames BN. 7-Methylguanine adducts in DNA are normally present at high levels and increase on aging: analysis by HPLC with electrochemical detection. *Proc Natl Acad Sci USA* 1988; **85**: 7467–7470.

53. Randerath K, Li D, Moorthy B, Randerath E. I-compounds endogenous DNA markers of nutritional status, ageing, tumour promotion and carcinogenesis. In *Postlabelling Methods for Detection of DNA Adducts*, edited by DH Phillips, M Castegnaro, H Bartsch. Lyon, France: IARC, 1993; **124**: 157–165.

54. Harman DH. The aging process: major risk factor for disease and death. *Proc Natl Acad Sci USA* 191; **88**: 5360–5363.

55. Ames BN, Shigenaga MB, Hagen TM. Oxidants, antioxidants, and the degenerative diseases of aging. *Proc Natl Acad Sci USA* 1993; **90**: 79915–7922.

56. Yu BP (ed). *Free Radicals in Aging*. Boca Raton, FL: CRC Press, Inc., 1993.

57. Shigenaga MK, Hagen TV, Ames BN. Oxidative damage and mitochondrial decay in aging. *Proc Natl Acad Sci USA* 1994; **91**: 10771–10778.

58. Poeggeler B, Reiter RJ, Tan D-X, Chen L-D, Manchester LC. Melatonin, hydroxyl radical-mediated oxidative damage, and aging: a hypothesis. *J Pineal Res* 1993; **14**: 151–168.

59. Du MQ, Carmichael PL, Phillips DH. Induction of activated mutations in the human c-Ha-ras proto-oncogene by oxygen free radicals. *Mol Carcinogenesis* 1994; **11**: 170–175.

60. Fraga CG, Shigenaga MK, Park J-W, Degan P, Ames BN. Oxidative damage to DNA during aging 8-hydroxy-2'deoxyganosine in rat organ DNA and urine. *Proc Natl Acad Sci USA* 1990; **87**: 4533–4537.

61. Turk PW, Laayoun A, Smith SS, Weitzman SA. DNA adduct 8-hydroxy-2'deoxyguanosine (8-hydroxyguanosine) affects function of human DNA DNA methyltransferase. *Carcinogenesis* 1995; **16**: 1253-l255.

62. Nair J, Barbin A, Guichard Y, Bartsch H. 1,N6-Etenodeoxyadenosine and 3, N4-ethenodeoxycytidine in liver DNA from human and untreated rodents detected by immunoaffinity/ ^{32}P-post-labeling. *Carcinogenesis* 1995; **16**: 613–617.

63. Harley CB, Vaziri H, Counter CM, Allsopp RC. The telomere hypothesis of cellular aging. *Exp Gerontol* 1992; **27**: 375–382.

64. Shay JW, Wright WE, Werbin H. Loss of telomeric DNA during aging may predispose cells to cancer (review). *Int J Oncology* 1993; **3**: 559–563.

65. Harley CB, Andrews W, Chiu CP, *et al.* Human telomerase inhibition and cancer. *Proc Amer Assoc Cancer Res* 1995; **36**: 671.

66. Wynford-Thomas D, Bond JA, Wyllie FS, Jones CJ. Does telomere shortening drive selection for p53 mutation in human cancer? *Mol Carcinogenesis* 1995; **12**: 119–123.

67. Lutz WK. Endogenous genotoxic agents and processes as a basis of spontaneous carcinogenesis. *Mutat Res* 1990; **238**: 287–295.

68. Ames BN, Gold LS. Endogenous mutagens and the causes of aging and cancer. *Mutat Res* 1991; **250**: 3–16.

69. Smith KC. Spontaneous mutagenesis. experimental, genetic and other factors. *Mutat Res* 1992; **277**: 139–162.

70. Vijg J, Gossen JA. Somatic mutations and cellular aging. *Comp Biochem Physiol* 1993; **104B**: 429–237.

71. Anisimov VN, Gvardina OE. N-Nitrosomethylures-induced carcinogenesis in the progeny of male rats of different ages. *Mutat Res* 1995; **316**: 139–145.

72. Berenblum I. Sequential aspects of chemical carcinogenesis. skin. In *Cancer — A Comprehensive Treatise*, edited by J Becker. New York: Plenum Press, 323–344, 1975.

73. Consensus Report. In *Mechanisms of Carcinogenesis in Risk Identification*, edited by H Vainio, PN Magee, DB McGregor and AJ McMichael. Lyon, France: IARC, 9–56, 1992.

74. Slaga TJ (ed). *Mechanisms of Tumor Promotion*. Vols 1–4. Boca Raton, FL: CRC Press, 1983/84.

75. Slaga TJ. Can tumor promotion be effectively inhibited? In *Models, Mechanisms and Etiology of Tumor Promotion*, edited by M Borzsonyi, NE Day, K Lapis, H Yamasaki. IARC Scientific Publication No. 56. Lyon, France: IARC, 497–506, 1984.

76. Stenback F, Peto R, Shubik P. Initiation and promotion at different ages and doses in 2200 mice. III. Linear extrapolation from high doses may underestimate low-dose tumour risks. *Br J Cancer* 1981; **44**: 24–34.

77. Ebbesen P. Papilloma development on TPA treated young and senescent mouse skin. In *Age-Related Factors in Carcinogenesis*, edited by A Likhachev, V Anisimov, R Montesano. IARC Scientific Publication No. 58. Lyon, France: IARC, 167–171, 1985.

78. Ward JM. Increased susceptibility of liver of aged F:344/Ncr rats to the effects of phenobarbital on the incidence, morphology, and histochemistry of hepatocellular foci and neoplasms. *J Natl Cancer Inst* 1983; **71**: 815–823.

79. Ward JM, Lynch P, Riggs C. Rapid development of hepatocellular neoplasms in aging male C3H/HeNcr mice given phenobarbital. *Cancer Lett* 1988; **39**: 9–18.

80. Reuber MD, Glover EL. Hyperplastic and early neoplastic lesions of the liver in Buffalo strain rats of various ages given. *J Natl Cancer Inst* 1967; **38**: 891–899.

81. Schulte-Hermann R, Timmermann-Trosiener I, Schuppler J. Promotion of spontaneous preneoplastic cells in rat liver as a possible explanation of tumor production by nonmutagenic compounds. *Cancer Res* 1983; **43**: 839–844.

82. Cuttley RC, Marsman DS, Popp JA. Age-related susceptibility to the carcinogenic effect of the peroxisome proliferator WY-14,643 in rat liver. *Carcinogenesis* 1991; **12**: 469–473.

83. Kraupp-Grasl B, Huber W, Taper H, Schulte-Hermann R. Increased susceptibility of aged rats to hepatocarcinogenesis by the peroxisome proliferator nafenopin and the possible involvement of altered liver foci occurring spontaneously. *Cancer Res* 1991; **51**: 666–671.

84. Anisimov VN. Effect of age on dose-response relationship in carcinogenesis induced by single administration of N-nitrosomethylurea in female rats. *J Cancer Res Clin Oncol* 1988; **114**: 628–635.

85. Anisimov VN. Age and dose-dependent carcinogenic effects of N-nitrosomethylurea administered intraperitoneally in a single dose to young and adult female mice. *J Cancer Res Clin Oncol* 1993; **119**: 657–664.

86. Anisimov VN. Effect of aging and interval between primary and secondary treatment in carcinogenesis induced by neonatal exposure to 5-bromodeoxyuridine and subsequent administration of N-nitrosomethylurea in rats. *Mutat Res* 1995; **316**: 173–187.

87. Lee G-H, Sawada N, Mochizuki Y, et al. Immortal epithelial cells of normal C3H mouse liver in culture: possible precursor populations for spontaneous hepatocellular carcinoma. *Cancer Res* 1989; **49**: 403–409.

88. Ogawa K, Onoe T, Takeuchi M. Spontaneous occurrence of gamma glutamyl transpeptidase-positive hepatocytic foci in 105-week-old Wistar and 72-week-old Fischer 344 male rats. *J Natl Cancer Inst* 1981; **67**: 407–412.

89. Ebbesen P. Reticulosarcoma and amyloid development in BALB/c mice inoculated with syngeneic cells from young and old donors. *J Natl Cancer Inst* 1971; **47**: 1241–1245.

90. Anisimov VN. Age-related mechanisms of susceptibility to cancer. In *Cancer in the Elderly. Treatment and Research*, edited by JS Fentiman, S Monfardini. Oxford, UK: Oxford Univ Press, 1–10, 1994.

91. Sobue T, Yamaguchi N, Suzuki T, et al. Lung cancer incidence rate for male ex-smokers according to age at cessation of smoking. *Jpn J Cancer Res* 13; **84**: 601–607.

92. Ershler WB. Mechanisms of age-associated reduced tumor growth and spread in mice. In *Geriatric Oncology*, edited by L Balducci, GH Lyman, WB Ershler. Philadelphia: Lippincott, 76–85, 1992.

93. Ershler WB. Explanations for reduced tumor proliferative capacity with age. *Exp Gerontol* 1992; **27**: 551–558.

94. Miller RA. Aging and cancer — another perspective. *J Gerontol* 1993; **48**: B8–B9.

95. Yancik R, Yates JW (eds). *Cancer in the elderly. Approaches to early detection and treatment*. New York: Springer, 1989.

96. Berrino F, Sant M, Verdecchia A, Capocaccia R, Hakulinen T, Esteve J (eds). *Survival of cancer patients in Europe*. EUROCARE Study. Lyon, France: IARC, 132, 1995.

97. Anisimov VN, Zhukovskaya NV, Loktionov AS, et al. Influence of host age on lung colony forming capacity of injected rat rhabdomyosarcoma cells. *Cancer Lett* 1988; **40**: 77–82.

98. Anisimov VN, Zhukovskaya NV, Loktionov AS, et al. *Host and donor age dependency of colony forming capacity of lung-affine rat rhabdomyosarcoma RA-2 cells*. Abstr. of The Int. Conf. on Tumor Microenvironment. Progression, Therapy and Prevention. Israel: Tiberias, 6, 1995.

99. McCullough KD, Coleman WB, Smith GJ, Grisham JW. Age-dependent regulation of the tumorigenic potential of neoplastically transformed rat liver epithelial cells by the liver micro-environment. *Cancer res* 1994; **54**: 3668–3671.

100. Larionov LF. *Cancer and Endocrine System*. Leningrad: Meditsina, 1938.

101. Ohno S, Nagai Y. Genes in multiple copies as the primary cause of aging. In *Genetic Effects of Aging*, edited by D Bergsma, DE Harrison, NW Paul. New York: Alan R. Liss, 501–514, 1978.

102. Anisimov VN. Blasomogenesis in persistent estrus rats. *Vopr Onkol* 1971; **8**: 67–75.

103. Teramoto S, Fukuchi Y, Uejima Y, Teramoto K, Orimo H. Influences of chronic tobacco smoke inhalation on aging and oxidant-antioxidant balance in the senescent-accelerated mouse (SAM)-P/2. *Exp Gerontol* 1993; **28**: 87–95.

104. Sacher GA. Life table modification and life prolongation. In *Handbook of the Biology of Aging*, edited by CE Finch and L Hayflick. New York: Van Nostrand Reinhold, 582–638, 1977.

105. Alexandrov SA. *Late Radiation Oathology of Mammals*. Fortschritte der Onkologie. Berlin: Band 6, Akademik-Verlag, 1982.

106. Golostchapov PV, Boitsova VP, Vorobjeva MI. *Comparative Analysis of Effectiveness of Chronic External Irradiation at Different Daily Doses*. Moscow: Central Research Institute Atominform, 1988.

107. Moskalev YI. *Late Effects of Ionizing Irradiation*. Moscow: Meditsina, 1991.

108. Beniashvili DSh, Bilanishvili VG, Menabde MZ. Low-frequency electromagnetic radiation enhances the induction of rat mammary tumors by nitrosomethyl urea. *Cancer Lett* 1991; **61**: 75–79.

109. Anderson LE. Biological effects of extremely low-frequency electromagnetic fields. *In vivo* studies. *Am Ind Hyg Assoc J* 1993; **54**: 186-196.

110. Loscher W, Mevissen M, Lehmacher W, Stamm A. Tumor promotion in a breast cancer model by exposure to a weak alternating magnetic field. *Cancer Lett* 1993; **71**: 75–81.

111. Anisimov VN, Zhukova OV, Beniashvili DS, Bilanishvili VG, Menabde MZ. Effect of light deprivation and electromagnetic fields on mammary carcinogenesis in female rats. *Adv Pineal Res* 1994; **7**: 231–236.

112. McLean J, Thansandote A, Lecueyer D, et al. A 60-Hz magnetic field increases the incidence of squamous cell carcinomas in mice previously exposed to chemical carcinogens. *Cancer Lett* 1995; **92**: 121–125.

113. Nikitina VM. *Effect of modulated electromagnetic fields induced by marine radio transmitters on aging of the organism*. Proc. Int. Conf. on Shipbuilding ISC, October 8–12, 1994; St. Petersburg, 1994; Sect. F., 60–66.

114. Morris SH. The genetic toxicology of 5-bromodeoxyuridine in mammalian cells. *Mutat Res* 1991; **258**: 161–188.

115. Lindahl T. DNA repair enzymes. *Ann Rev Biochem* 1982; **51**: 61–87.

116. Davidson RL, Broeker P, Ashman CR. DNA base sequence changes and sequence specificity of bromodeoxyuridine-induced mutations in mammalian cells. *Proc Natl Acad Sci USA* 1988; **85**: 4406–4410.

117. Potapenko AI. *Radiation-induced shortening of life span and natural aging in D. melanogaster*. Abstract of Diss Cand Biol Sci. Puschino. Institute of Biophysics of the USSR Acad Sci 1982.

118. Craddock VM. Shortening of the life span caused by administration of 5-bromodeoxyuridine to neonatal rats. *Chem-Biol Interact* 1981; **35**: 139–144.

119. Likhachev AJ, Tomatis L, Margison GP. Incorporation and persistence of 5-bromodeoxyuridine in newborn rat tissue DNA. *Chem-Biol Interact* 1983; **46**: 31–38.

120. Ward JM, Henneman JR, Osipova GY, Anisimov VN. Persistence of 5-bromo-2'-deoxyuridine in tissues of rats after exposure in early life. *Toxicology* 1991; **70**: 345–352.

121. Tapscott SJ, Lassar AB, Davis RL, Weintraub H. 5-Bromo-2' deoxyuridine blocks myogenesis by extinguishing expression of MyoD1. *Science* 1989; **245**: 532–53.

122. Weghorst CM, Henneman JR, Ward JH. Dose response of hepatic and DNA synthesis rates to continuous exposure of bromodeoxyuridine (BrdU) via slow-release -pellets or osmotic minipumps in male B6C3F1 mice. *J Histochem Cytochem* 1991; **39**: 177–182.

123. Napalkov NP, Anisimov VN, Likhachev AJ, Tomatis L. 5-bromo deoxyuridine-induced carcinogenesis and its modification by persistent estrus syndrome, unilateral nephrectomy, and X-irradiation in rats. *Cancer Res* 1989; **49**: 318–323.

124. Anisimov VN, Osipova GY. Effect of neonatal exposure to 5-bromo-2'-deoxyuridine on life span, estrus function and tumor development in rats — an argument in favor of the mutation theory of aging? *Mutat Res* 1992; **275**: 97–110.

125. Anisimov VN, Osipova GY. Life span reduction and carcinogenesis in the progeny of rats exposed neonatally to 5-bromo-2'-deoxyuridine. *Mutat Res* 1993; **295**: 113–123.

126. Anisimov VN. The sole DNA damage induced by bromodeoxyuridine is sufficient for initiation of both aging and carcinogenesis *in vivo*. *Ann NY Acad Sci* 1994; **719**: 494–501.

127. Anisimov VN. Carcinogenesis induced by neonatal exposure to various doses of 5-bromo-2'-deoxyuridine in rats. *Cancer Lett* 1995; **91**: 63–71.

128. Mikhelson VM. Diseases of DNA Repair and Their Relation with Carcinogenesis and Aging. *All-Union Institute for Medical Information Publ*. Moscow, 1983.

129. Lehmann AR. Ageing. DNA repair of radiation damage and carcinogenesis. Fact and fiction. In *Age-Related Factors in Carcinogenesis*, edited by A Likhachev, V Anisimov, R Montesano. IARC Scientific Publication No. 58. Lyon, France: IARC, 203–214, 1985.

130. Dilman VM. *Endocrinological Oncology*. Leningrad: Meditsina, 1983.

131. Alexandrov VA, Popovich IG, Anisimov VN, Napalkov NP. Influence of hormonal disturbances on transplacental and multigeneration carcinogenesis. In *Perinatal and multigeneration carcinogenesis*, edited by NP Napalkov, JM Rice, L Tomatis, H Yamasaki, IARC Scientific Publication No. 96. Lyon, France: IARC, 1989, 35–50.

132. Miller RA, Turke P, Chrips C, *et al*. Age-sensitive T-cell phenotypes covary in genetically heterogenous mice and predict early death from lymphoma. *J Gerontol* 1994; **49**: B255-B262.

133. Harrison DE. Potential misinterpretations using models of accelerated aging. *J Gerontol* 1994; **49**: B245.

134. Rudman D, Feller AG, Nagraj HS, *et al*. Effect of human growth hormone in men over 60 years old. *New England J Med* 1990; **323**: 1–6.

135. Vance ML. Growth hormone for the elderly? *New England J Med* 1990; **323**: 52–54.

136. Khansari DN, Gustad T. Effects of long-term, low-dose growth hormone therapy on immune function and life expectancy of mice. *Mech Ageing Develop* 1991; **57**: 87–100.

137. Moon HD, Simpson ME, Lee CH, Evans HM. Neoplasms in rats treated with pituitary growth hormone. III. Reproductive organs. *Cancer Res* 1950; **10**: 549–556.

138. Weindruch R, Gravenstein S. Cancer and aging. In *New Frontiers in Cancer Causation*, edited by OH Iversen. Washington, DC: Taylor & Francis, 321–332, 1993.

139. Dempsey JL, Pfeiffer M, Morley AA. Effect of dietary restriction on *in vivo* somatic mutation in mice. *Mutat Res* 1993; **291**: 141–14.

140. Reiter RJ, Tan D-X, Poeggeler B, *et al*. Melatonin as a free radical scavenger. Implications for aging and age-related diseases. *Ann NY Acad Sci* 1994; **719**: 1–12.

141. Anisimov VN, Khavinson VKh, Prokopenko VM. *Melatonin and epithalamin inhibit free radical oxidation in rats*. *Proc Russian Acad Sci* 1995; **343**: 551–559.

142. Vijayalaxmi, Reiter RJ, Meltz ML. Melatonin protects human blood lymphocytes for radiation-induced chromosome damage. *Proc Amer Assoc Cancer Res* 1995; **36**: 613.

143. Ubeda A, Trillo MA, House DE, Blackman CF. Melatonin-enhances junctional transfer in normal C3H/10T1/2 cells. *Cancer Lett* 1995; **91**: 241–245.

144. Anisimov VN, Khavinson VKh, Morozov VG. Twenty years of study on effects of pineal peptide preparation. Epithalamin in experimental gerontology and oncology. *Ann NY Acad Sci* 1994; **719**: 483–493.

145. Hirsch HR. Evolution of senescent. Natural increase of population displaying Gompertz or power-law death rates and constant of age-dependent maternity rates. *J Theor Biol* 1982; **98**: 321–346.

146. Gavrilov LA, Cavrilova NS. *The Biology of Life Span. A Quantitative Approach*. Chur. Switzerland: Harwood Acad. Publ., 1991.

147. Greenvald P, Sondik E (eds). *Cancer Control Objectives for the Nation 1985–2000*. Division of Cancer Prevention and Control, National Cancer Institute, U.S. Dept. of Health and Human Services, NCI Monographs No.2 1986.

148. Bauer ES. Cancer as a biological problem. In *Modern Problems of Theoretical Medicine*, edited by RE Jackson. Moscow: State Publ. House, *Biol Med Lit* 1936; **1**: 37–45.

9. Growth Factors, Oncogenes and Aging

J. Albert Fernandez-Pol

Introduction

The aims of this chapter are three. First, to contribute to the elucidation of some key concepts in the field of cancer and aging, such as growth factor-induced cell proliferation in malignant and senescent cells. Second, to show the complexity of these concepts, thereby demonstrating that simplicity and anticipation of findings is not possible in this area of research. Finally, the analysis of the main characteristics of a growth factor-induced gene, denoted Metallopanstimulin (MPS), and its use in the diagnosis of oncogenic processes will be summarized. Both the MPS mRNA and the MPS protein have been found to be present at abnormally high quantities in numerous different types of cancers. To the extent in which this chapter succeeds in clarifying some aspects of the complexity of this field, it should discourage the creation of oversimplified hypothesis of oncogenic processes *in vivo*, including those of the author. An astonishing example presented in this review is the expression of MPS-1 in malignant melanoma which offers an illustration of the extreme complexity of the oncogenic process *in vivo*.

The DNA sequence which encodes the MPS-1 protein has been previously described in detail (35–36). MPS-1 is a "zinc finger protein" (Figure 9.1) of subunit molecular weight of approximately 10,000-Dalton which because of its chemical and biological properties was originally designated as metallopanstimulin (35) since: 1) it forms a complex with metal ions such as zinc (*Greek: metallo*); 2) it has been detected in many different cell types (*Greek: pan = all*); and 3) it is associated with rapid cell proliferation (*Latin: stimulin*). Interestingly, when the MPS-1 protein is artificially overproduced by transformed cells, such as in Baculovirus infected cells, the MPS protein is released from the cells into the extracellular fluids (36). After our initial work on cloning and characterization of the MPS gene was published, a subsequent computer search of the Gene Bank revealed that the MPS-1 protein is homologous to the rat S27 ribosomal protein (28).

MPS-1 is a ribosomal protein, and many of its characteristics can be explained by this fact. It binds nucleic acid (36), is induced in cell growth states (35–36), and is decreased in senescent cells. All the molecular biology (sequence homology, biological actions, etc) and clinical data (histopathology, *in situ* hybridization, etc) are quite consistent with MPS-1 being a classical ribosomal protein in normal cells (35, 41). However, in addition to its role as a ribosomal protein, MPS-1 may have a variety of other natural or artificial activities which are more evident when the protein is overproduced by malignant cells or when experiments are performed with exogenously added recombinant MPS-1 protein, respectively. It is conceivable that overproduction of MPS-1 by malignant cells may lead to intra- and extra-cellular actions that are unrelated to ribosomal functions, such as (I) cytokine effects; (ii) alteration of transcription (e.g. by binding to cAMP response elements; 36); or (iii) even promotion of cellular transformation. While it is possible that a low molecular weight ribosomal protein such as MPS-1 can also function in the native state as an oncogene product, cytokine, or transcription factor, it is without precedent and has only been suggested by preliminary experiments. Proving in multiple reproducible ways that this particular ribosomal protein and MPS-1-like proteins can have an important role in cancer and can be used for practical purposes such as detection of cancer cells by immunohistopathology and detection of oncogenic processes in patients by serodiagnosis is documented in concise form in this review.

The biological properties of MPS-1 coincides well with the contention that MPS-1 is a good marker for cell proliferation and oncogenic processes. What could be a superior tissue marker for cellular proliferation than a ribosomal protein(s), when the ribosomal proteins reflect exactly the rate of protein synthesis related to grow stimulation, as can be found in classical textbooks of molecular biology (9)? Also, if the MPS-1(S27 ribosomal) protein and MPS-1-like proteins are released in the blood because of overproduction, intrinsic chemical properties (e.g. amphipathic characteristics), and/

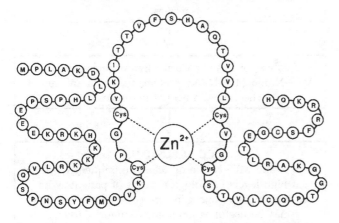

Figure 9.1 is a schematic representation of the MPS-1 protein showing the coordination of the zinc atom to cysteine residues.

or cancer cell destruction (apoptosis, necrosis), what could be a better marker for detection of cell activation and/or proliferative activity by serodiagnosis? If the ribosomal protein(s) MPS-1 or MPS-1-like proteins are released in the blood when overproduced in cancer cells, then a method for detecting cellular activity due to cell proliferation and/or oncogenic processes should be feasible.

Thus, we also describe here the unanticipated finding that there are immunoreactive forms of MPS-1 in the blood which were found by using specific protein sequences of MPS-1 as antigens in immunoassay procedures. None of these finding could be anticipated because of the complexity of the factors involved in the molecular and cellular systems active in oncogenesis such as growth factors, oncogenes, tumor-suppressor genes, and apoptosis.

Cancer, Growth Factors and Oncogenes

The cancer phenotype consists of several distinct characteristics such as indefinite proliferative life span, anchorage-independent growth, low growth factor requirements, invasion and metastasis; in addition, cancerous cells can synthesize their own growth factors, which leads to cell proliferation that is independent of the otherwise carefully regulated supply of growth factors and growth-related hormones (1–8, 11–13, 15).

As used in this review, "growth factors" refers to proteins and peptides that stimulate or promote cell division. Such growth factors are produced by virtually all types of tumors, and their involvement in cancer has been documented during the last 20 years in numerous scientific and medical articles (10–13, 15).

Growth factor independence and autonomous growth of cancer cells is due to the constitutive expression of growth factors, their membrane receptors, or intracellular signal pathways which ultimately leads to induction of DNA synthesis and cell division (7, 8, 15). The constitutively expressed growth factors, which function as transforming proteins in the neoplastic cell, may be encoded by oncogenes, or alternatively, their expression may be under the control of oncogenes (7).

A large number of different oncogenes have been identified, each encoding a specific protein that is involved in certain specific types of cancer (1–3, 7, 8). For example, the c-myc oncogene and its protein are involved in breast and colon carcinomas (7, 8), while the c-erbB-2 oncogene and its protein are involved in breast and ovarian carcinomas (14).

Many oncogenes enable continuous cell proliferation by either encoding the growth factor protein or inducing the expression of growth factor proteins which are secreted by the cells (7, 8, 15). The secreted proteins can interact with and stimulate growth-mediating receptors on the surfaces of the same cells that secreted the proteins. This self-stimulating property of cancerous cells has been termed "autocrine secretion" (11, 13, 15).

There are peculiar types of autocrine growth factors, produced by various normal and cancerous cells, which possess both growth stimulatory and inhibitory

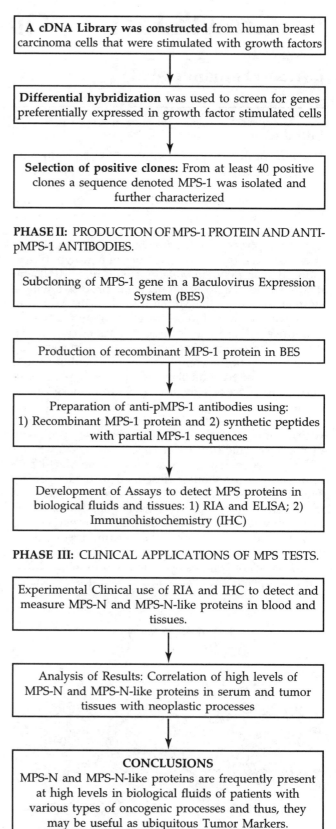

PHASE I: ISOLATION OF MPS-1 cDNA

A cDNA Library was constructed from human breast carcinoma cells that were stimulated with growth factors

Differential hybridization was used to screen for genes preferentially expressed in growth factor stimulated cells

Selection of positive clones: From at least 40 positive clones a sequence denoted MPS-1 was isolated and further characterized

PHASE II: PRODUCTION OF MPS-1 PROTEIN AND ANTI-pMPS-1 ANTIBODIES.

Subcloning of MPS-1 gene in a Baculovirus Expression System (BES)

Production of recombinant MPS-1 protein in BES

Preparation of anti-pMPS-1 antibodies using:
1) Recombinant MPS-1 protein and 2) synthetic peptides with partial MPS-1 sequences

Development of Assays to detect MPS proteins in biological fluids and tissues: 1) RIA and ELISA; 2) Immunohistochemistry (IHC)

PHASE III: CLINICAL APPLICATIONS OF MPS TESTS.

Experimental Clinical use of RIA and IHC to detect and measure MPS-N and MPS-N-like proteins in blood and tissues.

Analysis of Results: Correlation of high levels of MPS-N and MPS-N-like proteins in serum and tumor tissues with neoplastic processes

CONCLUSIONS
MPS-N and MPS-N-like proteins are frequently present at high levels in biological fluids of patients with various types of oncogenic processes and thus, they may be useful as ubiquitous Tumor Markers.

Chart 9.1 Main steps in the development of the mps-n test for detection of neoplastic processes

activities in the same molecule (13, 16–19). The growth response to these bifunctional growth factors is largely dependent on cell type and culture conditions (15). For example, transforming growth factor beta-1 (TGF beta-1) a 25,000 dalton disulfide-linked homodimer is mitogenic for many fibroblastic cell lines and growth inhibitory for diverse epithelial cell types including lung carcinoma, breast carcinoma, and prostatic carcinomas (15). One conspicuous attribute of TGF beta is that it affects the expression of a series of genes and oncogenes to either negatively or positively control their expression (15, 16, 19). Furthermore, there are unusual growth factors produced by viruses, such as the tat protein of the human immunodeficiency virus (HIV), a viral regulatory gene product, with growth stimulatory activity in certain cell types (20, 21).

Cellular aging

A fundamental characteristic of normal cells is their limited ability to proliferate in culture (22). Invariably, after an initial mitotic period in culture, normal cells from humans and most other species suffer a gradual decline in their ability to proliferate. Eventually, the decline becomes irreversible. This progression towards a lower activity state has been termed "cellular senescence" (22). Cellular senescence has been studied most often in cultures of human fibroblasts (e.g. WI-38 cells) (22). Numerous studies have indicated that cellular senescence in culture reflects aging *in vivo* (22). More recent studies have suggested that senescent fibroblasts are unable to proliferate, at least in part, because of selective repression of genes involved in transcriptional activity, such as a protooncogene designated as "c-fos" (22).

Zinc finger proteins

In the past several years, a series of discoveries revealed that many proteins contain metal ions, particularly zinc ions (Zn^{++}), that play fundamental roles in stabilizing specific protein conformations (23, 27). Many of these metalloproteins are involved in nucleic acid binding, gene regulation (23, 27), and enzymatic activity (23, 24). In addition, ribosomal proteins such as S27 (MPS-1) and S29 have zinc finger-like motifs (28).

Of particular interest for this review are the "zinc finger" metal ion binding proteins (23–28). The primary finding in this field came from the analysis of the sequence of the protein Transcription Factor III (TFIIIA) from *Xenopus laevis* (23). This sequence contains nine tandem imperfect repeats that have the consensus sequence (Phe,Tyr)-X-Cys-$X_{2,4}$-Cys-X_3-Phe-X_5-Leu-X_2-His-$X_{3,4}$-His-X_{2-6}, where X represents a nonconserved amino acid residue from 2 to 6 residues (23, 24). This sequence contains two cysteines and two histidines that form a complex with a single metal ion, particularly Zn^{++} (23,24). This structural domain was termed "zinc finger" (23, 25). The zinc finger domains function as the nucleic acid-binding regions of these regulatory molecules which are involved in the control of gene transcription (23–26). Subsequently, zinc finger motifs have been identified in numerous eukaryotic and viral proteins with transcriptional regulatory activity (23–27).

Molecular Biology of MPS-1 Gene Expression

Biotechnological advances such as differential hybridization of growth factor-induced cDNA libraries allowed us to identify genes associated with neoplastic growth and subsequently to develop isotopic and non-isotopic methods for measuring the protein products of these genes in biological fluids (Chart 1; Figures 9.2, 9.6). The biochemical and biological characteristics of one of such genes, denoted MPS, which was isolated by differential hybridization, are summarized in Tables 9.1, 9.4 and 9.5 and Figure 9.7.

Table 9.1 Summary of MPS-1 gene expression features.

Experiments	Results	Salient features[a] (Known or proposed)
Northern blot	0. 4kb mRNA	High levels in cancer cells
Western blot	10 kDal protein	High levels in cancer cells
Phosphorylation	Phosphoprotein	Required for action
Dimerization	Forms Dimers	Required for function (not known)
Gel shift	Binds CRE	Role in gene regulation (not known)
UV light activation	UV stimulates MPS-1 gene expression	Involved in DNA repair (not known)
In situ hybridization in mice embryos	Localizes in areas of cell proliferation	Role in embryogenesis

[a] Proposed features are based on indirect evidence and thus they are the subject of further investigation.

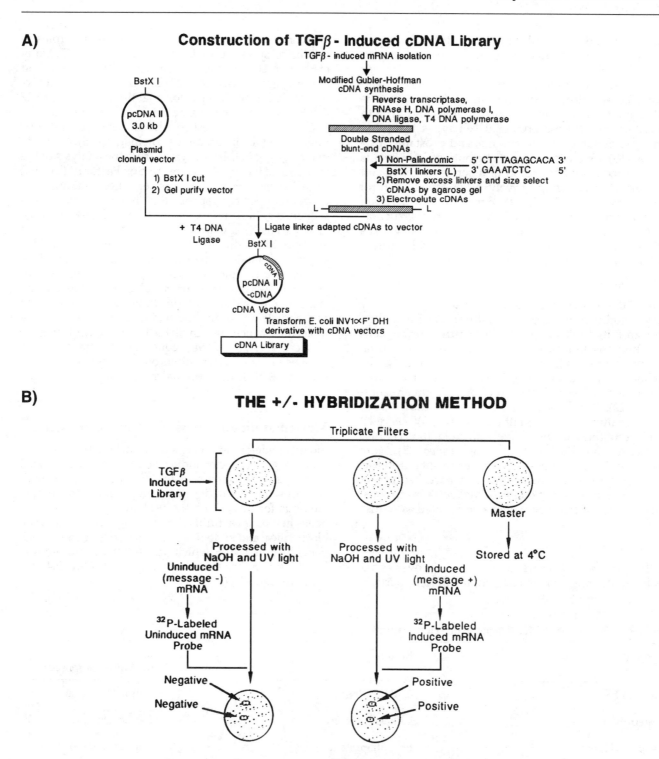

Figure 9.2 shows the construction and screening of the cDNA library from which the MPS-1 sequence was isolated. As shown in **Figure 9.2a**, human carcinoma cells were treated with transforming growth factor beta (TGFβ), in the presence of EGF, and their mRNAs were converted into cDNA. The various cDNA's were inserted into cloning plasmids, which were then used to transform E. coli cells to generate a library of numerous different cDNA sequences from which the MPS-1 sequence was isolated by differential hybridization. **Figure 9.2b** shows the +/− differential hybridization method. The cDNA library contained in E. coli cells was plated and triplicated using nitrocellulose filters lifts. Two filters were screened using two different sets of mRNA probes; one set (message +) was derived from mRNA from carcinoma cells that had been treated with TGFβ, and one set (message −) was derived from control cells that had not been treated with TGFβ. E. coli colonies containing cDNA which hybridized with the mRNA from treated cells, but which did not hybridize with the mRNA from untreated cells, were identified, isolated, and cloned. Those colonies were further analyzed, and one clonal colony contained a sequence that was later designanted as the MPS-1 cDNA sequence. The third of the triplicate filter lifts was stored as a master to preserve the colonies in the same spatial arrangement as the processed filters.

DNA Translation
MPS-1 cDNA

1		CG	ACC	TAC	GCA	CAC	GAG	AAC	ATG	CCT	CTC	GCA	AAG	GAT	CTC	CTT	CAT		47
1									M	P	L	A	K	D	L	L	H		9

48	CCC	TCT	CCA	GAA	GAG	GAG	AAG	AGG	AAA	CAC	AAG	AAG	AAA	CGC	CTG	GTG	95
10	P	S	P	E	E	E	K	R	K	H	K	K	K	R	L	V	25

96	CAG	AGC	CCC	AAT	TCC	TAC	TTC	ATG	GAT	GTG	AAA	TGC	CCA	GGA	TGC	TAT	143
26	Q	S	P	N	S	Y	F	M	D	V	K	C	P	G	C	Y	41

144	AAA	ATC	ACC	ACG	GTC	TTT	AGC	CAT	GCA	CAA	ACG	GTA	GTT	TTG	TGT	GTT	191
42	K	I	T	T	V	F	S	H	A	Q	T	V	V	L	C	V	57

192	GGC	TGC	TCC	ACT	GTC	CTC	TGC	CAG	CCT	ACA	GGA	GGA	AAA	GCA	AGG	CTT	239
58	G	C	S	T	V	L	C	Q	P	T	G	G	K	A	R	L	73

240	ACA	GAA	GGA	TGT	TCC	TTC	AGG	AGG	AAG	CAG	CAC	TAA	AAG	CAC	TCT	GAG	287
74	T	E	G	C	S	F	R	R	K	Q	H						84

288		TCA	AGA	TGA	GTG	GGA	AAC	CAT	CTC	AAC	AAA	CAC	ATT	TTG	GAT		329

Figure 9.3 shows the nucleotide sequence of the 329 bp fragment of plasmid ST1H2-pcDNA-II, containing the exon coding for the 84 amino acids of human MPS-1 and the 5' and 3' flanking regions. The deduced amino acid sequence is shown in one letter code. The translational initiation site ATG starts at nucleotide position 21 and the TAA termination signal begins at nucleotide 273. The underlined amino acid residues in regions 2–17, 41–55, and 67–84 correspond to three synthetic peptides designated A1, A2, and A3, respectively, that were utilized for antibody production. The numbers in each line refer to the nucleotide (upper) and amino acid (lower) positions. The methionine at position 21 constitutes the NH2-terminus.

The nucleotide sequence and deduced amino acid sequence of the MPS-1 gene is shown in Figure 9.3. The MPS sequence has a zinc finger motif (Figure 9.4), and it shows a significant homology to several transcriptionally active proteins including viral zinc finger proteins (Table 9.2; data not shown). It is noted that the MPS-1 protein has a zinc-finger like domain with four cysteins (Figure 9.1). Proteins with this motif generally bind to DNA as dimers (Table 9.1). How these motifs participate in binding to RNA, if indeed they do is not known.

Table 9.2 Comparison of the zinc finger structure, DNA interaction, and transacting activity of the MPS-1 protein with other zinc finger proteins.

c_x		
	c_4:	$c - x_2 - c - x_{13} - c - x_2 - c$
		$c - x_2 - c - x_{15} - c - x_2 - c$
	c_5:	$c - x_5 - c - x_9 - c - x_2 - c - x_4 - c$
	c_6:	$c - x_2 - c - x_6 - c - x_6 - c - x_2 - c - x_6 - c$

	Finger Type	Binds DNA *In vitro*	Transacting	Organism
GAL4 (PPRI/ARGRII/LAC9/qa-1f)	C6	+	+	Yeast
MPS-1 (ST1H2)	C4	+	+ (?)	Human/rat/mouse
E1A	C4	−	+	adenovirus
Steroid hormone Receptor Superfamily	C4+C5	+	+	human/rat/mouse/chicken

DNA binding activity is documented in Ref. 36. Trans-Acting activity was demonstrated in preliminary CAT assay analysis of COS-1 and PC-12 cell extracts which indicated enhancement of transcriptional activity induced by the MPS-1 protein (data not shown). The cells were cotransfected with the expression/activator (pMEP4-MPS-1) and reporter (pCRE-CAT) plasmids using the calcium phosphate method.

DNA Translation
MPS-1 cDNA

```
              29             38             47             56             65             74
5' ATG CCT CTC GCA AAG GAT CTC CTT CAT CCC TCT CCA GAA GAG GAG AAG AGG AAA
   Met Pro Leu Ala Lys Asp Leu Leu His Pro Ser Pro Glu Glu Glu Lys Arg Lys

              83             92            101            110            119            128
   CAC AAG AAG AAA CGC CTG GTG CAG AGC CCC AAT TCC TAC TTC ATG GAT GTG AAA
   His Lys Lys Lys Arg Leu Val Gln Ser Pro Asn Ser Tyr Phe Met Asp Val Lys

             137            146            155            164            173            182
   TGC CCA GGA TGC TAT AAA ATC ACC ACG GTC TTT AGC CAT GCA CAA ACG GTA GTT
  |Cys Pro Gly Cys| Tyr Lys Ile Thr Thr Val Phe Ser His Ala Gln Thr Val Val

             191            200            209            218            227            236
   TTG TGT GTT GGC TGC TCC ACT GTC CTC TGC CAG CCT ACA GGA GGA AAA GCA AGG
   Leu |Cys Val Gly Cys| Ser Thr Val Leu Cys Gln Pro Thr Gly Gly Lys Ala Arg

             245            254            263            272
   CTT ACA GAA GGA TGT TCC TTC AGG AGG AAG CAG CAC TAA 3'
   Leu Thr Glu Gly Cys Ser Phe Arg Arg Lys Gln His ***
```

Figure 9.4 shows the nucleotide sequence and deduced amino acid sequence of the region of ST1H2 cDNA coding for MPS-1. The deduced amino acid sequence is shown in the three letter code. The amino acid sequence for the zinc finger domain of MPS-1 is boxed at the zinc binding regions and underlined on the connecting region. Numbers above each line refer to the nucleotide position. The termination codon (TAA) is indicated by ***.

HYDROPHOBICITY INDEX

Index

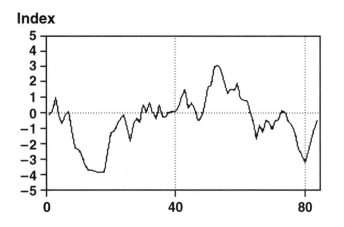

Figure 9.5 indicates the hydropathy profile of the MPS-1 84-kD protein. The horizontal axis represents amino acid residue number. A positive value on the vertical axis indicates that the corresponding residue is hydrophobic; a negative value indicates hydrophilicity. The residue window size used was six; the curve was generated by DNASIS (Hitachi).

As used herein, "metallopanstimulin" (MPS) is defined to include synthetic or naturally occurring proteins that have the following properties: (1) they have at least one zinc finger domain; (2) they are amphipathic (sufficiently soluble in both water and lipids to allow them to penetrate lipid membranes while remaining soluble in aqueous fluid) (Figure 9.5); (3) they are released or secreted from cancerous cells; (4) under certain experimental conditions they penetrate into the nucleus where they bind to specific sequences of DNA, identified as cAMP response elements (36). Thus, MPS proteins are zinc finger ribosomal proteins that can be experimentally shown to have a number of different functions (28, 35, 36).

Table 9.3 Presence of MPS-1 mRNA in cultured human malignant cell lines.

Cell type	Cell line
Breast carcinoma	MDA-MB-468, MDA-MB-231, BT-20
Prostate carcinoma	DU-145, PC-3
Melanoma	SK-MEL-28, RPMI-7951
Colon adenocarcinoma	LoVo
Lung carcinoma	A-549
Vulvar carcinoma	A-431
Fibrosarcoma	HT-1080
Neuroblastoma	LAN-5
Squamous cell carcinoma of skin	SCC-15

Cloning of MPS-1 (ST1H2.SEQ) Into the Baculovirus Transfer Vector pJVETL to Construct the Recombinant Expression Vector pJVETL-ST1H2/P17

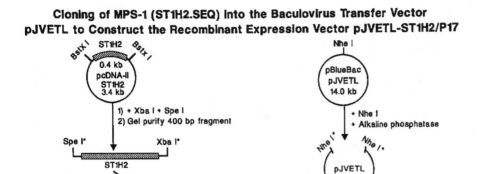

*Nhe I cut vector accepts cDNAs with Xba I and Spe I overhangs.
Nhe I site is not regenerated.

Figure 9.6 shows the cloning of the human MPS-1 (ST1H2) sequence into the baculovirus transfer vector pJVETL to construct the recombinant expression vector pJVETL-ST1H2/P17 which expressed two proteins: (1) the endogenous form of MPS-1, and (2) an additional protein which contained seventeen additional amino acid residues at the NH2 terminus.

Biological Characteristics of pMPS-1

1. Normal Proliferating Cell

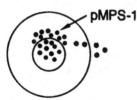

Extracellular
pMPS-1: Present at low levels (<10 ng/ml)

2. Benign Tumors

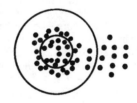

Extracellular
pMPS-1: Present at slightly elevated levels (10-30 ng/ml)

3. Malignant Tumors

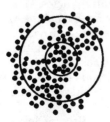

Extracellular
pMPS-1: Present in large quantities (30-2000 ng/ml)

4. Aging Cells

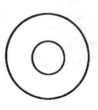

Extracellular
pMPS-1: Undetectable

Figure 9.7 Schematic representation of some of the biological characteristics of protein MPS-1 (pMPS-1). pMPS-1: refers to immunoreactive pMPS-1 and pMPS-1-like proteins detected by anti-R-MPS-1 antibodies in biological fluids. **1. In Normal proliferating cells**, pMPS-1 is produced and released in detectable amounts to the extracellular space. **2. In Benign tumors**, pMPS-1 is produced at higher levels than in proliferating normal cells and it is released in significant amounts to the extracellular space. **3. In Malignant tumors**, pMPS-1 is produced at much higher levels than in proliferating normal cells or benign tumors and it is is secreted/released to the extracellular space in abundant quantities. **4. In aging cells**, the synthesis of pMPS-1 is greatly reduced or absent and thus pMPS-1 is undectectable in extracellular fluids.

Table 9.4 Detection of MPS-1 mRNA and protein in human tissues.

Type of tissue	No of samples mRNA[1]/Protein[2]	Organ of origin
A. Carcinomas and sarcomas		
Carcinoma	52+++/+++	vulva, cervix, ovary, endometrium, colon, lung, bladder, liver, metastatic
Squamous cell carcinoma	35+++/+++	vulva, cervix, esophagus, lung
Adenocarcinoma	25++/++	cervix, ovary, endometrium, colon, prostate
Carcinoma *in situ*	9++/++	vulva
Serous carcinoma	5+/+	ovary
Papillary serous carcinoma	5++/++	endometrium
Sarcoma	4++/++	ovary, endometrium, metastasis
Melanoma	**2>+++/+++**	**vulva, metastasis**
Verrucous carcinoma	1++/++	vulva
Retroperitoneal liposarcoma	1+++/+++	retroperitoneal
Mucinous carcinoma	1+/+	ovary
Leiomiosarcoma	1++/++	ovary
Papillary carcinoma	1++/++	ovary
Papillary adenocarcinoma	1++/++	endometrium
Adenosqamous carcinoma	1++/++	endometrium
Clear cell carcinoma	1++/++	endometrium
Mixed mesodermal carcinoma	1+/+	endometrium
Mixed muellerian tumor	1+/+	endometrium
Ductal carcinoma	3+++/+++	breast
Inflammatory carcinoma	**1>+++/+++**	**breast**
B. Benign lesions		
Lichen sclerosus atrophicus	**1 –/–**	**vulvar skin**
Benign cysts	10ND/–	ovary, breast
Granuloma	1ND/+	lung
Leiomyoma	2ND/–	uterus
Fibroma	1ND/–	ovary
C. Normal tissues[3]	63 –/–	cervix, ovary, endometrium, myometrium, vagina, peritoneum, fallopian tubes, breast, rectal muscle, skin, small intestine, lymph node

[1] The MPS-1 mRNA was detected using a biotynilated single-stranded anti-sense DNA probe. [2] The MPS-1 protein was detected by immunohistochemical staining using anti-peptide A antibodies. Signals: (–) negative, (+) weakly positive, (++) positive, and (+++) strongly positive. The staining recorded refer to the that of the cancer cells, since the stoma cells were not significantly stained. As can be observed, there was an excellent correlation between MPS-1 mRNA and protein expression. [3] Note that although normal tissues are listed as (–), they showed staining (+ to +++) only in areas of normal cell proliferation. ND: Not done. Note that (i) vulvar melanoma, and breast inflammatory carcinoma had the highest levels of MPS-1 mRNA and protein detected; by Northern blot analysis the MPS-1 mRNA levels in these tissues were >80-fold normal levels; and (ii) lichen sclerosus atrophicus, a rare condition characterized by extremely low proliferation rates was negative for MPS-1 mRNA and protein in the usual areas of cell multiplication; these observations are highlighted by bold characters.

An important characteristic of the MPS-1 gene is that it has been shown to be transcribed into mRNA at abnormally high levels in a wide variety of cancerous cells (Refs. 35, 36, 37; Tables 9.3, 9.4 and 9.5). In addition, in a number of tumors studied to date, the quantity of MPS-1 mRNA present in the cells is a useful indicator of the aggressiveness and potential lethality of the malignancy (Figure 9.8; Table 9.4). Therefore, the MPS-1 protein offers a method of detecting and diagnosing a broad variety of cancers, as well as a method of assessing the level and aggressiveness of the treatment that will be required to combat the spread of a tumor in a specific patient.

It is of interest to mention here that embryologic studies in mice showed that the MPS-1 sequence is present in greater abundance in cells derived from the ectodermal layer than in those derived from endodermal or mesodermal layers (Figure 9.9). These results suggest that the MPS-1 sequence may be a marker for ectodermally-derived malignancies. Therefore, the embryologic studies also suggest that the MPS-1 cDNA and polypeptide sequences may provide a useful and widely applicable method of detecting the presence of a cancerous or pre-cancerous condition in a patient suspected of having numerous different types of cancer, regardless of which specific type of cancer is involved.

In addition, the widely different levels of MPS-1 mRNA or protein in various different tumors correlated well with the pathological degree of malignancy and growth rate of those tumors (Figure 9.8; Table 9.4). Therefore, the diagnostic methods presented elsewhere

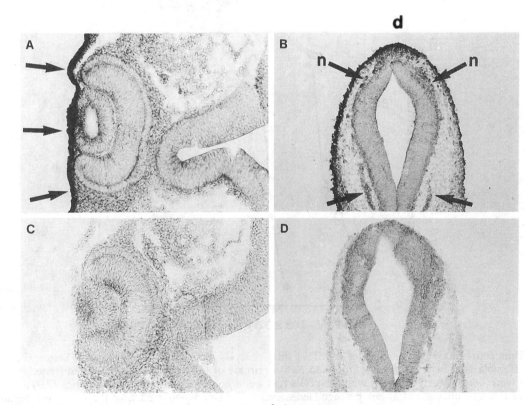

Figure 9.8 shows the MPS-1 mRNA level in various human carcinomas (O, ovarian carcinoma; C, carcinoma of the uterine cervix; E, endometrial carcinoma; VM, vulvar melanoma). The widely different levels of MPS-1 mRNA correlate with the pathological degree of malignancy and growth rate of the tumors. Ovarian carcinomas (samples 1–3) and carcinoma of the cervix (samples 4–6) were histologically well differentiated; endometrial carcinomas (samples 7 and 8) were highly invasive to myometrium. Sample number nine (VM) corresponds to a very fast growing malignant melanoma; the patient underwent vulvectomy at the time of sample collection and died 3 weeks later of wide-spread metastatic disease (see Reference 35).

Figure 9.9 MPS-1 mRNA expression in mice embryonic epithelia.

Mice embryos were 10-days old and were purchased from Novagene (Madison, WI). In situ hybridization was done using a biotinylated cDNA MPS-1 probe. A,C, parasagittal section shows the skin over the optic vesicle and optic nerve. B, D transverse section of the neural tube. A,B: biotinylated MPS-1 cDNA probe. C,D: Control, no MPS-1 cDNA probe; (Magnification: A,C, 200X; B, D 100X; reduced by 25%. Note that (1) the MPS- cDNA probe strongly labels the epithelia (skin) of the embryo (A, arrows); and 2) it also labels the neural crest (n, arrows; d, dorsal position) and ventral ganglia (open arrows); this observation is of interest, since melanomas which are neural crest derived showed strong MPS-1 mRNA expression, as shown elsewhere in this paper. These results show that the MPS-1 sequence is present in greater abundance in cells derived from the ectodermal layer than in those derived from endodermal or mesodermal layers.

A)

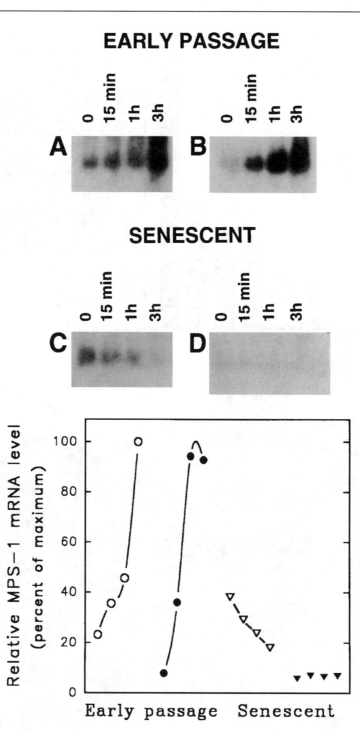

B)

Figure 9.10 Time course showing the changes in MPS-1 mRNA levels after addition of Fetal Calf Serum (FCS) in human WI-38 diploid fibroblasts at early passage (young) and at the extreme of their proliferative life-span (senescence). (a) WI-38 cells were used at early passage, when the cells had undergone < 20 population doublings (PD) and > 75% were capable of DNA synthesis, and at late passage (senescent; > 27 PDs), when < 20 % of the cells were capable of DNA synthesis, as determined by monoclonal anti-5-Bromo-2'deoxyuridine (BrdU) antibodies to detect BrdU incorporation in DNA (Cell Proliferation kit, Amersham, Arlington Heights, Illinois). WI-38 cells at early (PD, 19 and 20; A and B, respectively) and late passage (PD, 27 and 28; C and D, respectively) were plated at 1. 25 x 10^6 cells per 100-mm dishes in DME/F-12 plus 10% calf serum for 48 h. After rinsing with serum-free medium, the cells were maintained for 24 additional hours in synthetic serum free DME/F12+H medium. Subsequently, serum-deprived (control, time= 0) or 5% serum-stimulated (15 min, 1 h, and 3 h) early- and late- passage cells were analyzed for the abundance of MPS-1 mRNA. Aliquots of total RNA (20 ug per lane) were fractionated on agarose gels and transferred to a nylon membrane. The transcripts were detected by hybridization with ^{32}P-labeled MPS-1 cDNA probe and subsequent autoradiography. (b) The resulting autoradiogram was quantified by densitometric scanning and the relative abundance of the hybridization signal for each time point was plotted. (O), PD 19 ; (●), PD 20 ; (△), PD 27; and (▲), PD 28.

in this review can provide very useful and quickly available information on how aggressively a cancerous or pre-cancerous condition in a patient should be treated using chemotherapy, radiation therapy, or surgery.

Numerous experiments with human tissue culture cells and human pathological tissue specimens demonstrated that the MPS-1 mRNA and its encoded protein are expressed in normal cells to a much lesser degree than in premalignant or malignant tumor cells, and they are present at very low levels in senescent cells compared to young healthy cells.

The *in vitro* experimental results indicate that senescent human WI-38 fibroblasts express MPS-1 mRNA at lower levels than in their respective early passage cultures (Figure 9.10). Senescent cells also show striking, irreversible decreases in the expression of MPS-1 mRNA; this is manifested by the loss of MPS-1 mRNA inducibility by fetal calf serum and other growth factors (e.g. EGF, TGF alpha) which have been shown to induce MPS-1 mRNA in young human WI-38 fibroblasts. This loss results at least in part from a reduction in the production of the MPS-1 protein. Thus, reduction in MPS-1 production is associated with senescence and it may be one of the factors contributing to cellular aging. These results suggest that it may be possible to restore senescent cells to a replication-competent state by utilization of MPS-1 protein as an anti-aging factor, in combination with other critical factors that are involved in aging process.

It is interesting to note here that the rate at which a cell produces protein and thus the number of ribosomal units that are required, is linked closely to the rate of cell growth (9). For example, a change in growth conditions rapidly leads to an increase or decrease in the rate of synthesis of all ribosomal units (9). The mechanism of this coordinated regulation is due to the properties of ribosomal proteins related to their ability to act as translational repressors of their own synthesis (9). These universal properties of ribosomal proteins related to cell growth may make some of them, in particular those that might be released into the extracellular fluids by neoplastic cells, during the process of oncogenesis (1–7, 15), necrosis, or apoptosis (29), ideal for use as serum tumor markers. In fact, when the MPS-1 protein is artificially overproduced by transformed cells, such as Baculovirus transformed cells, the MPS-1 protein is released from the cells into the extracellular fluids (36). It should not be surprising that ribosomal proteins such as MPS-1 can be released from cancer cells into the extracelluar fluids. Several mechanisms may explain the release of MPS-1 and MPS-1-like proteins into extracellular fluids such as intrinsic chemical properties of MPS-1 (e.g. amphipatic properties (Figure 9.5) which conveys to the MPS molecule the ability to transverse cell membranes), necrosis, or possibly apoptosis (29). Even insoluble nuclear matrix proteins can be released from apoptotic cells in a soluble form and they can be detected in serum from cancer patients (30, 31).

It has been demonstrated that the MPS-1 protein is overproduced in cancer cells (35–37). The question is

what are the consequences of overproduction of MPS-1 if any, in addition to its standard ribosomal functions? It is conceivable that overproduction of MPS-1 by malignant cells may lead to intra- and extra-cellular actions that are unrelated to ribosomal functions, such as cytokine effects, interference with transcription (e.g. by binding to cAMP response elements; Ref. 36), promotion of transformation, or even toxic effects.

The results of some preliminary experiments with cultured cells exposed to recombinant MPS-1 seem to substantiate some of the points delineated above. We have studied the effects of MPS-1/P17 on the growth of human cultured cells. The ability of MPS-1/P17 to induce growth effects in culture cells was determined using MDA-468 human mammary carcinoma cells, SK-MEL-28 human melanoma cells, and WI-38 human normal diploid fibroblasts. The assay was performed on monolayer cells grown in Dulbecco-Vogt modified Eagle's medium supplemented with 5% fetal calf serum (v/v) as previously described (16). The MPS-1/P17 protein was produced in a baculovirus expression system (Figure 9.6; Ref. 36), purified from Sf9 insect cells by high-performance liquid chromatography (36), and it was added directly to the culture medium. The cell number was determined after trypsinization of cells on day 3 of culture by Coulter-counter measurements (16).

The MPS-1/P17 protein stimulated the growth of MDA-468 cells at 25 to 50 ng/mL. The stimulation of MDA-468 cell growth at 72 hours was 35% with 50 ng/mL MPS-1/P17 in comparison to control untreated cells.

The growth of SK-MEL-28 human melanoma cells was inhibited in a dose-dependent manner by 25 to 100 ng/mL MPS-1/P17. After 24 hours of exposure to MPS-1, SK-MEL-28 cells began to appear granular, numerous cells floated into the culture medium, many cells were destroyed and no mitotic cells were observed. After 72 hours of exposure to MPS-1/P17, the decrease in cell number of treated cells with respect to control untreated cells was about 33 % in cells treated with 100 ng/mL MPS-1/P17.

Under similar experimental conditions, no growth effects or cytotoxicity (as determined by cell granularity, floating or dead cells) was observed in WI-38 human diploid fibroblasts treated with 25 to 100 ng/mL MPS-1/P17.

These results suggest that the MPS-1/P17 protein is a bifunctional regulator of cell growth (13, 15) as indicated by the fact that MPS-1/P17 inhibits the growth of SK-MEL-28 cells, at concentrations similar to those that stimulate the growth of MDA-468 cells.

The unexpected growth stimulatory effect of a zinc finger proteins such as MPS-1/P17 is not without precedent. For example, the zinc finger tat protein of HIV, a viral regulatory gene product, can be released from infected cells as a biologically active protein and directly act as a growth stimulator of cells derived from Kaposi's sarcoma lesions (20).

While it is possible that a ribosomal protein such as MPS-1 can also function in the native state as a cytokine, oncogene or transcription factor, it is without precedent and has only been demonstrated in preliminary experiments. It might be that the molecular biology of certain ribosomal proteins such as MPS-1, and other ribosomal proteins that are known in great detail, may have a significant role in cancer previously unanticipated; except in certain instances (32).

In summary, as is the case with numerous proteins that are overproduced in many diseases, pathological effects of protein overproduction will eventually result that may be quite independent and unpredictable by the normal function of the protein.

Expression of MPS-1 mRNA and MPS-1 Proteins in Human Cancer

The MPS-1 cDNA was used to generate DNA and RNA probes to detect MPS-1 mRNA (35–37). Furthermore, the recombinant MPS-1 protein and chemical derivatives were used to generate polyclonal (36, 40) and monoclonal (data not shown) anti-MPS-1 antibodies. Both the DNA probes and the anti-MPS-1 antibodies were used to detect MPS-1 mRNA and MPS proteins, respectively, in various types of cultured cells and pathologic tissue specimens.

Table 9.3 indicates the presence of MPS-1 mRNA in exponentially growing cultured human malignant cell lines. Tissue culture experiments demonstrated that the level of MPS-1 mRNA was several-fold greater (from 3 to 15-fold) in human malignant cell lines than in normal human WI-38 diploid fibroblasts under the same experimental conditions (35, 36). Furthermore, experiments with pathologic tissue specimens demonstrated that the MPS-1 gene is expressed at high levels in numerous human cancers such as prostate, breast, brain, lung, and particularly melanomas (Table 9.4). In contrast, the MPS-1 gene is expressed at low levels in normal tissues (Table 9.4). Table 9.5 indicates the pres-

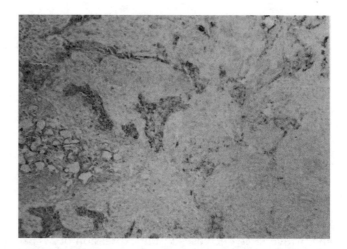

Figure 9.11 *In situ* hybridization with MPS-1 biotinylated DNA probe reveals that the MPS-1 mRNA is limited to the cytoplasm of cancerous cells and no staining is observed in the stroma. Pathological tissue specimen corresponds to patient 2J with ovarian carcinoma metastatic to omentum. *In situ* hybridization was done with biotin-labeled MPS-1 DNA probe. Darkly stained cells are both positive for MPS-1 mRNA and malignant. Tissues were subjected to standard *in situ* hybridization procedure. (Magnification X100)

ence of MPS-1 mRNA in peripheral blood of human patients with hematological malignancies.

The MPS-1 mRNA was detected using biotynilated single-stranded anti-sense DNA probe (Figure 9.11). The MPS-1 protein was detected by immunohistochemical staining using anti-peptide A antibodies; the MPS peptide sequences used for antibody production are underlined in Figure 9.3. As can be observed in Table 9.4, there is an excellent correlation between MPS-1 mRNA and protein expression.

The results of numerous immunohistochemistry experiments indicated that the MPS-1 antigen is a ubiquitous tumor marker which may be useful in the detection, prognosis and management of various types of neoplastic conditions. An illustrative example of the use of MPS in the study of human melanocytic lesions is presented in the following section.

The MPS Protein is a Useful Marker to Study Melanocytic Lesions at the Immunohistological Level

Although the detection and management of all forms of cancer is desirable, the detection of malignant melanoma is particularly challenging to the clinician. Often benign lesions are difficult to distinguish from malignant lesions. It is imperative, however, that malignant melanoma be detected early and reliably to improve survival rates.

Recently, immunohistochemical studies were conducted to examine the expression of MPS-1 protein in various types of benign and malignant melanocytic lesions (41). Protein antigen, detected with anti MPS-1

Table 9.5 Presence of MPS-1 mRNA in human hematological malignancies.

Type of malignancy	MPS-1 mRNA Negative	Positive
Presence of malignant cells in peripheral blood		
Chronic lymphocytic leukemia	0	3
Chronic myelogenous leukemia	0	2
Multiple myeloma	0	3
Lymphoma	0	3
Absence of malignant cells in peripheral blood (control)		
Melanoma	1	0
Small Cell lung carcinoma	1	0
Colon carcinoma	2	0

White blood cells were tested by Northern blot analysis with MPS-1 probe

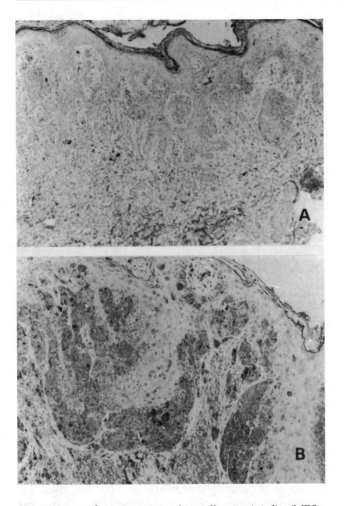

Figure 9.12 The expression of metallopanstimulin (MPS-1) in Melanocytic lesions. **A. Benign melanocytic lesion.** Melanocytic nevus, compound type. The patient is a 3 year old white girl with changing congenital nevus. Section shows nevus cell nests within the epidermis and dermis. "Droping off" is seen at the dermal-epidemal junction. **B. Malignant Melanocytic lesion.** Malignant melanoma superficial spreading type. The patient is a 65 year old white man with a shoulder lesion. Section shows a proliferation of atypical melanocytes in the dermis and epidermis. In areas, there is clear cell nesting as well as small basaloid cells consistent with intralesional transformation. Both sections A and B were identically processed for immunohistochemistry with anti-MPS-1 antibodies.

dermal melanocytic components were intensely and evenly stained. These findings were very similar to those seen in melanomas. These changes are an example of intense activation of the newly formed melanocyte population and not a sign of malignant transformation.

It is of interest to note that scar tissue generates large amounts of growth factors. Thus, growth factors may be responsible for both activation of melanocytic cells and intense expression of MPS observed in the biopsy. It will be appreciated that the histological features of these recurrent nevi were indistinguishable from melanomas, a phenomenon that often confounds the diagnostician. The correct diagnosis was made by reviewing the original melanocytic nevus.

In melanomas (Figure 9.12B), the staining patterns are more complex. While some melanomas stain evenly positive, others have remarkable variable expression of MPS. This seems to correlate, to some extent, with intralesional transformation (Figure 9.12B; and Ref. 5). The variability is so pronounced that some cells stain intensely positive in nests of cells staining moderately positive (Figure 9.13B). The scattered melanocytes migrating to the upper layers of the epidermis usually are intensely positive. Curiously, metastatic melanoma to lymph nodes shows only faint positivity in the limited sampling studied. A single example of melanoma metastatic to the skin was evenly and intensely positive in spite of its seemingly well differentiated, almost nevoid appearance. No gradient staining was present, as it should have been in the case of a benign nevus.

Macrophages in and around the area are intensely positive with a coarse, granular cytoplasmic pattern. Macrophages present in less intensely stained areas had less MPS content than those located in strongly stained areas. This was particularly true in nevi in which macrophages were rare or non-existent (Figure 9.12A). This finding tends to correlate with the near absence of apoptosis in nevi. On the other hand, the presence of MPS in macrophages of melanomas (Figure 9.12B) suggests direct phagocytosis of melanoma cell debris following apoptosis, a common phenomenon. Some melanocytes in melanomas show individual cells with similar patterns, supporting the concept of phagocytosis by melanoma cells.

As the above discussion points out, MPS is a useful marker for melanocytic lesions at the immunohistological level, providing important clues in the biological nature of melanocytic tumors not obtainable by other methods.

The MPS-N Antigen is a Ubiquitous Tumor Marker Which May be Useful in Early Detection, Prognosis and Management of Various Types of Benign and Malignant Oncogenic Processess

During the last 25 years, serum tumor markers have been intensely studied (33, 42). Numerous circulating antigens have been proposed as universal or organ-specific tumor markers for diagnosis, localization, and assessment of treatment. In the studies summarized in

antibodies was found in both benign and malignant melanocytic lesions. In benign lesions (Figure 9.12A), the staining was weak and in a gradient, the most superficial cells with nesting growth patterns were positive, particularly those within the epidermis. The stain intensity decreased as the melanocytes were located deeper in the dermis. Practically speaking, only type A melanocytes stain positive while the B and C types are negative.

Recurrent melanocytic nevi were also studied. MPS was nearly negative in the original untreated nevi. In the recurrent lesions, the regenerating epidermal and

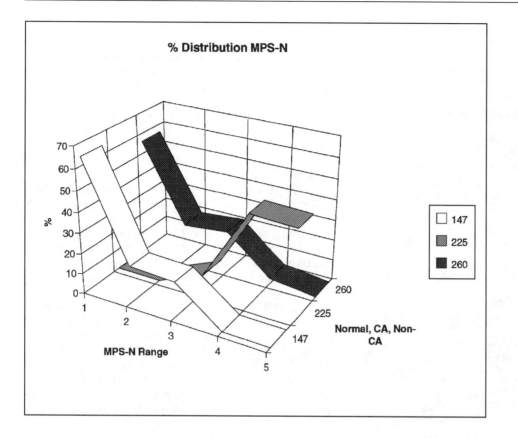

Figure 9.13 Percent Distribution of MPS-N values. The MPS-N ranges 1 to 5 correspond to those shown in Table 9.6, from left to right. Healthy subjects; Active cancerous disease; Non-malignant diseases. In the inset, the number of patients for each group is shown.

this review, MPS-N as a "universal or broad spectrum" tumor maker is defined as an antigen(s) found in abnormal concentrations in the blood of a large number of patients (> 80%) suffering form various forms of benign and malignant neoplastic processess. The results presented in this review demonstrate that the MPS-N antigen is a ubiquitous tumor marker which may be useful in early detection, prognosis and management of various types of benign and malignant neoplastic conditions.

It has been shown in a previous section that the MPS-1 DNA sequence and the protein can be used in diagnostic methods such as detection of malignant cells associated with several types of tumors. The development of a sensitive and specific radioimmunoassay (RIA) for MPS-N, using recombinant MPS-1 proteins (Figure 9.6; Ref. 36) and synthetic peptide technology (34), made it possible to detect the very low concentrations of MPS-N and MPS-N-like proteins in human blood and other body fluids (38–40). Thus, the MPS-N RIA provides a method for determining the presence of certain types of abnormal proliferative conditions and/or active oncogenic processes in patients.

A preliminary clinical study including 632 individuals separated in healthy subjects, active cancerous diseases, non-malignant diseases, and premalignant diseases has provided important information about the use of MPS-N in the detection of various types of cancer (40). The data from the clinical study is provided in Table 9.6 and also illustrated graphically in Figure 9.13. In general, the MPS-N test was found to be experimen-

tally useful in: 1) Detection of primary cancerous disease in previously undiagnosed individuals; and 2) Detection of cancer recurrence in previously diagnosed and treated patients. Since the MPS-N assay measures proteins common to various forms of cancer, including MPS-N and MPS-N like proteins in human serum, it is clearly not useful to determine tumor localization.

The MPS-N test may have significant importance in the detection of numerous types of undiagnosed common malignancies. As shown in Table 9.6, increased MPS-N levels have been detected with high frequency (>80% of the cases) in numerous types of common cancers such as prostate, colorectal, lung, neuroendocrine, leukemias, etc. Moreover, in patients having these types of cancers, MPS-N testing may have important value in monitoring metastatic or persistently active cancer, following chemotherapy, surgery, or radiotherapy. A persistent elevation in circulating MPS-N levels following treatment or increase in an otherwise lower level is indicative of recurrent or residual cancer and poor therapeutic response (33, 38). A declining MPS-N value is generally indicative of a good response to treatment and a favorable prognosis (Figure 9.14).

Serum MPS-N can also be elevated in active nonmalignant tumorigenic processes such as benign prostatic hypertrophy (BPH; Table 9.6) . It is conceivable that in a number of cases of BPH, MPS-N detects early cancer of the prostate, present in a field of neoplastic cells that was not detected by other means. Of course, it is also possible that MPS-N antigens are released by BPH cells that have not suffered malignant transformation. In-

Table 9.6 Distribution of MPS-N values: number of patients: 632.

	Number	Percent (ng/ml)				
		<7.0	7.0–10	10.01–20	20.01–50	>50.01
Healthy subjects						
Women (19–64 years)	20	70	20	10	0	0
Men (21–55 years)	20	65	10	25	0	0
Men (50–88 years)	107	62	20	18	0	0
Total	147	64	18	17	0	0
Cancerous diseases, active						
Genitourinary tract						
Prostate	126	1	<1	11	48	38
Bladder	6	0	0	0	33	66
Testicular	1	0	0	0	0	100
Gastrointestinal tract						
Esophageal	3	0	0	33	66	0
Pancreatic	1	0	0	0	0	100
Hepatoma	2	0	0	0	50	50
Colorectal	27	0	0	7	44	48
Lung cancer						
Epithelial malignancies	27	0	0	11	26	63
Head and neck region						
Epithelial malignancies	6	0	0	0	66	33
Central nervous system						
Primary neoplasms	1	0	0	0	0	100
Neuroendocrine origin	6	0	0	17	17	66
Leukemia and lymphoma	7	0	0	0	43	57
*Other malignancies**	12	0	0	0	58	42
Total	225	<1	<1	9	45	44
Nonmalignant diseases						
Benign prostatic hypertrophy	37	30	16	38	13	3
Hepatitis, B, C	18	83	5	11	0	0
Liver cirrhosis	4	100	0	0	0	0
Other	201	58	21	20	1	0
Total	260	56	19	21	3	<1
Premalignant disease						
Colorectal polyps	4	0	0	0	75	25

*Other malignancies: include cancer of unknown origins, squamous cell carcinomas, etc. See Reference 40.

flammatory conditions of the prostate, liver, intestine and colon were negative for MPS-N (Table 9.6, section on "Hepatitis, Cirrhosis, Other"). Finally, it is interesting to note here that four cases of premalignant colorectal polyps were positive for MPS-N antigen, suggesting that early diagnosis of premalignant proliferative conditions by measurement of MPS-N antigen in the serum may be feasible (Table 9.6).

In conclusion, the MPS-N test, which measures a unique serum antigen (s) common to a variety of oncogenic processes, provides the following clinically useful information: 1) First and foremost the MPS-N test narrows down the uncertainty zone concerning the presence or absence of an oncogenic process; 2) The MPS-N test may be useful to signal cases where further clinical investigation of oncogenic processes by a phy-

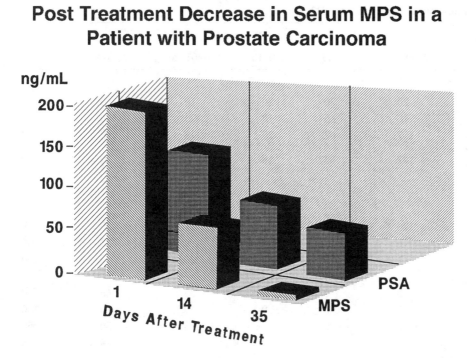

Post Treatment Decrease in Serum MPS in a Patient with Prostate Carcinoma

Figure 9.14 Monitoring serum levels of MPS-N antigen after successful therapy of a patient with prostate carcinoma. MPS, metallopanstimulin-N; PSA, prostatic specific antigen. Note the faster decline in serum MPS-N levels in comparison to the slower decrease in serum PSA levels.

sician is needed; 3) Thus, the MPS-N test is an indicator of potential clinical problems in the area of oncogenesis.

Conclusions and Future Prospects

The rate at which a cell produces protein and thus the number of ribosomal units that are required is linked closely to the rate of cell growth (9). Cancer cells somehow can subvert this system and overproduction of ribosomal proteins occurs. Many different human cancers overexpress the MPS-1 (S27 ribosomal) gene and that can be demonstrated by numerous different assays. Both, the MPS-1 mRNA and the MPS-1 protein are present in abnormally high concentrations in a wide variety of cancer cells. Therefore, they provide a method for detecting and diagnosing malignancy in many type of tumors. Assays using labeled DNA or RNA probes and antibodies that bind to MPS-1 mRNA and MPS-1 protein, respectively, have shown a high ability to distinguish between cancerous and noncancerous cells. Further analysis of this system promises to yield useful information for both understanding malignant transformation and use of MPS-1 and MPS-1-like antigens to aid in the early detection of cancer.

- The MPS-N antigen present in the blood does not meet some of the criteria for rating a protein as a perfect tumor marker (Table 9.7). Evidently, the MPS-N antigen is a non-specific tumor marker, since it is present in healthy subjects and it is produced by both benign and malignant tumors (Figure 9.7). However, the MPS-N antigen is sensitive (present in early stages; and present frequently in late stage), it can be use as management guide (the concentration reflects prognosis and it correlates with therapeutic resection), and analytically, the immunoassay

is quantitative and sensitive. Future world wide confirmatory reports will determine weather this test is acceptable to decrease the clinical uncertainty of the presence or absence of an oncogenic process.
- Finally, it is conceivable that the MPS-N tumor marker may be useful to detect numerous types of malignancies in early stages, thereby reducing the mortality from various types of cancers, and thus the enormous expenditures associated with the treatment of advanced cancer.
- *Note added concerning the MPS-N test*: In some serum samples of patients with active metastatic prostate cancer, we have recently identified authentic

Table 9.7 Rating a protein as a tumor marker.

- **Specificity**
  - Absent in health subjects
  - Exclusively produced by malignant tumors

- **Sensitivity**
  - Present in early stage
  - Present frequently in late state

- **Management guide**
  - Concentration reflects prognosis
  - Concentration correlates with therapeutic resection

- **Analytical**
  - Quantitative and sensitive assay

- **Confirmatory reports**
  - World wide acceptance

immunoreactive MPS-1 and antigens with sequence similarity to MPS-1. Thus, the immunoreactive substances detected by the MPS-N test do not accurately reflect the true levels of authentic immunoreactive MPS-1 in the circulation. Additional experimental and clinical studies are needed to determine with more precision the molecular profiles of MPS-N antigens in the sera of patients with metastatic prostate cancer and other cancers.

Acknowledgments

This work was supported by DVA Medical Center Research Funds. This review would not have been possible without the research work of Dennis J. Klos, Chemist, Paul D. Hamilton, Molecular Biologist, and Vera M. Schuette. The research contributions of Patricia Huygens, Visiting Professor, and Mariela Zirlinger, Chemist, both from the University of Buenos Aires, Argentina, are acknowledged. The contributions of Maria E. Fernandez-Pol, Computer Specialist, in patient data analysis is appreciated. The author thanks his collaborators in different areas for providing materials for this review: Gastrointestinal Cancer, Dany Ganger, M.D., Rush Presbyterian-St Luke's Medical Center, Chicago, IL; Gynecologic cancer, Francisco P. Xynos, M.D., St. Louis University; Melanocytic lesions, Daniel Santa Cruz, St. Johns' Mercy Medical center, Washington University, St. Louis, MO. Finally, the help of Dr. Daniel Santa Cruz in writing the section on melanoma is acknowledged.

References

1. Bishop JM. The Molecular Genetics of Cancer. *Science* 1987; **235**: 305–311.
2. Land H, Parada LF, Weinberg RA. Cellular Oncogenes and Multistep Carcinogenesis. *Science* 1983; **222**: 771–778.
3. Weinberg RA. Oncogenes, Antioncogenes and the Molecular Bases of Multistep Carcinogenesis. *Cancer Res* 1989; **49**: 3713–3721.
4. Klein G. The Approaching Era of the Tumor Suppressor Genes. *Science* 1987; **238**: 1539–1545.
5. Nowell PC. The Clonal Evolution of Tumor Cell Populations. *Science* 1976; **194**: 23–28.
6. Weinstein IB. The Origins of Human Cancer: Molecular Mechanisms of Carcinogenesis and Their Implications for Cancer Prevention and Treatment. *Cancer Res* 1988; **48**: 4135–4143.
7. Cooper GM. *Oncogenes*. Boston: Jones and Bartlett Publishers, pp. 1–302, 1990.
8. Brugge J, Brugge T, Curran E, Harlow, McCormick F (eds). *Origins of Human Cancer: A Comprehensive Review*. Cold Spring Harbor Laboratory Press, pp. 1–883, 1991.
9. Watson JD, Hopkins NH, Roberts JN, Steitz JA, Werner AM. *Molecular Biology of Gene Regulation*, 4th edition. Menlo Park: The Benjamin Cummings Publishing Co., pp. 494–496, 1988.
10. Saltiel AR. Signal transduction pathways as drug targets. *Scientific Amer Sci and Med 2* 1995; 58–67.
11. Goustin AS, Leof EB, Shipley GD, Moses HL. Growth Factors and Cancer. *Cancer Res* 1986; **46**: 1015–1029.
12. Carpenter G. Receptors for epidermal growth factor and other polypeptide mitogens. *Ann Rev Biochem* 1987; **56**: 881–914.
13. Sporn MB, Roberts AB, Wakefield LM, d de Crombrugghe B. Some recent advances in the chemistry and biology of transforming growth factor-beta. *J Cell Biol* 1987; **105**: 1039–1045.
14. Slamon DJ, Godolphin W, Jones LA, Holt JA, Wong SG, Keith DE, Levin WJ, Stuart SG, Udove J, Ullrich A, Press MF. Studies of the HER-2/neu proto-oncogene in human breast and ovarian cancer. *Science* (Wash. DC). 1989; **244**: 707–712.
15. Fernandez-Pol JA. Modulation of EGF receptor protooncogene expression by growth factors and hormones in human breast carcinoma cells. *CRC Critical Reviews in Oncogenesis* 1991; **2**: 173–185.
16. Fernandez-Pol JA, Klos DJ, Hamilton PD, Talkad VD. Modulation of epidermal growth factor receptor gene expression by transforming growth factor-beta in a human breast carcinoma cell line. *Cancer Res* 1987; **47**: 4260–4265.
17. Fernandez-Pol JA, Hamilton PD, Klos DJ. Transcriptional regulation of proto-oncogene expression by epidermal growth factor, transforming growth factor beta-1, and triiodothyronine in MDA-468 cells. *J Biol Chem* 1989; **264**: 4151–4156.
18. Fernandez-Pol JA, Klos DJ, Hamilton PD. Modulation of Transforming Growth Factor Alpha-Dependent Expression of Epidermal Growth Factor Receptor Gene by Transforming Growth Factor Beta, Triiodothyronine, and Retinoic Acid. *J Cell Biochem* 1989; **41**: 159–170.
19. Fernandez-Pol JA, Talkad VD, Klos DJ, Hamilton PD. Suppression of the EGF-dependent induction of c-myc proto-oncogene expression by transforming growth factor beta in a human breast carcinoma cell line. *Biochem Biophys Res Commun* 1987; **144**: 1197–1205.
20. Ensoli B, Barillari G, Salahuddin SZ, Gallo RC, Wong-Staal F. Tat protein of HIV-1 stimulates growth of cells derived from Kaposi's sarcoma lesions of AIDS patients. *Nature* 1990; **345**: 84–86.
21. Frankel AD, Pabo CO. Cellular uptake of the tat protein from human immunodeficiency virus. *Cell* 1988; **55**: 1189–1193.
22. Seshadri T, Campisi J. Repression of c-fos Transcription and an Altered Genetic Program in Senescent Human Fibroblasts. *Science* 1990; **247**: 205–209.
23. Berg JM. Metal-binding domains in nucleic acid-binding and gene regulatory proteins. *Prog Inorg Chem* 1989; **37**: 143–190.
24. Berg JM. Zinc fingers and other metal-binding domains. *J Biol Chem* 1990; **265**: 6513–6516.
25. Evans RM, Hollenberg SM. Zinc fingers; Gilt by association. *Cell* 1988; **52**: 1–3.
26. Berg JM. Zinc finger domains: hypothesis and current knowledge. *Annu Rev Biophys Biophys Chem* 1990; **19**: 405–421.
27. Johnson PF, McKnight SL. Eukaryotic transcriptional regulatory proteins. *Annu Rev Biochem* 1989; **58**: 799–839.
28. Chan Y-L, Suzuki K, Olvera J, Wool IG. Zinc finger-like motifs in rat ribosomal proteins S27 and S29.*Nuc Acids Res* 1993; **21**: 649–655.
29. Tomei LD, Cope O (eds). Apoptosis II: The molecular basis of apoptosis in disease. *Current Comm in Cell & Mol Biol* No. 8, pp. 1–421, 1994.
30. Miller TE, Beausang LA, Meneghini M, Lidgard G. Cell death and nuclear matrix proteins. In *Apoptosis II: The Molecular Basis of Apoptosis in Disease*, Current Comm. In *Cell & Mol Biol No 8*, Cold Spring Harbor Laboratory Press, pp. 357–376, 1994.
31. Miller TE, Beausang LA, Winchell LF, Lidgard GP. Detection of nuclear matrix proteins in serum from cancer patients. *Cancer Res* 1992; **52**: 422–427.
32. Thomas G, Novak-Hofer I, Martin-Perez J, Thomas G, Siegmann M. EGF-mediated phosphorylation of 40S ribosomal protein S6 in swiss mouse 3T3 cells. In *Cancer Cells 3/ Growth Factors and Transformation*, Cold Spring Harbor Laboratory, pp. 33–39, 1985.
33. Schwartz MK. Cancer Markers. In *Cancer: Principles and Practice of Oncology*, edited by VT DeVita Jr., S Hellman and SA Rosenberg, 4th Ed. Vol. 1. Philadelphia: J. B. Lippincott Co., pp. 531–542, 1993.
34. Grant GA (ed). *Synthetic Peptides*. New York: WH Freeman and Co., pp. 1–366, 1992.
35. Fernandez-Pol JA, Klos DJ, Hamilton PD. A Growth Factor-inducible gene encodes a novel nuclear protein with zinc-finger structure. *J Biol Chem* 1993; **268**: 21198–21204.
36. Fernandez-Pol JA, Klos DJ, Hamilton PD. Metallopanstimulin gene product produced in a Baculovirus expression system is a nuclear phosphoprotein that binds to DNA. *Cell Growth & Differentiation* 1994; **5**: 811–825.

37. Xynos FP, Klos DJ, Hamilton PD, Schuette V, Huygens P, Fenandez-Pol JA. Expression of Metallopanstimulin in Condylomata Acuminata of the Female Anogenital Region Induced by Papilloma Virus. *Anticancer Research* 1994; **4**: 773–786.

38. Fernandez-Pol JA, Klos DJ, Hamilton PD. The Evaluation of Metallopanstimulin as a novel tumor marker in sera of patients with prostatic carcinoma. *European J of Nuclear Medicine, Supp.* Vol. 21, No. 10, p. 94 (Abs), 1994.

39. Fernandez-Pol JA, Klos DJ. Metallopanstimulin as a novel tumor marker in sera of patients with prostatic carcinoma. *J Tumor Marker Oncology* 1995; **10**: 54 (Abs. 49).

40. Fernandez-Pol JA. Metallopanstimulin as a novel tumor marker in sera of patients with various types of common cancers: Implications for prevention and therapy. *Anticancer Research* 1996; **16**: 2177–2186.

41. Santa Cruz DJ, Hamilton PD, Klos DJ, Fernandez-Pol JA. Expression of Metallopanstimulin in Melanocytic lesions. Submitted for publication, 1997.

42. Klavins JV, Birkmayer GD, Pimentel E (eds). 12th International Conference on human tumor markers. *J Tumor Marker Oncology* 1995; **2**: 27–92.

10. Biologic Characteristics of Primary Breast Cancer in the Elderly

Maria Grazia Daidone, Antonella Luisi, Rosella Silvestrini
and Giovanni Di Fronzo

Introduction

A progressive increase in the average life expectancy has led to a marked increase in the absolute and relative frequencies of tumors in elderly patients. Such an increase will become mainly evident for specific age-related tumors, such as breast and prostate cancers. It has been foreseen, in fact, that by the end of the 20th century about 50% of newly diagnosed breast cancers each year will occur in elderly women (1).

In the last few decades, studies on breast cancer biology have been progressively intensified, and biologic information has substantially contributed to improve knowledge on the natural history of the disease, to define the clinical role of biologic markers such as hormone receptors, cell proliferation and ploidy (i.e., nuclear DNA content), and to give clinicians information for treatment decision making (2). However, such studies have been generally performed on tumors from relatively young patients who entered therapeutic clinical protocols. Conversely, tumors from elderly patients have been marginally investigated until now (3), so that available information has not been adequate to establish whether such cancers are biologically similar or different from those of younger women and even less information on whether the clinical outcome of the elderly patients could be improved by planning therapeutic protocols according to the biologic characteristics, as already done for patients under 70 years (4).

Study Design

On a series of more than 10,000 primary breast cancers admitted to the Istituto Nazionale Tumori of Milan during a 20-year period (1972 to 1992) we determined some biologic features, including cell proliferation, evaluated as the ^{3}H-thymidine labeling index (^{3}H-dT LI) (5), steroid receptors, evaluated by using the dextran-coated charcoal technique (5), and DNA ploidy, evaluated by flow cytometry (6). The relations among these biologic variables and between them and conventional pathologic factors were analyzed for the different age classes and compared in tumors from younger and older patients.

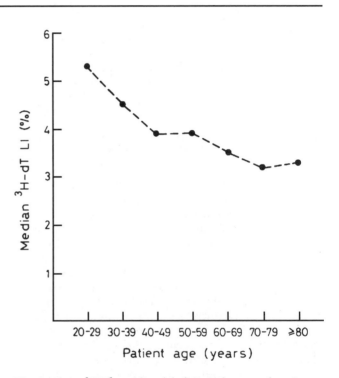

Figure 10.1 ^{3}H-Thymidine labeling index as a function of patient age.

Results

Basic Studies

The analysis performed on the overall series of more than 10,000 breast cancer patients showed that the fraction of tumor cells in the S-phase, as indicated by the ^{3}H-dT LI, progressively and consistently decreased with increasing patient age (Figure 10.1). In fact, the median ^{3}H-dT LI value of 5.5%, observed in tumors from the youngest patients, decreased as age increased, and reached a plateau around the value of 3% in tumors from patients over 70 years of age. Conversely, only a slight decrease in the frequency of aneuploid tumors (i.e., tumors with gross DNA abnormalities) was observed with increasing age (Figure 10.2), with the high-

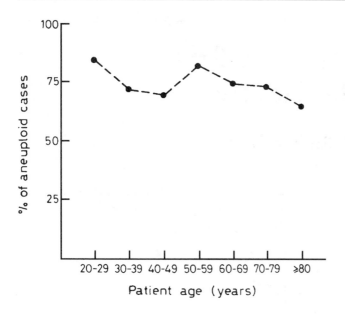

Figure 10.2 DNA ploidy as a function of patient age.

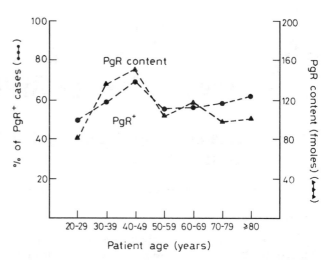

Figure 10.4 Progesterone receptor content and status as a function of patient age.

est frequency (80%) in patients younger than 30 years and the lowest value (70%) in patients older than 80 years. As regards to steroid receptors, a marked and direct age-related pattern was observed for estrogen receptors (ER), in terms of receptor presence and concentration (Figure 10.3). In fact, a progressive and relatively constant increase was observed in ER positivity from 65% in the youngest patients, to more than 80% in patients over 70 years of age. Such an increase was paralleled by an increase in ER content. In fact, the median value (which was around 40 fmol in premenopausal patients) dramatically increased from 3 to more than 4 times in patients older than 70 and 80 years, respectively. In contrast, the age-related behavior of progesterone receptor (PgR) was rather discontinuous, with a peak of positivity (75%) and the highest PgR

levels in tumors from patients aged 30–50 years, and a decrease to 50% positivity in tumors from older patients (Figure 10.4).

A significant association was observed between the biologic variables, except between ploidy and steroid receptors (Table 10.1). However, the agreement rate ranged for the different comparisons from 40 to 80% and was maximum between ER and PgR, intermediate for ^{3}H-dT LI and DNA ploidy, and poor for ^{3}H-dT LI and steroid receptors. In particular, cell proliferation was higher in steroid receptor-negative or aneuploid tumors than in steroid receptor-positive or diploid tumors, and PgR positivity was directly associated to the presence of ER. Moreover, the pattern of association between biologic variables was similar in patients younger or older than 70 years. Within the younger subset, no difference was observed for patients under or over 50 years of age.

With regards to the relation between biologic and pathologic factors, the biologic markers were generally independent of nodal involvement at the time of diagnosis (Table 10.2). This finding was consistent for patients under or over 70 years, except for a lower frequency of ER positive (ER+) tumors with an increased degree of nodal involvement in elderly patients. A similar type of relation was also observed between tumor size and biomarkers in the two age subgroups,

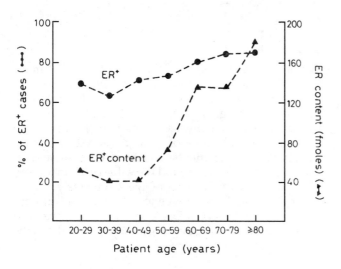

Figure 10.3 Estrogen receptor content and status as a function of patient age.

Table 10.1 Relation between biologic features according to patient age.

| | Percentage agreement in patients <70/≥70 yr | | |
	^{3}H-dT LI	ER	PgR
ER	51/55		
PgR	54/55	78/75	
Ploidy	63/62	44/42	50/46

Table 10.2 Relation between biologic and pathologic features according to patient age.

	Tumor size		Nodal involvement	
	<70 yr	≥70 yr	<70 yr	≥70 yr
^{3}H-dT LI	weak	weak	no	no
Ploidy	no	weak	no	no
ER	yes	yes	no	yes
PgR	yes	yes	no	no

and was consistent, with a weak relationship with ^{3}H-dT LI and a significant inverse relationship with steroid receptor positivity. Only the absence of a relation with DNA ploidy observed in younger patients became a trend in older patients.

Clinical Study

According to the guidelines previously proposed by some authors (4, 7), assessment of the clinical relevance of biologic markers might be carried out on substantial series of patients with an adequate follow-up and homogeneous for tumor stage and clinical treatment. Within the subset of elderly women, such requirements were fulfilled in a series of patients with node-positive tumors treated with tamoxifen for at least 1 year and with a median follow-up of 4 years. This case series of about 100 patients was completely characterized for ^{3}H-dT LI and steroid receptors, whereas information on DNA ploidy was available only on a limited number of cases.

Table 10.3 Univariate analysis of clinical outcome at 4 years.

Variable	Relapse	
	%	P
Tumor size (cm)		
≤2	37	ns
>2	30	
Positive nodes		
1–3	20	0.02
>3	43	
ER status		
+ve	30	0.001
−ve	77	
PgR status		
+ve	24	0.006
−ve	56	
^{3}H-dT LI		
Low	19	0.01
High	45	

The probability to relapse was unaffected by tumor size, whereas it was significantly related to the number of involved axillary lymph nodes, ER, PgR and ^{3}H-dT LI, although with a different discriminating power (Table 10.3). In particular, the relapse rate for patients with steroid receptor-negative tumors or patients with rapidly proliferating tumors was about twofold that of patients with steroid-receptor-positive tumors or those with slowly proliferating tumors. Moreover, the absence of ER was associated with the most unfavorable prognosis (3 out of 4 patients relapsing within 4 years of diagnosis), whereas a low proliferation rate identified the lowest risk subgroup of patients (only 1 out of 5 patients relapsing at 4 years), even within ER+ tumors (data not shown).

As already observed for tumors from younger patients (2), the integration of pathologic and biologic variables significantly improved predictive resolution for the low-risk patients, whereas it marginally contributed to the identification of high-risk patients. In fact, singly, good-prognosis markers identified patients with a 20–30% relapse rate at 4 years. In association, they provided more accurate prognostic information, with the best resolution for the association of low ^{3}H-dT LI and less than 3 positive nodes, which was able to identify a subgroup of patients with a 5% relapse rate within the overall series (Figure 10.5) as well as within ER+ tumors. Conversely, the single most powerful indicator of a poor prognosis was the absence of ER, which identified 77% of relapsing tumors.

The other markers did not give any additive prognostic information.

Discussion and Conclusions

In the past, the interest of clinicians in designing innovative therapeutic protocols has only rarely focused on breast cancer patients over 70 years of age. Such an attitude was due to the exclusion of elderly patients from randomized clinical trials for comorbid conditions and to spare them from the toxic side effects of systemic treatments. This latter belief also derived from the common, although still controversial, issue that

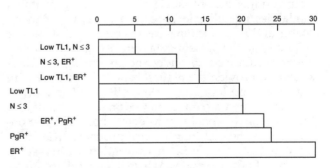

Figure 10.5 Identification of low-risk patients: probability of 4-year relapse according to the various biologic variables, singly or in combination.

elderly patients generally develop indolent disease, characterized by a lower responsiveness to treatment. However, against these statements, recent reports showed a worse survival rate for elderly patients than for younger patients with metastatic disease (8), and a significant benefit in disease-free survival after treatments using drugs with limited side effects (like tamoxifen) (9).

In consideration of these demonstrated or only hypothesized findings, there is a place for a renewal of scientific interest in a biologic characterization of breast cancers from elderly patients. In fact, as has already occurred for cancers in younger patients, biologic information on this subset of tumors could actually contribute to a better comprehension of the natural history of the disease in elderly patients, and possibly provide prognostic information and guidelines for treatment.

Overall, in our study, tumors in patients over 70 years of age showed a tendency towards a lower proliferative rate and a higher ER content than tumors from younger patients. Conversely, the incidence of aneuploid tumors determined by flow cytometry was similar to that observed for younger patients. The PgR content in tumors from patients over 70 years, although lower than that observed in tumors from patients under 50 years, did not differ from PgR content observed in tumors from patients aged 50–70 years. This last finding can be ascribed to the concomitant influence of menopausal status, since the absence of the estrogenic stimulus could be in part responsible for a low PgR expression.

In general, the relation patterns between the different biomarkers and the weak or even absent association with clinico-pathologic factors observed in tumors from elderly patients are in keeping with the results from similar analyses on tumors from younger patients. The absence of steroid receptors and the presence of aneuploid clones were associated with a rapid proliferation, and indirectly these findings should indicate that even for tumors from elderly patients, biologic aggressiveness could be defined on the basis of such features.

Cell proliferation and steroid receptors proved to be indicators of 4-year clinical outcome, and we now validated their predictive role already assessed in tumors from younger patients subjected to different treatment modalities, including local-regional (5, 10, 11), adjuvant chemical (12) or hormonal treatments (13). It should be stressed that the present data were obtained on elderly patients subjected to endocrine treatment, which is known to provide the highest benefit for tumors with hormone receptors and a slow cell proliferation (14, 15). However, a separate analysis on the subset of ER+ tumors, conventionally considered hormone responsive, again showed that the best prognosis was identified by low ^{3}H-dT LI in association with a small number of positive nodes. Whether slow cell proliferation can be considered specifically responsible for a

benefit from hormonal therapy or only a favorable prognostic indicator is still an open question.

All these data have been derived from retrospective analyses and need to be prospectively confirmed. However, particularly for elderly patients, for whom the cost benefit of treatments should be carefully assessed, it would seem reasonable to use biologic findings as a complement to clinico-pathologic features in a "risk-factor profile system" for treatment planning.

References

1. Baranovsky A, Myers MH. Cancer incidence and survival in patients 65 years of age and older. *Cancer* 1986; **36**(1): 26–41.
2. McGuire WL, Clark GM. Prognostic factors and treatment decisions in axillary-node-negative breast cancer. *N Engl J Med* 1992; **326**(26): 1756–61.
3. Valentinis B, Silvestrini R, Daidone MG, Coradini D, Galante E, Cerrotta AM, Abolafio G, Arboit L. 3H-Thymidine labeling index, hormone receptors, and ploidy in breast cancers in elderly patients. *Breast Cancer Res Treat* 1991; **20**(1): 19–24.
4. Silvestrini R, Daidone MG. Review of proliferative variables and their predictive value. In *Recent Results in Cancer Research 127*, edited by HJ Senn, RD Gelber, A Goldhirsch, B Thurlimann. Berlin-Heidelberg: Springer Verlag, **127**: 71–6, 1993.
5. Silvestrini R, Daidone MG, Luisi A, Boracchi P, Mezzetti M, Di Fronzo G, Andreola S, Salvadori B, Veronesi U. Biologic and clinicopathologic factors as indicators of specific relapse types in node-negative breast cancer. *J Clin Oncol* 1995; **13**(3): 697–704.
6. Silvestrini R, Daidone MG, Del Bino G, Mastore M, Luisi A, Di Fronzo G, Boracchi P. Prognostic significance of proliferative activity and ploidy in node-negative breast cancers. *Ann Oncol* 1993; **4**(3): 213–9.
7. McGuire WL. Breast cancer prognostic factors: evaluation guidelines (editorial, comment). *J Natl Cancer Inst* 1991; **83**(3): 154–5.
8. Yancik R, Ries LG, Yates JW. Breast cancer in aging women. A population-based study of contrasts in stage, surgery and survival. *Cancer* 1989; **63**(5): 976–81.
9. Castiglione M, Gelber RD, Goldhirsch A. Adjuvant systemic therapy for breast cancer in the elderly: completing causes of mortality. International Study Group. *J Clin Oncol* 1990; **8**(3): 519–26.
10. Meyer JS, Province M. Proliferative index of breast carcinoma by thymidine labeling: prognostic power independent of stage, estrogen and progesterone receptors. *Breast Cancer Res Treat* 1988; **12**(2): 191–204.
11. Tubiana M, Pejovic MH, Koscielny S, Chavaudra N, Malaise E. Growth rate, kinetics of tumor cell proliferation and long-term outcome in human breast cancer. *Int J Cancer* 1989; **44**(1): 17–22.
12. Silvestrini R, Daidone MG, Valagussa P, Di Fronzo G, Mezzanotte G, Mariani L, Bonadonna G. 3H-Thymidine-labeling index as a prognostic indicator in node-positive breast cancer. *J Clin Oncol* 1990; **8**(8): 1321–26.
13. Silvestrini R, Daidone MG, Mastore M, Di Fronzo G, Coradini D, Boracchi P, Squicciarini P, Salvadori B, Veronesi U. Cell kinetics as a predictive factor in node-positive breast cancer treated with adjuvant hormone therapy. *J Clin Oncol* 1993; **11**(6): 1150–55.
14. Meyer JS, Lee JY. Relationship of s-phase fraction of breast carcinoma in relapse to duration of remission, estrogen receptor contact, therapeutic responsiveness and duration of survival. *Cancer Res* 1980; **40**: 1890–96.
15. Paradiso A, Lorusso V, Tommasi S, Schittulli F, Maiello E, DeLena M. Relevance of cell kinetics to hormonal response of receptor-positive advanced breast cancer. *Breast Cancer Res Treat* 1988; **11**(1): 31–36.

11. Tumor-host Interactions, Aging and Tumor Growth

William B. Ershler

Introduction

Cancer is a geriatric disease. As described elsewhere in this text, over 50% of all cancers occur in the 13% of the population over 65 years old and this population sustains over 60% of all cancer deaths. Neoplastic transformation at the cellular level involves many of the same genetic and molecular pathways as normal cellular senescence. Cell immortalization and senescence reflect contrasting outcomes that involve similar metabolic and molecular pathways. In this chapter there is a discussion of certain of these common, clinically relevant principles relating cancer and aging. Additionally, host factors that influence the development and growth of cancer are discussed.

Biological Principles of Aging that may Relate to Tumor Growth

All normal mammalian cells have a finite life span determined by a complex interplay of replicative capacity, ability to maintain proliferative quiescence (e.g., in stage G_0 of the cell cycle) and the propensity to self destruct independent of cell age but in response to a variety of noxious stimuli. This latter process is by a series of genetically programmed events collectively termed apoptosis. Cancers arise when genetic or epigenetic events interfere with normal cellular senescence; cellular lifespan is extended and an anomalous collection of cells occurs.

In recent years one "epigenetic" mechanism has been postulated to be causally related to both cellular aging and cancer. DNA strands segregated into chromosomes are terminated at either end by common, repetitive DNA sequences termed telomeres. Telomere length shortens with each cellular division *in vitro*, and interestingly, *in vivo* as well. Blood cells and fibroblasts obtained from individuals of varying age also show shorter telomere length (1). Certain tumor cell lines have also been demonstrated to have shorter telomere length and in these cases, this has been related to end to end chromosomal hybridization and other signs of chromosomal instability (2). In contrast, the mechanism now proposed for the maintenance of telomere length (activation of an enzyme termed telomerase) may explain some of these phenomenon. Telomerase levels are elevated in germ line cells but are decreased in somatic cells (3). Another mechanism whereby cells might proliferate inappropriately is if the gene encoding telomerase is over-expressed, resulting in enhanced replicative capacity.

Dietary Restriction/Cancer/Aging

One common gerontologic experimental intervention that has repeatedly and robustly resulted in a reversal of selected biological markers of aging is the careful reduction in caloric intake (4). Evidence that certain tumors (or perhaps cancer in general) are related to primary aging processes can be forwarded based upon the observation from several laboratories in which the dietary restriction paradigm has demonstrated reduced appearance of primary and induced cancers and reduced tumor growth rates.

Explanations for the Increase in Tumor Incidence with Age

Carcinogenesis is a multistage process involving serial alterations of cellular genes. These include oncogenes and antiproliferative genes (antioncogenes), which modulate cell proliferation and genes which prevent apoptosis (as above). It is now understood that oncogenes encode proteins with a myriad of functions including growth factors, growth factor receptors, enzymes involved in the transduction of proliferative signals, DNA synthesis and replication (5). Similarly, antioncogenes encode cell proliferation or DNA-replication inhibiting proteins and apoptosis-preventing genes encode proteins which inhibit the activation of endonucleases which would otherwise disrupt the template function of DNA and result in cell death (6).

Another aspect of carcinogenesis relevant to aging is the abnormal differentiation of neoplastic cells. For example, in geriatric populations, acute leukemia is often preceded by a myelodysplastic syndrome. In many of these cases abnormalities of transcription factors (TF), and formation of fusion molecules from TF or TF-RNA are associated with differentiation inhibition (7). The responsible genetic abnormalities are largely unknown.

Different carcinogens may influence the process of transformation and progression at different steps. Consequently, carcinogens have been classified as early and late-stage carcinogens, or (more commonly) mutagens and promoters (8). These distinctions have practical implications because the effects of late-stage carcinogens (promoters), unlike those of early stage carcinogens (mutagens), may be reversible by environmental management and by chemoprevention (9).

The multistage nature of carcinogenesis has been demonstrated in experimental models with strong circumstantial support in human cancers. For example, for the case of colorectal cancer, Vogelstein and colleagues (10) described a sequence of genetic alterations leading from normal mucosal epithelium to invasive carcinoma. One step, the loss of the Familial Adenomatous Polyposis (FAP) gene on the 5th chromosome, is associated with hyperproliferation of the mucosal cells and formation of adenomatous polyps. Additional changes in the expression of the p53 gene on chromosome 18 and the DCC gene on chromosome 17 may lead to a more malignant phenotype. Likewise, in the case of brain tumors, loss of a portion of the 17th chromosome (17p) is seen in malignancy of all grades, whereas loss of chromosome 10 and of the genes encoding interferon receptors was found only in glioblastoma multiforme (11). These changes may provide the genetic basis for the transformation from indolent to more aggressive disease. Sequential genetic changes leading to more aggressive neoplasms have been reported in many other diseases, including breast, cervical, renal and lung cancer (12,13,14,15,16,17,18,19).

The interpretation of carcinogenesis as a multistage process presents at least two non-mutually exclusive explanations for the increasing incidence of cancer with age. The first and simplest is that the tissues of an older person will have, over time, sustained the serial stochastic events involved in carcinogenesis. Accordingly, the cancers more prevalent among the aged, such as prostate, colon or breast cancer, are those involving a greater number of steps. In contrast, this hypothesis would predict that tumors more common in young people (lymphoma, leukemia, neuroblastoma, etc.) would require fewer steps in the progression from normal to the malignant state.

The second hypothesis holds that age itself is a risk factor for cancer because the process of aging involves genetic events that are similar to those occurring during early carcinogenesis. Thus, the number of cells that would be susceptible to the effects of late stage carcinogens increases with age. Both experimental and clinical evidence support this theory. Cytogenetic and molecular changes observed in early carcinogenesis are also seen in cells maintained in long-term culture. These changes include formation of DNA adducts, DNA hypomethylation, chromosomal breakage and translocation (20,21). Also, the accumulation of iron commonly observed in some aging cells, may cause oncogene activation and antioncogene suppression (21,22). The likelihood of neoplastic transformation after exposure to late-stage carcinogens is higher in tissues from older animals than in those of younger animals, both in tissue culture and in cross-transplant experiments (23,24,25,26).

Epidemiological data for some cancers suggest that the susceptibility to late-stage carcinogens increases with age (27). The comparison between the incidence of melanoma and of squamous cell carcinoma (SCC) of the skin is particularly illustrative (28,29). Whereas, in the United States the incidence of melanoma plateaus at age 45 for women and 61 for men, the incidence of SCC continues to rise even beyond age 85. This is what might be predicted if there were more steps in the generation of SCC than in melanoma. However, the increased number of steps is not the total explanation because the incidence of SCC increases logarithmically with age (29). This suggests either the association of longevity with a genetic predisposition to SCC (unlikely) or, the increased susceptibility with-age to late-stage carcinogens. It should be underscored that both basic and clinical data suggest that there is an increased susceptibility and it may be tissue and organ specific. For example, skin epithelium, liver and lymphoid tissues, but not nervous or muscular tissues, show increased susceptibility to late-stage carcinogens in older rodents (30). Similarly, the incidence of melanoma, or mesothelioma in humans demonstrates an age-related plateau and, accordingly, does not support age-enhanced susceptibility to late-stage carcinogens for these tissues (27,28,29).

Other age-related factors which may increase the risk of cancer include reduced DNA repairing ability and decreased carcinogen catabolism (31,32). It has been proposed that these lead to an accelerated carcinogenic process with more rapid generation of cells susceptible to late-stage carcinogens (promoters) (33).

Finally, a discussion of cancer development and aging would not be complete without considering the importance of the decline in immunity and associated failure of "immune surveillance." It has long been proposed that the decline in immune function contributes to the increased incidence of malignancy. However, despite the appeal of such an hypothesis, scientific support has been limited, and the topic remains controversial (34,35). Proponents of an immune explanation point to experiments in which outbred strains of mice with heterogeneous immune functions were followed for their lifespan (36). Those who, early in life demonstrated better functions (as determined by a limited panel of assays available at the time on a small sample of blood) were found to have fewer spontaneous malignancies and a longer life, than those estimated to be less immunologically competent. Furthermore, it is difficult to deny that profoundly immunodeficient animals or humans are subject to a more frequent occurrence of malignant disease and it would stand to reason that others with less severe immunodeficiency would also be subject to more malignancy, perhaps less dramatically so. However, the malignancies associated with profound immune deficiency (such as with the Acquired Immune Deficiency Syndrome or after organ transplantation) are usually lymphomas, Kaposi's sarcoma or leukemia and not the more common malignancies of geriatric populations (lung, breast, colon and prostate cancers). Accordingly, it is fair to say that the question of the importance of age-acquired immune deficiency on the incidence of cancer in the elderly is unresolved. However, there is much greater consensus on the importance of the immune deficiency of aging on the clinical management of cancer including the problems associated with infection and disease progression.

Immune Senescence and Lymphomagenesis

Both old humans and mice have commonly exhibited a monoclonal gammopathy (paraprotein) in the last quartile of the life span (37,38,39,40). Indeed, 50% of B6 mice 24 months of age show monoclonal immunoglobulin (38). Radl (40) has defined four categories of age-associated monoclonal gammopathy: (a) myeloma or related disorders; (b) benign B-cell neoplasia; (c) immune deficiency, with T-cell loss greater than B-cell loss; and (d) chronic antigen stimulation. He speculates that the third category is by far the most common, and this imbalanced immune function is what is considered typical of immune senescence. In addition to the appearance of paraprotein, this same mechanism probably accounts for the age-associated occurrence of autoantibody (41). For example, antinuclear antibodies, rheumatoid factor, antimitochondrial antibodies, etc. are found with increasing frequency in late life, but these are considered of little clinical consequence (42). It is quite possible that immune senescence is initially associated with markers of aberrant immune regulation, such as paraproteinemia and/or autoantibody, and later contributes to the pathogenesis of lymphoma.

An abundant literature shows that lymphoma commonly and spontaneously occurs in old mice (e.g; 43,44,45,46,47,48). The vast majority of these are B-cell lymphomas (47,49,50). Pattengale and Frith described the immunomorphologic characteristics of 601 spontaneously occurring lymphoid neoplasms found in aged mice from many inbred strains (51). About 85% of these appeared histologically to be follicular center cell lymphomas with a small lymphocyte morphology (characteristic of a murine B-cell lymphoma). The B-cell phenotype was confirmed immunohistochemically in nearly all of these tumors.

In the commonly studied C57Bl/6 (B6) strain of mice, spontaneous lymphoma commonly occurs with advanced age. In Weindruch's experience in the dietary restriction/aging model (4), there was an incidence of lymphoma in 50–70% in four groups of *ad libitum* fed mice which lived out their natural life spans (46). Lymphoma incidence was not overtly affected by the animal's sex. In a life span study of B6 males, lymphomas occurred in 47% of mice fed ad lib (48). Not surprisingly, lymphoma incidence is much lower in studies where B6 mice are sacrificed prior to reaching truly old ages. For example, Frith *et al.* (49) found that several groups of male and female B6 mice killed for pathologic study between 17 and 23 months of age showed lymphoma incidences of 27% or less.

Histologically similar lymphomas also occur in states of more dramatic immune deficiency, such as organ or bone marrow transplant recipients who are pharmacologically immunosuppressed (52,53,54), children with severe combined immune deficiency (SCID) (55), and AIDS patients (56). In these clinical situations of profound immune deficiency, a curious lymphoproliferative disorder is frequently observed as an antecedent

of the lymphoma characterized by polyclonal B-cell proliferation followed by the development of a monoclonal immunoblastic lymphoma of B-cell type. It has been suggested that a defect in T-cell immunity results in an imbalanced (dysregulated) immunity, with the balance favoring B-cell proliferation. Nowhere is this more clear than in situations in which children with SCID developed lymphoma after partial immunological reconstitution by either bone marrow or thymus transplantation (57,58). Ultimately, from this polyclonal lymphoproliferative state, a single clone takes over and this may reflect another genetic change, as Weinberg (59) suggests, resulting in growth advantage.

The polyclonal lymphoproliferation may be considered a premalignant lesion or an early step in a multistep progression to overt lymphoma. The absence of immunoregulatory function, which is normally provided by competent T cells, may be reflected by an over expression of the oncogene *c myc*. This is suggested because *c myc* encodes a protein with DNA binding activity that presumably regulates cell growth and proliferation (60). Similarly, it is possible that over expression or alteration of *H ras*, often considered a complementary oncogene to *c myc* (59) may be sufficient to render a particular clone with a growth advantage and herald the appearance of monoclonal lymphoma.

Tumor "Aggressiveness" and Aging

There has been a long-held but incompletely documented clinical dogma that cancers in older people are "less aggressive" (Table 11.1). However, epidemiological data from tumor registries or large clinical trials have not been supportive. This may be because this type of data is confounded by special problems common to geriatric populations (e.g., comorbidity, "polypharmacy," physician or family bias regarding diagnosis and treatment in the elderly, and age-associated life stresses which may be as trivial as the inability to get to a medical center for treatment [61]). These factors may counter any primary influence that aging might have on tumor aggressiveness.

The imprecise term "tumor aggressiveness" encompasses several heterogeneous variables such as histologic grade, mitotic index, receptor status, tumor antigen profile, chromosomal abnormalities, presence and site

Table 11.1 Cancers reported to have reduced or altered patterns of growth with age.

Breast
Colon
Lung
Prostate
Renal

Tumors originating in these organs have been reported to have reduced tumor growth rates or longer survival in older patients. For a review of these reports, see reference 36.

of metastatic disease, and the presence or absence of tumor-controlling and/or tumor-promoting host factors (such as the interferons or tumor necrosis factor). We intuitively associate more aggressive tumor behavior with a poorer outcome and in most cases this association is valid. Nevertheless, for some aggressive tumors (such as large-cell lymphoma), the high mitotic index may actually render the tumor more responsive to cell cycle-specific chemotherapy. In contrast, less aggressive tumors with a low mitotic index may initially have a better prognosis, but are most resistant to chemotherapy and usually incurable once disseminated.

As alluded to above, the clinical data used to evaluate the relationship between tumor aggressiveness and age are confounded by other variables. For example, older patients are much more likely to suffer from comorbid conditions and have more limited access to health care (62). Furthermore, there is the issue of physician bias which may result in the failure to administer potentially effective therapy to older patients (61,63,64). Finally, data retrieved from death certificates are often fraught with inaccuracies, errors of omission, and inadequate documentation of competing morbidities (65).

Even data that compare the survival of patients of varying age who present with the same type and stage of tumor are subject to bias. For example, although 45% of new breast cancers are detected after the age of 65 (66), only 16% of mammograms are done in women over the age of 60 (67). This alone may explain why older patients with this disease present to their physician with more advanced disease (63,68,69). A similar age bias for cancer screening has been described for cervical cancer (67).

With the above caveats in mind, it is not difficult to understand why the clinical impression of less aggressive tumors in older patients has not been verified by epidemiologic investigation. In fact, epidemiologic investigation might suggest the opposite to be true. For example, one could interpret the recent SEER data to suggest that older patients present with more advanced disease and survive a shorter period after diagnosis. But for the reasons mentioned and until there is a prospective evaluation in which age bias is minimized, the data remain inconclusive.

There are, however, two tumors that bear special mention. The first is breast cancer, for which there is clearly the most controversy. There is evidence that breast cancer is more aggressive in young women (70), yet several reports indicate that the disease is diagnosed at a more advanced stage in older women (41,68,71) and still other reports are inconclusive in this regard (63,72). The survival data are even more contentious: some studies indicate that older women with breast cancer have a higher overall survival rate that younger women (73,74) while other studies report the opposite (75,76). However, pathological data suggest that breast carcinomas in elderly women have more "favorable" characteristics, such as a greater frequency of estrogen receptor positivity (77), a predominantly diploid rather than aneuploid chromosomal pattern (77,78), and a lower incidence of medullary and inflam-

Table 11.2 The effect of aging on the growth rate of experimental murine tumors.

Decreased Growth Rate in Older Mice	Reference
	B16 melanoma
Ershler et al. (89)	
Teratocarcinoma OTT60-50	Kubota et al. (107)
Line 1 alveolar carcinoma	Yuhas et al. (106)
Increased Growth Rate in Older Mice	
EMT6	Rockwell (108)
3-methylcholanthrene-induced sarcomas	Stjernsward (109)
UV light-induced sarcomas	Flood (28)

matory characteristics (64). Why these more favorable characteristics fail to translate into a more clearly demonstrable survival advantage is unclear. Perhaps it is related to the comorbidity issues mentioned above, or to the unproven speculation that older women are treated less aggressively (61,63,64).

The second specific tumor that bears mention is lung cancer. Unlike the situation for breast cancer, for lung cancer there is a clearly documented inverse relationship between patient age and tumor stage at the time of diagnosis (68,69,71,79,80,81). Older patients appear to have more squamous cell cancers (as opposed to adenocarcinoma, large-cell or small-cell variants [82]) Compared to the other histologic types, squamous cell carcinomas of the lung more typically present in a proximal location and are more likely to cause symptoms early. This may, in part, explain the curious inverse stage/age relationship observed for lung cancer (82). Other factors, such as age-associated obstructions in lymphatic drainage, may reduce the likelihood of tumor spread in elderly patients (79). Some workers have suggested that patients who are susceptible to aggressive tumors die after a shorter illness, and that the elderly represent a biologically select group (80).

We favor the concept that slower tumor proliferation is the result of physiologic restraints conferred by senescent tissues and that the phenomenon observed in lung cancer patients may be a general one. This concept is difficult to study in the highly heterogeneous population of elderly patients, but can be rigorously tested in animal models.

Providing Explanations for Reduced Tumor Growth with Age: Animal Models

There is experimental support for the hypothesis that there is reduced tumor aggressiveness with age. Data obtained from laboratory animals with a wide range of tumors under highly-controlled circumstances demonstrate slower tumor growth, fewer experimental metastases, and longer survival in the older cohorts (83,84,85,86).

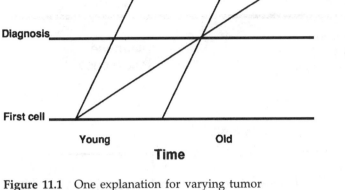

Figure 11.1 One explanation for varying tumor aggressiveness with age. Rates of tumor proliferation may play a role in the apparent slower growth of tumors. For example, if two tumors, one fast growing and one slow both arise at the same stage of life, the faster growing tumor would present clinically at a younger age. This model might explain why tumors arising in younger patients tend to be more aggressive, and why there is such great heterogeneity in tumor characteristics (such as aggressiveness) in older individuals.

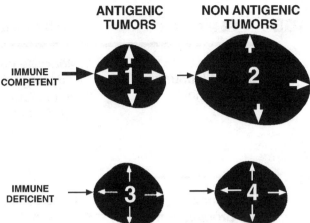

Figure 11.2 Immune forces, tumor antigenicity and age. This figure illustrates the proposed counter immune forces that might influence tumor growth. Shaded figures of different sizes reflect tumors growing at different rates. Tumors 2 and 4 represent poorly antigenic tumors, whereas 1 and 3 represent strongly antigenic tumors. The uppermost figures represent tumors in an immune competent (or young) host, while the figures below represent tumors in an immune deficient (or old) host. Strength of immune facilitating forces (for each tumor, the set of arrows within the tumor) and of immune suppressive forces (for each tumor, the left sided external arrow) are represented by the size of the arrows. The strongly antigenic tumors induce strong immune suppressive responses only in immune competent hosts, and tumor growth is therefore inhibited. Immune deficient hosts produce a weak immune suppressive response to a strongly antigenic tumor, and tumor growth is correspondingly greater. Poorly antigenic tumors induce little immune suppressive response in either immune competent or immune suppressed hosts. The immune competent host will produce a greater immune facilitating response, and tumor growth will be greater than in the immune suppressed host. This hypothesis would predict that in immune deficient (aged) hosts, with weakly antigenic tumors, the tumor growth would be slow compared to the growth of the same tumor in immune competent young hosts

What accounts for the age-associated changes observed in these experimental systems? One explanation derives from the understanding that the tumors, although histologically quite similar, may be biologically very different (seed vs soil) in old patients. For example, breast cancer cells are more likely to contain estrogen receptors, and yet leukemic cells more likely to harbor cytogenetic abnormalities in elderly patients with those disorders. Each of these associations has prognostic significance. Furthermore, there is the issue of the "time line" artifact (Figure 11.1) that implies that old patients (more so than young) may develop slow growing tumors on the basis of time required to develop such slow tumors. Such is, of course, consistent with the multistep hypothesis as discussed above.

It is probable that certain factors that influence tumor growth change with age. With this in mind, various endocrine, nutritional, wound-healing, and angiogenesis factors have been explored. For some tumors, age-associated changes in these factors have been correlated with reduced tumor growth (87,88,89,90,91). However, several early observations led to the seemingly paradoxical conclusion that immune senescence accounted for a large component of the observed reduced tumor growth with age. For example, B16 melanoma grows less well in congenitally immune deficient mice (92) and in young mice rendered T-cell deficient (85). Furthermore, when young, thymectomized, lethally irradiated mice received bone marrow or splenocytes from old donor mice, tumor growth was less than when the spleen or bone marrow was from young donor mice (84,85).

It is believed that competent immune cells provide factors that augment tumor growth under certain circumstances. If a tumor is only weakly antigenic, non-specific growth stimulatory factors provided by lym-

phocytes or monocytes may actually counteract the inhibitory forces provided by those same cells (because of the lack of tumor antigen). In this situation immune deficiency does not render a host more susceptible to aggressive tumor growth and spread; in fact immune deficiency renders a host more resistant because those cells are less likely to provide the non-specific stimulatory factors. This hypothesis is akin to the immune enhancement theory promoted several decades ago by Prehn and colleagues (93,94). Briefly stated in the context of cancer and aging; the positive growth, angiogenic and other tumor stimulatory signals produced nonspecifically by cells considered part of the immune system is less by cells from old animals. In other words, the "soil" is less fertile for aggressive tumor growth (Figure 11.2).

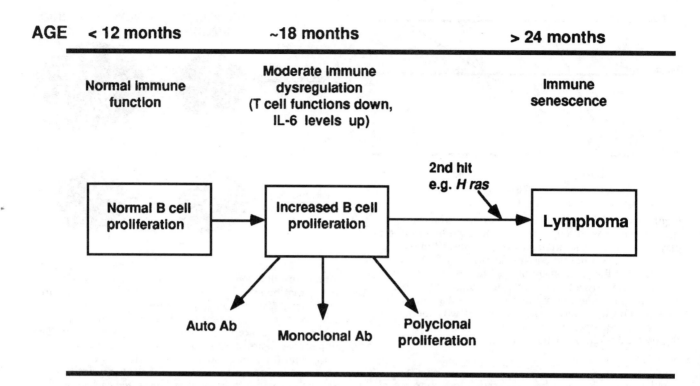

Figure 11.3 Proposed model of B cell lymphoma development in old C57Bl/6 mice. In this mouse strain a B cell Lymphoma develops in approximately 50% of mice by 24 months of age. The model suggests that the dysregulation of various cytokines (e.g., IL-6) contributes to the lymphoproliferation that is an antecedent to the monoclonal lymphoma.

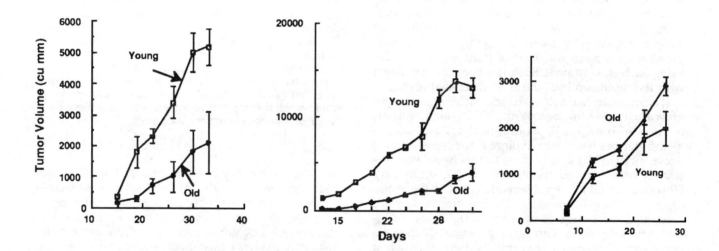

Figure 11.4   Panel A. Growth of B16 melanoma in young (2–4 mo.) and old (24 mo.) C57BL/6 mice. B16-F10 cells (10^5) were injected subcutaneously in the mice and the tumor size was measured I two dimensions every 3 days. Tumor volume is presented as mean ± SEM for groups of 10 mic (Modified from *J Natl Cancer Inst* 1984; **72**: 161–164).
Panel B. Growth of Lewis lung carcinoma growth after subcutaneous injection in young (2–3 mo.) and old (24 mo.) C57BL/6 mice of 10^5 tumor cells. Tumor size was measured in two dimensions approximately every two days and tumor volume is presented as mean ± SEM for groups of 10 mice. (Modified from *Cancer Res* 1984; **44**: 5677–5680)
Panel C. Growth of the fibrosarcoma S180 in young (2–4 mo.) and old (mo.) Balb/c mice. Cells (105) were injected subcutaneously and tumor size in two dimensions measured approximately every 3 days. This tumor, in contrast to the B16 melanoma and Lewis lung carcinoma, is highly antigenic and shows no significant growth advantage in young mice (W.B. Ershler, unpubl.). Tumor volume is presented as mean + SEM for groups of 10 mice.

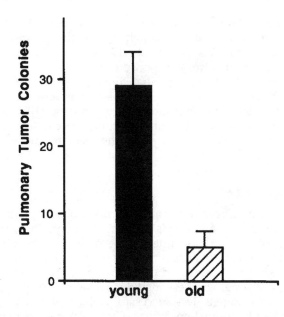

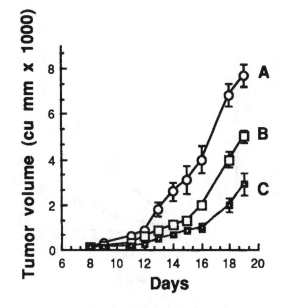

Figure 11.5 Formation of pulmonary tumor colonies in young (2–4 mo.) and old (24 mo.) C57BL/6 mice after intravenous injection of 10^5 B16 F1 cells into the lateral tail vein. Fourteen days later mice (10 per group) were sacrificed and the number of colonies (± SEM) counted. (Modified from *J Natl Cancer Inst* 1984; **72**: 161–164).

Figure 11.6 The effect of thymectomy and anti-T cell antiserum on the growth of B16-FI melanoma in young mice (24 mo.). Mice were thymectomized 8 weeks before inoculation of tumor cells (on day 0). Rabbit anti-q (anti-T cell) antiserum was injected twice (on days –7 and –4 **A**, sham thymectomized; **B**, thymectomized; **C**, thymectomized and injected with anti-q antiserum. Tumor volume is presented as mean + SEM for groups of 8 mice. (Modified from *Cancer Res.*1987; **47**: 3097–3100).

How can the data from experiments examining the influence of age on tumor growth be summarized? Some (perhaps most) models show a slower growth of tumors in older animals, whereas some others show a faster, more malignant growth. While data remains somewhat conflicting, it appears that the strongly immunogenic tumors have a growth advantage in older animals, while more poorly antigenic tumors may have a growth advantage in younger animals (Figure 11.2). The underlying mechanism for this is most probably related to senescence of the immune system. Before exploring immune senescence, some alternatives will be considered.

In the B16 murine melanoma model, hormonal factors clearly influence growth (87,95,96). The proposal that age-associated decreased secondary sex steroid levels may be the cause of decreased B16 growth was excluded by showing that B16 actually had increased growth in castrated young mice (87). This does however reveal the importance of considering hormonal influences in tumor models other than ones traditionally considered hormonally responsive.

Nutritional factors may also be important, as aging in mice brings about dietary changes such as decreased total food consumption (97). Dietary changes, especially calorie restriction, may have profound effects on the aging immune system. In mice, a 30% reduction in calories leads to a delay in immunesenescence (98) and prolonged survival (46). The effects of this on tumor growth and spread are as yet incompletely determined. We (86) and several others (4) have previously reported

that B16 melanoma grows more slowly in calorie restricted mice, and it is possible that the beneficial effects of undernutrition, which might occur spontaneously in old mice, might actually account for some of the observed "age-advantage" in certain of these models.

The ability of the body to heal wounds is decreased with age (99). Wound healing shares many characteristics of tumor growth and spread-cell localization with specific receptors, mitogenesis, tissue invasion, angiogenesis and extracellular matrix deposition. Changes in these factors with age may result in changes in tumor growth. Collagens are known to change with age, mainly demonstrating increased cross linking (100) without primary sequence alteration (101). Inhibition of-collagen deposition around tumors by administration of dehydroproline caused enhanced growth and invasiveness of B16 melanoma (83). Fibrosis surrounding B16 melanoma implants is enhanced in old mice (86). All of these "alternative" mechanisms deserve further study. What we will consider below, however, is how the immune system may act to enhance as well as inhibit the growth of tumors.

Immune Senescence and Tumor Growth

It has been proposed that competent immune cells provide factors that can augment tumor growth under

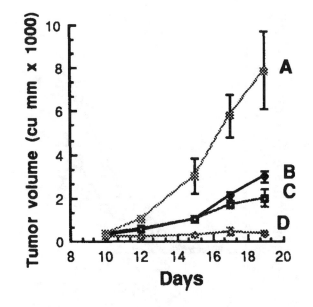

Figure 11.7 Growth of B16 melanoma in mice inoculated with splenocytes from old (24 mo.) or young (2–4 mo.) donor mice. Young mice (2–4 mo.) were thymectomized and 8 weeks later were lethally irradiated and given intravenous injections of 80×10^6 spleen melanoma cells from syngeneic young or old mice. Seventeen days later mice were inoculated with B16 cells subcutaneously (day 0). Tumor volume is presented as mean +SEM for groups of 6 mice. **A**, young controls; **B**, young, thymectomized, irradiated recipients of spleen cells from young donors; **C**, old (uninoculated) control mice; **D**, young, thymectomized, irradiated recipients of spleen cells from old donors. (Modified from *Cancer Res* 1987; **47**: 3097–3100).

certain circumstances (94). If a tumor is only weakly antigenic, nonspecific growth stimulatory factors provided by lymphocytes or monocytes may actually outweigh the inhibitory forces provided by those same cells (because of the lack of tumor antigen). In this situation, therefore, immune deficiency does not render a host more susceptible to aggressive tumor growth and spread, but in fact renders a host more resistant because those cells are less likely to provide the non-specific stimulatory factors (i.e., less fertile "soil").

Recently a large series of early stage breast cancer patients was reported in which predictive factors were determined that were associated with local relapse after breast conserving therapy (102). Local relapse was 21% in those under 40 years compared to 11% in those older. Multivariate analysis of 18 potential factors revealed four that significantly determined risk. These were: 1, unsatisfactory margin resections; 2, increasing histologic grade; 3, extensive intraductal cancer within the primary tumor; and 4, major lymphocyte stromal reaction (MCR). The latter factor may well pertain to the observed changes in tumor growth with advanced age. Compared with older patients, those younger than 40 years had tumors that more often exhibited MCR (36% vs 20%, p < .01). Although there are several other explanations for this finding, one plausible choice is

that these infiltrating host cells are a component of an inflammatory response which, indirectly, promotes tumor growth. It is likely that with age, a less rigorous cellular inflammatory response occurs.

One candidate tumor-enhancing cytokine would be lymphocyte-induced angiogenesis factor, believed to be important in the inflammatory response (103,104, 105). This factor may contribute to tumor vascularization (90) and its production has been shown to decline with age (91).

Conclusions

There is no doubt that cancer occurs more frequently in older people and this is a reflection of both the time it takes for a cell destined to become malignant to undergo the requisite events that render it both trans-formed and invasive and the physiologic changes that accompany aging. These include increased susceptibil-ity to carcinogens, less successful DNA repair mecha-nisms and immune senescence. These same factors may be held accountable for the decreased tumor "aggres-siveness" observed experimentally in rodent systems and possibly clinically for several of the common tumors (e.g., breast, prostate and lung carcinomas). There are several features of cancer and aging that are common and future research in either area is bound to shed light on the other.

References

1. Harley CB, Futcher AB, Greider CW. Telomeres shorten during aging of human fibroblasts. *Nature* 1990; **345**: 458–460.
2. Hastie ND, Allshire RC. Human telomeres: Fusion and interstitial sites. *Trends Genet Sci* 1989; **5**: 326–331.
3. De Lange T, Shiue L, Myers R, Cox DR, Naylor SL, Killery AM, Varmus HE. Structure and variability of human chromosome ends. *Mol Cell Biol* 1990; **10**: 518–527.
4. Weindruch R, Walford R. The retardation of aging and disease by dietary restriction. Springfield IL: Charles C. Thomas, 1988.
5. Weinberg RA. Oncogenes, antioncogenes and the molecular bases of multistep carcinogenesis. *Cancer Res* 1989; **49**: 3713–3721.
6. Korsemeyer SJ. Programmed cell death: Bc1-2. In *Important Advances in Oncology*, edited by VT DeVita, S Hellman, SA Rosenberg. J.B. Lippincott, 1993, 19–28.
7. Nichols J, Nimer SD. Transcription factors, translocation and leukemia. *Blood* 1992; **80**: 2953–2963.
8. Shields PG, Harris CC. Principles of carcinogenesis: Chemical. In *Cancer Principles & Practice of Oncology*, edited by VT DeVita Jr, S Hellman, SA Rosenberg, Fourth Edition. Philadelphia: J.B. Lippincott Co., pp. 200–212, 1993.
9. Meyskens FL. Strategies for prevention of cancer in humans. *Oncology* 1992; **6** (2,suppl): 15–24.
10. Vogelstein B, Fearon ER, Hamilton SR, *et al*. Genetic alterations during colorectal tumor development. *N Engl J Med* 1988; **319**: 525–532.
11. James CD, Carlbom E, Dumanskji JP, *et al*. Clonal genomic alterations in glioma malignancy stages. *Cancer Res* 1988; **48**: 5546–5551.
12. Boyle P, Leake R. Progress in understanding breast cancer: epidemiological and biological interactions. *Breast Cancer Res Treat* 1988; **11**: 91–112.
13. Harris IR, Lippman ME, Veronesi U, Willett W. Breast cancer. *N Engl J Med* 1992; **327**: 319–328, 390–398, 473–480.
14. Carney DN. Biology of small cell lung cancer. *Lancet* 1992; **339**: 843–846.

15. Correa P. Biochemical and molecular methods in cancer epidemiology and prevention: the path between the laboratory and the population. *Cancer Epidem Biomark Prev* 1993; **2**: 85–88.

16. Vineis P. Epidemiological models of carcinogenesis: the example of bladder cancer. *Cancer Epidem Biomark Prev* 1992; **1**: 149–154.

17. el Azouzi M, Chung RY, Farmer GE, *et al*. Lost of distinct regions on the short arm of chromosome 17 associated with tumorigenesis of human astrocytomas. *Proc Natl Acad Sci USA* 1989; **86**: 7186–7190.

18. Linehan WM, Gnarra JR, Lerman MI, *et al*. Genetic bases of renal cell cancer. In *Important Advances in Oncology*, edited by VT DeVita, S Hellman, SA Rosenberg SA. J.B. Lippincott, 47–70, 1993.

19. Franco EL. Prognostic value of human papilloma virus in the survival of cervical cancer patients: an overview of the evidence. *Cancer Epidemiol Biomark Prev* 1992; **1**: 499 504.

20. Anisimov VN. Age as a factor of risk in multistage carcinogenesis. In *Geriatric Oncology*, edited by L Balducci, GH Lyman, WB Ershler. J.B. Lippincott, 53–60, 1992.

21. Fernandez-Pol JA. Growth factors, oncogenes, antioncogenes and aging. In *Geriatric Oncology*, edited by L Balducci, GH Lyman, WB Ershler. J.B. Lippincott, 76–85, 1992.

22. Stevens RG, Jones DY, Micozzi MS, Taylor PR. Body iron stores and the risk of cancer. *N Engl J Med* 1988; **319**: 1047–1052.

23. Anisimov VN. Effect of age on dose-response relationship in carcinogenesis induced by single administration of N-methynitrosourea in female rats. *J Cancer Res Clin Oncol* 1988; **114**: 628–635.

24. Ward JM, Lynch P, Riggs C. Rapid development of hepatocellular neoplasms in aging male C3H/HeNcr mice given phenobarbital. *Cancer Lett* 1988; **39**: 9–18.

25. Ebbesen P. Reticulosarcoma and amyloid development in BALB/c mice inoculated with syngeneic cells from young and old donors. *J Natl Cancer Inst* 1971; **47**: 1241–1245.

26. Anisimov VN, Loktionov AS, Khavinson VK, Morozov VG. Effect of low molecular weight factors of thymus and pineal gland on life span and spontaneous tumor development in female mice of different age. *Mech Ageing Dev* 1989; **49**: 245–257.

27. Kaldor JM, Day NE. Interpretation of epidemiological studies in the context of the multistage model of carcinogenesis. In *Mechanisms of Environmental Carcinogenesis*, edited by JC Barrett, Vol 2. CRC press, 21–57, 1987.

28. Flood PM, Urban JL, Kripke ML, *et al*. Loss of tumor specific and idiotype specific immunity with age. *J Exp Med* 1980; **154**: 275–290.

28. Tantranond P, Karam F, Wang TY, *et al*. Management of cutaneous squamous cell carcinoma in an elderly man. *J Am Ger Soc* 1992; **40**: 510–512.

29. Glass AG, Hoover RN. The emerging epidemic of melanoma and squamous cell carcinoma of the skin. *JAMA* 1989; **262**: 2097–2100.

30. Matoha MF, Cosgrove JW, Atak JR, Rappoport SI. Selective elevation of the c-myc transcript levels in the liver of the aging Fischer 344 rat. *Biochem Biophys Res Commun* 1987; **147**: 1–7.

31. Bohr VA, Evans MK, Fornace AJ. Biology of disease: DNA repair and its pathogenetic implications. *Lab Invest* 1989; **61**: 143–161.

32. Balducci L, Wallace C, Khansur T, *et al*. Aging, nutrition and cancer, an annotated review. I- Diet, carcinogenesis and aging. *J Am Ger Soc* 1986; **34**: 127–136.

33. Randerath K, Reddy MV, Disher RM. Age- and tissue-related DNA modifications in untreated rats: Detection by 32P-postlabeling assay and possible significance for spontaneous tumor induction and aging. *Carcinogenesis* 1986; **7**: 1615–1617.

34. Ershler WB. The influence of an aging immune system on cancer incidence and progression. *J Gerontology* 1993; **48**: B3–B7.

35. Miller RA. Aging and Cancer: Another Perspective. *J Gerontology* 1993; **48**: B8–B10.

36. Covelli V, Mouton D, Majo V, Bouthillier Y, Bangazi C, Mevel JC, Rebessi S, Doria G, Biozzi G. Inheritance of immune responsiveness, life span and disease incidence in interline crosses of mice selected for high or low multispecific antibody production. *J Immunology* 1989; **142**: 1224–1234.

37. Radl J. Age-related monoclonal gammapathies: clinical lessons from the aging C57BL mouse. *Immunol Today* 1990; **11**: 234–236.

38. Radl J, SepersJM, Skvaril F, Morell A, Hijmans W. Immunoglobulin patterns in humans over 95 years of age. *Clin Exp Immunol* 1975; **22**: 84–90.

39. Radl J, Hollander CF, Van Den Berg P, De Glopper E. Idiopathic paraproteinemia. studies in an animal model — the ageing C57BL/KaLwRij mouse. *Clin Exp Immunol* 1978; **33**: 395–401.

40. Radl J, De Glopper E, Schuit HRE, Zurcher C. Idiopathic paraproteinemia. II. Transplantation of the paraprotein producing clone from old to young C57BL/KaLwRij mice. *J Immunol* 1979; **122**: 609–613.

41. Goodwin JS, Searles RP, Tring ASK. Immunological responses of a healthy elderly population. *Clin Exp Immunol* 1982; **48**: 403–410.

42. Kay MMB, Makinodan T. In *Clinical immunochemistry, Chemical and cellular bases and applications in disease*, edited by S Natelson, AJ Pesce, AA Dietz. Washington, DC: American Association for Clinical Chemistry, 192, 1978.

43. Smith GS, Walford RL, Mickey MR. Lifespan and incidence of cancer and other diseases in selected long-lived inbred mice and their F1 hybrids. *J Natl Cancer Inst* 1993; **50**: 1195–1213.

44. Cheney KE, Liu RK, Smith GS, Leung RE, Mickey MR, Walford RL. Survival and disease patterns in C57BL/6J mice subjected to undernutrition. *Exp Gerontol* 1980; **15**: 237 258.

45. Frith CH, Wiley LD. Classification and incidence of hyperplastic and neoplastic hemopoietic lesions in mice. *J Gerontol* 1981; **36**: 534–545.

46. Weindruch R, Walford RL. Dietary restriction in mice beginning at one year of age: effect on life span and spontaneous cancer incidence. *Science* 1982; **215**: 1415–1418.

47. Pattengale PK, Taylor CR. Experimental models of lymphoproliferative disease: The mouse as a model for human non-Hodgkin's lymphomas and related leukemias. *Am J Pathol* 1983; **113**: 237–265.

48. Bronson RT. Rate of occurrence of lesions in 20 inbred and hybrid genotypes of rats and mice sacrificed at 6 month intervals during the first years of life. In *Genetic effects on aging*, edited by DE Harrison. Caldwell, NJ: Telford Press, 279–357, 1990.

49. Frith CH, Highman B, Burger G, Sheldon WD. Spontaneous lesions in virgin and retired breeder BALB/c and C57BL/6 mice. *Lab Anim Sci* 1983; **33**: 273–286.

50. Pattengale PK, Frith CH. Immunomorphologic classification of spontaneous lymphoid cell neoplasms in female BALB/C mice. *J Natl Cancer Inst* 1983; **70**: 169–179.

51. Pattengale PK, Frith CH. Contributions of recent research to the classification of spontaneous lymphoid cell neoplasms in mice. *CRC Crit Revs Toxicol* 1986; **16**: 185 212.

52. Starzl TE, Penn I. Malignancies in renal transplant patients. *Transpl Rev* 1971; **7**: 112–122.

53. Penn I. Cancer as a complication of clinical transplantation. *Transpl Proc* 1977; **9**: 1121–1127.

54. Penn, I. Allograft transplant cancer registry. In *Immune deficiency and cancer; Epstein Barr virus and lymphoproliferative malignancies*, edited by DT Purtilo. New York: Plenum, 280–287, 1984.

55. Spector BD, Perry GS, Kersey JH. Genetically determined immunodeficiency diseases and malignancy: report from the Immunodeficiency-Cancer Registry. *Clin Immunol Immunopathol* 1978; **11**: 12–29.

56. Lipscomb H, Tatsumi E, Harada S, Sonnabend J, Wallace J, Yetz J, Davis J, McLain K. Metroka C, Tubbs R, Purtilo DT. Epstein-Barr virus, chronic lymphadenomegaly and lymphoma in male homosexuals with acquired immunodeficiency syndrome (AIDS). *AIDS Res* 1983; **1**: 59–66.

57. Borzy MS, Hong R, Horowitz SD, Gilbert E, Kaufman D, DeMendonca W, Oxelius VA, Dictor M, Pachman L. Fatal lymphoma after transplantation of cultured thymus in children with combined immunodeficiency disease. *N Engl J Med* 1979; **301**: 565–573.

58. Reece ER, Gartner JG, Seemayer TA, Joncas JH, Pagano JS. Epstein-Barr virus in a malignant lymphoproliferative disorder of B cells occurring after thymic epithelial transplantation for combined immunodeficiency. *Cancer Res* 1981; **41**: 4243–4248.

59. Weinberg RA. *Oncogenes and the Molecular Origins of Cancer.* Cold Spring Harbor Laboratory Press, 1989.

60. Leder P, Battey J, Lenoir G, Moulding C, Murphy W, Potter H, Stewart T, Taub R. Translocations among antibody genes in human cancers. *Science* 1983; **222**: 765–771.

61. Samet J, Hunt WC, Key C, Humble CG, Goodwin JS. Choice of cancer therapy varies with age of patient. *JAMA* 1986; **255**: 3385–3390.

62. Linden G. The influence of social class in the survival of cancer. *Am J Public Health* 1969; **59**: 267–274.

63. Mor V, Guadagnoli E, Masterson-Allen S, Silliman R, Glicksman AS, Cummings FJ, Goldberg RJ, Fretwell MD. Lung, breast and colorectal cancer: the relationship between extent of disease and age at diagnosis. *J Am Geriatr Soc* 1988; **36**: 873–876.

64. Allen C, Cox EB, Manton KG, Cohen HJ. Breast cancer in the elderly: current patterns of care. *J Am Geriatr Soc* 1986; **34**: 637–642.

65. Holmes FF. Clinical evidence for a change in tumor aggressiveness with age. *Semin Oncol* 1989; **16**: 34–40.

66. Robie PW. Cancer screening in the elderly. *J Am Geriatr Soc* 1989; **37**: 888–893.

67. Leventhal EA. The dilemma of cancer in the elderly. *Front Radiat Ther Oncol* 1986; **20**: 1–13.

68. Holmes FF, Hearne E. Cancer stage to age relationship: Implications for cancer screening in the elderly. *J Am Geriatr Soc* 1981; **29**: 55–57.

69. Goodwin JS, Samet JM, Key CR, Humble C, Kutvirt D, Hunt C. Stage at diagnosis of cancer varies with age of the patient. *J Am Geriatr Soc* 1986; **34**: 20–26.

70. Noyes RD, Spanos WJ, Montague ED. Breast cancer in women aged 30 and under. *Cancer* 1982; **49**: 1302–1307.

71. Mor V, Masterson-Allen S, Goldberg RJ, Cummings FJ, Glicksman AS, Fretwell MD Relationship between age at diagnosis and treatments received by cancer patients. *J Am Geriatr Soc* 1985; **33**: 585–589.

72. Rosen PP, Lesser ML, Kinne DW. Breast carcinoma at the extremes of age: A comparison of patients younger than 35 years and older than 75 years. *J Surg Oncol* 1985; **28**: 90–96.

73. Herbsman H, Feldman J, Seldera J, Gardner B, Alfonso AE. Survival following breast cancer surgery in the elderly. *Cancer* 1981; **47**: 2358–2363.

74. Sondik EJ, Young JL, Horm JW. (1987) NIH-publication No. 87-2789, Bethesda, MD, US Department of Health and Human Services.

75. Mueller CB, Ames F, Anderson GD. Breast Cancer in 3, 558 women: age as a significant determinant in the rate of dying and causes of death. *Surgery* 1978; **83**: 123–132.

76. Adami H-O, Malker B, Holmberg L, Persson I, Stone B. The relation between survival and age at diagnosis in breast cancer. *N Engl I Med* 1986; **315**: 559–563.

77. von Rosen A, Gardelin A, Auer G. Assessment of malignancy potential in mammary carcinoma in elderly patients. *Am J Clin Oncol* 1987; **10**: 61–64.

78. von Rosen A, Fallenius A, Sundelin B, Auer G. Nuclear DNA content in mammary carcinomas in women aged 35 or younger. *Am J Clin Oncol* 1986; **9**: 382–386.

79. Onuigbo WIB. Lung cancer, metastasis and growing old. *J Gerontol* 1962; **17**: 163–166.

80. Suen KC, Lau LL, Yermakow V. Cancer and old age. An autopsy study of 3,535 patients over 65 years old. *Cancer* 1974; **33**: 1164–1168.

81. Ershler WB, Socinski MA, Greene CJ. Bronchogenic cancer, metastases, and aging. *J Am Geriatr Soc* 1983; **31**: 673–676.

82. Teeter SM, Holmes FF, Mc Farlane MJ. Lung carcinoma in the elderly population: Influence of histology on the inverse relationship of stage to age. *Cancer* 1987; **60**: 1331–1336.

83. Ershler WB, Gamelli RL, Moore AL, Hacker MP, Blow AJ. Experimental tumors and aging: Local factors that may account for the observed age advantage in the B16 murine melanoma model. *Exp Gerontol* 1984; **19**: 367–376.

84. Ershler WB, Moore AL, Shore H, Gamelli RL. Transfer of age-associated restrained tumor growth in mice by old to young bone marrow transplantation. *Cancer Research* 1984; **44**: 5677–81.

85. Tsuda T, Kim YT, Siskind GW, DeBlasio A, Schwab R, Ershler WB, Weksler ME. Role of the thymus and T-cells in slow growth of B16 melanoma in old mice. *Cancer Research* 1987; **47**: 3097–3100.

86. Ershler WB, Berman E, Moore AL. B16 melanoma growth is slower, but pulmonary colonization is greater in calorie restricted mice. *J Natl Cancer Inst* 1986; **76**: 81–5.

87. Simon SR, Ershler WB. Hormonal influences on growth of B16 murine melanoma. *JNCI* 1985; **74**: 1085–1088.

88. Ershler WB. Guest Editorial: Why tumors grow more slowly in old people. *JNCI* 1986; **77**: 837–839.

89. Ershler WB, Stewart JA, Hacker MP, Moore AL, Tindle BH. B16 murine melanoma and aging: Slower growth and longer survival in old mice, *JNCI* 1984; **72**: 161–165.

90. Hadar E, Ershler WB, Kreisle RA, Ho S-P, Volk MJ, Klopp RG. Lymphocyte-induced angiogenesis factor is produced by L3T4+ murine T lymphocytes, and its production declines with age. *Cancer Immunol Immunother* 1988; **26**: 31–37.

91. Kreisle RA, Stebler B, Ershler WB. Effect of host age on tumor associated angiogenesis in mice. *JNCI* 1990; **82**: 44–47.

92. Fidler IJ, Gersten DM, Riggs CW. Relationship of host immune status to tumor cell arrest, distribution and survival in experimental metastases. *Cancer* 1977; **40**: 46–55.

93. Prehn RT, Lappe, MA. An immunostimulation theory of tumor development. *Transplant Rev* 1971; **7**: 26–30.

94. Prehn RT. The immune reaction as a stimulator of tumor growth, *Science* 1972; **176**: 170 175.

95. Proctor JW, Auclair BG, Stokowski L. Endocrine factors and the growth and spread of B16 melanoma. *J Natl Cancer Inst* 1976; **57**: 1197.

96. Proctor JW, Yammamura Y, Gaydos D, Matromatteo W. Further studies on endocrine factors and growth and spread of B16 melanoma. *Oncol* 1981; **38**: 102.

97. Greene EL. Handbook on genetically standardized mice. 2nd ed. Bar Harbor, Maine: Bar Harbor Time Publishing Co., 1977.

98. Weindruch RH, Kristie JA, Cheney KE, Walford RL. Influence of controlled dietary restriction on immunologic functioning and aging. *Fed Proc* 1979; **38**: 2007–2016.

99. Cohen BJ, Danon D, Roth GS. Wound repair in mice is influenced by age and antimacrophage serum. *J Gerontol* 1987; **42**: 295.

100. Miyahara T, Murai A, Tanaka T, Shiozawa S. Kameyama M. Age-related differences in human skin collagen: solubility in solvent, susceptibility to pepsin digestion, and the spectrum of solubilized polymeric collagen molecules. *J Gerontol* 1982; **37**: 651.

101. Miyahara T, Shiozawa S, Murai A. The effect of age on amino acid composition of human skin collagen. *J Gerontol* 1978; **33**: 498.

102. Kurtz JM, Jacquemier J, Amalric R, Brandone H, Ayme Y, Hans D, Bressac C, Spitalier J-M. Why are local recurrences after breast conserving therapy more frequent in younger patients? *J Clin Oncol* 1990; **8**: 591–598.

103. Sidky Y, Auerbach R. Lymphocyte-induced angiogenesis: A quantitative and sensitive assay of the graft vs. host reaction. *J Exp Medicine* 1975; **141**: 1084.

104. Sidky Y, Auerbach R. Response of the host vasculature system to immunocompetent lymphocytes. Effect of pre-immunization of donor or host animals. *Pro Soc Exp Biol Med* 1979; **161**: 174.

105. Auerbach R, Kubai L, Sidky YA. Angiogenesis induction by tumors, embryonic tissue and lymphocytes. *Cancer Research* 1976; **36**: 3435.

106. Yuhas JM, Pazimo NH, Proctor JO, Toya RE. A direct relationship between immune competence and the subcutaneous growth rate of a malignant murine long tumor. *Cancer Res* 1974; **34**: 722–728.

107. Kubota K, Kubota R, Talkeda S, Matsuzawa T. Effects of age and sex of host mice on growth and differentiation of teratocarcinoma OTT60-50. *Exp Gerontol* 1984; **16**: 371 384.

108. Rockwell S. Effect of host age on the transplantation, growth and radiation response of EMT6 tumor. *Cancer Res* 1981; **41**: 527–531.

109. Stjernsward J. Age-dependent tumor-host barrier and effect of carcinogen-induced immunodepression on rejection of isografted methylcholanthrene-induced sarcoma cells. *Natl Cancer Inst* 1966; **37**: 505–512.

12. Immunological Changes of Aging

Edith A. Burns and James S. Goodwin

Introduction

Immunologic function declines with age, as do most physiologic functions. As the reader will find by perusing other chapters in this volume, the incidence of many malignancies increases with increasing age, with greater associated mortality in adults over age 65 years. At the same time, the invasive characteristics of many cancers are often different in old adults compared to young adults. Are the age-related changes in immunity responsible, at least in part, for the changing epidemiology of malignancy with increasing age? This chapter will give a basic outline of the immune system, and then describe changes in the system attributed to aging.

Organization of the Immune System

The immune system classically has been divided into cellular and humoral components, with monocyte and granulocyte function treated separately. The cellular immune response, mediated primarily by T lymphocytes (or thymus-derived lymphocytes) rejects grafts of foreign tissues, kills virus-infected cells, protects against fungi and some intracellular parasites and bacteria, and modulates the immune response to prevent auto-immunity. It is also postulated to play a defensive role against the growth of tumors (Figure 12.1). The humoral immune system produces antibodies (manufactured by differentiated B cells, or bone marrow-derived lymphocytes) which are the main defense against bacteria and other infectious agents (Figure 12.2). Cells of the

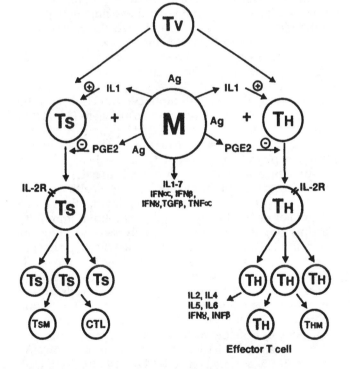

Figure 12.1 Model of cellular immunity. This component of the immune system provides protection against fungi, intracellular infectious invaders (viral, parasitic, bacterial), and is postulated to play a defensive role against the development of malignancy. Ag, antigen; CTL, cytotoxic T lymphocyte; IFN, interferon; IL, interleukin; IL-2R, interleukin-2 receptor; M, macrophage/monocyte; PGE2, prostaglandin E2; T_H, T helper (CD4+) lymphocyte; T_{HM}, T helper memory lymphocyte; T_S, T suppressor (CD8+) lymphocyte; T_{SM}, T suppressor memory lymphocyte; T_V, virgin T lymphocyte; TNF, tumor necrosis factor.

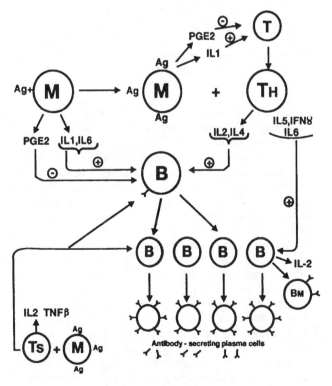

Figure 12.2 Model of humoral immunity. This component of the immune system is primarily involved in antibody production. Ag, antigen; B, B lymphocyte; B_M, B memory lymphocyte; IFN, interferon; IL, interleukin; M, macrophage/monocyte; PGE2, prostaglandin E2; T_H, T helper (CD4+) lymphocyte; T_S, T suppressor (CD8+) lymphocyte.

213

monocyte-macrophage series play an important regulatory role in both humoral and cellular immune responses, and a direct role in ingesting and/or killing foreign material. The distinction between cellular and humoral immunity is somewhat artificial because both B cells and T cells can participate in each reaction. For example, while T cells are the effectors of cellular immune responses, they are required for the great majority of humoral (antibody) responses. B cells can act as antigen-presenting cells in cellular immune responses, in addition to their antibody-producing function. Antibodies can be major participants in specific cytotoxic responses. As details of age-related changes in immunity become increasingly numerous, it may be easier to categorize them as qualitative or quantitative changes in cell populations, and production of or response to macromolecules rather than as changes in cellular versus humoral immunity.

General Evidence for the Importance of Decreased Immunity with Age

One of the major postulated roles of the immune system is protection against the development of malignancy. For example, the concept of "immune surveillance" proposes that the cellular immune system is the first defense against cancer, monitoring the body and eliminating new malignancies that are popping up every day (1,2). A corollary of this theory is that clinical cancer represents a failure of immune surveillance. Thus, elderly persons or other individuals with depressed immune function should have a higher incidence rate of malignancy. Recently, the lack of a generalized increase in most malignancies among immunosuppressed humans and experimental animals has thrown this theory into relative disrepute.

Although the epidemiologic data does not support the immune surveillance theory unconditionally, this does not mean that intact immune function is unimportant for continued health. The AIDS epidemic has highlighted the disastrous consequences of impaired immunity. While direct links between decreased immune responses and cancer in elderly persons have not been shown, a relation between depressed immunity and morbidity and mortality has been sought by looking for associations between abnormalities in a particular immune response and health status. Several studies have found a correlation between the response to delayed-type hypersensitivity skin tests and mortality. Elderly subjects who are anergic (responding poorly or not at all to a battery of antigens placed intradermally) have an increased risk of mortality compared to elderly subjects who respond vigorously to one or more of these antigens (3,4). In our studies of healthy elderly individuals in New Mexico, we found about a twofold higher mortality rate and a twofold higher incidence of pneumonia during 8 years of follow-up in the third of the group that was anergic at initial testing (4,5). The high incidence of anergy to delayed-type hypersensitivity skin testing seen in adults over 60 years of age (3,5,6), could represent

problems with antigen recognition, T-cell proliferation, lymphokine production, lymphocyte or monocyte chemotaxis, vascular responses to inflammatory mediators, or a multitude of other steps that are required to produce induration after an intradermal challenge with antigens.

Lymphocyte proliferation in response to mitogens is the *in vitro* correlate of delayed hypersensitivity skin testing. Decreased lymphocyte proliferation has also been associated with a significantly greater all-cause mortality rate among those with no response compared to those with a vigorous proliferative response (7). Another marker for disturbed immune status is the presence of circulating autoimmune antibodies. The presence of autoantibodies in a community-based study of Australian adults was associated with an increased risk of death due to vascular disease and cancer during 6 years of follow-up (8).

Changes in Immune Function with Age: Lymphocytes

T Lymphocytes

Although early reports of changes in the number of T cells with aging are variable, studies using monoclonal antibodies to specific T lymphocyte receptors have shown consistent increases in the number of "memory" T cells and declines in the number of "virgin" T cells in many species with advancing age (9,10).

One of the earliest age-related changes to be reported in qualitative T lymphocyte function was the decline in proliferative response to mitogens (3,7,11,12). Our study of 300 healthy elderly people showed a substantial decrease in response to all doses of the mitogen phytohemagglutinin (PHA) with age (5). PHA responses measured in 24 chronically ill elderly people were not different from those of the healthy group. Thus, age *per se*, and not an accompanying illness, was the major determinant of depressed cellular immunity in this population. Hyporesponsiveness to mitogens such as PHA is the sum of at least two deficiencies (11). First, the number of cells responding to mitogen is reduced in lymphocyte preparations from elderly persons. Second, the mitogen-responsive cells do not proliferate as vigorously as lymphocytes from young persons. In murine models, smaller percentages of T splenocytes from old mice respond to mitogenic stimulation by entering active phases of cell replication (13). This defect was noted on both CD4+ T helper cells and, to a lesser extent, on CD8+ T suppressor/cytotoxic cells. T helper cells from old mice are less capable of generating cytotoxic effector cells to participate in delayed hypersensitivity reactions (14). Cytotoxic lymphocytes from aged mice are less efficient at binding targets, though they appear to be equally effective in destroying their targets (15).

The role of T lymphocytes in supporting antibody production *in vitro* appears to change with increasing age. Lymphocytes from older subjects produce greater amounts of IgG and IgM when cultured with pokeweed

Table 12.1 Changes in T lymphocytes with age.

Decreased	Increased
Number of virgin (reactive) T cells	Number of memory T cells
Number of mitogen-responsive cells	T cell help for non-specific antibody production
Proliferative response	
Expression of early activation genes	
Sensitivity to activating signals	
Cytotoxic cell target-binding	
Help for generation of cytotoxic effector cells	

mitogen than lymphocytes from young control subjects (16), and old T cells are more capable than young T cells of supporting immunoglobulin production by either young or old B cells (17,18). This increased helper activity of old T cells is due, at least in part, to a failure of suppressor cell function (16).

Failure of suppressor T cells to provide tonic inhibition is a possible mechanism accounting for the increased incidence of autoimmune antibodies seen in aging. Healthy humans have circulating B cells that are programmed to differentiate into autoantibody-producing plasma cells (producing antinuclear, antithyroid, antimitochondrial and other antibodies). Suppressor T cells modulate these normal humoral immune responses and prevent the development of autoimmunity. Many investigators have reported an increase in the prevalence of positive tests for various autoantibodies with age, with a steep rise in prevalence around 70 years of age (5,19). The presence of elevated autoantibodies in elderly persons has been correlated to decreased T cell proliferation in response to the mitogen PHA (20) (i.e., the greater the proliferation of T cells to mitogens, the lower the level of autoantibodies). Studies of T suppressor cells in aging humans and mice have described decreased proliferation and suppressor function, and enhanced development of oral tolerance (16,21,22). Age-related changes in T lymphocytes are summarized in Table 12.1.

B Lymphocytes

Although the number of circulating B cells does not change appreciably with age (23), the ratios of surface immunoglobulins and class II molecule expression are altered (24). Early murine studies have shown age-related structural changes in B cell membranes (25). More recent studies have demonstrated that bone marrow precursor cells from old mice are impaired in their ability to generate B cells (26).

The functional ability of B cells to mount appropriate antibody responses does change with age (27). The distinction between antibody responses to T cell-dependent and T cell-independent antigens (often made in mice, but less clear in humans) is made on the basis of whether there is an absolute requirement for T cell

help in the antibody response. In experimental animal models, there is an 80% decrease in T-dependent antibody-forming cells in older animals (9). The accumulation of antiidiotypes (antibodies directed against other antibodies) with increasing age may also interfere with the production of specific antibody (28).

The ability to respond to a specific antigenic challenge with specific antibody production is decreased in aging (27). Serum antibody levels are significantly lower in older than in younger adults following *in vivo* immunization with influenza vaccine (29). Kishimoto *et al.*, studied specific anti-tetanus toxoid antibody production and found that B cells from adults over age 65 years made significantly less antibody than those from younger subjects (30).

We have also examined *in vitro* tetanus toxoid-specific antibody production by lymphocytes from elderly humans (31). Old adults had significantly lower serum levels of antibody to tetanus toxoid regardless of the time elapsed since the last booster immunization. *In vitro*, old adults had fewer numbers of B cells producing anti-tetanus toxoid antibody, and each cell produced significantly less antibody than the B cells from young adults. The estimated number of anti-tetanus toxoid precursor cells in the peripheral blood of the older subjects was more than a log magnitude lower than in younger subjects. Thus, the lack of precursor cells with the ability to respond to a specific antigen was primarily responsible for the decreased specific antibody production against tetanus toxoid (31). Immunizing the subjects with tetanus toxoid led to an increase in the numbers of B cells producing anti-tetanus toxoid antibody, but the old adults still had significantly fewer B cells producing specific antibody than did the young adults (32). Booster immunizations did not alter the mean amount of antibody produced per B cell for either age group. Decreased specific antibody synthesis in response to primary antigens (as well as secondary antigens) has been reported in older adults. Older subjects failed to maintain levels of specific IgG antibody after immunization with the primary antigen, flagellin, in contrast to levels maintained by young subjects (33).

Although most of the changes in antibody produc-

Table 12.2 Changes in B cells with age.

Decreased proportion of cells capable of clonal expansion

Decreased number of bone marrow precursors

Decreased number of T-dependent antibody-forming cells

Decreased specific antibody production to primary and secondary antigens

Decreased potency

tion described above are the result of declines in T lymphocyte function, there is some evidence for a decline in intrinsic B cell function. Findings from our laboratory and others suggest a diminished ability of purified B cells to respond to isolated T helper cells or to T cell-derived helper factors (17,34,35). This raises the possibility that the age-related changes in helper and suppressor T cell function might represent a homeostatic mechanism to maintain immunoglobulin production in the face of a failing B cell compartment. Age-related changes in B cell function are summarized in Table 12.2.

Macrophage Function

Macrophage function in aging is less well studied than that of other leukocyte subpopulations. Macrophages from old and young adults appear to produce similar levels of cytokines (36,37) and some differences in immune function between age groups may be modulated through changes in T and B cell responses to these substances. Recent studies however, have suggested that macrophage function may indeed be altered with aging. Wound healing, a process regulated by macrophages, was shown to take twice as long in old mice as in young mice (38). Adding peritoneal macrophages from young or old animals to wounds on old mice sped healing, but macrophages from young mice accelerated the healing process to a greater degree (38).

Bone marrow stem cells in senescence-accelerated mice seem to be defective in their ability to generate granulocyte-macrophage precursor cells (39). Defects in macrophage-T cell interactions in old humans have been described by Beckman *et al.*, who noted enhanced T cell responses when macrophages from old adults were replaced with other sources for activation, such as interleukin 2, or an activator such as phorbol 12-myristate 13-acetate (40). Because "old" macrophages effectively supported "young" T cells, the defect was postulated to lie in macrophage-T cell communication.

Aging at the cellular and molecular level has been described in a preceding chapter, so we shall only touch on these aspects of age-related change to the immune system briefly in the following sections.

Defects in Lymphocyte Ability to Repair DNA

T cells from old adults have X chromosomes that are more fragile than those from young adults (41), and certain sites on the X chromosome have been shown to be more sensitive to chemical insults. Humans over age 55 exposed to radiation have lymphocytes that mount poor cellular responses as opposed to humans exposed to radiation when under the age of 15 (42). Such differences may reflect the increased susceptibility of the aging immune system to radiation. When lymphocytes from old adults were exposed to irradiation *in vitro*, there were actually fewer breaks in double-stranded DNA, but the cells had a significantly reduced ability to repair the breaks compared to lymphocytes from young donors (43). The basal frequency of sister chromatic exchange, a measure of DNA damage, was ten times greater in lymphocytes from healthy old individuals than from newborns (44).

Defects in Lymphocyte Membrane Signal Transduction and Fluidity

Calcium mobilization is an indicator of membrane signal transduction in lymphocytes. Several laboratories have found an association between decreased calcium metabolism and defective proliferation in T cells from some mouse strains with old age (10,45). T lymphocytes that retain the ability to proliferate to mitogen have normal or enhanced mobilization of calcium compared to cells from young animals (46). Studies of human peripheral blood lymphocytes and isolated T cells have shown conflicting results, suggesting that decreased calcium mobilization is a factor in poor proliferation of some cell subpopulations but not others (9,22,47). Similarly, some studies have found no differences in membrane fluidity of lymphocytes from young versus old adults (48), while others have reported decreased fluidity of red blood cell membranes, which correlated to decreased immune responses in old adults (28).

Responses to Immunoregulatory Factors

Prostaglandins

Arachidonic acid metabolites, particularly the prostaglandins, have been strongly implicated in age-related changes in humoral immunity. Prostaglandin E2 is a feedback inhibitor of T cell proliferation in humans (49), and T cells from adults over 70 years of age are much more sensitive to inhibition by prostaglandin E2 (12,50). Prostaglandin E2 may play a role in some of the previously described age-related immune changes by interfering with the expansion of antigen-specific T cell helper clones. In addition to increased sensitivity to the inhibitory effects of prostaglandin E2, recent studies have shown increases in production of prostaglandin E2 by splenocytes from old mice compared to young mice (51). Increased sensitivity to prostaglandin E2 has been associated with impaired antibody production stimulated by a primary antigen (36). Removing monocytes (the source of prostaglandin E2 production) or adding drugs that blocked the production of prostaglandin E2 partially reversed the depressed response of older subjects (12,36). There does not appear to be a general increase in sensitivity to all immunomodulators with increasing age; for example,

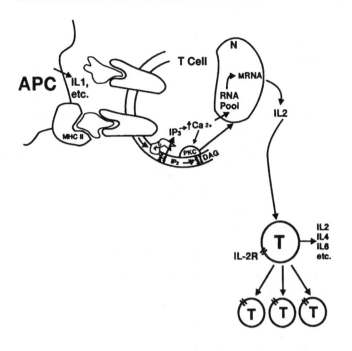

Figure 12.3 Steps in T cell activation. APC, antigen-presenting cell; Ca²⁺, calcium ion; DAG, diacylglycerol; IL, interleukin; IL-2R, interleukin-2 receptor; IP₂, inositol biphosphate; IP₃, inositol triphosphate; MHC II, major histocompatibility complex molecule; mRNA, messenger RNA; N, nucleus; PKC, protein kinase C; PLC, phospholipase C.

lymphocytes from subjects over 70 years of age actually are less sensitive to inhibition by histamine and hydrocortisone than are lymphocytes from young control subjects (50).

Interleukins

A complex set of interactions involving T cells and macrophages or other accessory cells results in the proliferative response of T cells to various stimuli. Mitogens such as PHA activate T cells by binding and cross-linking antigen receptors. This in turn activates phospholipase C, leading to cleavage of membrane phosphatidylinositol phosphates and liberation of inositol bisphosphate and diacylglycerol. The metabolite of inositol bisphosphate, inositol triphosphate, raises intracellular free calcium concentrations by releasing bound calcium from intracellular stores and by opening calcium channels. Diacylglycerol binds to and activates protein kinase C, which is further activated by the increased free calcium concentration. Protein kinase C activation leads to increased transcription and subsequent translation of the gene coding for interleukin-2 (also known as T-cell growth factor) and of receptors for interleukin-2 (Figure 12.3). Interleukin-2 is an example of an autocrine growth factor, produced by the same cells that respond to it. T cells bearing receptors for interleukin-2 that are exposed to interleukin-2 will then proliferate.

The accessory cells that cross-link T cell receptors secrete interleukin-1 and other monokines that provide additional signals necessary for complete activation of T cells (see Figure 12.3). The response to interleukin-2 has been extensively studied as one mechanism underlying the age-related defect in cellular immunity. Lymphocytes from old humans and animals demonstrate decreased production of interleukin-2 after mitogen stimulation, decreased density of interleukin-2 receptor expression, and decreased proliferation of these cells in response to interleukin-2 (52–56). Additional experiments in rodents suggest that the picture might be more complex, with specific defects in production of or sensitivity to interleukin-2 depending on the immunologic stimulus (57,58). Defects in the expression of messenger RNA for interleukin-2 have been described in lymphocytes from aged rats (59).

Interleukins 1 and 2 are important in the activation, recruitment and proliferation of T lymphocytes. Activated T cells go on to produce a variety of cytokines including B cell growth and differentiation factors such as interleukin-4 and interleukin-6. Age-related defects in lymphocyte production and response to other cytokines in aging, such as interleukin 1 and tumor necrosis factor, have been described (9,60). The stimulatory response seen when interleukin 4 is added to lymphocytes from young mice is not apparent in lymphocytes from old animals (61). The B cell proliferative response to interleukin 4 and anti-IgM is significantly lower in old mice than in young mice (622). We have shown that interleukin 4 production stimulated by specific antigen is lower in lymphocytes from old adults than lymphocytes from young adults (63). Lymphocytes from old adults are less sensitive to inhibition of specific antibody production when interleukin-4 is added early in the course of stimulation with specific antigen (63).

Several investigators have described elevated *in vivo* levels of interleukin-6 in old mice, monkeys, and adults (64,65). In another recent investigation, urinary levels of interleukin-6 were increased in old compared to young adults though circulating levels were similar in both ages (66). These findings were felt to be due to differential renal production or handling of interleukin-6 with age. Peritoneal macrophages from old mice produce higher levels of interleukin-6 than macrophages from young mice when stimulated with the mitogen lipopolysaccharide (67). Interleukin-6 levels are elevated in 24-hour, unstimulated culture supernates of lymphocytes from murine spleen and lymph nodes, and cultures of peripheral blood mononuclear cells from old humans compared to their young counterparts (64). Age-related changes in interleukins are summarized in Table 12.3.

As discussed in other chapters of this text, many of the macromolecules mentioned above play important roles in regulating tumor growth. Some of the characteristics of malignancies peculiar to older adults may result from altered production and/or sensitivity to these substances.

Table 12.3 Changes in interleukins with age.

Decreased	Increased
Expression of IL-2 mRNA	*In vivo* levels of IL-6
Proportion of cells expressing IL-2R	Non-specific stimulation of T-cell IL-4
High-affinity binding sites for IL-2	Non-specific stimulation of T-cell IFN gamma and IFN gamma mRNA
T cell production of IL-2	
T cell proliferative response to IL-2	
Specific antigen-stimulated IL-4 production	
B cell sensitivity to IL-4	

IL, interleukin; mRNA, messenger RNA; IL-2R, IL-2 receptor; IFN, interferon.

Stress, Immunity and Aging

The neurohumoral mediated effects of stress on the immune system have been well demonstrated in carefully controlled experiments with animals (68,69). Levels of cortisol and complement factors in primates are profoundly affected by a single stressful event (70). Studies in humans have demonstrated similar effects, though it is impossible to achieve the same degree of control as in animal studies. Clusters of illness (from the common cold to cancer) have been correlated to the occurrence of major life changes (71). Strong correlations have been demonstrated between loneliness and decreased proliferative responses of lymphocytes to mitogens, decreased natural killer cell activity, and impaired DNA splicing and repair in lymphocytes (71,72). We found that healthy old adults with a strong social support system (i.e., a close confidant) had significantly greater total lymphocyte counts, and a stronger mitogen-induced proliferation of lymphocytes than those without such a relationship (73). Indeed, being married has been correlated with lower mortality from any cause, in contrast to being single, widowed, or divorced (74).

Quasi experimental observations have also linked stress to depressed immune function and illness (75). Depressed lymphocyte proliferation in response to mitogens has been demonstrated after bereavement (76) although links between depressed immunity and depression are variable (77). The stress of final examinations has been correlated with the recurrence of herpes simplex type I cold sores and rises in serum antibody titers against the virus (78). Correlations have also been found between psychological factors and tumor progression in adults with cancer. Levy *et al.* found that women reporting more depression and apathy in response to breast cancer had poor natural killer cell function and were more likely to have positive axillary lymph nodes (79). Speigel *et al.* reported that women with metastatic breast cancer who participated in special emotional support therapy lived significantly longer than individuals with equivalent cancers who did not participate in such groups (80).

Old age is associated with a greater frequency of major life changes, such as loss of spouse or close friends, and changes in life-style due to retirement. Because of the decreased reserve in immune function with aging, elderly persons may be more sensitive to the effects of these stressful life events.

Unifying Theories

One of the earliest changes that occurs in the aging immune system is the involution of the thymus with subsequent loss of thymic hormone influences and declines in T cell function. The loss of thymic mass begins in adolescence, with a decrease in mass of up to 90% and a decreased output of thymic hormones (81). Thymectomy leads to the acceleration of normal age-related changes in immune function in mice, suggesting that thymic involution may indeed be a central aspect of age-related immunodeficiencies. Lymphocytes of old individuals exposed to thymic hormones either *in vivo* or *in vitro* evidence at least a partial restoration of immunity on a temporary basis (82,83).

Another theoretical explanation for age-related immune decline involves the role of cellular oncogenes and anti-oncogenes. The activation of oncogenes and loss of tumor suppressive genes has been associated with the progression of malignant lesions over long periods of time (84). These genes are postulated to play a role in the development of malignancies through regulation of cell growth and differentiation. Hybrid cells created from senescent cells and immortalized cell lines have finite life spans, a property felt to be controlled by anti-oncogenes (85). Thus, anti-oncogenes may play a role in immune senescence and contribute to tumor vulnerability.

Many of the age-related changes in immunity that have been described involve different systems and do not appear to be synchronized with each other (9,29). Defects can be seen at varying levels in different systems within a given individual. Immunomodulating substances may affect only some systems and not others. There are complex interactions between the nervous, endocrine, and immune systems, although no "global" mechanism has yet been found that might be the common underlying cause (86). It remains unclear that age-related declines in immunity are an independent risk factor for anything. As suggested in a recent review, in situations where immune mechanisms appear important for disease manifestation, age-related immune senescence may be of clinical significance (87). The few studies that link disordered immune function with subsequent morbidity and mortality are suggestive but far from conclusive. The above misgivings notwithstanding, we conclude with a brief discussion of the potential ways to stimulate a failing immune system in elderly persons.

Reversal of Age-Related Declines in Immune Function

Often the most intriguing scientific discoveries are those that are without obvious practical consequences. A prime example was the discovery by McCay and his colleagues in 1935 that caloric restriction of experimental animals markedly prolonged their life span (88). Restricting total caloric intake to 50–60% of what was required to maintain normal growth in adolescent mice, rats, and guinea pigs resulted in approximately 50% prolongation of the total life span of animals that survived the 6- to 12-month period of starvation. This interesting medical oddity received little attention over the next 3 decades until other investigators showed that the early starvation of experimental animals resulted in a preservation of normal immune function into old age (82). The potential benefits of lesser amounts of caloric restriction, supplemented with essential nutrients, is now being formally tested in primate models (89).

There has been a rapid accumulation of studies investigating links between nutrition and immune function (reviewed in 90,91). In contrast to studies on protein-calorie restriction, other nutritional deficiencies are generally associated with poor immune responses (90). Dietary supplementation with vitamins, trace elements, and calories has been associated with enhanced immune responses, better responses to vaccines, and fewer days of infectious illness in both nutritionally deficient and healthy elderly adults (92,93).

Much recent interest has been focused on antioxidants as potential anti-cancer and "anti-aging" treatments. Some of the most intriguing data involves the effects of vitamin E administration on immune function in old experimental animals and, more recently, in older men and women (94,95). For example, supplementation with 400 to 800 U of vitamin E in healthy elderly subjects resulted in enhanced responses to delayed-type hypersensitivity skin testing, and increased *in vitro* production of interleukin 2 (96,97). Vitamin E may cause these effects via inhibition of suppressive factors such as prostaglandin E2 (94).

The most dramatic demonstration of antioxidant effects on immunity was in a report by Chandra (93), who conducted a placebo-controlled, double-blinded trial of vitamin supplementation in healthy older men and women. Subjects in the experimental group received a multiple vitamin containing the recommended daily allowance for most vitamins with the exception of vitamin E and Beta carotene, which were at about four times the upper quartile of usual intakes. Vitamin supplementation was associated with marked increases in various parameters of immunity, and only half the number of days with infection and 60% of the days taking antibiotics during the one-year trial (93). If these remarkable results can be reproduced in other populations, it will have major implications for recommendations on appropriate intake of the antioxidant vitamins.

Given the association between thymic atrophy and the loss of immunocompetence with aging, one obvious group of strategies to reverse immune senescence has been exposing aging animals to thymic tissues or hormones (82). A variety of studies have indicated that in certain situations, injecting thymic tissue or hormones, or transplanting thymic tissue can lead to a restoration of some functions of an aging immune system (98,99). Various preparations of thymic hormones have been chemically synthesized or produced via recombinant DNA technology, and could be made available in large quantities if such preparations proved efficacious.

Other potential pharmacologic agents that might stimulate immune function include prostaglandin synthetase inhibitors, such as the nonsteroidal antiinflammatory drugs (NSAIDs). By reducing the production of the feedback inhibitor prostaglandin E2, NSAIDs stimulate immune responses (49). For example, we found that two completely anergic patients with adult-acquired immunodeficiency became responsive to delayed-type hypersensitivity skin testing when they were treated with the cyclooxygenase inhibitor indomethacin (100). Such therapeutic strategies might be especially relevant to elderly persons, because their T cells are more sensitive to inhibition by prostaglandin E2 (12). The use of prostaglandin synthetase inhibitors in aged individuals might also reduce increased autoantibody production (101), while stimulating the primary antibody response to new antigens (20).

Psychological interventions have been successful in reversing stress-induced suppression of immune function. Writing about traumatic events or participating in simple relaxation exercises has been associated with enhancement of the measured immune responses (102,103). The duration of effect has not been explored and the mechanisms underling such associations are not well understood.

The modes of immunostimulation discussed above are representative of the many therapies that have been proposed and/or tested. While it is difficult to justify medical intervention in a healthy individual with a disordered laboratory parameter, the studies of nutrition and immunity and stress and immunity, suggest the possibility of benign interventions that may have a significant impact on the health status of elderly individuals (93). Cancer and aging are both characterized by immunosuppression, and the combination of both conditions may have a synergistic effect on the morbidity and mortality associated with malignancy. Continued investigations into the mechanisms of age-associated immune decline, as well as tumor-associated immunosuppression may well lead to the development of successful interventions to prevent negative effects associated with the disordered immunity of aging.

References

1. Burnet FM. The concept of immunological surveillance. *Prog Exp Tumor Res* 1970; **13**: 1–27.
2. Thomas L. Reactions to homologous tissue antigens in relation to hypersensitivity. In *Cellular and Humoral Aspects of the Hypersensitivity States*, edited by HS Lawrence. New York, N.Y.: Hoeber-Harper, 529–532, 1959.
3. Roberts-Thompson IC, Whittingham S, Young-Chaiyud U, *et al.* Aging, immune response and mortality. *Lancet* 1974; **2**: 368–370.
4. Wayne S, Rhyne R, Garry P, *et al.* Cell mediated immunity as a predictor of morbidity and mortality in the aged. *J Gerontol* 1990; **45**: 45–49.
5. Goodwin JS, Searles RP, Tung KSK. Immunological responses of a healthy elderly population. *Clin Exp Immunol* 1982; **48**: 403–410.
6. Hess EV, Knapp D. The immune system and aging: a case of the cart before the horse. *J Chronic Dis* 1978; **31**: 647–649.
7. Murasko DM, Weiner P, Kaye D. Association of lack of mitogen-induced lymphocyte proliferation with increased mortality in the elderly. *Aging: Immunol Infect Dis* 1988; **1**: 1–6.
8. Ansbacher R, Keung-Yeung K, Wurster JC. Sperm antibodies in vasectomized men. *Fertil Steril* 1972; **23**: 640–643.
9. Miller RA. Aging and Immune Function. *Int Rev Cytol* 1991; **124**: 187–215.
10. Philosophe B, Miller RA. Diminished calcium signal generation in subsets of T lymphocytes that predominate in old mice. *J Gerontol* 1990; **45**: B87–B93.
11. Inkeles B, Innes JB, Kuntz MM, *et al.* Immunological studies of aging, III: Cytokinetic basis for the impaired response of lymphocytes from aged humans to plant lectins. *J Exp Med* 1977; **145**: 1176–1187.
12. Goodwin JS, Messner RP. Sensitivity of lymphocytes to prostaglandin E2 increases in subjects over age 70. *J Clin Invest* 1979; **64**: 434–439.
13. Ernst DN, Weigle WO, McQuitty DN, Rothermel AL, Hobbs MV. Stimulation of murine T cell subsets with anti-CD3 antibody: age-related defects in the expression of early activation molecules. *J Immunol* 1989; **142**: 1413–1421.
14. Vissinga C, Nagelkerken L, Sijlstra J, Hertogh-Huijbregts A, Boersma W, Rozing J. A decreased functional capacity of CD4+T cells underlies the impaired DTH reactivity in old mice. *Mech Ageing Devel* 1990; **53**: 127–139.
15. Gottesman SRS, Edington J. Proliferative and cytotoxic immune functions in aging mice. V. Deficiency in generation of cytotoxic cells with normal lytic function per cell as demonstrated by the single cell conjugation assay. *Aging: Immunol Inf Dis* 1990; **2**: 19–29.
16. Kishimoto S, Tomino S, Mitsuya H, *et al.* Age-related changes in suppressor functions of human T cells. *J Immunol* 1979; **123**: 1586–1592.
17. Rodriguez MA, Cueppens JL, Goodwin JS. Regulation of IgM rheumatoid factor production in lymphocyte cultures from young and old subjects. *J Immunol* 1989; **128**: 2422–28.
18. Crawford J, Oates S, Wolfe LA, Cohen HJ. An *in vitro* analogue of immune dysfunction with altered immunoglobulin production in the aged. *JAGS* 1989; **37**: 1141–46.
19. Delespesse G, Gausset PH, Sarfati M, *et al.* Circulating immune complexes in old people and in diabetics: correlation with autoantibodies. *Clin Exp Immunol* 1980; **40**: 96–102.
20. Hallgren H, Buckley C, Gilbertson V, *et al.* Lymphocyte phytohemagglutinin responsiveness, immunoglobulins, and autoantibodies in aging humans. *J Immunol* 1973; **111**: 1101–1107.
21. Grossmann A, Ledbetter JA, Rabinovitch PS. Reduced proliferation in T lymphocytes in aged humans is predominantly in the CD8+ subset and is unrelated to defects in transmembrane signaling which are predominantly in the CD4+subsets. *Exp Cell Res* 1989; **180**: 367–82.
22. Kawanishi H, Ajitsu S, Mirabella S. Impaired humoral immune responses to mycobacterial antigen in aged murine gut-associated lymphoid tissues. *Mech Ageing Devel* 1990; **54**: 143–61.
23. Makinodan T. Biology of aging: Retrospect and prospect. In *Immunology and Aging*, edited by T Makinodan, E Yunis. New York, N.Y.: Plenum Press, 1–8, 1977.
24. Subbarao B, Morris J, Kryscio RJ. Phenotypic and functional properties of B lymphocytes from aged mice. *Mech Ageing Devel* 1990; **51**: 223–41.
25. Callard R, Basten A, Blanden R. Loss of immune competence with age may be due to a qualitative abnormality in lymphocyte membranes. *Nature* 1979; **281**: 218–221.
26. Zharhary D. Age-related changes in the capability of the bone marrow to generate B cells. *J Immunol* 1988; **141**: 1863–69.
27. Delafuente JC. Immunosenescence: Clinical and pharmacologic considerations. *Med Clin North Amer* 1985; **69**: 475–486.
28. Cinader B, Thorbecke GJ. "Aging and the Immune System." Report on Workshop #94 held during the 7th international congress of immunology in Berlin on August 3, 1989. *Aging: Immunol Infect Dis* 1990; **2**: 45–53.
29. Ershler WB, Moore AL, Socinski MA. Influenza and aging: age-related changes and the effects of thymosin on the antibody response to influenza vaccine. *J Clin Immunol* 1984; **4**: 445–454.
30. Kishimoto S, Tomino S, Mitsuya H, *et al.* Age-related decrease in frequencies of B-cell precursors and specific helper T cells involved in the IgG anti-tetanus toxoid antibody production in humans. *Clin Immunol Immunopathol* 1982; **25**: 1–10.
31. Burns EA, Lum LG, Giddings BR, Seigneuret MC, Goodwin JS. Decreased Specific Antibody Synthesis by Lymphocytes from Elderly Subjects. *Mechs Aging Devel* 1990; **53**: 229–241.
32. Burns EA, Lum LG, l'Hommedieu GD, Goodwin JS. Decreased Humoral Immunity in Aging: *In vivo* and *in vitro* response to vaccination. *J Gerontology* 1993; **48**: B231–36.
33. Whittingham S, Buckley JD, Mackay IR. Factors influencing the secondary antibody response to flagellin in man. *Clin Exp Immunol* 1978; **34**: 170–178.
34. Ennist DL, Hones KH, St Pierre RL, Whisler RL. Functional analysis of the immunosenescence of the human B cell system: Dissociation of normal activation and proliferation from impaired terminal differentiation into IgM immunoglobulin-secreting cells. *J. Immunol* 1986; **136**: 99–105.
35. Whisler RL, Williams JW, Newhouse YG. Human B cell proliferative responses during aging. Reduced RNA synthesis and DNA replication after signal transduction by surface immunoglobulins compared to B cell antigenic determinants CD20 and CD40. *Mech Ageing Devel* 1991; **61**: 209–222.
36. Delfraissey J, Galanaud P, Wallon C, *et al.* Abolished *in vitro* antibody response in the elderly: exclusive involvement of prostaglandin-induced T suppressor cells. *Clin Immunol Immunopathol* 1982; **24**: 377–385.
37. Delfraissey JF, Galanaud P, Dormont J, Wallon C. Age-related impairment of the *in vitro* antibody response in the human. *Clin Exp Immunol* 1980; **39**: 208–214.
38. Danon D, Kowatch MA, Roth GS. Promotion of wound repair in old mice by local injection of macrophages. *Proc Natl Acad Sci USA* 1989; **86**: 2018–20.
39. Izumi-Hisha H, Ito Y, Sugkmoto K, Oshima H, Mori KJ. Age-related decrease in the number of hemopoietic stem cells and progenitors in senescence accelerated mice. *Mech Ageing Dev* 1990; **56**: 89–97.
40. Beckman I, Dimopoulos K, Xaioning X, Bradley J, Henschke P, Ahern M. T cell activation in the elderly: Evidence for specific deficiencies in T cell/accessory cell interactions. *Mech Ageing Devel* 1990; **51**: 265–76.
41. Esposito D, Fassina G, Szabo P, *et al.* Chromosomes of older humans are more prone to aminopterin-induced breakage. *Proc Natl Acad Sci USA* 1989; **86**: 1302–1306.

42. Akiyama M, Shou O-L., Kusunoki Y, *et al.* Age and dose related alteration of *in vitro* mixed lymphocyte culture response of blood lymphocytes from A-bomb survivors. *Rad Res* 1989; **117**: 26–34.

43. Mayer PJ, Lange CS, Bradley MO, Nichols WW. Age-dependent decline in rejoining of X-ray-induced DNA double-strand breaks in normal human lymphocytes. *Mutat Res* 1989; **219**: 95–100.

44. Melaragno MI, De Arruda Cardoso Smith M. Sister chromatid exchange and proliferation pattern in lymphocytes from newborns, elderly subjects and in premature aging syndromes. *Mech Ageing Devel* 1990; **54**: 43–53.

45. Miller RA, Philosophe B, Ginis I, *et al.* Defective control of cytoplasmic calcium concentration in T lymphocytes from old mice. *J Cell Physiol* 1989; **128**: 175–182.

46. Philosophe B, Miller RA. Calcium signals in murine T lymphocytes: Preservation of response to PHA and to an anti-Ly-6 antibody. *Aging: Immunol Infect Dis* 1990; **2**: 11–18.

47. Lustyik G, O'Leary JJ. Aging and the mobilization of intracellular calcium by phytohemagglutinin in human T cells. *J Gerontol* 1989; **44**: B30–B36.

48. Rivach DAJ, Rosen GM, Cohen HJ. Membrane protein organization of peripheral blood lymphocytes from healthy young and aged adults. *Mech Ageing Devel* 1988: **45**: 65–74.

49. Goodwin JS, Webb DR. Regulation of the immune response by prostaglandins: a critical review. *Clin Immunol Immunopathol* 1981; **15**: 116–132.

50. Goodwin JS. Changes in lymphocyte sensitivity to prostaglandin E, histamine, hydrocortisone, and X-irradiation with age: studies in a healthy elderly population. *Clin Immunol Immunopathol* 1982; **25**: 243–251.

51. Hayek MG, Meydani S, Meydani M, *et al.* Age differences in eicosenoid production of mouse splenocytes: effects on mitogen-induced T cell proliferation. *J Gerontol* 1994; **49**: B197–B207.

52. Negoro S, Hara H, Miyata S, *et al.* Mechanisms of age-related decline in antigen-specific T cell proliferative response: IL-2 receptor expression and recombinant IL-2 induced proliferative response of purified Tac-positive T cells. *Mech Ageing Devel* 1986; **36**: 223–241.

53. McElhaney JE, Beattie BL, Devine R, *et al.* Age-related decline in interleukin 2 production in response to influenza vaccine. *JAGS* 1990; **38**: 652–58.

54. Vissinga C, Hertogh-Huijbregts, Rozing J, *et al.* Analysis of the age-related decline in alloreactivity of CD4+ and CD8+ T cells in CBA/RIJ mice. *Mech Ageing Devel* 1990; **51**: 179–194.

55. Hara H, Tanaka T, Negoro S, *et al.* Age-related changes of expression of IL-2 receptor subunits and kinetics of IL-2 internalization in T cells after mitogenic stimulation. *Mech Ageing Dev* 1988; **45**: 167–175.

56. Nagel JE, Chopra RK, Powers DC, Adler WH. Effect of age on the human high affinity interleukin 2 receptor of phytohaemagglutinin stimulated peripheral blood lymphocytes. *Clin Exp Immunol* 1989; **75**: 286–91.

57. Ajitsu S, Mirabella S, Kawanishi H. *In vivo* immunologic intervention in age-related T cell defects in murine gut-associated lymphoid tissues by IL-2. *Mech Ageing Devel* 1990; **54**: 163–83.

58. Ernst DN, Weigle WO, Thoman ML. Retention of IL-2 production and IL-2 receptor expression by Peyer's patch T cells from aged mice. *Aging: Immunol Infect Dis* 1990; **2**: 1–9.

59. Wu W, Pahlavani M, Cheung HT, *et al.* The effect of aging on the expression of interleukin 2 messenger ribonucleic acid. *Cell Immunol* 1986; **100**: 224–231.

60. Bradley SF, Vibhagool A, Kunkel SL, Kauffman CA. Monokine secretion in aging and protein malnutrition. *J Leuk Biol* 1989; **45**: 510–514.

61. Udhayakumar V, Subbarao B, Seth A, Nagarkatti M, *et al.* Impaired T cell-induced T cell-T cell interaction in aged mice. *Cell Immunol* 1988; **116**: 299–307.

62. Thoman ML, Keogh EA, Weigle WO. *Aging: Immunol Infect Dis* 1988/1989; **1**: 245–253.

63. Burns EA, l'Hommedieu GD, Cunning J, Goodwin JS. Effects of Interleukin 4 on Antigen-specific Antibody Synthesis by Lymphocytes from Old and Young Adults. *Lymphokine and Cytokine Research* 1994; **13**(4): 227–231.

64. Daynes RA, Araneo BA, Ershler WB, *et al.* Altered regulation of IL-6 production with normal aging. *Journal of Immunology* 1993; **150**: 5219–30.

65. Ershler, W.B. Interleukin-6: A cytokine for gerontologists. *JAGS* 1993; **41**: 176–81.

66. Liao Z, Caucino JA, Schniffer SM, *et al.* Increased Urinary Cytokine Levels in the Elderly. *Aging: Immunol Infect Dis* 1993; **4**: 139–153.

67. Foster KD, Conn CA, Kluger MJ. Fever, tumor necrosis factor and interleukin-6 in young, mature and aged Fischer 344 rats. *Amer J Physiol* 1992; **262**: R211–15.

68. Ader R, Cohen N. Conditioned immunopharmacologic responses. In *Psychoneuroimmunology*, edited by R Ader. Orlando, FL: Academic Press Inc, 281–317, 1981.

69. Borysenko M, Borysenko J. Stress, behavior and immunity: animal models and mediating mechanisms. *Gen Hosp Psych* 1982; **4**: 59–67.

70. Rosenberg LT, Coe CL, Levine S. Complement levels in the squirrel monkey. *Lab Anim Sci* 1982; **32**: 371–372.

71. Minter RE, Patterson-Kimball C. Life events and illness onset: a review. *Psychosomatics* 1978; **19**: 334–339.

72. Glaser R, Thorn BE, Tarr KL, *et al.* Effects of stress on methyltransferase synthesis: an important DNA repair enzyme. *Health Psych* 1985; **4**: 403–412.

73. Thomas PD, Goodwin JM, Goodwin JS. Effect of social support on stress-related changes in cholesterol level, uric acid level and immune function in an elderly sample. *Am J Psych* 1985; **142**: 735–737.

74. Goodwin JS, Hunt WC, Kay CR, *et al.* The effect of marital, treatment and survival of cancer patients. *JAMA* 1987; **255**: 3125–3130.

75. Andersen BL, Kiecolt-Glaser JK, Glaser R. A biobehavioral model of cancer stress and disease course. *Amer Psychol* 1994; **49**: 389–404.

76. Schleifer SJ,Keller SE, Camerino M, *et al.* Suppression of lymphocyte function following bereavement. *JAMA* 1983; **250**: 374–377.

77. Stein M, Miller AH, Trestman RL. Depression, the immune system, and health and illness. *Arch Gen Psychiatry* 1991; **48**: 171–177.

78. Glaser R, Kiecolt-Glaser JK, Speicher CE, *et al.* The relationship of stress and loneliness and changes in herpes virus latency. *J Behav Med* 1985; **8**: 249–260.

79. Levy SM, Herberman RB, Maluish AM, Schlien B, Lippman M. Prognostic risk assessment in primary breast cancer by behavioral and immunological parameters. *Health Psych* 1985; **4**: 99–113.

80. Speigel D, Bloom HC, Kraemer JR, Gottheil E. Effect of psychosocial treatment on survival of patients with metastatic breast cancer. *Lancet* 1989; Oct. 14: 888–911.

81. Lewis V, Twomey J, Bealmear P, *et al.* Age, thymic function and circulating thymic hormone activity. *J Clin Endocrinol Metab* 1978; **47**: 145–152.

82. Hirokawa K, Utsuyama M, Kasai M, *et al.* Aging and immunity. *Jap Soc Path* 1992; **42**: 537–548.

83. Effros RB, Casillas A, Walford RL. The effect of thymosin-1 immunity to influenza in aged mice. *Aging: Immunol Infect Dis* 1988; **1**: 31–40.

84. Ershler WB. The influence of an aging immune system on cancer incidence and progression. *J Gerontol* 1993; **48**: B3–B7.

85. Ferluga J. Potential role of anti-oncogenes in aging. *Mech Ageing Devel* 1990; **53**: 267–75.

86. Fabris N. A neuroendocrine-immune theory of aging. *Intern J Neurosci* 1990; **51**: 373–375.

87. Ershler WB. The influence of an aging immune system on cancer incidence and progression. *J Geron* 1993; **48**: B3–B7.

88. McCay C, Crowell M, Maynard L. The effects of retarded growth upon the length of life span and upon the ultimate body size. *J Nutr* 1935; **10**: 63–79.

89. Kemintz JW, Weindruch R, Roecker EB, Crawford K, *et al.* Dietary restriction of adult male rhesus monkeys: Design, methodology, and preliminary findings from the first year of study. *J Gerontol* 1993; **48**: B17–B26.

90. Chandra RK. Nutrition is an important determinant of immunity in old age. *Prog Clin Biolog Res* 1990; **326**: 321–334.

91. Burns EA, Goodwin JS. Aging: Nutrition and Immunity. In *Diet, Nutrition and Immunity*, edited by RA Forse, SJ Bell, GL Blackburn. CRC Press: Boca Raton, p. 57–72, 1994.

92. Chandra RK, Puri S. Nutritional support improves antibody response to influenza vaccine in the elderly. *Brit Med J* 1985; **291**: 709.

93. Chandra RK. Effect of vitamin and trace-element supplementation on immune responses and infection in elderly subjects. *Lancet* 1992; **340**: 1124–27.

94. Meydani M. Vitamin E. *Lancet* 1995; **345**: 170–175.

95. Meydani SN, Hayek M. Vitamin E and immune response. In *Proceedings of international conference on nutrition and immunity*, edited by RK Chandra. St. John's, Newfoundland: ARTS Biomedical Publishers and Distributors, 105–28, 1992.

96. Meydani SN, Barklund PM, Liu S, *et al.* Vitamin E supplementation enhances cell-mediated immunity in healthy elderly subjects. *Am J Clin Nutr* 1990; **52**: 557–563.

97. Meydani, SN, Leka L, Loszewski R. Long-term vitamin E supplementation enhances immune response in healthy elderly. *FASEB J* 1994; **8**: A274.

98. Duchateau J, Servais G, Vreyens R, *et al.* Modulation of immune response in aged humans through different administration modes of thymopentin. *Surv Immunol Res* 1985; **4**(suppl 1); 94–101.

99. Ershler WB, Moore AL, Hacker MP, *et al.* Specific antibody synthesis *in vitro*, II. Age-associated thymosin enhancement of anti-tetanus antibody synthesis. Immunopharmacol 1984; **8**: 69–77.

100. Goodwin JS, Bankhurst A, Murphy S, *et al.* Partial reversal of the cellular immune defect in common variable immunodeficiency with indomethacin. *J Clin Lab Immunol* 1978; **1**: 197–199.

101. Cueppens J, Rodriguez M, Goodwin JS. Nonsteroidal anti-inflammatory drugs inhibit the production of IgM rheumatoid factor *in vitro*. Lancet 1982; **1**: 528–531.

102. Pennebaker JW, Kiecolt-Glaser JK, Glaser R. Disclosure of traumas and immune function: health implications for psychotherapy. *J Consult Clin Psych* 1988; **56**: 239–245.

103. Kiecolt-Glaser JK, Glaser R, Williger D, *et al.* Psychosocial enhancement of immunocompetence in a geriatric population. *Health Psych* 1985; **4**: 25–41.

13. Clinical Evidence for Changes in Tumor Aggressiveness with Age

Frederick F. Holmes

Introduction

Age is the most important risk factor for cancer. Cancer incidence at age 80 is nearly 250 times as great as at age 8. While it is trite to say that a group of 80 year olds is much more diverse than a group of 8 year olds, nonetheless, uniformity is a characteristic of youth and diversity a characteristic of old age. On this basis alone it is likely that there is diversity among cancers afflicting the elderly. A critical question, for which there is no answer at present, is whether or not old people have old tumors. Some neoplastic cell lines are immortal, seemingly having escaped aging altogether. Whether or not tumors age, hosts age, particularly in regard to immunocompetence. Tumor growth is obviously a product of intrinsic cellular factors as well as host factors, some of which may be humoral and, thus, affect tumors directly.

To confound matters it is difficult to separate the intrinsic properties of any cancer from the defenses of its host. More than 70 years ago Sistrunk and McCarty studied the contributions of cellular differentiation, hyalinization, fibrosis, and lymphocytic infiltration to prolonged survival in breast cancer. They thought that lymphocytic infiltration was not the most important factor but rather cellular differentiation and hyalinization (1). Even those who have attempted to focus specifically on host factors influencing the growth of tumors in humans have found that the degree of differentiation of tumors is intimately related to expression of host factors (2).

Ershler has characterized host factors as the "soil" and the tumor itself as the "seed" (3). Let us see if an old seed germinates differently than a young seed. To do this one can view the tumor in terms of stage and growth, intrinsic aspects of histology, and survival of the host.

Stage and Growth

The relationship between age and cancer stage at the time of diagnosis was described by Holmes and Hearne in 1981 (4). They found increasing age to be significantly related to increased stage at diagnosis in cancer primary to breast, cervix, endometrium, ovary, and urinary bladder and to a lesser significance in kidney and stomach. In colorectal cancer there was no relationship and in lung cancer there was a significant inverse relationship of stage to age. In 1986 Goodwin,

Table 13.1 Relationship of stage at diagnosis of common cancers to increasing patient age: Studies of Holmes and Hearne (4) and of Goodwin et al. (5).

Site	Holmes & Hearne	Goodwin et al.
Breast	increase	increase
Cervix	increase	increase
Colon	—	neutral
Colorectum	neutral	—
Endometrium	increase	increase
Gallbladder/Liver	—	neutral
Kidney	increase	neutral
Lung	decrease	decrease
Melanoma	—	increase
Ovary	increase	increase
Pancreas	—	decrease
Prostate	—	neutral
Rectum	—	decrease
Stomach	—	decrease
Thyroid	—	increase
Urinary Bladder	increase	increase

et al. studied 15 varieties of cancer and found breast, cervix, endometrium, melanoma, ovary, thyroid, and urinary bladder more likely to be diagnosed at an advanced stage with increasing age, and no trend of stage with age for colon, gall bladder/liver, kidney, or prostate. For cancers primary to lung, pancreas, rectum, and stomach there was an inverse trend, with lung being highly significant (5). The data for these two studies are shown in Table 13.1. The methods of analysis were not the same but the results are generally concordant.

Another view of the relationship of stage to age may be obtained by reviewing large autopsy studies. An early study cataloged locations of metastases in 1,000 consecutive cancer cases in a large metropolitan hospital without more than a general reference to age as a potential factor influencing numbers and distributions of metastases (6). In an autopsy series of 3,535 patients over 65 years of age, Suen and colleagues noted that cancer tended to metastasize less frequently in the elderly. They found this in cancers primary to breast, colon, kidney, lung, pancreas, prostate, rectum, stomach, urinary bladder, and uterus. Numbers of cases were small in the oldest age groups and no statistical analysis was reported. Another finding of note from their study was that the number of cancers newly diagnosed at autopsy increased as a percentage of all cancers by age, from 20.7% in the 66 to 75 age group to 36.2% in those 86 and older (7). Studying gastric cancer in Japan, Esaki et al. found peritoneal involvement to be less in older patients but no difference in hepatic involvement between the elderly and those younger (8).

This raises the possibility that many cancers in the elderly may be relatively indolent and not cause symptoms during the life of the patient. McFarlane and co-workers, in their autopsy study make this point (9). Some think that these autopsy-discovered cancers tend to be more differentiated than those diagnosed during life. In focusing on particular cancers, an autopsy study of 1,828 renal adenocarcinomas in Japan found considerable decrease in number of metastases with age generally and in organs usually bearing metastases, specifically (10). Much the same phenomenon was demonstrated by Ershler and colleagues in lung cancer (11).

The magnitude of the decreasing stage with increasing age trend in lung cancer is considerable. A study of 22,874 lung cancer cases showed local stage disease in 13.9% of those less than 54 years of age, 19.2 % in those 55 to 64, 21.4% in those 65 to 74, and 25.4% in those 75 and older (12). Quite apart from other considerations this makes routine screening for curable lung cancer in the elderly a much more attractive possibility than in the middle-aged. At least part of the reason for the stage to age trend in lung cancer is the changing balance of histologies with age shown in a study of 9,062 histologically confirmed lung cancer cases by Teeter and colleagues (13). Squamous cell carcinoma increased from 26% to 40% of the total cases between ages 40 and 80 and adenocarcinoma and small cell carcinoma declined proportionately with large cell carcinoma unchanged. The proportion of staged cases with local disease increased from 27% to 54% for squamous cell carcinoma between ages 40 and 80, with smaller but statistically significant increases for all other histologies but large cell carcinoma.

Yancik and her colleagues focused on SEER data for 125,000 women with breast cancer to study the relationship of age to stage and survival. They found women presenting with distant disease or unstaged disease more likely to be elderly (14). Growth rates for breast cancer are highly variable. Spratt et al. found an inverse relationship between patient age and tumor size at mammographic diagnosis. Mean tumor diameter for those younger than 70 was 13 mm and for those older was 9 mm. There were no age differences in doubling times or growth rates. None of Spratt's observations reached statistical significance (15). Other studies have shown age-related lead time differences and Pelikan and Moskowitz have created mathematical models to study mammographic screening using numbers that presume slower tumor doubling in older women (16).

One other factor of stage to age relationships deserves mention. Where a cancer arises in a particular organ may be of importance. In 1977 Rhodes, et al. described a shift from distal to proximal subsite origin of colorectal cancer during the preceding three decades (17). In 1985 Butcher, et al., of this same group, identified increasing age and female gender as two factors at least in part responsible for this interesting phenomenon (18). In this vein elderly women are more likely to have medial and central breast cancers than younger women (19). Right sided colon cancers cause symptoms later than those near the rectum and medial breast cancers are more likely to spread to lymph nodes within the chest than lateral cancers.

Intrinsic Aspects of Histology

Scrutiny of chemically stained small pieces of tumor tissue under the microscope has been common practice for over a hundred years. Yet, even the most clever pathologist can't determine the age of the patient by microscopic examination of his or her cancer. The relations of cancer histology to age have not received much attention over the years. In 1950 Lees and Park surveyed the extant literature and studied hundreds of cases of their own. They concluded that histologic indicators of cancer aggressiveness or indolence did not appear to be a function of patient age with the possible exception of carcinoma of the lung (20). On the other hand indolent cancers may be more common in the young than the old at sites such as ovary (21).

Carcinoma of the cervix and its precursor states are uniquely available to histologic study through exfoliative cytology. An atypical Papanicolaou cervical smear in a woman over age 60 is 16 times more likely to lead to a diagnosis of invasive cancer than one in a woman less than 30 (22). Some think that in situ carcinoma of the cervix often has a distinctive cytological appearance in the elderly characterized by a large number of keratinizing cancer cells with a variable admixture of lesser numbers of third type cells of Graham (23). In addition there is evidence for a slowly evolving cervical cancer in young women and a more rapidly evolving one in older women (24, 25).

Much of the study of the relationship of cancer histology to age has been pursued with breast cancer. The distributions of the various histologic types of breast cancer are different when older women are compared with middle-aged and younger women (26). Most breast cancers, regardless of age, are infiltrating duct carcinomas. A higher histologic grade is most common in the youngest breast cancer patients as are inflammatory and medullary breast cancers. Infiltrating lobular and colloid carcinomas were found to be especially common among the elderly (19, 27). Breast cancers in elderly women are more likely to be diploid and, thus, relatively slow growing (28). Yancik's very large study

Table 13.2 Relationship of increasing age to increasing histologic grade for common carcinomas, Cancer Data Service, 1982–1987.

Type of carcinoma	Number	Significance of increasing age/grade trend, P value
Breast	2,303	NS
Colorectum	5,140	<0.01
Lung	3,660	<0.001
Ovary	520	NS
Prostate	4,596	<0.001
Stomach	534	NS
Urinary bladder	2,037	<0.01

Table 13.3 SEER five-year relative survival rates (percent) for all sites and stages combined, 1974–1983 (38).

Age Group	All	Male	Female
All	48.8	42.0	55.0
0–54	59.2	48.3	66.6
55–64	47.9	40.1	55.7
65–74	44.7	40.8	49.2
75+	39.9	38.6	41.1

of 125,000 women with breast cancer found medullary carcinoma to decrease and mucinous carcinoma to increase with age. Other histologies changed little with aging (14).

Identifying cellular components by methods other than microscopy has been a burgeoning field in the past several decades. Perhaps the best example of the utility of these techniques in neoplasia is the quantification of estrogen and progesterone receptors in breast cancer cells. Repeatedly, an increasing likelihood of the presence of estrogen receptor protein has been correlated with increasing age and mean concentration increases with age as well. This association is independent of all of the other breast cancer risk factors (29, 30). The same seems to be true for progesterone receptors also and a higher survival rate in patients with estrogen and with progesterone receptor positivity has been demonstrated (31). It seems likely that, at least in part, this phenomenon is related to cellular differentiation.

For many years it has been known that there is a relationship of histologic grading to survival in cancer (1, 32). People with higher grade cancers, that is cancers that are less differentiated, have shorter survivals than those with lower grade cancers. This has no particular relationship to size of the primary tumor but it has great prognostic value when the issues of screening and likelihood of cancer cure are addressed (33). Using unpublished data from the Cancer Data Service, the regional cancer registry for Kansas and western Missouri, it is possible to compare distributions by age for differentiated and undifferentiated histologies for common carcinomas. The results of this simple chi-square analysis are shown in Table 13.2. The numbers of cases are large so the differences may have more apparent significance than clinical significance. Nonetheless there does seem to be a trend towards less differentiation with increasing age for colorectum, lung, prostate, and urinary bladder. No difference is seen for breast, ovary and stomach, but the numbers of cases are smaller in the latter two sites.

In thyroid cancer, patient age at diagnosis can be combined with sex and histologic grade to create a

highly significant prognostic scoring system. In this system, male gender, higher age, and higher histologic grade were related to decreased survival in papillary thyroid carcinoma (34).

Prostate carcinoma is the quintessential cancer of older men, usually indolent but often aggressive and lethal. The contrast between those two extremes has only recently prompted an explanation. Whittemore et al. believe that the tumor volume of Gleason low-grade latent prostatic cancer per patient is directly related to the chance of transformation to Gleason high-grade cancers which will threaten life. They calculate that one may expect 0.024 high-grade cancers per year per cubic centimeter of low-grade latent cancer volume. If true, this observation has great import for the understanding of prostate cancer in older men (35).

Survival of the Host

The final arbiter in the study of the biology or natural history of human cancer is duration of survival of the patient who bears the cancer. Survival analysis is difficult to do well, particularly in the elderly. By necessity we compute survival from the time of diagnosis and not from the time the cancer actually started with a cell or cells beginning a course of malignant growth. If you read only the last 100 pages of a 400 page novel can you really understand the story? Computing survival in elderly populations is fraught with considerable hazard. Competing mortalities, a sharply rising mortality curve, inaccuracy of death certificate data, recent improvements in survival in the oldest age groups, and lack of accurate national bench mark statistics conspire to flaw any computation of survival of elderly cancer patients. In spite of this, survival comparisons of elderly with middle-aged and young cancer patients have been attempted.

Summary articles tell us that survival in elderly cancer patients varies with the site and that there seems to be little agreement among authors even for specific sites (36, 37). SEER five-year relative survival rates for all sites and all stages combined show that there is a general decline by age for both sexes as shown in Table 13.3 (38). This is confounded by the different distributions of cancer sites by age groups and the fact that older people are often treated less aggressively than those younger (39, 40).

In lung and colon cancer there are data establishing that elderly patients do just as well as those who are younger if they are acceptable candidates for surgery. Their survival is comparable to younger patients. In lung cancer Kirsh found a 30% absolute five-year survival rate in 55 patients over age 70 (41). Sherman and Guidot compared the results in thoracotomy for lung cancer in 64 patients older than 70 with 75 younger than 70. Operative mortality was increased in the older age group (9.4% vs 4.0%) but there was no significant difference in survival between the two age groups (42). Even the results of chemotherapy of small cell carcinoma of the lung in the elderly are encouraging in one study (43). A study of colon cancer found five-year survival of 156 patients 80 years of age or older at the time of surgical treatment to be better than survival in younger patients (44).

In the acute leukemias, lymphomas, and Hodgkin's disease advanced age is related to decreasing chance of remission and decreased survival overall (37, 45, 46, 47). Sadly, this remains true in acute myelocytic leukemia and the paradox of the inverse relationship of age to survival has recently been examined (48, 49). In multiple myeloma the aged patient does at least as well with comparable response rates and survival equal to or better than younger patients (50–52).

Probably studies of the relationship of age to survival in breast cancer have equaled in number such studies in all other sites of cancer combined. This may be because this is a very common cancer with long survival also common. Early studies seemed to indicate that older women survived longer with this disease than those middle-aged or younger (1, 53). Very long survival, even in the untreated state, and very late recurrence make the study of survival in breast cancer difficult (32, 54). However, small and occasionally significant differences in survival have been reported comparing younger and older women in various cohorts over recent decades (26). Though estrogen receptor (ER) positive cancers are increasingly common with increasing age and ER positivity is associated with improved survival, the survival differential between patients with ER positive tumors and those with ER negative tumors seems to lessen as age increases (55). Comparing the extremes of age, those less than 35 with those older than 75, Rosen and associates found no significant difference in recurrence or survival (19). In a surgical series of 780 breast cancer patients, Herbsman and associates found absolute survival the same or better with increasing age when patients were stratified by stage and absolute survival strikingly increased as age at diagnosis increased (56).

In 1978 Mueller and associates identified age as a significant determinant in the rate of dying and causes of death in 3,558 breast cancer cases. Using cancer registry data from an upstate New York hospital and life-table analysis focusing on deaths from breast cancer, they found breast cancer lethality to increase directly with increasing age (57). The validity of their study was questioned by Newcombe and Hillyard who thought their estimation of deaths from breast cancer in their greater than 70 age group was inflated by a factor of three (58). This is illustrative of the difficulty in accurately computing survival from cause of death data in the elderly.

In 1983 Hibberd and colleagues published long term survival data of 2,019 New Zealand women with histologically proven breast cancer diagnosed in New Zealand between 1950 and 1954, representing an estimated 80% of the breast cancer cohort of those years for that country. They found no apparent relation between age and excess mortality except that the very youngest cohort (60 women who were aged 20 to 34 at diagnosis) had virtual flattening of the survival curve after 10 years whereas none of the other cohorts did (59).

Adami and associates have studied survival in two large breast cancer populations in Sweden, 12,319 diagnosed between 1959 and 1963 and 57,068 diagnosed between 1960 and 1978. Because cancer registration in Sweden is virtually complete these data are of high quality. They found relative survival to decline markedly after age 49 with women older than 75 having the worst survival. Unfortunately they did not stratify the data for stage at diagnosis (60, 61). Analyzing survival of 78,405 white females diagnosed with breast cancer in America between 1974 and 1983 the SEER group found consistently decreased percent relative survival out to seven years when those younger than 50 were compared with those 50 and older. When these patients were stratified by stage, three and five year survival were apparently better for the older women in stages I and II and the younger women for stages III and IV. However, the only statistically significant difference was at the 0.05 level at five years for stages I and II (38).

It may be possible to resolve these conflicting results, at least in part. Survival analysis in breast cancer without stratification by stage has limited value. Stage increases with age and thereby worsens survival for older women (4, 5). Two studies have identified a subgroup of elderly women with relatively indolent low-stage breast cancer who have reduced excess mortality (62, 63). It seems possible that there is heterogeneity in low-stage breast cancer in the elderly, perhaps from more favorable histologic patterns (19, 26–28).

The Meaning and Importance of These Trends

The studies and data presented do not support a simple and single trend for change in tumor aggressiveness with increasing age. In that cancer is not a single disease but a collection of diseases this should be no surprise. There seems to be diversity even within a single site, for example breast. Because cancer incidence rises steeply with age and because there are so many cases in older people, one-half of all cancers diagnosed in the United States are in the one-eighth of the population age 65 and older, the sheer volume of cases would suggest the possibility of diversity. Beyond this one must recognize the fact that old people of a given age are far less homogeneous that those who are younger.

Thus, though there is a general trend for increasing stage at diagnosis with increasing age for most common sites of cancer, colon, gall bladder / liver, prostate, and perhaps kidney show no such trend at all. In lung cancer there is a strongly significant trend for decreasing stage with age and this is at least partly explained by changing distributions of common histologies with age. Evidence is not present for increasing histologic grade with age for carcinomas primary to the breast, ovary, and stomach but it is present for colorectum, prostate, urinary bladder, and even the lung. Though in lung this seems to contrast the stage to age trend. A study of nearly 5,000 prostate cancers showed a highly significant increase in histologic grade with increasing age, even in locally confined disease (64). In relative survival for all sites of cancer there is a general decline with age but differences emerge when specific sites are stratified by stage. However, in acute leukemia in the elderly a recent study shows that survival still has not improved, a striking contrast to the remarkable improvement in survival in children (46, 48, 65).

In many respects the phenomenon of change in tumor aggressiveness with age can best be illustrated by breast cancer. Though stage at diagnosis increases with age there is not a corresponding increase in histologic grade with age. However, the distribution of various histologies changes with age and the proportion of both estrogen and progesterone receptor positive tumors increases with age. The meaning of these trends may become clear when one considers the final arbiter, survival, stratified by stage and age. Older women survive longer than those younger when low stage disease is examined and the reverse is true for high stage disease.

So it seems that those who believe that slow-growing tumors are associated with old age are correct as are those who believe that rapidly growing tumors are associated with old age. Site and stage are two important determinants. It would seem that groups of old tumors are just as diverse as groups of old people.

Present and Future Considerations

The prevalence of cancer in the elderly part of our population and its contribution to overall mortality has been studied and the possibility is raised that cancer could become the preeminent cause of death in the United States (66). Breast cancer offers the best immediate opportunities to stratify older patients by disease growth patterns so that screening and treatment may be practiced on a sound biological basis (67, 68). The cancer site that will offer the best future opportunities to stratify screening and treatment by age is probably prostate. Carter has presented evidence that, in prostate cancer, multiple malignant events are necessary for a normal cell to give rise to a fully malignant cancer cell (69). Further he has proposed a scheme to calculate velocity of growth of prostate cancer based on serial

PSA values (70). This will provide a better biological basis for understanding the behavior of prostate cancer in old men who might, on the basis of those findings, be spared over-zealous screening and treatment. Sadly, similar understanding in other common cancers of the elderly is lacking and does not seem to be immediately forthcoming.

References

1. Sistrunk WE, MacCarty WC. Life expectancy following radical amputation for carcinoma of the breast: a clinical and pathologic study of 218 cases. *Ann Surg* 1922; **75**: 61–69.

2. Di Paola M, Angelini L, Bertolotti A, *et al.* Host resistance in relation to survival in breast cancer. *Br Med J* 1974; **4**: 268–270.

3. Ershler WB. Why tumors grow more slowly in old people. *JNCI* 1986; **77**: 837–839.

4. Holmes FF, Hearne E. Cancer stage-to-age relationship. implications for cancer screening in the elderly. *J Am Geriatr Soc* 1981; **29**: 55–57.

5. Goodwin JS, Samet JM, Key CR, *et al.* Stage at diagnosis of cancer varies with the age of the patient. *J Am Geriatr Soc* 1986; **34**: 20–26.

6. Abrams HL, Spiro R, Goldstein N. Metastases in carcinoma: analysis of 1,000 autopsied cases. *Cancer* 1950; **3**: 74–85.

7. Suen KC, Lau LL, Yermakov V. Cancer and old age. A n autopsy study of 3,535 patients over 65 years old. *Cancer* 1974; **33**: 1164–1168.

8. Esaki Y, Hirayama R, Katsuiku H. A comparison of patterns of metastasis in gastric cancer by histologic type and age. *Cancer* 1990; **65**: 2086–2090.

9. McFarlane MJ, Feinstein AR, Wells CK, *et al.* The 'epidemiologic necropsy.' Unexpected detections, demographic selections, and changing rates of lung cancer. *JAMA* 1987; **258**: 331–338.

10. Saitoh H, Shiramizu T, Hida M. Age changes in metastatic patterns in renal adenocarcinoma. *Cancer* 1982; **50**: 1646–1648.

11. Ershler WB, Socinski MA, Greene CJ. Bronchogenic cancer, metastases, and aging. *J Am Geriatr Soc* 1983; **31**: 673–676.

12. O'Rourke MA, Feussner JR, Feigl P, *et al.* Age trends of lung cancer stage at diagnosis: implications for lung cancer screening in the elderly. *JAMA* 1987; **258**: 921–926.

13. Teeter SM, Holmes FF, McFarlane MJ. Lung carcinoma in the elderly population: influence of histology on the inverse relationship of stage to age. *Cancer* 1987; **60**: 1331–1336.

14. Yancik R, Ries LE, Yates JW. Breast cancer in aging women: a population-based study of contrasts in stage, surgery, and survival. *Cancer* 1989; **63**: 976–981.

15. Spratt JA, vonFournier D, Spratt JS, Weber EE. Mammographic assessment of human breast cancer growth and duration. *Cancer* 1993; **71**: 2020–2026.

16. Pelikan S, Moskowitz M. Effects of lead time, length bias, and false-negative assurance on screening for breast cancer. *Cancer* 1993; **71**: 1998–2005.

17. Rhodes JB, Holmes FF, Clark GM. Changing distribution of primary cancers in the large bowel. *JAMA* 1977; **238**: 1641–1643.

18. Butcher D, Hassanein K, Dudgeon M, *et al.* Female gender is a major determinant of changing subsite distribution of colorectal cancer with age. *Cancer* 1985; **56**: 714–716.

19. Rosen PP, Lesser ML, Kinne DW. Breast carcinoma at the extremes of age: a comparison of patients younger than 35 years and older than 75 years. *J Surg Oncol* 1985; **28**: 90–96.

20. Lees JC, Park WW. The malignancy of cancer at different ages: a histological study. *Br J Cancer* 1949; **3**: 186–197.

21. Richardson GS, Scully RE, Nikrui N, *et al.* Common epithelial cancer of the ovary. *N Engl J Med* 1985; **312**: 415–424.

22. Shingleton HM, Partridge EE, Austin JM. The significance of age in the colposcopic evaluation of women with atypical Papanicolaou smears. *Obstet Gynecol* 1977; **49**: 61–64.

23. Gard PD, Fields MJ, Noble EJ, *et al.* Comparative cytopathology of squamous carcinoma in situ of the cervix in the aged. *Acta Cytol* 1969; **13**: 27–35.

24. Ashley DJ. Evidence for the existence of two forms of cervical carcinoma. *J Obstet Gynaec Brit Comm* 1966; **73**: 382–389.

25. Hakama M, Penttinen J. Epidemiological evidence for two components of cervical cancer. *Br J Obstet Gynaecol* 1981; **88**: 209–214.

26. Schottenfeld D, Robbins GF. Breast cancer in elderly women. *Geriatrics* 1971; **26**: 121–131.

27. Allen C, Cox EB, Manton KG, *et al.* Breast cancer in the elderly. Current patterns of care. *J Am Geriatr Soc* 1986; **34**: 637–642.

28. von Rosen A, Gardelin A, Auer G. Assessment of malignancy potential in mammary carcinoma in elderly patients. *Am J Clin Oncol* 1987; **10**: 61–64.

29. McCarty KS, Silva JS, Cox EB, *et al.* Relationship of age and menopausal status to estrogen receptor content in primary carcinoma of the breast. *Ann Surg* 1983; **197**: 123–127.

30. Elwood JM, Godolphin W. Oestrogen receptors in breast tumors: associations with age, menopausal status and epidemiological and clinical features in 735 patients. *Br J Cancer* 1980; **42**: 635–644.

31. Szakacs JG, Arroyo JG, Girgenti AJ. Assessment of results of estrogen and progesterone receptor assays performed in a community hospital. *Ann Clin Lab Science* 1986; **16**: 266–273.

32. Bloom HJG, Richardson WW, Harries EJ. Natural history of untreated breast cancer (1805–1933). Comparison of untreated and treated cases according to histological grade of malignancy. *Brit Med J* 1962; **2**: 213–221.

33. Meyers FJ. Tumor biology in explanation of the failure of screening for cancer and in determination of future strategies. *Am J Med* 1986; **80**: 911–916.

34. Akslen L. Prognostic importance of histologic grading in papillary thyroid carcinoma. *Cancer* 1993; **72**: 2680–2685.

35. Whittemore AS, Keller JB, Betensky R. Low-grade, latent prostate cancer volume: predictor of clinical cancer incidence? *J Natl Cancer Inst* 1991; **83**: 1231–1235.

36. Peterson BA, Kennedy BJ. Aging and cancer management. Part I: Clinical observations. *Ca* 1979; **29**: 322–332.

37. Lipschitz DA, Goldstein S, Reis R, *et al.* Cancer in the elderly: basic science and clinical aspects. *Ann Intern Med* 1985; **102**: 218–228.

38. Sondik EJ, Young JL, Horm JW: *1986 annual cancer statistics review*. NIH Publication No. 87-2789. Bethesda, U.S. Department of Health and Human Services, 1987.

39. Samet J, Hunt WC, Key C, *et al.* Choice of cancer therapy varies with age of patient. *JAMA* 1986; **255**: 3385–3390.

40. Mor V, Masterson-Allen S, Goldberg RJ, *et al.* Relationship between age at diagnosis and treatments received by cancer patients. *J Am Geriatr Soc* 1985; **33**: 585–589.

41. Kirsh MM, Rotman H, Bove E, *et al.* Major pulmonary resection for bronchogenic carcinoma in the elderly. *Ann Thorac Surg* 1976; **22**: 369–373.

42. Sherman S, Guidot CE. The feasibility of thoracotomy for lung cancer in the elderly. *JAMA* 1987; **258**: 927–930.

43. Clamon GH, Audeh MW, Pinnick S. Small cell lung carcinoma in the elderly. *J Am Geriatr Soc* 1982; **30**: 299–302.

44. Calabrese CT, Adam YG, Volk H. Geriatric colon cancer. *Am J Surg* 1973; **125**: 181–184.

45. Sorensen JT, Gerald J, Bodensteiner D, Holmes FF. Effect of age on survival in acute leukemia. *Cancer* 1993; **72**: 1602–1606.

46. Baudard M, Marie JP, Cadiou M, Viguie F, Zittoun R. Acute myelogenous leukaemia in the elderly: retrospective study of 235 consecutive patients. *Br J Haem* 1994; **86**: 82–91.

47. Peterson BA, Pajak TF, Cooper MR, *et al.* Effect of age on therapeutic response and survival in advanced Hodgkin's disease. *Cancer Treat Rep* 1982; **66**: 889–898.

48. Stone RM,, Berg DT, George SL, Dodge RK, Raciucci PA, Schulman P, Lee EJ, Moore JO, Powell BL, Schiffer CA. Granulocyte-macrophage colony-stimulating factor after initial chemotherapy for elderly patients with primary acute myelogenous leukemia. *N Engl J Med* 1995; **332**: 1671–1677.

49. Hamblin TJ. Disappointments in treating acute leukemia in the elderly. *N Engl J Med* 1995; **332**: 1712–1713.

50. Ludwig H, Fritz E, Friedl HP. Epidemiologic and age-dependent data on multiple myeloma in Austria. *J Natl Cancer Inst* 1982; **68**: 729–733.

51. Holmes FF. *Aging and cancer*. Berlin/New York: Springer-Verlag, 1983.

52. Cohen HJ, Silberman HR, Forman W, *et al.* Effects of age on responses to treatment and survival of patients with multiple myeloma. *J Am Geriatr Soc* 1983; **31**: 272–277.

53. Daland EM. Untreated cancer of the breast. *Surgery Gynecol and Obstet* 1927; **44**: 264–268.

54. Sutton M. Late recurrence of carcinoma of breast. *Brit Med J* 1960; **2**: 1132–1134.

55. Croton R, Cooke T, Holt S, *et al.* Oestrogen receptors and survival in early breast cancer. *Br Med J* 1981; **283**: 1289–1291.

56. Herbsman H, Feldman J, Seldera J, *et al.* Survival following breast cancer surgery in the elderly. *Cancer* 1981; **47**: 2358–2363.

57. Mueller CB, Ames F, Anderson GD. Breast cancer in 3,558 women: age as a significant determinant in the rate of dying and causes of death. *Surgery* 1978; **83**: 123–132.

58. Newcombe RB, Hillyard JW. Age and death in breast cancer. *Surgery* 1980; **87**: 599–600.

59. Hibberd AD, Horwood LJ, Wells JE. Long term prognosis of women with breast cancer in New Zealand: study of survival to 30 years. *Br Med J* 1983; **286**: 1777–1779.

60. Adami H-O, Malker B, Meirik O, *et al.* Age as a prognostic factor in breast cancer. *Cancer* 1985; **56**: 898–902;

61. Adami H-O, Malker B, Holmberg L, *et al.* The relation between survival and age at diagnosis in breast cancer. *N Engl J Med* 1986; **315**: 559–563.

62. Langlands AO, Pocock SJ, Kerr GR, *et al.* Long-term survival of patients with breast cancer: a study of the curability of the disease. *Br Med J* 1979; **2**: 1247–1251.

63. Christiansen HD, Holmes FF, Scott TE, *et al. Age and survival in breast cancer.* Proceedings of the Annual Meeting of the American Geriatric Society, 1983.

64. Borek D, Butcher D, Hassanein K, Holmes F. Relationship of age to histologic grade in prostate cancer. *The Prostate* 1990; **16**: 305–311.

65. Whitely R, Hannah P, Holmes F. Survival in acute leukemia in elderly patients, no improvement in the 1980s. *J Am Geriatr Soc* 1990; **38**: 527–530.

66. Manton KG, Wrigley JM, Cohen HJ, Woodbury MA. Cancer mortality, aging and patterns of co-morbidity in the United States: 1968 to 1986. *J Gerontol (Social Sciences)* 1991; **46**: S225–234.

67. Peer PGM, van Dijck JAAM, Hendriks JHCL, Holland R, Verbeek ALM. Age-dependent growth rate of primary breast cancer. *Cancer* 1993; **71**: 3547–3551.

68. Silliman RA, Balducci L, Goodwin JS, Holmes FF, Leventhal EA. Breast cancer care in old age: what we know, don't know, and do. *J Natl Cancer Inst* 1993; **85**: 190–199.

69. Carter HB, Piantadosi, Isaacs JT. Clinical evidence for and implications of the multistep development of prostate cancer. *J Urology* 1990; **143**: 742–746.

70. Carter HB, Pearson JD. PSA velocity for the diagnosis of early prostate cancer: a new concept. *Urologic Clinics of North America* 1993; **20**: 665–670.

14. Morbid Anatomy of Aging

Giorgio Stanta

Introduction

Aging is associated with a progressive restriction in the functional reserve of many organ systems and with the development of many coexisting diseases. Functional restriction and comorbidity generate a series of clinical challenges for the practitioner. Common clinical questions include: does a new symptom herald the presence of a new disease or does it represent instead an exacerbation of a chronic disease or an expected progression of preexisting organ disfunction? How will this older person with already compromised respiratory function tolerate the additional stress of an upper respiratory infection or of anemia? Which one of many comorbidities is causing a progressive deterioration in the patient's condition? How prevalent are occult malignancies and what is the value of screening older persons for cancer? Pathology may provide a key to many of these questions, by defining the common age-related changes at the level of different organs and tissue, by establishing the causes of death of older individuals in the presence of multiple pathologies, by discovering unsuspected conditions which might have caused the death of an older person.

The interest in the pathology of aging has been rekindled by the difficulties to establish precise diagnoses in the elderly, in spite of all the recently available sophisticated technologies. Diseases in elderly patients often lack those symptoms and signs that may guide physicians to a certain diagnosis. And expert pathologists can attest that even after autopsy it may prove difficult to define the cause of death in elderly people. In the age of molecular biology, morbid anatomy can still be important to distinguish normal and pathological events of aging.

In this chapter we review the literature concerning morbid pathology of aging, that dates back more than 20 years (1–10) and we contribute our own casistic. A detailed review of the pathology of aging is beyond the scope of this chapter. Rather, we will highlight those aspects which are of interest to the interactions of aging and cancer.

Non Neoplastic Pathology of the Aging

The incidence of chronic degenerative diseases increases with age. These diseases are generally systemic and cause lesions in multiple organs and apparatus. A classical example of these diseases is arteriosclerosis, which causes myocardial fibrosis, nephrosclerosis and atrophy of many organs.

Table 14.1 Chronic and degenerative lesions commonly found at the autopsy of persons aged 80 and older.

A. Cardiovascular lesions

Coronary arteries: the degree of sclerosis is generally lesser than seen in younger olds (aged 65–75) (11)

Severe myocardial fibrosis (1,3)

Cardiac amyloid (1)

B. Pulmonary lesions

Panacinar emphysema (5)

Bronchiectasis (5)

C. Genit.-Urinary Lesions

Nephrosclerosis (3)

Chronic pyelonephritis (6)

Renal Infarctions (6)

D. Digestive Lesions

Sigmoid diverticulosis

Hepatic atrophy without fibrosis or other specific lesions (6)

E. Skeleton

Osteoporosis

Acute diseases are present in any age and can not be considered characteristic of the elderly. Nevertheless some of these are more common among old people and may be especially severe in the extreme ages of life when they become relevant causes of death. Bronchopneumonia is a typical example of an acute illness which is often lethal in the elderly.

In Table 14.1 are summarized the degenerative conditions commonly found at autopsy in elderly individuals.

Cardiovascular System

Most octogenarians and nonagenarians present atherosclerosis of the major arteries with atheromas and thrombi that sometimes obstruct the vessel lumen. These lesions are usually localized at the take-off of major vessels from the aorta (11–13), and are of varying severity. Two third of the nonagenarians present se-

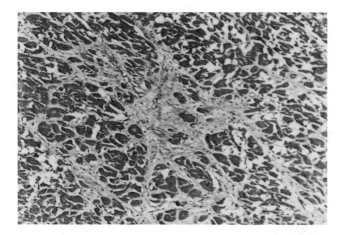

Figure 14.1 Myocardial fibrosis.

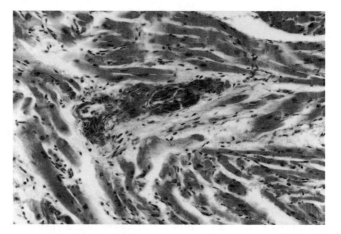

Figure 14.2 Amyloidosis of the heart.

vere atherosclerosis (3). In other cases, however, atherosclerosis is minimal even in persons of this age. Selective changes are seen in different vessels in persons of different ages. The observation of the coronary artery is very instructive. In older persons the degree of intimal fibrous thickening with stenosis of the coronary vessels appears related to the degree of intimal fibrosis in the aorta (3), but in the centenarians the pattern somehow changes. From our and others' experience (5) the degree of sclerosis and arterial obstruction is lesser in the coronaries than in the aorta of persons aged 100 and older. The changes observed in the cerebral vessels parallel the changes of the coronary artery and are generally less severe than in the aorta. This relative preservation of the integrity of coronary and cerebral vessels is selective: the atherosclerosis of other vessels, such as the femoral arteries becomes more severe with age, even after age 100, and closely parallel the degree of intimal fibrosis of the aorta.

Myocardial fibrosis is one of the most important pathological finding in aging (Figure 14.1) and is an extremely relevant condition in contributing to death of octogenarians and nonagenarians (1,3,11,13). In our centenarian case study myocardiosclerosis was moderate in 35% of the cases, marked in 42% and severe in 12%. Fibrosis was confined to the left ventricle, mostly localized to the anterior and posterior wall and to the septum. The areas of more severe fibrosis generally correspond to the most severe obstructive lesions of coronary vessels. This association suggests a predominately ischemic pathogenesis of myocardial fibrosis. Also the wall of the right ventricle of the elderly shows anatomical signs of a decreased contractile efficiency with the presence of adipocytes between the muscle fibers. These idiopathies may give origin to the pattern of the so called right ventricle lipomatosis (5). Myocardial scars from previous myocardial infarction are often seen and may also contribute to a cardiac failure.

Amyloidosis of the heart is another characteristic of the elderly. We found amyloid in 12% of our cases (Figure 14.2), but other studies report the presence of cardiac amyloidosis in over 30% of centenarians (5).

Myocardial atrophy was evident in 23% of our centenarian cases. In this population we did not find any case of real cardiac hypertrophy, with increased heart weight (5). As reported by other authors (5) we did not find a real case of brown atrophy, which is associated with severe malnutrition rather than directly with the aging process.

Degenerative processes of the cardiac valves are also common. In association with cardiomyopathy these valvular lesions may contribute to a chronic heart failure. A calcified ring or fibrous thickening at the mitral or aortic level is a frequent finding in the elderly (5).

Respiratory System

In our area bronchopneumonia is the final cause of death in only 2.5% of people over 65 years, but it represents 20% of the causes in people over 95 and 30% in centenarians. Usually pneumonia may be considered the final cause of death, a complication of other evident contributory diseases, like an hip fracture with immobilization of the patient; sometimes it is apparently the only cause of death. The lesion is usually focal but it may involve an entire pulmonary lobe or more. It is often reported that most of the pneumonias of the elderly are "ab ingestis" lesions. The rare occurrence of foreign body granulomas in our and in others' case studies (5) does not confirm this hypothesis. Perhaps the causes of the high frequency of bronchopneumnia include immunesenescense and stagnation of secretions from poor cough reflex and decreased strength of respiratory muscles. Emphysema and bronchiectasis are common and may also play an important role in the occurrence of pneumonia (5). The presence of emphysema (Figure 14.3) was described in over 70% of the nonagenarians examined (3) and in only 20% of centenarians (5). The lesions vary in severity and tend to increase in frequency particularly among people over 80 years of age, together with bronchiectatic changes.

A fibrous pleuritis with pleural adhesions is present in more than one third of the people over 90 years of age.

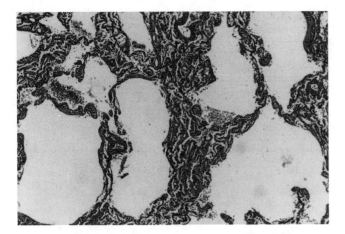

Figure 14.3 Emphysema.

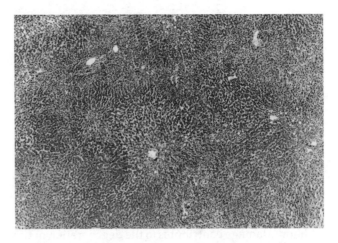

Figure 14.4 Normal histological structure of the liver in a centenarian.

Pulmonary tuberculosis caused the death of three centenarians out of 99 examined. In one more case the disease was detected but it was not related to the cause of death. None of the cases was suspected before death.

Digestive Tract

The most frequent lesion of the digestive tract in the elderly is diverticulosis of large bowel that involves sigmoid colon in about 40% of the people over 80 years of age (3,14). Complications of diverticulosis in very old people are not very frequent. In our case study of centenarians only one case out of 99 showed perforation of a diverticulum. The peritonitis that followed caused the death of the patient.

The liver is remarkably well preserved throughout old ages. In centenarians the liver appears moderately atrophic, but always with a normal histological structure (Figure 14.4) (6). The microscopical findings of an high number of binucleated cells and the alteration of the nuclear/cytoplasmic ratio are considered specific histological changes of the senile liver (15).

Fatty changes and congestion are frequently observed as a consequence of final respiratory and cardiac failure. Chronic primary lesions of the liver like chronic hepatitis and cirrhosis are quite frequent autopsy findings in the younger age groups of elderly (65–80), but they are uncommon in the extreme ages of life.

We found a marked atrophy of the pancreas in one third of centenarians and lithiasis of the gallbladder in 15% of the cases.

Genitourinary Lesions

Most very old people have atrophic kidneys with macroscopic scars and multiple retention cysts. Atrophy mainly involves the cortex, while the medulla presents interstitial fibrosis (Figure 14.5). The renal arterioles show hyaline thickening. Signs of chronic pyelonephritis and previous infarctions are often present. All these lesions generally worsen with age.

In 253 autopsy examinations of prostate gland in elderly males over 80 years of age, 92 hyperplastic glands, 21 latent adenocarcinomas and 16 aggressive tumors were found (1). The testis show atrophy of the spermatic ducts and moderate hyperplasia of the Leydig cells. In females there is a marked atrophy of uterus and of ovaries with loss of germinal follicles.

Other Organs

Characteristic of aging is also the pathology of other organs, including degenerative lesions of bones, joints, and brain. These pathologies are very well studied and do not add much to our knowledge of the mechanisms of death in the older person. On the other side acute cerebrovascular accidents, like strokes and hemorrhages, are frequently found as main or contributory cause of death at autopsy. Also, the aging process of the skin and the pressure ulcers contribute significantly to the elderly pathology.

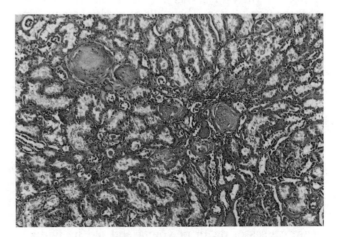

Figure 14.5 In the aging kidney, the cortex is atrophied while the medulla presents interstitial fibrosis.

Characteristic Pattern of Non-Neoplastic Pathology in the Extreme Ages of the Life Span

There are many autopsy studies about the pathology in the extreme ages of life (2,3,5–9). Chronic lesions, characteristic of the aging process, are more frequent and severe in nonagenarians and centenarians. Arteriosclerosis among chronic degenerative diseases particularly characterizes the aging process. The localization of the atheromas in the elderly is not uniform. In centenarians the lesions in aorta and femoral arteries are more severe than in cerebral and coronary vessels (5). Many of the characteristic pathologies found in extremely aged people are related to arteriosclerosis of the major and the small arteries. The consequent chronic ischemic damage contributes to the degeneration of the other organs which is associated with the aging process. Myocardial fibrosis, nephrosclerosis and atrophy of the organs are the outcomes. The heart efficiency as pump is decreased by fibrosis and the possible association with myocardial atrophy and amyloidosis. The respiratory system is damaged by a panacinar emphysema to which are associated bronchiectatic changes and stagnation of secretions. In such a critical situation bronchopneumonia or cardiac failure are the frequent fatal outcomes.

Characteristics of the oldest old (nonagenarians and centenarians) include atrophy and fibrosis of most parenchymal organs and adipose atrophy. Organ dysfunction is a common consequence of these changes. The absence of pathologic changes in the liver is also characteristic of centenarians (6). No signs of chronic hepatitis or fibrosis of any origin are usually detected in very old people even after microscopical examination. On the contrary these lesions are common findings in autopsies of the younger age groups. Cardiac and pancreatic fibrosis is in average more severe in centenarians than in people between 75 and 85 years of age. Prevalence of arteriolosclerosis of kidney and brain vessels is also different in the two age groups. The wall of the kidney arterioles is clearly thicker in centenarians than in people of 75–85 years of age as expected. The opposite is the case in the cerebral and coronary circulation. The walls of cerebral small arteries are as average thinner in the centenarians than in persons aged 70–85.

From this review we may identify two distinct pathological patterns in the old and in the oldest old. Among persons aged 65–90 chronic diseases are more prominent, whereas among the oldest old the most prevalent lesion is diffuse organ atrophy. The selective sparing of cerebral and coronary circulation among the centenarians suggests that preservation of these circulatory beds may represent a precondition to advanced aging.

Causes of Death in the Elderly

Many dfferences emerge from the comparison of the main causes of death of young and old individuals. There are also many differences among different sub-

Table 14.2 Causes of death in the oldest old in the Trieste area.*

	Over 95		Over 65	
	Rank Order	%	Rank order	%
Cardiovascular	1	21.4	1	31.6
Pneumonia	2	20	9	2.4
Cerebrovascular	3	19	3	13.3
Neoplasia	4	9.5	2	26.1
Accident	5	10.2	6	3.4
Atherosclerosis	6	8.4	4	4.0
Digestive diseases	7	3.7	8	2.7
Tuberculosis	8	1.8	13	0.1
Urological	9	1.8	12	0.6
Septicemia	10	0.5	14	0.1
COPD	11	0.5	5	3.4

COPD = Chronic Obstrucfive Pulmonary Diseases

*Data from the Trieste Tumor Registry.

groups of elderly, particularly between the youngest old (over 65) and the oldest old (over 90) (Table 14.2). Malignant neoplasms are the first cause of death among people under 65 years of age, but they become the second cause after cardiovascular diseases in people over 65, the fourth cause in nonagenarians and only the fifth one in centenarians (16). Cardiovascular diseases are the second most common cause of death in the people under 65, but they become the first one in the elderly, up to age 99. However, after age 90, cardiovascular diseases become a less common cause of death, while accidents (mainly hip fractures) become more prevalent. In centenarians cardiovascular diseases are the second cause of death, while bronchopneumonia is by far the first cause and it accounts for one third of all the deaths (7,10). In some cases bronchopneumnia is the only evident cause of death, in others it is the final cause associated with other contributory causes. One of the most frequent contributory causes is the hip fracture with immobilization of the patients and final bronchopneumonia.

Cerebrovascular diseases are the third cause of death in the elderly in any age sub-group, but they are decreasing again in frequency in centenarians. In our experience they account for almost 20% of the deaths among nonagenarians, but only for 10% in centenarians.

Another condition deserves some attention: cirrhosis is one of the most frequent causes of death in the area of Trieste in people under 65 years of age. It is at the fourth place in the rank order of the causes of death and it is mostly related with alcohol abuse. On the contrary in people over 65 cirrhosis is at the tenth place

Table 14.3 Comparison of cancer incidence in the youngest and the oldest old. (>85/<65 incidence ratio).*

Males	Ratio	Females	Ratio
Prostate	203.0	Pancreas	49.3
Pancreas	50.2	Bladder	34.8
Stomach	31.6	Colon	34.4
Colon	28.4	Stomach	34.1
Kidney	21.4	Gallbladder	32.8
Liver	18.3	Rectum	15.8
Esophagus	16.7	Kidney	13.2
Rectum	16.6	Lung	11.9
Bladder	16.4	NHL	7.9
NHL	15.8	Breast	4.5
Pleura	14.6	Ovary	2.9
Lung	10.5	Endometrium	2.8
Melanoma	10.5	Melanoma	2.4
		Cervix	1.9

and its frequency decreases more and more with age and it becomes extremely rare in people over 95 years of age.

In the extreme ages of life contributory causes of death must be considered in addition to the main causes (7,10). In this group in fact the death may not be ascribed to just one final cause. Heart, pulmonary and renal conditions contribute together to a critical situation, and any acute stress overimposed to these chronic conditions may precipitate end-organ failure and lead to a rapid death. Sometimes the contribution of many causes is so relevant that even the autopsy examination fails to identify a well defined cause of death (7,9,10). In these cases a pattern of a general atrophy of the organs with moderate myocardial fibrosis and nephrosclerosis and with a limited, focal inflammation of the lung is found. The single lesion can not justify the death that can be explained only with the contribution of all the chronic lesions together.

Agreement between clinical diagnosis and autopsy diagnosis for the main causes of death is quite good even in centenarians with a correspondence of about 70% (17). The correspondence is lower in malignant tumors and acute diseases.

Latent and Undiagnosed Tumors

Latent and undiagnosed tumors are more frequent in elderly than in young people. This because the tumors of any anatomical site are more common in people over 65 years and also because in the oldest age groups the diagnosis is more difficult. The lower aggressiveness of malignant tumors in very old people also contributes to the latency. A well known biological problem is latent cancer of the prostate that presents a very high prevalence in the glands removed at autopsy in the elderly (18).

In our necropsy series we discovered more than two early (but macroscopically evident) gastric cancer every 1000 autopsies in people over 70 years of age (19). The prevalence of undiagnosed colorectal cancers increased from about three cases per 1000 autopsies in people between 60 and 70 years, to 9 cases / 1000 in people over 80 years of age (20). On the contrary, for breast cancer the cases discovered only at autopsy seem to decrease in the more advanced age (21).

Studies of comparison between death certificate and autopsy show that false negative death certificate for malignant tumors are more common in elderly. In males the agreement for lung cancer decreases from 70% in people under 60 years to 40% in those over 85 years. In females over 85 with lung cancer there is a complete agreement only in 17% of the cases (22). The same trend is present in many other tumors. Correspondence for ovary tumors, for example, is complete in almost 80% of the cases in the younger age groups, but decreases to 30% in women over 80 years of age (23). Considering all together the malignant tumors of any anatomical site in people over 75 years of age the false negative death certificates are around 40% of all the compared cases (24).

Malignant Tumors in the Extreme Ages

Although the prevalence of malignant tumors increases with age, there are variations among different tumors. The reports of tumor registries provide an important database of the incidence of neoplasia in the different age groups in different countries. For the oldest old, tumor registries proved inadequate. As tumor registries underestimate the actual incidence of cancer in the oldest old, it would be helpful to estimate the incidence of false-negative diagnoses in this population of patients, to calculate the real incidence of tumors in the oldest ages. Autopsy studies in the elderly may allow this estimate.

The Tumor Registry of Trieste obtains autopsy information in over 60% of all the deaths of the area (25), so the occurrence of tumors in a very old population can be evaluated. The median age for all the tumors in both sexes is 71 years that is higher than the age of the population surveyed by S.E.E.R. (67.9 years). The median age for cancers of large bowel, stomach, kidney, liver, gallbladder and pancreas is higher than the median age of the SEER population. In our area, the median age of prostate cancer is 76, of pancreatic cancer in women is 78.

In a series of 99 autopsies of centenarians 17 cases of malignant tumor were found (16). Only 5 of these cases were correctly diagnosed and in only 7 out of 17 the tumor was the main cause of death. Only in four of the seven fatal tumors, the cause of death was directly related to the metastatic spreading of the neoplasia (a rectal adenocarcinoma, a pancreatic tumor and two breast cancers). In the other three tumors no distant metastases were found and the cause of death were: an hemorrhage in a gastric cancer, the obstruction of the extrahepatic biliary ducts in a gallbladder tumor and a bronchopneumonia "ab ingestis" in a destruent carcinoma of the nasal sinuses. Surprisingly other infiltrative, usually aggressive tumors, like three stomach cancers, one colonic adenocarcinoma, two adenocarcinomas of the small intestine, two adenocarcinomas of the gallbladder, a ductal carcinoma of the breast, a small cell carcinoma of the lung, a melanoma and a hepatocarcinoma did not give origin to macroscopic metastases. In the tumors with metastatic spreading the number of anatomical sites involved by the metastases was always low (from one to three) and always localized only to the liver, the lung and to the distant lymph nodes.

Causes of Death and Comorbidity in Cancer

Establishing the cause of death in the elderly with cancer may be a very complicated task. The contributory effect of the multiple comorbidities is often very important. Elderly people treated for a tumor may die with a recurrence, but this recurrence may not represent the main cause of death. An infection, a stroke, an episode of cardiac failure, or even a second primary malignant tumor can be the main final cause of death. In the death certificate the initial neoplasia is very often considered the main cause, even when the neoplasia is contributory of death only in a marginal way or it is completely unrelated. When a second primary cancer is present in the elderly, it is often diagnosed as a metastasis of the first neoplasm.

In our experience there is a clear difference between the causes of death of women aged 65 and older, and of younger women, who underwent mastectomy for breast cancer (26). Among women under 65 over 60% of the women died directly for the tumor, among those aged 65 and older, cancer was the direct cause of death in only 36% of cases. In the other cases the main cause of death was unrelated to the tumor. A thorough analysis of the existing pathology was necessary to dissect the effect of recurrences, of antineoplastic therapy, and of comorbidity in causing the patient's death (27). The survival was quite different in the two age groups. In our case study only 9% of the women who underwent mastectomy for cancer under 65 years of age died in the first year after surgery, while this percentage was 38% for women aged 65 and over. Also, 52% of the younger women, but only the 24% of those older, survived 5 years and longer after mastectomy. The differences in survival were mostly related to comorbidty in the elderly (28). In the older group of patients bronchopneumonia was the main cause of death in over 16% of the cases and a pulmonary embolism in over 10%; heart failure in 9% and stroke in 6%. Surprisingly a second primary tumor was the cause of death in around 10% of the cases regardless of the age at mastectomy (26).

The contribution of concurrent non neoplastic causes to the death in the elderly with cancer is even more evident in centenarians. As already described above only seven out of 17 cancers found in a group of centenarian were the cause of death. In the ten cases left the cause was related to non-neoplastic conditions, such as bronchopneumonia, stroke, heart failure. The role of the malignant tumor was judged to be only contributory in most of the cases.

Cancer Spreading

Frequency and localization of the metastases may change for the same tumor with the age of the patient. The number of anatomic sites found at the autopsy in women died for breast cancer is different depending on the age at the mastectomy (29). The average number of metastasized sites is over 3 in women mastectomized under 55 years of age, it becomes 2.5 in those between 55 and 65, 1.9 in the group 65–75 and 1.6 in those over 75. The localization pattern of the metastases also change with the age (26). Localization to the endocrine organs is more frequent in the younger group. Involvement of the skin and lymph nodes is more common among women who underwent mastectomy in advanced age. In our case study the average age at the mastectomy is 52 years for those with a metastasis to the ovary and 66 for those with skin metastases. Even the frequency of metastases to the classic anatomical sites changes with the age. In women mastectomized under 65 years liver metastases are found in over 55% of the cases, lung metastases in 42% and pleura metastases in 33% of the cases. In women that were treated for breast cancer over 65 years of age the frequencies of metastases in the same sites were respectively 27%, 29% and 22%.

Conclusions

Autopsy studies reveal a changing pathology between the younger old and the oldest old. In the younger old (up to age 90), the predominant changes appear related to atherosclerosis; after that age, and especially among the centenarians, the predominant pathology is organ atrophy.

The incidence of malignant tumors increases with age up to around age 85 and seems to decline after age ninety. Likewise, malignant tumors acquire a more indolent course in the oldest old (lesser number of metastases, lower incidence of life-threatening metastases). The incidence of occult malignant tumors appears negligible after age 85.

The interactions of end-organ atrophy and lower cancer prevalence are unknown. An open and extremely important question is whether reversal of the aging process may lead to more and more aggressive malignant neoplasms.

References

1. Mulligan RM. Geriatric pathology: autopsy findings in three hundred fifty-six persons eighty years of age and older. *AMA Arch Path* 1990; **69**: 9–42.
2. Howell TH. Causes of death in nonagenarians. *Geront Clin* 1963; **5**: 139–143.

3.   Howell TH. Multiple pathology in nonagenarians. *Geriatrics* 1963; **18**: 899–902.
4.   Hofman WI. The pathologist and the geriatric autopsy. *J Am Geriatr Soc* 1975; **23**: 11–13.
5.   Ishii T, Stemby NH. Pathology of centenarians. I. The cardiovascular system and lungs. *J Am Geriatr Soc* 1978; **26**: 108–115.
6.   Ishii T, Stemby NH. Pathology of centenarians. II. Urogenital and digestive system. *J Am Geriatr Soc* 1978; **26**: 391–396.
7.   Ishii T, Sternby NH. Pathology of centenarians. III: Osseus system, malignant lesions, and causes of death. *J Am Geriatr Soc* 1978; **26**: 529–533.
8.   Ishii T, Hosoda Y, Maeda K. Cause of death in the extreme aged. *Age Ageing* 1980; **9**: 81–89.
9.   Kohn RR. Cause of death in very old people. *JAMA* 1982; **247**: 2793–2797.
10.   Puxity JAH, Horan MA, Fox RA. Necropsies in the elderly. *Lancet* 1983; **i**: 1262–1264.
11.   Pomerance A. Pathology of the heart in the tenth decade. *J Clin Path* 1968; **21**: 317.
12.   Howell TH, Piggot AP. Morbid anatomy of old age. *Geriatrics* 1951; **6**: 85.
13.   Howell TH, Piggot AP. Morbid anatomy of old age. Part VII. Cardiovascular lesions. *Geriatrics* 1955; **10**: 428.
14.   Manousos ON, Truelove SC, Lumbsden K. Prevalence of colon diverticulosis in general population of Oxford area. *Brit Med J* 1967; **3**: 762.
15.   Tauchi H. On the fundamental morphology of senile changes. *Nagova J Med Sci* 1961; **24**: 97.
16.   Stanta G, Cavallieri F, Campagner L. Cancer of the oldest old: what we have learned from autoptic studies. *Clin Ger Med* 1997; **13(1)**: 55–68.
17.   Paterson DA, Dorovitch MI, Farquhar DL, Cameron HM, Currie CT, Smith RG, MacLennan WJ. Prospective study of necropsy audit of geriatric inpatient deaths. *J Clin Pathol* 1992; **45**: 575–578.
18.   Guileyardo JM, *et al*. Prevalence of latent prostate carcinoma in two U.S. populations. *JNCI* 1980; **65**: 311.
19.   Stanta G, Sasco AJ, Riboli E, Cocchi A, Rossitti P. Prevalence of gastric cancer in a large necropsy series. *Lancet* 1986; **i**: 624.
20.   Delendi M, Gardiman D, Riboli E, Sasco AJ. Latent colorectal cancer found at necropsies. *Lancet* 1989; **i**: 1331–1332.
21.   Giarelli L, Stanta G, Delendi M, Sasco AJ, Riboli E. Prevalence of female breast cancer observed in 517 unselected necropsies. *Lancet* 1986; **ii**: 864.
22.   Delendi M, Riboh E, Peruzzo P, Stanta G, Cocchi A, Gardiman D, Sasco AJ, Giarelli L. Comparison of diagnoses of cancers of the respiratory system on death certificates and at autopsy. In *Autopsy in epidemiology and medical research*, edited by E Riboli, M Delendi. Lyon: IARC, 55–62, 1991.
23.   Di Bonito L, Stanta G, Delendi M, Peruzzo P, Gardiman D, Cocchi A, Patriarca S, Giarelli L. Comparison between diagnoses on death certificates and autopsy reports in Trieste: gynaecological cancers. In *Autopsy in epidemiology and medical research*, edited by E Riboli, M Delendi. Lyon: IARC, 63–71, 1991.
24.   Stanta G, Cavallieri F, Peruzzo P, Delendi M, Pavletic N, Giarelli L. Death certificate autopsy diagnosis comparison in elderly with malignant tumors. In *Recent advances in aging science*, edited by E Baregi, IA Gergely, K Rajczi. Bologna: Monduzzi, 1993.
25.   Parkin DM, Muir CS, Whelan SL, Gao YT, Ferlay J, Powell J. Cancer incidence in five continents Volume VI — IARC Scientific Publication No. 120, Lyon, 1992.
26.   Stanta G, Campagner L, Cavallieri F. Breast cancer spreading, survival and causes of death. In preparation.
27.   Cho SY, Choi HY. Causes of death and metastatic patterns in patients with mammary cancer. *Am J Clin Path* 1980; **73**: 232–234.
28.   Mueller CB, Ames F, Anderson GD. Breast cancer in 3,558 women: age as a significant determinant in the rate of dying and causes of death. *Surgery* 1978; **83**: 123–132.
29.   Viadana E, Cotter R, Pickren JW, Bross IDJ. An autopsy study of metastatic sites of breast cancer. *Cancer Res* 1973; **33**: 179–181.

15.   Apoptosis, Chemotherapy and Aging

David E. Fisher

Historical

The formal recognition that apoptotic death was a distinct entity which differed from other forms of cell death, was made in 1972 by a group of British pathologists studying the appearance of a variety of tissue types under growth/exposure conditions. Their striking observation was that rather than all cells appearing uniform, certain cells appeared to undergo changes which were highlighted by condensation of the nucleus, cell shrinkage, and eventual fragmentation (1). The term apoptosis was coined from the Greek for "falling apart." (Although there are numerous controversies in the field of apoptosis research, probably none is so fierce as the question of whether the second P is pronounced aloud!)

Subsequent to its original formal description, apoptotic death became widely recognized throughout biology, both among toxin-exposed cells, and throughout normal development. Since it occurs in normal development, it has been generally accepted that apoptosis may play a genetically encoded role in tissue homeostasis. If life in a multicellular organism represents a dynamic equilibrium between cell populations which are proliferating and others which are dying, apoptosis would be the metabolic opposite of mitosis leading to demise rather than division and proliferation. Though only preliminarily, models such as these have given rise to the notion that mechanisms in apoptosis may be central to the process of cellular senescence, and ultimately the aging process. However, the mechanistic means by which death at the unicellular level can produce aging within a multicellular organism remains uncertain. Apoptosis has also been called "programmed cell death" because it is destined to occur during development (1, 2, 3). Semantic distinctions have been made between the description of apoptotic death in development ("programmed") as compared to apoptotic death following toxin exposure, since the latter was a response to the environment rather than the direct result of the execution of a development program. Nonetheless, within the field of cancer biology apoptotic death has been found to play roles in two major areas: tumorigenesis and therapeutics. As described below, loss of apoptosis may play significant roles in the establishment of continuously propagating cell lineages. Moreover, loss of apoptosis-mediating molecules (through deletion or mutation) may disarm a suicide response to certain toxic exposures including antineoplastic agents. In this way the presence or absence of intact apoptosis

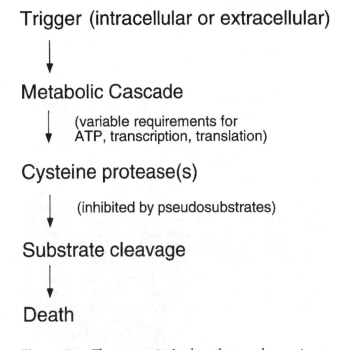

Trigger (intracellular or extracellular)

↓

Metabolic Cascade

↓ (variable requirements for ATP, transcription, translation)

Cysteine protease(s)

↓ (inhibited by pseudosubstrates)

Substrate cleavage

↓

Death

Figure 15.1   The apoptosis death pathway schema. A variety of intra- or extracellular triggers lead to a metabolic cascade whose energy requirements may vary depending on cell type and specific apoptosis trigger. Cystein proteases of the ICE family become activated and cleave a variety of substrates to produce death.

machinery may profoundly determine sensitivity to chemotherapeutics.

The Suicide Pathway

The emerging biochemistry of apoptotic cell death appears to involve a common metabolic pathway. This pathway is initiated by a "trigger". Apoptotic triggers are diverse and can include factors from the environment (such as toxins, drugs, or radiation) or factors within a cell (such as aberrant oncogene expression, mutation of certain genes, or changes in cell adhesion or growth factor properties). As outlined in Figure 15.1, subsequent to initiating the apoptotic cascade, a series of biochemical events occurs, much of which are not well characterized at this time. While it is assumed that the events which respond to the apoptotic trigger are energy requiring activities, it is difficult to ascertain even the energy dependency of apoptosis, because

Apoptosis

1. cell shrinkage................................... cell swelling
2. nuclear condensation......................... diffuse nuclear staining
3. cell,nuclear fragmentation.................. cell swelling
4. phagocytosis by non-phagocytic........ phagocytosis by normally
   or phagocytic cells   phagocytic cells
5. lacks inflammatory component........... inflammatory component
6. no release of lysosomal contents....... release of lysosomal contents
7. endonucleolytic internucleosomal...... random DNA cleavage
   DNA fragmentation
8. activation of cysteine proteases..........activation of numerous autolytic proteases
9. often involvement of individual cells....involvement of masses of cells
10. occurs in normal development..........always pathologic
   or pathologic circumstances

Necrosis

Figure 15.2 Contrasted features of apoptosis and necrosis.

manipulations which alter ATP availability or production may in themselves trigger apoptosis. Similarly, it was long felt that apoptosis requires active gene transcription and translation. However, other studies have suggested that apoptosis in certain cases may proceed rapidly even in the presence of transcriptional inhibitors such as actinomycin D or translational inhibitors such as cycloheximide (4, 5). It is difficult however to be certain that apoptosis despite high doses of cycloheximide is not "cycloheximide-induced," rather than resistant to the inhibition of translation.

While mediators of the apoptotic trigger produce a metabolic cascade which is poorly understood at present, a common target appears to be the activation of proteases which utilize cysteine at their active sites (6, 7). The cysteine proteases in turn cleave target proteins to result in the presumed final death blow. While it is clear that most biochemical details of apoptosis remain to be elucidated, apoptotic death differs from necrosis in that the cell is thought to play an active role in its own demise. Thus the apoptotic trigger *activates* a specific (suicide) metabolic program while necrotic triggers *inactivate* metabolic pathways producing death by default.

Assays for Apoptosis

The "gold standard" for the identification of apoptotic cells is cellular morphology. Using either electron microscopy or light microscopy, it is possible to distinguish the features of cells undergoing apoptosis from those dying by other means. As shown in Figure 15.2, apoptosis can be distinguished by a number of morphologic criteria. Apoptotic death typically involves individual cells, whereas necrosis is frequently the result of massive tissue injury (such as from burning or ischemia). While necrotic death is thought to result purely from environmental insults, apoptotic death is more often thought of as death "from the inside out." Plasma membrane integrity is lost early in necrosis, but late in apoptosis. Correspondingly, necrotic cells typically swell, whereas apoptotic cells typically shrink. Inflammation typified by the presence of neutrophils is usually significant among necrotic tissues whereas inflammation is minimal in the context of apoptosis.

Phagocytosis occurs by macrophages only in the case of necrotic cells whereas an interesting feature of apoptotic cells is that they tend to be phagocytized by surrounding cells which are generally not phagocytic. Thus it is not uncommon to see apoptotic tumor cells undergoing phagocytosis by surrounding viable non macrophage tumor cells. The other morphologic feature which is easily recognizable in apoptosis is chromosomal condensation leading to intensely stained nuclei. Fluorescent DNA interchelating dyes are frequently used to stain cells undergoing apoptosis. The nucleus is typically small, brightly stained, and frequently fragmented into small bodies, which when broken away from the intact cell are called "apoptotic bodies".

The biochemical hallmark of apoptosis is endonucleolytic DNA cleavage into fragments of 100 Kilobase pairs down to ~150 base pairs in length. This cleavage likely represents the activity of calcium and magnesium dependent endonucleases, and reflects internucleosomal cleavage. This leaves 150–200 base pair units representing the length of individual histone-bound nucleosomes. While DNA fragmentation is one of the hallmarks of apoptosis, its detection is not always simple. Numerous examples of clear morphologic apoptosis have been found to lack the "DNA ladder" of 150 bp DNA fragments. Though DNA ladders are easily visualized by simple agarose gel electrophoresis, the presence of DNA cleavage down to 50–100 kb DNA fragments fails to produce a DNA ladder, despite this extensive DNA fragmentation. Therefore, pulse-field gell electrophoresis may be employed to visualize these larger cleavage fragments in apoptosis.

A series of stains have also been developed to aid in the identification of cells undergoing DNA fragmentation. These stains utilize enzymes (such as deoxynucleotidyl terminal tranferase or the Klenow fragment of E. coli DNA polymerase) to enzymatically incorporate nucleotide analogs onto the ends of DNA molecules (8). In cells undergoing DNA fragmentation, the concentration of free DNA ends becomes extremely high, producing high levels of nucleotide analog incorporation. A variety of different analogs have been used, typically as part of a "sandwich" staining protocol to produce either fluorescent, colored, or radioactive signals within the cell. These methods have been applied to histologic analysis of tissues, as well as the study of cells in culture. They provide an advantage over gel electrophoresis that apoptosis may be quantitated within a population, both with respect to the intensity of DNA fragmentation in a given cell and the number of cells undergoing apoptosis in a given population. For these analyses the use of a fluorescent activated cell sorter has been of considerable importance. Caution must be taken, however, because the incorporated nucleotide analogs need not reflect apoptotic DNA fragmentation, but rather nonspecific DNA degradation during necrosis. Therefore morphologic features should be utilized as confirmation of apoptotic death.

While DNA fragmentation accompanies apoptosis, it should be noted that it is probably not causative, but rather an indication of apoptosis. A mutant exits ("nuc-1") in the nematode C. elegans in which DNA fragmentation is impeded. This mutant is nonetheless efficient at apoptosis during development (9, 10). Furthermore, Fas mediated apoptosis has been shown to occur even in the absence of a cell nucleus or DNA fragmentation (11). DNA fragmentation could be advantageous during apoptosis to minimize the propagation of dangerous nucleic acids, such as viral genomes. Therefore it is plausible that DNA fragmentation is not in itself the "final death blow," although additional studies are needed (since the degradation may be incomplete).

More recent markers of apoptosis are protease cleavage products. The best characterized of these is the enzyme poly ADP ribose polymerase (PARP) (12,13). PARP is an enzyme which is cleaved by cysteine proteases at a specific site in a fashion which is easily detected using antibodies on Western blots. This biochemical feature of apoptosis appears to be fairly universal for mammalian cells, although it is not known whether PARP is an effector of apoptosis or simply a marker of cells undergoing apoptosis. It seems unlikely to be an essential mediator of apoptosis because ADP ribosylation-deficient mice develop essentially normally (14). As more substrates of cysteine proteases are identified, additional such indicators of apoptosis will presumably be measurable.

Apoptosis in Development and Aging

With the recognition that apoptosis is a discrete death process, it has been recognized in the normal development of virtually every organ system in the body. One striking example is the nervous system in which approximately three-fold more neurons exist at birth than in adulthood — approximately two thirds dying probably from apoptosis in response to the presence or absence of specific trophic or toxic cell: cell connections. The immune system is replete with examples of apoptosis. Thymic selection and deletion of T cells, and B cells, all appear to involve the induction of apoptosis. While the specific triggers of apoptosis in each case remain uncertain, one pathway, the Fas pathway, has

been determined to play a major role in the deletion of autoreactive peripheral T cells.

The Fas trigger of apoptosis is a membrane receptor protein with some sequence homology to the tumor necrosis factor (TNF) alpha receptor (15). Both Fas and the TNF alpha receptor are stimulated upon ligand binding to initiate a metabolic cascade which ends in apoptotic death. While the biochemical mechanisms underlying this pathway are incompletely understood, both of these receptors contain a homologous peptide motif within the cytoplasmic tails. This motif has been termed the "death" domain, and biochemical studies are underway to examine the consequences of protein interactions in this region. Subsequent protein phosphorylation is likely to play a role in mediating the signaling pathway which ultimately activates ICE-like proteases and subsequent apoptotic death. Strong evidence that the Fas pathway is involved in deletion of autoreactive T cells was obtained with the recognition that two mouse strains with severe autoimmune pathologies contain mutations in either the Fas receptor or its ligand, which is also a membrane associated protein (15). These two mouse strains, *lpr* and *gld,* are animal models for autoimmune diseases such as Lupus. Other examples of apoptosis in development include hormone dependent tissues such as breast epithelial tissue which undergoes involution following lactation. These and numerous other hormone dependent cell proliferation events have been found to involve apoptosis under the condition of hormone deprivation. It is interesting that hormonal therapies of various malignancies may similarly kill via hormone dependent apoptosis. In fact, given the clinical efficacy of hormonal therapies in cancer (including anti-estrogins, anti-androgens and high dose glucocorticoid therapies), the potency of apoptosis induction as an antineoplastic strategy is quite evident.

Several additional important examples of apoptosis include responses to various environmental insults such as UV irradiation and infection by foreign pathogens. Following UV irradiation, a cell may either undergo cycle arrest and DNA repair or alternatively die. While the factors which determine the decision between these two pathways remain uncertain, this choice between repair versus death is pivotal in both tumorigenesis and cancer therapy (see below). Similarly, in the case of viral infections it is clear that apoptosis is frequently triggered. It is interesting that a number of anti-apoptotic gene products have been isolated from virally infected cell systems. It appears that many viruses express anti-apoptotic genes to prevent the death of their host cells, thereby permitting more efficient viral replication or latency phases. These anti-apoptotic factors such as Crm A from Cow Pox virus, have been highly informative with regard to the biochemical mechanism of apoptosis induction by cysteine proteases (see below).

Genetic Systems in the Study of Apoptosis

The most extensively studied system for the study of apoptotic differentiation involves the nematode C.

elegans. Studies on these primitive worms, pioneered by Horvitz at Massachusetts Institute of Technology, suggested C. elegans was ideal for the study of cell death during development because each cell lineage was mapped in its entirety throughout development (16, 17). During C. elegans hermaphrodite development, 1090 cells are generated, but 131 die by apoptosis. A series of C. Elegans Death genes (CED) have been isolated which influence the efficiency of death in these 131 cells. Two such mutants, CED 3 and CED 4, allow all 131 cells to survive. These mutations imply that the genes themselves are pro-apoptotic. In contrast, an additional gene, CED 9, is anti-apoptotic. CED 9 loss-of-function mutations result in more than 131 cells dying. Gain-of-function produces more than 131 extra living cells. The functions of these various CED genes played a major role in the initial biochemical characterization of apoptosis modulators. While CED 4 lacks any clear sequence homologies, CED 3 was found to represent a homolog of the mammalian enzyme Interleukin 1 beta converting enzyme (ICE), a cysteine protease (18). From this observation has come the further identification of apoptosis-inducing cysteine proteases. The CED 9 gene, an anti-apoptotic factor, was found to share several sequence motifs with the BCl-2 family of oncogenes (19). With the subsequent demonstration that BCl-2 could substitute for CED 9 in CED 9 mutant worms (20), the link had been clearly established between apoptosis during primordial development and the genesis of human malignancy.

A more recently described system amenable to the genetic analysis of apoptosis has been the study of the fruitfly, Drosophila. Several genes have been identified whose loss decreases cell death; that is, excessive cells survive following fly development. Two such genes are *reaper* and *hid* (hid involution defective) (21, 22). The Reaper protein has been proposed to carry a "death domain", homologous to that found in the cytoplasmic tail of the Fas receptor. The hid-triggered apoptosis pathway has been shown to be inhibitable by anti-apoptotic factors which disrupt cysteine proteases, suggesting that common apoptotic mechanisms function through evolution from worms to flies to mammals.

Apoptosis and Tumorigenesis

The first clear connection between human malignancy and modulators of apoptosis came following the identification of the molecular participants in the translocation occurring in follicular lymphoma (23, 24, 25). In this tumor, a translocation occurs between chromosomes 18 and 14 in nearly 100% of cases, and places the BCl-2 gene under the transcriptional regulation of the immunoglobulin heavy chain gene. This constitutive expression appears to contribute critically to establishment of the neoplastic phenotype.

The biological consequences of dysregulated BCl-2 over expression were revealed in studies involving growth factor-dependent hematopoietic cell lines into which the BCl-2 gene had been transfected (26, 27).

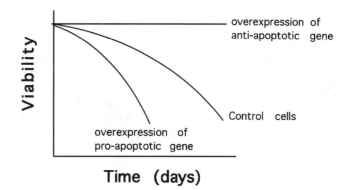

Figure 15.3 Assay to measure the action of apoptosis-regulating genes transfected into target cells. Control cells die with reproducible kinetics upon removal of a critical growth factor. Overexpression of anti-apoptotic genes (such as bcl-2) produces enhanced viability, whereas overexpression of pro-apoptotic genes (such as Bax) accelerate death.

In such cells (see Figure 15.3) the removal of a critical growth factor results in apoptotic death over a defined time course. It was discovered however that stable expression of BCl-2 (by gene transfection) had a profound protective effect against this apoptosis. Importantly, the resulting cells did not grow *faster* than cells in the presence of growth factor. However, when growth factor was removed, the cells continued to survive rather than die with rapid kinetics. These studies suggested that BCl-2 may encode an "immortalization" phenotype and that it may function by antagonizing the apoptotic machinery. Biochemical studies of BCl-2 suggested that it was capable of forming oligomers via several short domains which were highly conserved between species. These domains, called BCl-2 homology domains (BH1 and BH2), appeared to play a central role in the ability to form dimers or higher order protein complexes. With this information in hand, it was of significant interest to search for potential dimerization partners. Using a variety of methodologies including affinity chromatography, co-immunoprecipitation, degenerate PCR, and yeast two hybrid screens, a number of additional Bcl-2 family member proteins have been identified. These additional factors also mostly contain homologous BH 1 and BH2 motifs, and are likely to form protein: protein complexes among each other and/or with BCl-2. In each case, the newly identified BCl-2 family members have been studied in comparable growth factor-dependent cell lines to examine their influences over apoptotic death. Several of these factors have been shown to be protective, similar to BCl-2, while others appear to actually accelerate apoptotic death in response to growth factor deprivation. For example the Bax protein was found to accelerate apoptotic death in this experiment (28). The Bcl-X factor (29) was found to exist in two splice forms. The long form (Bcl-XL) was protective against apoptosis, whereas the short form

(BC1-XS) was pro-apoptotic, similar to Bax. Currently, there are numerous BCl-2 family members including BCl-2, Bcl-X, Bak, Bak2, Bak3, Bax, Bcl-H, and others. One caveat to these studies is that the normal function of these factors remains uncertain. For example, it is imaginable that transfection of any gene into a cell may have either a protective or an exacerbating effect on a measured phenotype, particularly if the phenotype is simply cell survival. Further support for a normal role of bcl-2 family members in regulating apoptosis comes from mice with targeted overexpression or loss-of-function mutations in bcl-2. For example, bcl-2 over-expression targeted to lymphoid cells results in excessive survival of B cells (30) and leads to development of B cells lymphomas (31, 32). In contrast, mice engineered with a "knock-out" of bcl-2 display dramatic lymphocyte apoptosis and cell death in a variety of organ systems, presumably due to altered cell death inhibition (33, 34, 35, 36). Probably the best evidence that these factors truly play a role in the regulation of apoptosis remains the fact that they retain the BCl-2 homology motifs and that BCl-2 itself is overexpressed analogously in follicular lymphoma. It is unclear at this time whether any of the factors other than BCl-2 are genetically aberrant in human malignancies.

Mechanistically, a model has been proposed (37) to explain the BCl-2 family effect on regulation of apoptosis. In this "rheostat model," at one extreme dimers may form between pro apoptotic factors, such as Bax. At the other extreme dimers may form between anti-apoptotic factors, such as BCl-2. In the center, heterodimers may form between these two factors. Thus, depending on the relative abundance of either pro- or anti-apoptotic BCl-2 family members, the net activity may be either protective or permissive of the apoptotic process. Importantly, it remains to be seen whether the function of BCl-2 family members is active or passive in regulating apoptosis. A recently obtained mouse knockout of the Bax gene (38) revealed substantial lymphoid hyperplasia as well as germ cell hypoplasia. This mixed cell proliferation/cell death phenotype thus far suggests a somewhat complex relationship for Bax in regulating apoptosis *in vivo*. Are these factors critical elements within the pathway or are they extraneous factors capable of regulating an existing pathway?

Another important system involving the genetic analysis of apoptosis involves the p53 gene. Humans with the hereditary condition Li-Fraumeni syndrome contain germ line mutation or deletion of one of their two p53 genes (39). These individuals are at very high risk for the development of a variety of malignancies, usually at early age, (childhood or young adulthood). In these cases, it has been observed that the tumors have mutated the remaining wild type allele, thereby explaining the high frequency of malignancy through only a single mutational event rather than inactivation of both alleles. The p53 gene has also been studied within mice. Animals nullizygous for p53 ("knockout") display normal development, but develop tumors in 100 percent of cases within the first year of life (40). These genetic observations clearly implicate p53 as a significant tumor suppressor gene in mouse as well as in man. Additionally, the availability of mice containing the homozygous deletion of the p53 gene has allowed for mechanistic analysis of its role in cancer cell regulation (see below).

Other fascinating examples of genetic systems which demonstrate regulated apoptosis are the mechanisms utilized by viruses to inactivate the apoptotic machinery of host cells. Examples of this include the Adenovirus ElB gene, the human papillomavirus E6 protein, the cowpox virus CrmA protein, and the Baculovirus-encoded gene p35. In each of these cases, genes have been identified which functionally disable the apoptosis pathway presumably to perpetuate a more efficient viral life cycle within the infected cell. The fact that several of these apoptosis inhibitors utilize common intracellular targets suggests the importance of those targets in the normal apoptosis pathway (see below).

Piecing Together the Apoptosis Pathway

The biochemical pathway which has emerged to result in apoptosis can be described schematically as depicted in Figure 15.1. Apoptosis is initiated by a specific trigger. As described below, an apoptotic trigger can be either extracellular (from the environment such as through radiation or drug exposures) or intracellular (as with dysregulated oncogene expression). Subsequent to triggering apoptosis, a series of events occur which probably differ for each specific trigger. For example, in the case of Fas dependent apoptosis, the subsequent events likely involve a signaling cascade which initiates at the cytoplasmic tail of the Fas receptor and may involve phosphorylation events and other second messengers. In other cases, the subsequent biochemistry of triggering remains unknown. It is likely that various regulators of apoptosis, such as the BCl-2 family of factors, modify the biochemical cascade which bridges the trigger with the later effector stages of the pathway. Based on studies using the CED-3 gene from C. elegans (18) it has emerged that cysteine proteases are potent effectors of apoptosis. A mammalian homologue of CED-3, Interleukin 1-beta Converting Enzyme (ICE), is a protease which utilizes cysteine at its active site, shares sequence homology with CED-3, and is capable of inducing apoptosis when overexpressed in a cell (41). Subsequently it has been shown that other related cysteine proteases are also able to induce apoptosis, presumably through their proteolytic enzymatic activity (41, 42, 43, 44). A number of anti-apoptotic factors derived from viruses have recently been shown to function through the competitive inhibition of cellular cysteine proteases (41, 45, 46, 47, 48, 49). For example, the baculovirus protein p35 has been shown to block apoptosis and compete with intracellular substrates of cysteine proteases (49), thereby effectively inhibiting these enzymes.

If cysteine proteases are major enzymatic effectors of apoptosis, the identity of their substrates will be important in understanding the death pathway. In addition to ICE, other cysteine proteases have been shown to be capable of cleaving certain substrates which are associated with the presence of apoptosis in a cell population. For example the enzyme CPP32 (also called YAMA or Apopain, (6, 48)) has been shown to be capable of specific cleavage of the substrate poly-ADP-ribose-polymerase (PARP). PARP is cleaved at a specific site in apoptotic cells (12) and the identity of its cleavage enzyme may be important in unraveling its role in apoptosis. At this time however, it is uncertain whether PARP cleavage represents a causative event in the apoptosis pathway or represents a marker for apoptosis.

Chemotherapy and the Induction of Apoptosis

One of the most important medical implications of apoptotic death is its role in the therapy of human malignancy. It has been recognized for a number of years (3) that tumor samples either following treatment or even without treatment may contain significant numbers of morphologically apoptotic cells. Moreover, it has been increasingly clear that the presence of certain molecular genetic aberrations may correlate with poor prognosis in a fashion which could reflect the "disabling" of an apoptotic pathway. Perhaps the most striking such molecular association has been made with the p53 tumor suppresser gene.

P53 was originally identified as a protein which co-immunoprecipitated with the T antigen oncoprotein in SV40-transformed cells (50, 51). Its function as a tumor suppresser gene became clear with the observation that mutations or deletions in p53 are probably the most common genetic alteration in human cancer (52). In addition, germ line mutations in p53 have been identified in the familial cancer predisposition syndrome Li-Fraumeni Syndrome (39). While affected individuals carry constitutive mutations in one p53 allele, their tumors display aberrations in both alleles.

A molecular connection between p53 and apoptosis was made in 1991 (44) with the observation that over expression of p53 induced massive apoptosis in a myeloid leukemia cell line. Subsequently it was demonstrated that radiation-induced apoptosis of thymocytes was dependent upon the presence of p53 and did not occur in mice "knocked out" for the p53 gene (53, 54).

P53's normal functions have suggested certain tumor-specific activities. A series of studies on cell cycle regulation (55, 56, 57) suggested that p53 regulates entry of cells into S phase in response to DNA damage such as irradiation. Since p53 is a DNA binding transcription factor (58, 59), it was assumed that this cell cycle regulation may involve the transcription of specific target genes. One such gene, p21, was shown to be transcriptionally regulated by p53 and capable of impeding entry into S phase through the ability to bind and inactivate cyclin dependent kinases (60, 61, 62). A "knockout" of p21 has recently been achieved in the mouse, and demonstrates partial loss of the p53-dependent G1/S checkpoint (63). However, a partial

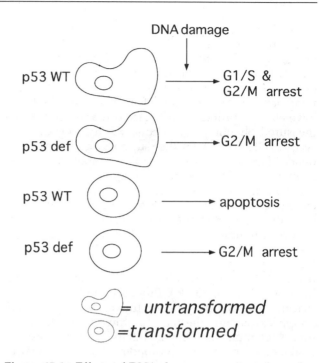

Figure 15.4 Effects of DNA damage on untransformed cells (top two) and ocogenically transformed cells (lower two). Low doses of irradiation induce 2 checkpoints in normal cells: one a G1/S and one at G2/M. P53 deficient cells selectively lose the GI/S checkpoint, but do not necessarily enter apoptosis from low doses of radiation, whereas p53 deficient transformed cells remain radioresistant to apoptosis induction.

checkpoint still remains, suggesting that p21 may only be modulating a portion of p53's cell cycle activity. Furthermore, thymic irradiation in these mice produces apoptosis, suggesting that this p53 dependent apoptosis does not require p21. The suggestion that p53 may not produce apoptosis via its transcriptional activity has been previously made, based on studies demonstrating that p53-dependent apoptosis could occur in the presence of high doses of actinomycin D, where gene transcription was non-specifically inhibited (4, 5). Since radiation causes p53 to alter the cell cycle (in normal cells), it was of interest to examine whether p53's ability to induce *apoptosis* would also respond to this trigger, particularly within oncogenically transformed cells.

Utilizing fibroblast cells derived from either wild type or p53 knockout mice, Lowe *et al.* (65) generated oncogene transformed cells which were genetically matched except for the presence or absence of wild type p53. Using these cells, the authors demonstrated that whereas untransformed fibroblasts would arrest growth in response to DNA damaging radiation or drugs, transformed, p53 wild type cells would enter apoptosis (65). This observation suggested a mechanism by which a therapeutic window could be achieved during anti-cancer therapy (64). If a drug produced apoptosis in transformed cells, but cell cycle arrest in normal cells, it would display tumor-specific toxicity via apoptosis (see Figure 15.4). Note that the normal response to DNA damage is cycle arrest at both a G1/S checkpoint as well as a G2/M checkpoint. The selective loss of a G1/S checkpoint which accompanies p53 deficiency renders the cell sensitive to the accelerated accumulation of DNA errors just prior to genome replication. The additional key observation by Lowe and colleagues was that lack of p53 in matched transformed cells was associated with resistance to the induction of apoptosis by the identical anticancer treatments (65). This cell system was then studied in a solid tumor nude mouse model (66) and demonstrated that solid tumors containing p53 were highly — radiation and drug — sensitive while those lacking p53 were resistant. Moreover, in p53 wild type tumors treated repetitively with radiation, but ultimately achieving radioresistance, acquired p53 mutations could be identified (66). Thus, apoptosis was suggested to play a major role in determining the efficacy of anticancer therapies, and p53 emerged as a major regulator of this therapy-induced apoptotic response.

In the field of radiation oncology, it was long recognized that one means by which a tumor cell could become radioresistant could be through an enhanced ability to repair DNA damage. Recent results with p53 and its modulation of apoptosis have suggested an alternative model (64) in which an important determinant of radiation resistance is the ability to trigger apoptotic rather than non-apoptotic cell death. This suggestion has sparked significant interest in understanding the biochemical mechanisms by which p53 triggers apoptosis, with the hope of exploiting this pathway in the induction of apoptotic death by better anticancer agents.

The specific chemotherapy families which have been suggested to induce apoptotic death in a p53-dependent fashion include antimetabolites, alkylaters, anthracyclines, topoisomerase inhibitors, and a continuously growing list of other factors. One important question will be to determine whether agents exist which induce apoptosis independently of the presence or absence of wild type p53. Specifically, it would be of interest to know whether non-DNA damaging agents such as microtubule targeted drugs produce toxicity which is p53 dependent as well. Furthermore, it will be important to determine whether mechanisms exist to restore wild type p53 activity to cells harboring p53 mutations. Attempts to achieve this result could involve use of viral vectors (67, 68, 69), although delivery of such vectors to all tumor cells is a potential problem. The attractiveness of p53 and its regulation of apoptotic death involves its tumor cell selectivity. P53 deficient mice display no developmental abnormalities (70) with the exception that malignancies develop within the first year of life. P53's activity thus appears to be tumor cell specific and is likely to involve carefully regulated expression of the protein. A better understanding of its normal biochemical activities may provide important clues to restoring its apoptotic pathway in human tumor cells.

Another important anticancer strategy will be the identification of agents capable of inducing tumor-selective, p53-independent apoptosis. With the availability of genetically defined mice and cells, reagents should allow for the identification of such drugs if the appropriate pathways exist within a p53-deficient cell. Among the potentially interesting targets along these lines, are radiation sensitisors which have been suggested to enhance apoptotic death under conditions where radiation is ineffective.

Other apoptosis-modulating factors also represent potential drug targets for anticancer therapy. For example, inhibition of BCl-2 activity could substantially lower the threshold for the induction of apoptosis. A variety of studies have demonstrated that over expression of BCl-2 may render a cell relatively drug resistant (71). Thus, inhibition of endogenous BCl-2 may be therapeutically advantageous. It must be noted, however, that such BCl-2 inhibition may have more systemic effects as well, since the BCl-2 knockout mouse demonstrates increased apoptotic death in a wide variety of organ systems (36). Perhaps other BCl-2 family members will be found to display tissue-type specificity, and perhaps tumor cell specificity.

Finally, the tumor selective induction of apoptosis which occurs in cells transformed by dominant oncogenes such as Myc (72), suggests that dominant oncogene activity sensitizes a cell to the induction of apoptosis. While loss of other apoptosis modulators may neutralize this sensitization, a better biochemical understanding of these events may allow for enhanced targeting of these tumor-specific pathway. For example, Myc over expression (which occurs in a significant fraction of human tumors) triggers apoptosis in cells which are deprived of certain critical growth factors. These growth factors have been identified using defined growth conditions (73), and thereby demonstrate a connection between extracellular growth factor availability and nuclear oncogene activity. The accessibility of growth factor receptors on the plasma membrane coupled to a better understanding of how its signaling may clash with Myc over expression (to produce apoptosis) provides a new opportunity to potentially trigger oncogene-selective apoptosis from the cell surface. Similarly adhesion dependent apoptosis (74) as well as Fas and TNF receptors may offer extracellular targets for apoptosis isolation in tumor cells. Tumor cell-selective toxicity will, however, have to be established to be therapeutically useful.

Future Prospects

A considerable body of knowledge has accumulated regarding some of the key mechanistic steps in the induction of apoptosis. Much of this information has been derived from studies of primitive organisms, but is exciting because of the apparent biochemical parallels in mammalian and human systems. Enhanced capabilities at blocking apoptosis, for example with inhibitors to cystine proteases, may hold promise for diseases of excessive cell death, such as neurodegenerative, rheumatologic, or other inflammatory conditions. The recognition that apoptotic death occurs in human cancer therapy has suggested important mechanisms for anticancer therapy success as well as failure. Critical regulators of apoptosis induction by chemotherapeutics have been successfully correlated with prognosis in a large number of human malignancies. An important implication of these observations is that chemotherapeutic agents may produce tumor cell death not by "strangulating" the cell through extreme disruption of metabolism but may neatly induce a cell to commit suicide through the induction of apoptosis. With this understanding, coupled to an increased understanding of the biochemistry of apoptosis, it appears likely that future generations of cancer therapeutics will focus on manipulating the apoptotic pathway. Many important questions remain, particularly with regard to the cancer cell-specific apoptosis pathway. However the efficiency of apoptotic death once it has been triggered and the clinical evidence that such death is prognostically important in human cancer suggest that apoptosis-directed therapies may offer significant promise in the future.

References

1. Kerr JFR, Wyllie AH, Currie AR. Apoptosis: A basic biological phenomenon with wide-ranging implications in tissue kinetics. *Br J Cancer* 1972; **26**: 239–257.
2. Raff MC. Social controls on cell survival and cell death. [Review]. *Nature* (London) 1992; **356**: 397–400.
3. Wyllie AH, Kerr JF, Currie AR. Cell death: The significance of apoptosis. *Int Rev Cytol* 1980; **68**: 251–306.
4. Caelles C, Helmberg A, Karin M. p53-dependent apoptosis in the absence of transcriptional activation of p53-target genes. *Nature* 1994; **370**: 220–223.
5. Wagner AJ, Kokontis JM, Hay N. Myc-mediated apoptosis required wild-type p53 in a manner independent of cell cycle arrest and the ability of p53 to induce *p21wafl/cip*. *Genes and Dev* 1994; **8**: 2817–2830.
6. Nicholson DW, Ali A, Thornberry NA, Vaillancourt JP, Ding CK, Gallant M, Gareau Y, Griffin PR, Labelle M, Lazebnik YA, Munday NA, Raju SM, Smulson ME, Yamin TT, Yu VL, Miller DK. Identification and inhibition of the ICE/CED-3 protease necessary for mammalian apoptosis. *Nature* 1995; **376**: 37–43.
7. Tewari M, Dixit VM. Fas- and TNF-induced apoptosis is inhibited by the poxvirus *crmA* gene product. *J Biol Chem* 1995; **270**: 3255–3260.
8. Gavrieli Y, Sherman Y, Ben-Sassoon A. Identification of programmed cell death *in situ* via specific labeling of nuclear DNA fragmentation. *J Cell Biol* 1992; **119**: 493–501.
9. Ellis RE, Jacobson DM, Horvitz HR. Genes required for the engulfment of cell corpses during programmed cell death in Caenorhabdtitis elegans. *Genetics* 1991; **129**: 79–94.
10. Hevelone J, Hartman PS. An endonuclease from Caenorhabditis elegans: partial purification and characterization. *Biochemical Genetics* 1988; **26**: 447–461.
11. Schulze-Osthoff K, Walczak H, Droge W, Krammer PH. Cell nucleus and DNA fragmentation are not required for apoptosis. *J Cell Biol* 1994; **127**: 15–20.
12. Lazebnik YA, Kaufmann SH, Desnoyers S, Poirier GG, Earnshaw WC. Cleavage of poly(ADP-ribose) polymerase by a proteinase with properties lice ICE. *Nature* 1994; **371**: 346–347.
13. Oberhammer FA, Hochegger K, Froschl G, Tiefenbacher R, Pavelka M. Chromatin condensation during apoptosis is accompanied by degradation of lamin A + B, without enhanced activation of cdc2 kinase. *J Cell Biol* 1994; **126**: 827–837.
14. Wang ZQ, Auer B, Stingl L, Gerghammer H, Haidacher D, Schweitger M, Wagner EF. Mice lacking ADPRT and poly (ADP-ribosyl)ation develop normally but are susceptible to skin disease. *Genes and Dev* 1995; **9**: 509–520.
15. Nagata S, Golstein P. The Fas death factor. *Science* 1995; **267**: 1499–56.
16. Hengartner MO, Horvitz HR. Programmed cell death in Caenorhabditis elegans. [Review]. *Curr Opin Gen & Dev* 1994; **4**: 581–586.
17. Horvitz HR, Shaham S, Hengartner MO. The genetics of programmed cell death in the nematode Caenorhabditis elegans. [Review]. Cold Spring Harbor Sym. on Quan. *Biol* 1994; **59**: 377–385.
18. Yuan J, Shaham S, Ledoux S, Ellis MH, Horvitz. The C. elegans cell death gene ced-3 encodes a protein similar to mammalian interleukin-1 β-converting enzyme. *Cell* 1993; **75**: 641–652.
19. Hengartner MO, Horvitz HR. C. *elegans* cell survival gene ced-9 encodes a functional homolog of the mammalian proto-oncogene BCl-2. *Cell* 1994; **76**: 665–676.
20. Hengartner MO, Ellis RE, Hovitz HR. Caenorhahditis elegans gene ced-9 protects cells from programmed cell death. *Nature* 1992; **356**: 494–499.
21. Golstein P, Marguet D, Depraetere V. Homology between Reaper and the cell death domains of Fas and TNFR1. *Cell* 1995; **81**: 185–186.
22. Grether ME, Abrams JM, Agapite J, White K, Steller H. The head involution defective gene of Drospophila melanogaster functions in programmed cell death. *Genes and Dev* 1995; **9**: 1694–1708.
23. Bakhshi A, Jensen JP, Goldman P, Wright JJ, McBride OW, Epstein AL, Korsmeyer SJ. Cloning the chromosomal breakpoint of the t(14:18) human lymphomas: Cloustering around JH on chromosome 14 and near a transcriptional unit on 18. *Cell* 1985; **41**: 889–906.
24. Cleary ML, SDS, Sklar J. Cloning and structural analysis of cDNAs for BCl-2 and a hybrid bcl-2/immunoglobulin transcript resulting from the t(14: 18) translocation. *Cell* 1986; **47**: 19–28.
25. Tsujimoto Y, Gorham J, Cossman J, Jaffe E, Croce CM. The t(14;18) chromosome translocations involved in B cell neoplasms result from mistakes in VDJ joining. *Science* 1985; **229**: 1390–1393.
26. Hockenbery D, Nunez G, Milliman C, Schreiber RD, Korsmeyer S. BCl-2 is an inner mitochondrial membrane protein that blocks programmed cell death. *Nature* 1990; **348**: 334–336.
27. Vaux DL, Cory S, Adams TM. BCl-2 promotes the survival of haemopoietic cells and cooperates with *c-myc* to immortalize pre-B cells. *Nature* 1988; **335**: 440–442.
28. Oltvai ZN, Millman CL, Korsmeyer SJ. BCl-2 heterodimerizes *in vivo* with a conserved homolog, Bax, that accelerates programmed cell death. *Cell* 1993; **74**: 609–619.
29. Boise LH, Gonzalez-Garcia M, Postema CE, Ding L, Lindsten T, Turka LA, Mao X, Nunez G, Thompson C. bcl-x, a BCl-2 related gene that functions as a dominant regulator of apoptotic death. *Cell* 1993; **74**: 597–608.
30. Nunez G, Hockenbery D, McDonnell TJ, Sorensen C M, Korsmeyer SJ. Bcl 2 maintains B cell memory. *Nature* 1991; **353**: 71–73.
31. McDonnell TJ, Deane N, Platt FM, Nunez G, Jaeger U, McKearn JP, Korsmeyer SJ. bcl-2-immunoglobulin transgenic mice demonstrate extended B cell survival and follicular lumphoproliferation. *Cell* 1989; **57**: 79–88.
32. McDonnell TJ, Korsmeyer SJ. Progression from lymphoid hyperplasia to high grade malignant lymphoma in mice transgenic for the t (14: 18). *Nature* 1991; **349**: 254–256.
33. Kamada S, Shinto AA, Tsujimura Y, Takahashi T, Noda T, Kitamura Y, Kondoh H, Tsujimoto Y. BCl-2 deficiency in mice leads to pleiotropic abnormalities. Accelerated lymphoid cell death in the thymus and spleen, polycystic kidney, hair hypopigmentation, and distorted small intestine. *Cancer Rsch* 1995; **55**: 354–359.
34. Nakayama K, Nakayama K, Negishi I, Kuida K, Sawa H, Loh DY. Targeted disruption of BCl-2 alpha beta in mice-occurrence of grey hair, polycystic kidney disease, and lymphocytopenia. *Proc Natl Acad Sci* 1994; **91**: 3700–3704.
35. Nakayama KE, Nakayama K, Negishi I, Kuida K, Shinkai Y, Louie MC, Fields LE, Lucas PJ, Stewart V, Alt FW, Loh DY. Disappearance of the lymphoid system in BCl-2 homozygous mutant chimeric mice. *Science* 1993; **261**: 1584–1588.

36. Veis DJ, Sorenson CM, Shutter JR, Korsmeyer SJ. BCl-2 deficient mice demonstrate fulminant lymphoid apoptosis, polycyctic kidneys, and hypopigmented hair. *Cell* 1993; **75**: 229–240.

37. Korsmeyer SJ, Shutter JR, Veis DJ, DEM, Oltvai ZN. Bcl-2/Bax: a rheostat that regulates an anti-oxidant pathway and cell death. *Sem in Cancer Biol* 1993; **4**: 327–332.

38. Knudson CM, Tung K, Brown G, Korsmeyer SJ. Bax deficient mice demonstrate lymphoid hyperplasia but male germ cell death. *Science* 1995; **270**: 96–99.

39. Malkin D, Li FP, Strong LC, Fraumeni JF, Nelson CE, Kim DH, Kassel J, Gryka MA, Bischoff FZ, Tainsky MA, SH F. Germline p53 mutations in a familial syndrome of breast cancer, sarcomas, and other neoplasms. *Science* (Washington DC) 1990; **250**: 1233 1238.

40. Shimamura A, Fisher DE. p53 in life and death. *Clin Cancer Rsch* 1996; **2**: 435–440.

41. Miura M, Zhu H, Rotello R, Hartwieg EA, Yuan J. Induction of apoptosis in fibroblasts by IL-1,B-converting enzyme, a mammalian homolog of the C. *elegans* cell death gene *ced-3*. *Cell* 1993; **75**: 653–660.

42. Munday NA, Vaillancourt JP, Ali A, Casano FJ, Miller DK, Molineaux SM, Yamin TT, Yu VL, Nicholson DW. Molecular cloning and pro-apoptoic activity of ICErel-II and ICErel-IKII, members of the ICE/CED-3 family of cysteine precesses. *J Biol Chem* 1995; **270**, 15870–15876.

43. Wang L, Miura M, Gergeron L, Zhu H, Yuan J. *Ich-l* an ICE/ *ced-3-related* gene, encodes both positive and negative regulators of programmed cell death. *Cell* 1994; **78**: 739–750.

44. Yonish-Rouach E, Resnitzky D, Lotem J, Sachs L, Kimchi A, Oren M. Wild type p53 induces apoptosis of myeloid leukaemic cells that is inhibited by interleukin-6. *Nature* 1991; **352**: 345–347.

45. Komiyama T, Ray CA, Pickup DJ, Howard AD, Thornberry NA, Peterson EP, Salvesen G. Inhibition of interleukin-1~ converting enzyme by the cowpox virus serpin CrmA. *J Biol Chem* 1994; **269**: 19331–19337.

46. Ray CA, Black RA, Kronheim SR, Greenstreet TA, Sleath PR, Salvesen GS, Pickup DJ. Viral inhibition of inflammation: Cowpox virus encodes an inhibitor of the interleukin-l,B converting enzyme. *Cell* 1992; **69**: 597–604.

47. Sugimoto AP, Friesen PD, Rothman JH. Baculovirus *p35* prevents developmentally programmed cell death and rescues a *ced-9* mutant in the nematode *Caenorabditis elegans*. *EMBO J* 1994; **13**: 2023–2028.

48. Tewari M, Quan LT, O'Rourke K, Desnoyers S, Zeng Z, Beidler DR, Poirier G, Salvesen GS, Dixit VM. Yama/CPP32~, a mammalian homolog of CED-3, is a CrmA-inhibitable protease that cleaves the death substrate poly(ADP-ribose) polymerase. *Cell* 1995; **81**: 801–809.

49. Xue D, Horvitz HR. Inhibition of the *Caenorhabditis elegans* cell-death protease CED-3 by a CED-3 ceavage site in baculovirus p35 protein. *Nature* 1995; **377**: 248–251.

50. Lane DP, Crawford LV. T antigen is bound to a host protein in SV40 transformed cells. *Nature* (Lond.) 1979; **278**: 261–263.

51. Linzer DI, Levine AJ. Characterization of a 54K dalton cellular SV40 tumor antigen present in SV40-transformed cells and uninfected embryonal carcinoma cells. *Cell* 1979; **17**: 43–52.

52. Harris CC, Hollstein M. Clinical implications of the p53 tumor-suppressor gene. *NEJ of Med* 1993; **329**: 1318–1327.

53. Clarke AR, Purdie CA, Harrison DJ, Morris RG, Bird CC, Hooper ML, Wyllie AH. Thymocyte apoptosis induced by p53-dependent and independent pathways. *Nature* 1993; **362**: 849–852.

54. Lowe SW, Schmitt EM, Smith SW, Osborne BA, Jacks T. p53 is required for radiation-induced apoptosis in mouse thymocytes. *Nature* 1993; **362**: 847–849.

55. Kastan MB, Onyekwere O, Sidransky D, Vogelstein B, Craig RW. Participation of p53 protein in the cellular response to DNA damage. *Cancer Res* 1991; **51**: 6304–6311.

56. Kastan MB, Zhan Q, El-Deiry WS, Carrier F, Jacks T, Walsh WV, Plunkett BS, Vogelstein B, Fomace AJ. A mammalian cell cycle checkpoint pathway utilizing p53 and GADD45 is defective in ataxia-telangiectasia. *Cell* 1992; **71**: 587–597.

57. Kuerbitz S, Plunkett B, Walsh W, Kastan M. Wildtype p53 is a cell cycle checkpoint determinant following irradiation. *Proc Natl Acad Sci USA* 1992; **89**: 7491–7495.

58. Kern SE, Pietenpol JA, Thiagalingam S, Seymour A, Kinzler KW, Vogelstein B. Oncogenic forms of p53 inhibit p53-regulated gene expression. *Science* (Washington DC) 1992; **256**: 827–830.

59. Vogelstein B, Kinzler KW. p53 function and dysfunction. *Cell* 1992; **70**: 523–526.

60. El-Deiry WS, Tokino T, Velculescu VE, Levy DB, Parsons R, Trent JM, Lin D, Mercer WE, Kinzler KW, Vogelstein B. *WAF1*, a potential mediator of p53 tumor suppression. *Cell* 1993; **75**: 817–825.

61. Harper JW, Adami GR, Wei N, Keyomarsi K, Elledge SJ. The p21 Cdk interacting protein Cipl is a potent inhibitor of G1 cyclin-dependent kinases. *Cell* 1993; **75**: 805–816.

62. Xiong Y, Hannon GJ, Zhang H, Casso D, Kobayashi R, Beach D. p21 is a universal inhibitor of cyclin kinases. *Nature* (Lond.) 1993; **366**: 701–704.

63. Deng C, Zhang P, Harper WJ, Elledge SJ, Leder P. Mice lacking p21 $^{CIP1/WAF1}$ undergo normal development, but are defective in G1 checkpoint control. *Cell* 1995; **82**: 675–684.

64. Fisher DE. Apoptosis in cancer therapy: crossing the threshold. *Cell* 1994; **78**: 539–542.

65. Lowe SW, Ruley HE, Jacks T, Houseman DE. p53-dependent apoptosis modulates the cytotoxicity of anti-cancer agents. *Cell* 1993; **74**: 957–967.

66. Lowe LW, Bodis B, McCarthy A, Remington LH, Ruley E, Fisher D, Houseman DE, Jacks T. p53 can determine the efficacy of cancer therapy *in vitro*. *Science* (Washington DC) 1994; **266**: 807–810.

67. Asai A, Miyagi Y, Sugiyama A, Gamanuma M, Hong SH, Takamoto S, Nomura K, Matsutani M, Takakura K, Kuchino Y. Negative effects of wild-type p53 and s-Myc on cellular growth and tumorigenicity of glioma cells. Implication of the tumor suppressor genes for gene therapy. *J of Neuro-Oncol* 1994; **19**: 259–268.

68. Runnebaum IB, Kreienberg R. p53 trans-dominantly suppresses tumor formation of human breast cancer cells mediated by retroviral bulk infection with marker gene selection: an expeditious *in vitro* protocol with implications towards gene therapy. *Hybridoma* 1995; **14**: 153–157.

69. Zhang WW, Fang X, Mazur W, French BA, Georges RN, Roth JA. High efficiency gene transfer and high-level expression of wild-type p53 in human lung cancer cells mediated by recombinant adenovirus. *Cancer Gene Therapy* 1994; **1**: 5–13.

70. Donehower LA, Harvey M, Slagle BL, McArthur MJ, Montgomery CA, Butel JS, Bradley A. Mice deficient for p53 are developmentally normal but susceptible to spontaneous tumors. *Nature* 1992; **356**: 215–221.

71. Reed JC. BCl-2 family proteins: regulators of chemoresistance in cancer. *Toxicology Letters* 1995; **82–83**: 155–158.

72. Evan GI, Wyllie AH, Gilbert CS, Littlewood TD, Land H, Brooks M, Waters CM, Pen LZ, Hancock DC. Induction of apoptosis in fibroblasts by c-myc protein. *Cell* 1992; **69**: 119–128.

73. Harrington EA, Bennett MR, Fanidi A, Evan GI. c-Myc-induced apoptosis in fibroblasts is inhibited by specific cytokines. *EMBO J* 1994; **13**: 3286–3295.

74. Ruoslahti E, Reed JC. Anchorage dependence, integrins, and apoptosis. *Cell* 1994; **77**: 477–478.

16. Physiology of Aging: Relevance to Symptoms, Perceptions and Treatment Tolerance

Edmund H. Duthie, Jr.

Introduction

Aging is associated with anatomic and structural changes which have implications for physiologic function. Clinicians need to be aware of the physiologic changes that occur in association with the aging process. Since disease occurrence is so ubiquitous in late life, physiologic changes may be the result of disease (pathophysiology) and this can further confound the care of the elderly patient.

When reviewing the topic of aging physiology a few principles need to be kept in mind. First, most physiologic processes change gradually over time. Figure 16.1 is a classic depiction of physiologic decrement over time in groups of subjects (1). Decline in physiologic function can be shown to begin in early adulthood and gradually progress into the middle years and beyond. It is also noteworthy that for some of the measures shown in Figure 16.1 that reevaluation of physiologic function in more recent years, using stricter criteria for heath, can sometimes show that previously described

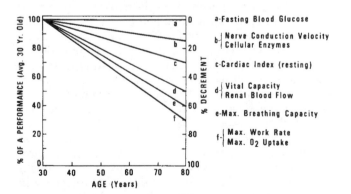

AGE DECREMENTS IN PHYSIOLOGICAL PERFORMANCE

Figure 16.1 Age decrements in physiological performance. Average values for 30-year-old subjects taken as 100%. Decrements shown are schematic. (a) Fasting blood glucose, (b) Nerve conduction velocity and some cellular enzyme activities, (c) Resting cardiac index, (d) Vital capacity and renal blood flow, (e) Maximum breathing capacity, (f) Maximum work rate and maximum oxygen uptake (ref. 1).

decrements are no longer found. The decline in cardiac output with age may be a case in point. Early reports noted a decline in cardiac output (2), but later studies (3,4) have not verified this result. Subjects with occult nondetectable heart disease could account for the earlier findings.

Another important point about aging physiology is the variability of measures. In older subjects, it appears that a wide range for the variable being measured will be found compared to younger subjects. As a corollary, though the mean value of a measure may decline, among individual subjects the value may decline, remain static, or even increase over time. This has been shown most impressively for changes in creatinine clearance (5). Lipsitz and Goldberger have expanded further on the analysis of physiologic changes in senescence to point out that even beyond genetic background, diet, and activity there are factors at work which mitigate toward variability in physiologic function in later life (6). Also, key to aging appears to be the reduced capacity to adapt to stress. Therefore, measurements of a variable at rest (e.g. heart rate or serum glucose) may not show much difference among subjects of varying ages, but with stress (exercise or glucose infusion) impressive differences can be noted to occur. This has led to the suggestion that with age, there is a loss of complexity among organ system functions leading to an impairment in the ability of the organism to adapt to stress.

This chapter will review physiologic changes occurring in later life and highlight the relevance these changes have for oncologic practice. The approach will be to follow the order of the usual physical examination and comment upon changes in the systems as they are examined. Some changes (e.g. eyesight/hearing) will be commented upon under neurosensory changes rather than during the "head and neck" examination. Some areas of physiologic change (e.g. immunology or hematopoietic system) will not be addressed in this section, since they are covered elsewhere in this text.

Body Composition and Aging

At the beginning of the clinical encounter the clinician will obtain a height, weight and inspect the body habitus of the patient. Serial measurements of weight

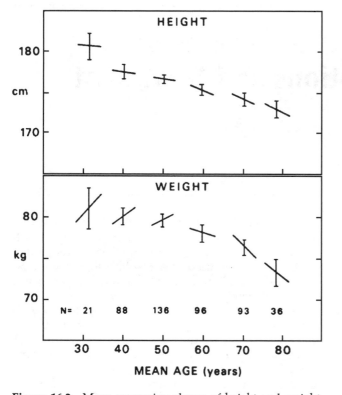

Figure 16.2 Mean regression slopes of height and weight on age determined from serial measurements on the same subjects (normal males) over a period of 8 years. The vertical line represents ±1 standard deviation of the mean value (ref. 1).

are particularly important in oncologic practice. Both cross sectional (point in time assessment of subjects of varying ages) and longitudinal analyses (serial measurement of the same subject over time) show changes in height and weight with age (Figure 16.2) (1). Loss of height is likely related to changes in the intervertebral disc. Buckwalter, *et al.* note that "no musculoskeletal tissue undergoes more dramatic age-related changes than the intervertebral disc" (7). Table 16.1 lists the changes that are seen in aged subjects and which contribute to height loss with age. From age 20 to late life a man may loose 4.0 centimeters of height and a woman 6.8 centimeters (8). Calculations for body surface area should rely on measured height since older patients may not be aware of height loss and will report heights that are erroneous, based upon what patients recall their height to be when younger.

Table 16.1 Intervertebral disc changes with age.

Fissure and cracking of disc

Decrease in proteoglycans and water concentration

Increase in non-collagenous protein concentration

Loss of viable cells in-central regions

Decrease in number of arteries supplying the disc region

Excessive loss of height in late life may be the result of osteoporosis with compression of vertebral bone causing pathologic height loss.

In regard to body weight, Figure 16.2 does demonstrate a weight plateau through mid adult life with a gradual decline in weight in the later decades (age 70 and beyond). Associated with this weight change are important changes in body composition. With age there appears to be a decline in the percent of body mass that is lean mass (9,10). Body water seems to remain constant or decline slightly with age, and there is a shift of water from intra to extracellular space. Body fat mass and percent body weight that is composed of fat increase through adulthood into senescence. Studies using CT scanning suggest that fat is "internalized" in older persons, i.e., it is not subcutaneous in the extremities but rather is intra-abdominal and infiltrated within and between muscles (11). Mechanisms to explain these changes have included diet, sedentary life styles, and hormonal changes. For example, exercise programs have been shown to increase muscle mass even in frail older nursing home residents (12). Growth hormone replacement in growth hormone deficient older subjects has resulted in some loss of fat and gain in lean mass (13). This suggests age related changes in body composition may be due to loss of growth hormone with advancing age in some people.

No matter what the precise mechanism for changes in body composition with advancing age, the implications for clinical practice are important. For example, lipid soluble drugs will have a greater volume of distribution and altered pharmacokinetics just as water soluble agents will have a smaller volume of distribution, higher concentration for a given drug dose and changed pharmacokinetics.

Vital Signs and Autonomic Function

Histologic studies of the myocardium show that there is a decrement of pacemaker cells in older subjects and connective tissue infiltration in the area of the SA node (14). Likewise, a loss of Purkinje fibers is seen in the bundle of HIS (14). These anatomic changes do not seem to produce major changes in resting heart rate. Data are conflicting whether resting heart rate remains constant or declines with aging (15). From the clinical perspective, even if heart rate does decline with age, the decline is modest. Detection of bradycardia, particularly symptomatic bradycardia should not be attributed to aging, but rather cardiac disease. Respiratory variation of heart rate and spontaneous variations in heart rate over a 24 hour period are diminished with aging. Even more impressive is the reduction of heart rate in response to catecholamine stimulation or exercise as subjects age (Figure 16.3) (16). The reduction of maximal heart rate with aging is not due to a decline of circulating catecholamines or excessive vagal tone. Rather, there appears to be severe blunting of beta adrenergic receptor response in healthy older individuals (17). The oncologist caring for the geriatric patient may find, therefore, that stress or fear will not

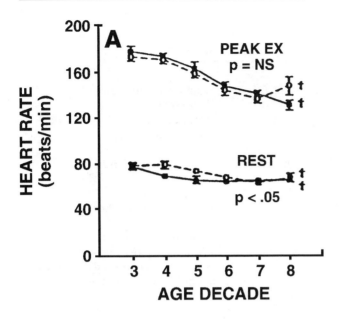

Figure 16.3 Heart rate plotted by age decade at rest and at peak exercise (Peak ex) in males (■) and females (□). † Significant age regressions within gender at rest or peak effort. P values indicate gender differences by analysis of variances (ref. 16).

produce the same degree of pulse elevation among older patients as occurs in younger patients.

Blood pressure is known to change with aging. Arteriosclerosis is the age related change in the arterial blood vessels. In the aorta and other large vessels, elastic fibers are fractured and unrolled with aging. Simultaneously, calcium is deposited along with collagenous matrix (18). These changes cause vessels to become "stiff." As a result the arterial pulse is forceful in the geriatric patient. This can be true even in conditions where one might expect a reduction of pulse amplitude such as significant aortic stenosis. Smaller arteries and arterioles demonstrate hyaline degeneration within the media and a decrease in the lumen to wall ratio and overall cross-sectional area of the lumen with aging (18). The effect of these changes is to produce an increase in systemic vascular resistance with

Table 16.2 Determinants of blood pressure and changes with aging.

Factor	age related change
Peripheral vascular resistance	increased
Plasma catecholamines	no change/increased
Alpha receptor response	no change
Beta receptor response	decreased
Baroreceptor response	decreased
Plasma renin	decreased
Sodium excretion	decreased/decreased

aging. Table 16.2 outlines the various influences on blood pressure and changes seen with aging. When populations are studied to examine the changes in blood pressure with age, it appears that systolic pressure steadily rises throughout adult life, while the diastolic pressure reaches a mid life plateau. Interestingly, these changes have not been documented in all human populations, but seem to be true for Western Europe, North America and other industrialized nations. In later life, blood pressure elevation continues to be a risk factor for cardiovascular morbidity and mortality.

One troublesome area in the clinical arrestment of blood pressure in the geriatric patient in the issue of "pseudohypertension." This entity is felt to be the false measurement of an elevated blood pressure in the face of a normal intra arterial pressure (19). Pseudohypertension may be the result of excessive arteriosclerosis that causes the brachial artery to be poorly compressible when the sphygmomanometer is applied, so that a falsely elevated reading is obtained. Patients with pseudohypertension may show little target organ change from their elevated blood pressure and be very sensitive to the blood pressure lowering effect of antihypertensive agents. Attempts to clinically differentiate pseudohypertensives from true hypertensives without resorting to the direct measurement of inter arterial blood pressure have not been particularly successful.

Also important in blood pressure determination of geriatric patients is the measurement of orthostatic blood pressure. Despite factors that might predispose to orthostasis (Table 16.2: e.g., decrease in baroreceptor sensitivity, decreased arterial compliance, decreased renal sodium conservation, decreased renin), studies indicate that blood pressure should not decline significantly (20mm Hg systolic or greater) when geriatric patients go from the supine to the upright position (20) Orthostatic blood pressure drop is found commonly in geriatric patients and requires an explanation. It is good practice to measure orthostatic blood pressure in all geriatric oncology patients at baseline. Abnormalities need to be pursued and follow up examination can be indexed against the baseline determination.

Temperature is another key vital sign assessed in geriatric medicine practice. Core body temperature does not appear to change as a function of age (21). Heat or cold stress may not be as well tolerated by older subjects, and older patients are more prone to heat illness or hypothermia during times of environmental stress (22). Debate exists whether it is generalizable that older patients have less ability to mount a febrile response to an infection (23). There certainly are older patients who show little or no temperature elevation from infection or in the presence of tumor.

Respiratory rate is the other vital sign measured routinely on patient assessments. There is no clear evidence that resting respiratory rate changes as a function of age. With hypoxia or hypercapnic stress, however, older subjects respond with a diminished respiratory response (24).

Table 16.3 Age associated skin changes*.

Component	Anatomic or functional change	Impacted function
Epidermis		
Keratinocytes	decreased proliferation	wound healing; vitamin D_3
melanocytes	decreased 10% per decade	photoprotection; color
Langerhans cells	decreased up to 40%	delayed hypersensitivity reactions; immune recognition
Basement membrane zone	flattens, reducing the dermo-epidermal interface	epidermal-dermal adhesion
Dermis		
fibroblasts	decreased collagen elastin synthesis	tensile strength elasticity
microvasculature	decreased vascular area	thermoregulation and inflammatory response
mast cells	decreased	immediate hypersensitivity reactions
neural elements	decreased by one-third	sensation, pain threshold
Subcutis		
fat	decreased	insulation and mechanical protection
Appendages		
eccrine glands	decreased number and output	thermoregulation
apocrine glands	decreased number and output	unknown
sebaceous glands	increased size and decreased output	unknown
hair follicles	decreased number and growth rate	cosmetic

*Source: Chuttani and Gillcrest (25)

Skin

Although not traditionally viewed as a physiologic system, the skin is one of the areas of the body where aging is clinically manifest. The barrier function of the skin is particularly important in oncologic practice. Chuttani and Gilchrest have reviewed this topic in great detail (25). Table 16.3 is a summary of age associated skin changes with the anatomic or functional changes and the implications for function. Clearly, wrinkling of the skin occurs with aging. Hair loss occurs and graying of the hair is seen as the result of melanocyte loss and decreased melanocyte activity. The impact of these changes on chemotherapy or radiotherapy induced alopecia and recovery in geriatric patients is not well studied. Wound healing is reported to be affected by age and may be due to a muted inflammatory response, change in skin metabolic responses, and diminished rates of capillary in growth. This has important implications for the surgical patient or patient receiving radiation with secondary skin involvement.

Age related skin changes effect the endocrine function of the skin. Less vitamin D3 is present in the skin of older subjects and the skin of older people is less able to produce vitamin D3 than the skin of younger people. These changes in vitamin D production as well as reduced sunlight exposure of some older patients may presage the occurrence of vitamin D deficiency among certain older patients with resultant osteomalacia.

Cellular and biochemical changes of the skin effect the skin's tensile strength and elasticity. As a result, the assessment of skin turgor as a measure of hydration in geriatric patients is not as valid as it might be in younger patients. Microvascular changes of skin blood vessels may relate to the ability to dissipate or conserve heat in late life. Additionally, thinning of blood vessel walls and loss of subcutaneous fat in areas such as the dorsum of the hand can predispose to easy bruisability in some of older patients. Furthermore, loss of subcutaneous fat in areas such as the heel of the foot results in less mechanical protection to that area and propensity for injury (i.e., pressure ulceration).

Respiratory System

The bedside examination of the chest and lungs does not change much with aging. Older persons who are dyspneic or have a cough generally have underlying pathology to account for their symptoms. There are, however, important anatomic changes in the chest wall, lung, and central nervous system (CNS) that have implications for respiratory physiology and clinical practice. Figure 16.4 summarizes the physiologic changes that occur with aging. Total lung capacity remains constant. Residual-volume, the amount of air in the lung at maximal expiration, increases with age as does

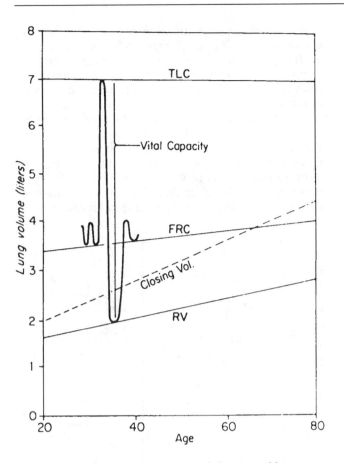

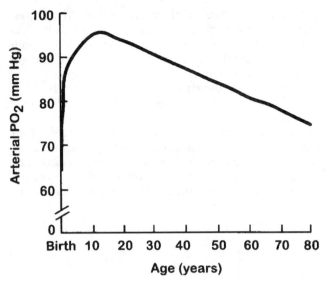

Figure 16.5 Arterial PO_2 as a function of age from birth to 80 yrs. (ref: Murray JF. *The Normal Lung.* Philadelphia, PA: Saunders, 1976.)

Figure 16.4 The effect of age on subdivision of lung volume: TLC = total lung capacity, FRC = functional residual capacity, RV = residual volume. (ref. Tockman MS. *Aging of the Respiratory System.* In *Principles of Geriatric Medicine and Gerontology Third Edition,* edited by WR Hazzard, EL Bierman, JP Blass, WH Ettinger, JB Halter. New York, NY: McGraw-Hill Inc., pp. 557, 1994.)

the functional residual capacity, the amount of air in the lung after a quiet expiration. Since vital capacity, maximum amount of air expired after maximal inspiration is the difference between total lung capacity and residual volume, it is inevitable that vital capacity will decline with age as the residual volume increases. The closing volume, the volume of the lung at which the dependent airways begin to close, also is higher in older subjects.

These just described changes have been detailed and reviewed by Sparrow and Weiss (26). In addition, these authors elaborate further upon changes in flow rates with advancing age. The forced vital capacity (FVC), forced expiratory volume in one second (FEV-1) and forced expiratory flow between 25% and 75% of the vital capacity (FEF 25-75) all decline with age. Regression equations have been developed and published so that pulmonary function laboratories may use the appropriate reference values when testing aged subjects (27). These changes in physiologic function relate in part to declining strength in respiratory muscles with age, an age-related increase in pleural elastin leading to increased elastic load on respiratory mus-

cles, stiffening of the chest wall due to changes in the rib cage (e.g. calcification of rib articulations) and loss of lung elastic recoil with increase in lung compliance.

Measurement of blood gases is important in oncologic practice. Figure 16.5 depicts the decline in arterial PO2 in adulthood. One regression equation that has been employed to calculate the impact of aging on PO2 is:

$$PaO2 = 100.0{-}0.323 \ (age)$$

Since alveolar PO2 remains constant with age, the Aa gradient widens as patients grow older. The PCO2 does not appear to undergo any significant age related change, but the diffusing capacity for carbon monoxide (DLCO) does decrease. These blood gas changes may result from observed distributional changes in ventilation with age and a mismatch of ventilation and perfusion. A decline in alveolar capillary surface area with increasing age also plays a role. As mentioned earlier (vide supra), hypoxia and hypercapnia fail to elicit the same response in respiratory rates in older subjects as compared to the young, i.e., the old seem less sensitive. It has also been reported that older subjects perceive shortness of breath less intensely than the young. Other changes with age in the respiratory system include a decline in cough, laryngeal reflexes and a slowing of mucous velocity (26). It remains speculation whether these latter mentioned changes result in a predisposition to aspiration or pneumonia in aged patients.

Cardiac Function and Exercise

Aging results in changes in the heart and vascular system. Blood vessel changes were described earlier. In the heart, the interventricular septum thickens as well as the left ventricular free wall, with greater thickening of the septum. The heart mass as indexed against the body mass increases in older women (28). These finding can be seen on echocardiography as well as at autopsy. This change in muscle mass may be the result of increased aortic impedance, due to structural changes in the aorta. On microscopic examination, pigment deposition (lipofuscin) within myofibrils has been reported and an increase of connective tissue at localized sites (29). Valvular changes have also been noted with aging. The mean circumference for each of the four cardiac valves increase progressively throughout life (28). Valve leaflet thickness increases with aging. Calcification of the aortic valve, mitral annulus, and mitral valve are seen commonly in the hearts of older people.

Mitral annulus calcification is more prevalent among elderly women. Although these valvular changes are evident on echocardiography, it is not clear that they result in any functional disturbance. Changes in the conducting system were alluded to in the discussion of pulse.

Lakatta has detailed the functional properties of the senescent myocardium (15). Although early reports note a decline in cardiac performance with advancing age, more recent studies do not support this finding. The more recent reports probably reflect better ability to screen for subclinical cardiac disease and exclude affected subjects from research studies. Figure 16.6 is a

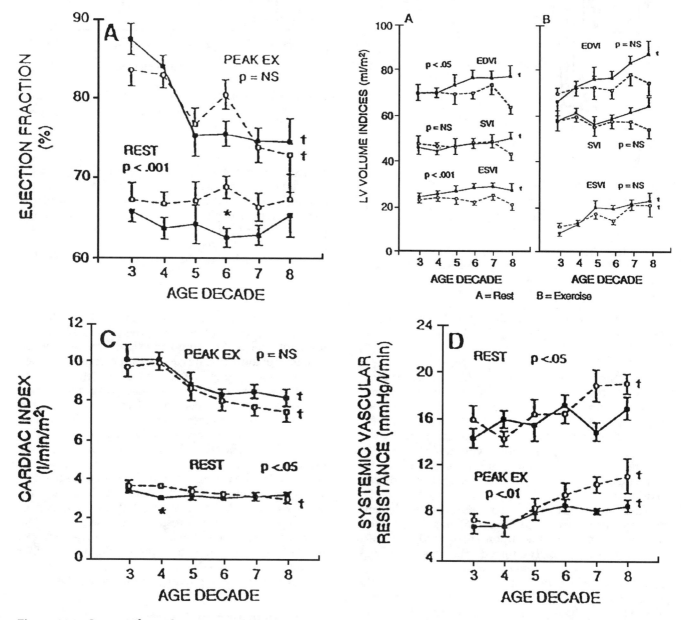

Figure 16.6 Systemic hemodynamic variables plotted by age decade at rest and peak exercise (Peak Ex) in males (■) and females (□). *Significant gender differences for individuals decades adjusted for multiple comparison. † Significant age regressions within gender at rest or peak effort. P values indicate gender differences of variance.
LV = left ventricular volume
EDVI = end-diastolic volume index
SVI = end-systolic volume index
(Ref. 16)

series of studies examining subjects of different ages and various physiologic parameters at rest, with exercise and by gender (16). In men the end systolic volume index (ESVI), end diastolic volume index (EDVI), and the stroke volume index (SVI) increase with age at rest; this is not seen in women. Resting ejection fraction (EF) and cardiac index (CI) show no change in men; in women the EF is stable, but the CI declined 16% from the third to eighth decade. Peripheral vascular resistance does increase in both sexes with aging at rest, while the resting heart rate declines slightly. The gender differences appear to be the result of differences in fitness levels. It is interesting, therefore that since cardiac output is the product of stroke volume and heart rate, that older men maintain cardiac output by compensating for a mild heart rate reduction with increased stroke volume which is due to an increase of end diastole volume ("preload"). Figure 16.6 also examines cardiac functional changes with aging during exercise. In older men with exercise, the end diastolic volume index (EDVI) rises compared to the young. For men and women the stroke volume indices (SVI) are comparable with exercise and age while the end systolic volume index (ESVI) is greater for older subjects of both sexes with exercise compared to the young. The ejection fraction with exercise increases markedly in younger subjects. This increase is not seen in exercising older men and women. Similarly, although heart rate and cardiac index increase in both old and young with exercise, older men and women do not have the same degree of heart rate or cardiac index (CI) elevation that is seen in the young.

In summary then, at rest cardiac function does not appear to change much with aging. With the stress of exercise, older subjects are less able to augment cardiac function as much as younger subjects. This lack of comparable response to exercise is the result of age associated decreases in heart rate, a relative reduction in myocardial contractile reserve, and a relatively greater increase in impedance of left ventricular ejection. All of these factors could be related to blunted adrenergic responsiveness that is seen with aging (17).

Maximum oxygen consumption (VO2max) achieved during exercise reflects cardiac and pulmonary factors as well as local tissue oxygen delivery, extraction, and utilization. When measured in subjects of different ages, VO2 max declines with advancing age (15). This remains true when the data are controlled for weight, lean body mass, and training effects. This decline is likely the result of changes in cardiac output, respiratory reserve, and loss of skeletal muscle fitness with aging. Skeletal muscle metabolism does not appear to account for the decline in VO2 max. Although maximal performance with exercise is greater in young adulthood than in senescence, older patients can exercise and should exercise to minimize decrements in physiologic function with aging. Symptoms of cardiac dysfunction in late life are the result of disease and need evaluation and explanation. Cardiac disease remains the number one cause of death even into the ninth decade.

Gastrointestinal Function

The evaluation of the gastrointestinal system begins at the mouth. This is particularly important in oncologic practice since geriatric cancer patients may have mucositis or other oral complaints. The teeth and gums do undergo aging changes with gingival recession, pulp recession inside individual teeth, and an increase in tooth brittleness (30). The ability to efficiently chew food declines with aging (31). Salivary function, on the other hand, is preserved into late life (32). Xerostomia (dry mouth) is generally the result of drugs, radiation therapy, or disease (e.g. Sjogren's syndrome).

Studies of taste sensation show that the threshold for detecting taste is greater in late life, i.e., older subjects do not have as acute a sense of taste as younger subjects (33). However, the meaning of these studies for clinical practice is unclear since the stimuli for taste are present in much greater concentrations in the routine diet than experienced in the laboratory environment where thresholds are being examined. Overall, the ability to taste is preserved with advancing age in ordinary day to day life. It should be noted, however, that the same is not true for olfaction. The identification and recognition of odor decline dramatically with age (33). Therefore, disturbance in taste should suggest some pathologic process in the geriatric patient. A decline in olfaction is more difficult to sort out in regard to whether the change is due to disease (e.g. upper respiratory infection). Complete loss of smell (anosmia) should not be attributed to aging, though defining a precise etiology may be elusive.

Swallowing is a complex function requiring intact sensory, voluntary motor and involuntary motor functions. Shaker has reviewed the effect of aging on swallowing and esophageal motor function (34). Data are lacking regarding consistent changes in oromotor function that change with age. Measurement of upper esophageal sphincter pressure has yielded conflicting results making generalizations difficult. In the pharynx, the peristaltic pressure wave amplitude and duration seem to be greater in elderly subjects compared to young subjects. These changes in pressure may be needed to overcome a reduced cross sectional area of the deglutitive upper esophageal sphincter opening in elderly patients.

Older studies suggested changes in esophageal motor function termed "prebyesophagus." More recent data suggest that primary esophageal peristalsis induced by swallowing does not necessarily change with age. Secondary peristalsis (initiated in response to local esophageal stimuli) is either absent or inconsistent, and significantly less frequent in old subjects compared to the young (35). This loss of secondary peristalsis may result in impairment of esophageal volume clearance, and predispose to esophageal and supra esophageal complications of reflux among older patients. Also noted in this study was less relaxation of the lower esophageal sphincter in response to esophageal distention among the old subjects (35). Resting lower esophageal sphincter pressure has been reported to be stable with aging but in response to swallowing, the sphincter may not completely relax consistently in the oldest subjects (those aged 90 and above). Symptoms of dysphagia, choking or odynophagia in older patients need evaluation and should not be attributed to aging.

In regard to gastric function, it has been traditionally thought that acid production declines with age. On closer scrutiny, investigators excluding subjects with diseases such as atrophic gastritis, H. pylori infestation, and controlling for body composition have found that basal acid output and maximal/stimulated acid outputs are preserved into later years (36). It may even be the case that there is a significant increase of acid output with aging. The clinician must keep in mind, however, that diseases such as atrophic gastritis are exceedingly common in late life, may affect 40% or more of persons aged 80 and over, and result in decreased secretion of acid (37).

Evaluation of the literature on gastric motility and aging is plagued with the same problems of subject selection as acid output. Since motility is affected by acid, studies must control for achlorhydria since this condition has been shown to delay gastric emptying. Many reports do not comment on whether achlorhydria is present or absent among subjects. Therefore, there are contradictory reports on gastric motility and age. Holt has summarized this motility literature and states "overall, these studies lead to the conclusion that by the best nuclear medicine techniques that examine passage of both solid and liquid meals, gastric emptying of food is little reduced as a function of age, though gastric emptying of the liquid part of a meal may be slightly delayed" (36).

Important in clinical practice is the ability of the gastric mucosa to protect itself. Arthritis is the number one chronic illness seen in older persons, and is frequently treated with aspirin and nonsteroidal anti-inflammatory agents which can influence gastric mucosal protection. Unfortunately this remains an evolving area of research, and there are little data on prostaglandin concentration or synthesis in the upper gastrointestinal tract. Animal studies do suggest that experimentally induced gastric injury causes more severe injury and reduced healing in senescent research animals (36). Older patients do have an appreciable risk of gastrointestinal hemorrhage when treated with nonsteroidal agents.

Small intestine physiology in humans represents a challenge to investigators due to the inaccessibility of the small bowel. Controversy exists whether any significant morphologic changes occur in the intestinal mucosa with aging. In regard to absorption, carbohydrate digestion seems unimpaired by aging. However, intestinal monosaccharide absorption does seem reduced with age (36). This may be due to a change in intestinal receptor density or affinity for actively absorbed substrates. This reduction in carbohydrate absorption is unlikely to result in malnutrition in healthy older patients. Protein absorption is less well studied than carbohydrate absorption and data from humans are not sufficient enough to make generalizations. For fat absorption, there is little evidence that major changes in intestinal lipid transport occur with age (36).

For iron and minerals: sodium, potassium, zinc and copper appear to be absorbed effectively into late life. Iron has been reported to have altered absorption, but more recently this finding has been called into question and it is believed that iron absorption is intact in healthy older subjects (36). Calcium, on the other hand, does have impaired absorption with advancing age. Since achlorhydria, vitamin D deficiency, and dietary calcium or fiber intake can all influence calcium absorption, these must be factored into interpretation of studies examining calcium absorption. When these factors are considered, it still does appear that aging is associated with a reduced calcium absorption (36). As a result, recommendations have been made for older persons to increase dietary calcium intake.

Vitamin absorption has been examined as a function of age. Thiamine, niacin, folate, vitamin B12, vitamin K, and vitamin A all seem to be absorbed without difficulty in healthy older persons. Vitamin D absorption does appear to be impaired (36). Small intestinal transit time appears unaffected by age.

As far as colonic structure and function, it is well known that colonic diverticuli are seen with increasing frequency as patients age. Although constipation is common in later life, it does appear that this is a pathologic state and that colonic transit time is not affected by aging. Manometric anorectal study shows that rectal distention may be associated with higher pressures and decreased basal and squeeze anal pressures in elderly volunteers compared to young volunteers. These findings might contribute to the risk of fecal incontinence among geriatric patients (38).

Pancreatic function has been assessed closely in animal and humans. A number of physiologic changes such as reduced responsiveness of secretion to exogenous stimuli, a delay in responsiveness of pancreatic growth to proliferative signals, and an impaired or delayed response of pancreatic enzyme synthesis to changes in nutrient substrate uptake have all been reported to occur with aging (36). None of these, however, is sufficient to cause clinical manifestations of pancreatic exocrine dysfunction in geriatric patients.

Table 16.4 outlines the influence of age on hepatic structure and function. The clinical examination is not sensitive enough to reliably demonstrate the decline in hepatic size/weight in geriatric patients. The reduction of hepatic blood flow in older patients may result in diminished first pass metabolism of drugs. Hepatic synthetic capacity is well maintained into late life and changes in serum albumin are modest and probably not of much clinical importance. Serologic measures of enzymes found in liver cells appear to have similar reference ranges for younger and geriatric patients.

Endocrine Aspects of Aging

After consideration of the abdomen and gastrointestinal system, the clinician will often examine the genitalia.

Table 16.4 Effects of aging on liver physiology*.

Liver variable	Aging effect
liver size	decreased
hepatic blood flow	decreased
BSP, galactose elimination	decreased
microsomal drug metabolism	normal to decreased
glucuronidation	probably unchanged
Glutathione	may be deceased
serum albumin	slightly decreased
routine liver chemistries	normal

*Source: Russell (37).

This raises issues of endocrine aspects of aging as well as renal physiology. The endocrine system will be dealt with first followed by consideration of the kidneys and urinary tract.

Elderly women have evidence of estrogen loss with vaginal, uterine, ovarian, and breast atrophy. Bone loss is accelerated with estrogen depletion. Although menopause is initially associated with marked elevation of follicle stimulating hormone (FSH) and luteinizing hormone (LH), data are conflicting whether these gonadotropins remain elevated or decline, particularly after age 60 (39). After menopause FSH increases to a greater extent than LH. Therefore the ratio of FSH to LH is greater than 1 in the postmenopausal state, as opposed to premenopause when it is less than 1 (40). The administration of luteinizing hormone-releasing hormone (LHRH) to older women still produces a surge of LH and to a lesser extent FSH (40).

Estradiol levels are, of course, markedly depressed in the elderly postmenopausal women. Estrone levels, which in premenopausal women are lower than estradiol levels, exceed estradiol levels in late life (41). The source of estrone appears to be the extra glandular aromatization of adrenal androstenedione by adipose tissue, bone, muscle, skin and brain. As more data become available confirming the benefits of estrogen replacement in late life regarding reduced cardiovascular morbidity and mortality as well as beneficial effects on bone, oncologists caring for elderly women are likely to find significant numbers of their patients on estrogen replacement therapy.

The physical examination of the older man's genitalia does not show significant change from earlier in life. Pubic hair thins and greys. The prostate gland does enlarge. Although testicular size may not change with age, histologic examination does show a drop in the percentage of seminiferous tubules containing sperm; atrophy of the seminiferous tubules with thickening of the tunica propria and basement membrane; loss of Sertoli cells and spermatids per Sertoli cell; and a loss of Leydig cells (42). Conflicting data have been reported regarding what happens to serum testosterone with aging in men. Since there is considerable variability among men in regard to testosterone levels, it is difficult to interpret the studies. In a recent review, Nelson states that both free and total serum testosterone levels decline with advancing age (39). Discrepant reports may be due to subject selection and variability in the timing and rate of age-related decline of testosterone in men. Even if a decline in serum testosterone is noted with age, the occurrence of frank hypogonadism requires clinical evaluation and should not be ascribed to old age. Studies are ongoing to document the benefits and risks of androgen replacement in geriatric male patients.

Estradiol levels have been reported to generally decrease less with age in men than serum testosterone. This means that the estradiol: testosterone ratio may increase with age (39). There is speculation that this ratio shift may relate to prostatic hyperplasia in late life. At the level of the pituitary, LH pulse frequency has been reported to remain normal in older men, but the frequency of high amplitude LH pulses, as well as total LH pulse height and the total area under the LH pulses are significantly decreased in elderly men (43). Stimulation of the pituitary with luteinizing hormone releasing hormone (LHRH) yields similar results in young and elderly men. These data suggest that diminution of testosterone plasma levels with aging are more likely due to primary testicular failure than central causes.

Analysis of gonadal function naturally leads to a consideration of general pituitary function with aging. The ability of the pituitary to secrete gonadotropins has just been described for men and women. Growth hormone (GH) has been extensively studied and reviewed as a function of aging (44). GH decrement between the ages of 20 and 80 years ranges between 30 and 50%. A parallel decline in insulin-like growth factor-1 (IGF-1) has also been reported. IGF-1 is a hepatic protein whose synthesis is dependent upon growth hormone. A significant number (40%-50%) of patients aged 70 and over have evidence of profound growth hormone depletion. Studies continue to examine the risks and benefits of replacing growth hormone in deficient elderly people. Beneficial effects might include improved lean body mass content, decreased body fat mass, increased muscle mass/strength, improved exercise capacity, and improved bone density (13). The pituitary does seem to be able to respond to growth hormone releasing hormone (GHRH) in older subjects, though there are conflicting results whether the response is as brisk as that seen in younger subjects (45).

Regarding prolactin secretion and aging, studies are variable in their results showing no change, decreased serum levels, or increased basal/stimulated levels of the hormone in older subjects (46).

Also produced in the pituitary gland is adrenocorticotropic hormone (ACTH). ACTH secretion is pulsatile and complex. Human studies have not taken this into full consideration and reports of increased or unchanged secretion with aging need further follow up (47). The pituitary remains responsive to corticotropin releasing hormone (CRH) in late life (48). At the level of the adrenal gland, Nelson in a review of 19 studies notes that plasma cortisol levels are generally unchanged in late life, though occasional reports do note increased plasma levels in aging individuals. When these increases are noted, they are relatively small (39). The most plentiful adrenal steroid found in the serum is dehydroepiandrosterone (DHEA) and its sulfate. Although abundant, the precise role of this weak androgen is unknown in human physiology. What is noteworthy for the care of geriatric patients is a marked decline of plasma DHEA concentration with aging (39). Epidemiologic studies have linked depressed DHEA levels to higher risk of breast cancer, higher risk of cardiovascular disease, and higher all cause mortality. This has led to an interest in human trials of DHEA to assess benefits and side effects of this agent.

Yet another pituitary hormone is thyroid stimulating hormone (TSH). TSH levels seem to be stable throughout life. Basal pituitary secretion of TSH increases somewhat in older persons and pituitary response to thyrotropic releasing hormone (TRH) has yielded conflicting results with decreased, unchanged, or increased TSH responses (48). With aging there is fibrosis, decreased follicular cellularity and size, and increased microscopic nodularity of the thyroid gland. Despite these anatomic changes, serum levels of T4 and T3 generally appear stable with advancing age. Both hyper and hypothyroidism have increased frequency in geriatric patients and can be difficult to diagnose due to atypical manifestations and nonspecific symptoms.

In close anatomic proximity to the thyroid gland are the parathyroid glands. Throughout life, the reference range for serum calcium level determination does not change appreciably. Careful research studies indicate that there may be a slight decline in serum calcium with aging (49). Whether this is the result of a slight decline in serum albumin with age or a true decline due to depression of ionized calcium is disputed. Serum parathyroid hormone (PTH) has been shown to be higher in older persons, particularly older women than in younger persons (48). This elevation may be due to diminished clearance of PTH associated with declining glomerular filtration rate with aging. Reduced calcium absorption due to intestinal effects of aging as well as slight reduction in serum albumin may cause a decline in ionized serum calcium in late life which, in turn, results in increased secretion of PTH.

Since the prevalence of diabetes is known to increase with advancing age, any consideration of endocrine function and aging must include some mention of pancreatic endocrine function. Modest anatomic changes of the pancreas have been described with aging and include some atrophy, increased incidence of tumors, and deposition of amyloid material and lipofuscin granules (50). Halter has reviewed the area of carbohydrate metabolism and aging in depth (51). From this review a number of important points about aging and pancreatic endocrine function emerge.

When fasting levels of glucose are measured in healthy subjects of varying ages, values appear to be stable and perhaps a minor clinically insignificant rise may occur. With the administration of glucose either orally or intravenously, significant differences are seen among subjects of differing age. In young adulthood the rise in plasma glucose is not as high or sustained as long as seen in late life. This impairment in glucose homeostasis is not due to defective insulin release since measured insulin levels are comparable for the young and old. These differences must be accounted for when interpreting glucose tolerance results in geriatric patients. The National Diabetes Data Group criteria for diabetes have factored these age related changes into the standards used to made a diagnosis for diabetes (52).

Therefore, a diagnosis of diabetes is made when the fasting plasma glucose is greater than or equal to 140 mg/dl on two occasions. Alternatively, if the patient has classic diabetes symptoms, random hyperglycemia, a fasting plasma glucose of <140 mg/dl and a one hour and two hour plasma glucose level ≥200 mg/dl after a 75 g glucose load, a diagnosis of diabetes is also possible. Impaired glucose tolerance is diagnosed when patients have a normal fasting plasma glucose, but one hour after a 75g glucose load the plasma glucose is ≥200 mg/dl and at two hours the value is 140–200 mg/dl.

Extensive studies have been done to determine the mechanism for altered glucose homeostasis with age (51). As mentioned previously insulin response does not seem impaired. Insulin action beyond the level of the insulin receptor appears to be where the problem lies with glucose metabolism and aging. There is not much evidence that glucagon changes with age and in any way mediates the change in glucose metabolism seen with age. Since growth hormone may decline with age, its action could not explain the age related rise in plasma glucose with a challenge. Also, thorough plasma cortisol may increase subtly with age, this rise does not seem sufficient enough to account for the observed glucose differences in young and old after glucose challenge. As alluded to earlier in the discussion of blood pressure (Table 16.2), plasma norepinephrine levels and norepinephrine release increase with aging. Although it does not appear that these increased resting levels have much effect on basal glucose levels, with catecholamine infusion (epinephrine), greater hyperglycemia is seen among older subjects than for the young when simultaneous glucose administration occurs.

The clinical importance of the above mentioned issues for the oncologist is multifaceted. First, diabetes is a common comorbidity among geriatric oncologic patients and must be factored into treatment strategies. Secondly, geriatric patients without a history of diabetes may have hyperglycemia induced more easily than young subjects as the result of stress, use of glucose infusion during intravenous therapy or total parenteral nutrition, and the administration of drugs (e.g., glucocorticoids) in the course of treatment of a malignancy.

Changes in body composition described previously (i.e., loss of lean mass and accumulation of adipose) and sedentary lifestyle may also predispose older persons to the development of diabetes.

To conclude this section on endocrine function and introduce the discussion of renal function, there should be some mention of salt and water metabolism with aging. Arginine vasopressin (AVP) is a peptide hormone produced in the hypothalamus and released from the posterior pituitary. AVP levels have been reported to decline, remain steady, and increase in the resting state with advancing age (53). When AVP is stimulated using osmotic (saline infusion) or pharmacologic stimuli (e.g. metoclopromide injection) older subjects appear to have less inhibition of AVP release and loss of alcohol suppressive effect compared to the young subjects (53). Curiously, when AVP release is stimulated by blood volume/blood pressure using overnight dehydration and the stress of acute upright positioning, the response is not exaggerated as just noted for osmotic/pharmacologic stimuli. Therefore AVP response to osmotic stimuli with aging is exaggerated while to volume/pressure stimuli it is blunted. The blunting may be the result of diminished baroreceptor sensitivity (Table 16.2) noted with aging. Although there is an increase in AVP response to osmotic stimuli, there appears to be relative resistance to the effect of AVP at the level of the kidney in late life (54).

Reference values for serum electrolytes do not appear to be effected by aging. However, the hormonal systems governing sodium balance and blood pressure do appear to change. Plasma renin values are consistently lower when measured in older subjects and compared to the young (54). Not surprisingly, plasma and urinary concentration of aldosterone are similarly depressed. Furthermore, it has been reported that atrial natriuretic factor (ANF) levels are higher for older subjects than younger ones (54). The net effect of these changes is that older patients may have difficulty retaining sodium/salt than their younger counterparts. There is evidence that with sodium restriction, healthy older patients with intact renal function are less able to effectively conserve sodium (54).

There are a number of clinical implications to these physiologic changes in water/salt metabolism. The geriatric oncology patient who is placed on a sodium restricted intake, given hypotonic fluid, given agents that provoke AVP (e.g., narcotics or metoclopramide), and who is stressed (e.g., fearful, in pain, or post op) is at risk for the development of hyponatremia due to problems with faulty sodium retention and exaggerated AVP response, despite peripheral AVP resistance. Another scenario is the geriatric oncology patient who is salt/water deprived (e.g., NPO for diagnostic studies or anorectic) more rapidly becomes dehydrated due to lesser ability to conserve salt and water through the renin/angiotensin/aldosterone system as well as a less effective renal sodium concentrating mechanism. Further compounding this situation is what appears to be a physiologic decline with thirst with aging that may make correction of water loss more difficult for the

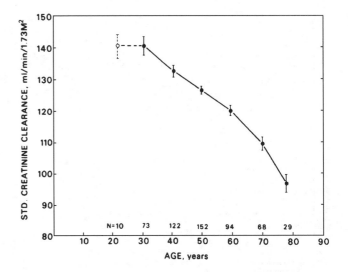

Figure 16.7 Cross sectional difference in standard creatinine clearance with age. The number of subjects in each age group is indicated above the abscissa. Values plotted indicate mean ± S.E.M. (ref: Rowe JW, Andres R, Tobin JD, Norris AH and Shock NW. The Effect of Age on Creatinine Clearance in Men: A Cross-Sectional and Longitudinal Study. *J Gerontol* 1976; **31**: 155–163.).

aged patient (55). Finally, with the depressed renin aldosterone response plus decline in glomerular filtration rate with aging (*vide infra*), the oncologist must be on guard for the subtle development of hyperkalemia in aged patients associated with the use of nonsteroidal antiinflammatory agents, potassium sparing agents, beta blockers, or angiotensin converting enzyme (ACE) inhibitors.

Renal Function

There is little on the bedside examination that alerts clinicians to the important changes that occur in renal function with age. Even laboratory measurements of electrolytes, blood urea nitrogen, serum creatinine or urinanalysis do not readily convey age related changes in renal physiology.

Lindeman has summarized anatomic changes in the kidneys over the lifespan (56). Renal mass declines 1% per year. The loss of mass is primarily from the renal cortex. The number of glomerular tufts per unit area as well as the number of glomerular and tubular cells decreases. Large renal arteries undergo sclerotic change in their walls. Sclerotic glomeruli increase with advancing age so that at age 40 less than 5% of the total glomeruli are sclerotic while 10–30% of the total are sclerotic by the eighth decade. The mesangium of the glomerulus takes up a greater percentage of glomerular volume and the glomerular basement membrane thickens in older subjects.

Glomerular filtration rate has been shown to decline as a function of age whether estimated by inulin or creatinine clearance (54) (Figure 16.7). This decline is important to the clinician who must take this into

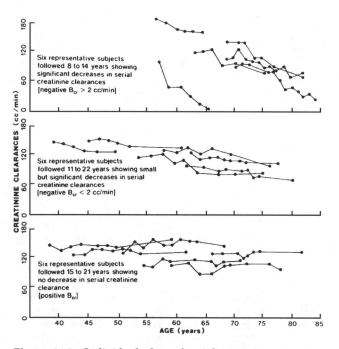

Figure 16.8 Individual plots of serial creatinine clearances vs. age in years for representative subjects (ref. 5).

Table 16.5 Age related changes in micturition.

Parameter	Age related change
bladder capacity	decreased
post void residual volume	increased
Involuntary bladder contraction	common
bladder outlet/urethral resistance	decreased in women
prostate size	increased in men

assessment of bladder functioning (57). Due to a smaller capacity bladder some older persons may need to void more frequently. When checking geriatric patients for residual volume after voiding as much as 100 ml of urine may be obtained without there being any significant pathology. Involuntary bladder contractions can be documented on cystometrographic studies and their significance is not always clear due to poor correlation of these contractions with clinical symptoms. Estrogen levels, injury and anatomic realignment of the urethra from childbirth, and deconditioning may all contribute to a reduction of resistance to urine flow in the elderly woman. As alluded to earlier, prostate growth may be the result of changing estrogen: testosterone ratio with advancing age in men.

Although these changes may predispose to the development of urinary incontinence in elderly patients, the occurrence of incontinence should be viewed as a disease process and investigated for an underlying etiology. The oncologist must be aware that agents which affect autonomic function (e.g., anticholinergics or alpha blockers) can affect bladder/urethral function (e.g., urinary retention or laxity of the internal urethral sphincter). Also, use of agents such as diuretics may precipitate incontinence in patients with small bladder capacities, weakened urinary outlet, and who have difficulty ambulating to the toilet.

account when dosing patients with drugs that are affected by renal excretion (e.g. methotrexate or aminoglycosides). Unfortunately the serum creatinine concentration does not reflect the drop in creatinine clearance with the expected rise in creatinine level. This is due to the fact that with age there is a loss of lean body mass and, therefore, a decline in creatinine production.

Figure 16.8 makes the point that on longitudinal follow up one-third of healthy geriatric subjects have no decrease in creatinine clearance. This suggests that the age related decline in glomerular filtration rate demonstrated in cross sectional studies may not be the inevitable consequence of age, but rather may reflect subclinical nondetectable renal disease (5). Estimates of creatinine clearance need to recognize this variation so that appropriate clinical monitoring and serum drug levels are also used as guides to therapy of the geriatric patient.

Other changes in renal function with age include a decrease in renal plasma flow; a decrease in tubular maximum transport for PAH and glucose; a decrease in concentrating ability probably due to a decline in medullary hypertonicity; a decline in maximum diluting ability due to nephron loss; a reduced ability to excrete an acid load (54). Under basal conditions pH, pCO_2 and bicarbonate are similar in old and young subjects. However, in the face of an acid load, older patients take longer to correct acidosis and don't buffer/excrete acid as effectively as the younger person.

Since urinary incontinence is seen commonly among geriatric patients, it is important to consider the physiology of micturition in late life. Table 16.5 lists some of the changes seen in the lower genitourinary tract with age that can affect micturition and the clinical

Musculoskeletal Function

As the examination proceeds, the limbs and joints are next considered. Sarcopenia is the term that has been used to describe the loss of muscle mass. With advancing age, muscle mass has been shown to decline (58). This loss of mass is due to muscle fiber loss, particularly type ll (fast twitch) muscle fibers and a reduction in the size of muscle fibers. Clinical evaluation does not always readily show this loss due to replacement of muscle with fat and connective tissue. Although not known for sure, it is speculated that this loss of muscle is related to a slowly progressive neurogenic process (i.e., loss of motor neurons in the spinal cord).

When muscle strength is measured as a function age, data suggest that strength peaks between the second and third decade, plateaus until age 45–50 and then declines 12–15% per decade until the eighth decade (59). Some muscle groups tested have included the quadriceps, plantar/dorsal foot flexors, upper extremity muscle groups, and hand grips. Although these changes in strength are significant and well documented, the clinician must be aware that these measurements of strength are carefully recorded using sophisticated instruments that give precise values for force. The finding of clinically detectable weakness or atrophy should be evaluated so that myopathy or neuropathy is excluded. Attributing clinically significant weakness or atrophy to age without prior evaluation will likely result in missed diagnoses.

Though sedentary lifestyle and inactivity accelerate and accentuate loss of muscle mass and strength, there still does appear to be an aging effect to account for these losses that is independent of disease. Additionally, since muscle mass is an important determinant of basal oxygen consumption, it is not surprising that basal metabolic rate declines with advancing age (60). There is also speculation that with loss of muscle mass, there is less ability to generate heat through shivering and less body insulation from the cold, which may predispose older persons to hypothermia (61).

Osteoarthritis is the number one chronic illness which occurs in late life. Geriatric patients will often have evidence on physical examination of this condition particularly in the hips, knees, feet, hands, and spine. With normal aging articular cartilage undergoes changes with decline in chondrocyte cell density once maturity is reached; a decline in chondrocyte ability to synthesize proteoglycans; decrease in cartilage stiffness, fatigue resistance, and strength; decline in water content; change in proteoglycan composition and amount of keratin/chondroitin sulfate (7). Together, these cellular and biochemical changes may alter the stability and mechanical properties of the cartilage matrix and interfere with matrix turnover to replace degraded molecules. The relationship between age related changes in cartilage and the occurrence of osteoarthritis is not completely understood and is the subject of active investigation.

Another major component of the extremity evaluation is the bone. Unfortunately, bone does not readily lend itself to clinical examination and plain radiographs are insensitive to many changes that occur in bone. Loss of bone mass is felt to be an inevitable consequence of age (62). This loss is accelerated by the menopause. Bone mass in late life is related to the complex interaction of factors such as genetics, race, exercise, nutrition (calcium intake) and habits (smoking, alcohol use, caffeine intake). Although deficits in calcium intake, change in vitamin D metabolism, and decline in estrogen in women and possibly androgen in men have traditionally been thought to mediate this bone loss, more recent studies have also implicated local factors in bone and cytokines as playing a role. Some considerations have included an age related stimulation of pluripotential stem cells to form osteoclasts through colony forming units for the granulocyte macrophage series (GFU-GM); interleukin-1 and tumor necrosis factor-alpha (TNF-) increasing in later life and mediating bone resorption; prostaglandin secretion by bone cells in late life stimulating osteoclastic bone resorption (62).

Table 16.6 Age related changes in neuroanatomy and neurochemistry.

Variable	Age Effect
Brain weight	decrease
Ventricular volume	increase
Neuronal number esp	decrease
superior temporal neocortex	
locus ceruleus	
substantia nigra	
Neurofibrillary changes esp	increase
parahippocampus	
anterior olfactory nucleus	
Synapse number esp	decrease
frontal cortex	
Biochemical markers	
choline acetyl transferase	decrease
esp in hippocampus and temporal neocortex	
dopamine esp in caudate	decrease

From the clinical standpoint, the treating oncologist must be aware that chemotherapy regimens that cause gonadal failure may accelerate physiologic bone loss. Agents such as steroids can also aggravate age related decline in bone loss. Immobility associated with poor performance status has a similar impact of augmenting physiologic loss of bone. Measures should be employed so that hormonal replacement be given to patients if appropriate, nutrition be optimized to promote adequate intake of vitamin D and calcium, and a program of exercise be encouraged.

The Nervous System

It has been stated that post mitotic tissues (e.g., neural, muscular, myocardial) are impacted the greatest by the effects of aging. The area of the neurobiology of aging and neural change associated with aging is large and has recently been reviewed by Katzman (63). Some highlights of age related changes in the central nervous system are listed in Table 16.6. These changes result in the occurrence of atrophy on imaging studies such as computerized tomography (CT) or magnetic resonance-imaging (MRI) in geriatric patients.

From the physiologic perspective, higher cortical function remains intact into late life. Mental status should be assessed in all geriatric patients and those with abnormalities should be investigated. Verbal ability seems well maintained throughout life. Timed tasks requiring speed in processing information or measuring reaction time do appear to be effected by aging with delayed performance. Short term memory and recall don't appear to be as well maintained in late life as compared to earlier years.

On assessment of cranial nerve function in older patients there are important changes in eyesight and hearing that must be considered. "Presbyopia" results from change in the lens with age so that accommodation is impaired and reading becomes more difficult. Other changes in the eye include a shrinking of the pupillary orifice and diminished ability to dilate the pupil; yellowing of the lens; decrease in visual evoked response with decreased amplitude and increased latency (63). In addition to having problems with near vision, geriatric patients may have difficulty functioning in low light; have problems functioning due to glare from light; have subtle changes in seeing objects colored blue-green; and have some difficulty with depth perception.

"Presbycusis" is the term used to describe hearing loss in elderly people. In countries such as the U.S., there appears to be a loss of the ability to hear high frequency sounds in late life. Additionally, speech understanding may be impaired through more central changes. Auditory evoked responses have been described to change with age and show a decrease in amplitude and increased latency (63).

Motor assessment was outlined in the musculoskeletal section. Sensation should remain intact with aging though threshold for sensation, particularly vibration, has been described to decline with age (63).

Gait and balance are reported to change with age. Healthy older persons have a shorter step length, lift their feet less, and are more flexed at the hips, knees, and elbows (64). On measures of balance the elderly subject appears to sway more and appear to be less stable when balance is perturbed. Falls are a major problem for elderly patients and although neural aging may serve as a risk factor, the physician should sort out environmental factors or diseases that might be causing a fall rather than ascribing the fall to aging.

Conclusion

With the passage of time, changes in anatomy and function occur in patients. These physiologic changes should be factored into the assessment of the geriatric patient with cancer. Changes in body composition and renal function will influence pharmacotherapy. Loss of reserve in some systems (e.g. cardiac, respiratory, endocrine, musculoskeletal) may make patients more vulnerable to adverse consequences of treatment. The impressive reserve in most physiologic systems, however, does allow for reasonable organ system function into senescence, particularly in the resting or unstressed state. Physiologic dysfunction at baseline assessment will frequently be the result of disease, either oncologic or some comorbidity.

Acknowledgements

Supported in part by NIH Grant #AG12210: "Causes of Lean Body Mass Atrophy in Aging Men and Women," and VAMC-Milwaukee Medical and Research Services "The author wishes to acknowledge Ms. Karen Hartzell for her invaluable assistance in preparing this manuscript."

References

1. Shock NW "Energy Metabolism, Caloric Intake and Physical Activity of the Aging". In *Nutrition In Old Age. X Capital Symposium Swedish Nutrition Foundation*, edited by LA Larson. Almquist and Wiksell Uppsala, 1972.

2. Brandfonbrener M, Landowne M, Shock NW. Changes in Cardiac Output with Age. *Circulation* 1955; **12**: 557–566.

3. Port S, Cobb R, Coleman RE, Jones RH. Effect of Age On the Response of the Left Ventricular Ejection Fraction to Exercise. *N Engl J Med* 1980; **301**: 1113–1117.

4. Rodeheffer RS, Gerstenblith G, Becker LC, Fleg JL, Weisfeldt ML, Lakatta EG. Exercise Cardiac Output is Maintained With Advancing Age in Healthy Human Subjects: Cardiac Dilatation and Increased Stroke Volume Compensate for a Diminished Heart Rate. *Circulation* 1984; **69**: 203–213.

5. Lindeman RD, Tobin JD, Shock NW. Longitudinal Studies on the Rate of Decline in Renal Function with Age. *J Am Geriatr Soc* 1985; **33**: 278–285.

6. Lipsitz LA, Goldberger AL. Loss of Complexity and Aging. Potential Applications of Fractals and Chaos Theory to Senescence. *JAMA* 1992; **267**: 1806–1809.

7. Buckwalter JA, Woo SL-Y, Goldberg VM, Hadley ED, Booth F, Oegema TR, Eyre DR. Soft-Tissue Aging and Musculoskeletal Function. *J Bone and Joint Surg* 1993; **75-A**: 1533–1548.

8. Sorkin JP, Muller DC, Andres R. Change In Height With Aging: Effects On Body Mass Index and On Weight-For-Height Guidelines. *Gerontologist* 1995; **35** (special issue 1): 206(abstract).

9. Novak LP. Aging, Total Body Potassium, Fat-Free Mass and Cell Mass in Males and Females Between Ages 18 and 85 Years. *J Gerontol* 1972; **27**: 438–443.

10. Bruce A, Andersson M, Arvidsson B, Isaksson B. Body Composition. Prediction of Normal Body Potassium, Body Water and Body Fat in Adults on the Basis of Body Height, Body Weight and Age. *Scand J Clin Lab Invest* 1980; **40**: 461–473.

11. Borkan GA, Hults DE, Gerzof SG, Robbins AH, Silbert CK. Age Changes in Body Composition Revealed By Computed Tomography. *J Gerontol* 1983; **38**: 673–677.

12. Fiatarone MA, Marks EC, Ryan ND, Meredith CN, Lipsitz LA, Evans WE. High-Intensity Strength Training In Nonagenarians. Effects on Skeletal Muscle. *JAMA* 1990; **263**: 3029–3034.

13. Rudman D, Feller AG, Nagraj HS, Gergans GA, Lalitha PY, Goldberg AF, Schlenker RA, Cohn L, Rudman IW, Mattson DE. Effects of Human Growth Hormone in Men Over Age 60 Years Old. *N Engl J Med* 1990; **323**: 1–6.

14. Davies MJ. Pathology of the Conduction System. In *Cardiology In Old Age*, edited by F Caird, JLC Dall, RD Kennedy. New York, NY: Plenum Press, 57–80, 1976.

15. Lakatta EG. Cardiovascular System. In *Handbook of Physiology Section 11: Aging*, edited by EJ Masoro. Oxford, England: Oxford University Press, 413–474, 1995.

16. Fleg JL, O'Connor F, Gerstenblith G, Becker LC, Clulow J, Schulman SP, Lakatta EG. Impact of Age on the Cardiovascular Response To Dynamic Upright Exercise in Healthy Men and Women. *J Appl Physiol* 1995; **78**(3): 890–900.

17. Lakatta EG Deficient Neuroendocrine Regulation of the Cardiovascular System With Advancing Age in Healthy Humans. *Circulation* 1993; **87**: 631–636.

18. Williams L, Lowenthal DT. Hypertension in the Elderly. *Cardiovascular Clinics* 1992; **22**: 49–61.

19. Messerli FH, Ventura HO. Osler's Maneuver and Pseudohypertension. *N Engl J Med.* 1985; **312**: 1548–1551.

20. Smith JJ, Porth CJM. Age and Response to Orthostatic Stress. In *Circulatory Response To Upright Posture*, edited by JJ Smith. Boca Raton, FL: CRC Press, 121–139, 1990.

21. Keilson L, Lambert D, Fabian D, Thebarge J, Ackerson T, Palomaki G, Turgeon W. Screening For Hypothermia in the Ambulatory Elderly: The Maine Experience. *JAMA* 1985; **254**: 1781–1784.

22. Collins KJ, Exton-Smith AN. Thermal Homeostasis In Old Age. *J Am Geriatr Soc* 1983; **31**: 519–524.

23. Fedullo AJ, Swineburne AJ. Relationship of Patient Age to Clinical Features and Outcome For In-Hospital Treatment of Pneumonia. *J Gerontol* 1985; **40**: 29–33.

24. Kronenberg RS, Drage CW. Attenuation of the Ventilatory and Heart Rate Response to Hypoxia and Hypercapnia with Aging in Normal Men. *J Clin Invest* 1973; **52**: 1812–1819.

25. Chuttani A, Gilchrest BA. Skin. In *Handbook of Physiology Section 11: Aging*, edited by EJ Masoro. Oxford, England: Oxford University Press, 309–324, 1995.

26. Sparrow D, Weiss ST. Respiratory System. In *Handbook of Physiology Section 11: Aging*, edited by EJ Masoro. Oxford, England: Oxford University Press, 475–483, 1995.

27. Enright PL, Kronmak RA, Higgins M, Schenker M, Haponik EF. Spirometry Reference Values For Women and Men 65 to 85 Years of Age. *Am Rev Respir Dis* 1993; **147**: 125–133.

28. Kitzman DW, Scholz DG, Hagen PT, Ilstrup DM, Edwards WD. Age Related Changes in Normal Human Hearts During the First 10 Decades of Life Part ll (Maturity): A Quantitative Anatomic Study of 765 Specimens From Subjects 20 to 99 Years Old. *Mayo Clin Proc* 1988; **137**–146.

29. Kohn RR. Heart and Cardiovascular System. In *Handbook of the Biology of Aging*, edited by CE Finch, L Hayflick. New York, NY: Van Nostrand, Reinhold Co., 281–317, 1977.

30. Lloyd P, Shay K. Dental Pain in the Elderly. *Age* 1987; **10**: 70–80.

31. Baum BJ, Booner L. Aging and Motor Function; Evidence for Altered Performance Among Old Persons. *J Dental Research* 1983; **2**: 2–6.

32. Wolff A, Fox PC, Ship JA, Atkinson JC, Macynski AA, Baum BJ. Oral Mucosa Status and Major Salivary Gland Function. *Oral Surg Oral Med Oral Pathol* 1990; **70**: 49–54.

33. Weiffenbach JM, Bartoshur CM. Taste and Smell. *Clin Ger Med* 1992; **8**: 543–555.

34. Shaker R, Lang IM. Effect on the Deglutitive Oral, Pharyngeal and Esophageal Motor Function. *Dysphagia* 1994; **9**: 221–228.

35. Ren J, Shaker R, Kusano M, Podvrsan B, Metwally N, Dua KS, Sui Z. Effect of Aging on the Secondary Esophageal Peristalsis: Presbyesophagus Revisited. *Am J Physiol* 1995; G772–G779.

36. Holt PR. The Gastrointestinal Tract. In *Handbook of Physiology Section 11: Aging*, edited by EJ Masoro. Oxford, England: Oxford University Press, 505–554, 1995.

37. Russell RM. Changes in Gastrointestinal Function Attributed to Aging. *Am J Clin Nutr* 1992; **55**: 1203S-1207S.

38. Bannister JJ, Abovzekry L, Read NW. Effect of Aging On Anorectal Function. *Gut* 1987; **28**: 353–357.

39. Nelson JF. The Potential Role of Selected Endocrine Systems in Aging Processes. In *Handbook of Physiology Section 11: Aging*, edited by EJ Masoro. Oxford, England: Oxford University Press, 377–394, 1995.

40. Odell WO. The Menopause. In *Endocrinology Volume 3 Second Edition*, edited by LJ DeGroot. Philadelphia, PA: W.B. Saunders Harcourt Brace Johanovich, Inc. 2009–2018, 1989.

41. Marshburn PB, Carr BR. The Menopause and Hormone Replacement Therapy. In *Third Edition Principles of Geriatric Medicine and Gerontology*, edited by WR Hazzard, EL Bierman, JP Blass, WH Ettinger, JB Halter. New York, NY: McGraw Hill, Inc., 867–878, 1994.

42. Merry BJ, Holehan AM. Aging of the Male Reproductive System. In *Physiological Basis of Aging and Geriatrics Second Edition*, edited by PS Timiras. Boca Raton, FL: CRC Press, 171–178, 1994.

43. Vermeulen A. Clinical Review 24: Androgens in the Aging Male. *J Clin Endocrinol Metab* 1991; **73**: 221–224.

44. Rudman D, Shetty KR. Unanswered Questions Concerning the Treatment of Hyposomatotropism and Hypogonadism In Elderly Men. *J Am Geriatr Soc* 1994; **42**: 522–527.

45. Corpas E, Harman SM, Blackman MR. Human Growth Hormone and Aging. *Endocr Rev* 1993; **14**: 20–39.

46. Shetty KR, Duthie EH. Anterior Pituitary Function and Growth Hormone Use in the Elderly. *Endocrinology and Metabolism Clinics of North America* 1995; **24**: 213–231.

47. Terry LC, Halter JB. Aging of the Endocrine System. In *Third Edition Principles of Geriatric Medicine and Gerontology*, edited by WR Hazzard, EL Bierman, JP Blass, WH Ettinger, JB Halter. New York, NY: McGraw Hill, Inc., 791–805, 1994.

48. Blackman MR. Aging. In *Endocrinology Volume 3 Second Edition*, edited by W De Groot. Philadelphia, PA: WB Saunders Harcourt Brace Johanovich, Inc., 2348–2366, 1989.

49. Chapuy MC, Durr F, Chapuy P. Age-Related Changes in Parathyroid Hormone and 25 Hydroxycholecalciferol Levels. *J Gerontology* 1983; **38**: 19–22.

50. Timiras PS. The Endocrine Pancreas and Carbohydrate Metabolism. In *Physiological Basis of Aging and Geriatrics. Second Edition*, edited by PS Timiras. Boca Raton, FL: CRC Press, 191–199, 1995.

51. Halter J. Carbohydrate Metabolism. In *Handbook of Physiology Section 11: Aging*, edited by EJ Masoro. Oxford, England: Oxford University Press, 119–146, 1995.

52. National Diabetes Data Group. Classification and Diagnosis of Diabetes Mellitus and Other Categories of Glucose Intolerance. *Diabetes* 1979; **28**: 1039–1057.

53. Miller M. Hormonal Aspects of Fluid and Sodium Balance In the Elderly. *Endocrinology and Metabolism Clinics of North America* 1995; **24**: 233–253.

54. Lindeman RD. Renal and Urinary Tract Function. In *Handbook of Physiology Section 11: Aging*, edited by EJ Masoro. Oxford, England: Oxford University Press, 485–503, 1995.

55. Philips PA, Rolls BJ, Ledingham JJG, Forsling ML, Morton JJ, Crowe MJ, Wollner L. Reduced Thirst After Water Deprivation In Healthy Elderly Men. *N Engl J Med* 1984; **311**: 753–759.

56. Lindeman RD. Renal Physiology and Pathophysiology of Aging. *Contrib to Nephrology* 1992; **105**: 1–12.

57. Brocklehurst JC. The Bladder. In *Textbook of Geriatric Medicine and Gerontology Fourth Edition*, edited by JC Brocklehurst, RC Talis, HM Fillit. New York, NY: Churchill Livingstone, 629–646, 1992.

58. Lexell J. Human Aging, Muscle Mass and Fiber Type Composition. *J Gerontol* 1995; **50A**: 11–16.

59. Hurley B. Age, Gender and Muscular Strength. *J Gerontol* 1995; **50A**: 41–44.

60. Tzankoff SP, Norris AH. Longitudinal Changes In Basal Metabolism In Man. *J Appl Physiol* 1978; **45**: 536–539.

61. Kenney WL, Buskirk ER. Functional Consequences of Sarcopenia; Effects On Thermoregulation. *J Gerontol* 1995; **50A**: 78–85.

62. Kalu DN. Bone. In *Handbook of Physiology Section 11: Aging*, edited by EJ Masoro. Oxford, England: Oxford University Press, 395–412, 1995.

63. Katzman R. Human Nervous System. In *Handbook of Physiology Section 11: Aging*, edited by EJ Masoro. Oxford, England: Oxford University Press, 325–344, 1995.

64. Murray MP, Kory RC, Clarkson BH. Waling Patterns in Healthy Old Men. *J Gerontol* 1969; **24**: 169–178.

17. Practical Proposals for Clinical Protocols in Elderly Patients with Cancer

Martine Extermann and Lodovico Balducci

Introduction

The goal of this chapter is to review some principles of clinical research in elderly patients with cancer. In the process, we will examine the tools that may be used in this research. These tools may have widespread clinical applications in providing individualized treatment to the older cancer patient.

Older cancer patients are different from those who are younger because they have shorter life expectancy and higher prevalence of comorbid conditions, functional limitations, emotional, cognitive and socio-economic restrictions. Clinical trials of older persons must take into account each of these factors in defining individual patient profiles which may affect both the goals of treatment and the type of intervention planned.

In the following discussion we will explore the issues of external validity of clinical research in older individuals, choice of research end-points, assessment of functional status, comorbidity and quality of life in geriatric oncology protocols, and mathematical analysis of data from older individuals, including mathematical models.

External Validity

Clinical studies in the elderly are particularly prone to selection bias. A major characteristic of the older population is diversity. Hence, the risk that clinical trials involve only a particularly healthy fringe of this population and that the results of these trials be not generalizable to the older population at large. Patients referred to tertiary care centers are generally selected for what concerns comorbidity and function. Patients with other diseases or poor performance status are most likely treated in a primary care center. Medications taken for other conditions may influence the course of cancer (eg: aspirin, coumarinic anticoagulants). Patients with comorbidities may be more sensitive to the complications of the tumor and of antineoplastic treatment. Financial bias is also becoming increasingly important, especially in countries without universal insurance coverage. An increasing number of patients cannot afford care in a tertiary care center because of no or partial insurance coverage and limited income. Predictably, further selection will occur as an effect of managed care. Older persons are less likely than younger ones to receive aggressive cancer treatment, even after stratification for comorbidity (1–4). Elderly patients are also less likely than younger ones to be referred to specialized practitioners, such as medical oncologists (3). These biases are not always avoidable, and may themselves be the object of future studies.

It is particularly important to establish the part of the physician and that of the patient in the decision to limit cancer care (3–7). These biases should be carefully accounted for in the analysis of the results, when one wants to establish the applicability of these results to the general population of older cancer patients. Comorbidity, an independent predictor of survival in elderly patients (8–9), should be graded independently from performance status. In addition to overall mortality, disease-specific mortality should be reported. The general type of patients seen by the center should be described, as well as data allowing to evaluate the external validity of the study. Such data may include: the proportion of eligible patients included/excluded from the study, the proportion of eligible/non-eligible patients with the disease, and the level of dependence of the study population.

The elements allowing to assess external validity of a study are summarized in Table 17.1.

Table 17.1 Data that should be reported in clinical trials involving older individuals, to establish the external validity of the study.

External validity assessment

Functional status

Comorbidity
- Qualitative
- Quantitative

Overall Mortality

Disease-specific mortality

Overall population of the institution(s) where the studies are conducted.

Enrolled/non-enrolled patients

Eligible/ineligible patients

Level of dependence of individual patients.

Table 17.2 Alternative study end-points in the older cancer patient.

Overall survival

Disease-free survival

Tumor response rates

Cancer-related survival

Cancer-unrelated survival

Active life-expectancy

Symptom reduction (eg. pain)

Quality of life

Choice of End-Points

The treatment of elderly patients raises issues about study end-points that are specific to their age group. The cure of the cancer may not increase survival, due to competing causes of death. Therefore, overall survival may not always represent the "gold standard" of treatment effectiveness and alternative end-points should be examined (Table 17.2). One of these is the distinction between cancer-related and unrelated mortality. Comorbidity level is highly variable in the elderly population, and can lead to some 10–20 fold changes in annual death rate (10). An endpoint with major impact on the patient's quality of life and on the cost of patient care to the society is active life expectancy. This term refers to the length of time during which the patient is able of independent living (11–12).

Certain tumors, more prevalent in the elderly, may not lead to measurable lesions, as it is the case in metastatic prostate cancer, or locally advanced pancreatic cancer. In such setting, assessment of symptoms evolution, such as pain, can prove a highly sensitive and relevant end-point (13–15). More generally, quality of life is an important end-point that should be assessed, although it may not be directly related to tumor response.

Comorbidities

Comorbidities significantly influence life-expectancy in elderly persons. For persons in their sixties or seventies, they can increase the non-cancer mortality 10–20 fold (10). Practically, in our opinion, patients with a tumor that has a median tumor-specific survival of 2 years or longer should be stratified for comorbidity upon enrollment in clinical trials. Comorbidity may influence not only the patient's survival but also pharmacokinetics of antineoplastic agents and tolerance to treatment. Comorbidity levels should be graded independently from functional status. In elderly patients, comorbidity is an independent predictor of survival (8–9) and of risk of hospitalization (16). Regarding the impact of comorbidity in older cancer patients, few information is presently available from prospective therapeutic trials as these studies have generally selected patients in good general condition. Epidemiologic or retrospective studies are fraught by confounding factors, such as uncontrolled reductions in treatment intensity (1,3), and underreporting of comorbidity.

Probably, cohort studies represent the most powerful setting to explore the impact of comorbidity on treatment and survival of older cancer patients. It is essential to grade comorbidity according to objective scales, to have interpretable data that establish the impact of comorbidity on treatment and survival. As the list of possible comorbidities is practically unending, several approaches have been taken to select clinically significant conditions, to group these conditions into specific categories of disease, and to attribute a relative weight to each condition and to each category of diseases. This process has generated various comorbidity scales, which are summarized in Table 17.3.

The Charlson Comorbidity Scale

The Charlson comorbidity scale was constructed from the one year mortality data of patients admitted to a medical hospital service. The relative risk of death associated with several conditions was assessed. Any comorbidity implying relative risk >1.2 was used in the scale and weighted, leading to a scale with 19 diseases weighted from 1 to 6 points. The scale has been validated retrospectively and prospectively, as well as in medical data bases (17–20). The Charlson scale is valid in predicting mortality risk over a period of a few weeks to 10 years in conditions ranging from breast cancer to spine surgery (17–19). It is correlated also with such outcomes as postoperative complications, length of hospital stay, discharge to a nursing home (19). As the relative risk of death varies with age as well as with comorbidity, a version of the scale combining

Table 17.3 Some characteristics of four clinical comorbidity scales. "Validated" refers to formal validation (see text for references).

Scales Type	Charlson Comorbidity (+age)	CIRS and var. Comorbidity	ICED Comorbidity+function	Kaplan/ Feinstein Comorbidity
Correlation with mortality	+	+		+
Correlation with other outcomes	+	+	+	
Validated in cancer patients	+		+	+
Validated in the elderly	+	+	+	

age and comorbidities was also designed (18). The Charlson Scale is easy to use. Potential limitations include the fact that the scale ignores numerous comorbidities that may be relevant in designing the treatment of cancer patients, such as hematopoietic disorders other than malignancies, polyneuropathy, or moderate renal dysfunction.

The Cumulative Illness Rating Scale

The Cumulative Illness Rating Scale (CIRS) (21), and its variants (9,22) have a structure analogous to the WHO toxicity scale, well known to medical and radiation oncologists. This scale classifies comorbidities by organ systems (13 or 14 according to the version), and grades each condition from 0 (no problem) to 4 (severely incapacitating or life-threatening condition). Scores may be summarized in different ways, with comparable results. The scale encompasses both potentially lethal and non-lethal comorbid conditions. The CIRS has good inter-rater (Kendall's W >.82) reliability and correlates well with post-mortem findings (23). An adaptation for geriatric patients (CIRS(G)) has been developed with pluridisciplinary defined scoring guidelines (24). The CIRS(G) version has also good inter-rater reliability and face validity (22). In an institutionalized elderly population, the CIRS scores correlated with mortality, acute hospitalization, medication usage, abnormal laboratory test results and functional disability. In addition, the CIRS showed good divergent validity vis a vis functional disability in predicting mortality and hospitalization (9). In another study on geriatric outpatients, comorbidity measured by CIRS and IADL were the only variables which could independantly predict mortality (8). In a third study, the CIRS has been shown to correlate with ADL, IADL, patient morale, duration of hospitalization, number of medications, survival in a geriatric outpatient population, but showed no significant improvement over ADL in a logistic regression model predicting survival. CIRS and age predicted acute care hospitalization duration, ADL and IADL predicted use of nursing home services (16).

More complicated to grade than the Charlson scale, the scale requires good familiarity with the scoring criteria. With training, it may become a quick instrument to use.

The Index of Coexistent Disease

The Index of Coexistent Disease (ICED) (25) includes two parts: one for the assessment of comorbidity, the other for the assessment of functional impairment. Comorbidity and functional impairment are independently scored and the two scores are combined in an index with four levels of severity. The inter-rater agreement is 90% (25). The ICED scores are positively correlated with severe hospital complications, length of stay after hip surgery (25). In a retrospective study, the ICED scale was correlated with patterns of care in breast and prostate cancer patients (1, 26), with incidence of complications and length of hospital stay in surgical patients (25). The functional component of the

ICED may allow the rater to assess both comorbidity and function with a single instrument and to forgo other measurements, such as ADL, IADL and ECOG performance status in a comprehensive geriatric assessment. However, the equivalence of the ICED and other forms of functional assessment has not been yet established. The difficulties related to the use of ICED and CIRS are comparable.

The Kaplan-Feinstein Scale

The Kaplan-Feinstein scale focuses on diseases that may compromise a patient's long-term survival (27). Several conditions are graded from 0 to 3, and categorized according to involvement of specific organs, presence of specific functional disabilities, and of alcohol-related diseases. The worst score in each category is utilized as summary score. This scale positively correlated with 5 years mortality in diabetic patients (27). In patients with prostate cancer, this scale predicted 5-year survival, and in a multivariate analysis remained an independent variable besides stage and tumor-related symptoms. In the same study, ADL were not an independent prognostic factor (28). The Kaplan-Feinstein scale has also been used in a retrospective series of breast cancer patients and was found to have a good discriminative power for 10 year mortality (17). The Kaplan-Feinstein scale is more complex than the Charlson scale but simpler than CIRS and ICED.

Other indexes based on physiological measures rather than categorization of clinical disease are also available and may be useful in certain settings, such as studies of in-hospital survival or short-term outcome of hospitalized patients. We cite as examples: Apache III, Support, Smith (29–31). A comparison of different instruments would be most desirable for the practitioners, but unfortunately only few and limited studies have addressed this issue. The Kaplan-Feinstein and the Charlson scales were compared in breast cancer patients and gave very similar results in terms of patient classification and prediction of 10 year mortality (17). The main limitation of this study, from our standpoint at least, was the inclusion of a large number of young breast cancer patients: more than 30% of patients were under 40. Not surprisingly 80% of the patients assessed with the Kaplan-Feinstein scale and 86% of those assessed with the Charlson scale fell in the "no comorbidity" category. Another study compared the performance of the Charlson, Charlson adapted to databases, Kaplan-Feinstein, ICED and Smith indexes in predicting the risk of hospital readmission of hospitalized patients. All instruments failed to predict readmission (32).

Thus, the practitioner is faced with a number of instruments, all of which have reasonable validity. At present, the choice of the most appropriate instruments can be based on two criteria: simplicity to use and special needs of specific practice settings. In our geriatric oncology clinic, we elected to use both the Charlson Scale and the CIRS(G) as part of the comprehensive geriatric assessment (CGA). The Charlson scale because of its simplicity, the CIRS(G) because it offered a wider variability on a sample of older cancer patients and does not overlap the other elements of our CGA. We are currently comparing the performance of these assessment tools, in terms of predicting survival, loss of independence, tolerance of antineoplastic treatment, and quality of life for our patients.

Comprehensive Geriatric Assessment

A multidimensional assessment of the older person, capable to evaluate several areas of potential interventions, has been utilized for several years in geriatric practice. The Comprehensive Geriatric Assessment (CGA) complemented by appropriate geriatric follow-up has proved helpful in prolonging the survival and improving the opportunity to live at home for older individuals (33). The CGA may be performed both at home or in the hospital setting. The specific contribution of CGA to the management of treatment of elderly cancer patients is largely unexplored. Seemingly CGA may provide important leads for therapeutic choices, mostly in the palliative setting.

The basic core of CGA includes medical history and physical examination, and appropriate scales for the assessment of Activities of Daily Living (ADL), Instrumental Activities of Daily Living (IADL), cognition, and depression, and a form of evaluation of social support. The CGA entails a multidisciplinary approach to the older patient. The assessment team must include a physician with geriatric orientation, a nurse or nurse practitioner, and a social worker. The team is most often complemented by a clinical pharmacist, a dietician, a physical therapist, a gerontopsychologist or any specialty needed (34–37).

A practical approach to the use of the CGA in elderly cancer patients is discussed in other chapters of this volume (38–39).

The relative relevance of the tumor stage, CGA, and comorbidity for the prognosis and therapeutic strategy of an elderly cancer patient is an area of active research in our program and in other institutions (40).

Quality of Life

A main concern of physicians treating elderly cancer patients is preservation of quality of life. Elderly patients have a highly variable functional reserve. In some situations the antineoplastic treatment may overtax this limited reserve and compromise the survival and the quality of life of older individuals more than cancer itself. The risk of losing personal independence due to symptoms of cancer or complications of oncological treatment is much higher among older than among younger individuals. Thus, the effects of both cancer and cancer treatment on quality of life may be much deeper in the older population.

It should be emphasized that quality of life is an important prognostic factor in cancer patients, in addition to being a major end point of medical intervention. Self-perceived health is in fact a predictor of death in the general population or even "medically healthy"

elderly individuals (41–42). In lung cancer patients, Quality of life was found predictive of survival, independently of tumor stage and performance status (43–46). Similar results have been found in breast cancer (7). Whether these results are influenced by some low-level comorbidity is unknown.

The definition of quality of life has been quite diverse in the literature (47–49). A reliable definition of quality of life is especially important for elderly patients undergoing a comprehensive geriatric assessment, as other dimensions such as performance status or functional status are analyzed on separate scales. Quality of life can be conveniently defined as "patients' appraisal of and satisfaction with their current level of functioning as compared to what they perceive to be possible or ideal" (50). More technically quality of life may be defined: "a multidimensional construct encompassing perceptions of both positive and negative aspects of dimensions such as physical, emotional, social, and cognitive functions, as well as the negative aspects of somatic discomfort and other symptoms produced by the disease or its treatment" (51). Clearly, an assessment of quality of life is patient-centred. Indeed, it has been shown that there is a low correlation between patient's own estimate of quality of life and those provided by the physician or the caregiver (51–53). The caregiver or the physician tend to underestimate the quality of life of severely ill patients (53). Therefore, every effort should be made to have quality of life measures obtained directly from the patient.

A plethora of quality of life scales have been created during the last 15 years and have been reviewed elsewhere (43,44,49,54). A list of scales frequently used in oncology includes: the FLIC (55), the CARES (56), the EORTC-30 (57), the FACT (58), the SF-36 (59), the LASA (60). The SF-36 has also norms for the general population with age stratification, which is certainly an advantage in a geriatric population. Some scales exist in many languages (eg. EORTC-30, FACT), which may be useful for international studies. Some scales also have complementary subscales specific to certain tumors (EORTC-30, FACT).

There is no absolute rule for the choice of a particular Quality of life scale. A scale adapted to the patient population and the type of question addressed in the study should be selected among the scales with which the investigators are familiar. The assessment of quality of life in older individuals is dealt with in another chapter of this volume (61).

Mathematical Methods

Aging is highly individualized. Consequently, elderly cancer patients represent a very diverse population, whose assessment in terms of functional reserve, comorbidity, emotional and cognitive function, and socioeconomic conditions is problematic. Chronologic age is a poor predictor of individual age-related changes and there are no reliable biological or physiological markers of extent of aging in individual situations. The diversity of aging is a major obstacle to the recruitment of a representative sample of older individuals into clinical trials and the major limit to the use of clinical studies in clinical practice. This diversity represents also a major therapeutic challenge as it mandates individualized treatment plans, which cannot be tested in large clinical trials. Furthermore, the ability of human mind to integrate complex prognostic data has limits (62). This complexity of data is particularly common in medical decisions involving older individuals. Meta-analysis of different clinical trials may allow firmer conclusions of the value of prognostic factors and the effectiveness of therapeutic interventions in older persons with cancer. Decision analysis models may help estimate individual benefits and risks of different courses of action and to calculate the cost-effectiveness of specific interventions. We should emphasize, however, that the reliability of mathematical methods is predicated upon the reliability of clinical data. Thus, a uniform and comprehensive evaluation of the older patient is essential to the applications of these methods.

Meta-Analysis

Meta-analysis has proved a powerful tool in the acquisition of knowledge from clinical studies (33, 63–64). It is particularly useful in establishing trends from inconclusive studies, and for this reason may become an important way to obtain information about older patients. The use of meta-analysis in the elderly population encounters however certain hurdles. Of these, diversity represent probably the major challenge. One should therefore pay a very careful attention to the way patients have been selected for studies. For example, the setting of the study may play a role, as demonstrated by Stuck et al., in the case of CGA (33). Stratification of study populations in each trial, by comorbidity or functional level, could certainly increase the reliability of meta-analysis in the elderly.

Decision Analysis

The term "decision analysis" refers to an ensemble of mathematical methods trying to consider in a systematical way and ponder the elements that influence (medical) decision making. They allow evaluating the accuracy of diagnostic procedures, interpreting the meaning of positive or negative results of a procedure in a specific patient, modelling complex patient problems in order to select the most appropriate approach.

The management of elderly patients involves very complex clinical decisions, implying the consideration of multiple factors, cancer-related or not. Even when we limit ourselves to cancer alone, a prognostic estimation is a difficult exercise. For example, estimates given for the 10 year survival of breast cancer patients by trained oncologists varied on a range of 20–50% for each of 3 hypothetical cases (62). Physicians were basing their judgement on few variables and the addition of more variables, such as tumor grade or proliferation markers, was only adding to the dispersion of opin-

ions. We can thus postulate that having to integrate information on comorbidities would lead to an even greater dispersion of prognostic estimates and hence treatment options. Computer databases may prove useful in this respect. There is also a large space opened for decision help programs. For the moment, the bases for such programs are limited by the scarcity of discriminant information on elderly cancer patients with comorbidities. As data accrue, carefully designed, controllable decision analysis models could prove of great help for every day practice. Several tools are available for these projects, such as decision trees, Markov models, classification and regression trees (CART), neural networks (65).

An essential aspect of decision analysis is the estimate of the expected value of different interventions. The expected value generally integrates objective outcomes, such as prolongation of survival, cost, and relief of symptoms, with personal perceptions of those outcomes, such as the desirability to live longer at the price of loss of function or pleasure. Several methods have been proposed for estimating the expected value of clinical outcomes. Of these, the "trade-off" and the "standard bargaining" methods have become particularly popular.

Trade-off methods are methods that propose an exchange between two options. Eg " Suppose that you can live 10 years in your present condition and that I could offer you a lesser number of years in perfect health, how many years of life in perfect health would you be willing to exchange for 10 years in the present condition?". In the "standard bargaining techniques" the patient is asked to state how many chances of the worst outcome (generally death) he/she is willing to take to reverse the present condition of misery. "An example of standard bargaining technique is the following: "Chemotherapy may relieve your cancer pain, but involves a risk of dying. How many chances of dying are you willing to accept, to relieve your current pain?" These methods are widely used in decision analysis for including quality of life in the models. They are also used for comparing the different estimates of the same situation by different persons. These situations may include global estimates of quality of life, or willingness to receive treatment under specific conditions (5,6,52,54). These techniques may prove very valuable in estimating the expected value of certain outcomes by specific cohorts of elderly patients.

Cost-Effectiveness

As we are living in a cost-conscious environment, this domain will sustain an intense development in the coming years. Cost-effectiveness refers to the cost of the outcome of specific interventions. Cost-effectiveness may be expressed as cost per additional year of life, cost per life saved, cost per quality of life-adjusted year of survival. Cost effectiveness may be examined from the point of view of a medical center (charges generated by the treatment), of the patient (charges of treatment and loss of gain), and of the society (costs and productivity). Interestingly, a recent study on projected Medicare expenditures from 1990 to 2020 showed that only 3.2% of the increase in costs would be due to improved life-expectancy beyond 65 years, while 74.3% would be due to the larger size of the original cohort of persons and 22.5% to an increase in the proportion of that cohort expected to survive to 65 years of age (66). However, Medicare covers only 5% of nursing home care, which represent 20% of total health care expenditure in the United States. Nursing home care spending increases with age (66). Therefore, a particularly interesting point will be to incorporate evaluations of the cost of cancer treatment into the more general issue of preventing institutionalization. In this perspective, some treatments may prove more cost-effective or even cost-saving in the elderly, when compared to younger patients. Survival evaluation should also include, when relevant, quality of life correction, especially if the intent of the treatment is palliative. One should also realize that, while cost-effectiveness concerns may play an important part in societal or insurance budget decisions, the care of the individual patient should always be aimed at the best reasonable care to improve survival and quality of life. At individual levels, cost-effectiveness studies should be aimed at choosing the most cost-effective method to achieve the same results. From a research point of view, cost-effectiveness studies could emphasize domains where there is a need to develop cheaper techniques or approaches. One should also keep in mind that charges are a highly volatile data and that any analysis refers to a certain time and location. A comprehensive consideration of all possible charges (such as eg. time lost by the family) is also extremely difficult (67). However, cost-effectiveness analyses may prove a very useful tool in identifying what are the major influences on the cost of a treatment (eg. duration of hospitalization, treatment of complications, cost of a specific procedure, nursing home care) and help focus on them as study- or cost-intervention-goals. They could also help discriminating the costs of treating cancer from the costs of aging itself.

Conclusions

Clinical research in older cancer patients requires clarification of research goals and comprehension of the diversity of the older population. Survival of older individuals may be compromised by alternative causes of death and may not represent the most reliable endpoint of clinical trials. Alternative end points of relevance include disease-free survival, cancer-related mortality, preservation of independence and of quality of life. Multidimensional geriatric evaluation (including comorbidity) of older cancer patients in clinical trials and in clinical practice may allow meaningful comparisons of different studies and meta-analysis of these studies, as well as assessment of the validity of community practices.

Meta-analysis techniques and cohort studies appear as the most effective methods to study cancer in the elderly, because they may comprehend and account for the diversity of the older population.

Abundant tools are available that are fitted to afford the challenge of developing solid bases to treat elderly cancer patients with therapies best tailored to their personal conditions. As other authors of this book mentioned, the elderly are the fastest growing segment of Occidental populations. They deserve an important and sustained high quality research effort. Also in oncology.

References

1. Greenfield S, Blanco D, Elashoff RM, Ganz P. Patterns of care related to age of breast cancer patients. *JAMA* 1987; **257**: 2766–70.
2. Obrist R, Honegger HP, Pichert G, Senn HJ. Physician's attitudes in the treatment of elderly patients with aggressive NHL. *Ann Oncol* 1992; **3**(suppl 5): 123.
3. Newcomb PA, Carbone PP. Cancer treatment and age: patient perspectives. *J Natl Cancer Inst* 1993; **85**: 1580–4.
4. Bergman L, Dekker G, van Kerkhoff EHM, Peterse HL, van Dongen JA, van Leeuwen FE. Influence of age and comorbidity on treatment choice and survival in elderly patients with breast cancer. *Breast Cancer Res Treat* 1991; **18**: 189–198.
5. Slevin ML, Stubbs L, Plant HJ, et al. Attitudes to chemotherapy: comparing views of patients with cancer with those of doctors, nurses, and general public. *Brit Med J* 1990; **300**: 1458–60.
6. Bremnes RM, Andersen K, Wist EA. Cancer patients, doctors and nurses vary in their willingness to undertake cancer chemotherapy. *Eur J Cancer* 1995; **31A**: 1955–9.
7. Coates A. Who shall decide? *Eur J Cancer* 1995; **31A**: 1917–8.
8. Keller BK, Potter JF. Predictors of mortality in outpatient geriatric evaluation and management of clinic patients. *J Gerontol* 1994; **49**: M246–251.
9. Parmelee PA, Thuras PD, Katz IR, Lawton MP. Validation of the Cumulative Illness Rating Scale in a geriatric residential population. *J Am Geriatr Soc* 1995; **43**: 130–7.
10. Satariano WA, Ragland DR. The effect of comorbidity on 3-year survival of women with primary breast cancer. *Ann Intern Med* 1994; **120**: 104–110.
11. Rogers A, Rogers RG, Belanger A. Longer Life but worse health? Measurement and dynamics. *Gerontologist* 1990; **30**: 640–9.
12. Liu X, Liang J, Muramatsu N, Sugisawa H. Transitions in functional status and active life-expectancy among older people in Japan. *J Gerontol* 1995; **50B**: S383–94.
13. Reyno LM, Egorin MJ, Eisenberger MA, Sinibaldi VJ, Zuhowski EG, Sridhara R. Development and validation of a pharmacokinetically based fixed dosing scheme for suramin. *J Clin Oncol* 1995; **13**: 2187–95.
14. Andersen JS, Burris HA, Casper E, et al. Development of a new system for assessing clinical benefit for patients with advanced pancreatic cancer. *Proc Annu Meet Am Soc Clin Oncol* 1994; **13**: A1600.
15. Rothenberg ML, Burris HA, Andersen JS, et al. Gemcitabine: effective palliative therapy for pancreas cancer patients failing 5-FU. *Proc Annu Meet Am Soc Clin Oncol* 1995; **14**: A470.
16. Waldman E, Potter JF. A prospective evaluation of the cumulative illness rating scale. *Aging (Milano)* 1992; **4**: 171–8.
17. Charlson ME, Pompei P, Ales K, McKenzie CR. A new method of classifying prognostic comorbidity in longitudinal studies: development and validation. *J Chron Dis* 1987; **40**: 373–383.
18. Charlson M, Szatrowski TP, Peterson J, Gold J. Validation of a combined comorbidity index. *J Clin Epidemiol* 1994; **47**: 1245–51.
19. Deyo RA, Cherkin DC, Ciol MA. Adapting a clinical comorbidity index for use with ICD-9-CM administrative databases. *J Clin Epidemiol* 1992; **45**: 613–9.
20. D'Hoore, Sicotte C, Tilquin C. Risk adjustment in outcome assessment: the Charlson Comorbidity Index. *Meth Inform Med* 1993; **32**: 382–7.

21. Linn BS, Linn MW, Gurel L. Cumulative Illness Rating scale. *J Am Geriatr Soc* 1968; **16**: 622–6.

22. Miller MD, Paradis CF, Houck PR, *et al*. Rating chronic medical illness burden in geropsychiatric practice and research: application of the Cumulative Illness Rating Scale. *Psychiatry Res* 1992; **41**: 237–48.

23. Conwell Y, Forbes NT, Cox C, Caine ED. Validation of a measure of physical illness burden at autopsy: the Cumulative Illness Rating Scale. *J Am Geriatr Soc* 1993; **41**: 38–41.

24. Miller MD, Towers A. *A manual of guidelines for scoring the cumulative illness rating scale for geriatrics.* (CIRS-G). Pittsburgh, May 1991.

25. Greenfield S, Apolone G. *Assessment of comorbidity: the Index of Coexistent Disease* (ICED). (manual) Boston, Milan, 1990.

26. Bennett CL, Greenfield S, Aronow H, Ganz P, Vogelsang N, Elashoff RM. Patterns of Care Related to age of men with prostate cancer. *Cancer* 1991; **67**: 2633–41.

27. Kaplan MH, Feinstein AR. The importance of classifying initial co-morbidity in evaluating the outcome of diabetes mellitus. *J Chron Dis* 1974; **27**: 387–404.

28. Clemens JD, Feinstein AR, Holabird N, Cartwright S. A new clinical-anatomic staging system for evaluating prognosis and treatment of prostatic cancer. *J Chron Dis* 1986; **39**: 913–28.

29. Knaus WA, Wagner DP, Draper EA, *et al*. The Apache III prognostic system. *Chest* 1991; **100**: 1619–36.

30. Knaus WA, Harrell FE, Lynn J, *et al*. The SUPPORT prognostic model. *Ann Intern Med* 1995; **122**: 191–203.

31. Smith DM, Norton JA, McDonald CJ. Nonelective readmissions of medical patients. *J Chron Dis* 1985; **38**: 213–24.

32. Waite K, Oddone, Weinberger M, Samsa G, Foy M, Henderson W. Lack of association between patients' measured burden of disease and risk for hospital readmission. *J Clin Epidemiol* 1994; **47**: 1229–1236.

33. Stuck AE, Siu AL, Wieland D, Adams J, Rubenstein LZ. Comprehensive geriatric assessment: a meta-analysis of controlled trials. *Lancet* 1993; **342**: 1032–6.

34. Stuck AE, Aronow HU, Steiner A, *et al*. A trial of annual in-home comprehensive geriatric assessments for elderly people living in the community. *New Engl J Med* 1995; **333**: 1184–9.

35. Silverman M, Musa D, Martin DC, Lave JR, Adams J, Ricci EM. Evaluation of outpatient geriatric assessment: a randomized multi-site trial. *J Am Geriatr Soc* 1995; **43**: 733–40.

36. Reuben DB, Borok GM, Wolde-Tsadik G, *et al*. A randomized trial of comprehensive geriatric assessment in the care of hospitalized patients. *N Engl J Med* 1995; **332**: 1345–50.

37. Landefeld CS, Palmer RM, Kresevic DM, Fortinsky RH, Kowal J. A randomized trial of care in a hospital medical unit especially designed to improve the functional outcomes of acutely ill older patients. *N Engl J Med* 1995; **332**: 1338–44.

38. Overcash J. The case for a Geriatric Oncology Program in a cancer center. In *Comprehensive Geriatric Oncology*. In press.

39. Repetto L, Granetto C, Venturino A, Simoni C, Gianni W, Santi L. Prognostic evaluation of the older cancer patient. In *Comprehensive Geriatric Oncology*.

40. Monfardini S, Ferrucci L, Fratino L, Del Lungo I, Serraino D, Zagonel V. Validation of a multidimensional evaluation scale for use in elderly cancer patients. *Cancer* 1996; **77**: 395–401.

41. Kaplan GA, Camacho T. Perceived health and mortality: a nine-year follow-up of the human population laboratory cohort. *Am J Epidemiol* 1983; **117**: 292–304.

42. Schoenfeld DE, Malmrose LC, Blazer DG, Gold DT, Seeman TE. Self-rated health and mortality in the high-functioning elderly-a closer look at healthy individuals: MacArthur study of successful ageing. *J Gerontol* 1994; **49**: M109–115.

43. Ruckdeschel JC, Piantadosi S. Quality of life in lung cancer surgical adjuvant trials. *Chest* 1994; **106**(S6): 324S–328S.

44. Kaasa S, Mastekaasa A, Lund E. Prognostic factors for in-operable NSCLC, limited disease: the importance of patient's experience of disease and psychosocial well-being. *Radiother Oncol* 1989; **15**: 235–242.

45. Ganz PA, Lee JJ, Siau J. Quality of life assessment: an independent prognostic variable for survival in lung cancer. *Cancer* 1991; **67**: 3131–35.

46. Fleishman SB, Kosty M, Herndon J. Quality of life predicts survival in advanced NSCLC: a cancer and leukemia group B study (8931). *Proc ASCO* 1994; **13**: 431.

47. Gill TM, Feinstein AR. A critical appraisal of the Quality of life measurements. *JAMA* 1994; **272**: 619–26.

48. Guyatt GH, Cook DJ. Health status, Quality of life, and the individual. *JAMA* 1994; **272**: 630–1.

49. Cella DF, Tulsky DS. Measuring Quality of life today: methodological aspects. *Oncology (Huntingt.)* 1990; **4**: 29–38.

50. Osoba D. Lessons learned from measuring health-related Quality of life in oncology. *J Clin Oncol* 1994; **12**: 608–16.

51. Slevin ML, Plant H, Lynch D, Drinkwater J, Gregory WM. Who should measure quality of life, the doctor or the patient? *British Journal of Cancer* 1988; **57**: 109–112.

52. Pearlman RA, Uhlman RF. Quality of life in chronic diseases: perceptions of elderly patients. *J Gerontol* 1988; **43**: M25–30.

53. Tsevat J, Cook EF, Green ML, *et al*. Health values in the seriously ill. *Annals of Internal Medicine* 1994; **122**: 514–20.

54. Spilker B, Molinek FR, Johnson KA, Simpson RL, Tilson HH. Quality of life bibliography and indexes. *Med Care* 1990; **28**(S12): DS1–77.

55. Schipper H, Clinch J, McMurray A, *et al*. Measuring the Quality of life of cancer patients: the functional living index-cancer: development and validation. *J Clin Oncol* 1984; **2**: 472–483.

56. Schag CAC, Heinrich RL. Development of a comprehensive Quality of life measurement tool: CARES. *Oncology* (Huntingt.) 1990; **4**: 135–8.

57. Aaronson NK, Ahmedzai S, Bergman B, *et al*. The European Organization for Research and Treatment of Cancer QLQ-C30: a Quality of life Instrument for use in international clinical trials in oncology. *J Natl Cancer Inst* 1993; **85**: 365–376.

58. Cella DF, Tulsky DS, Gray G, *et al*. The functional assessment of cancer therapy scale: development and validation of the general measure. *J Clin Oncol* 1993; **11**: 570–9.

59. Ware JE, Donald Sherbourne C. The MOS 36-item short form health survey (SF-36). *Medical Care* 1992; **30**: 473–83.

60. Selby PJ, Chapman JAW, Etazadi-Amoli J, *et al*. The development of a method for assessing Quality of life in cancer patients. *Br J Cancer* 1984; **50**: 13–22.

61. Ganz PA. Quality of life considerations in the older patient. In *Comprehensive Geriatric Oncology*. In press.

62. Loprinzi CL, Ravdin PM, De Laurentiis M, Novotny P. Do American oncologists know how to use prognostic variables for patients with newly diagnosed primary breast cancer? *J Clin Oncol* 1994; **12**: 1422–6.

63. Early Breast Cancer Trialists' Collaborative Group. Systemic treatment of early breast cancer by hormonal, cytotoxic, or immune therapy. *Lancet* 1992; **339**: 1–15.

64. Prostate Cancer Trialists' Collaborative Group. Maximum androgen blockade in advanced prostate cancer: an overview of 22 randomised trials with 3283 deaths in 5710 patients. *Lancet* 1995; **346**: 265–9.

65. Miles BJ, Kattan MW. Computer modelling of prostate cancer treatment. A paradigm for oncologic treatment? *Surg Oncol Clin N Am* 1995; **4**: 361–73.

66. Lubitz J, Beebe J, Baker C. Longevity and Medicare expenditures. *New Engl J Med* 1995; **332**: 999–1003.

67. Gulati SC, Bitran JD. Cost-effectiveness analysis: sleeping with an enemy or a friend? *J Clin Oncol* 1995; **13**: 2152–4.

18. Quality of Life Considerations in the Older Cancer Patient

Patricia A. Ganz

Introduction

Since the ancient philosophers (1), Western societies have been concerned about the well-being of individuals. From the individual perspective and the philosophical tradition, the concept of quality of life includes the idea of happiness, as well as an individual's ability to pursue activities that are personally and subjectively valued. From a societal perspective, quality of life concerns such things as the quality of housing, the environment, jobs, and community services, and their availability to members of the society. Using quality of life as viewed from the societal perspective, individual countries can be compared at a single point in time, and the well-being of individuals in the society can be monitored over time. Philosophers and demographers have examined both of these aspects of quality-of-life and well-being for some time. However, it is only during the past two decades that these considerations have been applied to health-related issues.

Quality of life considerations have been brought to the forefront of health care research in the late twentieth century as a result of the convergence of several important factors. These include 1) prolonged life expectancy, from the eradication of many infectious diseases and the successful treatment of other conditions, e.g., diabetes, kidney failure; 2) the appearance of many new chronic diseases, e.g., arthritis, heart disease, cancer and HIV; 3) the increasing cost and toxicities of some treatments; 4) and the concern about health outcomes beyond mortality. Coincident with these circumstances has been an emerging science of outcomes assessment (2), which borrows extensively from concurrent methodologic advances in the social sciences, enabling the quantification and evaluation of the quality of life outcomes of diseases and their treatments. In this chapter, we will have an opportunity to examine the intersection of these events from the perspective of cancer in the elderly.

There are numerous textbooks and reviews that devote considerable time to the examination of quality-of-life assessment (3,4,5,6,7). This chapter cannot cover all of the important topics that a reader may be interested in, and therefore, reference will be made to more detailed texts. However, this chapter will provide sufficient information to allow discussion of critical issues relevant to older persons with cancer, including the definition and conceptualization of quality of life; methods of measuring quality of life; the role of quality of life assessment in the elderly cancer patient; common cancers in the elderly, including the most important quality-of-life issues for each, special aspects of quality of life in the elderly; and future directions for research and application.

Definition and Conceptualization of Quality of Life

Definition and History

Although most of us intuitively understand what the phrase "quality of life" connotes, it has been exceedingly difficult for social scientists, health services researchers and clinicians to define precisely. Often "quality of life" is used by the authors of scientific papers without explicit definition, and a wide range of variables are used as measures of quality of life (QL) (from physiologic indicators such as weight loss, to standardized psychologic measures of emotional distress) (8). "Quality of life" has been a frequently abused catch phrase; however, there is growing consensus about its definition. Two research groups have proposed definitions: 1) "Quality of life is the subjective evaluation of life as a whole" (9). 2) Quality of life "refers to patients' appraisal of and satisfaction with their current level of functioning compared to what they perceive to be possible or ideal" (10). The first definition emphasizes the subjectivity of the measurement, as well as the importance of a global assessment or summary score. The second definition also highlights the subjectivity of quality of life assessment, as well as the preference or value given to the person's current health state. For example, two people with the same disability may place a different value on their current health state. Conceptually, both of these definitions contribute to our understanding of the phrase "quality of life," however they do not necessarily indicate how one should measure it.

Many recent reviews and papers have focused on the evolving conceptualization of quality of life (QL) (11,12,13,14). While the concept of QL has broad, general meaning based on its roots in ancient philosophical works (15), contemporary definitions and measurement strategies derive from historical efforts designed to measure the well-being of the population using social indicators such as general satisfaction and happiness, as well as satisfaction with housing, employment, income, etc. (16,17,18), as well as from the World Health

Table 18.1 Historical Aspects of Health-Related Quality of Life Assessment

World Health Organization Definition of Health, 1948

Functional Health Classification Schemes

(e.g., N.Y. Heart Association, Arthritis, Karnofsky Performance Status (1940–1950)

Social Indicators Research the Great Society (1960s)

The RAND Health Insurance Experiment (1970s)

Patient's Rights Movement (1980s)

Organization (WHO) definition of health as a "state of complete physical, mental, and social well-being and not merely the absence of disease" (19). While the WHO definition was considered impossible to operationalize and measure at the time of its publication, contemporary QL assessment tools focus on these three critical dimensions of health and QL. Current conceptualization of QL as measured in relationship to disease and treatment is called health-related quality of life (HRQL), as it tends to limit the focus to dimensions of QL that are directly affected by health and/or disease states (12,20). (See Table 18.1 for highlights of the history of QL assessment).

One of the first major research efforts directed at measuring the health and well-being of individuals occurred three decades ago when Lester Breslow and colleagues studied a population sample in Alameda County, California (2). In their work, they adopted the WHO definition of health to guide their assessment of the population, focusing on the physical, emotional and social dimensions of well-being. Although they examined some social indicators in their study sample, the main thrust of their work was on the self-reported evaluation of the three dimensions of well-being. These early QL researchers demonstrated the feasibility and reliability of asking people about these dimensions of HRQL.

In oncology practice, the Karnofsky Performance Status scale (22) was an early tool that was developed to measure the functional performance of cancer patients. The scale was developed by clinicians primarily to collect and record information that was thought to be important for diagnosis, treatment, and clinical response. Although widely accepted clinically, the reliability of clinically-rated scales like the Karnofsky tends to be poor (23), which limits their use for monitoring health care outcomes and QL. Although the Karnofsky Performance Status scale correlates highly with the physical functioning dimension of QL questionnaires in some studies, it does not seem to correlate well with overall measures of quality of life in cancer patients (24). The measure is limited further by being *clinician* rather than *patient*-rated . However, it has the advantage of being brief, acceptable in the clinical setting, and having a clear relationship to other important clinical variables such as mortality (22,23).

Early in the 1980s, Spitzer and colleagues developed a tool specifically to evaluate the quality of life of cancer patients (25). This instrument contains a uniscale for the global evaluation of QL, along with separate components that evaluate the physical and emotional aspects of QL. This latter 10 point scale is appealing because of its simplicity, as well as the ease with which it can be rated by an observer. For this reason, it was extensively used in cancer research during the 1980s (e.g., the National Hospice Study). However, during the past decade there was growing consensus that QL should be rated by the patient rather than by a clinician or proxy (26). Thus, many new tools have been developed to capture the patient's own assessment of QL. The National Cancer Institute has had two workshops (1990 and 1995) on the topic of QL assessment in clinical trials (27), and now each of the clinical trials cooperative groups has clinical investigators and staff devoted to consideration of inclusion of QL endpoints in clinical treatment trials. In addition, many pharmaceutical companies are routinely including QL measures as part of the evaluation of new drugs. Recently, improvements in QL, (including pain and symptom relief), have been acknowledged as being relevant endpoints in the new drug approval process.

Multi-dimensionality of QL

Most experts in this field perceive QL as a multidimensional construct that includes several key dimensions (13,14,20,28,29). These include **physical functioning** (performance of self-care activities, functional status, mobility, physical activities, and role activities such as work or household responsibilities); **disease and treatment-related symptoms** (specific symptoms from the disease such as pain or shortness of breath, or side effects of drug therapy such as nausea, hair loss, impotence or sedation); **psychological functioning** (anxiety or depression that may be secondary to the disease or its treatment); social functioning (disruptions in normal social activities). Additional considerations in the evaluation of QL may include spiritual or existential concerns, sexual functioning and body image, and satisfaction with health care. Figure 18.1 represents one author's conceptualization of the dimensionality of QL (30).

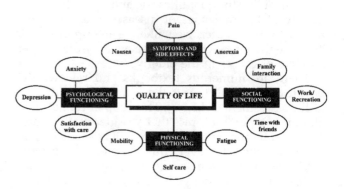

Figure 18.1 The multidimensional aspects of the quality of life construct. Adapted from reference 30.

Whenever possible, HRQL should be assessed by the patient (8,31) and should reflect the evaluation of a number of dimensions affecting his/her life at that moment. Although the specific dimensions that are the most satisfactory or unsatisfactory at any point in time may vary, the individual's QL may in fact remain stable or change depending on how these dimensions fluctuate and interact. For this reason, some have argued that both the component dimensions of QL as well as a global assessment should be considered (32). Therefore, in the research or clinical setting, one should always ask what specific dimensions of QL are likely to be affected, and choose a QL tool based on its content relevance to the questions of interest.

Measurement of QL

Data Collection Methods

Although there is consensus that QL should be assessed by the patient, there are a variety of ways in which this information can be obtained. The clinical interview (using structured questions from a validated instrument) is the most comprehensive approach in that it allows participation of the greatest number individuals (e.g., those who cannot read or write, those with visual impairment or frailty). However, the personal interview is more costly in personnel and time, and there may be some bias introduced through in-person interaction. Interviews can be conducted in-person or by telephone, and can assure less missing data. For geriatric research, the clinical interview is a standard approach for a variety of reasons, but often because of the frailty of the target population.

In contrast, most of the research on QL in cancer patients has focused on self-administered questionnaires. This has occurred primarily because of an interest in the inclusion of QL assessments in clinical trials, where extensive personnel for conduct of interviews is unavailable. The advantages of the self administered format include: limited need for personnel to collect data, more accurate responses for sensitive information, administration at a time and place that are convenient for the patient. However, there are important limitations to self-administered instruments which include a requirement for literacy and language translation, familiarity with completion of pencil and paper tests, and the increased likelihood of missing data. In addition, very ill patients (e.g., Karnofsky score less than 60), may have difficulty completing more than the briefest scales (33).

Ideally, a combination of these two approaches should be used in the assessment of QL in cancer patients. One can start with the self-administered format, and reserve the structured research interview for those patients who are unable to complete the written form without assistance. Even when a self-administered format is used, however, it is important to review all questionnaires for missing data. Thus, the combination of the two approaches can lead to the greatest efficiency in terms of data completeness and personnel

time. In the Medical Outcomes Study, which included a sizeable portion of outpatients over 65 years of age, their fairly lengthy survey was self-administered by the majority of subjects, with telephone interview required in the remainder (34). While in general, results from self-report and telephone interviews are similar, there can be some variation, especially on sensitive topics, and researchers should track the mode of administration. In research studies with older cancer patients, an attempt should be made to collect the data in a single systematic format. If resources permit, the interview may be the best approach to ensure inclusion of all eligible older patients.

Choice of Instruments

In the field of QL assessment there is a tension between using instruments that are highly specific to the research or clinical question at hand (e.g., a unique toxicity for a treatment), versus use of a tool that has been widely used with other samples of cancer patients or patients with other chronic conditions (e.g., diabetes, arthritis, heart disease). The debate revolves around the use of generic measures or cancer specific/cancer site and phase specific tools (see Table 18.2). In considering the geriatric cancer patient, one must also consider a whole body of geriatric assessment tools as an additional reference point (e.g., Mini-Mental Status Exam, the Geriatric Depression Scale). However, for the purpose of this discussion, we will focus on scales that have been used in a broad range of populations.

Generic instruments such as the RAND measures (34,35,36), the Dartmouth COOP charts (37), the Duke scales (38), all have considerable value if one wishes to compare the general impact of differing diseases/conditions on HRQL. From a policy standpoint, this may be important in terms of preventing discrimination against cancer patients, as their functional status and quality of life may exceed patients with other chronic conditions (39). On the other hand, the information obtained from these scales often lacks the sensitivity to detect impairments from cancer treatments (40,41).

In contrast, the cancer-specific QL instruments (e.g., FLIC, EORTC, CARES, FACT) that have been developed during the past decade have high reliability and validity, and are responsive to changes from treatments (42). In addition, they are more likely to capture the known toxicities and concerns related to cancer treatment. Therefore, they should be a preferred choice in the comparative evaluation of cancer treatments. However, one must recognize that each of these generic cancer-specific instruments may need to be supplemented with disease-specific modules (e.g., for breast cancer, prostate cancer, leukemia, etc.) or condition-specific questions that target specific QL issues (e.g., pain, nausea, sexual functioning). Thus, in designing a QL assessment, one must carefully define the expected impacts of the disease and its treatment on QL, and use a battery of assessment tools that are likely to reflect these effects.

In considering how to assess QL in the geriatric cancer patient, one must follow the same general prin-

Table 18.2 Examples of HRQL Instruments Used with Cancer Patients

Generic Health Status Measures

Sickness Impact Profile (SIP)

RAND Health Insurance Experiment Measures

Medical Outcomes Study (MOS) Instruments

Nottingham Heath Profile

Psychosocial Adjustment to Illness Scale (PAIS)

Dartmouth COOP Charts

Generic Cancer-Specific Instruments

Quality of Life Index (Spitzer)

Quality of Life Index (Padilla and Grant)

Functional Living Index — Cancer (FLIC)

European Organization for Research and Treatment of Cancer Quality of Life Questionnaire (EORTC-QLC)

Cancer Rehabilitation Evaluation System (CARES)

Functional Assessment of Cancer Therapy (FACT)

Cancer Site-Specific Instruments

Breast Cancer Chemotherapy Questionnaire

Linear Analogue Self-Assessment (LASA) for Breast Cancer

Performance Parameter (Head & Neck)

Site-specific modules for the FACT and the EORTC-QLQ

Symptom-Oriented Scales

Rotterdam Symptom Checklist

Symptom Distress Scale (McCorkle)

Memorial Pain Assessment Card

Morrow Assessment of Nausea and Emesis (MANE) Scale

ciples as for other populations; however, special issues may arise in very frail elderly samples, especially those who are not routinely included in clinical trials because of other exclusion criteria. Relatively little research has been conducted with this group of cancer patients and it is unclear whether other chronic conditions (e.g., arthritis, heart and pulmonary disease) will overwhelm any specific contribution made by the cancer. This is clearly an area ripe for further research, and is beginning to receive attention from several (43,44) investigators.

Role of QL Assessment in Cancer Treatment

QL assessment can be used for a variety of purposes: to describe the impact of cancer and its treatment on patients; to compare the outcome of different treatments in clinical trials; to identify unanticipated benefits or toxicities of treatment; to inform future treatment planning through modification of aspects which detract from QL. Information gained from prior QL research can help inform treatment decisions. For example, multiple studies have shown that overall QL, and most of its dimensions, differ little among women who choose mastectomy over lumpectomy in the primary treatment of breast cancer (45). Therefore, a woman who is considering alterative surgical treatments for breast cancer can be reassured that her subsequent adjustment will not be dependent on the type of surgery she receives. However, since research has shown that there is much more body image disruption from mastectomy compared to lumpectomy (46), a woman who expresses concerns about her body image should be encouraged to consider a lumpectomy.

Several studies have also demonstrated that QL is an important prognostic factor for survival (33,47). While this should not be the only variable used in considering whether a patient should receive aggressive cancer therapy, assessing patient-rated QL could help physicians determine more systematically when only palliative care should be offered. In this regard, there is mounting evidence that physicians regularly ignore the advanced directives or expressed wishes of patients regarding end-of-life support (48). Regular evaluation of a patients QL over time can capture functional deterioration, which physician's poorly assess (31). Physician reluctance to engage in discussions with seriously ill patients are likely to be enhanced by more objective and quantified measures of outcome. Although these issues are relevant to all cancer patients, they are particularly salient for the elderly who are responsible for the majority of cancer deaths.

Common Cancers in the Elderly and Important QL Concerns

Breast Cancer

Breast cancer is the most common cancer in women in Western industrialized countries. The disease has a bimodal distribution with the greatest incidence in older women (49). Older women are diagnosed with breast cancer at a more advanced stage, and this probably directly results from less frequent screening for breast cancer (mammography and physical exam) (50,51). Once diagnosed, there are additional differences in the patterns of care for older versus younger women with breast cancer (52,53,54,55). All of these factors contribute to a poorer overall survival for older women with breast cancer (49).

In a recent review of breast cancer care in old age (43), the authors point out that there is considerable variation in the care of older women with breast cancer (e.g., lumpectomy without radiation therapy, inconsistent use of tamoxifen; omission of axillary lymph node dissection). These variations in care may have a substantial impact on QL as well as survival, yet they

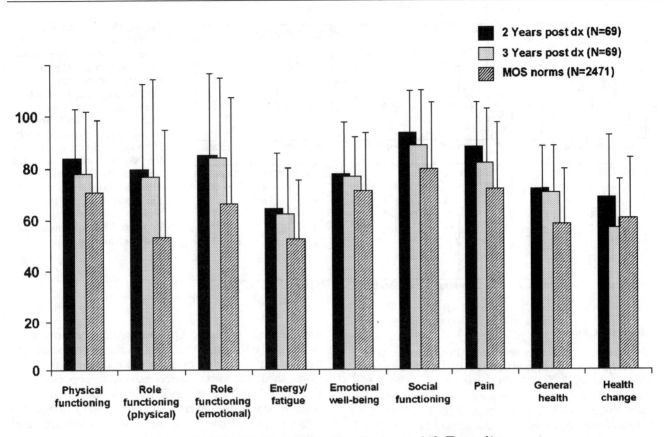

RAND 36-Item Health Survey 1.0 Results

Figure 18.2 RAND 36-Item Health Survey results in breast cancer survivors who are two and three years since diagnosis compared to non-cancer outpatients. Breast cancer data from reference 41 and non-cancer outpatients data from 36. Data presented are mean and one standard deviation (bar) for each scale.

have not been studied systematically. Indeed, little is known about whether patients are actually consulted as these decisions are made, or whether physicians have assumed patient preferences (e.g., more frequent use of mastectomy over lumpectomy in older women). There is an emerging interest in studying alternative treatment strategies for older women with breast cancer (e.g., omission of axillary node dissection). Whenever possible, these therapeutic studies should be coupled with evaluation of QL outcomes.

Although there is a growing literature on QL in breast cancer patients, few studies have examined the relationship of age to QL. In a series of reports from a longitudinal cohort study (N=227) of newly-diagnosed breast cancer followed in the first year after surgery, we have demonstrated better adjustment in older women with breast cancer (56), and in a predictive model for psychosocial distress in the year after breast cancer, women older than 55 years fared better (57). These findings are consonant with the literature (39), and suggest that older women are resilient, in spite of increasing physical limitations that occur with age. Other variables that may be important include social support and co-morbid conditions. However, as is generally the case, QL cannot be predicted and should

be assessed directly by the patient. Therefore, although, in general, older women adapt well to breast cancer, some may not.

With the increasing use of generic measures of QL, such as the RAND and MOS measures, we will begin to be able to compare the well-being of cancer patients to the general population of outpatients and individuals with specific other chronic conditions. In a study of long-term breast cancer survivors, we used the RAND 36-item health survey 1.0 to evaluate QL in 2 and 3 year breast cancer survivors (41). Compared to outpatients with chronic medical conditions, the breast cancer survivors were functioning at a higher level (range about .5 SD for most subscales) (See Figure 18.2). These findings would argue that breast cancer survivors have comparatively high levels of functioning, similar to other non-cancer outpatients visiting medical offices. On the other hand, in this same report which used the CARES (58), we demonstrated a substantial number of ongoing rehabilitation concerns, especially in the area of body image and sexual functioning (41). These latter observations point to the greater sensitivity of a cancer-specific measure in capturing disease-specific concerns that are not readily assessed in a general population measure of QL.

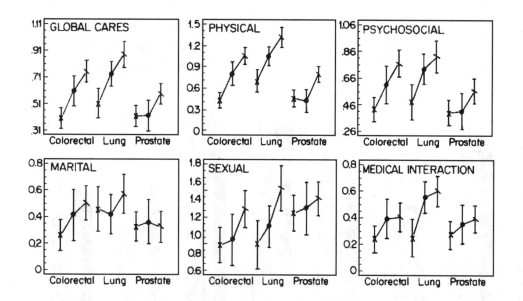

Figure 18.3 Mean global CARES and CARES summary scale scores (with 95% confidence intervals) for three cancer sites (colorectal, lung, prostate) according to extent of disease. The 'x' indicates the mean value for patients who have no evidence of disease, the '●' indicates mean value for patients with limited disease, and the '\' indicates the mean value for patients with extensive disease. Reprinted from reference 60 with permission.

Colorectal Cancer

Colorectal cancer ranks second to lung cancer as the most frequent cause of cancer death in the United States, (with more than 55,000 deaths anticipated in 1995) (59). It affects men and women equally, and is a particular health threat in the aging population. In contrast to breast cancer, which is often diagnosed at a localized or regional stage, colorectal cancer is diagnosed at a localized stage in only 37% of cases, and in 19% of cases it is metastatic at the time of diagnosis (59). Relatively few clinical trials have studied QL among colorectal cancer patients. As a common disease affecting the elderly, colorectal cancer has largely been neglected.

In our own work evaluating the CARES, we have studied a group of patients with colorectal cancer and have compared them to patients with lung and prostate cancer (60). All of the patient samples were older (mean for colorectal 62.6 years with range of 28–89 years; mean for lung 61.6 years with range of 23–87 years; mean for prostate 69.0 years with range of 43–90 years). In a group of comparisons of patients with no evidence of disease, localized disease and metastatic disease, colorectal cancer patients fared better than patients with lung cancer in many dimensions of QL, but poorer than prostate cancer patients, except in the area of sexual functioning (Figure 18.3). This findings might be anticipated based on the more severe physical symptoms associated with lung cancer and the specific sexual problems associated with prostate cancer.

In a separate study focusing on adult cancer survivors, we examined the long term QL of 117 colorectal cancer survivors using the CARES (61). Predictors of QL (as measured by the CARES) in this sample of patients included Karnofsky Performance Status, type of hospital in which treatment was received (private hospital most favorable), gender (males had more favorable QL), and work status (better QL for those who were not working). In contrast to the lung and prostate cancer survivors, colorectal cancer survivors

experienced improved QL the greater the time since diagnosis, with improvements in the psychosocial dimension of QL. However, in spite of these observations, these colorectal cancer survivors reported continuing rehabilitation concerns in a number of areas (e.g., worry about cancer recurrence, body image disruption, sexual dysfunction, at work concerns, and financial/insurance issues) (61).

Lung Cancer

Lung cancer is the most common cause of cancer mortality in both men and women and is common in the elderly (59). Survival is poor in this cancer primarily due to advanced stage of disease in patients at diagnosis, and the limited survival benefit from chemotherapy and radiation therapy. Chemotherapy for this disease is quite toxic, and thus it may contribute to poorer quality of life, especially in patients with minimal or no response to treatment. Although several meta-analyses support a modest improvement in survival from chemotherapy in advanced non-small cell lung cancer (62,63), many clinicians and patients are concerned about the QL benefits of treatments. This remains an important area for continuing investigation in clinical trials.

Several studies have demonstrated that patient-rated QL in lung cancer patients provides additional prognostic information beyond performance status and other biologic variables (33,64). This has been demonstrated with a variety of QL measures, including the FLIC. In a study we completed, there was also a suggestion that social support (as measured by marital status) moderated the effects of poorer QL on prediction of survival (33). In our study that compared the CARES in patients with colorectal, lung and prostate cancer (see above)(60), lung cancer patients demonstrated the poorest physical functioning at all phases of illness, and the metastatic lung cancer patients had substantially more impairment in overall quality of life, physical functioning, psychological functioning, and marital functioning than patients with metastatic prostate cancer (see Figure 18.3) (60). In our examination of lung cancer survivors (average age 62.38 years) (61), QL was predicted by Karnofsky Performance Status only (compare to colorectal cancer patients discussed earlier), suggesting that the physical impact of the disease, treatment, and perhaps co-existent pulmonary disease, have a major impact on QL in lung cancer survivors (61).

Prostate Cancer

Prostate cancer is primarily a disease of aging men, and now is the leading cancer in men (59). The recent increase in new prostate cancer cases is due largely to the expansion of population screening with the prostatic specific antigen (PSA) blood test. Major controversies exist related to the benefits of PSA screening with respect to mortality, the survival benefit of treatment in men older than 70 years, and the morbidity associated with surgery and radiation, compared with observation. All of these controversial areas are the subject of clinical trials, and many ongoing studies include QL assessments. Specific QL issues include: 1) the psychological impact of a false positive screening test, along with the physical and psychological morbidity of diagnostic tests; 2) the sexual and urinary dysfunction associated with radical prostatectomy surgery; 3) the sexual, urinary and bowel dysfunction associated with radiation therapy for prostate cancer; 4) the psychological and overall QL impact of watchful waiting as a treatment strategy for prostate cancer.

As it may be many years before the QL results from on-going clinical trials are reported, it may be useful to look at some existing information on QL in prostate cancer patients. In our study of colorectal, lung and prostate cancer patients (60), our sample included 288 prostate cancer patients (see above age distributions). Patients who were disease-free or only had a local recurrence had similar assessments in all dimension assessed by the CARES. Patients with advanced metastatic prostate cancer experienced poorer overall QL as well as poorer physical and psychosocial functioning. Interestingly, sexual functioning was impaired in all phases of the illness and was substantially worse than the lung and colorectal cancer patients (see Figure 18.3). As noted earlier, in spite of being older the prostate cancer patients in general had a better QL in most dimensions than patients with the other types of cancer.

In our study of the prostate cancer survivors (61), significant predictors of QL included Karnofsky Performance status (higher score more favorable), medical co-morbidity and time since diagnosis (both associated with poorer QL). Psychiatric co-morbidity was also associated with poorer QL. There was a trend favoring treatment in a private hospital setting and an association with better QL. This sample of survivors was on average 69.5 years and the long-term survivors were on average 73.44 years. Therefore, in this aging sample of prostate cancer patients there may be substantial interaction between cancer and other chronic illnesses (61).

In another cross-sectional study of prostate cancer survivors treated for localized prostate cancer, we examined the QL of patients receiving surgery, radiation therapy, or observation in comparison to age matched non-cancer controls (40). In this study we used a generic measure of QL (RAND 36-item Health survey), two cancer-specific QL instruments (CARES-SF and the FACT), and a newly developed condition specific measure targeting urinary, sexual and bowel function (40). On average, the patients were more than 5 years since diagnosis of prostate cancer, and were elderly (surgery patients were mean age 69.7; radiation therapy patients were mean age 76.2; observation patients were mean age 75.2; control group were mean age 72.5). Other demographic and medical history variables were comparable across all four groups. The QL evaluation found no difference on the RAND measure among the four groups, with the exception of lower emotional role functioning in the observation prostate cancer patients. For the two cancer-specific QL tools, the only significant difference between the cancer patients and controls occurred in sexual functioning, which was poorer in the cancer patients than controls, and in medical interaction (e.g., communication with doctors and nurses) which was somewhat poorer in the surgically treated and observation groups. Overall, these cancer patients looked similar to their age-matched, non-cancer controls in most dimensions of QL (40).

An added value from this study, however, was the sensitivity of the new condition specific measure (40), in detecting treatment-related differences in functioning. Sexual functioning was poorest in the surgery group (significantly worse than observation and control), and observation patients were worse than control subjects. Urinary functioning was also poorest in the surgery group, and was significantly worse than the irradiation, observation and control groups. Bowel functioning was most impaired in the irradiation group, as might have been predicted. We concluded that "Physicians interacting with prostate cancer patients should advise them that treatment is unlikely to affect general health-related QL, but it may be associated with clinically significant changes in sexual, urinary, or bowel function. Any survival gain from surgery or radiation must be balanced with expected decrements in some areas of function and bother" (40).

Special Aspects of QL in the Older Cancer Patient

Often there have been assumptions made about the QL impact of cancer and its treatment on older patients. These include the belief that older patients suffer more side effects from treatment or have more difficulty adjusting to a cancer diagnosis. As indicated earlier, the elderly are quite heterogeneous and one cannot assume that chronologic age is the primary factor affecting functioning or well-being. In a study by Kahn and colleagues (65), 300 matched pairs of adult patients with cancer and their physicians were interviewed concerning the effects of disease and treatment on the patients' QL. The physicians overestimated the problems of the elderly cancer patients, while in actuality younger patients reported more difficulties. These authors suggest that physicians need to become more sensitized to the individualized, personal nature of their patients' QL and the factors that may shape or modify it (65). Thus, it is critical that health care providers assess the individual patient's QL; there is no room for paternalistic decision-making for older adults simply because of their age.

Where side effects of cancer treatment have been examined (e.g., nausea and vomiting), older patients often fare better than younger patients, requiring less anti-emetic therapy (66). Some side effects, such as diarrhea (and resultant dehydration), may be more of a problem in the older cancer patient receiving chemotherapy. Pain is an important symptom that may detract from QL (67,68), and care should be given to provide adequate education and treatment for this problem. Although pain research specific to the elderly is sparse (69,70), older persons with cancer are the majority of those cared for in hospice programs, where excellent palliative care is a primary goal.

Several studies have documented better mental health in the elderly in general, with consistent findings among older cancer patients (39). Life experiences, as well as familiarity with the health care setting, allow older cancer patients to cope with a cancer diagnosis with more resiliency. With fewer responsibilities to juggle (e.g., child care, work), as well as awareness that this is a disease experience their peers have had, older cancer patients often are not as distressed as younger cancer patients. A specific issue for the elderly, however, may be their need for assistance of various types. In a detailed study of determinants of need and unmet need among cancer patients residing at home, Mor and colleagues (71) found that physiological factors (metastases, disease stage, and functional status) were associated with the need for assistance in the areas of personal care, instrumental tasks, and transportation. Also, older age (over 65) and low income predicted need for help with personal care, and women were more likely than men to report illness-related need for assistance with instrumental tasks and transportation. Unmet need was primarily associated with the patients' social support system (71). Again, there may be considerable variation in the degree of social support among elderly cancer patients, and this may influence the patient's functioning and well-being. Health care providers should include evaluation of social support when considering treatment decisions as well as the patient's subjective assessment of well-being.

Conclusions and Future Directions

Although the majority of cancer patients are over age 60 years, the elderly are not always adequately represented in clinical trials or quality of life research. In particular, patients with co-morbid conditions or physiologic abnormalities of aging (e.g., decreased renal function) usually are excluded from clinical treatment trials. Therefore, it may be difficult to extrapolate information obtained in clinical trials to the general elderly population. There is increasing awareness of the need for effectiveness studies (examination of what clinical practices work in the real world) to determine which treatments are best for the general community of older cancer patients. Similarly, QL studies in older cancer patients should be conducted under these circumstances to better understand their values and estimation of QL. These studies are particularly necessary because of the exclusion of these patients from usual clinical cancer research.

Beyond research, considerable improvement in patient care will likely occur with the advancement of the outcomes movement and the integration of QL assessments into routine care (2). Unfortunately, the tools that have been developed to monitor outcomes among groups of patients do not as yet have the precision to monitor all dimensions of HRQL accurately in clinical practice (72). If nothing else, an acknowledgment of the value of the patient's own subjective assessment of well-being must remain central to any considerations about cancer treatment, and physicians may use information derived from research studies to help them identify important areas for inquiry in their conversations with their patients (73). Most importantly, patients care about these issues, and therefore physicians and other health care providers must include consideration of HRQL issues in treatment planning for older cancer patients.

References

1. Calman KC. Definitions and Dimensions of Quality of Life. In *The Quality of Life of Cancer Patients*, edited by NK Aaronson, J Beckman. New York: Raven Press, 1–9, 1987.
2. Ellwood PM. Shattuck Lecture. Outcomes management: A technology of patient experience. *The New England Journal of Medicine* 1988; **318**: 1549–1556.
3. Aaronson NK, Beckmann J. *The Quality of Life of Cancer Patients*. New York: Raven Press, 1987.
4. McDowell I, Newell C. *Measuring Health: A guide to Rating Scales and Questionnaires*. New York: Oxford University Press, 1987.
5. Tchekmedyian NS, Cella DF. Quality of life in current oncology practice and research. *Oncology* May 1990; **4**(5 Supplement).
6. Tchekmedyian NS, Cella DF, Winn RT. Economic and quality of life outcomes in oncology. *Oncology* November 1995; **9**(11 Supplement).
7. Osoba D. *Effect of Cancer on Quality of Life*. Boca Raton, Florida: CRC Press, 1991.
8. Hollandsworth JG Jr. Evaluating the impact of medical treatment on the quality of life: a five year update. *Social Science and Medicine* 1988; **26**: 425–434.
9. De Haes JCJM. Quality of life: Conceptual and theoretical considerations. In *Psychosocial Oncology*, edited by M Watson, S Greer, C Thomas. Oxford: Pergamon Press, pp. 61–70, 1988.
10. Cella DF, Cherin EA. Quality of life during and after cancer treatment. *Comprehensive Ther* 1988; **14**(5): 69–75.
11. Cella DF, Tulsky DS. Quality of life in cancer: Definition, purpose, and method of measurement. *Cancer Investigation* 1993; **11**(3): 327–336.
12. Guyatt GH, Feeny DH, Patrick DL. Measuring health-related quality of life. *Annals of Internal Medicine* 1993; **118**: 622–629.
13. Aaronson NK. Quality of life: What is it? How should it be measured. *Oncology* 1988; **2**: 69–74.

14. De Haes JCJM, Van Knippenberg FCE. The quality of life of cancer patients: A review of the literature. *Soc Sci Med* 1985; **20**: 809–817.

15. Aristotle. *Ethics*. Harmondsworth, England: Penguin Books, 1976.

16. Andrews FM, Withey SB. *Social Indicators of Well Being: Americans' Perception of Life Quality*. New York: Plenum, 1976.

17. Campbell A. Subjective measures of well-being. *American Psychologist* 1974; **31**: 117–124.

18. Campbell A. *The Sense of Well-being in America: Recent Patterns and Trends*. New York: McGraw-Hill, 1981.

19. World Health Organization. *Constitution in Basic Documents*. Geneva: World Health Organization, 1948.

20. Ware JE Jr. Conceptualizing disease impact and treatment outcomes. *Cancer* 1984; **53** (Supplement): 2316–2323.

21. Breslow L. A quantitative approach to the World Health Organization definition of health: Physical, mental and social well-being. *International Journal of Epidemiology* 1972; **1**: 347–355.

22. Karnofsky DA, Burchenal JH. The clinical evaluation of chemotherapeutic agents in cancer. In *Evaluation of Chemotherapeutic Agents*, edited by CM Macleod. New York: Columbia University Press, 1949, 199–205.

23. Patrick DL, Deyo RA. Generic and disease-specific measures in assessing health status and quality of life. *Medical Care* 1989; **27**: S217–S232.

24. Adams AG, Britt DM, Godding PR, *et al*. Relative contribution of the Karnofsky Performance Status scale in a multi-measure assessment of quality of life in cancer patients. *Psycho-Oncology* 1995; **4**: 239–246.

25. Spitzer WO, Dobson AJ, Hall J, *et al*. Measuring the quality of life of cancer patients. *Journal of Chronic Diseases* 1981; **34**: 585–597.

26. Moinpour CM. Quality of life assessment in Southwest Oncology Group Trials. *Oncology* (May 1990) **4**: 79–89.

27. Nayfield SG, Hailey BJ. Quality of Life Assessment in Cancer Clinical Trials. *Report of the Workshop on Quality of Life Research in Clinical Trials* held July 16–17, 1990. Bethesda, MD: U.S. Dept. of Health and Human Services, Public Health Service, NIH.

28. Patrick DL, Erickson P. Assessing health-related quality of life for clinical decision making. In *Quality of Life: Assessment and Application*, edited by SM Walker, RM Rosser. Lancaster: MTP Press Limited, 9–49, 1988.

29. Schipper H, Clinch J, McMurray A, Levitt M. Measuring the quality of life of cancer patients: The Functional Living Index — Cancer: Development and validation. *J Clin Oncol* 1984; **2**: 472–483.

30. Tcheckmedyian NS, Hickman M, Sian J, *et al*. Treatment of cancer anorexia with megestrol acetate: impact on quality of life. *Oncology* 1990; **4**: 185–92.

31. Slevin ML, Plant H, Lynch D, *et al*. Who should measure quality of life, the doctor or the patient? *British Journal of Cancer* 1988; **57**: 109–112.

32. DeHaes JCJM, van Knippenberg FCE. Quality of life instruments for cancer patients: Babel's tower revisited. *Journal of Clinical Epidemiology* 1989; **42**: 1239–1241.

33. Ganz PA, Haskell CM, Figlin R, *et al*. Estimating the quality of life in a clinical trial of metastatic lung cancer using the Karnofsky Performance Status and the Functional Living Index — Cancer (FLIC). *Cancer* 1988; **61**: 849–856.

34. Stewart AL, Ware JE. Measuring function and well-being. *The Medical Outcomes Study Approach*. Durham: Duke University Press, 1992.

35. Ware JE, Sherbourne CD. The MOS 36-Item Short-Form Health Survey (SF-36): I. Conceptual framework and item selection. *Medical Care*; **30**: 473–483, 1992.

36. Hays RD, Sherbourne CD, Mazel RM. The RAND 36-Item Health Survey 1.0. *Health Economics* 1993; **2**: 217–227.

37. Nelson E, Wasson J, Kirk J, *et al*. Assessment of function in routine clinical practice: Description of the COOP chart method and preliminary findings. *J Chronic Disease* 1987; **40**(Suppl): 55S–63S.

38. Parkerson GR, Broadhead WE, Tse CJ. The Duke Health Profile: A 17-item measure of health and dysfunction. *Medical Care* 1990; **28**: 1056–1072.

39. Cassileth BR, Lusk EJ, Strouse TB, Miller DS, Brown LL, Cross PA, Tenaglin AN. Psychosocial status in chronic illness. *New England Journal of Medicine* 1984; **311**: 506–511.

40. Litwin MS, Hays RD, Fink A, Ganz PA, Leake B, Leach GE, Brook RH. Quality-of-life outcomes in men treated for localized prostate cancer. *JAMA* 1995; **273**: 129–135.

41. Ganz PA, Coscarelli A, Fred C, Kahn B, Polinsky ML, Petersen L. Breast cancer survivors: Psychosocial concerns and quality of life. *Breast Can Res and Treat* (in press).

42. Cella DF, Bonomi AE. Measuring quality of life: 1995 update. *Oncology* 1995; **9**(11 Supplement): 47–60.

43. Silliman RA, Balducci L, Goodwin JS, Holmes FF, Leventhal EA. Breast cancer care in old age: What we know, don't know, and do. *Journal of the National Cancer Institute* 1993; **85**: 190–9.

44. Goodwin JS, Hunt WC, Samet JM. Determinants of cancer therapy in elderly patients. *Cancer* 1993; **72**: 594–601.

45. Kiebert GM, de Haes JCJM, van de Velde CJH. The impact of breast-conserving treatment and mastectomy on the quality of life of early-stage breast cancer patients: A review. *J Clin Oncol* 1991; **9**: 1059–1070.

46. Ganz PA, Schag CAC, Lee JJ, Polinsky ML, Tan S-J. Breast conservation versus mastectomy: Is there a difference in psychological adjustment or quality of life in the year after surgery? *Cancer* 1992; **69**: 1729–1738.

47. Coates A, Gebski V, Bishop JF, Jeal PN, Woods RL, Snyder R, Tattersall MH, Byrne M, Harvey V, Gill G. Improving the quality of life during chemotherapy for advanced breast cancer. A comparison of intermittent and continuous treatment strategies. *New England Journal of Medicine* 1987; **317**(24): 1490–5.

48. The Support Principal Investigators. A Controlled trials to improve care for seriously ill hospitalized patients. The Study to Understand Prognoses and Preferences for Outcomes and Risks of Treatments (SUPPORT). *JAMA* 1995; **274**: 1591–1598.

49. Yancik R, Ries LG, Yates JW. Breast cancer in aging women: A population-based study of contrasts in stage, surgery, and survival. *Cancer* 1989; **63**: 976–981.

50. Fox SA, Murata PJ, Stein JA. The impact of physician compliance on screening mammography for older women. *Arch Intern Med* 1991; **151**: 50.

51. Celentano DD, Shapiro S, Weisman CS: Cancer preventive screening behavior among elderly women. *Preventive Medicine* 1982; **11**: 454.

52. Greenfield S, Blanco DM, Elashoff RM, Ganz PA. Patterns of care related to age of breast cancer patients. *JAMA* 1987; **287**: 2766–2770.

53. Silliman RA, Guadagnoli E, Weitberg AB, Mor V. Age as a predictor of diagnostic and initial treatment intensity in newly diagnosed breast cancer patients. *Journal of Gerontology: Medical Sciences* 1989; **44**: M46–50.

54. Allen C, Cox EB, Manton, KG, *et al*. Breast cancer in the elderly. Current patterns of care. *Journal of the American Geriatrics Society*. 1986; **34**: 637.

55. Chu J, Diehr P, Feigl P, *et al*. The effect of age on the care of women with breast cancer in community hospitals. *Journal of Gerontology* 1987; **42**: 185.

56. Ganz PA, Lee JJ, Sim M-S, Polinsky ML, Schag CAC: Exploring the influence of multiple variables on the relationship of age to quality of life in women with breast cancer. *Journal of Clinical Epidemiology* 1992; **45**: 473–486.

57. Ganz PA, Hirji K, Sim M-S, Schag CAC, Fred C, Polinsky ML. Predicting psychosocial risk in patients with breast cancer. *Medical Care* 1993; **31**(5): 419–431.

58. Schag CAC, Heinrich RL. Development of a comprehensive quality of life measurement tool: CARES. *Oncology* 1990; **4**(5): 135–138.

59. Wingo PA, Tong T, Bolden S. Cancer statistics, 1995. *CA: A Cancer Journal for Clinicians* 1995; **45**: 8–30.

60. Ganz PA, Schag CAC, Lee JJ, Sim M-S. The CARES: A generic measure of health-related quality of life for cancer patients. *Quality of Life Research* 1992; **1**: 19–29.

61. Schag CAC, Ganz PA, Wing DS, Sim M-S, Lee JJ. Quality of life in adult survivors of lung, colon, and prostate cancer. *Quality of Life Research* 1994; **3**: 127–141.

62. Souquet PJ, Chauvin F, Boissel JP, Cellerino R, Cormier Y, Ganz PA, Kaasa S, Pater JL, Quoix E, Rapp E, Tumarello D, Williams J, Woods BL, Benard JP. Polychemotherapy in advanced non small cell lung cancer: Ameta-analysis. *TheLancet* 1993; **342**: 19–21.

63. Non-small Cell Lung Cancer Collaborative Group. Chemotherapy in non-small cell lung cancer: A meta-analysis using updated data on individual patients from 52 randomized clinical trials. *Brit Med J* 1995; **311**: 899–909.

64. Kaasa S, Mastekaasa A, Lund E. Prognostic factors for patients with inoperable non-small cell lung cancer, limited disease. The importance of patients' subjective experience of disease and psychological well-being. *Radiotherapy and Oncology* 1989; **15**: 35.

65. Kahn SB, Houts PS, Harding SP. Quality of life and patients with cancer: A comparative study of patient versus physician perceptions and its implications for cancer education. *Journal of Cancer Education* 1992; **7**(3): 241–9.

66. Nerenz DR, Love RR, Leventhal H, Easterling DV. Psychosocial consequences of cancer chemotherapy for elderly patients. *Health Services Research* 1986; **20**(6 Pt 2): 961–76.

67. Hillier R. Control of pain in terminal cancer. *British Medical Bulletin* 1991; **46**(1): 279–91.

68. Stein WM, Miech RP. Cancer pain in the elderly hospice patient. *Journal of Pain and Symptom Management* 1993 **8**(7): 474–82.

69. Portenoy RK. Pain management in the older cancer patient. *Oncology* 1992; **6**(2 Suppl): 86–98.

70. Ferrell BR, Ferrell BA, Ahn C, Tran K. Pain management for elderly patients with cancer at home. *Cancer* 1994; **74**(7 Suppl): 2139–46.

71. Mor V, Allen SM, Siegel K, Houts P. Determinants of need and unmet need among cancer patients residing at home. *Health Services Research* 1992; **27**(3): 337–60.

72. McHomey CA, Tarlov AR. Individual-patient monitoring in clinical practice: Are available health status surveys adequate? *Qualify of Life Research* 1995; **4**: 293–307.

73. Ganz PA. Impact of quality of life outcomes on clinical practice. *Oncology* 1995; **9**(11 Suppl): 61–65.

19. Social Support and the Elderly Cancer Patient

Cleora S. Roberts

Introduction

The elderly person diagnosed with cancer must deal with many changes in psychological and social functioning along with the physical health problems. The social support system, which is believed to buffer the stress of illness for patients of all ages (1–2), is a critical factor for the aging as they simultaneously experience increased need for and decreased availability of such support (3). The aging process can be accompanied by retirement, financial worries, changes in living arrangements and bereavement in response to loss of spouse, other family members or friends. All of these changes or losses pose threats to the patient's social support system.

There is considerable research evidence that older cancer patients suffer fewer negative psychosocial consequences than younger patients (4–7). Various explanations have been offered. Mor, Allen and Malin argued that older individuals may cope better because they have few competing demands such as jobs or children in their lives (8). McMillan found that older patients reported lower intensity of pain and physical symptoms, which are sources of emotional distress (9). Others have pointed out that seniors have more experience in dealing with illness and the medical setting (4,10). Massie and Holland observed that older patients have different health expectations which, coupled with more experience in coping with life stresses, prepare them to confront a cancer diagnosis with less surprise and anger (11).

Although a correlation between advancing age and better psychosocial adaptation to cancer has been demonstrated, the relationship between the two variables is not a strong one. Further, as Kane observed, there is tremendous variability among older people and their social situations (12). Roberts, Cox and Reintgen reported that older breast cancer patients who were experiencing significant life stressors prior to their diagnosis had higher levels of psychological distress (13). They stressed the importance of looking beyond age differences (older versus younger patients) and looking instead at specific life circumstances of older patients as predictors of their adjustment to cancer.

Defining Social Support

Although the term "social support" is widely used by health professionals, agreement as to its specific defi-

nition is lacking. In general, social support has been defined and measured using one of two different approaches (3). Objective measures attempt to quantify an individual's social interactions by assessing the size and density of one's social networks. Objective definitions of social network could include reliance on relatives, frequency of contact with friends or family, or memberships in social organizations such as churches or neighborhood groups. Alternately, social support has been defined subjectively and focuses on the person's perception and evaluation of the adequacy of his or her social relationships. Some researchers have concluded that the subjective measure of perceived adequacy of support is more predictive of positive outcome than objective measures of availability of support (14).

Wortman (15) reviewed the literature on social support and the cancer patient and identified five types of social support: (1) expression of positive affect or caring, (2) agreement with one's beliefs and feelings, (3) encouragement of open expression of beliefs and feelings, (4) provision of material aid and (5) inclusion in a network of mutual or reciprocal help. Wortman suggested that social support assessments of cancer patients should look at both emotional support and tangible aid (transportation to treatment appointments, help with household chores, assistance with medications).

Effects of Social Support

There are two hypotheses as to how social support operates in relation to health and mental health outcomes. One posits that social support has a stress buffering effect (2) while the other claims a direct or main effect. Ryan and Austin postulate that direct and buffering effects of social support may function simultaneously and that a balance between the person's needs and available resources is the critical factor in health outcomes (3).

Although most researchers have explored the role of social support in quality of life during illness, some have focused on social support and mortality rates. In a sample of over 1,000 Chinese subjects aged 70 or over, subjects who were widowed or never married had a 2.3 fold risk of dying compared with married subjects (16). Additionally, subjects with higher social support (defined as integration into the community, larger networks and participation in family and social activities) had lower mortality rates. Helsing *et al.* (17) found that widowed males who remarried had lower mortality rates, but widowed females who remarried did not show different mortality rates. Vernon and Jackson also found inconsistent findings in their review of literature on social support and mortality rates (18).

Having reviewed definitions and hypothesized mechanisms of social support we will now examine research on the role of social support in four areas of management of cancer in older adults: (1) Prevention, screening and early detection, (2) Treatment, (3) Psychosocial adaptation and (4) Responses of family caregivers.

Role of Social Support in Cancer Prevention, Screening and Early Detection

Suarez *et al.* found that older Mexican-American women rated as having strong social networks were more likely to participate in cancer screening programs. Specifically, the women with close friends were more likely to have mammography and pap smear screening (19). Kang and Bloom (20) noted that Black Americans suffer higher cancer mortality rates believed to be associated with less frequent use of cancer detection tests. They examined the association of social network size with utilization of cancer screening tests among Black Americans aged 55 or older and concluded that social support was a predictor of use of mammography and occult blood stool examinations. Similarly, Richardson *et al.* (21) found that women at high risk of breast cancer by virtue of having a twin diagnosed with breast cancer were somewhat more likely to receive mammography if they were supported by their family to do so.

It is unclear what role social support plays in determining how soon a symptomatic patient seeks cancer treatment. Whereas Berkanovic (22) found that lack of social support was related to patient delay in seeking treatment, Samet *et al.* (23) reported that social support was not a significant factor in careseeking among a sample of elderly New Mexican residents.

Moritz and Satarino (24) studied 444 breast cancer patients age 55 or older to determine what factors were associated with being diagnosed at local versus advanced disease stage. Living arrangements were found to be a rather strong predictor with women living alone being more likely to be diagnosed earlier at the local stage while women living with a spouse were twice as likely to be diagnosed with advanced disease. For married women the health of the husband was an important factor in that women with healthy husbands were less likely to be diagnosed with advanced disease while women with husbands in poor health were more likely to have advanced disease. In a study involving both men and women, however, married subjects were more likely to be diagnosed with a local stage of cancer (25).

Social Support and Cancer Treatment

It is generally believed that social support is a critical variable in aiding recovery from illness. After reviewing public health and nursing literature on this topic. Ryan and Austen concluded that lack of social support is associated with longer hospitalizations and negative emotional and cognitive changes in the elderly (3). In a similar vein Berkman and colleagues found that severely ill cancer patients who lived with a spouse were less likely to be placed in long-term care facilities (26).

Based on their findings Goodwin *et al.* (27) expressed concern that patients with poor social support networks may not receive maximal treatment because of lack of assistance in areas of transportation, medication reminders and treatment decision-making. These researchers discovered that elderly cancer patients with lower levels of social support and limited access to transportation were less likely to receive definitive cancer treatments, particularly radiation therapy. In their study, patients who drove or lived with a driver were more than four times as likely to receive radiation treatment. They did not provide data analyses by gender, but it seems likely that the non-drivers were disproportionately female.

Older persons who move, perhaps upon retirement, and later are diagnosed with cancer are deprived of their former social networks as a resource. Goodwin and colleagues (28) found that recent migrants to New Mexico, the site of their study, had increased risk for poor social support for at least ten years after moving. They pointed to the important implications for sunbelt states which have a large influx of elderly migrants.

Larson *et al.* (29) analyzed the relationship between social support (measured as size and strength of the social network) and functional status of elderly lung cancer patients undergoing radiation therapy. Surprisingly, subjects with lower social support perceived themselves to have higher functional status or quality of life. The authors offer the possible interpretation that subjects with fewer social support resources may feel they have to be more self-reliant and functionally independent. In comparing functional responses to a course of therapy in their mostly male sample, patients over 65 years did not have more therapy-related problems than the younger cohort. They caution that chronological age is not sufficient to judge a patient's ability to undergo curative or palliative treatment regimens. These same researchers (30) examined the effect of social support on a slightly younger sample (age 61 and over) which included breast (42%) and lung cancer (58%) patients and found almost no relationship between social support and functional status. Although the authors do not address the issue, the conflicting findings of the two studies may be related to gender. The majority of the lung cancer patients were males, whereas the second sample included breast cancer patients and presumably the majority were females.

Mor *et al.* (31) examined cancer patients' needs and unmet needs for assistance with personal care (e.g., bathing), instrumental activities (preparing meals), transportation and home health tasks (including high tech care such as infusion therapy.) In this longitudinal study the prevalence of need for personal care increased at three and six month follow-up. Approximately one third of patients reporting need for assistance at one baseline or follow-up did not have enough help. Patients older than 65 were 1.3 times more likely to have a personal assistance need. Seventeen percent of those with need for transportation had an unmet need at some point, a finding which may well affect treatment compliance. Married patients reported more help with personal care and household tasks. The presence of children living nearby also protected patients from having unmet needs. The data suggested that the burden of care as the illness progressed weakened informal supports such as help from neighbors over time.

Psychosocial Adaptation

A number of studies have demonstrated a positive correlation between social support and enhanced psychological adjustment in cancer patients. Specifically, breast cancer patients with higher levels of support have fewer adjustment problems (32–34). Social support was found by Ell and colleagues (35) to be a significant, though modest, predictor of psychological and functional adaptation in a sample of breast, lung and colorectal cancer patients with an average age of 61 years. Patients with stronger supports also had a higher personal sense of control and more positive psychological well-being. Persons who relied upon religion also described their support systems as being stronger. As in other studies, older patients in this sample were found to have less psychological distress.

Halstead and Fernsler explored coping strategies of long-term cancer survivors (more than five years) and compared coping styles of elderly and middle-aged survivors (36). They reported that the older survivors were more likely to use and benefit from supportant strategies ("talked problem over with family and friends") as well as optimism ("tried to think positively") and palliative strategies ("tried to keep busy"). In this sample spiritual coping strategies were identified as helpful by 68% of the subjects and use of support systems was described as helpful by 42%.

Some authors have cautioned that the relationship between social support and psychosocial adjustment to illness, although generally presumed to be causal, may in fact be correlational only. Wortman pointed out that a poorly adjusted person is less likely to possess, establish, or benefit from a strong support system (15). A study by Roberts and colleagues found that when the patient personality variable of social desirability was controlled for, the relationships between social support and well-being were not as strong (37). Roberts et al. concluded that patients who are highly socialized and have strong self esteem may cultivate more satisfying social relationships and possess stronger coping mechanisms which protect them from distress. Kessler and McLeod also suggest that the patient's mental health may be the causal variable which leads to establishment of a good support system or that patient well-

being and social support operate in a web of mutual influence (38).

Role of Family and Social Network in Providing Care for Cancer Patients

Growing numbers of elderly cancer patients mandate greater understanding of the impact of age on cancer management. It is necessary to focus on the social support systems of this expanding cohort (39, 40), particularly in a climate of dehospitalization of cancer care which places demands on family members to manage illness and treatment side effects (31, 41). In addition to focusing on patients' needs, health care professionals must be aware of the special needs and stressors placed on caregivers, who are most frequently spouses or family members. A growing number of researchers have studied the stress experienced by caregivers of cancer patients.

Oberst et al. studied 47 family members of cancer patients, average age 61, receiving radiation therapy (41). Caregivers reported more stress over time as the patient experienced greater fatigue as radiation therapy progressed. Caregivers reported they expended greatest time and effort in providing transportation and emotional support. Interestingly the older caregivers saw their situation as more benign than did younger caregivers. The authors suggest that older persons may be more accepting of and better prepared to cope with the illnesses that accompany aging. Caregivers with poor health, less education and fewer financial resources reported greater stress.

Kurtz et al. also found that older caregivers of cancer patients were less depressed than their younger counterparts and perceived caregiving as being less disruptive to their lives (42). These older caregivers also reported receiving more support from friends. As the patient's illness progressed, caregivers in the Kurtz study experienced higher levels of depression and a greater impact on their own health. However, caregivers did not report a corresponding increase in support from friends during this more stressful period. In drawing conclusions, Kurtz et al. cite the findings of Vachon et al. whose widowed subjects reported that during their spouse's terminal cancer illness, family and friends withdrew "leaving the couple to face a social death long before the physical death occurred." p. 1152 (43).

Given et al. (44) examined caregiving spouses' reactions in a sample of 159 subjects, of whom 75% were female. The patients, who had a mean age of 74, had primary diagnoses of cancer, stroke, Alzheimer's and Parkinson's diseases, emphysema, diabetes or heart disease. Spousal caregivers were assessed in four domains: negative emotional reactions, feelings of responsibility for the patient, feelings of abandonment by family, and impact of caregiving on daily schedules. Negative or antisocial patient behaviors, seen less frequently in cancer patients, were correlated with negative responses by caregivers. Caregivers who perceived adequate affective and tangible support from family members reported more positive emotional reactions to their role.

Grobe *et al.* interviewed 30 terminally ill cancer patients (median age 63 years) and 28 family members to learn what services they thought were needed (45). Patients expressed greater need for help with symptoms and medical services whereas families mentioned need for respite care, emotional support, and recreation for the family members as well as more visits by the physician. The authors conclude that the cancer patient's family warrants increased attention during the patient's terminal stage and that greater communication between patients and families is needed.

Welch-McCaffrey emphasized that cancer strikes all members of the family and should be viewed as a family disease (46). She delineates several issues elderly couples must confront while coping with anxiety regarding treatment outcome. Remarried older adults may have lost a previous spouse to cancer and experience acute revival of those memories which influence negative expectations regarding the present spouse's cancer experience.

Most studies of cancer patients and their caregivers tend to assume that the two groups are mutually exclusive when, in fact, caregivers are sometimes patients and vice versa. Older caregivers may be more challenged physically in caring for an ill spouse or sibling and themselves may be characterized as hidden patients. Cancer patients may be caring for a spouse in poor health. Also, it is not uncommon for patients in their sixties or seventies to be caring for frail elderly parents. Persons in these dual roles of patient and caregiver require additional attention to address their complex psychosocial needs and stressors. Boyle points out that cancer patients who, as former caregivers, are grieving the death of family and friends to cancer and other illnesses may find it difficult to feel positive about their own chances for recovery (47). Boyle contends that patients whose spouse lost a battle with cancer may experience survivor guilt and feel obligated to "give up."

A Word of Caution about Social Support

Some investigators have found that the presence of a social support system is not a guarantee of patient benefit. Further, certain behaviors by family or friends may actually have adverse effects for the patient. Revenson *et al.* found that supportive behaviors may actually increase negative mood and decrease self-esteem in the cancer patient and hypothesized that these behaviors during periods of disability may highlight the person's inability to reciprocate that support (48). Wortman and Dunkel-Schetter observed that family and friends may hold negative feelings about the patient's illness but believe they should remain positive and cheerful in the patient's presence (49). Such behavior precludes open communication by the patient about his or her concerns about the disease and its effects.

Role of the Physician and Health Caregivers in Addressing Social Support System of the Older Adult with Cancer

Assessment

Mor, Allen and Malin point out that as cancer care becomes increasingly dehospitalized, the nursing and clerical staff in physician's offices may need to screen for and refer patients to community resources for unmet social service needs (8). They suggest that screening tools be used in oncologist's office or outpatient settings to identify patients in need of social services and referral to appropriate agencies in the community. Kane and Kane have developed questionnaires for multidimensional assessment of older patients (50). These checklists and questionnaires inquire about the patient's psychological well-being as well as their social relationships and the help they receive from others. Family members are also queried about their ability and readiness to assume caregiving tasks.

Welch-McCaffrey advocates that four categories of assessment questions be asked of the primary family support person (46). These questions relate to the caregiver's perception of the cancer crises and how it has affected the caregiver, communication skills, immediate needs and asking how the staff can be of help.

Referral to Social Support Systems

If assessment determines that the patient's natural social support system is weak or unable to fulfill patient needs, the health care team should consider referral to "artificial" support systems. Three resources should be considered. Volunteer organizations such as the American Cancer Society can provide information and assistance with concrete social service needs such as transportation. Also, local chapters of the American Cancer Society sponsor peer support counseling programs such as Reach For Recovery for breast cancer patients and Man-to-Man for prostate cancer patients. Area hospitals may be co-sponsors of these activities or have their own support programs. Professionally led group therapy programs may be available. Spiegel, Bloom and Yalom found that patients with metastatic breast cancer who met weekly for group therapy for one year had better mood and more adaptive coping than a control group (51). In a follow-up study, Spiegel and colleagues reported that support group members survived longer that the control group (52). These research findings have been widely reported and have stimulated the formation of many new support groups for cancer patients. The third and final resource to be considered for the older cancer patient is individual counseling, preferably with a social worker or other mental health professional with experience with oncology patients. Some older patients may reject such a referral as they consider it a stigma to "need" psychological help. Anticipating this reaction, some physicians refrain from making referrals to mental health agencies and thus deprive the patient of potentially beneficial treatment.

Based on my experience in medical settings with patients in need of mental health services, I recommend the following approach. A brief inquiry about a history of treatment for depression or questions about current symptoms of depression should be made. If the answers indicate presence of depressive illness, the physician should recommend consultation with a psychiatrist for evaluation (or a mental health professional who works in collaboration with psychiatrists), explaining that treatments such as counseling and/or medications are very effective in most cases of depression. It is best to recommend a particular professional with whom you are familiar and convey your confidence in working with that person on the patient's behalf. When done in a straightforward and optimistic manner, many patients, particularly those suffering from severe or unremitting depression, will accept the referral immediately. Some patients may feel hurt, insulted or rejected by the suggestion and will ask, "do you really think I need it?" My recommended response is "I believe you can continue to handle the stresses of cancer without counseling. At the same time, counseling could help you and your family and improve your overall quality of life, and I would like to see you take advantage of it." If the patient continues to voice resistance, you can suggest they think it over and let you know if they want you or your staff to arrange an appointment. Some patients will mull this over for several weeks or months before deciding to follow-up with the referral. Many patients need reassurance that your relationship with them will not be diluted or changed by their receiving psychological care.

This discussion of the role of social support of the care of the older cancer patient would not be complete if we omit the role of medical caregivers. Some investigators have conceptualized support from the health care team as a very important type of social support (53). For example, Roberts *et al.* discovered that the physician's use of interpersonal skills and provision of information during the cancer diagnostic interview was a significant predictor of a breast patient's subsequent psychological adjustment, whereas, social support from family and friends was not (54). These and similar findings underscore the importance of the physician and allied health professionals' use of a biopsychosocial model in caring for the older adult cancer patient.

References

1. Cobb S. Social support as a moderator of life stress. *Psychosom Med* 1976; **38**: 300–314.
2. Hammer M. Cored and "extended" social networks in relation to health and illness. *Soc Sci & Med* 1983; **17**: 404–411.
3. Ryan MC, Austin AG. Social supports and social networks in the aged. *Image* 1989; **21**: 176–180.
4. Ganz PA, Schag CC, Heinrich RL. The psychosocial impact of cancer on the elderly: A comparison with younger patients. *J Am Geriatr Soc* 1985; **33**: 429–435.
5. Cassileth BR, Lusk TB, Strouse DS, Miller LL, Brown PA, Cross PA, Tenaglia AN. A comparative analysis of six diagnostic groups. *N Engl J Med* 1984; **311**: 506–511.
6. Maisiak R, Gams R, Lee E, Jones B. The psychosocial support status of elderly cancer outpatients. *Prog Clin Biol Res* 1983; **120**: 395–403.
7. Roberts CS, Rosetti C, Cone D, Cavanagh D. The psychosocial impact of gynecologic cancer: A descriptive study. *J Psychosoc Oncol* 1992; **10**: 101–10.
8. Mor V, Allen S, Malin M. The psychosocial impact of cancer on older versus younger patients and their families. *Cancer* 1994; **74**: 2118–27.
9. McMillan SC. The relationship between age and intensity of cancer-related symptoms. *Oncol Nurs Forum* 1989; **16**: 237–241.
10. Edlund B, Sneed NV. Emotional responses to the diagnosis of cancer: Age-related comparisons. *Oncol Nurs Forum* 1989; **16**: 691–7.
11. Massie MJ, Holland JC. The older patient with cancer in special issues in psychological management of cancer. In *Handbook of Psyoncology*, edited by JC Holland, JH Rowland. New York: Oxford University Press, 444–452, 1990.
12. Kane, RA. Psychological and social issues for older people with cancer. *Cancer* 1991; **68**: 2514–18.
13. Roberts CS, Cox CE, Reintgen D. The psychological impact of breast cancer on older women. *Cancer Control* 1994; **1**: 367–71.
14. Ell K. Social networks, social support and health status. *Soc Serv Rev* 1984; **58**: 133–45.
15. Wortman CB. Social support and the cancer patient: Conceptual and methodological issues. *Cancer* 1984; **63**: 2339–60.
16. Ho SC. Health and social predictors of mortality in an elderly Chinese cohort: *Am J Epidemiol* 1991; **133**: 907–20.
17. Helsing KJ, Szklo M, Comstock GW. Factors associated with mortality after widowhood. *Am J Public Health* 1981; **71**: 802–9.
18. Vernon SW, Jackson GL. Social support, prognosis and adjustment to breast cancer. In *Aging, Stress and Health*, edited by KS Markides, CL Cooper. New York: John Wiley and Sons, 165–98, 1989.
19. Suarez L, Lloyd L, Weiss N, Rainbolt T, Pulley L. Effect of social networks on cancer screening behavior of older Mexican-American women. *J Natl Cancer Inst* 1994; **86**: 775–9.
20. Kang SH, Bloom JR. Social support and cancer screening among older Black Americans. *J Natl Cancer Inst* 1993; **95**: 737–42.
21. Richardson JL, Mondrus GT, Deapen D, Mack TM. Future challenges in secondary prevention of breast cancer for women at high risk. *Cancer* 1994; **74**: 1474–81.
22. Berkovic E. Seeking care for cancer relevant symptoms. *J Chronic Dis* 1982; **35**: 727–34.
23. Samet JM, Hunt WC, Lerchen ML, Goodwin JS. Delay in seeking care for cancer symptoms: A population-based study of elderly New Mexicans. *J Natl Cancer Inst* 1988; **80**: 432–8.
24. Moritz DJ, Satariano WA. Factors predicting stage of breast cancer at diagnosis in middle aged and elderly women: The role of living arrangements. *J Clin Epidemiol* 1993; **46**: 443–54.
25. Goodwin JS, Hunt WC, Key CR, Samet JM. The effect of marital status on stage, treatment and survival of cancer patients. *JAMA* 1987; **258**: 3125–30.
26. Berkman B, Stolberg C, Calhoun J, Parker E, Stearns N. Elderly cancer patients: Factors predictive of risk for institutionalization. *J Psychosoc Oncol* 1983; **1**: 85–100.
27. Goodwin JS, Hunt WC, Samet JM. Determinants of cancer therapy in elderly patients. *Cancer* 1993; **72**: 594–601.
28. Goodwin JS, Hunt WC, Sarnet JM. A population-based study of functional status and social support networks of elderly patients newly diagnosed with cancer. *Arch Intern Med* 1991; **151**: 366–70.
29. Larson PJ, Lindsey AM, Dodd, MJ, Brecht ML, Packer A. Influence of age on problems experienced by patients with lung cancer undergoing radiation therapy. *Oncol Nurs Forum* 1993; **20**: 473–80.
30. Lindsey AM, Larson PJ, Dodd MJ, Brecht ML, Packer A. Comorbidity, nutritional intake, social support, weight, and functional status over time in older cancer patients receiving radiotherapy. *Cancer Nurs* 1994; **17**: 113–124.
31. Mor V, Masterson-Allen S, Houts P, Siegel K. The changing needs of patients with cancer at home: A longitudinal view. *Cancer* 1992; **69**: 829–38.
32. Northouse LL. Social support in patients' and husbands' adjustment to breast cancer. *Nurs Res* 1988; **37**: 91–5.
33. Funch DP, Mettlin C. The role of support in relation to recovery from breast surgery. *Soc Sci Med* 1982; **16**: 91–8.

34. Lichtman RR, Taylor SE, Wood JV. Social support and marital adjustment after breast cancer. *J Psychosoc Oncol* 1987; **5**: 47–74.

35. Ell KO, Mantell JE, Hamovitch MB, Nishimoto RH social support, sense of control, and coping among patients with breast, lung, or colorectal cancer. *J Psychosoc Oncol* 1989; **7**: 63–89.

36. Halstead MT, Fernsler JI. Coping strategies of long-term cancer survivors. *Cancer Nurs* 1994; **17**: 94–100.

37. Roberts CS, Cox CE, Shannon V, Wells N. A closer look at social support as moderator of stress in breast cancer. *Health Soc Work* 1994; **19**: 157–64.

38. Kessler RC, McLeod JD. Social support and mental health in community samples. In *Social Support and Health*. Academic Press, Inc., 219–40.

39. Yancik R. Frame of reference: Old age as the context for the prevention and treatment of cancer: *Perspectives on Prevention and Treatment of Cancer in the Elderly*. New York: Raven Press, 5–17, 1983.

40. Yancik R, Ries LG. Caring for elderly cancer patients: Quality assurance considerations. *Cancer* 1989; **64**: 335–41.

41. Oberst MT, Thomas SE, Gass KA, Ward SE. Caregiving demands and appraisal of stress among family caregivers. *Cancer Nurs* 1989; **12**: 209–15.

42. Kurtz ME, Given B, Kurtz JC, Given CW. The interaction of age, symptoms and survival status on physical and mental health of patients with cancer and their families. *Cancer* 1994: **74**: 2071–8.

43. Vachon M, Freeman K, Formo A, Rogers J, Lyall W, Freeman S. The final illness in cancer: The widow's perspective. *Can Med Assoc J* 1977; **117**: 1151–3.

44. Given B, Stommel M, Collins C, King S, Given CW. Responses of elderly spouse caregivers. *Res Nurs Health* 1990; **13**: 77–85.

45. Grobe ME, Ahmann DL, Ilstrup DM. Needs assessment for advanced cancer patients and their families. *Oncol Nurs Forum* 1982; **9**: 26–30.

46. Welch-McCaffrey D. Family issues in cancer care: Current dilemmas and future directions. *J Psychosoc Oncol* 1988; **1**: 199–210.

47. Boyle DM. Realities to guide novel and necessary nursing care in geriatric oncology. *Cancer Nurs* 1994; **17**: 125–136.

48. Revenson TA, Wollman CA, Felton BJ. Social supports as stress buffers for adult cancer patients. *Psychosom Med* 1983; **45**: 321–31.

49. Wortman CB, Dunkel-Schetter D. Interpersonal relationships and cancer: A theoretical analysis. *J Soc Issues* 1979; **35**: 120–55.

50. Kane RA, Kane RL. *Assessing the elderly: A practical guide to measurement*. Lexington, MA: DC Heath, 1981.

51. Spiegel D, Bloom JR, Yalom I. Group support for patients with metastic cancer. *Arch Gen Psych* 1981; **38**: 527–33.

52. Spiegel D, Bloom JR, Krawmer HC, Gottheil E. Effect of psychosocial treatment on survival of patients with metastic breast cancer. *Lancet* 1989; **2**: 888–91.

53. Hermann JF. Psychosocial support: Interventions for the physicians. *Semin Oncol* 1985; **12**: 466–71.

54. Roberts CS, Cox CE, Reintgen DR, Gibertini M, Baile W. Influence of physician communication on newly diagnosed breast patients' psychological adjustment and decision making. *Cancer* 1994; **74**: 157–64.

20. Prognostic Evaluation of the Older Cancer Patient

Lazzaro Repetto, Cristina Granetto, Antonella Venturino, Ricardo Rosso, Walter Gianni and Leonardo Santi

The majority of patients seen in the practice of oncology are older individuals. Aging is a major risk factor for cancer: more than 50% of all new neoplasms and more than 60% of all cancer deaths occur in persons aged 65 and older.

In the last two decades cancer-related mortality has declined for persons under 50, but has increased for those who are older (1,2). This disturbing observation may reflect the scarce information related to cancer prevention and cancer treatment in the aged. Only recently have older individuals been recognized as a group of persons at high risk for developing cancer and dying of cancer. This chapter explores the influence of age on the prognosis and the management of cancer.

Definition of the Problem

The scarcity of information related to cancer and age is a multifaceted problem with multiple causes. These include the diversity of the geriatric population, the limited understanding of the biology of aging, the current perception of the elderly as frail and dependent individuals, the poor comprehension that older patients and their family have of clinical research, and the scarcity of clinical trials specifically designed for the aged.

Any discussion of aging must acknowledge the diversity of the older population. Seemingly, this diversity implies different tolerance of the complications of cancer and of cancer treatment and mandates individualized management, tailored to individual differences in functional reserve, life expectancy, motivation, social support and possibly other factors not yet defined. Every practicing oncologist has observed individuals in their 80s tolerate without excessive toxicity at full dose-intensity chemotherapy regimens that proved too toxic for persons in their 60s.

Aging is multidimensional and involves changes in physical, emotional, cognitive and social areas. In addition, the prevalence and the severity of comorbidity and of disability increases with age. The combination of these factors likely influences the outcome of cancer treatment, but a prognostic model incorporating these factors into useful clinical predictions is still wanted.

Previous clinical trials provide little clue as to the influence of age on the prognosis of cancer (3). Cancer treatment in the aged is unexplored, with the exception of few studies involving breast cancer, acute leukemia, and lymphomas. In the past, the majority of persons over 65 were excluded from clinical trials on the basis of their age, and are still excluded today on the basis of their functional status. The management of older individuals with cancer is modeled on the treatment of younger persons, rather than being derived from clinical trials focused primarily on the elderly. Even when direct data on the management of cancer in the elderly exist, these data were extracted from studies involving the general population. As a rule, only individuals in excellent performance status and with negligible comorbidity are enrolled in clinical trials of cancer treatment. Thus, these studies may have included only a small fringe of the older population and the conclusions of these studies may not be applicable to the majority of older persons. This point was highlighted by Begg and Carbone, who compared effectiveness and complications of cytotoxic chemotherapy in individuals older than 70 and in younger individuals enrolled in 19 randomized trials of cancer treatment run by the Eastern Cooperative Oncology Group (4). These authors found that the incidence of chemotherapy-related toxicity was similar for older and younger patients, with exception for myelotoxicity, which was more frequent and more severe among the elderly. They also reported that older individuals constituted only 13% of the enrollees and unlikely represented the older population at large. If the trial patients were representative of the general population, approximately 30%–40% of them would have been over 70, reflecting the prevalence of cancer in persons of different ages.

An ageistic bias by health care providers was likely a cause for excluding older individuals from clinical trials, but another possibility should be explored, i.e. poor acceptance of clinical trials by older individuals. The reluctance of older individuals to seek specialized medical care and the reluctance of their families to accept aggressive forms of treatment for an elderly relative may explain in part the poorer outcome of cancer in the elderly and the limited participation of the elderly in clinical research (5).

According to recent reports, less than 50% of older individuals with cancer are referred to specialistic care throughout Western Europe (6). Many of the reasons preventing a higher referral rate are not evidence-based (Table 20.1), and reflect common prejudices related to age. A reversal of this referral pattern may improve the outcome of cancer in older individuals.

Table 20.1 Causes of delay in medical referral of older patients with cancer

Fatalistic attitude by patients and physicians

Therapeutic nihilism

Social Isolation

Limited financial resources

Inadequate information

Poor functional status from comorbid conditions

Poor perception and understanding of new symptoms by patient and family

Clearly, the issues related to the management of cancer in the elderly are very important and very timely, given the progressive expansion of the older population, the continuous improvement in the function of older individuals, the progressive prolongation of mean life-expectancy, the advances in diagnosis and treatment of cancer, and the development of new insights of the biology of aging. The aim of this chapter is to analyze these differences and to propose a reliable prognostic evaluation system, capable of accounting for the diversity of aging. We outline some important evolving issues concerning prognostic evaluation and treatment decisions in elderly cancer patients. Current instruments of functional evaluation are illustrated and their role in clinical practice is discussed.

Prognostic Assessment of Elderly Patients: Limitations of Chronologic Age and Performance Status

Two opposite trends occur in the management of older individuals, and may compromise their outcome. Undertreatment from excessive fear of therapeutic complications and overtreatment from overestimate of the risk of cancer death may be equally devastating. It is clear that older cancer patients are at increased risk of complications from antineoplastic therapy (7), and it is also clear that inadequate treatment of the older patients may fail to provide the desired cancer control (8).

The first step for avoiding both under and over treatment is to try to define individual parameters which may predict tolerance of treatment. Aging is characterized by a progressive reduction in the functional reserve of several organs and systems (2). Thus, the aged may have reduced tolerance of conditions of stress even when he/she is able to carry on daily activities without particular difficulties. The elderly is the individual capable of maintaining homeostasis in "non stressed" circumstances, but at increased risk of losing independence, developing serious illnesses, and even dying, when faced by stress (9). A well known example of reduced functional reserve is the fact that older individuals tolerate elective surgery remarkably well, but are at increased risk of death and serious compli-

cations from emergency surgery. In a review of several surgical studies, McGinnis et al., concluded that the same surgical options for the management of colorectal cancer should be offered to all individuals, irrespective of age, in the absence of serious comorbidity (10). Likewise, the morbidity of mastectomy is similar in older and younger women, in the absence of concurrent serious diseases (11).

Radiation therapy is frequently used instead of surgery, in patients who are poor surgical candidates, but the information related to effectiveness and toxicity of radiotherapy in the aged is very limited. Zachariah et al., assessed the effects of external beam irradiation in 36 patients aged 80–94, affected by various types of cancer (12). These included persons with poor functional status. The authors concluded that radiotherapy was well tolerated by the majority of patients and that frailty did not represent a contraindication to treatment. Thus, the role of radiation therapy in the management of frail older individuals will likely expand, especially in the management of cancer of the chest and of the head and neck. Hanks et al., evaluated the effects of radiotherapy in 2210 men with prostate cancer and did not find any difference in toxicity and effectiveness between patients over 70 and younger individuals (13). Olmi et al., reviewed the cases of 2060 persons over 70 treated with external beam irradiation for different neoplasms and found that these patients tolerated with minimally increased complication rate the same treatment strategies in use for younger individuals (14). The effects of chemotherapy were studied by Begg and Carbone (4). Despite some increase in myelotoxicity, chemotherapy was overall well tolerated by individuals over 70. Thus, these studies indicate that more than one treatment option is available to the aged with cancer and treatment withdrawal is seldom justified. This conclusion is emphasized by the observation that cancer is often lethal for older individuals, even when the course of the disease appears more indolent (15), and that the life-expectancy of the Western population is in continuous expansion (9). At age 85 the life expectancy is 7 years for women and 5.5 years for men (9).

Clearly, chronologic age is an inadequate predictor of treatment-related complications and more precise prognostic factors are wanted (16). In patients under 65, Performance Status (PS), is a powerful predictor of therapeutic response, toxicity, and outcome (17). The prognostic value of PS may fade with increasing age. In older individuals, PS is likely affected by chronic diseases and disability and may not reflect the influence of cancer on the organism. Thus PS appears helpful in older individuals without comorbidities, but is inadequate for the prognostic assessment of elderly patients with serious comorbidity. PS has another important limitation, as it represents a physician's measure and does not account for the subjective psychosocial aspects of life, that assume greater importance in the aged. For many older persons, the activities of daily living (ADL), and the instrumental activities of daily living (IADL) may be more informative than PS (18).

Table 20.2 Functional assessment of the older person

Instrumental activities of daily living (ADL)	Activities of daily living (ADL)
Cooking	Transfer
Cleaning	Bathing and grooming
Laundry	Toileting
Use of telephone	Dressing
Use of transportation	Feeding
Managing money	Appropriate behavior
Taking medications	

In addition, ADL and IADL are reliable indices of rehabilitative potential and life-expectancy (Table 20.2). Particular attention should also be paid to the emotional and the socioeconomic status of the older person with cancer. These factors condition both treatment compliance and personal support (6).

Clearly, the diversity of the older population is reflected in the multiple and different factors which may influence the final outcome of treatment. The adoption of an uniform evaluation of older individuals treated in clinical trials is essential to establish the prognostic value of different factors.

In the following discussion we explore the management of specific diseases in the elderly, as examples of the complexity of age-related factors which may influence therapeutic decisions.

Management of Specific Diseases in the Elderly

To illustrate the complexity of cancer management in the aged and the specific information necessary in this age group we will review the current knowledge related to four common neoplasms.

Breast

The optimal management of breast cancer in older women has not been well defined, though 50% of breast cancer occurs in women aged 65 and over. The inadequacy of prognostic assessment may account in part for lack of more precise information.

Several retrospective studies indicated that the treatment of breast cancer varies with the age of the patient (5, 19–22). Martin *et al.*, observed that the use of surgery decreased, while the use of radiation therapy and hormonal therapy as primary treatment of localized breast cancer increased with the age of the patient (19). These authors observed that the percentage of women who did not receive any treatment at all also increased with age. Sometimes the patient's general medical conditions supported the physician's decision for a less aggressive form of management than surgery. In many cases, however, unconventional treatment was adopted without apparent reason. Seemingly, overestimate of the risk of surgical complications related to age and comorbidity influenced the physician decision to forgo curative surgery. The stage of the disease had not a role in the treatment decision, as the stage of disease at presentation was similar in women of different ages (23–24). The NCI SEER program examined the influence of advanced age on presentation of breast cancer in 125,000 women (25). This survey concluded that: 1. The incidence and the mortality of breast cancer increased with age; 2. There was a tendency to utilize more conservative surgery in older women; 3. Surgery was well tolerated by older women in good general health; 4. The incidence of comorbidity, limitations in functional status, social isolation and financial restrictions increased with age and complicated the treatment-related decisions in these women. The authors suggested that older breast cancer patients may require special evaluation to account for the physiologic, medical and social changes related to aging . To explore this approach we review in some details three important issues which pertain to the treatment of older patients. These include modification of the doses of cytotoxic agents based on functional status and comorbidity, alternative measurements of outcome, and competitive causes of death.

At the Istituto Nazionale per la Ricerca sul Cancro in Genova, Italy, we explored a treatment strategy which may take into account decline in functional status and comorbidity. We treated patients with metastatic breast cancer with mitoxantrone, and we varied the doses of the drug according to the PS and the number of comorbid conditions. The dose was reduced one level for PS ≥ 2 and/or for ≥ 2 comorbid conditions. Twenty-seven patients, median age 77 years (range 68–86) with progressive metastatic disease received a median of 5 courses of treatment (range 1–9). The basal dose was 10 mg/m2, and this was escalated to 14 mg/m2 in 17 patients. At the lower dose we observed 4 PR and 4 cases of disease stabilization; median response duration was 6 months and median survival 8 months. We could not demonstrate any difference in the degree of toxicity experienced by patients with poor performance status and multiple comorbidity and healthier patients. We concluded that our treatment strategy allowed the majority of older women to receive chemotherapy with acceptable risk of complications (26).

Christopher *et al.*, examined an alternative end point to survival in older women with breast cancer, an endpoint that might reflect comorbid conditions and functional status (27). These authors defined "active life expectancy" as the expected duration of functional well-being, and found "active life-expectancy" a more relevant end-point of cancer treatment than survival in older patients. Active life-expectancy reflects independence in the activities of daily living and may even be a surrogate for quality of life. Unfortunately, this study did not address the "utility", i.e. the personal perception of "active life expectancy" by individual patients. The utility value is crucial to establish the validity of this end-point in clinical trials.

Another complicating factor in sorting out the most appropriate management of breast cancer in older women, is represented by competitive causes of death. Castiglione *et al.*, conducted a trial of adjuvant treatment with tamoxifen in 320 women with operable breast cancer aged 66 to 80 (28). Patients were randomized to tamoxifen (20 mg/d) and low-dose prednisone for one year or no treatment. After 96 months of follow-up the authors found that tamoxifen lessened the risk of breast cancer recurrences but did not affect the overall patient survival, due to competitive causes of death. The incidence of deaths unrelated to breast cancer was 10% in the control group and 24% in the tamoxifen group. Of the women who had died in the tamoxifen group, 9% had no evidence of breast cancer. A similar study, involving 181 elderly women, was conducted by Cummings *et al.* (29). Twenty-two percent of the deaths occurring during 10 years of follow up were not cancer-related and were equally distributed between cardiovascular and cerebrovascular diseases.

Lung

The incidence of lung cancer peaks during the seventh decade of life; approximately 1 of 3 patients with lung cancer is over 65 (30–31). Similarly to breast cancer, the use of any form of antineoplastic treatment decreases with patient's age. In 2406 lung cancer patients, Crawford *et al.*, observed that 31.4% of those younger than 55, but only 14.9% of those older than 74 underwent curative surgery.

The standard treatment for localized non-small cell lung cancer (NSCLC) is surgery (31), for small cell lung cancer (SCLC) is systemic chemotherapy associated with radiation to the chest (32). Treatment options for elderly patients with NSCLC are similar to those of younger patients. For patients with unresectable or inoperable disease, palliation of symptoms is the main goal of treatment.

The information related to the tolerance of combined chemo-radiotherapy by elderly patients with SCLC is scarce, because people over 65 were excluded from most studies. Sorensen and Hansen suggested that the benefits of treating SCLC are inferior for older than for younger patients (33).

Comorbidity and inadequate treatment may account in part for the poorer outcome of older patients. Findlay *et al.*, compared aggressive treatment with vincristine, cyclophosphamide and doxorubicin and gentler treatment consisting of radiotherapy alone, single agent chemotherapy or combination chemotherapy at reduced doses in elderly patients with SCLC (34). They found increased response rate, and increased incidence of therapeutic complications for patients receiving more aggressive treatment. The overall differences in survival were negligible, which is not surprising, given the rapidly lethal nature of the disease, even for patients who experience a complete remission. To prevent the excessive risk of therapeutic complications, Carney *et al.*, explored the role of etoposide as single agent and in combination in elderly patients with SCLC. Carboplatin and oral etoposide in combination yielded results similar to those previously reported for more

aggressive treatment. The advantages of oral etoposide included excellent compliance, easy administration and low toxicity.

It is important to underline that age should not determine the treatment strategy even in the case of lung cancer. Several studies indicate that the stage of NSCLC at presentation tends to be less advanced in older individuals (30,35). The risk of cancer surgery even for patients in their 80s, is not substantially increased when serious comorbidity is not present (31).

Lymphoma

Approximately 60% of all cases of non-Hodgkin's Lymphoma (NHL) occur in persons aged 65 and older (36–37). Chemotherapy is the primary and most active form of treatment for NHL; in some forms of lymphoma, such as the large-cell diffuse lymphomas, chemotherapy may induce a cure rate approaching 50% (38). Older patients may achieve prolonged disease control with an adequate treatment (39). O'Reilly *et al.*, reviewed different forms of treatment of patients over 60 with diffuse large cell lymphoma and observed a complete remission of the disease in at least one third of the patients (40–42). Despite these encouraging results, age over 60 appears a poor prognostic factor for patients with large cell lymphoma (41–42). The International Non-Hodgkin's Lymphoma Prognostic Factors Project involved 16 Institutions and Cooperative Groups from the United States, Canada, and Europe. In this large study, the response rate to chemotherapy was similar for younger and older individuals, but the duration of complete remission was shorter for persons aged 60 and older (41). The complete remission rate for low risk patients under 60 was 92% and 91% for those aged 60 and over. High risk patients achieved a complete remission rate of 46% if they were under 60 and 36% if older. The relapse-free survival at two years for patients at low risk of recurrence was 88% for those under 60 and 75% for those older; for high risk patients under 60 years the relapse free survival was 61% and 47% for those older. The 2 year survival was respectively 90% and 80% for patients at low risk, and 37% and 31% for those at high risk. These observations were supported by several other studies. Vose *et al.*, reported a 62% five year survival for patients under 60 and 34% for older patients (43). Interestingly, the response rate and the duration of complete response was similar in both age groups, but competitive causes of death accounted for the higher mortality of older patients. In this study comorbidity represented a cause of death comparable to lymphoma and to antineoplastic treatment, for older patients (44). Tirelli *et al.* observed a higher incidence of severe (WHO grade 3 and 4, 22%) and lethal (11%) toxicity in unselected patients over 70 with diffuse large cell lymphoma treated with chemotherapy regimens of common use in younger individuals (45). To avoid these serious and frequent complications, chemotherapy regimens of high dose intensity but shorter duration have been investigated in older lymphoma patients, with encouraging results (39, 46–48). These data em-

Table 20.3 Comorbidity in Different studies

Author(s)	P#/age	Arthritis	HBP	CVD	RD
Bergman (20)	200/>55	–	17%	6.3%	6.3%
Satariano (54)	340/>55	19.9%	7.1%	9.5%	–
Lindsey (pc)	45/61–86	53.3%	48.9%	42.2%	22.2%
Repetto (58)	138>70	37.0%	31.9%	23.2%	12.3%

CVD= cardiovascular diseases
HBP= High blood pressure
pc = personal communication
RD = Respiratory diseases

phasize once more the need to assess older patients individually, prior to enrollment in any form of treatment plan.

Prostate

Prostate cancer is the second leading cause of cancer death among men and is, above all, a cancer of elderly persons.

The management of prostate cancer is an important model to study the effects of life-expectancy on therapeutic decisions. Chodak *et al.*, analyzed 10 non-randomized studies of patients with clinically localized prostate cancer managed with observation and hormonal treatment upon progression (50). The survival of patients with well and moderately differentiated prostate cancer (Grade 1 and 2) was similar to the expected survival of a general population of men of similar ages. They concluded that watchful waiting was a reasonable option for patients with localized prostate cancer, especially those whose life-expectancy was 10 years or less. These results were supported by Fleming *et al.*, who compared watchful waiting and radiotherapy in the management of men with localized prostate cancer and found similar survival for the two treatment groups (51). In the perspective of these studies, the comparison of the benefits between treatment and watchful waiting is extremely important for patients with limited life-expectancy.

Comorbidity

Several studies indicated that the stage at diagnosis and the treatment of cancer may vary with the age of the patients (52). Comorbidity, whose prevalence increases with age, represents one of the most visible factors of difference in the presentation of cancer between younger and older individuals. The most frequent comorbid conditions in the elderly with cancer are summarized in Table 20.3 and include diabetes mellitus, cardiovascular, renal or respiratory diseases, hypertension, arthritis, and dementia. These conditions may influence the management of the older patient in several ways. They may lessen the benefits of treatment by shortening the patient's life expectancy and enhancing the risk of therapeutic complications; they

may also affect the natural course of cancer, and may cause a delay in diagnosis by masking symptoms of cancer with other symptoms or complains (53). To assess the importance of these effects, Satariano studied the prevalence of comorbidity in older women with breast cancer (54). The most frequent conditions included arthritis, hypertension, cataract, heart disease, varicose veins, diabetes mellitus, osteoporosis and stroke. Two or more conditions were observed in 45% of women aged 60 to 69; 61% of those aged 70 to 79 and 70% of those aged 80 years and older. As expected, the risk of dying of causes unrelated to cancer increased with the number of comorbid conditions. He also assessed the prevalence of comorbid conditions in elderly men with different types of cancer and found that two or more conditions were present in 35% of those aged 60–69, 47% of those 70–79 and 53% of those over 80. The author concluded that comorbidity affects breast cancer diagnosis, treatment and prognosis, and suggested the need for more research aimed at defining and grading comorbidity. Presently, we know very little how the number and types of comorbid conditions influence cancer screening practice and staging modalities or how they influence treatment choices, response to treatment, and survival. In a study of the Netherlands Cancer Institute the authors analyzed the primary treatment and the survival of 611 patients 55 year and older with breast cancer. Differences in treatment between younger and older breast cancer patients were observed: hormonal therapy as the only form of treatment was frequently given to patients older than 75 years with early stage disease, while the therapy most frequently used in younger women was surgery, followed by radiotherapy. It was observed that these differences were mostly attributed to the age-related factors, such as comorbid diseases and weak physical conditions, which are more common in the oldest and are responsible for the lower survival (8).

Comorbidity may affect the presentation and recognition of symptoms and delay the diagnosis of cancer in several ways. Cancer-related symptoms may be attributed to other health problems or dismissed as normal aspect of aging (54). Also, early symptoms of cancer may be hidden by more significant symptoms related to other immediate health problems. The older person affected by comorbid conditions may accept a certain degree of pain and discomfort as a consequence of chronic diseases and may be late in recognizing the appearance of symptoms and signs of cancer. Likewise, the caregiver of the older demented person may not be aware of early symptoms and signs of cancer, and may be inclined to ascribe these symptoms and signs to chronic diseases.

Comorbidities may lessen treatment efficacy. This is particularly important in elderly patients in whom "frailty" should be regarded as the primary constraint in the use of cancer therapy (6).

Any type of cancer-related interventions in older persons, both diagnostic and therapeutic, must take into account physiologic changes and coexisting pathology. A variety of studies indicate that older people are less likely than younger people to receive definitive cancer therapy: an increasing prevalence of comorbidities may explain only in part the age - related decline in treatment intensity (5). It is important to emphasize once more that many practitioners are reluctant to administer and many patients are reluctant to receive aggressive anticancer treatment even when comorbidity is minimal or absent. Chronologic age is often predictive of treatment after adjusting for comorbidity and stage of disease: Greenfield and his colleagues (55) found that while a higher comorbidity level was associated with a lower likelihood of receiving an appropriate therapy, older age was an independent risk factor for not receiving appropriate therapy. Even among patients with little or no comorbidity who were diagnosed with early stage cancer, only 83% of patients aged 70 and over received appropriate treatment, in contrast to 95.6% of those aged 50 to 69.

On the other hand, some of the less aggressive treatments represent an appropriate response to frail, older patients unable to tolerate the rigors of diagnostic testing and treatment (56). The key-point remains to recognize in advance patients who are likely to benefit from cancer treatment, taking into account life expectancy, and to avoid aggressive therapy in patients at high risk for toxicities.

It is important to realize that chemotherapy may provide valuable palliation even when survival benefits may be small. In older men with hormone-resistant prostate cancer, for example, currently available chemotherapy is unlikely to affect survival or symptom control. Chemotherapy with mitoxantrone plus prednisone showed a good tolerability and some beneficial effects on disease-related symptoms and quality of life of patients, even if it is not the most active treatment according to the standard criteria of response evaluation (57).

Research in the area of measurement of comorbidity is needed: it is necessary to establish the severity of comorbid diseases and to determine whether comorbid conditions are antecedent, concurrent or subsequent to the diagnosis of cancer (54).

To explore the hypothesis that only selected groups of older patients with cancer are referred for treatment to specialized cancer centers, we studied the prevalence and the severity of comorbidity, the education, and the income of older individuals with and without cancer. The majority of cancer patients in Italy are referred to specialized cancer centers for any type of oncologic treatment. We compared three groups of subjects: cancer patients aged 70 and older; cancer patients under 70, and a third group of non-cancer patients over 70 (Table 20.4). The two groups of cancer patients were from the Istituto Nazionale Per La Ricerca Sul Cancro in Genova, while non-cancer patients were from geriatric or general medicine clinics at the University of Genova and at the University of Rome. We observed that older patients with cancer were overall healthier than those without cancer. Also, cancer patients were better educated and had higher income. The prevalence of 4 or more comorbid diseases was

Table 20.4 Age, social status, functional status, and comorbidity in elderly cancer patients (pt) compared to young neoplastic and elderly non-neoplastic population.

	Neoplastic pt 50–69	Neoplastic pt ≥70	Non-neoplastic pt ≥70
Number:	177	138	278
Median age:	62	74	79
Age range:	50–69	70–103	70–110
Living conditions:			
family	152 (84%)	84 (61%)	200 (72%)
alone	18 (12%)	25 (18%)	36 (13%)
institution	7 (6%)	29 (21%)	42 (16%)
Education:			
≥ senior high	45 (25%)	24 (17%)	32 (12%)
junior high	35 (20%)	33 (23%)	38 (14%)
elementary	92 (52%)	74 (54%)	181 (65%)
illiterate	5 (3%)	4 (6%)	27 (9%)
ECOG PS			
0	161 (91%)	97 (70%)	42 (15%)
1	11 (6%)	30 (22%)	99 (36%)
≥2	5 (3%)	11 (8%)	137 (49%)
Comorbidities			
0	26 (15%)	17 (12%)	–
1–2	75 (42%)	60 (43%)	29 (10%)
3–4	60 (34%)	36 (26%)	89 (32%)
>4	16 (9%)	25 (18%)	160 (57%)

much higher among the non-cancer patients than among the cancer patients (57.6% vs 18.1%). Also, none of the patients without cancer and 17% of those with cancer was free of comorbid conditions.

Our results support the observation that only a selected population of elderly cancer patients is referred for specialized care (58). Possibly, comorbidity may account for this pattern of referral.

Quality of Life (QL)

According to WHO, health is a state of physical, mental and social well-being, including absence of disease (59). According to Satariano, in assessing health, it is important to distinguish disease, that's the presence of a diagnosed condition, and illness, that refers to the functional limitations and disabilities resulting from that condition (60).

In recent years, there has been a growing interest in broadening the evaluation criteria employed in cancer clinical trials beyond the traditional measures and endpoints of therapeutic outcome (tumor response, time to progression and disease-free and overall survival). New measures and endpoints include the impact of the disease and its treatment on the physical, psychological and social function of the patient (61). From these new approaches emerged the concept of QL and the measurement of QL has recently been proposed as a component of clinical trials research.

A number of reviews have indicated both the importance of measuring quality of life in the medical assessment and the increase in published reports containing QL evaluation.

QL refers to those aspects of life and human function considered essential for living fully. Global evaluation of QL generally focused on a composite of physical, emotional, social and economic factors that are influenced by the physical sequelae of disease (62). QL in cancer care may be seen as a more comprehensive evaluation of treatment outcome, that includes the patient's own assessment of that outcome.

Unlike performance status, QL is a subjective assessment of treatment outcome: some authors observed that patient perception of symptoms and well-being may more accurately reflect disease status and psychologic factors may play an important role in survival. Unfortunately, psychosocial indicators are rarely used in clinical trials as many physicians hesitate to apply them for lack of experience. This may be explained in part by a low familiarity with such soft issues, but probably more often by the fact that most physicians are focused on cure rather than palliation or supportive care.

QL may expand the scope of clinical trials. While QL data do not supplant traditional end points of survival, response and toxicity, they add new information related to the patient's perspective, which includes perception of toxicity, impact of treatment on emotion, on social relationships, on work, on self perception and more in general on enjoyment of one's life (63). QL has also been used as an independent prognostic factor. QL information may suggest new and more individualized interventions, aimed to optimize the treatment of individual patients.

By its own nature QL is a subjective measurement and should be assessed by the patients themselves. Historically, "subjective assessment" has most often been undertaken by the physician, who rated patients' physical conditions and subjective toxicities such as nausea and vomiting. A poor agreement has been found between patients' ratings and physician's ratings (64).

In 1986, the European Organization for Research and Treatment of Cancer (EORTC) Study Group on QL initiated a research program (EORTC protocol 15861) with the long-term goal of developing an integrated measurement system for evaluating the QL of cancer patients participating in clinical trials.

A multidimensional core questionnaire was generated to cover basic QL domains, including physical, emotional and social functioning and global QL (65).

Additional disease-specific measurement modules were developed to cover disease and treatment-related issues in more details. The first generation 36-item core questionnaire, the EORTC QLQ-C36, was developed in 1987, but it was revised in some areas and a refined,

second version consisting of 30 questions was validated within an EORTC study. The result of this evaluation lent support to the QLQ-C30 as a reliable and valid measure of the QL of cancer patients in international clinical trials. The EORTC QLQ C-30 is a 30 item questionnaire composed of multi-item scales and single items that reflect QL as a multidimensional construct. It incorporates 5 functional scales (physical, role, cognitive, emotional and social), 3 symptom scales (fatigue, pain, and nausea and vomiting) and a global health and QL scale. The remaining single items assess additional symptoms commonly reported by cancer patients (dyspnea, appetite loss, sleep disturbance, constipation and diarrhea) as well as the perceived financial impact of the disease and treatment. The EORTC QLQ-C30 has good validity and reliability (61).

The questionnaire was well accepted by patients: it required 11–12 minutes to complete. In most cases patients were able to complete the questionnaire without assistance. QL assessment was administered before, during and immediately after the end of treatment, was found to reflect the patient's clinical status and to change over time.

The assessment of QL may be particularly helpful in the management of older patients. As the survival benefits of treatment wane with shrinking life-expectancy, improvement of QL becomes the main treatment goal (66). The clinical information in this area is very limited and somehow controversial. Mckenna described several clinical situations suggesting that older individuals, when faced by serious diseases and severe illnesses, usually prefer improved quality over quantity of life; they may be less interested in a trade-off of months or years of life in exchange for the side effects of cancer treatment, especially when cure is impossible (68). On the contrary, a recent study conducted by Yellen at al (67), does not support this observation. The authors interviewed 244 cancer patients of different ages about their acceptance of hypothetical treatments with different levels of expected toxicities and survival gain. No effect of age or stage of the disease was observed on acceptance of chemotherapy-related toxicity. The patients studied by Yellen et al., had been referred to tertiary care center and may not be reflective of the general geriatric population. Mostly, these studies emphasize once more the diversity of older individuals and the need of an individual assessment taking quality of life into account when planning cancer treatment.

Cancer may restrict the autonomy of the elderly and these restrictions may generate new suffering. Caregivers may interpret this suffering as fear of death and may be eager to prolong life at any cost, misunderstanding the patient's priorities. An open discussion of the patient's goals and desires together with the family and the most likely caregivers may dissipate this misunderstanding and allow a more relaxed climate of cooperation between caregivers and health care providers. Whenever possible, this conversation should be held immediately after the diagnosis of cancer, when death is not yet imminent and judgement is not clouded by intervening and conflicting emotions. This discussion is essential to preserve the quality of life of the older patients and to achieve reasonable therapeutic successes.

The instruments to measure QL in clinical trials have been used both in younger and older individuals, but validation in older individuals is wanted. Several potential problems with current instruments suggest the need for modifications or for new tools. First of all older individuals may have physical difficulties, such as poor vision and poor hearing, especially the oldest old, that prevent adequate understanding of the questionnaires. They also may require more time for the completion of the test, due to slower cognitive processes. Second, the instruments of current use are tuned to the QL of younger adults, and include measurements of scarce interest to the elderly, while they may exclude items of special interest to the aged. Several cancer centers, including ours, are trying to formulate individualized tools for the measurement of QL in older individuals.

Comprehensive Geriatric Assessment (CGA)

Aging is multidimensional and involves the functional, the cognitive, the emotional and the socioeconomic domains. As changes in each of these domains may affect treatment plans, it is particularly important to develop an uniform method for assessing these changes including comorbidity, functional limitations, socioeconomic status, emotional stability, and cognition. CGA is currently the most reliable instrument to recognize unsuspected comorbid conditions, to identify areas of physical, social and emotional dysfunction and possibly to estimate life expectancy (68). CGA allows inclusive therapy plans and long-term follow-up of individual patients (68). An uniform CGA adopted in all industrial countries would be highly desirable, for obtaining epidemiological and prognostic data related to the influence of aging on cancer. CGA should also include special attention to the stress of the caregiver, which may determine further treatment plans and may suggest the need for caregiver support. Parr (personal communication, Gerontological Society of America, Los Angeles, California, November 17, 1995) found that the caregivers of older cancer patients reported quite often more severe stress than the patient him/herself. This observation is of particular concern as the caregiver of older persons is most often an older spouse.

Although CGA itself does not require specific instruments and scales, the use of easy-to-administer, well validated instruments, encompassing the major domains of geriatric assessment, makes the process more reliable and considerably easier to apply in the daily clinical practice; moreover, it allows the collection of homogenous information and facilitates the communication among health care providers.

The assessment of ADL is a cornerstone of CGA. The first assessments and classifications of ADL as functional index were performed in the fifties: Katz's scale

Table 20.5 Prognostic assessment of the older cancer patient: elements of age-weighing.

Area	Instruments
Functional Status	ADL/IADL
Nutrition	Serum albumin, transferrin triceps skin fold
Emotional status	Geriatric Depression Scale
Cognitive function	Mini Mental Status
Social and economic status	Income
	Living conditions
	Caregiver

of activities of daily living (ADL) (69) and Lawton's scale of instrumental activities of daily living (IADL) (70) became a fundamental tool in geriatric evaluation as they permit to assess skills of older people to live fully independently in the community. Simultaneously the focus of geriatric medicine became preservation of active life (or compression of morbidity), rather than prolongation of life.

Successively, more complex systems of evaluation were developed, inclusive of both ADL-IADL (Table 20.5) assessment and psychosocial, economic and emotional issues. Such programs usually have several goals, which include increasing the patient's level of functioning, improving diagnosis and treatment, achieving more appropriate institutional placement, reducing the use of institutional services and generally increasing the overall quality of care delivered to elderly patients (71). These programs are geared to specific purpose and may differ from each others: for example, some programs are designed for outpatients assessment service, whereas others are targeted to community-dwelling elderly patients or to patients recently discharged from hospital. Nevertheless, all geriatric assessment programs share many common characteristics: all of them provide multidimensional evaluation, using one or more sets of instruments to quantify functional ability, functional status, physical health and social function (72).

In 1989, in a Consensus Conference sponsored by the Department of Veterans Affairs, the National Institute on Aging and the Robert Wood Johnson Foundation, the definition of CGA was established: "A multidimensional, interdisciplinary patient evaluation that leads to the identification of patient's problems and the development of a plan for resolving these problems" (73).

The endpoints of CGA concern four major categories: physical health, function, care utilization and satisfaction with care and quality of life (74).

Several non-controlled and controlled clinical trials have been conducted to establish the benefits and costs of CGA, but the results about effectiveness and cost-effectiveness are inconclusive (75). A meta-analysis of 28 controlled trials of CGA was performed in 1993, with the purpose of identifying CGA program characteristics associated with favorable outcomes. The 28 studies included 4959 subjects assigned to one of five different types of CGA and 4912 controls. CGA programs were classified as: hospital geriatric evaluation and management unit; inpatients geriatrics consultation service; home assessment service; hospital home assessment service and outpatient assessment service. The results indicate that certain types of CGA have a significant effect on mortality, living conditions, and patients' physical and cognitive status. For example, the hospital geriatric evaluation and management unit decreased early mortality by approximately 35%. In particular, programs with control on medical recommendation and extended ambulatory follow-up are more likely to be effective. In this meta-analysis, the importance to improve the processes of CGA is underlined, in order to develop more efficient interventions for elderly diseases.

A major factor which appears to influence the outcome of a CGA program is patients' selection. An NIH Consensus Development Conference on CGA, held in October 1987, concluded that comprehensive geriatric assessment is effective for selected older persons: in general, the elderly persons most likely to benefit from assessment are those with some disabilities that may require institutionalization, those in the lower socio-economic groups, those who have inadequate primary medical care and those with poor social support networks (72). CGA may permit the recognition of those frail elderly, who have an increased risk to develop treatment related toxicities and loss of functional independence. In oncology practice there is no study employing CGA in the clinical management of elderly patients. Older people are still evaluated with inadequate parameters, such as PS and biochemical assessment of renal and liver functions while a CGA may reveal unsuspected conditions which can interfere with cancer treatment, reveal unexpected social and rehabilitative needs and provide information on life expectancy, quality of life and treatment tolerance. The application of CGA should be encouraged and evaluated in prospective clinical trials to confirm that CGA may help in improving the approach and care of older cancer patients. In a Senior Oncology Program at the H. Lee Moffitt Cancer Center in Tampa, Florida, a CGA is applied to all older patients evaluated. In approximately 37% of patients over 70 malnutrition was detected and unnecessary polypharmacy eliminated; in 14% of cases social intervention was required, and caregiver-related problem were detected in 28% of cases. In collaboration with the CRO-Aviano we are conducting a prospective study of CGA in the practice of oncology. All new patients aged 65 and over are assessed with a CGA. Diagnostic and management-related decisions, therapeutic responses, the incidence of cancer-related and unrelated mortality are reported to the results of the CGA. The goals of our study involve a CGA based prognostic scale.

The main obstacles to a more widespread use of CGA in clinical practice are manpower, time and cost (W. Applegate, personal communication, Gerontological Society of America, 1995, Los Angeles, California, November 17, 1995). An abbreviated version of the CGA has been explored in several USA nursing homes, for the initial assessment of the residents. Preliminary results indicate that this abbreviated version, which can be administered in less than 30 minutes, provide as much information as older more cumbersome methods of CGA (Beghe' C., personal communication, Gerontological Society of America, Los Angeles, California, November, 17, 1995.)

Conclusions

The prognosis of older persons with cancer may be influenced by several aspects of aging. As aging is highly individualized, the instruments to assess the prognosis of older cancer patients must be fine-tuned to individual differences.

Due to scarce participation of older patients in clinical trials of cancer treatment, the information on prognosis is still limited, but some general considerations are in order:

A diffuse ageistic prejudice may prevent adequate treatment of older individuals; this prejudice is not limited to the health care providers, but involves even patients and their families. A wide based educational effort may allow a more appropriate treatment of cancer in the older person and may provide at the same time needed information on treatment outcome.

Comorbidity is an important prognostic factor, as it may determine the life-expectancy of the patients, the tolerance of treatment and the quality of life.

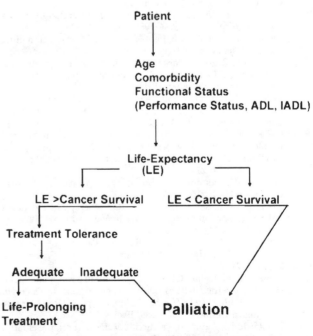

Figure 20.1 Algorithm for the treatment of older cancer patients at the Istituto Nazionale per la Ricerca sul Cancro, Genova.

Functional status is an important prognostic factor; in older individuals with chronic disabling diseases that are not life-threatening, ADL may provide a more reliable estimate of outcome and treatment tolerance, than performance status (PS).

Quality of life of older individuals is both a prognostic factor and an endpoint of management.

The CGA of frail elderly may improve their prognosis by identifying undetected conditions and unexpected medical, rehabilitative, nutritional and social needs. A time-sparing, abbreviated version of CGA may be easily applied in clinical practice, without unnecessary economic and time burden.

Several areas of research in this field are still widely open. They include influence of chronic diseases and chronic medications on myelotoxicity and other organ-related toxicities of antineoplastic therapy, individualized assessment of QL in the elderly, prognostic importance of the different components of CGA, value of abbreviated CGA, and cancer prognosis in the oldest old, i.e. of patients over 80 or 85.

In Figure 20.1 we present the algorithm of current use at our institution, in the management of older cancer patients. In this algorithm we try to integrate tumor and patient-related characteristics.

References

1. Monfardini S, Tirelli U, Serraino D, Fentiman I. After 65, cancer has a different impact on life expectancy in men and women. *Eur J Cancer* 1991; **27**(8): 1065–1066.
2. Cohen HJ. Biology of aging as related to cancer. *Cancer* 1994; **74**: 2092–2100.
3. Kennedy BJ. Needed: clinical trials for older patients. *J Clin Oncol* 1991; **9**: 718–720.
4. Begg B, Carbone PP. Clinical trials and drug toxicity in the elderly. The experience of the Eastern Cooperative Oncology Group. *Cancer* 1983; **2**: 1986–1992.
5. Samet J, Hunt WC, Key C, *et al.* Choice of cancer therapy varies with age of patient. *JAMA* 1986; **255**: 3385–3390.
6. Monfardini S, Chabner B. Joint NCI-EORTC Consensus meting on neoplasia in the elderly. *Eur J Cancer* 1991; **27**(5): 653–654.
7. Balducci L, Beghè C, Parker M, Chausmer A. Prognostic evaluation in geriatric oncology: problems and prospectives. *Arch Gerontol Geriatr* 1991; **13**: 31–41.
8. Bergman L, Dekker G, van Leeuwen FE, *et al.* The effect of age on treatment choice and survival in elderly breast cancer patients. *Cancer* 1991; **67**: 2227–2234.
9. Cohen HJ. Geriatric principles of treatment applied to medical oncology: an overview. *Sem Oncol* 1995; **22** (1), suppl. 1: 1–2.
10. McGinnis LS. Surgical treatment options for colorectal cancer. *Cancer* 1994; **74**: 2147 2150.
11. Fleming ID, Fleming MD. Breast cancer in elderly women. *Cancer* 1994; **74**: 2160–2164.
12. Zachariah B, Casey L, Balducci L. Radiotherapy of the oldest old cancer patients: a study of effectiveness and toxicity. *J Am Ger Soc* 1995; **41**: 793–795.
13. Hanks GE, Hanlon A, Owen JB, *et al.* Patterns of radiation treatment of elderly patients with prostate cancer. *Cancer* 1994; **74**: 2174–2177.
14. Olmi P, Ausili-Cefaro GP. G.R.O.G.: risultati e commento dello studio prospettico della radioterapia nell'anziano. In *Tumori in eta senile*, edited by GA Cefaro, P Olmi. Gruppo di Radioterapia Oncologica Geriatrica, 151–188, 1995.
15. Monfardini S, Aapro M, Ferrucci L, *et al.* Cancer in the elderly. *Eur J Cancer* 1993; 29A,**16**: 2325–2330.
16. Beghe' C, Balducci L. Geriatric oncology: perspectives from decision analysis. A review. *Arch Gerontol Geriatr* 1990; **10**: 141–162.
17. Balducci L. Cancer and age. *Recent progresses in gerontology*, 1990.
18. Balducci L, Cox CE, Greenberg H, *et al.* Management of cancer in the older aged persons. *Cancer Control* 1994; **1** (2): 132–137.
19. Martin LM, le Pechoux C, Calitchi E, *et al.* Management of breast cancer in the elderly. *Eur J Cancer* 1994; 30A,**5**: 590–596.
20. Bergman L, Kluck HM, van Leenewen FE, *et al.* The influence of age on treatment choice and survival of elderly breast cancer patients in South-Eastern Netherlands: a population-based study. *Eur J Cancer* 1992; 28A,**8/9**: 1475–1480.
21. Silliman RA, Guadagnoli E, Weitberg AB *et al.* Age as a predictor of diagnostic and initial treatment intensity in newly diagnosed breast cancer patients. *J Gerontol* 1989; **44**: 46–50.
22. Fentiman IS, Tirelli U, Monfardini S. Cancer in the elderly: why so badly treated? *Lancet*; 1990; **335**: 1020–1022.
23. Mor V, Guadagnoli E, Silliman RA, *et al.* Influence of old age, performance status, medical and psychosocial status on management of cancer patients. In *Cancer in the elderly. Approaches to early detection and treatment*, edited by R Yancik, JW Yates. New York: Springer Publishing Company, 127–146, 1989.
24. Goodwin J, Samet J, Key C, *et al.* Stage at diagnosis of breast cancer varies with the age of the patients. *J Am Ger Soc* 1986; **34**: 20–26.
25. Yancik R, Ries LB, Yates JW. A population-based study of contrasts in stage, surgery and survival. *Cancer* 1989; **63**: 976–981.
26. Repetto L, Simoni C, Venturino A, *et al.* Mitoxantrone in elderly women with advanced breast cancer: a phase II study. *Anticancer Res* 1995; **15**(5B): 2297–2300.
27. Christopher ED, Hillner BE, Smith TJ, *et al.* Should the elderly receive chemotherapy for node-negative breast cancer? A cost-effectiveness analysis examining total an active life-expectancy outcomes. *J Clin Oncol* 1993; **11**(4): 777–782.
28. Castiglione M, Gelber RD, Goldhirsch A. Adjuvant systemic therapy for breast cancer in the elderly: competing causes of mortality. *J Clin Oncol* 1990; **8**(3): 519–526.
29. Cummings FJ, Gray R, Tormey DC, *et al.* Adjuvant tamoxifen versus placebo in elderly women with node-positive breast cancer: long-term follow-up and causes of death. *J Clin Oncol* 1993; **11**: (1): 29–35.
30. Teeter SM, Holmes FF, McFarlane J. Lung carcinoma-influence of histology on the inverse relationship of stage to age. *Cancer* 1987; **60**: 1331–1336.
31. Crawford J, O'Rourke MA, Cohen HJ. Age factors in the management of lung cancer. In *Cancer in the elderly. Approaches to early detection and treatment*, edited by R Yancik, JW Yates. New York: Springer Publishing Company, 177–203, 1989.
32. Carney DN, Byme A. Etoposide in the treatment of elderly/poor prognosis patients with small-cell lung cancer. *Cancer Chemother Pharmacol* 1994; **34** (suppl.): S96–S100.
33. Sorensen JB, Hansen HH. Recent advances in diagnosis and treatment of small cell and non-small cell lung cancer. *Current Opinion in Oncology* 1994; **6**: 162–170.
34. Findlay MPN, Griffin AM, Raghavan D, *et al.* Retrospective review of chemotherapy for small cell lung cancer in the elderly: does the end justify the means? *Eur J Cancer* 1991; **27** (12): 1597–1601.
35. Holmes FF, Hearne E. Cancer stage-to-age relationship: implications for cancer screening in the elderly. *J Am Ger Soc* 1981; **29**: 55–57.
36. Carbone A, Tirelli U, Volpe R, *et al.* Non-Hodgkin's lymphoma in the elderly: a retrospective clinicopathologic study of 50 patients. *Cancer* 1986; **57**: 2185–2189.
37. Anderson T, Chabner B, Young RC, *et al.* Malignant lymphoma. The history and staging of 473 patients at the National Cancer Institute. *Cancer* 1982; **50**: 2693–2707.
38. Inanc SE, Onat H. Brief weekly chemotherapy for elderly patients with intermediate-grade or high-grade non-Hodgkin's lymphoma. *J Natl Cancer Inst* 1993; **85**.
39. O'Reilly SE, Connors JM, Howdle S, *et al.* In search of an optimal regimen for elderly patients with advanced-stage diffuse large-cell lymphoma: results of a phase II study of P/DOCE chemotherapy. *J Clin Oncol* 1993; **11**: 250–2257.

40. Dixon DO, Neilan B, Jones SE, *et al*. Effect of age on therapeutic outcome in advanced diffuse histiocytic Lymphoma. *J Clin Oncol* 1986; **4**: 295–305.

41. Shipp M. Prognostic factors in aggressive non-Hodgkin's lymphoma. Who has "high risk" disease?. *Blood* 1994; **83**: 1165–1173.

42. Shipp M, Harrington D, Cabanillas F, *et al*. Development of a predictive model for aggressive lymphoma: the International NHL prognostic factors project. *Proc Am Soc Clin Oncol* 1992; **11**: 319 (abstr 1084).

43. Vose JM, Armitage JO, Weisemburger DD, *et al*. The importance of age in survival of patients treated with chemotherapy for aggressive non Hodgkin's lymphoma. *J Clin Oncol* 1988; **6**: 1838–1844.

44. Martelli M, Guglielmi C, Coluzzi S, *et al*. P-VABEC: a prospective study of a new weekly chemotherapy regimen for elderly aggressive non-Hodkin's lymphoma. *J Clin Oncol* 1993; **11**: 2362–2369.

45. Tirelli U, Zagonel V, Serraino D, *et al*. Non-Hodgkin's lymphomas in 137 patients aged 70 years or older: a retrospective european organization for research and treatment of cancer lymphoma group study. *J Clin Oncol* 1988; **6**(11): 1708–1713.

46. Tirelli U, Zagonel V, Errante D, *et al*. A prospective study of a new combination chemotherapy regimen in patients older than 70 years with unfavorable non-Hodgkin's lymphoma. *J Clin Oncol* 1992; **10**: 28–236.

47. McMaster ML, Johnson DH, Greer GP, *et al*. A brief-duration combination chemotherapy for elderly patients with poor-prognosis non-Hodgkin's lymphoma. *Cancer* 1991; **67**: 1487–1492.

48. Sweetenham JW, Mead GM, Whitehouse JMA. Intensive weekly combination chemotherapy for patients with intermediate-grade non-Hodgkin's lymphoma. *J Clin Oncol* 1991; **9**: 2202–2209.

49. Catalona WJ. Management of cancer of the prostate. *N Engl J Med* 1994; **331**(15): 996–1004.

50. Chodak GW, Thisted RA, Gerber GS, *et al*. Results of conservative management of clinically localized prostate cancer. *N Eng J Med* 1994; **330**: 242–248.

51. Fleming C, Wasson JH, Albertsen PC, *et al*. A decision analysis of alternative treatment strategies for clinically localized prostate cancer: Prostate Patient Outcomes Research Team. *JAMA* 1993; **269**: 2650–58.

52. Yancik R, Ries LG. Cancer in the aged. An epidemiologic perspective on treatment issues. *Cancer* 1991; **68**: 2502–2510.

53. Bergman L, Dekker G, van Kerkhoff EHM, *et al*. Influence of age and comorbidity on treatment choice and survival in elderly patients with breast cancer. *Breast Cancer Res and Treat* 1991; **18**: 189–198.

54. Satariano WA. Comorbidity and functional status in older women with breast cancer: implications for screening, treatment and prognosis. *J Gerontol* 1992; **47**: 24–30.

55. Greenfield S, Blanco DM, Elashoff RM, Ganz PA. Patterns of care related to age of breast cancer patients. *JAMA* 1987; **20**: 2766–70.

56. Silliman RA, Balducci L, Goodwin JS, *et al*. Breast cancer in older age: what we know, don't know and do. *J Natl Cancer Inst* 1993; **85**: 190–199.

57. Moore MJ, Osoba D, Murphy K, *et al*. Use of palliative endpoints to evaluate the effects of mitoxantrone and low-dose prednisone in patients with hormonally resistant prostate cancer. *J Clin Oncol* 1994; **12**: 689–694.

58. Repetto L, Vercelli M, Simoni C, *et al*. Comorbid conditions among elderly cancer patients. *Annals Oncology* 5 suppl. 1994, abstr.288.

59. WHO: the first ten years of the World Health Organization. Geneva: WHO, 1958.

60. Satariano WA, Ragheb NE, Dupuis MH. Comorbidity in older women with breast cancer: an epidemiologic approach. In *Cancer in the elderly. Approaches to early detection and treatment*, edited by R Yancik, JW Yates. New York: Springer Publishing Company, 71–107, 1989.

61. Aaronson NK, Ahmedzai S, Bergman B, *et al*. for the European Organization for Research and Treatment of Cancer Study Group on Quality of Life: the European Organization for Research and Treatment of Cancer QLQ-C30: a quality of life instrument for use in international clinical trials in oncology. *J Natl C Inst* 1993; **85**: 365–376.

62. Mor V, Allen S, Malin M. The psychosocial impact of cancer on older versus younger patients and their families. *Cancer* 1994; **74**: 2118–2127.

63. McMillen Moinpour C, Feigl P, Metch B, *et al*. Quality of life end points in cancer clinical trials: review and recommendations. *J Natl Cancer Inst* 1989; **81**: 485–495.

64. Slevin ML, Plant H, Lynch D, *et al*. Who should measure quality of life: the doctor of patient? *Br J Cancer* 1988; **57**: 109–112.

65. Bergman B, Aaronson NK, Ahmedzai S, *et al*. The EORTC QLQ-LC13: a modular supplement to the EORTC core quality of life questionnaire (QLQ-C30) for use in lung cancer clinical trials. *Eur J Cancer* 1994; **30**(A)5: 635–642.

66. McKenna RJ. Clinical aspects of cancer in the elderly: treatment decisions treatment choices and follow-up. *Cancer* 1994; **74**: 2107–2117.

67. Yellen SB, Cella DF, Leslie WT. Age and clinical decision making in oncology patients. *J Natl Cancer Inst* 1994; **86**: 1766–1770.

68. Balducci L. Do we need geriatric oncology? *Cancer Control* 1994; **1**(2): 1–5.

69. Katz S, Ford AB, Moskowitz RB, *et al*. The index of ADL: a standardized measure of biological and physical function. *JAMA* 1963; **185**: 914–919.

70. Lawton MP, Brody EM. Assessment of older people: self-monitoring and instrumental activities of daily living. *Gerontologist* 1969; **9**: 179–186.

71. Rubinstein LZ, Josephson KR, Wieland GD, *et al*. Effectiveness of a geriatric evaluation unit: a randomized clinical trial. *N Engl J Med* 1984; **311**: 1664–74.

72. Rubinstein LZ. Comprehensive geriatric assessment. In *Moderator. New issues in geriatric care*, edited by DH Solomon. *Ann Int Med* 1988; **108**: 718–732.

73. Consensus Conference: the future of geriatric assessment. *J Am Ger Soc* 1991; **39**: 1S–59S.

74. Beghè C, Robinson B. Comprehensive geriatric assessment: diagnostic, therapeutic and prognostic value. *Cancer Control* 1994; **1**(2): 121–125.

75. Stuck AE, Siu AL, Wieland GD, *et al*. Comprehensive geriatric assessment: a meta-analysis of controlled trials. *Lancet* 1993; **342**: 1032–1036.

Appendix

To facilitate the understanding of our approach to older persons with cancer, we offer here a number of case studies.

Case 1

A 92 year old resident of a nursing home was found to have a 2 cm nodule in her left breast, by a nursing assistant, during her daily bath. The patient had been institutionalized for 23 months, due to dementia (MMS score 16), agitation, and severe osteoarthritis. She had history of atrial fibrillation for several years, treated with digoxin 0.125 mg every other day and coumadine, 2 mg at alternate days. She was dependent in all ADLs. A mammogram revealed a mass 1 × 2 cm in diameter, with poorly defined margins.

The patient weighted 42 kg and had atrophy of facial and palmar muscles. She was unable to follow commands and gave only generic responses to specific questions. In addition to severe arthritis of her hands, knees and feet, she had a irregular heart beat, with a central heart rate of 89/min.

A biopsy was recommended, but refused by the patient and by her son. The patient became very agitated at the mention of the biopsy and required sedation with haloperidol.

It was decided to follow the patient with serial physical exams at monthly intervals.

Eight months later the patient died of a respiratory infection: the size of the tumor had not significantly enlarged.

Comments

The first question we faced in this case concerned the need of a biopsy. In a woman of this age, a breast mass with poorly defined margin is highly suggestive of breast cancer, yet a biopsy was indicated, especially to rule out carcinoma "*in situ*" or unusual neoplasms (medullary carcinoma, cystosarcoma phylloides, lymphoma).

The second question concerned the need to obtain a court authorization for the procedure, in view of the lack of cooperation from patient and family. This decision involved considerations of life expectancy, quality of life, treatment effectiveness. Clearly, this woman had a limited average life expectancy that could be estimated between 6 months and 2 years, as calculated from age, comorbidity, and poor functional status; clearly, the cancer was not causing any symptoms and could be closely followed; in the case of the most common forms of breast cancer (infiltrating ductal carcinoma) one could have expected a 30–40% chances of local progression, causing discomfort, over the following two years. The chances of disseminated metastases, causing the patient death within two years were negligible (as estimated from the treatment trial of the Breast Cancer Campaign published in 1991 in the British Journal of Surgery). The only disease that might have undergone a more rapid progression would have been a high grade lymphoma, and the chances of this neoplasm were 1–2%. Furthermore, treatment of breast cancer would have involved at least a partial mastectomy. Though such procedure may be performed under local anesthesia, in ordinary circumstances, it would have required general anesthesia in the case of an uncooperative and agitated patient, and general anesthesia would have been associated with substantial risk. In the case of lymphoma, the treatment with high dose chemotherapy would have not been tolerated by this patient with poor performance status and malnutrition. Thus, a biopsy would have not probably helped us at this stage of management.

The third decision concerned the possibility to institute medical treatment with tamoxifen, which is effective in approximately 60% of women over 70 in delaying the progression of the disease for at least two years. The main risk of tamoxifen, deep vein thrombosis, in a woman over 70 and virtually immobilized, might have been offset by the ongoing treatment with coumadine.

We felt that serial physical exams were the only intervention necessary at that time; should we have disease progression and risk of local complications, we might have been able to enroll the cooperation of the son for surgery or we might have started the tamoxifen treatment at that time.

Case 2

A 83 year old previously fully independent woman was found by her daughter confused and dehydrated. The daughter, who lived in a close city, was concerned because she had not heard from the patient for more than a week. The patient was a retired homemaker and a widow. She had had three previous pregnancies and no other significant medical history, except for a hysterectomy thirty years earlier. She was taking no prescription drugs, nor over the counter medications. She used to travel, to prepare her own meals, and to conduct a very active social life.

On admission to the hospital she weighted 46 kg, and had a blood pressure of 85/50 when lying. Upon sitting, the blood pressure was undetectable. The turgor of the skin was markedly decreased. The CBC was normal, the BUN 47 mg/dl, the serum creatinine 2.4 mg/dl, serum sodium 152 Meq, serum K 5.3 mEq, and the serum albumin 3.1 gm/dl.

After fluid resuscitation the patient became more alert and reported she had been unable to eat any solid food during the past week, and she also had a poor fluid intake due to nausea and vomiting. Abdominal CT revealed a gastric mass. Esophagogastroscopy revealed high degree of gastric obstruction, and the biopsy of the mass revealed large cell lymphoma, diffuse.

Total parenteral nutrition was immediately instituted and the patient was treated with low doses of doxorubicin (15 mg/m2) and cyclophosphamide (300 mg/m2)IV. After approximately three weeks the patient symptoms had subsided and she was able to ingest a full liquid diet. Treatment with cyclophosphamide, doxorubicin, vincristine and prednisone at full doses caused a complete remission of her disease. Recently the patient celebrated her 86th birthday.

Comments

This case illustrates two important points. First, rapid decline of performance status in elderly patient should not be interpreted as a contraindication to treatment. Owing to a limited functional reserve, older individuals are susceptible to rapid changes in performance status, when faced by stress. This lady with a highly treatable malignancy had been fully independent until one week prior to admission. Her function prior to the onset of her acute condition was a more reliable guide to treatment than her function at the time of hospital admission.

Second, low doses of chemotherapy had been well tolerated even when the patient was severely debilitated, and set the stage for her prompt recovery. Though more tolerable drugs, such as mitoxantrone or navelbine may be active in older persons with large cell lymphoma, doxorubicin appears still as the mainstay treatment. As demonstrated by investigators from Vancouver (O'Reilly *et al.*) even low doses of doxorubicin may be effective in this disease. Some form of treatment is almost always advisable in curable malignancies associated with a short survival when left untreated. The average life expectancy of this lady, prior to the diagnosis of lymphoma, was approximately ten years; with an untreated lymphoma she could have hardly survived one more month. Furthermore, the neoplasm had caused a very rapid deterioration of her quality of life. Though cure is obtainable in only 30% of the patients, a therapeutic response would have controlled the present symptoms and would have restituted her autonomy to this lady.

Another important consideration is that social support was essential to the proper management of this lady, whose independence was severely curtailed by her disease. This possibility of rapid deterioration is typical of the aged and is the reason why we use proactively a CGA in all patient aged 75 and over.

Case 3

A 71 year old man presented to us with diagnosis of small cell lung cancer, limited disease, involving the left lower stem bronchus, the ipsilateral mediastinum and the left supraclavicular lymph nodes. The patient had lost approximately 8 kg in weight over the past three months and was able to perform with some difficulties his daily activities. He was post coronary bypass surgery and now had a history of stable angina well controlled with nitrates and Ca^{++} channel blockers. He also had history of moderate chronic pulmonary obstructive disease.

Past medical history included two motor vehicular accidents.

He had been divorced 20 years and he lived alone; two adult daughters lived in the neighborhood and took turns in caring for him with daily visits.

On physical exam the patient was alert but kind of uncooperative: showed a flat affect and gave slow response to questions. He was 1m 72 cm tall and weighted 61 Kg (< 80% ideal body weight); the triceps skin fold was reduced by 17%. A 4 × 7 cm mass was palpable on the left supraclavicular area. Breath sounds were almost absent on left lower lobe. Neurologic exam was intact.

CGA revealed a 13/15 items positive geriatric depression scale. He was ADL independent, but needed assistance in grocery shopping, meal preparation and managing money. He spent most of his time at home, watching television and quite often skipped meals. Both daughters clearly expressed no interest in providing frequent transportation to the hospital and in managing potential complications of chemotherapy or radiotherapy.

We recommended treatment with amitriptyline 25 mg at night and oral etoposide 50 mg twice daily for three weeks out of four, with weekly monitoring of CBC.

The patient expired 7 months later from a cerebral accident likely due to brain metastases. During the first two months of treatment he had gained some weight and improved his range of activities. Eventually, however, he failed to keep his clinic appointments and discontinued the chemotherapy.

Comments

The optimal treatment of this patient would have involved combination chemotherapy (cisplatin/etoposide) with radiation therapy to the chest and the brain. However, the patient had a borderline performance status, which might have made the treatment particularly hazardous. Furthermore, he lacked the social support to receive appropriate treatment and to respond in a timely fashion to the complications of treatment.

We opted then to manage his depression with a mild antidepressant and to institute low dose chemotherapy which was effective and reasonably safe under the circumstances. The initial effects were improvement of performance status and mood, but the social situation prevented the patient from receiving more aggressive and effective treatment, despite these encouraging signs.

Another important aspect of this case is diagnosis of depression in older individuals. Though the prevalence of depression increases with the age of the population, it may be very difficult to obtain adequate history from older persons, especially older men who lack communicative skills. In this circumstances the Geriatric Depression Scale is very valuable.

This case is a good example of how the CGA may assist in the management of older individuals. Without CGA the patient's emotional, functional, and social problems might have never emerged and the patient might have received inappropriately toxic treatment.

Case 4

A 95 year old woman, who managed a "prank shop", developed over three months severe back pain, anorexia, and lost 5 kg of weight. The pain was exacerbated by movements of the trunk. Radiograph of the back revealed osteoarthritis of the thoracic and lumbar spine. An abdominal CT showed a 7 × 9 cm mass in the body of the pancreas. Laboratory work showed a serum albumin of 2.8 gm/dl. CA19-9 was 167 mg/dl.

A fine needle aspiration biopsy showed a adenocarcinoma.

The patient was fully alert and independent, until the pain developed and she was living now with an adult daughter and her husband. Two other children lived close and were very supportive. She had been a widow for 45 years.

CGA showed that the patient had been ADL and IADL independent until recently. Her Mini mental status score were normal and so was the geriatric depression scale. Originally she thought her pain was due to arthritis and did not seek immediate medical attention.

She was not interested in any form of life-prolonging treatment for a cancer that was clearly incurable, and only asked for pain relief.

Initially she was treated with radiation therapy to the pancreas and low doses of fluorouracil, but severe nausea and vomiting mandated frequent interruptions of treatment. Also, oral morphine was poorly tolerated, because of nausea and vomiting.

A nerve block with alcohol was unsuccessful, but the placement of an intrathecal catheter, with intermittent administration of morphine at low doses produced a complete relief of symptoms, without side effects. She died at home 4 months later.

This case illustrates the trial and error approach in the management of the oldest old. The unusual response of this patient to radiotherapy and oral morphine was unexpected. Seemingly, it indicates that the gastric mucosa in the aged is often atrophic and poorly tolerant of radiation injury. It also suggests that the half life of opiate medications is prolonged and this prolongation is associated with more frequent and unpleasant complications. It should be highlighted that the excellent social support of this lady allowed us to experiment different forms of treatment. When such support is not present a nerve block should probably represent the most effective form of management.

Another important point of this case is the delay in diagnosis, as the back pain was initially ascribed to ingravescing osteoarthritis.

Case 5

A 76 year-old man had diagnosis of stage II prostate cancer, three years prior to referral to our center. He was treated with external beam irradiation of the prostate. One year later his serum PSA, which had dropped to 2.2 ng/ml six months after irradiation, risen to 12 ng/ml. Bone scan and pelvic CT were negative for tumor. The patient was treated with orchiectomy and flutamide. The patient was referred to us for increasing bone pain in his back, which failed to improve after two months of flutamide withdrawal.

The patient was a retired salesman; he lived with his wife of 45 years and had two married children who lived out of town. He was fully independent in his ADL and IADL, and used to travel and to play golf.

Past medical history included appendectomy.

Current medications included hydrochlorothiazide for hypertension.

Physical exam showed a well developed and nourished man, in no acute distress, alert, intelligent and cooperative. Beside for pain in his thoracic and lumbar spine, exacerbated by movements, his physical exam was normal.

Serum PSA was 88 ng/dl; alkaline phosphatase 451 IU. CBC showed a WBC of 8800/ul, Hemoglobin 11.9 gm/dl platelet 574000/ul.

Bone scan was widely positive in the axial and appendicular skeleton.

We treated the patient with mitoxantrone 12mg/m2 IV every three weeks and after three treatments the pain had all but disappeared; the serum PSA was 17 ng/ml. The treatment was interrupted at that point to allow the patient to take a cruise with his wife.

Comments

Several options were available for the management of this extremely healthy gentleman with metastatic prostate cancer. They included external beam irradiation to the spine, radioactive strontium, and other forms of chemotherapy, such as estramustine in combination with etoposide or navelbine, cisplatin, cyclophosphamide. We felt that external beam irradiation probably was inadequate, in view of diffuse bony metastases, and radioactive strontium might have compromised our ability to treat him later with chemotherapy, whereas strontium may have represented a most valuable option at a later time. The cyclic administration of mitoxantrone appeared more convenient for this healthy patient with no transportation problems than the daily administration of multiple tablets.

This case illustrates how cytotoxic chemotherapy may represent valuable palliation for older patients with metastatic cancer. We had similar experience with older women with metastatic breast cancer treated with mitoxantrone.

Case 6

A 79 year old woman was referred to us for management of breast cancer metastatic to the bones, which caused severe pain. One year earlier, the patient had a left modified radical mastectomy for an infiltrative adenocarcinoma which had a diameter of 2.3 cm, was poor in hormone receptor, was grade 3 histologically, and had a high proliferation rate. 0/14 lymph nodes were involved by the tumor. The patient refused adjuvant chemotherapy and received adjuvant tamoxifen 20 mg/daily.

The past medical history was positive for a cerebrovascular accident in the region of the right middle cerebral artery, which resulted in hemiparesis. The patient also had history of hypertension and chronic renal insufficiency.

She lived with her husband of 56 years and received daily assistance from a married daughter. She was unable to take bath by herself and was able only to take few steps at a time. The geriatric depression scale revealed scored 5/16 and the Mini mental status scored 24.

The CT of the abdomen revealed hepatic metastases, the radio nuclide bone scan was widely positive, the MRI of the brain revealed brain atrophy, compatible with the patient age.

We treated the patient with mitoxantrone IV 12 mg/m2 every three weeks. The patient developed severe neutropenia and neutropenic fever after the first course of treatment. Despite a dose reduction to 9 mg/m2, the patient developed sepsis and expired after the second course of treatment.

Comment

This case is mainly presented to illustrate how chemotherapy even in small doses may be very toxic to some elderly patients with poor performance status and with dependent ADLs. In retrospect, after the severe complications following the first treatment, supportive care only might have been more advisable for this patient.

21.   Nutrition, Cancer and Aging

Jeanne Hudson

Introduction

This chapter reviews the interaction of cancer and nutrition in carcinogenesis, cancer prevention, and cancer treatment. These interactions are particularly important in older patients who are at increased risk for nutritional disorders. Nutrient deficiencies in the elderly may occur. Various causes include abnormalities in energy metabolism due to chronic illnesses, suboptimal oral intake, chronic use of a laxative interfering with fat-soluble vitamin absorption, and limited financial and transportation resources. In an older cancer patient, nutrient deficits may heighten the risk of poor outcome in the treatment course. Silver estimated that malnutrition occurs 0 to 15% in ambulatory geriatric outpatients, 35 to 65% in acute-hospitalized older adults, and 25 to 60% in institutionalized older adults (1). The incidence of mortality in malnourished older adults is well documented (2). Various reports have indicated that 40 to 80% of cancer patients develop some clinically detectable malnutrition (3–4). Warren noted that cachexia was associated most frequently with carcinoma of the stomach (45%), breast with extensive lung and liver involvement (33.1%), and large bowel (22%); bladder and prostate cancers were associated with the least incidence (5). Cancer patients are considered at higher nutritional risk because of the potential to develop one or more nutritional problems during treatment.

Diet and Carcinogenesis

Carcinogens are substances producing cancer in man or animals. Carcinogenesis has three phases: initiation (normal cell is irreversibly changed by mutagen), pro-
motion (initiated cells turn into benign tumor cells), and progression (further mutations occur until tumor cell invades tissue and metastase) (6). Ames and his colleagues have proposed the HERP (human exposure/rodent potency) index to estimate possible cancer toxicity associated with various substances and food items on human beings (7–8). It has been cautioned by many researchers that animal bioassays and *in vitro* studies provide clues to which carcinogens and mutagens may be contributing to human cancers; but tests on animals are expensive and the animal to human correlations are difficult to ascertain. Food compounds may contain both inhibitors and enhancers of carcinogenesis. Some of the possible food enhancers include smoked, salted, and pickled foods that may cause gastric and esophageal cancers. Nitrates may be found in vegetables and drinking water; but are also used in the process of pickling, salting, and curing of foods in the form of sodium and potassium nitrates. Nitrosamines are present in tobacco and tobacco smoke. Studies have shown a causal role of stomach and esophageal cancers with the frequent intake of smoked and fried foods (9). Some nutritional substances may be synergistic with viruses that play a role in cancer development (10). Aflatoxin (a mold found in peanuts, wheat and corn) eaten by a person with hepatitis B virus is associated with a high incidence of liver cancer in certain populations (11). Alcohol has been directly associated with oral, esophageal, gastric and possibly colorectal cancers. Chronic alcohol use has been associated with malnutrition and nutrient deficiencies. Dietary fat may play a role in causing cancer of the colon, rectum, breast, and prostate. Increased body weight has been associated with post menopausal breast and endometrial cancer (12). Possible inhibitors of carcinogenesis currently being stud-

Table 21.1   Vulnerability of the elderly to dietary carcinogens.

Increased Vulnerability	
Decreased ability to repair chemically induced DNA injury	Gastric hypochloridria
Decreased ability to dispose of intracellular free radicals	Decreased dietary ingestion of vitamins, fiber, and trace elements
Constipation	Waning immunologic defenses

Decreased Vulnerability	
Decreased ability for interaction between carcinogens and DNA	Decreased ability to metabolically activate the carcinogens
Decreased enteric absorption of carcinogens	Decreased cellular proliferative activity

ied include vitamins C, A, E, selenium, and dietary fiber (refer to section on the role of diet in cancer prevention in this chapter). Vulnerability to dietary carcinogens may be both increased and decreased in the elderly (Table 21.1) (13).

Role of Diet in Cancer Prevention

Doll and Peto estimate that between 20–60% of cancers in the United States are related to dietary factors (14). It has been proven that reducing fat intake may reduce the risk of cancers of the colon, rectum, breast, and prostate (15–17). Both the American Cancer Society and the National Cancer Institute agree that fat intake should be less than thirty percent of a person's total caloric intake. At the same time, increasing fruits and vegetables in diet may act as agents which inhibit the carcinogenic process against cancers of the lung, colon, rectum, bladder, oral cavity, stomach, cervix, and esophagus. A high fiber diet (i.e., whole grain cereals and breads, vegetables, fruits) may decrease the risk of colon cancer. Whether the fiber is soluble or insoluble type, most studies suggest increasing the amount of total fiber per day (18). Phytochemicals show promise as a new nutritional approach to fighting cancer. Phytochemicals are chemicals found in plants. Scientists are still unsure which specific compounds in fruits, vegetables, grains, seeds, and nuts may help prevent cancer. There are over 500 known carotenoids. Beta-carotene is the most well-known but other carotenoids include alpha-carotene, lutein, and lycopene (19). Phytoestrogens are attracting the interest of health professionals. Isoflavonoids, genistein and daidzein are found in soy foods which may lower the risk of cancer, cardiovascular disease, osteoporosis, and menopausal problems. Genistein, a weak estrogen has been shown to inhibit a wide range of cancer cells *in vitro* studies and in several animal studies by competing with estradiol for estrogen receptors, consequently functioning as an antiestrogen. Table 21.2 is a list of a few of the phytochemicals and their food sources (20–21).

NHANES II survey reported that only nine percent of the subjects consumed the National Cancer Institute (NCI) recommended five or more servings of fruits or vegetables per day (22). The NCI and most medical professionals will agree that the "Five A Day Program" is one of the best recommendations for cancer prevention. The "Five A Day Program" recommends eating five servings of fruits and vegetables a day: one rich in vitamin A; one rich in vitamin C; one high in fiber; and cruciferous vegetables several times during the week. With the help of various health organizations, nutritional counseling, and the media, the public has been made aware of some of the more appropriate dietary changes needed. Americans have decreased consumption of red meats. increased consumption of poultry, reversed amount of whole milk to skim milk consumption, increased fruit and selected vegetable consumption (Table 21.3).

Table 21.2 Phytochemicals.

Phytochemical	Food source
Genistein	soybeans
Flavones	dried beans
Indoles and isothiocyanates	cruciferous vegetables
Phytic acid	grains
Caffeic acid	fruits
Ellagic acid	grapes, strawberries, raspberries
Limonene	citrus fruit peel
Allyl sulfides and other allium compounds	garlic, onions, leeks, and chives
Betacarotene	sweet potatoes, carrots, cantaloupe
Lycopene	tomato, pink grapefruit, watermelon
Monterpenes	oils for citrus fruits, nuts, seeds

Cancer and Malnutrition

Cancer may promote malnutrition in different ways. First, cancer may cause dysfunction of the digestive system (i.e., dysphagia, maldigestion, and malabsorption). Second, cancer may result in abnormalities in protein, lipid, and carbohydrate metabolism. Third, cancer treatment itself may be a cause of malnutrition. Radiation, chemotherapy, and surgery are the current treatment options/combinations presented to patients. Nutritional status can be affected by the location of the cancer, the cancer treatment chosen, poor nutritional status prior to treatment, and emotional stress. Various side effects may occur with the different treatment options. Table 21.4 illustrates the nutritional complications of radiation. Radiation to the brain may occasion-

Table 21.3 Per capita consumption of major food commodities: 1970 to 1992.

Commodity	1970	1992
Red meat, total (boneless, trimmed weight)	131.7#	114.1#
Poultry products (boneless weight)	33.8#	60.1#
Plain whole milk	213.5#	81.4#
Plain low fat milk	29.8#	99.3#
Fresh fruits, total	79.1#	98.7#
Selected fresh vegetables	88.1#	109.3#

From Statistical Abstract of the United States 1994, 114th edition.

Table 21.4 Nutritional consequences of radiation therapy.

Irradiated region	Nutritional consequence
Brain	Nausea and vomiting
	Elevated blood sugar secondary to steroids
	Dysgeusia (taste alterations)
	Dysosmia (distortion of normal smell)
Oral cavity	Dysegusia
	Hypogeusia (blunting of taste sense)
	Mucositis
	Xerostomia (dry mouth)
	Thick saliva
	Dysphagia
	Chewing impairment
	Taste fatigue
Upper esophagus and thorax	Mucositis
	Esophagitis
	Stomatitis
	Loss of appetite
	Dysphagia
	Esophageal stricture
	Weight loss
	Hypergeusia (excessive acuteness of taste sense)
Gastrointestinal tract/abdomen	Nausea and vomiting
	Stomatitis
	Malabsorption
Pelvis/prostate	Chronic diarrhea
	Constipation
	Bloating
	Flatulence
	Lactose intolerance
	Rectal bleeding
	Dehydration
	Electrolyte imbalance

Table 21.5 Nutritional consequences of chemotherapy.

Leukopenia	Electrolyte abnormalities
Nausea	Anorexia
Vomiting	Xerostomia
Diarrhea	Dysgeusia
Mucositits	Constipation
Stomatitis	Lactose intolerance

tube placement, or TPN (total parenteral nutrition) may be necessary to prevent malnutrition.

Chemotherapy affects both normal and malignant tissue cells. Table 21.5 shows some of the side effects seen depending on dosage, chemotherapy agent(s) used and number of cycles given of each drug. If a person is in good nutritional status, tolerance of chemotherapy and its side effects may be less severe. Nausea occurs with a majority of chemotherapy agents used. Ability to eat, chew, and swallow may diminish due to mucositis, esophagitis, and glossitis; nutritional status will decrease and may lead to malnutrition if not treated early.

Nutritional Assessment

Nutritional assessment of the older adult includes evaluation of (1) physiological data; (2) medical, social, and dietary history information; and (3) clinical assessment. Physiological data includes anthropometrics and biochemical information. Particularly important are height and weight data. Stated heights and weights are often erroneous. Height decreases with age because of possible postural changes and bone disease (23). There are alternate height measurements that can be used if an older adult cannot stand erect or without assistance (i.e., knee height, total arm length, recumbent height) (24–26). Weight history and current weights help in evaluating a patient's nutritional status. As little as 5 to 10% loss of usual body weight can have a negative impact on survival and influence the prognosis (27). For correct chemotherapy dosing, it is essential to have accurate height and actual current body weight to figure body surface area. Changes in weight must be viewed with caution since they are susceptible to a variety of factors and diseases (i.e., amount of clothing worn, if the client ate or drank prior to weighing, edema, cancer cachexia, etc.). Important changes in body composition occurs with age. This includes a decrease in total body water to approximately forty-five percent of body weight and increase in body fat. Dehydration is often missed while evaluating an older adult. Dehydration may be partially due to decreased osmoreceptor capacity of older people which assists in signaling thirst sensation (26). Decreased fluid intake may interfere with medication absorption, distribution, metabolism, and excretion by the body. Overhydration or dehydration status can affect nutritional assessment (i.e., accu-

ally cause nausea and vomiting; but frequency is low. Steroids used for long periods of time may cause hyperglycemia. Radiation to the oral cavity, upper esophagus/thorax, and gastrointestinal tract/abdomen have a high incidence of side effects. If the client is unable to eat adequate amounts of food to meet nutritional needs, nutritional supplements, possible feeding

Table 21.6

Biochemical measures	Affected by Age	Comments
Albumin	no	Reliable index of malnutrition. Affected by hydration status, stress, trauma or altered liver functions.
Transferrin	yes	Affected by increased tissue iron stores
Pre-albumin	no	Response to repletion not studied well
Hemoglobin/hematocrit	no	Maintained well
Red blood cell count	no	Maintained well
Iron	no	Maintained well
Ferritin	yes	Abnormally high in the elderly
Serum B-12	no	Reliable index of B-12 deficiency
Glucose	possible	FBG level may have a higher baseline value in the elderly
Total lymphocyte count	no	Decreases with malnutrition and increases with stress or sepsis
Skin text anergy panel	yes	Incidence of anergy increases with age
Creatinine height index	yes	Alterations in kidney function in the elderly
Cholesterol	no	Recommend monitoring regularly. Low levels are associated with increased mortality
Thyroid hormones	no	Aging decreases production of thyroid hormone but is counterbalanced by decreased thyroid hormone degradation

rate weight, laboratory levels). Several biochemical assays are used to assess nutritional status (Table 21.6).

Reviewing medical, social, and dietary history data are essential. Co-morbid medical conditions, alternative medical therapies, medication use (both prescription and over-the-counter drugs), febrile status, and use of alcohol will compromise nutritional status. Social history involves evaluating the living situation, depression, stress from coping with the cancer, fatigue, and should be triggers to health professionals that nutritional intake may be affected. If an older adult needs meals, health professionals should consider the functional level and/or the financial status of each individual. The dietitian can offer possible solutions and community resources to help improve nutritional intake (refer to Nutrition Intervention section). Assessment of dietary history (typical 1–2 day intake) would help assess an older adult's calorie, protein, and other nutrient status. The Harris-Benedict formula is recommended for calculating energy requirements for an older adult since it considers age as one of the variables (Table 21.7).

Current Recommended Dietary Allowances (RDAs) do not acknowledge different nutrient requirements for persons over 65 years of age compared with younger persons. Current RDAs group age 51+ together (30).

Table 21.7 Equations for predicting caloric requirements.

In males	$BEE(kcal/day) = 66 (13.7 \times W) + (5 \times H) - (6.8 \times A)$
In females	$BEE(kcal/day) = 655 (9.6 \times W) + (1.7 \times H) - (4.7 \times A)$

W = weight in kilograms; H = height in centimeters; A = age in years

Source: From *A Biometric Study of Basal Metabolism in Man* by J.A. Harris and F.G. Benedict. (1919). Washington D.C.: Carnegie Institute of Washington, Publ. No. 279.

BEE reflects the caloric needs in the resting, fasting, and unstressed state (29):
    For weight maintenance: $BEE \times 1.15$–1.3
    For weight anabolism: $BEE \times 1.5$

For calculating protein requirements: Divide Ideal Body Weight (IBW) by 2.2 = kg of IBW
For protein maintenance: Multiply 0.8–$1.4g \times$ kg of IBW
For protein anabolism: Multiply $1.5g \times$ kg of IBW

Table 21.8 National Research Council: Diet and Health, 1989.

1. Reduce total fat intake to 30% or less of calories. Reduce saturated fatty acid intake to less than 10% of calories and dietary cholesterol to less than 300 mg daily. Polyunsaturated fatty acid intake should stay about the present 7% of calories (and not be above 10% of calories in individuals).

2. Every day eat five or more servings of a combination of vegetables and fruits, especially green and yellow vegetables and citrus fruits. Also, increase intake of starches and other complex carbohydrates by eating six or more daily servings of a combination of breads, cereals, and legumes.

3. Maintain protein intake at moderate levels (no more than twice the RDA).

4. Balance food intake and physical activity to maintain appropriate body weight. All healthy people should maintain physical activity at a moderate level.

5. The Committee does not recommend alcohol consumption. For those who do drink, limit consumption to two standard drinks a day. Pregnant women and women attempting to conceive should avoid alcoholic beverages.

6. Limit total daily salt (sodium chloride) intake to 6 g or less. Salty and highly processed salty, salt-preserved, and salt-pickled foods should be consumed sparingly.

7. Maintain adequate calcium intake.

8. Avoid taking dietary supplements in excess of the RDA in any one day.

9. Maintain an optimal intake of fluoride, particularly during the years of primary and secondary tooth formation.

Ryan *et al.* found 37–40% of 65+ year old men and women had oral intake of less than two-thirds the RDAs (31).

Nutritional Intervention

If an older adult has either financial constrains or limited mobility, possible solutions would include recommending Home-Delivered Meal program (a.k.a. Meals-On-Wheels), Congregate Eating Centers, frozen TV dinners, or restaurants that deliver meals to one's home. The Congregate and Home-Delivered Meal nutrition programs provide one-third of the RDAs (Recommended Dietary Allowances). For the older adults with financial burdens, the Food Stamp Program may offer assistance by decreasing the financial restraints and providing adequate nutrients. To inquire about the Food Stamp Program, call the Health & Rehabilitative Services: Department of Information and Referral phone number in the county where the client lives. The department will be able to provide information and eligibility requirements of the program. Food supplements (i.e., Ensure, Sustacal, etc.) are being strongly advertised through the media today for both healthy and ill adults. These supplements are meant as an addition to an inadequate diet to meet daily nutritional requirements and not as a complete meal replacement.

Nutritional counseling should be given early on in the therapy to help decrease the severity of the side effect(s) of the various treatment options. If a client is compliant but has persistent weight loss even with nutritional counseling, megestrol acetate is recommended. Megestrol acetate has been shown to improve appetite and food intake in 3 placebo-controlled randomized trials in advanced cancer patients with anorexia and cachexia (32–34). Clients whose disease is not considered end stage disease; but are not responding to nutritional counselings or megestrol acetate should be considered for possible feeding tube placement. It needs to be emphasized that it is up to the health care professional to state objective positive and negative points of options; but the decision of a feeding tube should be left up to the client.

Summary

Recognizing and treating the older patient with cancer can be a significant challenge. Changes in body composition, socioeconomic issues, and nutritional status must be evaluated in the older adult along with disease state(s). Eating a well-balanced diet and consuming the optimal nutrients needed remains the best recommendations for reducing cancer risk. The National Research Council recommends the following guidelines to reduce cancer risk (Table 21.8).

The American public has made some positive changes in eating habits; but not to the standards as hoped. Ryan reported that the older adult population still does not meet even two-thirds of the RDAs in daily needs. It is up to the health care professionals to inform and educate the public on facts and guidelines that have been found fundamentally sound. The keys to preventing nutritional depletion from cancer are nutritional screening and early nutritional intervention.

References

1. Silver AJ. Malnutrition. In *Geriatrics Review Syllabus. A Core Curriculum in Geriatric Medicine. Book I/Syllabus and Questions*, edited by JC Beck. New York: American Geriatrics Society, 1991.

2. Morley JE. Anorexia in older patients: Its meaning and management. *Geriatrics* 1990; **45**, 59–66.

3. Kern KA, Norton JA. Cancer cachexia. *JPEN* 1988; **12**: 286–298.

4. Ollenschlager G, Viell B, Thomas W, Konkol K, Burger B. Tumor anorexia: causes, assessment, treatment. *Recent Results Cancer Res* 1991; **121**: 249–259.

5. Warren S. The immediate causes of death in cancer. *Am J Med Sci* 1932; **184**: 610–615.

6. Pariza MW. Diet, cancer, and food safety. In *Modern nutrition in health and disease*, edited by ME Shils, JA Olson and M Shike. Philadelphia: Lea Febiger, 1994.

7. Ames B, *et al. Does Nature Know Best? Natural Carcinogens in American Food*. Revised ed. New York: American Council on Science and Health, 1992.

8. Ames BN, Magaw R, Gold LS. Ranking possible carcinogenic hazards. *Science* 1987; **236**: 271–280.

9. Wu-Williams AH, *et al.* Lifestyle, workplace, and stomach cancer by subsite in young men of Los Angeles County. *Cancer Res* 1990; **50**: 2569–2576.

10. Meyskens FL, Jr. Strategies for prevention of cancer in humans. *Oncology* 1992; **6** (suppl): 15–24.

11. VanRensburg SJ, *et al. Br J Cancer* 1985; **51**: 713.

12. Weinstein IB. Cancer prevention: Recent progress and future opportunities. *Cancer Research (suppl.)* 1991; **51**: 5080s–5085s.

13. Balducci L, Wallace C, Khansur T, Vance RB, Thigpen JT, Hardy C. Nutrition, cancer, and aging: An annotated review. *JAGS* 1986; **34**: 127–136.

14. Doll FRS, Peto R. *The causes of cancer*. New York: Oxford University Press, 1981.

15. Bal DG, Foerster SB. Dietary strategies for cancer prevention. *Cancer* 1993; **72** (Suppl.): 1005–1010.

16. Kritchevsky D. Dietary guidelines. *Cancer* 1993; **72** (Suppl.): 1011–1014.

17. Herbert V, Subak-Sharpe GJ. Mount Sinai School of Medicine. *Complete book of nutrition*. New York: St. Martin's Press, 1990

18. Slattery ML, Sorenson AW, Mahoney AW, *et al.* Diet and colon cancer: Assessment of risk by fiber type and food source. *J Natl Cancer Inst* 1988; **80**: 1474–1480.

19. Mangels AR, Holden JM, Beecher GR, Forman MR, Lanza E. Carotenoid content of fruits and vegetables: An evaluation of analytic data. *JADA* 1993; **93**: 284–296.

20. Steinmetz KA, Potter JD. Vegetables, fruit, and cancer. I. Epidemiology. *Cancer Causes Control* 1991; **2**: 325–357.

21. Steinmetz KA, Potter JD. Vegetables, fruit, and cancer. II. Mechanisms. *Cancer Causes Control* 1991; **2**: 427–442.

22. Patterson BH, Block G, Rosenberger WF, *et al.* Fruit and vegetables in the American diet: Data from the NHANES II survey. *Am J Public Health* 1990; **80**: 1443–1449.

23. Kuczmarski RJ. Need for body composition information in elderly subjects. *Am J Clin Nutr* 1989; **50**: 1150–1157.

24. Roubenoff R, Wilson PWF. Advantage of knee height over height as an index of stature in expression of body composition in adults. *Am J Clin Nutr* 1993; **57**: 609–613.

25. Haboubi NY, Hudson PR, Pathy MS. Measurement of height in the elderly. *JAGS* 1990; **38**: 1008–1010.

26. Gray DS, Crider JB, Kelley C, Dickinson LC. Accuracy of recumbent height measurement. *JPEN* 1985; **9**: 712–715.

27. Chlebowski RT. Nutritional support of the medical oncology patient [Monograph]. *Hematol Oncol Clin North Am* 1991; **5**: 147–160.

28. Abrams WB, Beers MH, Berkow RB. *Merck manual of geriatrics*. Whitehouse Station, New Jersey: Merck Co, Inc., 1995.

29. Bloch AS. *Nutrition management of the cancer patient*. Rockville, MD: Aspen Publishers, 1990.

30. *Recommended daily allowances*. (10th ed.) Washington DC: National Academy Press, 1989.

31. Ryan AS, Craig LD, Finn SC. Nutrient intakes and dietary patterns of older Americans: A national study. *J Gerontol Med Sci* 1992; **47**: M145–150.

32. Loprinzi CL, Ellison NM, Schaid DJ, *et al.* Controlled trial of megestrol acetate for the treatment of cancer anorexia and cachexia. *J Natl Cancer Inst* 1990; **82**: 1127–1132.

33. Bruera E, Macmillan K, Kuehn N, *et al.* A controlled trial of megestrol acetate on appetite, caloric intake, nutritional status, and other symptoms in patients with advanced cancer. *Cancer* 1990; **66**: 1279–1282.

34. Tchekmedyian NS, Hariri L, Siau J, *et al.* Megestrol acetate cancer anorexia and weight loss [Abstract]. *Proc Am Soc Clin Oncol* 1990; **9**: 336.

22. Chemoprevention of Cancer in the Elderly

Susan E. Minton and Gail L. Shaw

Introduction

Advancing age is associated with an increased incidence of cancer. During 1986–90, the total cancer incidence per 100,000 in persons aged 65 and over was approximately ten times higher than in younger persons. Total cancer incidence between 1973 and 1990 in the older population increased 1.5% per year, compared to 0.7% for those under the age of 65. Melanoma, non-Hodgkin's lymphoma, lung, prostate, brain, kidney, liver, breast, esophagus, and ovary cancers all demonstrated an increased incidence in those 65 and older between 1973 and 1990. In 1973 the cancer related death rate was 16% and rose to 26% in 1990 in persons 65 and older. Over two-thirds of deaths from cancer occur in persons 65 and older (1). With the rising incidence of and mortality from cancer, the geriatric population stands to benefit significantly from advances in chemoprevention. This field can potentially have a dramatic clinical impact on the reduction of invasive cancer in the elderly.

The process of carcinogenesis is characterized by multiple genetic events at the molecular level. During the early part of the twentieth century, it was discovered that the process of tumorigenesis could be interrupted by specific chemical agents. These initial experiments in rodent models used a locally directed approach with chemopreventive agents demonstrating suppression of skin tumor growth. These early agents were highly toxic and could not be applied in human trials. In the 1970's, Wattenberg showed that dietary antioxidants were potentially protective against carcinogenesis, ushering in the field of chemoprevention. Epidemiologic studies provide the basis for many of the potentially beneficial dietary components that have been studied. As our understanding of the biology of carcinogenesis has increased, potential targets for intervention to block or reverse the process have been identified. More than 20 classes of chemical agents that block mutagenic carcinogenesis or inhibit epithelial proliferation have been discovered (2).

Vitamin A was first recognized in the early 1900s and later named in 1920 (3). Wolbach and Howe subsequently demonstrated that a vitamin A deprived diet in rats was associated with gastrointestinal, respiratory, and urogenital epithelial metaplasia (4). In 1941, Abels et al. conducted the first studies that showed an association with vitamin A deficiency and human malignancy, particularly in the gastrointestinal tract (5). Sporn et al. used the term chemoprevention during an early investigation in 1976 evaluating the protective effects of vitamin A (6). Since then, the most extensively studied agents for chemoprevention have been vitamin A and the retinoids. Retinoids prevent proliferation of many different malignant cell lines possibly through alteration of the cell growth cycle. Aggregation of cells in G1 phase of the cell cycle retards their entry into S-phase (7–11). The mechanism for inducing differentiation in normal and neoplastic tissue is less clear. Retinoids have a broad range of activity including control of enzymes, growth factors, binding proteins, membrane function, genomic expression, immune function, extracellular activity, and possibly oncogene activation (12). The generic term, retinoid, encompasses both natural and synthetic compounds that have similar biological activities to vitamin A. Clinical trials have been designed using vitamin A (retinol) and its esters, β-all trans retinoic acid (vitamin A acid, or tretinoin), 13-cis-retinoic acid (isotretinoin, or Accutane), and an aromatic ethyl ester derivative of retinoic acid (etretinate, or Tegison). One of the most recently studied synthetic retinoids is N-(4-hydroxyphenyl) retinamide (4HPR, or Fenretinide) which is less toxic than the other vitamin A analogues. Fenretinide has the ability to concentrate in the granular and fat tissue of the breast making it an ideal drug for chemoprevention studies in breast cancer. Retinoids have demonstrated activity in such premalignant lesions as oral leukoplakia, bronchial metaplasia, actinic keratoses, and cervical dysplasia as well as bladder, gastric, and breast cancer (12).

Chemoprevention is designed to decrease cancer incidence with the ultimate goal of reducing cancer-related mortality. In this chapter we plan to review the chemoprevention clinical trials of specific solid tumors that are the most relevant to the geriatric population.

Methodology of Chemoprevention Clinical Trials

The ideal endpoints for trials of chemopreventive agents are cancer incidence and mortality. Prospective trials require large sample sizes and long duration of follow-up since on a population level cancer is still a rare event and most cancers are believed to develop biologically over decades. It is not feasible to test each prospective chemopreventive agent with this degree of rigor due to the time and expense involved. One approach to this problem has been the use of high risk populations for the evaluation of new interventions. Defined populations with an increased risk of the cancer of interest will have a greater number of observations (newly diagnosed cancers) over a shorter period of follow-up, resulting in a smaller sample size for the study population. Examples of such populations include patients with resected stage I non-small cell lung cancer who have a 1–3% chance per year of developing a second primary lung cancer, or patients with definitively treated early stage head and neck cancer who have a 3–7% chance per year of developing a second primary head and neck cancer. The elderly are another example of a high risk population, since two-thirds of all cancers are diagnosed in persons aged 65 and older. Consequently, study of this population should yield results with a more economic study design.

The other approach in defining endpoints in chemoprevention studies has been to move the measurable event from the individual (cancer incidence) to the cellular level in the form of molecular events. Biomarkers are measurable events at the cellular level which may reflect changes in cell proliferation, differentiation, transformation or carcinogenesis. Biomarkers include genetic, cellular, histologic, biochemical, and pharmacologic markers which serve as an intermediate endpoint in the spectrum of events that occur during the carcinogenic process (13). Examples of such markers include gene mutations, nuclear changes measured by micronuclei and nuclear ploidy, and proliferation measures done by thymidine labeling index and immunohistochemical detection (Proliferating Cell Nuclear Antigen (PCNA), Ki67 antibody). Cellular differentiation is measured by phenotypic expression of cells in the mature state versus the immature state. Ornithine decarboxylase and cyclo-oxygenase activity are select biochemical markers. Biomarker endpoints have been extensively studied in colon, head and neck, and lung cancer. Several premalignant lesions have been identified and include adenomas, leukoplakia, cervical dysplasia, bronchial squamous metaplasia, and actinic keratoses.

Colon Cancer

There is a histopathologic progression from hyper proliferation of the colon to adenomas with varying degrees of malignant potential, and finally adenocarcinoma. The malignant potential of adenomas correlates with the histopathologic type (tubular, tubulovillous, villous), size (>1 cm), and severity of dysplasia. Tubular adenomas are much more common and usually smaller than villous adenomas. Tubular adenomas are fairly evenly distributed throughout the bowel and 25% are multiple. Villous adenomas concentrate in the rectum and have 8 to 10 times greater risk of becoming malignant compared to tubular adenomas. Almost half of polyps that are larger than 2 cm are malignant (14). Vogelstein et al. have identified several molecular markers of colon carcinogenesis (15). Figure 22.1 depicts where some of these specific molecular changes may occur in the progression from adenoma to invasive colon cancer.

Chemoprevention trials in colorectal cancer have concentrated on adenomatous polyp regression and

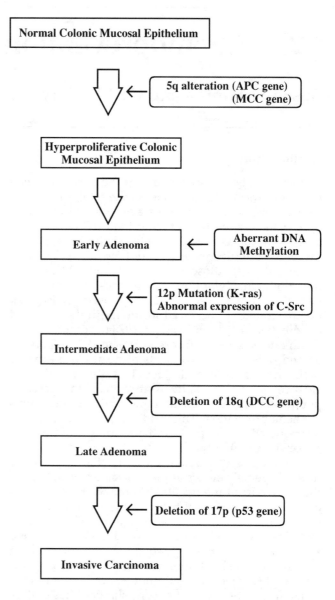

Figure 22.1 Molecular sequence of alterations in colon carginogenesis.
Abbreviations. FAP gene, familial adenomatous polyposis; genetic changes seen in sporadic colon cancers: MCC gene, mutated colon cancer; DCC gene, deleted in colon cancer.

mucosal proliferation indices such as thymidine labeling index, and immunohistochemical detection by PCNA and Ki67 as intermediate endpoint markers. Most recently ornithine decarboxylase and cyclo-oxygenase activity are being evaluated in trials using piroxicam and eflornithine (DFMO). None of these intermediate endpoint markers have proven to be accurate predictors of future cancer development. Continued biomarker characterization should lead to future phase III trials that are more cost effective because of shorter follow-up time.

Nonsteroidal antiinflammatory agents (NSAIDs), which inhibit colorectal carcinogenesis in rodent models (16–19), have been evaluated in several published ongoing trials for their potential in colon cancer prevention. The mechanism of inhibition is hypothesized to be through the arachidonic acid cycle, since NSAIDs, including aspirin, piroxicam and sulindac, inhibit cyclo-oxygenase. Prostaglandins, synthesized in the arachidonic acid cycle, are believed to play a role in tumorigenesis (20,21). Thun *et al.* prospectively assessed 635,031 cancer-free adults by questionnaire for risk factors including aspirin use. Follow-up was conducted from 1982 through 1988. Mortality was decreased in frequent aspirin users for cancers of the colon, rectum, esophagus and stomach. Mortality was 40% lower in the group using 16 or more aspirin a month for at least one year compared to nonusers, and the greater reduction in mortality was seen with 10 or more years of aspirin use (22).

A recent report from the Nurses' Health study evaluated 89,446 female nurses between the ages of 30 and 55 by mailed questionnaire between 1980 and 1992. Regular aspirin use was defined as consumption of 2 or more aspirin a week. Colorectal cancer risk was decreased among women who took aspirin for 10 or more consecutive years. This decreased risk was statistically significant in women taking aspirin for more than twenty years (23). This report is similar to the prospective cohort study in male health professionals that reported a lower risk for incidence of total and advanced colorectal cancer with regular use of at least two aspirin per week (24). The United States Physicians' Health Study conducted a phase III randomized trial using 325 mg of aspirin every other day (25). They reported no significant reduction in colon cancer during the first six years of use.

Aspirin may inhibit adenomas in the early stages of the proliferation process as seen in animal models, which would explain the long duration of aspirin use required to see a significant decline in incidence of colon cancer. Most large cohort epidemiologic studies have reported an association between aspirin use and decreased risk of colon cancer (22–24,26–30). One exception is a report of a cohort of 22,781 residents of a retirement community in California with a median age of 73. Aspirin use was ascertained by mailed questionnaire, and after 6.5 years of follow up there was a slight increase in colon cancer risk (31). The only prospective, randomized trial has short follow-up, and data from previously reported epidemiologic studies would suggest that at least ten years treatment duration is needed.

More recently other NSAIDs have been tested in chemoprevention of colon cancer. There are now two positive randomized phase ll trials using sulindac in patients with familial adenomatous polyposis (32,33). The most recent trial showed a significant decrease in both mean polyp number and mean polyp diameter, in comparison with placebo (33). Piroxicam has been shown to suppress rectal mucosal prostaglandin E2 levels and is currently being evaluated in a randomized trial in patients with previously resected adenomas using prostaglandin E2 and labeling index as end points (34). It is unknown whether polyp regression varies

with malignant potential. The polyps that regress may be ones that had low to no risk of malignant transformation or may have regressed spontaneously. The unresponsive polyps could possess the greatest potential for transformation. Unfortunately polyp regression is not maintained upon discontinuing the NSAID, and because of incomplete polyp inhibition these therapies will not replace colonoscopic surveillance and polyp excision, limiting their clinical usefulness.

Initial data from animal models have found that dietary calcium decreases both bile acid induced mucosal damage and suppresses epithelial cell proliferation that can potentially lead to colon cancer (35). Epidemiologic studies demonstrated a protective influence using dietary calcium (36). Chemoprevention trials using calcium have assessed crypt cell proliferation rates measured by labeling index as their end point. Four randomized prevention trials of calcium evaluated patients with previously resected sporadic adenomas (37,38), previous colon cancer (39), and familial polyposis (40), and found no significant suppression of epithelial cell proliferation. The most recently published trial measured the distribution of proliferating cells in the crypts of the colonic mucosa of sporadic adenoma patients (38). Although there was no change in the proliferation index in the calcium arm, there was a statistically significant difference in the distribution of proliferating cells within the crypts of the colonic mucosa. Calcium supplementation normalized the distribution of proliferating cells possibly by accelerating the cellular proliferation and differentiation phase lower in the crypt, thereby decreasing exposure of proliferating cells at the surface to injury from bile acids. The only randomized trial that demonstrated a decrease in epithelial cell proliferation rates evaluated only 20 patients and analysis did not include all patients (41).

Six randomized trials have evaluated antioxidant vitamins with inconsistent results on reduction of adenoma recurrence (42–47). A recent trial reported by Greenberg and his colleagues (47) was the largest, evaluating 864 patients in a two by two factorial design. Treatment arms consisted of placebo, 25 mg/d of beta carotene, 1 g/d of vitamin C, 400 mg/d of vitamin E, and a combination of beta-carotene, and vitamins C and E. The four-year clinical trial showed no benefit in reduction of adenomas in the treatment arms. Other dietary factors in fruits and vegetables may have influenced decreased cancer rates in previous epidemiologic studies.

Currently there are trials in prevention of colon cancer evaluating exciting new agents such as DFMO and oltipraz. Oltipraz is an antioxidant that is structurally related to dithiolthione, and has been used previously in the treatment of schistosomiasis. Diets comprising cruciferous vegetables, which contain oltipraz, have been associated with a decreased risk of cancer in both human and animal studies. Further preclinical testing in animals has shown oltipraz to be an effective agent against tumors in the colon. Oltipraz acts on enzymes that catalyze electrophilic detoxification and reduce

Table 22.1 Chemoprevention colon cancer randomized trials in progress.

Study Group	Agent	Population	Endpoint
CLGB	Aspirin	Resected Dukes' A-C colon ca	Adenoma recurrence
DMS	Folic Acid/Aspirin	Resected adenomas	Adenoma recurrence
ECOG	Folic Acid	Resected adenomas	Adenoma recurrence
SWOG	Calcium	Resected Stage 0/I/II colon ca	Adenoma recurrence/SPT
UARIZ	Wheat bran fiber	Resected adenomas	Adenoma recurrence/LI
UCI	DFMO	Resected adenomas	Polyamine content/LI
DMS	Calcium	Resected adenomas	Adenoma recurrence
LUMC	Beta-carotene	Resected colon ca, adenomas, normal	Cell proliferation/Polyamine content
MIBH	Acarbose	Resected adenomas	Fiber poly-saccharide content
NCCTG	Sulindac	Resected adenomas	Adenoma recurrence
UARIZ	Piroxicam	Resected adenomas	PGE_2/LI
UMN	Calcium	Resected adenomas	LI
UUMC	Sulindac	Adenomas	Adenoma regression/PGE_2/LI

Abbreviations:CLGB, Cancer and Leukemia Group B; DMS, Dartmouth Medical Center; ECOG, Eastern Cooperative Oncology Group; SWOG, Southwest Oncology Group; UARIZ, University of Arizona, Arizona Cancer Center; UCI, University of California Irvine Clinical Cancer Center; LUMC, Loyola University Medical Center; MIBH, Mary Imogene Bassett Hospital and Clinics; NCCTG, North Central Cancer Treatment Group; UMN, University of Minnesota Hospital and Clinic; UUMC, University of Utah Medical Center, Huntsman Cancer Institute; SPT, second primary tumor; LI, labeling index; PGE2, prostaglandin E.

glutathione. With increased dietary intake, oltipraz stimulates glutathione transferases as well as the P-450 system, thus improving carcinogen elimination (48). Phase I studies are currently being conducted in individuals who are at increased risk of developing colon cancer. DFMO is an irreversible inhibitor of ornithine decarboxylase (ODC). ODC is an enzyme involved in the biosynthesis of polyamines, which are thought to play a role in normal cell differentiation and proliferation. During malignant transformation, polyamines are increased in association with increased cell proliferation. Preclinical testing has demonstrated DFMO to have chemopreventive activity in rat bladder, rat mammary glands, rat colon, and mouse skin (49). Currently there is a phase IIb prevention trial testing the effect of DFMO on colonic mucosa in patients with a history of adenomas using colonic mucosal polyamine content and crypt cell proliferation indices as endpoint biomarkers. Table 22.1 lists current phase II and III colon

cancer chemoprevention trials. Table 22.2 refers to selected agents now being evaluated for toxicity and efficacy.

Head and Neck Cancer

Head and neck cancer in heavy smokers is associated with a high incidence of local recurrence and second primary tumors (SPTs) in the upper aerodigestive tract (UADT). This is attributed to the phenomenon of field carcinogenesis, which is the result of chronic exposure of the UADT to environmental carcinogens in cigarette smoke and may progress to multiple foci of intra epithelial neoplasia throughout the exposed field. Molecular studies of biopsy specimens from the UADT in smokers at high risk for head and neck, and lung cancer demonstrate multiple genetic abnormalities such as p53 mutations, 3p deletions, and aneuploidy through the exposed epithelial field. Field carcinogenesis is thought to develop from the progression of initially transformed premalignant lesions (50–52). Chung *et al.* demonstrated discordant p53 mutations in second primary cancers arising in patients with primary head and neck malignancies using the single strand conformation polymorphism technique, providing molecular evidence for the independent nature of these events in field cancerization (53).

Oral leukoplakia is a premalignant lesion of the aerodigestive tract that is a tobacco related precursor of squamous cell carcinoma. Oral leukoplakia has

Table 22.2 Chemoprevention agents under study in colon cancer.

Oltipraz
Glycyrrhetinic acid
Ibuprofen
Fish oil

Table 22.3 Current chemoprevention randomized trials in head and neck cancer.

Study Group	Agent	Population	Endpoint
EORTC	Vitamin A/N-Acetylcysteine	Resected early stage head and neck cancer	SPTs
ECOG	13-CRA	Resected Stage I/II head and neck cancer	SPTs
MDA	Vitamin E	Oral leukoplakia	LKP
MDA	13-CRA/β-carotene/Vitamin A	Oral leukoplakia	LKP
RTOG	13-CRA	Resected Stage I/II head and neck cancer	SPTs
SWOG	β-carotene	Resected Stage I/II head and neck cancer	SPTs
NCOG	13-CRA	Resected Stage I/II head and neck cancer	SPTs
UARIZ	β-carotene	Oral leukoplakia	LKP
Yale	β-carotene	Resected Stage I/II head and neck cancer	SPTs

Abbreviations: EORTC, European Organization of Research and Treatment of Cancer; ECOG, Eastern Cooperative Oncology Group; MDA, M.D. Anderson; RTOG, Radiation Therapy Oncology Group; NCOG, Northern California Oncology Group; SWOG, Southwest Oncology Group; UARIZ, University of Arizona, Arizona Cancer Center; SPTs, second primary tumors; 13 CRA, 13-Cis retinoic acid; LKP, leukoplakia.

served as an excellent model for determining various intermediate biomarkers and agents for chemoprevention of head and neck cancer (53–55). Early single arm studies in oral premalignancy have used selenium, beta-carotene, α-tocopherol, and retinoids with positive results (56–63). Retinoids are the only agents that have been shown to be active in randomized trials. The initial trial evaluated isotretinoin treating 44 participants with 1 to 2 mg/kg/day for three months. They reported both clinical and histologic response rates of 67% (p=.0002) and 54% (p=.01) in the isotretinoin group compared to placebo response rates of 10%. However, there was a significant amount of toxicity associated with this dose of isotretinoin, and a majority of the patients relapsed within 2 to 3 months of completing treatment (60). These results led to a second trial evaluating 70 patients at a dose of 1.5 mg/kg/d for 3 months followed by 9 months of maintenance therapy in initial responders with either 0.5 mg/kg/d of isotretinoin or 30 mg/d of beta-carotene (61). Although, the beta-carotene arm had a 55% disease progression, the maintenance therapy appeared to decrease relapse rates seen in the first trial with progression of disease seen in only 8% of the isotretinoin arm. Response continued during long term therapy in 33% of the patients on isotretinoin and 10% on beta-carotene. The isotretinoin maintenance arm produced low grade toxicity consisting of reversible dermatitis, cheilitis, conjunctivitis, and hypertriglyceridemia. Two other small randomized, placebo controlled trials testing vitamin A (62) and retinamide (63) in patients with oral premalignancy have shown significant response rates. Another maintenance trial evaluating fenretinide for 12 months compared with no treatment after resection of premalignant oral lesions shows similar relapse rates (6%) to the isotretinoin maintenance trial (64). The placebo relapse rate was 30%. These trial results with retinoids are promising but do not conclusively show long term inhibition of malignancy.

Lotan and colleagues demonstrated that retinoids upregulated retinoic acid receptor (RAR) expression in leukoplakia lesions (65). RAR expression in oral premalignant lesions was determined using in situ hybridization techniques to detect mRNAs of RARs. During isotretinoin therapy, the increasing level of RAR expression was seen in 16 of 20 lesions that responded clinically. Similarly, Lippman *et al.* (66) studied p53 protein pattern of expression in oral premalignancy, and its association with retinoid response. An inverse relationship was found between the initial levels of accumulated protein in the biopsy specimens and response to isotretinoin. However, during treatment isotretinoin did not affect the level of p53 expression.

SPTs are the leading cause of death after resection of early-stage head and neck cancer. Because of the positive studies with retinoids in oral premalignant lesions, adjuvant trials using isotretinoin were initiated. A phase III adjuvant trial using high dose isotretinoin randomized patients after definitive treatment of head and neck cancer to receive either isotretinoin 50–100 mg/m²/d or placebo for one year. After a median follow-up of 32 months, isotretinoin significantly reduced the incidence of SPTs (p=.005) (67). Isotretinoin had no influence on recurrence rate, perhaps confounded by the numerous locally advanced head and neck cancer patients who were included in the trial and at high risk for disease recurrence. During a repeat analysis at 55 months of median follow-up, the overall incidence of SPTs as well as the incidence of aerodigestive tract SPTs were still decreased in the isotretinoin arm (p=.04 and p=.008 respectively) (68). Table 22.3 lists the randomized chemoprevention trials in head and neck cancer in progress.

Lung Cancer

Lung cancer is the leading cause of death from cancer in both men and women overall and above the age of

35 in the United States. Between the ages of 60 to 79, 1 in 15 men and 1 in 28 women will develop lung cancer (69). Cigarette smoking, including passive smoking, accounts for at least 80 percent of the cases. Recent progress in cellular biology of lung cancer has increased our understanding of the mechanisms involved in tumor development. Further understanding of the biology of lung cancer may elucidate molecular targets for chemopreventive agents.

There are a number of cytogenetic abnormalities in lung tumors. Nearly all cases of small cell lung cancer (SCLC) and the majority of non-small cell lung cancer (NSCLC) have genetic aberrations in chromosome region 3p (70). Allelic loss from chromosomes 13 and 17 is also seen. The genetic change most frequently identified in lung cancer is the p53 gene mutation (71). There are many other genetic changes that activate proto-oncogenes.

K-ras oncogene activation has been demonstrated in adenocarcinoma of the lung, and is most frequently seen in smokers (72–74). Thus far K-ras oncogene expression has been correlated with a poor survival and resistance to chemotherapy in *in vitro* cell lines (72,73). MYC oncogenes are present in SCLC, and c-erb-β-2 genes have been demonstrated in both NSCLC and SCLC (72,75,76). Future studies of early tumorigenesis in lung cancer focusing on these genetic changes may help identify targets for chemopreventive agents.

Monoclonal antibodies are now being evaluated in the early detection of lung cancer by immunostaining bronchial epithelial cells shed in sputum (77). Tockman and colleagues archived sputum specimens from the Johns Hopkins University Lung Project and stained them with monoclonal antibodies specific for SCLC and NSCLC. They reported a 90% accuracy in detecting lung cancer 2 years before clinical onset by using monoclonal antibody staining of the sputum specimens (78). The Lung Cancer Early Detection Working Group and the Eastern Cooperative Oncology Group are currently sponsoring a prospective study obtaining annual induced sputum samples for monoclonal antibody staining in resected stage I NSCLC patients. The endpoint is second primary lung cancer. Results of this study will hopefully validate the findings from the previous archival study. Inherited variation in the ability to metabolize various carcinogens may contribute to the differential risk of lung cancer among tobacco users. Aryl hydrocarbon hydroxylase inducibility, debrisoquine metabolism, and glutathione-s transferase mu activity have been examined with conflicting results (79–85). Elucidation of the role of metabolic polymorphisms in carcinogen activation and inactivation may provide a mechanism to modulate the risk of carcinogen induced lung cancer.

Chemoprevention strategies in lung cancer are a logical extension from experience gained in previous head and neck cancer research. The effect of tobacco related carcinogenesis on the field of the upper aerodigestive tract, or field cancerization, is common between lung, and head and neck cancer (86,87). This similarity, and potential for SPTs among both types of

cancer patients, is the reason that retinoids are now being evaluated for prevention of lung cancer. Premalignancy trials have centered on sputum atypia and bronchial dysplasia. These studies are based on previous work in both lung and head and neck cancer showing multiple genetic abnormalities in premalignant epithelial lesions.

Several trials have now been published in premalignant lung cancer. An initial uncontrolled trial by Misset *et al.* (88) evaluating 25 mg/day of etretinate in heavy smokers for six months reported a reduction in the mean bronchial metaplasia index from 34.57% before treatment to 26.96% after. Two randomized trials of retinoids were conducted in heavy smokers. Arnold *et al.* (89) evaluated reversal of metaplasia in sputum samples after treatment with etretinate for six months and found no significant difference in response between the etretinate and the placebo group. Lee *et al.* used bronchoscopy to evaluate bronchial epithelial metaplasia reversal with isotretinoin treatment for six months and found a similar reduction in metaplasia index in both treatment and placebo groups (54.3% and 58.8% respectively) (90). Reduction of metaplasia index was seen in participants from both groups who quit smoking. Another placebo controlled randomized trial treated 73 smokers with metaplasia determined by sputum cytology with folic acid and vitamin B12 for four months (91). This trial reported a significant improvement in dysplasia in the treatment group (p=.02). However, the small sample size and other criticisms of the methods and analysis limit the implications of this study.

Currently, there is a trial looking at various premalignant markers in high risk patients following smoking cessation. Table 22.4 lists various biomarkers under evaluation for the early detection of lung cancer. The identification of more precise intermediate end-

Table 22.4 Biomarkers under investigation in lung cancer chemoprevention biomarkers.

Markers of genetic mutation
  Micronuclei
  Oncogene expression
  DNA analysis

Markers of Histologic Change
  Squamous metaplasia/dysplasia
  Sputum atypia

Markers of cellular proliferation
  Proliferating cell nuclear antigen
  Epidermal growth factor receptor
  Retinoic acid receptor
  Transforming growth factor-β
  Ornithine decarboxylase activity

Table 22.5 Chemoprevention lung cancer trials in progress.

Study Group	Agent	Population	Endpoint
EORTC	Vitamin A/N-Acetylcystein	Resected early stage NSCLC	SPTs
Intergroup	13-CRA	Stage I NSCLC	SPTs
UCHSC	13-CRA	Smokers/cured NSCLC	Lung cancer

Abbreviations: EORTC, European Organization of Research and Treatment of Cancer; UCHSC, University of Colorado Cancer Center; 13-CRA, 13-Cis-retinoic acid; NSCLC, non-small-cell lung cancer; SPTs, second primary tumor.

points will facilitate the development of chemopreventive agents to target specific preneoplastic molecular events.

Retinoid treatment in prevention of SPTs, in contrast to premalignant lung cancer trials, has shown positive results. Pastorino *et al.* randomized 307 patients who had complete resections of stage I NSCLC to either 300,000 IU of retinyl palmitate or to no treatment for 12 months (92). With a median observation of 46 months, time to development of SPTs in the aerodigestive tract was significantly longer in the treatment arm (p=0.045).

The alpha-tocopherol, beta-carotene cancer prevention study was a primary chemoprevention trial which enrolled over 29,000 male smokers between the ages of 50 to 69 in Finland (93). This randomized, double-blind, placebo controlled trial used a two by two factorial design to assign treatment with 50 mg/d of alpha-tocopherol, 20 mg/d of beta-carotene, both or placebo with a follow-up of 5 to 8 years. The beta carotene arm showed a statistically significant 18 percent increased risk of lung cancer, with no change in the alpha-tocopherol group.

The beta-carotene and retinol efficacy trial (CARET) is a six center phase III randomized, double-blind, placebo controlled trial which is testing the effect of 25,000 IU Vitamin A and 30 mg beta-carotene/day in preventing lung cancer in 14,420 heavy smokers as well as 4,010 workers exposed to asbestos. Interim analysis of the CARET trial was conducted in January 1996 and demonstrated a 28% increase in lung cancer incidence in the beta-carotene arm (94). The surprising finding of an increased lung cancer risk in these two trials suggests that a dietary supplement cannot provide all the elements in yellow and green leafy vegetables which confer protective benefits in epidemiologic studies. Furthermore, there may be a harmful interaction in smokers taking the beta-carotene supplement contributing to the increased risk. There are several large ongoing randomized trials evaluating agents in the high risk heavy smoker population. Table 22.5 shows the current large scale trials being conducted for the chemoprevention of lung cancer.

Breast Cancer

Breast cancer is the most common cancer and the second leading cause of death from cancer in women in the United States. There will be an estimated 185,700 new cases and 44,560 deaths from breast cancer in 1996

in the United States. Women from the ages of 60 to 79 have a one in fifteen chance of developing breast cancer with a one in eight lifetime risk (69).

Contralateral breast cancer develops in approximately 10% of all women with previous breast cancer (95). Most of the data in prevention of contralateral breast cancer is from the adjuvant breast cancer trials using tamoxifen. Over 30,0000 women have been evaluated from 40 randomized adjuvant trials (96). Tamoxifen use reduced the odds of developing a contralateral breast cancer by 39%. Tamoxifen is more effective when used for a longer duration as evidenced by a 53% reduction in the annual odds of developing a contralateral breast cancer after 2 years of tamoxifen use compared to a 26% reduction with less than 2 years of tamoxifen use (97). The optimal duration of tamoxifen therapy remains controversial.

There are now several large scale tamoxifen studies going on in high risk women for the primary prevention of breast cancer. The National Surgical Adjuvant Project for Breast and Bowel Cancer (NSABP) is the American trial comprised of 288 centers throughout the United States and Canada consisting of 16,000 women ages 35–78 who are at a twofold or greater risk of breast cancer than women in the general population. There are United Kingdom and Italian trials that are similar. Risk is determined by a model reported by Gail *et al.* (98) using risk factors of age, number of first-degree relatives with breast cancer, number of benign breast biopsies, presence of atypical hyperplasia, age of menarche, and age at delivery of first child. Based on previous data from adjuvant tamoxifen trials, each study is estimated to reduce the incidence of breast cancer by 33%. The combined results from all three trials may detect a 20–25% reduction in mortality (97). The trial design also included analysis of myocardial infarction and bone fracture incidence. Although all women age 60 and over are eligible for trial participation, 72% of the first 3791 patients recruited are under the age of 60 years and have a five fold risk over the general population (99).

The Italian National Cancer Institute conducted a large scale, placebo controlled trial of fenretinide at 200 mg/d in the prevention of contralateral breast cancer (100). Eligible patients included those between the ages of 33 and 68 with a previous history of operable T1–2 breast cancer without axillary lymph node involvement, local recurrence, or distant metastasis. The study was recently closed with slightly less than 3000 patients secondary to a fall off in accrual, probably due to the results of adjuvant trials showing benefit of chemotherapy and tamoxifen in node negative breast cancer. Fenretinide therapy results in a fall in serum retinol levels which can result in impaired dark adaptation. Administration with a three-day drug holiday monthly avoids ocular toxicity. Fenretinide accumulates in the breast and its mechanism of action is thought to be associated with inducing decreased levels of insulin-like growth factor-l (IGF-I) (101). Estrogen dependent growth of human breast cancer cells *in vitro* is inhibited by fenretinide, and it may have a stronger inhibition potential than tamoxifen.

The combination of fenretinide and tamoxifen is being evaluated in both high risk populations for primary breast cancer prevention and in patients with a previous history of breast cancer for contralateral disease prevention. Data for synergistic activity comes from human breast cancer cell lines, animal mammary carcinoma models, and clinical studies in metastatic breast cancer patients (102,103). Tamoxifen and fenretinide have been shown to decrease circulating levels of IGF-I. When administered alone the IGF-I levels have decreased by 29% with tamoxifen, 18% with fenretinide, and 36.1% in combination (104). IGF-I has been used as an intermediate endpoint marker in early pilot studies.

Although these agents appear relatively safe when used alone, a key issue will be to determine long term toxicity during co-administration. Short term toxicity determination in phase I/II studies in metastatic breast cancer patients has demonstrated no significant adverse side effects. Fenretinide at a daily dose of 200 mg causes impaired dark adaptation in approximately 25% of patients (105). These ocular symptoms are reversible upon interruption of the drug. Tamoxifen is associated with an increased risk of endometrial cancer that is dose dependent, with the highest risk noted at 40 mg/d (106,107). In animal models an increased incidence of liver cancer has been noted, but no significant increase has been seen thus far in human clinical studies (108). There are sporadic cases of retinal toxicity on tamoxifen (109). Efficacy in combination with the least amount of toxicity will have to be determined for chemoprevention in healthy patients.

Luteinizing hormone-releasing hormone (LH-RH) has been suggested as a chemoprevention approach in breast cancer because of its suppressive effects on ovarian hormone production (110). It is estimated that bilateral ovariectomy at the age of 35 is associated with a 60% decreased risk of breast cancer (111). A pilot study employing LH-RH has added hormone replacement therapy to minimize bone loss and changes in lipid levels seen in postmenopausal women. Table 22.6 lists several of the current randomized trials.

Cervical Cancer

Cervical cancer remains the second most common malignancy in women worldwide. There will be an expected 15,700 new cases and 4,900 deaths from

Table 22.6 Current randomized chemoprevention trials in breast cancer.

Study Group	Agent	Population	Endpoint
ITA-MIL	Fenretinide	Resected Stage I/II breast cancer	CTRLSPT CTRLSPT
NCI	Fenretinide/ tamoxifen	High risk*	Primary BC
NSABP	Tamoxifen	High risk*	Primary BC
UKCCCR	Tamoxifen	High risk*	Primary BC
UUMC	Tamoxifen	Proliferative breast disease	Primary BC

Abbreviations: ITA-MIL, European Institute of Oncology; NCI, National Cancer Institute; NSABP, National Surgical Adjuvant Breast and Bowel Project; UKCCCR, United Kingdom Coordinating Committee on Cancer Research; UUMC, University of Utah Medical Center; CTRLSPT, contralateral second primary tumor; BC, breast cancer.

*risk factors of age, number of first-degree relatives with breast cancer, number if benign breast biopsies, presence of atypical hyperplasia, age of menarche, and age at delivery of first child.

cervical cancers in the U.S. in 1996 (69). The peak age of incidence of carcinoma of the cervix is between 48 and 55 years (112,113). There are now 600,000 new cases of squamous intra epithelial lesions per year in the U.S. (114). Despite aggressive screening in the U.S. with pap smear testing, cervical cancer and squamous intra epithelial lesions remain important health problems for women. Increasing age is associated with an increased risk of progression of disease from carcinoma in situ to invasive cancer (115), and a lower rate of regression of cervical intra epithelial neoplasia (116).

Ninety percent of cervical cancer cases are associated with Human Papilloma Virus (HPV) expression (117). In addition, most of the epidemiologic risk factors for cervical cancer are associated with HPV infection (118). Although HPV prevalence falls sharply with increasing age from a peak in the late teens to early twenties, the prevalence of HPV DNA in women with cervical cancer remains elevated with increasing age. Other epidemiologic risk factors may be important in the geriatric population including age, immune status, or failure of intracellular control mechanisms (119).

Case control studies have shown an inverse relationship between a high dietary intake of beta-carotene and folic acid and the risk of cervical cancer. Several epidemiologic studies evaluating serum levels of beta-carotene have shown an inverse relationship with cervical neoplasia (120). Furthermore, exfoliated cervical epithelial cells were found to have a lower level of beta-carotene in patients who had cervical dysplasia compared with controls (121).

Experimental data suggests that vitamin A and its derivatives inhibit HPV associated proliferation. Retinoic acid has been shown to antagonize the action of the E6 and E7 oncogenes which have been implicated in the pathophysiology of HPV induced cervical dysplasia. HPV proteins E6 and E7 bind to and interfere with tumor suppressor gene products (122), and are thought to be important in malignant transformation of cervical epithelium. Transcription of the E6 and E7 HPV genes and the transformation of human keratinocytes by HPV 16 were found to be inhibited by retinoic acid (123).

Several clinical trials have been published from the University of Arizona on the use of topical retinoic acid in preinvasive cervical lesions. Based on a phase I study, a dose of 0.372% retinoic acid cream was delivered to the cervix by a collagen sponge inserted into a cervical cap. Four consecutive days of treatment were followed by two days every three months for a period of one year. The complete response rate in this trial was 50% (124). A randomized prospective study was then completed evaluating 301 women with moderate to severe cervical intra epithelial neoplasia and demonstrated a 43% complete regression rate using locally applied all-trans-retinoic acid to the cervix, compared to a complete regression rate of 27% in the placebo group (p=.041). The difference was significant only in the moderate dysplasia group, and minimal cervical intra epithelial lesions were not evaluated (125). Two randomized trials of oral folate and one of beta-carotene as chemopreventive agents in preinvasive cervical lesions have shown no enhancement of regression of these lesions (126,127). Several randomized trials utilizing a local treatment approach with interferon have not demonstrated any significant activity (128–132).

There has been little progress in the treatment of advanced squamous cell carcinoma of the cervix. No survival benefit has been demonstrated for cervical cancer in the adjuvant, neoadjuvant, recurrent, or metastatic setting. This lack of survival benefit with chemotherapy, along with the hundreds of thousands of deaths in women worldwide yearly from cervical cancer, accents the urgent need for effective early therapeutic interventions during the preinvasive disease state. Successful prevention of progression of preneoplastic lesions could reduce the frequency of invasive surgical procedures needed as well as the overall morbidity and mortality from cervical cancer.

Uterine Cancer

The incidence of endometrial cancer rose dramatically to a peak about 1975, then rapidly declined. This change in incidence coincided with the increased use of estrogen replacement therapy (ERT) in the late 1960's and early 1970's (133,134). After this association was recognized from case-control studies, a cyclic estrogen progesterone regimen was adopted by most physicians by the mid-1980's. Estrogen is a potent stimulant of endometrial tissue growth and induces endometrial hyperplasia, anaplasia, carcinoma in situ, and eventually invasive carcinoma when used in an unopposed fashion. Progesterone reverses the stimulatory growth

process caused by estrogen through differentiation and maturation, and converts proliferative endometrium into secretory endometrium (135).

Although an increased incidence of uterine cancer is associated with estrogen therapy, the addition of a progesterone results in no increased incidence of this cancer (136). Gambrell and others (137) found that postmenopausal women on estrogen-progesterone combination hormone replacement therapy (HRT) had a lower incidence of endometrial cancer than untreated women. In this large study the relative incidence of endometrial cancer was 245 per 100,000 among untreated women, 390 per 100,000 among women treated with estrogen alone, and 49 per 100,000 among women treated with both estrogen and progesterone (137).

The effects of estrogen and progesterone on heart disease risk factors as well as endometrial hyperplasia were evaluated in the Postmenopausal Estrogen/Progestin Interventions Trial (PEPI) (138). PEPI was a 3-year, multicenter, randomized, double-blind, placebo-controlled trial of 875 healthy postmenopausal women ages 45 to 64. Participants were randomized to one of five treatments in 28 day cycles: (1) placebo, (2) 0.625 mg/d conjugated equine estrogen (CEE), (3) CEE plus medroxyprogesterone acetate (MPA) 10 mg/d for the first 12 days, (4) CEE plus MPA 2.5 mg/d, or (5) CEE plus micronized progesterone (MP) 200 mg/d for the first 12 days. Cardiovascular disease risk endpoints included high-density lipoprotein cholesterol (HDL-C), systolic blood pressure, serum insulin, and fibrinogen. Hormonal therapies decreased mean low-density lipoprotein cholesterol (0.37 to 0.46 mmol/L) and increased mean triglyceride (0.13 to 0.15 mmol/L) compared with placebo. More substantial increases occurred in fibrinogen levels in the placebo group than treatment groups. Differences in the various treatment arms were not statistically significant. There was a significantly increased risk of adenomatous or atypical hyperplasia (34% versus 1%), and hysterectomy (6% versus 1%) in the unopposed estrogen group not seen in other treatment groups. Although unopposed estrogen was associated with the highest levels of HDL-C, the unacceptably high rate of endometrial hyperplasia limits its use to those women who have had a hysterectomy. CEE plus MP had the most favorable effect on cardiovascular risk factors including HDL-C without increasing the risk of endometrial hyperplasia (138).

Whitehead et al. (139) showed that duration is a more important factor than the actual dosage of progesterone in inducing a secretory endometrium. The optimal type, dose, and duration of progesterone in reversing estrogen mediated endometrial carcinoma has not been established. It has been suggested that the lowest possible dose of progesterone be used in order to produce the desired effects on the endometrium without promoting possible adverse effects on risk of heart disease and breast cancer. Because of these issues long term use of HRT for postmenopausal women remains controversial.

The Women's Health Initiative opened in the fall of 1993, and is a randomized trial with 57,000 postmenopausal women. The effects of a low fat, high fiber diet, HRT, and calcium supplementation on the prevention of cancer, cardiovascular disease, and osteoporosis are being evaluated. This study includes a prospective examination of 100,000 women for risk factors and predictors for the subsequent development of disease (140).

The use of combination oral contraceptives (OCs) has consistently been reported in case control studies to decrease the risk of endometrial cancer by about 50% (141). The Centers for Disease Control and the National Institute of Child Health and Human Development sponsored the Cancer and Steroid Hormone Study which showed a 0.5 relative risk for endometrial cancer in combination OC users compared to nonusers. This protection occurred in women who used oral contraception for at least one year, and the protection persisted for women who discontinued using OCs 15 years before participation in the study (142).

Ovarian Cancer

Ovarian cancer is the fourth most common cause of death in women in the United States. The death rate from ovarian cancer each year is higher than cervical and endometrial cancer combined. The age-adjusted cancer death rate has risen steadily in the last 25 years in the United States. There will be an estimated 26,700 new cases of ovarian cancer and 14,800 deaths in the United States in 1996 (69). The incidence in women ages 40 to 44 is 15.7 per 100,000 and rises to 54 per 100,000 in women ages 75 to 79. Approximately 1 in 70 women will develop ovarian cancer in their lifetime.

There are several studies demonstrating that women who have taken OCs have a reduced risk of ovarian cancer (143–145). The risk of ovarian cancer clearly decreases with increasing duration of OC use, and this effect seems to be independent of parity. Protection appears to be long lasting. In the Cancer and Steroid Hormone Study, women on OCs for 10 years or more had one-half the risk of nonusers. This protective effect was independent of histologic type of ovarian cancer and persisted for several years after discontinuation (146). The inhibition of ovulation by OCs may be the mechanism of the protective benefit, since the chronic trauma of ovulation on the ovary is hypothesized to be a promoter of carcinogenesis. An analysis of case control studies found that women over the age of 55 had a larger percentage risk reduction associated with OC use than younger women, perhaps due to the early high-potency contraceptive formulations used by these older women (147) .

Little data is available on ovarian cancer risk in association with ERT. In general most available data indicate that there is no difference in risk with exception of endometrioid tumors of the ovary (148). Cramer *et al.* (149) found a higher incidence of endometrioid tumors in women who used estrogens compared to nonusers. In another study, an excess risk of ovarian cancer was shown with any use of menopausal estrogens (150). These tumors are histologically similar to adenocarcinoma of the endometrium. The effects of HRT on ovarian cancer risk are unknown. It has been suggested that ovarian cancer risk is associated with endocrine dysfunction, and is a result of accumulated exposure to gonadotropins. Further understanding of the mechanisms of the development of ovarian cancer will aid in identifying drugs that may modulate ovarian tumor growth and act as chemopreventive agents.

Prostate Cancer

Prostate cancer is the second leading cause of cancer death among men in the United States. Approximately 1 in 8 men will develop prostate cancer between the ages of 60 to 79. There will be 317,000 estimated new cases of prostate cancer for 1996, and 41,400 men are expected to die from prostate cancer in 1996 (69). Prostate cancer is the most common cancer found in men over the age of 40. Thus far treatment for early stage, localized prostate cancer with radical prostatectomy or radiation therapy has not shown significant survival benefit over age matched controls. Recently, a morphologic precursor for prostate cancer has been described and termed prostate intra epithelial neoplasia (PIN). It is estimated that this lesion is present in prostatic tissue at least ten years prior to the onset of invasive carcinoma, and of the two grades identified, the low grade may begin as early as the third decade of life in men (151). Animal models have suggested that PIN progression is testosterone dependent. Testosterone is converted to 5a-dihydrotestosterone (DHT) by 5a-reductase. DHT is the major androgen in the prostate which mediates prostate proliferation. Finasteride (Proscar) inhibits the enzyme testosterone 5a-reductase, which thereby lowers the intraprostatic level of DHT, without lowering serum testosterone. Lowered levels of DHT in the prostate results in inhibition of cell proliferation (152). Finasteride has been used with success in the treatment of prostatic hypertrophy with an excellent safety profile (153). *In vivo* rat and human models have shown tumor inhibition with low levels of DHT in the presence of 5a-reductase inhibitors (152). The prostate cancer prevention trial (PCPT) is a large-scale, double-blind, randomized multicenter trial investigating finasteride versus placebo for the chemoprevention of prostate cancer in men aged 55 and older. Eighteen thousand men will be randomized to treatment with finasteride 5 mg/d versus placebo for 7 years (154). Prostate cancer incidence at 7 years and overall survival will be assessed. The trial will also evaluate the utility of following patients on 5α-reductase inhibitors with prostate specific antigen (PSA) because of the known effects of reducing PSA.

Studies in rat models have shown a chemoprotective effect with the use of 4-HPR or fenretinide, a synthetic vitamin A derivative (155). Initial testing in patients with localized prostate cancer who refused surgery or radiation shows that 100 mg of 4 HPR taken three times a day with meals for six months followed by 100 mg of 4-HPR taken twice a day for the duration of the study is a relatively well tolerated regimen (156). Twenty-one of the 29 treated patients reported side effects, although the majority reported only mild side effects including gastrointestinal upset and minor vision changes. Moderate side effects of dermatitis, gastrointestinal upset, and double vision occurred in 13.7%, causing transient interruption of therapy. Two patients withdrew from the study secondary to severe nausea and an exacerbation of asthma. The prostate specific antigen (PSA) velocity of the treated group was greater than the control group after adjusting for cancer stage, perhaps explained by data from a previous study which demonstrated that retinoic acid induced PSA secretion in a cancer cell line (157). These results suggest that PSA will not be a reliable endpoint marker to follow in future chemoprevention studies. A phase ll trial using 4 HPR in high risk males that are biopsy negative for prostate cancer and have PSA levels greater than or equal to 4 ng/ml is currently in progress.

DFMO is an enzyme activated irreversible inhibitor of ornithine decarboxylase (ODC), an early enzyme in the synthetic pathway of polyamines, which have epithelial growth promoting effects. ODC is found at high levels in the prostate. DFMO has greater activity in ODC inhibition in the prostate than in other tissues, making it a promising new agent for future prostate chemoprevention trials (158).

The high incidence of prostate cancer in the geriatric population is of major concern. Coupled with the slow growth rate of prostate cancer, and the extensive amount of time needed for follow-up to determine response rates and differences in survival, surrogate endpoint biomarkers are urgently needed in prostate cancer. PIN appears to be the noninvasive premalignant lesion of prostate cancer, and will likely be investigated in future chemoprevention trials.

Bladder Cancer

Bladder cancer is the fourth most common type of cancer in men in the United States (69). Most recently a proposed model of multi-step carcinogenesis of premalignant lesions was reported. Usually superficial bladder tumors will be papillary, with a high recurrence rate and a low potential for progression to invasive disease. Carcinoma in situ is a high grade, aneuploid lesion with a high propensity to progress to invasive disease. Figure 22.2 shows the proposed schema of progression (159). By gaining a better understanding of the many cytogenetic changes that have been elucidated in the development of bladder cancer, we may be able to determine those at higher risk of carcinoma in situ development. Figure 22.3 shows a hypothetical model of the genetic changes that occur, and as we learn new data on such genetic changes this model will be modified (160). Molecular studies now show that altered retinoblastoma (Rb) gene determines a poorer prognosis in bladder cancer. Deletion of chromosome 9 seems to be a very early event in the

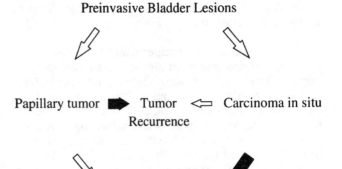

Preinvasive Bladder Lesions

Papillary tumor → Tumor ⇐ Carcinoma in situ
Recurrence

Invasive Bladder Cancer

Figure 22.2 Proposed model of bladder carcinogenesis.

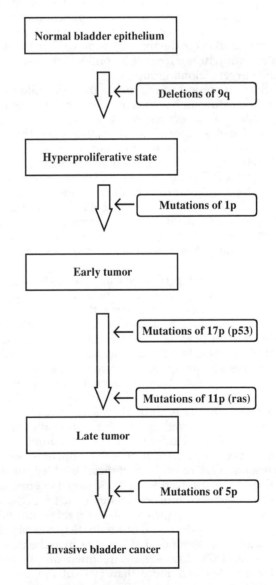

Normal bladder epithelium

← Deletions of 9q

Hyperproliferative state

← Mutations of 1p

Early tumor

← Mutations of 17p (p53)

← Mutations of 11p (ras)

Late tumor

← Mutations of 5p

Invasive bladder cancer

Figure 22.3 Hypothetical model for genetic aberrations that occur during the process of malignant transformation to invasive bladder cancer.

multi-step carcinogenic process and is being tested as an early detection marker for recurrence of bladder cancer.

The recurrence rate of superficial bladder cancer is a significant problem with new tumors developing in approximately 50% of all patients after surgical removal of a superficial bladder tumor. Intravesical bacillus Calmette-Guerin (BCG), a live attenuated tuberculosis organism, is the most active agent against superficial bladder tumors. It is not clear how BCG mediates its antitumor effect, although it may be through the local inflammatory response produced by intravesical BCG. Several randomized trials have now been done evaluating BCG for prophylaxis against future tumor occurrence after transurethral resection (TUR). Herr et al. conducted one of the largest of these trials and demonstrated a significant reduction in tumor recurrence compared to the control group (161). The BCG group had a tumor frequency of 3.6 per patient pre-treatment as compared to 0.7 per patient post-treatment. Prolongation of the disease free interval by intravesical BCG is demonstrated by 63% of the BCG treated group tumor free at 60 months compared to 5% of the surgery alone group.

Other intravesical agents such as thiotepa, mitomycin C, and doxorubicin have been evaluated for inhibition of bladder tumor recurrence. BCG has been shown to be significantly superior to doxorubicin and thiotepa in randomized trials for prevention of recurrence (162,163), and a meta-analysis of randomized trials for prophylaxis found the reduction of recurrence was 8% for thiotepa, 10% for doxorubicin, 12% for mitomycin C, and 42% for BCG (164). Furthermore, the reduction in recurrence is maintained with immunotherapy using BCG in contrast to a recurrence rate similar to surgery alone after five years in the chemotherapy groups.

The pattern of progression of disease has been documented in patients with superficial bladder tumors treated with BCG (165). During the first five years following treatment with BCG, relapses are primarily confined to the bladder. However, after five years such recurrent tumors usually appear outside the bladder, in the prostatic or upper tract uroepithelium. Future studies must concentrate on agents that protect the entire uroepithelium, and will likely be systemic.

In the late 1970s animal models showed that isotretinoin and etretinate inhibited transitional cell carcinoma of the bladder (166). Three randomized trials have been conducted testing the retinoid etretinate in patients with resected superficial bladder tumors. All three trials used a dose of 25–50 mg/d of etretinate and had extensive mucocutaneous toxicity. Pederson et al. randomized 73 patients with recurrent noninvasive bladder tumors to 50 mg/d of etretinate versus placebo and found no significant difference in reduction of recurrence (167). However, the treatment duration was only 8 months and more than 50% of the patients dropped out of the study. Seventeen patients withdrew from the study secondary to severe mucocutaneous toxicity. A second trial had to decrease the dose of etretinate from 50 to 25 mg/d because of similar toxicity. This trial evaluated 30 patients, 15 of whom received treatment, and found a recurrence rate of 60% for the etretinate group versus 86% for the control group (168). The third randomized trial, lasting two years, was done at multiple centers with 86 patients who also required dose reductions again done from the initial 50 mg/d secondary to toxicity. Recurrence rates were higher in the placebo group than the etretinate group at 3 months (40% versus 29%), 12 months (55% versus 35%), and 24 months (56% versus 29%) (169). Thus far data is mixed and these studies have small numbers with short term follow-up. The National Bladder Cancer Cooperative Group (NBCCG) trial of isotretinoin starting at 0.5 mg/kg/d and increasing to 1 mg/kd/d at 4 weeks, in patients with recurrent superficial bladder tumors, was closed prematurely because of toxicity. Toxicity consisted of cheilosis, conjunctivitis, pruritus, joint and eye pain and flashing lights (170).

Fenretinide has shown significant activity against bladder cancer in rodents and is less toxic than etretinate or isotretinoin. Fenretinide has been evaluated in a phase II Italian trial using DNA flow cytometry as an intermediate endpoint (171). Twelve patients with previously resected superficial bladder cancer were treated with 200 mg/d of 4-HPR and were compared to 17 nonrandomized controls. At four-month intervals patients had bladder washings done with DNA ploidy assessment on the cells. With a median follow-up of 12 months in the treatment group a decrease from 58% to 45% in the percentage of aneuploid cells was observed, in contrast to an increase from 41% to 59% in the control group. All patients with pretreatment abnormal cytology regressed to normal after 4-HPR. The control group had an increase in the rate of cytologic abnormalities during the follow-up period. Side effects included impaired adaption to darkness in 4 patients and dermatologic abnormalities including photodermatitis, rash, desquamation, and pruritus.

DFMO has shown significant activity in N-methyl-N-nitrosourea induced rat bladder tumors (172–174). A recent pilot study was completed evaluating 76 patients with resected superficial bladder cancer (175). In a Phase I trial, patients were randomized to 125 mg/d, 250 mg/d, 500 mg/d, or 1000 mg/d of DFMO for one year. Overall, DFMO was well tolerated with no significant toxicity. Only mild side effects such as nausea, tinnitus, diarrhea, stomatitis, peripheral neuropathy, and lethargy were documented even at doses of 1000 mg/d. DFMO is now being studied in a phase ll trial for chemoprevention of bladder cancer. Other agents including oltipraz, tumor necrosis factor, interleukin 2, interferon, suramin, and bropirimine are being tested in humans for toxicity and efficacy. Table 22.7 lists selected ongoing phase II and III trials in superficial bladder cancer.

Skin Cancer

Retinoids affect proliferation and differentiation of the epidermis. They decrease sebum production, inhibit keratinization, and accumulate in the skin. Many skin

Table 22.7 Selected randomized chemoprevention bladder cancer trials in progress.

Study Group	Agent	Population	Endpoint
EORTC-GUTCCG	BCG/EPI	CIS bladder ca	Regression/recurrence
EORTC-GUTCCG	BCG/EPI BCG-INH	Ta/T1 papillary bladder ca	Recurrence
UKMRC	Glycine/Etoglucid/Mitomycin	Superficial bladder ca	Recurrence
SWOG	Mitomycin/BCG	Superficial bladder ca	Recurrence

Abbreviations: EORTC, European Organization of Research and Treatment of Cancer; GUTCCG, Genito-Urinary Tract Cancer Cooperative Group; UKMRC, United Kingdom Medical Research Council; SWOG, Southwest Oncology Group; BCG, bacillus Calmette-Guerin; EPI, epirubicin

diseases are associated with hyperkeratinization, and have been successfully treated with 13-cis-retinoic acid. Vitamin A deficiency in animals and in epidemiologic human studies has shown an inverse association between plasma retinol or beta carotene and the development of cancer. All-trans-retinoic acid was the first retinoid tested after vitamin A showing an inhibition of skin papillomas and carcinomas in mice (176).

Actinic keratoses are premalignant skin lesions with a low transformation rate to nonmelanoma skin cancer. Bollag and Ott used 0.1% and 0.3% topical retinoic acid cream on 60 actinic keratoses, and reported a complete regression in 40% and partial response in 45% (177). Similar responses have been reported by others (178,179). Two small randomized trials using 75 mg/d of oral etretinate found positive results in a study population with actinic keratoses. Moriarty et al. used a double-blind, placebo controlled crossover design with 50 patients, and found an 84% response rate in the etretinate group compared to only 5% response rate in the control group (180). Watson et al. conducted a double-blind, placebo controlled, crossover trial with only 15 patients, and reported a response in 14 of the 15 patients (181). During the first four months off etretinate one patient improved, one progressed, and seven remained stable. Despite these initial significant response rates, neither trial addresses long term response or relapse rates off therapy. Kraemer and associates treated five patients with xeroderma pigmentosum at risk for basal cell carcinoma with 2 mg/kg/d of isotretinoin for 2 years (182). They demonstrated a reduction in skin cancer occurrence while on therapy which was not maintained off therapy.

The retinoid skin cancer prevention (SKICAP) trials are a set of double-blind, placebo controlled large clinical trials testing retinoids (183). The SKICAP-actinic keratoses trial involved 2,297 patients who were treated with 25,000 IU/d of oral retinol for 5 years. This trial demonstrated a significant decrease in the incidence of squamous cell, but not basal cell skin cancers. The SKICAP-squamous cell carcinoma/basal cell carcinoma (S/B) trial involved 525 patients who were treated with daily supplementation of 25,000 IU of retinol or 5 or 10 mg of 13-cis-retinoic acid for three years. The incidence of second primary skin cancer was not reduced with either intervention. Two phase III randomized trials in patients with a previous history of nonmelanoma skin cancers tested 50 mg/d of beta-carotene (184), and 10 mg/d of isotretinoin (185), and did not find a significant reduction in the recurrence rate.

Current studies include the double-blind, randomized nonmelanoma skin cancer prevention trial testing low and high dose selenium in patients with a previous history of either squamous cell or basal cell carcinoma. This study was based on previous data from epidemiologic studies showing an association between individuals with low plasma levels of selenium and an increased risk of skin cancer (186). The study has accrued approximately 1300 patients to receive selenium enriched brewer's yeast versus brewer's yeast placebo.

Conclusion

The important general concepts in chemoprevention are antimutagenesis and antiproliferation. Many of the present agents used in current chemoprevention trials such as retinoids, DFMO, and NSAIDs all are thought to act by growth inhibition. The ideal chemopreventive agent should act early in the multi-step carcinogenic process, prior to the onset of carcinoma. Continuing research in molecular biology and cellular growth processes hopefully will lead to the discovery of early targets for these agents. The determination of intermediate end points that correlate with incidence of cancer will significantly decrease the time needed to complete chemoprevention trials. Thus far no definitive intermediate end point biomarkers have been established.

Retinoids have demonstrated significant activity in cervical, oral, lung, skin, bladder, and breast cancer. Randomized published trials have shown retinoids to reverse oral, skin, and cervical premalignant lesions, primary skin cancers, and SPTs in head and neck, and lung. Several important large scale trials are now in progress to define a potential role for the use of finasteride in prostate, beta-carotene and retinol in lung, and tamoxifen in breast cancer prevention.

Supported by the Cancer Institute of the Chinese Academy of Medical Sciences and the National Cancer Institute, the General Population Trial randomized over 30,000 individuals by a slightly varied factorial design to test various vitamins and minerals in primary chemoprevention of cancer. The trial began in 1986 and treatment lasted for five years. Participants received various combinations of retinol, zinc, riboflavin, niacin, vitamin C, molybdenum, beta-carotene, vitamin E, and selenium at doses one to two times the United States recommended daily allowance. The beta-carotene, vitamin E, and selenium combination showed an overall 13% reduction in the cancer death rate. Gastric cancer had the most dramatic reduction in mortality. The results of this trial have stimulated a lot of interest in this micronutrient combination, but may be of limited value in a more nourished population that is not deficient in these supplements.

There are two ongoing large scale chemoprevention trials in progress to reduce overall cancer incidence. The Physicians' Health Study was started in 1982 and is comprised of male physicians in the United States testing beta-carotene and aspirin in the prevention of cancer and cardiovascular disease. The Womens' Health Study cohort was established in 1976, when 121,701 U.S. female nurses between the ages of 30 and 55 answered a questionnaire concerning risk factors for breast cancer and cardiovascular disease in association with beta-carotene, vitamin E, and aspirin use. Both studies have published the results of aspirin usage and the incidence of colon cancer as mentioned in the colorectal section of this chapter. Interim analysis of the Physician's Health Study showed no effect on lung cancer risk with beta-carotene use. This cohort is primarily comprised of nonsmokers in contrast to the CARET and ATBC trials. The results of these trials will be determined only after many years of follow-up, but have a potentially dramatic impact on public health.

Chemoprevention is not yet a standard approach in the clinical setting. However, the growing progress in positive randomized chemoprevention clinical trials establishes the feasibility and value of this field. Cancer chemoprevention is currently being investigated in populations at high risk of certain neoplasms. Improvement in molecular techniques will increase our detection of high risk individuals who have the best chance of benefiting from chemoprevention strategies. In the future we may be able to apply the results of these high risk studies to the geriatric population. The impact that chemoprevention treatments can have on the morbidity and mortality of cancer makes it an exciting new branch of oncology.

References

1. Ries LAG, Miller BA, Hankey BF, Kosary CL, Harras A, Edwards BK. *SEER Cancer Statistics Review, 1973–1991*: Tables and Graphs, National Cancer Institute. NIH Pub. No. 94–2789. Bethesda, MD, 1994.
2. Wattenburg LW. Prevention, therapy, basic science and the resolution of the cancer problem. *Cancer Res* 1993; 53: 5890–96.
3. Drummond JC. The nomenclature of the so-called accessory food factors (vitamins). *Biochem J* 1920; 14: 660.
4. Wolbach SB, and Howe PR. Tissue changes following deprivation of fat soluble vitamin A. *J Exp Med* 1925; 42: 753–77.
5. Abels JC, Gorham AT, Pack GT, et al. Metabolic studies in patients with cancer of the gastrointestinal tract. I. Plasma Vitamin A levels in patients with malignant neoplastic disease, particularly of the gastrointestinal tract. *J Clin Invest* 1941; 20: 749–64.
6. Sporn MB, Dunlop NM, Newton DL, et al. Prevention of chemical carcinogenesis by vitamin A and its synthetic analogs (retinoids). *Fed Proc* 1976; 35: 1332–38.
7. Gallagher RE, Chang CS, and Schwartz EL. (Abstract) Metabolism of retinoic acid (RA) by wild type (wt) and RA-resistant HL-60 cells: marked effect of serum. *Blood* 1986; 68(suppl 1): 188a.

8. Marth C, Mayer I, and Daxenbichler G. Effect of retinoic acid and 4 hydroxytamoxifen on human breast cancer cell lines. *Biochem Pharma Col* 1984; 33: 2217–21.
9. Traganos F, Higgins PJ, Bueti C, et al. Effects of retinoic acid versus dimethylsulfoxide on friend erythroleukemia cell growth. II. Induction of quiescent nonproliferating cells. *JNCI* 1984; 73: 205–18.
10. Yen A, Reese SL, and Albright KL. Control of cell differentiation during proliferation II Myeloid differentiation and cell cycle arrest of HL-60 promyelocytes preceded by nuclear structural changes. *Leuk Res* 1985; 9: 51–71.
11. Craig RW, Frankfurt OS, Sakagami H, et al. Macromolecular and cell cycle effects of different classes of agents inducing the maturation of human myeloblastic leukemia (ML-1) cells. *Cancer Res* 1984; 44: 2121–29.
12. Lippman SM, Kessler JF, and Meyskens, FL Jr. Retinoids as Preventive and Therapeutic Anti-cancer Agents (Part 1). *Cancer Treat Rep* 1987; 71: 391–405.
13. Pillai R, Garewal HS, Wood S, Watson RR. Biological monitoring of cancer chemoprevention. *J Surg Oncol* 1992; 51: 195–202.
14. Cohen AM, Misky BD, Schilsky RL. Colon Cancer. In *Cancer Principles and Practice of Oncology*, edited by VT Devita Jr, S Hellman, SA Rosenberg. Philadelphia: J.B. Lippincott, 929–77, 1993.
15. Fearon ER, Vogelstein B. A genetic model for colorectal tumorgenesis. *Cell* 1990; 61: 759–67.
16. Craven PA, DeRubertis FR. Effects of aspirin on 1,2-dimethyl hydrazine-induced colonic carcinogenesis. *Carcinogenesis* 1992; 13: 541–6.
17. Pollard M, Luckert PH. Effect of indomethacin on intestinal tumors induced in rats by the acetate derivative of dimethylnitrosamine. *Science* 1981; 214: 558–9.
18. Reddy BS, Maruyama H, Kelloff G. Dose-related inhibition of colon carcingenesis by dietary piroxicam, a nonsteriodal anti-inflammatory drug during different stages of rat colon tumor development. *Cancer Res* 1987; 47: 5340–6.
19. Moorghen M, Ince P, Finney KJ, Sunter JP, Appleton DR, Watson AJ. A protective effect of sulindac against chemically-induced primary colonic tumors in mice. *J Pathol* 1988; 156: 341–7.
20. Kelloff GJ, Boone CW, Cromwell JA, et al. Chemopreventive drug development: Perspectives and progress. *Cancer Epidemiol Biomarkers Prev* 1994; 3: 85–98.
21. Marnett LJ. Aspirin and potential role of prostaglandins in colon cancer. *Cancer Res* 1992; 52: 5575–89.
22. Thun MJ, Namboodiri MM, Heath CW Jr. Aspirin use and reduced risk of fatal colon cancer. *N Engl J Med* 1991; 325: 1593–6.
23. Giovannucci E, Egan KM, Hunter DJ, et al. Aspirin and the risk of colorectal cancer in women. *N Engl J Med* 1995; 333: 609–614.
24. Giovannucci E, Rimm EB, Stampfer MD, Colditz GA, Ascherio A, Willett WC. Aspirin use and the risk of colorectal cancer and adenoma in male health professionals. *Ann Intern Med* 1994; 121: 241–46.
25. Gann PH, Mason JE, Glynn RJ, Buring JE, Hennekeus CH. Low dose aspirin and incidence of colorectal tumors in a randomized trial. *J Natl Cancer Inst* 1993; 85: 1220–4.
26. Kune GA, Kune S, Watson CF. Colorectal cancer risk, chronic illnesses, operations, and medications: Case control results from the Melbourne Colorectal Cancer Study. *Cancer* 1988; 48: 4399–404.
27. Rosenburg L, Palmer JR, Zauber AG, Warshauer ME, Stalley PD, Shapiro S. A hypothesis: Nonsteroidal anti-inflammatory drugs reduce the incidence of large-bowel cancer. *J Natl Cancer Inst* 1991; 83: 455–8.
28. Suh O, Mettlin C, Petrelli NJ. Aspirin use, cancer, and polyps of the large bowel. *Cancer* 1993; 72: 1171–7.
29. Peleg II, Maibach HT, Browns H, Wilcox CM. Aspirin and nonsteriodal anti-inflammatory drug use and the risk of subsequent colorectal cancer. *Arch Intern Med* 1994; 154: 394–9.
30. Schreinemachers DM, Everson RB. Aspirin use and lung, colon, and breast cancer incidence in a prospective study. *Epidemiology* 1994; 5: 138–46.
31. Paganini-Hill A, Chao A, Ross RK, Henderson BE. Aspirin use and chronic diseases: A cohort study of the elderly. *BMJ* 1989; 299: 1247–50.

32. Labayle D, Fischer D, Vielh P, *et al*. Sulindac causes regression of rectal polyps in familial adenomatous polyposis. *Gastroenterology* 1991; **101**: 635–39.

33. Giardiello FM, Hamilton SR, Krush AJ, *et al*. Low-dose aspirin and incidence of colorectal tumors in a randomized trial. *J Natl Cancer Inst* 1993; **85**: 1220–24.

34. Earnest DL, Hixson LJ, Fennerty MB, *et al*. Inhibition of prostaglandin synthesis: Potential for chemoprevention of human colon cancer, *Cancer Bull* 1989; **43**: 561–68.

35. Newmark HL, Wargovich MJ, Bruce WR. Colon cancer and dietary fat, phosphate, and calcium: A hypothesis. *J Natl Cancer Inst* 1984; **72**: 1323–5.

36. Bostick RM, Potter JD, Sellers TA, *et al*. Relation of calcium, Vitamin D, and dairy food intake to incidence of colon cancer among older women. The Iowa Women's Health Study. *Am J Epidemiol* 1993; **137**: 1302–17.

37. Baron JA, Tosteson TD, Wargovich MJ, *et al*. Calcium supplementation and rectal mucosal proliferation: A randomized controlled trial. *J Natl Cancer Inst* 1995; **87**: 1303–7.

38. Bostick RM, Fosdick L, Wood JR, *et al*. Calcium and colorectal epithelial cell proliferation in sporadic adenoma patients: A randomized double-blinded, placebo-controlled clinical trial. *J Natl Cancer Inst* 1995; **87**: 1307–15.

39. Gregorie RC, Stern HS, Yeung KS, *et al*. Effect of calcium supplementation on mucosal cell proliferation in high risk patients for colon cancer. *Gut* 1989; **30**: 376–82.

40. Stern HS, Gregorie RC, Koshtan H. Long-term effects of dietary calcium on risk markers for colon cancer in patients with familial polyposis. *Surgery* 1990; **108**: 528–533.

41. Wargovich MJ, Isbell G, Shabot M, *et al*. Calcium supplementation decreases rectal epithelial cell proliferation in subjects with sporadic adenoma. *Gastroenterology* 1992; **103**: 92–97.

42. Bussey HJR, DeCosse JJ, Deschner EE, *et al*. A randomized trial of ascorbic acid in polyposis coli. *Cancer* 1982; **50**: 1434–39.

43. McKeown-Eyssen G, Holloway C, Jazmaji V, *et al*. A randomized trial of vitamins C and E in the prevention of recurrence of colorectal polyps. *Cancer Res* 1988 **48**: 4701–4705.

44. DeCosse JJ, Miller HH, Lesser ML. Effect of wheat fiber and vitamins on rectal polyps in patients with familial adenomatous polyposis. *J Natl Cancer Inst* 1989; **81**: 1290–97.

45. Paganelli GM. Biasco G, Brandi G, *et al*. Effect of vitamins A,C, and E supplementation on rectal cell proliferation in patients with colorectal adenomas. *J Natl Cancer Inst* 1992; **84**: 47–51.

46. Roncucci L, Donato PD, Carati L, *et al*. Antioxidant vitamins or lactulose for the prevention of the recurrence of colorectal adenomas. *Dis Colon Rectum* 1993; **36**: 227–34.

47. Greenberg ER, Baron JA, Tosteson TD, *et al*. A clinical trial of antioxidant vitamins to prevent colorectal adenoma. *N Engl J Med* 1994; **331**: 141–7.

48. Baghei D, Doeltz MK, Fay JR, *et al*. Database of inhibitors of carcinogenesis. *J Environ Sci Health* 1988; **C6**: vii–xviii, 262–403.

49. Kelloff GJ, Boone CW, Crowell JA, *et al*. Chemopreventive drug development: Perspectives and progress. *Cancer Epidemiol Biomarkers & Prev* 1994; **3**: 85–98.

50. Shin DM, Kim J, Ro JY, *et al*. Activation of p53 gene expression in premalignant lesions during head and neck tumorigenesis. *Cancer Res* 1994; **54**: 321–326.

51. Lee JS, Kim Sy, Hong WK, *et al*. Detection of chromosomal polysomy in oral leukoplakia, a premalignant lesion. *J Natl Cancer Inst* 1993; **85**: 1951–54.

52. Sozzi G, Miozzo M, Tagliabue E, *et al*. Cytogenetic abnormalities and over expression of receptors for growth factors in normal bronchial epithelium and tumor samples of lung cancer patients. *Cancer Res* 1991; **51**: 400–4.

53. Chung KY, Mukhopadhyay T, Kim J, *et al*. Discordant p53 gene mutations in primary head and neck cancers and corresponding second primary cancers of the upper aerodigestive tract. *Cancer Res* 1993; **53**: 1676–83.

54. Boone CW, Kelloff GJ, Steele VE. Natural history of intraepithelial neoplasia in humans with implications for cancer chemoprevention strategy. *Cancer Res* 1991; **52**: 1651–59.

55. Slaughter DP, Southwick HW, Smejkal W. Field cancerization in oral stratified squamous epithelium: clinical implications of multicentric origin. *Cancer* 1953; **6**: 963–68.

56. Silverman S, Renstrup G, Pindborg JJ. Studies in oral leukoplakias: Ill. Effects of vitamin A comparing clinical, histopatholigic, cytologic and hematologic responses. *Acta Odont Scand* 1963; **21**: 271–92.

57. Stich HF, Rosin MP, Hornby AP, *et al*. Remission of oral leukoplakia and micronuclei in tobacco/betel quid chewers treated with beta carotene and beta-carotene plus vitamin A. *Int J Cancer* 1988; **42**: 195–99.

58. Garewal HS, Meyskens FL, Killen D, *et al*. Response of oral leukoplakia to beta-carotene. *J Clin Oncol* 1990; **8**: 1715–20.

59. Benner SE, Winn RJ, Lippman SM, *et al*. Regression of oral leukoplakia with α-tocopheral: A community clinical oncology-program chemoprevention study. *J Natl Cancer Inst* 1993; **85**: 44–47.

60. Hong WK, Endicott J, Itri LM, *et al*. 13-cis-retinoic acid in the treatment of oral leukoplakia. *N Engl J Med* 1986; **315**: 1505–5.

61. Lippman SM, Batsakis JG, Toth BB, *et al*. Comparison of low-dose isotretinoin with beta carotene to prevent oral carcinogenesis. *N Engl J Med* 1993; **328**: 15–20.

62. Stich HF, Hornby AP, Mathew B, *et al*. Response of oral leukoplakias to the administration of vitamin A. *Cancer Lett* 1988; **40**: 93–101.

63. Han J, Lu Y, Sun Z, *et al*. Evaluation of N-4-(hydroxycarbophenyl) retinamide as a cancer prevention agent and as a cancer chemotherapeutic agent. *In Vivo* 1990; **4**: 153–60.

64. Costa A, Formelli F, Chiesa F, *et al*. Prospects of chemoprevention of human cancers with the synthetic retinoid fenretinide. *Cancer Res* 1994; **54**(7 suppl): 2032s–2037s.

65. Lotan R, Xu XC, Ro JY, *et al*. Decreased retinoic acid receptor β inhuman oral premalignant lesions and its induction by retinoic acid *in vivo*. *Proc Annu Meet Am Soc Clin Oncol* 1994; **13**: A472.

66. Lippman SM, Shin DM, Lee JJ, *et al*. p53 and retinoid chemoprevention of oral carcinogenesis. *Cancer Res* 1995; **55**: 16–9.

67. Hong WK, Lippman SM, Itri LM, *et al*. Prevention of second primarytumors with isotretinoin in squamous-cell carcinoma of the head and neck. *N Engl J Med* 1990; **323**: 795–801.

68. Benner SE, Pajak TF, Lippman SM, *et al*. Prevention of second primary tumors with isotretinoin in squamous cell carcinoma of the head and neck: Long term follow-up. *J Natl Cancer Inst* 1994; **86**: 140–41.

69. Parker SL, Tong T, Bolden S, Wingo PA. Cancer Statistics 1996. *Ca Cancer J Clin* 1996; **46**: 5–27.

70. Carney DN. Lung cancer biology. *Curr Opin Oncol* 1991; **3**: 288.

71. Iggo R, Galter K, Bustek, *et al*. Increased expression of mutant forms of p53 oncogene in primary lung cancer. *Lancet* 1990; **335**: 675.

72. Brennan J, O'Connor T, Makuch RW, *et al*. MYC family DNA amplifications in 107 tumors and tumor cell lines from patients with small cell lung cancer treated with different combination chemotherapy regimens. *Cancer Res* 1991; **51**: 1708.

73. Mitsudomi T, Steinberg SM, Oie HK, *et al*. Ras gene mutations in non-small cell lung cancer are associated with shortened survival irrespective of treatment intent. *Cancer Res* 1991; **51**: 4999.

74. Slebos RJ, Kibbelear RE, Dalesio A, Kooistra A, *et al*. K-ras oncogene activation as a prognostic marker in adenocarcinoma of the lung. *New Engl J Med* 1990; **323**: 561.

75. Weiner DB, Nordberg J. Robinson R, *et al*. Expression of the new gene-encoded protein (p185neu) in human non-small cell carcinoma of the lung. *Cancer Res* 1990; **50**: 421.

76. Kern JA, Schwartz DA, Nordberg JE, *et al*. p185neu expression in human lung adenocarcinoma predicts shortened survival. *Cancer Res*, 1990; **50**: 5184.

77. Shaw GL, Mulshine JL. Monoclonal antibodies for early cytologic detection of lung cancer. *Seminars in Thoracic and Cardiovascular Surgery* 1993; **5**: 201–9.

78. Tockman MS, Gupta PK, Meyers JD, *et al*. Sensitive and specific monoclonal antibody recognition of human lung cancer antigen or preserved sputum cells: A new approach to early lung cancer detection. *J Clin Oncol* 1988; **6**: 1685–93.

79. Law RM, Hetzel MR, Idle JR. Debrisoquine metabolism and genetic predisposition to lung cancer. *Br J Cancer* 1989; **59**: 686.

80. Siedergard J, Peron RW, Markowitz MM, *et al.* Isoenzyme (5) of glutathione transferral (class mu) a marker for the susceptibility to lung cancer with a follow-up study. *Carcinogenesis* 1990; **11**: 33.

81. Kellerman G, Shaw CR, Lylen-Kellerman M. Aryl hydrocarbon hydroxylase inducibility and bronchogenic carcinoma. *N Engl J Med* 1973; **289**: 934–37.

82. McLemor TL, Martin RR, Busbee DL, *et al.* Aryl hydrocarbon hydroxylase activity in pulmonary macrophages and lymphocytes from lung cancer and non-cancer patients. *Cancer Res* 1977; **37**: 1175–81.

83. Idle JR, Mahgoub A, Angelo MM, *et al.* The metabolism of [^{14}C] debrisoquine in man. *Br J Clin Pharmacol* 1979; **7**: 257–66.

84. Duche JC, Joanne JC, Barre J, *et al.* Lack of relationship between the polymorphism of debrisoquine oxidation and lung cancer. *Br J Clin Pharmacol* 1991; **31**: 533–36.

85. Shaw GL, Falk RT, Deslauriers J, *et al.* Debrisoquine metabolism and lung cancer risk. *Cancer Epidemiol Biomarkers & Prev* 1995; **4**: 1–8.

86. Lippman SM, Hong WK. Not yet standard: retinoids versus second primary tumors. *J Clin Oncol* 1993; **11**: 1204–7.

87. Lippman SM, Spitz MR. Intervention in the premalignant process. *Cancer Bull* 1991; **43**: 473–573.

88. Misset JL, Mathe G, Santelli G, *et al.* Regression of bronchial epidermoid metaplasia in heavy smokers with etretinate treatment. *Cancer Detect Prev* 1986; **9**: 167–70.

89. Arnold AM, Browman GP, Levine MN, *et al.* The effect of the synthetic retinoid etretinate on sputum cytology: Results from a randomized trial. *Br J Cancer* 1992; **65**: 737–743.

90. Lee JS, Lippman SM, Benner SE, *et al.* Randomized placebo controlled trial of isotretinoin in chemoprevention of bronchial squamous metaplasia. *J Clin Oncol* 1994; **12**: 937–45.

91. Heimberger DC, Alexander B, Birch R, *et al.* Improvement in bronchial squamous metaplasia in smokers treated with folate and vitamin B12. Report of a preliminary randomized, double-blind intervention trial. *JAMA* 1988; **259**: 1525–30.

92. Pastorino V, Infante M, Maioli M, *et al.* Adjuvant treatment of stage I lung cancer with high dose vitamin A. *J Clin Oncol* 1993; **11**: 1216–22.

93. The Alpha-Tocopherol, Beta Carotene Cancer Prevention Study Group. The effect of vitamin E and beta carotene on the incidence of lung cancer and other cancers in male smokers. *N Engl J Med* 1994; **330**: 1029–35.

94. Smigel K. Beta Carotene Fails to Prevent Cancer in Two Major Studies; CARET Intervention Stopped. *J Nat Cancer Inst* 1996; **88**: 145.

95. Kinne DW. Special therapeutic problems: Management of the contralateral breast. In *Breast Diseases*, edited by JR Harris, S Hellman, B Henderson. Philadelphia: J.B. Lippincott, 827–34, 1991.

96. Early Breast Cancer Trialists' Collaborative Group. Systemic treatment of early breast cancer by hormonal, cytotoxic, or immune therapy. 133 randomized trials involving 31,000 recurrences and 34,000 deaths among 75,000 women. *Lancet* 1992; **339**: 71–85.

97. Gray R. Tamoxifen: How boldly to go where no women have gone before. *J Natl Cancer Inst* 1993; **85**: 1358–1360.

98. Gail MH, Brinton LA, Byar DP, *et al.* Projecting individualized probabilities of developing breast cancer for white females who are being examined annually. *J Natl Cancer Inst* 1989; **81**: 1879–96.

99. NSABP Breast Cancer Prevention Trial (BCPT): a progress report. *Proc Am Soc Clin Oncol* 1993; **12**: 69.

100. Veronesi U. DePalo G, Costa A, *et al.* Chemoprevention of breast cancer with retinoids. *J Natl Cancer Inst Monogr* 1992; **12**: 93–7.

101. Torrisi R, Pena I, Orengoma, *et al.* The synthetic retinoid fenretinide lowers plasma IGF-1 levels in breast cancer patients. *Cancer Res* 1993; **53**: 4769–71.

102. Fontana JA, Interaction of retinoids and tamoxifen on the inhibition of mammary carcinoma cell proliferation. *Exp Cell Biol* 1987; **55**: 136–44.

103. Ratko TA, Detrisac CJ, Dinger MN, *et al.* Chemopreventative efficacy of combined retinoid and tamoxifen treatment following surgical excision of a primary mammary cancer in female rats. *Cancer Res* 1989; **49**: 4472–76.

104. Cobleigh MA, Oleske DM, Nickerson T, Pollak M. IGF-1 levels in stage IV breast cancer treated with tamoxifen (tam) and fenretinide (fen). *Proc Annu Meet Am Assoc Cancer Res* 1995; **36**: a1462.

105. Decensi A, Torrisi R, Polizzi A, *et al.* Effect of the synthetic retinoid fenretinide on dark-adaptation and ocular surface. *J Clin Oncol* 1993; **11**: 474–77.

106. Moon RC, Minn I, Benson AB III, *et al.* Phase I/II trial of tamoxifen with or with without fenretinide, an analog of vitamin A, in women with metatstatic breast cancer. *J Clin Oncol* 1993; **11**: 474–77.

107. Fornander T, Rutqvist LE, Cedermark B, *et al.* Adjuvant tamoxifen in early breast cancer: Occurrence of new primary cancer. *Lancet* 1989; **1**: 117–20.

108. Williams GM, Latzopoulos MJ, Djordjevic MV, *et al.* The triphenylethylene drug tamoxifen is a strong liver carcinogen in the rat. *Carcinongenesis* 1993; **14**: 315–317.

109. Pavlidis NA, Petris C, Briassoulis E, *et al.* Clear evidence that the long term, low dose tamoxifen treatment can induce ocular toxicity. *Cancer* 1992; **62**: 2961–4.

110. Pike MC, Ross RK, Lobo RA, *et al.* LHRH agonists and the prevention of breast and ovarian cancer. *Br J Cancer* 1989; **60**: 142–8.

111. Trichopaulius D, MacMahon B, Cole P. Menopause and breast cancer risk. *J Natl Cancer Inst* 1972; **48**: 605–13.

112. Cramer DW, Cutler SJ. Incidence and histopathology of malignancies of the female genital organs in the United States. *Am J Obstet Gynecol* 1974; **118**: 443–60.

113. Barber HRK. Incidence, prevalence, and median survival rates of gynecologic cancer. In *Modern concepts of gynecologic oncology*, edited by JR Van Nagell, HRK Barber. Boston: John Wright PSG, 1–19, 1982.

114. Mitchell MF, Hittelman WN, Hong WK, Lotam R, Schottenfeld D. The natural history of cervical intraepithelial neoplasia: An argument for intermediate endpoint biomarkers. *Cancer Epidemiol Biomarkers & Prev* 1994; **3**: 619–26.

115. Coppleson LW, Brown BW. Observation on a model of the biology of carcinoma of the cervix: a poor fit between observation and theory. *Am J Obstet Gynecol* 1975; **122**: 127–36.

116. Stern E, Neely PM. Dialysis of the uterine cervix: incidence of regression, recurrence and cancer. *Cancer* 1964; **17**: 508–12.

117. McCance DJ, Campion MJ, Clarkson PK, Chesters PM, Jenkins D, Singer A. Prevalence of human papilloma virus type 16 DNA sequences in cervical intraepithelial neoplasia and invasive carcinoma of the cervix. *Br J Obstet Gynaecol* 1985; **92**: 1101–5.

118. Jones CJ, Brinton LA, Hamma, RI, *et al.* Risk factors for *in situ* cervical cancer: Results from a case-control study. *Cancer Res* 1990; **50**: 3657–62.

119. Mandelblatt J, Richart R, Thomas L, *et al.* Is Human papillomavirus associated with cervical neoplasia in the elderly? *Gynecologic Oncology* 1992; **46**: 6–12.

120. Palan PR, Ramsey SL, Mikhail M, *et al.* Decreased plasma beta carotene levels in women with uterine cervical dysplasia and cancer. *JNCI* 1988; **80**: 454–5.

121. Palan PR, Mikhail MS, Basa J, Ramsey SL. Beta-carotene levels in exfoliated cervico-vaginal epithelial cells in cervical intraepithelial neoplasia and cervical cancer. *Am J Ob Gyn* 1992; **167**: 1899–1903.

122. Hatch KD. Pre-invasive cervical neoplasia seminars. *Oncology.* 1994; **21**: 12–16.

123. Khan MA, Jenkins GR, Tolleson WH, Creek KE, Pirisi L. Retinoic acid inhibition of human papilloma virus type 16-mediated transformation of human keratinocytes. *Cancer Res* 1993; **53**: 905–09.

124. Graham V, Surwit ES, Weiner S, *et al.* Phase II trial of beta-all-trans retinoic acid for cervical intraepithelial neoplasia delivered via a collagen sponge and cervical cap. *West J Med* 1986; **145**: 192–95.

125. Meyskens FL, Surwitt E, Moon TE, *et al*. Enhancement of cervical intraepithelial neoplasia II (moderate dysplasia) with topically applied all-trans-retinoic acid: A randomized trial. *J Natl Cancer Inst* 1994; **86**: 539–43.

126. Butterworth CE, Hatch KD, Soong SJ, *et al*. Oral folic acid supplementation for cervical dysplasia: A clinical intervention trial. *Am J Obstet Gynecol* 1993; **166**: 803–9.

127. DeVet HCW, Knipschild PG, Willebrand D, *et al*. The effect of beta carotene on the regression and progression of cervical dysplasia: A clinical experiment. *J Clin Epidemiol* 1991; **44**: 273–283.

128. Byrne MA, Moller BR, Taylor-Robinson D, *et al*. The effect of interferon on human papillomaviruses associated with cervical intraepithelial neplasia. *Br J Obstet Gynecol* 1986; **93**: 1136–44.

129. Yliskoski M, Canteel K, Syrjanen K, *et al*. Topical treatment with human leukocyte interferon of HPV 16 infections associated with cervical and vaginal intraepithelial neoplasia. *Gynecol Oncol* 1990; **36**: 353–57.

130. Frost L, Skajaak, Huidman LE, *et al*. No effect of intralesional injection of interferon on moderate cervical intraepithelial neoplasia. *Br J Obstet Gynecol* 1990; **97**: 626–630.

131. Dunham AM, McCartney JC, McCance DJ, *et al*. Effects of perilesional injection of alpha-interferon on cervical intraepithelial neoplasia and associated human papillomavirus infection. *J R Soc Med* 1990; **83**: 490–92.

132. Bornstein J, Ben-David Y, Atad J, *et al*. Treatment of cervical intraepithelial neoplasia and invasive squamous cell carcinoma by interferon. *Obstet Gynecol Surv* 1993; **48**: 251–60.

133. Walker AM, Jick H: Declining rates of endometrial cancer. *Obstet Gynecol* 1980; **56**: 733.

134. Weiss NS, Szekely DR, Austin DF. Increasing incidence of endometrial cancer in the United States. *N Engl J Med* 1976; **294**: 1259.

135. Gambrell RD Jr, Bagnell CA, Greenblatt RB. Role of estrogens and progesterone in the etiology and prevention of endometrial cancer. *Am J Obstet Gynecol* 1983; **146**: 696.

136. Persson I, Adami HO, Bergkuist L, *et al*. Risk of endometrial cancer after treatment with estrogens alone or in conjunction with progestogens: Results of a prospective Study. *Br Med J* 1989; **298**: 147–51.

137. Gambrell RD Jr. Use of progestogen therapy. *Am J Obstet Gynecol* 1987; **156**: 1304.

138. Writing Group for the PEPI Trial. The effects of estrogen/progestin regimens on heart disease risk factors in postmenopausal women. The Postmenopausal Estrogen/Progestin Interventions (PEPI) Trial. *JAMA* 1995; **273**: 199–208.

139. Whitehead MI, Townsend PT, Pryse-Davis J, *et al*. Effects of various types and dosages of progestogens on the postmenopausal endometrium. *J Reprod Med* 1982; **27**: 539–47.

140. Greenwald P, Kelloff G, Burch-Whitman C, Kramer BS. Chemoprevention. *Ca Cancer J Clin* 1995; **45**: 31–49.

141. Bernstein L, Ross RK, Henderson BE. Relationship of hormone use to cancer risk. *J Natl Cancer Inst Monogr* 1992; **12**: 137–47.

142. Centers for Disease Control Cancer and Steroid Hormone Study. Oral contraceptives and the risk of ovarian cancer. *JAMA* 1983: **249**: 1596.

143. Casagrande JT, Louie EW, Pike MC, Roy S, Ross R, Henderson BE. "Incessant ovulation" and ovarian cancer. *Lancet* 1979; **2**: 170–3.

144. Weiss NS, Lyon JL, Liff JM, Vollmer WM, Darling JR. Incidence of ovarian cancer in relation to the use of oral contraceptives. *Int J Cancer* 1981; **28**: 669–71.

145. Rosenberg L, Shapiro S, Stone D, *et al*. Epithelial ovarian cancer and combination oral contraceptives. *JAMA* 1992; **247**: 3210–2.

146. Centers for Disease Control Cancer and Steroid Hormone Study. The reduction in risk of ovarian cancer associated with oral contraceptive use. *N Engl J Med* 1987; **316**: 650–5.

147. Whittemore AS. Personal characteristics relating to risk of invasive epithelial ovarian cancer in older women in the United States. *Cancer* 1993; **71**(2 Suppl): 558–65.

148. Kelsey JL, Hildreth NG. *Breast and Gynecologic cancer epidemiology*. Boca Raton, FL: CRC, 1983.

149. Cramer DW, Hutchinson GB, Welch WR. Determinants of ovarian cancer risk I. Reproductive experiences and family history. *JNCI* 1983; **71**: 711–16.

150. Weiss NS, Lyon JL, Krishnamurthy S, *et al*. Non-contraceptive estrogen use and the occurrence of ovarian cancer. *J Natl Cancer Inst* 1982; **68**: 95.

151. Bostick DG. Prostatic Intraepithelial Neoplasia (PIN): Current concepts. *J Cell Biochem* (Suppl.) 1992; **16H**: 10–19.

152. Isaacs JT. Hormonal balance and the risk of prostatic cancer. *J Cell Biochem* (suppl) 1992; **16H**: 107–8.

153. Gormley GJ. Chemoprevention strategies for prostate cancer: The role of 5α-reductase inhibitors. *J Cell Biochem* (suppl)1992; **16H**: 113–17.

154. Brawley OW, Ford LG, Thompson I, *et al*. 5-alpha-reductase inhibition and prostate cancer prevention. *Cancer Epidemiol Biomarkers Prev* 1994; **3**: 177–82.

155. Pollard M, Luckert PH, Sporn MB. Prevention of primary prostate cancer in Lobund-Wistar rats by 4-hydroxyphenyl-retinamide. *Cancer Res* 1991; **51**: 3610–3616.

156. Evan R, Goldfischer HL, Gornik DB, *et al*. Evaluation of the toxicity and effects on PSA velocity of 4-HPR in men with localized prostate cancer. *Proc Am Soc Clin Oncol* 1995; **14**: 241.

157. Fong CJ, Sutkowski DM, Braun EJ, *et al*. Effect of retinoic acid on the proliferation and secretory activity of androgen-responsive prostatic carcinoma cells. *J Urol* 1993; **149**: 1190–4.

158. Kadnom, D. Chemoprevention in Prostate Cancer: the role of difluoromethylorinithine (DFMO). *J Cell Biochem* (Suppl) 1992; **16H**: 122–27.

159. Fradet Y, Lafleur L, LaRue H. Strategies of chemoprevention based on antigenic and molecular markers of early and premalignant lesions of the bladder. *J Cell Biochem* (Suppl) 1992; **161**: 85–92.

160. Sandberg M. Chromosome changes in early bladder neoplasms. *J Cell Biochem* (Suppl) 1992; **161**: 76–9.

161. Herr HW. Intravesical therapy: A critical review. *Urol Clin North Am* 1987; **145**: 399–404.

162. Martinez-Pineiro JA, Leon JJ, Martinez-Pineiro L Jr, *et al*. Bacillus Calmette-Guerin versus doxorubiuin vs. Thiotepa: a randomized prospective study in 202 patients with superficial bladder cancer. *J Urol* 1990; **143**: 502–6.

163. Lamm DL, Blumenstein BA, Crawford ED, *et al*. A randomized trial of intravesical doxorubicin and immunotherapy with bacille Calmette Guerin for transitional cell carcinoma of the bladder. *N Engl J Med* 1991; **325**: 1205.

164. Herr HW. Transurethral resection and intravesical therapy of superficial bladder tumors. *Urol Clin North Am* 1991; **81**: 525.

165. Herr HW, Wartinger DD. BCG therapy for superficial bladder cancer. A 10-yearfollow-up. *J Urol* 1992; **147**: 1020–23.

166. Sporn MB, Squire RA, Brown CC, *et al*. 13-cis-retinoic acid: Inhibition of bladder carcinogenesis in the rat. *Science* 1977; **195**: 487–89.

167. Pederson H, Wolf H, Jensen SK, *et al*. Administration of a retinoid as prophylaxis of recurrent noninvasive bladder tumors. *Scand J Urol Nephrol* 1984; **18**: 121–23.

168. Alfthan D, Tarkkanen J, Grohn P, *et al*. Tigason (etretinate) in prevention of recurrence of superficial bladder tumors. *Eur Urol* 1983; **9**: 6–9.

169. Studer UE, Biedermann C, Chollet D, *et al*. Prevention of recurrent superficial bladder tumors by oral etretinate: Preliminary results of a randomized, double-blind, multi-center trial in Switzerland. *J Urol* 1984; **131**: 1469–72.

170. Prout GR, Barton BA. 13-cis-retinoic acid in chemoprevention of superficial bladder cancer. *J Cell Biochem* (Suppl) 1992; **161**: 148–52.

171. Decensi A, Bruno S, Giaretti W. Activity of 4-HPR in superficial bladder cancer using DNA flow cytometry as an intermediate endpoint. *J Cell Biochem* (Suppl) 1992; **161**: 139–47.

172. Matsushima M, Yagishita T, Ando K, *et al*. Inhibition by sulfur containing compounds of rodent vesical carcinogen-induced urinary ornithine decarboxylase (ODC) activity and bladder carcinogenesis. XIII International Cancer Congress 1982; 606.

173. Nowels K, Homma Y, Seidenfeld J, Oyasu R. Prevention of inhibition effects of alpha-difluoromethylornithine on rat urinary carcinogenesis by exogenous putrescine. *Cancer Biophys* 1986; **8**: 257–63.

174. Homma Y, Ozono S, Numata I, *et al*. Inhibition of carcinogenesis by alpha-difluoromethylornithine in heterotopically transplanted rat urinary bladders. *Cancer Res* 1985: **45**: 648–52.

175. Loprinzi CL, Messing E, O'Fallon J, *et al*. Pilot evaluation of difluoromethylornithine (DFMO): Doses for use in prospective chemoprevention trials. *Proc Annu Meet Am Soc Clin Oncol* 1995; **14**: A346.

176. Bollag W. Vitamin A and retinoids: From nutrition to pharmacotherapy in dermatology and oncology. *Lancet* 1983; **1**: 860–63.

177. Bollag W, and Ott F. Vitamin A acid in benign and malignant epithelial tumors of the skin. Acta Dermatol Venereol (Stockh)suppl 1975; **74**: 163–66.

178. Belisario JC. Recent advances in topical cytotoxic therapy of skin cancer and pre-cancer. In *Melanoma and skin cancer: Proceedings of the International Cancer Conference*, Sydney, 1972; 349–65.

179. Kligman AM, Thorne EG: Topical therapy of actinic keratosis with tretinoin. In *Retinoids in Cutaneous Malignancy*, edited by R Marks. Cambridge, MA: Blackwell Scientific, 66–73, 1991.

180. Moriarty M, Dunn J, Darragh A, *et al*. *Etretinate in treatment of actinic keratosis: A double blind crossover study*. Lancet 1982; 364–65.

181. Watson AB. Preventative effect of etretinate therapy on multiple actinic keratosis. *Cancer Detect* 1986; **9**: 161–65.

182. Kraemer KH, DiGiovanna JJ, Moshell AN, *et al*. Prevention of skin cancer in xeroderma pigmentosum with the use of oral isotretinoin. *N Engl J Med* 1988; **318**: 1633–37.

183. Moon TE, Cartmel B, Levine N, *et al*. The Arizona Skin Cancer Study Group. Chemoprevention and Etiology of Non-melanoma Skin Cancers. Program and Abstracts, 17th Annual Meeting of the American Society of Preventive Oncology, Tuscon. AZ, March 20–23, 1993.

184. Greenberg ER, Baron JA, Stukel TA, *et al*. A clinical trial of beta carotene to prevent basal-cell and squamous-cell cancers of the skin. *N Engl J Med* 1990; **323**: 789–95.

185. Tangrea JA, Edwards BK, Taylor PR, *et al*. Long-term therapy with low-dose isotretinoin for prevention of basal cell carcinoma: A multi center clinical trial. *J Natl Cancer Inst* 1992; **84**: 328–32.

186. Clark LC, Patterson BH, Weed DL, *et al*. Design issues in cancer chemoprevention trials using micronutrients: Application to skin cancer. *Cancer Bull* 1991; **43**: 519–24.

23. A Practical Approach to the Screening of Asymptomatic Older Persons for Cancer

Lodovico Balducci and Patricia P. Barry

Introduction

Secondary prevention of cancer is aimed at the individual in whom the disease has begun but symptoms have not yet appeared, in order to diagnose and treat early disease and/or prevent spread. Secondary prevention is a reasonable strategy for cancer control in the aged in whom primary prevention, aimed at the individual who has not yet developed the disease, may no longer be feasible. Screening the asymptomatic population at risk may be justified if it enables diagnosis at an asymptomatic or preclinical phase and if treatment at this stage leads to a longer life or reduced morbidity for those individuals whose disease is thereby detected (Figure 23.1) (1–4).

Decisions related to screening asymptomatic older persons for cancer should be individualized according to the most beneficial and effective approach for each patient (5). This chapter will review the basic principles of cancer screening, age-related implications and existing data regarding effectiveness and likelihood of benefit to the patient.

Principles of Cancer Screening

In order to justify screening, specific criteria must be fulfilled (6): (1) the disease must have a significant effect on quality or quantity of life, (2) acceptable methods of treatment must be available, (3) the disease must have an asymptomatic period during which detection and treatment significantly reduce morbidity and/or mortality, (4) treatment in the asymptomatic period must yield a therapeutic result superior to that obtained by delaying treatment until symptoms appear, (5) tests must be available at a reasonable cost to detect the condition in the asymptomatic period, and (6) the incidence of the condition must be sufficient to justify the costs of screening.

Table 23.1 Important characteristics of a screening test for cancer.

Safety
Low cost
High predictive value, both positive (PV+) and negative (PV–)*
Specificity
Sensitivity

*Note: The predictive value varies greatly with the disease prevalence in the screened population.

Characteristics of an ideal screening test include safety and low cost, as well as acceptability to the patient and physician (Table 23.1). Risks of morbidity, beyond the mild and temporary discomfort of blood drawing and rectal or pelvic examination, should be absent, as should the risk of long-term complications from exposure to radiation or other harmful effects.

Results of screening tests should be valid, reliable, and reproducible. The validity of the test depends on its ability to correctly identify persons with preclinical disease as test-positive and those without preclinical disease as test-negative. Risks of screening include the consequences of false results (7). A false positive test can trigger an extensive workup which is unnecessary, expensive, and hazardous and which can lead to adverse emotional reactions. A false negative test may foster an unwarranted sense of security and lead to neglect of warning symptoms with delay in appropriate care.

Appropriate interpretation of test results requires a knowledge of the characteristics of both the test and the disease. Although "sensitivity" and "specificity" are terms often used to describe the accuracy of tests,

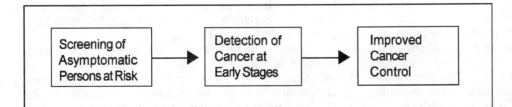

Figure 23.1 Assumptions underlying secondary prevention through screening.

Screening of Asymptomatic Persons at Risk → Detection of Cancer at Early Stages → Improved Cancer Control

these two parameters are calculated by using the test in a population in which the disease status is known, with "sensitivity" indicating the percentage of patients with the disease who have a positive test and "specificity" indicating the percentage of patients without the disease who have a negative test. In an individual patient, however, the disease status is unknown. The ability of the test to diagnose disease in this case depends also upon the pretest probability, or the prevalence of the disease in the patient population. The "positive predictive value" (PV+) is the percentage of patients with a positive test who have the disease; the "negative predictive" (PV–) is the percentage of patients with a negative test who do not have the disease (8). In screening, it is virtually impossible to obtain precise measurements of PV–; thus, PV+ is the parameter which best reflects the performance of a screening test. The PV+ of most common screening tests should improve with the increasing age of the population screened, due to the rising prevalence of cancer (9).

The goal of cancer screening is the reduction of cancer-related mortality. Prolonged survival and higher prevalence of early stage cancers in those patients whose cancer was diagnosed at screening, compared with those whose cancer was symptomatic, are not proof of effectiveness. Such end points are affected by lead time, length time, and overdetection bias (2). Lead-time bias occurs when screening prolongs the length of time during which a person is aware of cancer, rather than a person's actual survival. Length-time bias occurs when only slow-growing tumors, whose natural history is unlikely to be altered by early diagnosis, are detected at screening, while more aggressive tumors, for which early detection would be desirable, are not detected. Overdetection bias occurs when cancers which would never become clinically significant are detected by screening.

The aging of the population may influence both the performance of screening tests and the goals of screening. As previously noted, the PV+ of screening tests may improve with the increasing age of the population, due to higher prevalence of the disease. In addition, the sensitivity of some tests may be altered as a result of physiological or anatomic changes of aging. For example, physical examination of the breast may become more accurate in the detection of breast masses because of atrophy of the mammary tissue. Since the growth of some tumors (breast cancer, lung cancer) may be slower in the elderly (1), a longer time interval between screening examinations may be appropriate, with benefits in terms of cost and convenience.

With the aging of the population, competing causes of death may limit the benefits of reduction in cancer mortality. Life expectancy, a function of age and comorbid conditions (7), may limit the benefits of screening and determine the reality of preventing premature cancer death. Recently, A. Siu, M.D., has established a correlation between functional status and life expectancy (personal communication, April 1993): in a population of persons over 65 years, the two-year mortality was 8% for fully independent individuals, 16% for those

dependent in one to three activities of daily living (ADLs), 31% for those dependent in three to six ADLs, and 40% for those totally dependent and institutionalized. Screening may also affect the quality of life of the older person (10–12), even if early detection of malignancies is not associated with improved survival of older persons. For example, early detection of breast cancer may prevent the development of painful and unsightly local masses; early detection of rectal cancer may avoid the need for colostomy.

Overview of the Effects of Screening on the Control of Common Neoplasms

Screening of asymptomatic individuals for cancer of the breast, cervix, colorectum, prostate and lung will be reviewed, and current practices in persons aged 65 years and over will be examined.

Breast Cancer

Several studies have assessed the effectiveness of serial mammograms, physical examination of the breast by a physician (PBE), and breast self examination (BSE) in early detection of and mortality from breast cancer. Five prospectively controlled and four historically controlled trials investigated the value of serial mammography with or without PBE (Table 23.2) (13–24). With two exceptions (17,23,24), these studies showed a 20% to 30% reduction in breast cancer related mortality for woman aged 50 to 65 years. Improvement in mortality was first seen five to seven years after the initial examination. In four studies of women aged 65 to 70 years, a reduction in breast cancer-related mortality occurred from screening (15,17,18,21). Two studies (only one of which was prospectively controlled) included women up to age 75 years; a reduction in the number of breast cancer deaths could not be conclusively demonstrated in this age group (15–21). Important considerations include determination of the optimal interval between serial mammograms, how long to continue mammograms, and the value of PBE (13). A reasonable approach might include mammography every one or two years for women aged 50 to 75 years, and yearly PBE for all women over 50 years. In selected circumstances, such as women with a life expectancy of at least five years, mammographic screening could be extended beyond age 75 years (2,25). Although the value of PBE without mammography has never been conclusively demonstrated, physician examination is advisable for a number of reasons. Some cases of breast cancer which escape mammographic detection are diagnosed with PBE, and the sensitivity of PBE may improve with the increasing age of the patient. PBE can be incorporated into any office visit and can be a more convenient method of screening than mammography, especially for frail, older women.

Effectiveness of BSE was examined in 11 studies without conclusive results (26). Failure was due to inadequate performance of the examination and poor compliance with the recommended schedule. An intensive education program may improve the perform-

Table 23.2 Clinical trials of screening asymptomatic women for breast cancer.

Trial	Intervention	Number of Subjects	Age Groups (years)	Percentage of Reduction of Cancer Mortality
HIP (14)	M + PBE yearly × 4	62,000	40–64 60–64	23 21
Tabar (15)*	M every 24–33 month	163,000	40–74 50–69 70–74	31 39 Trend
UK (16)*	M Biennially × 7 PBE yearly × 7	237,000	45–64	24
Malmo (17)*	M every 18–24 months	42,000	45–69 55–69	4 20
BCDDP (21)+	M + PBE yearly × 5	238,000	35–74 50–59 59–74	20 24 26
Nijmegen (18)+	M yearly	30,000	35–70 55–69	50 52
Florence (19)+	M + PBE every 30 months	15,000	40–70	47
Utrecht*	M + PBE every 6 months × 4	15,000	50–64	30
CNBSS(23,24)*	M + PBE yearly × 5	89,835	40–49 50–60	NR 3

BCDDP = Breast Cancer Detection Demonstration Project
CNBSS = Canadian National Breast Cancer Screening Study
HIP = Health Insurance Plan
M = Mammography
NR = No reduction
PBE = Physical Breast Examination
UK = United Kingdom
* = prospective controlled study
+ = historically controlled study

ance of BSE in selected cases, but it is unlikely to be beneficial to the majority of women. BSE may heighten awareness of breast cancer risk, but it should be clearly understood that BSE is not a substitute for mammography and PBE.

Cervical Cancer

Serial examinations of cervical cytology have reduced by 70% the mortality from cervical cancer among sexually active women up to age 40 years, but data for older women are inconclusive. In one study a reduction in mortality was obtained for women aged 65 years and older who had undergone at least one examination of cervical cytology within the previous 10 years (27). Serial Pap smears are advisable for older women who are sexually active and for those who failed to undergo earlier screening, at least every three years to age 65 to 70 years (8). The test is safe and inexpensive, and the incidence and death rate of cervical cancer among older women are increasing.

Colorectal Cancer

Techniques for colorectal cancer screening include serial fecal occult blood testing (FOBT) and serial proctosigmoidoscopy. In a randomized, controlled study from the University of Minnesota, annual FOBT of persons

aged 50 to 80 years reduced the risk of death from
colorectal cancer by 33% over a period of 13 years (28).
The decline in cancer mortality began three years after
the initial examination and became progressively
greater. Biennial FOBTs were not as effective. Competing causes of death may limit the benefits of FOBT for
older persons. A recent large case-control study has
also demonstrated reduction in mortality as a result of
screening by sigmoidoscopy (29).

Annual FOBTs are indicated for elderly persons aged
70 years and older with a life expectancy of three years
or longer (30). Proctosigmoidoscopy every three to five
years may be considered as an additional screen, although the cost is high, and is particularly recommended for persons with a family history of colorectal
cancer or colorectal polyps.

Lung Cancer

The effectiveness of serial chest radiographs and sputum cytology in the reduction of death from lung cancer
was examined in three randomized prospective trials,
from the Johns Hopkins Oncology Center, Memorial
Sloan-Kettering Cancer Center, and the Mayo Clinic
(31). All subjects were smokers, and all had yearly
chest radiographs. In addition, the intervention group
received periodic examinations of sputum cytology. At
the end of the five years, the number of lung cancer
deaths in all three studies was similar in the control
group and in the experimental group. In none of the
studies was the control group unscreened, as all underwent serial chest radiography. In the Sloan-Kettering
trial, the five-year survival of patients diagnosed with
lung cancer was 35%, which is a threefold increase over
the figures for the general population; therefore, it is
possible that yearly chest radiography was of some
benefit.

Prostate Cancer

Serial rectal examinations and serial determinations of
circulating levels of prostate specific antigen (PSA) have
been proposed to screen asymptomatic men for prostate cancer. In several studies, the sensitivity of the
rectal examination was inadequate to detect early prostate cancer and to affect the death rate (32). In one
recent report only 20% of asymptomatic patients whose
prostate cancer was detected with rectal examination
had localized disease amenable to resection (33).

In contrast, PSA is a very sensitive test for prostate
disease. According to Catalona et al., (34) the PV+ was
24% for values of 4 to 9 μg/L and 61% for higher values;
the combination of rectal examination and PSA further
improved the detection rate of early prostate cancer. In
an American Cancer Society study, the overall PV+ of
PSA was 61% (35). The PV+ may be improved by
considering causes of increased PSA levels other than
cancer. Although many of these are transient (urinary
tract infection, acute prostatitis, acute urinary retention), benign prostatic hypertrophy (BPH) is chronic
and is the most common. Calculation of the PSA "density" (the concentration of PSA/g of prostatic tissue,
estimated at physical examination), has been proposed

to distinguish between BPH and prostate cancer (36).
Another important parameter is the rate of rise of PSA
levels over time. In the American Cancer Society study,
yearly increments of ≥ 1 μg/L had a PV+ of 40% for
prostate cancer (37).

In terms of PV+, cost-benefit, and safety, determination of PSA is very close to an ideal screening test.
However, the value of early diagnosis of prostate cancer in elderly men is unclear. The majority of men aged
80 years and older harbor a prostate cancer which is
diagnosed only at autopsy. In one American study, one
British study, and two Swedish studies, the survival of
patients aged 70 years and older with early prostate
cancer receiving no immediate treatment was comparable to the survival of age-matched men without
prostate cancer. Only a minority of these patients died
of cancer (38). For younger men, it is unclear whether
immediate treatment with surgery or radiation therapy
has an impact on survival. Gerber and Chodak (39)
calculated that the number of patients who would
benefit from screening with PSA is equivalent to the
number of patients who would die from complications
of radical prostatectomy, should the screening of all
men aged 50 years and older be implemented. One
strategy proposed is to determine PSA and perform
rectal examination in all men aged 50 years and older
and evaluate further if either is abnormal (32).

Other Neoplasms

Several screening strategies have been proposed for
epithelial cancer of the ovary and for endometrial cancer,
although data are not conclusive. In particular, it would
be desirable to detect ovarian cancer at early stages,
when it is curable surgically. Though uncommon,
ovarian cancer is generally diagnosed at advanced
stages, when it is uniformly fatal. Monoclonal antibody
to the CA 125 antigen and transvaginal sonography are
promising screening tests which have high specificity.
Screening for ovarian cancer is complicated by the low
prevalence of the disease, which markedly reduces the
PV+ of the tests. Screening must be targeted to those
with specific risk factors such as family history, not
simply performed on all older women (40). Serial examinations of vaginal or endometrial cytology have
failed to influence the mortality of endometrial cancer
(41); at present, routine screening of asymptomatic older
women not on estrogen cannot be recommended.

Age Related Barriers to Screening

Several age related barriers to screening have been
identified in studies of breast cancer screening (Table
23.3) (42–44): similar barriers may exist for detection of
other neoplasms as well. A recent survey indicated that
the use of screening mammography by women aged
65 to 74 years increased almost 50% in some areas in
the United States between 1985 and 1990 (45). These
encouraging results were probably due to a number of
factors, including more effective public education, aging
of a cohort of better educated women instructed in
health maintenance, and increased support by primary

Table 23.3 Age-related barriers to screening.

A. Patient Related	B. Provider Related
Lack of information	Lack of information
Lack of incentive	Lack of incentive
Cost	Volume load
Accessibility	Lack of Training
Transportation	Equipment and quality control

Table 23.4 Screening-related recommendations promulgated by different professional and voluntary organizations in the United States.

	ACS	AGS	USPSTF
Mammography			
Interval	Yearly[a]	Biennially	Biennially
Upper age	No limit[a]	85	75
FOBT			
Interval	Yearly[b]	Yearly	NR[c]
Upper age	No limit[b]	85	NR
Cervical Pap			
Interval	2–3 years after two negative tests	2–3 years	2–3 years
Upper age	No limit	75	75
PSA	Yearly[d]	NR	NR

ACS = American Cancer Society
AGS = American Geriatric Society
USPSTF=United States Preventive Service Task Force
NR = No recommendations

[a]This is also the recommendation of the National Cancer Institute (NCI) and the American College of Obstetrics and Gynecology

[b]This is also the recommendation of the NCI

[c]This position may be changed in view of new data

care physicians. In a study by Fox *et al.*, (46) recommendation by primary care physicians for yearly mammography was the single most important factor affecting compliance of women aged 65 years and older. Physicians are a major factor in encouraging health maintenance for elderly patients.

A number of strategies, such as personalized letters as reminders of deadlines, laminated pocket cards listing the dates of future sessions, use of mobile units, and the enrollment of volunteers willing to accompany older persons through the process, may facilitate the screening of asymptomatic older persons for cancer (13). Cooperative oncology groups are testing several of these strategies to improve cancer diagnosis among the aged.

Conclusions and Recommendations

Secondary cancer prevention appears to be an important strategy for the control of cancer in the aged. In the absence of adequate data, its real impact cannot be evaluated. Of necessity, many recommendations for screening of older patients are based on circumstantial evidence of effectiveness and inspired by common sense (47). Not surprisingly, the recommendations of various professional and voluntary organizations differ somewhat (Table 23.4).

Screening programs involving serial mammograms and PBE for breast cancer, annual FOBT for colorectal

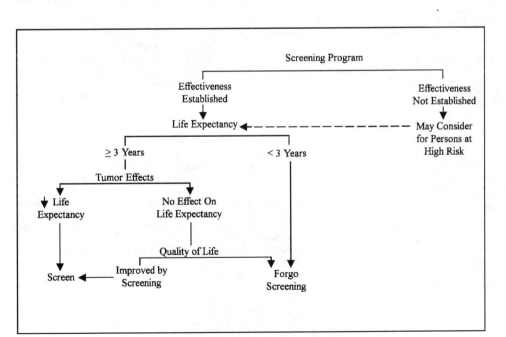

Figure 23.2 Algorithm for deciding who is a good screening candidate among persons aged 75 years and older.

cancer, and targeted serial examinations of Pap smears for cervical cancer are effective and should be conducted in older persons. The value of screening for lung cancer remains unproven and for prostate cancer has not been conclusively demonstrated.

From existing data, it is reasonable and realistic to recommend screening of asymptomatic persons up to age 75 years with annual PBE and mammography for women, cervical Pap smear every three years for sexually active women and women who were sexually active prior to age 65 years and did not undergo regular screening, and yearly FOBT. The algorithm in Figure 23.4 provides guidelines for individualized screening programs for persons over 75 years.

Screening recommendations will continue to evolve with advances in several areas predicted for the near future and benefits which include prolonged life and active function for men and women of all ages.

Acknowledgement

Reprinted with permission of *Cancer Control: Journal of the Moffitt Cancer Center*, H. Lee Moffitt Cancer Center and Research Institute, publisher.

References

1. Ershler WB, Balducci L. Cancer and aging. *N Engl J Med* 1994; in press.

2. Smart CR. Screening and early cancer detection. *Semin Oncol* 1990; **17**: 456–63.

3. Lerman C, Rimer B, Engstrom PF. Reducing avoidable cancer mortality through prevention and early detection regimens. *Cancer Res* 1989; **49**: 4955–62.

4. Balducci L, Cox C, Greenberg H, *et al*. Management of cancer in the older aged person. *Cancer Cont: JMCC* 1994; **1**(2): 132–137.

5. Beghe' C, Balducci L. Geriatric oncology: perspectives from decision analysis: a review. *Arch Gerontol Ger* 1990; **10**: 141–62.

6. Riegelman RK, Povar GJ. *Putting Prevention into Practice*. Boston, Mass: Little, Brown & Co., 1988.

7. Lerman C, Trock B, Rimer BK, *et al*. Psychological and behavioral implications of abnormal mammograms. *Ann Intern Med* 1991; **114**: 657–61.

8. Riegelman RK, Hirsch RP. *Studying a Study and Testing a Test*. 2nd ed. Boston, Mass: Little, Brown & Co., 151–63, 1989.

9. Lyman GH. Decision analysis: a way of thinking about health care in the elderly. In *Geriatric Oncology*, edited by L Balducci, GH Lyman, WB Ershler. Philadelphia, PA: JB Lippincott Co., 5–14, 1992.

10. Balducci L. Management of cancer in older patients: perspectives on quality of life. *Drugs Aging* 1994; in press.

11. Applegate W, Deyo R, Kramer A, *et al*. Geriatric evaluation and management: current status and future research directions. *J Am Geriatr Soc* 1991; **1**(suppl): 2–7.

12. Guyatt GH, Feeny DH, Patrick DL. Measuring health-related quality of life. *Ann Intern Med* 1993; **118**: 622–9.

13. Silliman RA, Balducci L, Goodwin JS, *et al*. Breast cancer care in older age: what we know, don't know, and do. *JNCI* 1993; **85**: 190–9.

14. Schapiro S, Venet W, Strax P, *et al*. Ten to 14 year effect of screening on breast cancer mortality. *JNCI* 1982; **69**: 349–55.

15. Tabar L, Fagerberg G, Day NE, *et al*. Breast cancer screening and natural history: new insights from results of screening. *Lancet* 1992; **339**: 412–4.

16. First results in mortality reduction in the UK trial of early detection of breast cancer. UK trial of early detection of breast cancer group. *Lancet* 1988; **2**: 411–6.

17. Andersson I, Aspegren K, Janzon L, *et al*. Mammographic screening and mortality from breast cancer: the Malmo mammographic screening trial. *Br Med J* 1988; **297**: 943–8.

18. Verbeek AL, Hendriks JH, Holland R, *et al*. Mammographic screening and breast cancer mortality: age-specific effects in Nijmegen project. *Lancet* 1985; **1**: 865–6.

19. Palli D, Del Turco MR, Buiatti E, *et al*. A case control study of the efficacy of a non- randomized breast cancer screening program in Florence, Italy. *Int J Cancer* 1986; **38**: 501–4.

20. Collette HJ, Day NE, Rombach JJ, *et al*. Evaluation of screening for breast cancer in a non-randomized study (the DOM project) by means of a case-control study. *Lancet* 1984; **1**: 1224–6.

21. Morrison AS, Brisson J, Khalid N. Breast cancer incidence and mortality in the Breast Cancer Detection Demonstration Project. *JNCI* 1988; **80**: 1540–7.

22. Roberts MM, Alexander FE, Anderson TJ, *et al*. Edinburgh trial of screening for breast cancer: mortality at seven years. *Lancet* 1990; **335**: 241–6.

23. Miller AB, Baines CJ, To T, *et al*. Canadian National Breast Cancer Screening Study: 1. Breast cancer detection and death rates among women aged 40 to 49 years. *Can Med Assoc J* 1992; **147**: 1459–76.

24. Miller AB, Baines CJ, To T, *et al*. Canadian National Breast Cancer Screening Study: 2. Breast cancer detection and death rates among women aged 50 to 59 years. *Can Med Assoc J.* 1992; **147**: 1477–88.

25. Mandelblatt JS, Wheat ME, Monane M, *et al*. Breast cancer screening for elderly women with and without comorbid conditions. *Ann Intern Med* 1992; **116**: 722–30.

26. O'Malley MS, Fletcher SW. Screening for breast cancer with breast self-examination. *JAMA* 1987; **257**: 2196–2203.

27. Celentano DD, Klassen AC. The impact of aging on screening for cervical cancer. In *Geriatric Oncology*, edited by L Balducci, GH Lyman, WB Ershler. Philadelphia, PA: JB Lippincott Co., 105–17, 1992.

28. Mandel JS, Bond JH, Church TR, *et al*. Reducing mortality from colorectal cancer by screening for fecal occult blood. *N Engl J Med* 1993; **328**: 1365–71.

29. Selby JV, Friedman GD, Quesenberry LP Jr. A case-control study of screening sigmoidoscopy and mortality from colorectal cancer. *N Engl J Med* 1992; **1326**: 653–7.

30. Wagner JL, Herdman RC, Wadhwa S. Cost effectiveness of colorectal cancer screening in the elderly. *Ann Inter Med* 1991; **115**; 807–17.

31. Strauss GM, Gleason RE, Sugarbaker DJ. Screening for lung cancer reexamined. *Chest* 1993; **103**.337S–341S.

32. Garnick MB. Prostate cancer: screening, diagnosis and management. *Ann Intern Med* 1993; **118**: 804–18.

33. Catalona WJ, Smith DS, Ratliff TL, *et al*. Detection of organ confined prostate cancer is increased through prostate-specific antigen-based screening. *JAMA* 1993; **270**: 948–54.

34. Catalona WJ. Smith DS, Ratliff TL, *et al*. Measurement of prostate specific antigen in the serum as a screening test for prostate cancer. *N Engl J Med* 1991; **324**: 1156–61.

35. Mettlin C. The status of prostate cancer early detection. *Cancer* 1993; **72**: 1050–5.

36. Benson MC, Whang IS, Pantuck A, *et al*. Prostate specific antigen density: a means of distinguishing benign prostatic hypertrophy and prostatic cancer. *J Urol* 1992; **147**: 815–6.

37. Carter HB, Pearson JD, Metter EJ, *et al*. Longitudinal evaluation of prostate-specific antigen levels in men with and without prostate disease. *JAMA* 1992; **267**: 2215–20.

38. Johansson JE, Adami HO, Andersson SO, *et al*. High 10-year survival rate in patients with early untreated prostatic cancer. *JAMA* 1992; **267**: 2191–6.

39. Gerber GS, Chodak GW. Routine screening for cancer of the prostate. *JNCI* 1991; **83**: 329- 35.

40. Schapira MM, Matchar DB, Young MJ. The effectiveness of ovarian cancer screening: a decision analysis model. *Ann Intern Med* 1993; **118**: 838–43.

41. Averette HE, Steren A, Nguyen HN. Screening in gynecological cancers. *Cancer* 1993; **72**: 1043–9.

42. Mandelblatt J, Traxler M, Lakin P, *et al*. Mammography and Papanicolaou smear use by elderly poor black women. *J Am Geriatr Soc* 1992; **40**: 1001–7.

43.   Caplan LS, Wells BL, Haynes S. Breast cancer screening among older racial/ethnic minorities and whites: barriers to early detection. *J Gerontol* 1992; **47**(special issue): 101–10.

44.   Weinberger M, Saunders AF, Bearon LB, *et al.* Physician-related barriers to breast cancer screening in older women. *J Gerontol* 1992; **47**(special issue): 111–7.

45.   Fletcher SW, Harris RP, Gonzales JJ, *et al.* Increasing mammography utilization: a controlled study. *JNCI* 1993; **85**: 112–20.

46.   Fox SA, Murata PJ, Stein JA, The impact of physician compliance on screening mammography for older women. *Arch Intern Med* 1991; **151**: 50–6.

47.   Robie PW. Cancer screening in the elderly. *J Am Geriatric Soc* 1989; **37**: 888–93.

24. Cancer Screening in the Older Person

Kathryn L. Edmiston and Mary E. Costanza

Introduction

Cancer is the second leading cause of death in the United States and more than 65% of all cancer deaths occur in patients over the age of 55 (1). As the population ages, the magnitude of the cancer problem is likely to dramatically increase in the coming decades. Since the incidence of many common cancers including lung, breast and prostate increases in the older adult years, this is a population at high risk for the development of cancer. Appropriate measures for cancer prevention and the use of selected tools for cancer screening may have its greatest impact on the older adult population.

Prevention

Any discussion of cancer screening would be incomplete without acknowledging the fact that we screen for disease because we cannot prevent it. Primary prevention by the elimination of cancer causing behaviors is perhaps the most effective way to reduce mortality due to cancer in the older adult population. Many common cancers are clearly related to specific carcinogens. Of all the specific risks associated with the development of cancers, tobacco is the most important. Deaths from tobacco use are estimated to exceed 190,000 per year. Ninety percent of lung cancers deaths are due to tobacco use (1). For women, the death rate from lung cancer has now begun a logarithmic ascent since 1960 (2). Smoking cessation leads to an immediate drop in morbidity, followed shortly by a drop in lung cancer mortality. Thus patients of any age who smoke should be advised of the increased frequency of developing lung cancer, as well as other cancers of the aerodigestive tract. Death from tobacco related noncancer causes is also substantial; chief among these are cardiovascular disease (heart attack and stroke), peripheral vascular disease, and obstructive lung disease. Since the benefits of smoking cessation are immediate, patients who smoke should be provided with the tools and support they need to stop smoking or tobacco use.

Other ways to prevent cancer (and therefore obviate the need for screening) may not be as clear cut as the tobacco story. Many common cancers seem related to diet or other life style behaviors. Some of these behaviors may be impossible to change in later life. Some behaviors may have been important to change but only in early life. For example, age at first live birth confers a lifelong decrease in breast cancer incidence and mortality. Unfortunately, the opportunity to avail one's self of the benefit of this life style change evaporates by about age 25 (3). Other lifestyle changes may effect cancer development although perhaps not as clearly as tobacco use cessation. Dietary changes such as adopting the Mediterranean diet may decrease the incidence of colon cancer, if the individual survives for several years (4). A diet low in fat, high in vegetables and fiber as recommended by the National Cancer Institute (5) and the American Cancer Society (ACS) (6) may have immediate benefits for lowering cholesterol and improving bowel regularity, two major concerns for many older Americans. Again, the most dramatic returns on adopting a healthy life style will no doubt be seen if these behaviors are adopted well in advance of older age.

Screening

Cancer screening is defined as the use of diagnostic studies to identify cancer in *asymptomatic* individuals. People who present to their physician with symptoms should undergo appropriate diagnostic testing, not screening. For cancer screening to be meaningful, it should result in an improvement or better outcome than if one did not screen. Thus, screening for acute leukemia is not recommended because for the stages at which we can detect it, there is no additional benefit than waiting until symptoms occur. On the other hand there are many cancers for which screening seems to provide a benefit, either by reducing cancer specific mortality or reducing morbidity (for example the need for lesser surgery).

The gold standards for measuring the utility of cancer screening are randomized clinical trials comparing disease specific mortality in a screened population to that of an unscreened population. A useful screening test is one that results in lower disease specific mortality in the screened population. Although all cancer screening tests do not necessarily result in decreased disease specific mortality, diagnosis in the early stages of disease before symptoms become apparent is important for most types of cancer. Since patients with advanced cancer often have a poor outcome, screening may also be recommended if it results in a stage shift with the screened population having earlier stage disease than the unscreened population. This stage shift may result in the need for less aggressive, less disabling and more successful cancer treatment.

In addition to its ability to detect potentially curable or treatable cancer, the "perfect" cancer screening tool would have the following characteristics (7). First, it must be sensitive with a low rate of false negative results. False negative results may falsely reassure the patient and symptoms may be ignored resulting in a delay in diagnosis. Secondly, it must be specific with a low false positive rate so that only patients with the disease are identified by the screening tests. False positive results usually require additional testing resulting in increased cost, discomfort, risks and psychological distress in the patient. Finally, cancer screening tests which are proven to be useful must be readily available and acceptable to the population for whom it is useful. Physicians caring for patients who are likely to benefit from screening must recognize the utility of the test and be prepared to recommend it to their patients. Patient compliance is increased if the test is affordable and safe, and needs to be repeated infrequently and if they are educated about the potential benefits of the screening.

The application of screening guidelines to the older adult is fraught with difficulties. The high rate of chronic comorbid conditions and mortality due to these conditions may mask the benefits of screening in an otherwise healthy population of older adults. Diagnosis of cancer in an asymptomatic individual who cannot tolerate intervention for that cancer or who is likely to succumb to comorbid disease before the cancer becomes symptomatic is unlikely to benefit from screening. For the general practitioner, knowing how much comorbidity and mortality there might be in the patient's near future is often the most difficult determination to make. There is frequently an overestimate of morbidities and probable mortality by those who group "over 65" as a uniform cohort. This is inappropriate when considering screening. Chronological age is the least important factor when deciding about the usefulness of screening an individual (8). Yet chronological age remains one of the most frequently used indicators for the appropriateness or inappropriateness of screening (9).

Other factors which confound the apparent utility of screening in older people are physiologic changes which affect the screening test itself. In breast cancer screening, the change is for the better. Mammography becomes a more sensitive test as the patient ages (10–12). Mammary glandular tissue atrophies and is replaced with fat making the discrimination between normal and cancerous tissue easier. On the other hand, in cervical cancer screening, advanced age may make collecting the pap specimen difficult as the vaginal tissues may be atrophied (13).

Even more difficult in evaluating the utility of cancer screening in the older population is the fact that most screening studies have included only younger patients. For example none of the mammography trials collected sufficient data on women over 69, in spite of the fact that at least half the breast cancers occur in women 65 and older (14)! This is true for other cancer screening trials as well.

Another difficulty in interpreting the utility of screening in the older adult, is the fact that screening tools may detect disease with a different natural history than that seen in younger individuals. For breast cancer, the disease does not appear to be biologically less aggressive in the older adult (15–17). Age at diagnosis does not appear to be an important prognostic factor for breast cancer. The 5 and 10 year survival rates for older adult women with breast cancer are approximately equivalent to a younger group. Prostate cancer, in contrast, seems quite different. The disease seems far more virulent when diagnosed in younger men (<50) while many older men die *with* prostate cancer not *of* prostate cancer (18).

Cancer screening is generally recommended when screening has been demonstrated to result in decreased disease specific morality in the screened population. This stringent standard for screening may not apply as readily to older adults. As mentioned, studies of screening utility have infrequently, if ever, included individuals in their seventies, eighties and certainly not older. To demand that studies demonstrate reduction in mortality for the elderly is a demand for which there is no data. This is different than the situation in breast cancer screening in young women. In this instance, there is evidence that screening women under the age of 50 does not result in reduction in breast cancer mortality (14). Much of what can be said about cancer screening in the elderly is, at best, an extrapolation from evidence obtained from women 50–69 (19). Unless there is some reason to believe that the screening test is likely to be less specific or less sensitive in the older person or that the older individual would be unable to tolerate the prescribed diagnostic therapeutic test and live long enough to enjoy the benefits of screening, we see no reason to stop screening. By specifically ignoring chronologic age as the most important factor in discontinuing screening we are unfortunately adding to the burdens of the primary care physician. However, we believe that individualized physician judgement is necessary to identify the appropriate time to stop cancer screening.

While mortality reduction is the acid test for screening utility, this endpoint may not be the most salient benefit for some older people. As patients age, there may be greater emphasis on quality of life not quantity of life. Therefore screening studies may be useful in the older adult population if they result in earlier disease requiring less aggressive therapy or alternatively prevent debilitating complications from advanced cancer.

Screening Guideline Policies

Cancer screening guidelines are published by a number of professional groups including the American Cancer Society (ACS) (20), the US Preventive Services Task Force (USPSTF) (21), the American College of Physicians (ACP) (22), the Canadian Task Force (CTF) (23), the American Academy of Family Physicians (AAFP) (24). Other groups such as the American College of Obstetrics and Gynecology (ACOG) (25), American Urological Association (AUA) (26), the American College of Radiology (ACR) (27) have published disease specific screening guidelines in their areas of interest.

Cancer screening guidelines have recently come under great scrutiny as third party payers seek to balance costs and benefits. Not surprisingly, many payors give credence only to screening recommendations that have been based on solid evidence for cause specific reduction in mortality...the bottom line in screening economics. Most medical organizations such as those listed above have different policies about the level of evidence needed to recommend various screening tests. The most economically conservative guidelines demand reduction in cause specific mortality to be demonstrated by studies of high scientific merit, *viz.* prospective randomized trials with large numbers of screens preferably corroborated by several different groups. Less conservative organizational guideline policies accept evidence of stage reduction, even though stage reduction may not necessarily be associated with a decrease in cause specific mortality (the so called lead time bias). This bias occurs when a disease is diagnosed earlier in a patient's life at an earlier stage but the identification of the disease does not result in longer life but only a longer time with the diagnosis known. Other organizations believe that reduction in morbidity is sufficient to recommend screening.

The controversies which result from the acceptance of different guidelines are often confusing to patient and doctor alike. For example, these controversies have prompted vehement debate regarding prostate cancer screening. The current screening tools (prostate specific antigen and transrectal ultrasound) diagnose many cancers of the prostate at an early stage. But as yet, there is no evidence that treatment of screen-detected cancers will result in a decrease in clinical disease and a decrease in the mortality from prostate cancer (28).

Another example based on differences in the demand for evidence-based guidelines are the current recommendations of the USPSTF (29) and those of the National Cancer Institute (30) regarding mammography screening in women 70 and older. There is no direct evidence at all in women 70 and older. The most conservative guidelines come from the USPSTF. It recommends screening from ages 50–69. Beyond 69, the USPSTF stresses that no benefit is known and it cannot recommend (or not recommend mammography). The NCI Screening guidelines review panel emphasizes that while there is no evidence of benefit (no studies have been done) they could see no reason not to continue to screen as long as a woman's health was not overly compromised.

Differences in guidelines which rest on the discretion of the recommending body where the evidence is weak or not conclusive is exemplified again by mammography recommendations. The proper interval for screening has not definitely been determined by scientific studies. There have been no trials which study whether one or two years is the best interval. A panel reviewing all randomized trials conducted concluded that there was no difference in mortality reduction within the interval of 12 and 33 months (19). The government through its Medicare program decided that a two year interval gave the best cost effectiveness and accordingly pays for screening mammogram in all women over 65 at two year intervals. On the other hand the ACS, decided that one year would continue

to be recommended although they did acknowledge that it was not proven that annual interval was not proven to be better (20).

Thus, policies set by different organizations depend on many criteria, not just on the most rigorous scientific evidence of utility. Individual physicians need to understand how these guidelines come to be and what type of evidence supports them. As an aid to understanding their recommendations, both the USPSTF and NCI have published the criteria underlying their screening recommendations. Interestingly, the NCI has recently disclaimed all recommendations, taking instead the nonpolitical position of reviewing the evidence for or against various cancer screens and commenting on the scientific value of the evidence leaving the conclusions about what the most appropriate guideline might be up to the special medical organizations (31).

This area will no doubt become more political as managed care organizations have begun to recommend their own intervals. Such activities need to be monitored as the drive toward bottom line economics may obscure real benefits. In addition to managed care policies, one should be aware that many advocacy groups are pushing for their own guidelines. In Massachusetts for example, due to the efforts of committed advocates, a bill was passed which mandates that all insurance companies doing business in Massachusetts pay for yearly screening mammogram in all women 40 and over. There is no upper limit above which screening will not be paid for.

There are unique dangers of promulgated guidelines for the older population. It is highly likely that the demand for evidence based recommendations will escalate, since payors are likely to support only the most conservative guidelines. We must remember that there is very little evidence of any kind concerning cancer screening in the elderly. Therefore, the demand for evidence based guidelines will exclude the older population unless studies are begun and unless the old become advocates for themselves. Indeed several older women's groups are quite vocal in what they perceive to have been a prejudice against them on the part of the Medicare reimbursement schedule for mammography.

What is the individual practitioner to recommend? The following commentary reviews guidelines and strategies for cancers in which there is some evidence of utility.

Breast Cancer

Breast cancer is the most common cancer in women and is the second leading cause of cancer death in women. The American Cancer Society estimates that there will be 185,700 cases of breast cancer diagnosed in 1996 and 44,500 deaths will occur (1). One of the single most important risk factors for the development of breast cancer is increasing age. At the beginning of the 20th century, fewer than 1 in 10 Americans was over the age of 55 and only 1 in 25 was over 65 years old. By 1989, 1 in 5 Americans was over 55 years old and 1 in 8 was greater than 65. Between 1989 and 2050, the population over the age of 85 is expected to increase from 1 to 5%. Older adult women now outnumber older adult men by 3:2. For the over 85 age group, women outnumber men 3:1 (32). Since there continues to be an age-specific increase in the incidence of breast cancer well into the 8th decade of life, the changing demographics of the US population is likely to result in a continuing increase in the numbers of breast cancers diagnosed each year (33).

Screening tools for the early detection of breast cancer include mammography, clinical breast exam (CBE) and breast self exam (BSE). There is abundant evidence from at least six large clinical trials that demonstrate a reduction in mortality in women over the age of 50 undergoing screening mammography (14,34,35). Meta-analysis of all of these trials show a significant and consistent reduction in mortality (up to 30%)(36). Eligibility criteria differed in each trial with some trials limited to women from 50–69 years old at trial entry and others including women as young as 40 and as old as 74 at trial entry. None of the trials included women over the age of 74 so data for screening this particular subgroup is lacking. Although the results in women ages 40–49 at study entry have not shown a significant reduction in mortality due to breast cancer, all of these other trials demonstrate a 20–50% reduction in mortality at 5–10 years of follow-up (14,37,33). Compliance in these trials with screening studies was variable but was markedly less in older women. The techniques for mammography as well as the frequency of screening varied. Some trials used 2 views of each breast while others used single view mammography. Even the studies with screening intervals of 24–33 months demonstrated a significant reduction in breast cancer mortality in the screened group. Half of these trials also included periodic CBE as part of the screening recommendations.

Although CBE and BSE are usually recommended for breast cancer screening in all age groups after the age of 20, direct evidence supporting such recommendations is scarce. Many professional groups have published recommendations for breast cancer screening. Specific recommendations in women over the age of 70 are often lacking.

Although the data is scarce, there are compelling reasons to continue to screen healthy women after the age of 65. The life expectancy of women at age 65 is an additional 12 years and for women over the age of 75 an additional 8.5 years. Morbidity and mortality due to breast cancer takes its greatest toll in this group. Although women over the age of 65 represent only 14% of the female population fully 45% of invasive breast cancers occur in this group. More than 32% of deaths due to breast cancer occur in women over 75 (1).

Mammography is more accurate for detecting breast cancer in older women (10–12). Since the prevalence of breast cancer in this group is higher than in younger women, the positive predictive value (PPV) of mammography in older women would be expected to be higher. Indeed in a retrospective study of screening mammography the PPV was greater in women over 65 compared to women 50–64 (20 vs 12%) and the breast cancer detection rate was 50% higher than for women 50–64. Comparable numbers of Stage 0 and 1 breast cancers were seen in the two age groups (15). Since, the most important predictor of prognosis in women with breast cancer is stage at diagnosis, it might be expected that the benefits of screening might be as great or greater in this age group.

For many women in older age groups, maintenance of quality of life may be a far greater priority than prolongation of survival. Women over the age of sixty five who are diagnosed with breast cancer will almost always receive some type of local treatment, either lumpectomy, mastectomy or radiation therapy (39,40). Screening and diagnosis of early breast cancer may provide more options for local treatment (35). With the widespread use of adjuvant hormonal therapy, women may be rendered disease free for a substantial period of time after diagnosis and treatment for early stage breast cancer (41,42). Minimizing treatment related morbidity has been a focus of breast cancer research in the older age groups. The efficacy of tamoxifen alone in women over 75 with breast cancer has been reported (43,44). Tamoxifen alone may not be adequate for local control. An ongoing study is underway to compare lumpectomy plus tamoxifen to lumpectomy plus radiation and tamoxifen in women over 70 years old with early stage breast cancer.

There may be detrimental effects on quality of life due to screening. Fear and anxiety may result from borderline abnormalities which are detected or by abnormalities which require further testing and biopsy. A decision analysis model suggests that the detrimental effects of screening in this regard offset the potential benefits in the over 85 age group but not in the 65–84 year old group even if there are comorbid conditions such as hypertension or congestive heart failure (45). Further prospective studies are clearly needed to investigate quality of life issues. Even though a woman may be destined to die of breast cancer, the morbidity associated with unnecessarily advanced breast cancer may be substantial. While death may not be averted by screening, untreated local disease may cause pain, infection and disfigurement. Axillary metastases can lead to disabling lymphedema and brachial plexopathy with pain and weakness in the affected upper extremity. These problems can be avoided by "early" detection.

Recommendations of Other Groups

The American Cancer Society (20), American College of Obstetrics and Gynecology (25) recommend routine annual screening after the age of 50 without an upper age recommended to discontinue screening. The American Academy of Family Physicians (24), the American College of Physicians (22), the Canadian Task Force (23) and the USPSTF (21) recommend annual or biannual screening up to 69 or 75. The best interval between mammograms remains uncertain. Medicare will currently reimburse for biennial screening mammograms in women over 65. Data from some of the screening trials suggest that intervals of 24–33 months may be sufficient to maintain the benefit of mammography. The need to repeat the examination less frequently has obvious benefits in terms of reducing the costs associated with screening.

Summary

In summary there is little direct data regarding the benefits of screening mammography in women over 65. Nonetheless, there are powerful reasons to expect that mammography will be at least as useful in older women as younger women for detecting early stage breast cancer. We recommend that mammographic screening in older women should continue at regular 1–2 year intervals. The decision to stop screening at any specific time should be individualized based on each patient's comorbid problems and life expectancy.

Prostate Cancer

Prostate cancer is the most common non-skin cancer occurring in men and is the second leading cause of cancer death in men. The ACS estimates that there will be 317,000 new cases diagnosed in 1996. Forty one thousand deaths will occur in 1996 due to prostate cancer (1). The only known risk factors for prostate cancer are advancing age, family history, and being African American. Since there are currently no known means to prevent the occurrence of prostate cancer, efforts are currently directed at early diagnosis when disease is confined to the prostate. Prognosis is dramatically affected by stage at diagnosis. Since prostate cancer confined to the prostate is rarely symptomatic, up to 40% of cases of prostate cancer are diagnosed after regional or distant spread has occurred (46). Once cancer has spread beyond the prostate to the seminal vesicles, pelvic lymph nodes, and other structures the prognosis is poor. Distant disease with spread to bones, lung and liver is never curable with standard treatment.

The incidence of prostate cancer begins to increase dramatically in the 6th decade; 1 in 6 men age 60–79 will develop prostate cancer compared to 1 in 78 for men 40–59 (47). Over half the deaths due to prostate cancer occur in men over 75. Although prostate cancer is a significant cause of morbidity and mortality, the natural history of prostate cancer may be indolent. In autopsy series, 30% of men over 50 will be found to have histologic evidence of cancer in the prostate (48,49). This indicates a disease prevalence far higher than clinically seen and suggests that some of these cancers are biologically unimportant and never progress to clinical disease. With expectant therapy of clinical stage A prostate cancer (incidentally discovered in biopsies done for other reasons), only 2–10% of patients will have progressed at five years with 16% progressing 10 years after diagnosis (50, 51). The risk of progression increases with more advanced stage of disease at diagnosis.

Since prostate cancer is common and a significant cause of morbidity and mortality, an effective screening test could have a major impact on the general health of the older adult male population. Unfortunately data in this regard is lacking. Screening tools for the early diagnosis of prostate cancer include digital rectal examination (DRE) and prostate specific antigen (PSA). The role of transrectal ultrasound will also be discussed.

A DRE performed at the time of routine physical examination has a number of potential advantages and disadvantages. Its role in screening for colorectal cancer will be discussed later. The posterior and lateral aspects of the prostate gland are accessible to the examining finger. Since most prostate cancers occur in the peripheral zone which is not usually palpated on DRE, a high false negative rate is expected. In addition, by definition the earliest stage prostate cancer (Stage A) is non-palpable and cannot be detected on DRE. The reported cancer detection rate for "screening DRE" varies widely in the literature. This may be related the population being studied and the skill of the examiner. Cancer detection rates for screening DRE by a urologist in men 55–70 are 1.4% with 6.0% abnormal DRE compared to.34 for screening DRE in men 50–60 with 20% abnormal DRE performed by a generalist (52,53). In some series the patients may be referred to a urologist for symptoms thought to be due to benign prostatic hypertrophy and so do not truly represent a screened population. Since the prevalence of disease would be higher in these symptomatic patients, the value of DRE will be overestimated. The age of the screened population may also affect the potential value of DRE. Although DRE may detect prostate cancer, there is little data to support that earlier stage disease with a more favorable prognosis is detected. In Thompson's series of 2627 DRE, 3.24% of the population had prostatic nodules. Biopsy revealed cancer in 17/55 and although clinical staging suggested early stage disease, pathologic staging revealed more advanced disease with spread beyond the capsule in 66% of patients who underwent pathologic staging (54). Although direct survival data is lacking, the high false positive rate and low positive predictive value make it unlikely that DRE will substantially reduce mortality due to prostate cancer. In the ACS-National Prostate Cancer Detection Project (ACS NPCDP), 2,425 men underwent DRE, serum PSA and transrectal ultrasonography (TRUS). Criteria for biopsy included a suspicious DRE or hypoechoic lesions on US >5 to 7 mm in two dimensions. Five patients with a normal DRE and TRUS had PSA > 10ng/ml and further evaluation led to the diagnosis of cancer. DRE alone was abnormal in 2.7% of volunteers. Of the forty patients who underwent biopsy 22.5% were found to have prostate cancer. When the DRE was negative, TRUS was found to be abnormal in 10% of volunteers. The positive predictive value of an abnormal TRUS in the face of a normal DRE is 8.9%. These results indicate that the DRE has a low false positive rate but at the expense of a high false negative rate. In contrast TRUS is neither sensitive nor specific in this population. Interestingly when analyzed by age cohort, the positive predictive value of DRE and TRUS decrease (12.5 and 10.4% respectively) in the older age group 66–70. Although most of the screen-detected cancers were clinically early stage (A-B1), the results of surgical staging are not presented (53,55). Efforts to focus on high risk populations and other screening modalities may improve prostate cancer detection.

Prostate specific antigen (PSA) is a glycoprotein secreted by prostatic epithelium which can be easily measured in serum. PSA was identified as a potential screening tool for prostate cancer when it was noted to be elevated in men with metastatic prostate cancer and to decrease in patients who respond to treatment. Although it is usually elevated in men with metastatic disease it is normal in 14–27% of men with localized prostate cancer and may be elevated in benign conditions (56,58). These are some of the limitations of using PSA for routine screening. Nevertheless, PSA appears to be a more favorable screening tool than prostatic acid phosphatase (PAP) since PAP is rarely elevated in patients with localized disease and frequently negative even in patients with widespread disease (59).

Although PSA has been widely studied as a potential screening tool for the early detection of prostate cancer, no randomized trial has demonstrated its efficacy in reducing mortality due to prostate cancer, (52,60,63). Many of the studies reported in the literature are difficult to interpret as screening studies since symptomatic patients and patients referred to urologists are frequently included in the analyses. The estimated sensitivity and specificity of the tests may be inaccurate since men with negative tests do not routinely undergo biopsy and the period of follow-up may be short. The use of PSA alone for screening is not routinely recommended. In healthy cohorts, the positive predictive value of PSA is only 28–30% resulting in unnecessary testing and expense in 2/3 of the patients with an elevated PSA (64,66). False positive PSA results occur predominantly in patients with BPH and 25–46% of such patients will have falsely elevated PSA levels. Although PSA testing alone is not sufficient for screening, the sensitivity and specificity of PSA testing may be increased when combined with the results of other screening tests. When DRE, TRUS, and PSA are abnormal, the positive predictive value of an abnormal test increases dramatically. Attempts to improve the sensitivity and specificity of PSA testing have examined the rate of change (67), the PSA density (68) and age-adjusted reference ranges (69,70). Further refinement of PSA testing may lead to more favorable results in the future (71,72).

Although there is no direct data to indicate that prostate cancer screening leads to decreased disease specific mortality, the data is encouraging that further study is necessary. Reference has already been made to the variable natural history of prostate cancer. Given this variable natural history of prostate cancer, it is possible that screening with any technique may detect a high frequency of latent disease that would be unlikely to cause symptoms or death due to prostate cancer (73). If cancers that are detected by screening are indolent tumors, diagnosis by screening has significant disadvantages both to the patients and society. Treatment of early stage prostate cancer may be associated with significant morbidity. Patients who undergo radical prostatectomy face a significant risk of impotence, urethral stricture and urinary incontinence. Although these risks may be lower with external beam radiation they are not inconsequential particularly if survival is not favorably affected. There is limited data to suggest that cancers detected by PSA screening may be more aggressive (60,74,75). Approximately 35% of cancers detected through PSA screening have adverse prognostic features such as extracapsular extension, large volume disease and poorly differentiated histology. The potential public health costs of treating indolent disease are enormous. Decision analysis of screening methods for prostate cancer suggest that there is little benefit to screening when adverse outcomes of treatment were considered (71).

Recommendations of Other Groups

At present only the ACS (20), AUA (26) and ACR (27) recommend routine screening. The ACS recommends annual DRE beginning at age 40 and PSA annually after age 50. Earlier routine screening is recommended for high risk groups. The USPSTF (21) did not find any evidence to support routine screening for prostate cancer and recommends that patient education material regarding pros and cons of screening be provided to interested patients.

Summary

There is no definitive data to indicate a survival benefit for prostate cancer screening. Many features of prostate cancer such as the high prevalence of asymptomatic disease in the elderly population confound the potential benefits of down staging. The potential costs and associated morbidities of treating indolent disease and obtaining further diagnostic workup for false positive results may prove to be worthwhile if future studies demonstrate a survival advantage for screened patients. In the meantime, we do not recommend routine screening for prostate cancer. We do recommend providing patients with written material outlining the pros and cons. Reimbursement for routine screening may not be routinely covered and is not covered for Medicare recipients. Any patient electing to undergo screening should also be informed about potential out of pocket expenses.

Colorectal Cancer

Colorectal carcinoma (CRC) is the second leading cause of cancer death in the United States. An estimated 143,500 new cases of CRC will be diagnosed in the US in 1996 and 44,900 deaths will occur (1). Nearly all cases of CRC are diagnosed after 50 years of age unless the patient is in a high risk group such as those with a history of familial polyposis or ulcerative colitis. The highest probability of developing CRC is in the 6th and

7th decades. The prognosis for patients with CRC depends on the extent of disease. Patients with advanced disease have a dismal prognosis with 5 year survival rates of only 6%. In contrast, patients with localized or regional disease have a much more favorable prognosis. There are three widely accepted screening tools for the early detection of CRC: digital rectal examination (DRE), fecal occult blood testing (FOBT) and flexible sigmoidoscopy.

Digital rectal examination is generally performed as part of a complete routine physical examination. The utility of DRE for the early detection of CRC has not been studied in controlled clinical trials. DRE will detect only cancers that are within 7–8 cm of the anal verge which accounts for less than 25% of all CRC and therefore is of limited value in screening for CRC.

Screening for fecal occult blood is usually accomplished though the detection of a pseudoperoxidase reaction on paper slide impregnated with guaiac. The slide can be prepared in the physician's office or by the patient at home and developed in the office. False positive results may be obtained due to the presence of red meat in the diet or the consumption of fruits and vegetables containing peroxidase. Patients should be counseled to avoid these substances prior to testing to lower the risk of a false positive result. Since nonsteroidal anti inflammatory agents may cause gastric irritation with bleeding these should also be avoided prior to testing. When the FOBT is positive, colonoscopy should be performed to rule out a CRC or to detect and remove precancerous polyps (76,77).

The results of five clinical trials in healthy persons over 50 years old have supported the beneficial role of FOBT in the early detection of CRC (78,79). At initial screen, 1–2.4% of tests will be positive. Approximately 30% of patients with a positive test will be found to have CRC or polyps. The false positive rate is 60% due to diet, non-malignant conditions or medication. Despite the high false positive rate, 70–80% of patients with CRC in the screened population will have Duke's A and B disease compared to 30–40% in the control group. The stage shifts seen in these trials suggests that as the data matures a survival benefit may be seen. One trial to date has shown a 43% reduction in mortality in the group screened with FOBT in addition to sigmoidoscopy (78).

Approximately 30% of CRC will be missed despite FOBT (80–82). This may occur because the cancer is not bleeding or bleeds only intermittently or small amounts of blood may be below the limits of detection of currently available methods. Multiple studies are underway in an attempt to improve the sensitivity of FOBT or by using immunological detection methods or a combination of methods (82).

Sigmoidoscopy is the third screening tool for primary and secondary prevention of CRC. The use of the 60 cm flexible sigmoidoscope allows visualization to the proximal end of the sigmoid colon. Forty to sixty five percent of CRC and 65–75% of adenomatous polyps occur within reach of the 60 cm flexible sigmoidoscope. Sigmoidoscopy allows the removal of adenomatous polyps which are known precursors to invasive CRC. Patients who are found to have polyps on screening sigmoidoscopy have a high frequency of additional adenomas elsewhere in the colon and should undergo full colonoscopy. Colonoscopic polypectomy results in a lower than expected incidence of CRC according to the data of the National Polyp Study Workgroup (83). Exceptions may include patients with very small (< 1 cm), single tubular adenomas who may not be at increased risk for subsequent cancer.

Although there are very few randomized clinical trails of screening sigmoidoscopy there is ample data from recent case control studies to support its routine use. In case control studies, sigmoidoscopy has been shown to reduce the risk of death due to CRC within reach of the sigmoidoscope (84,85). Similarly data has been published recently which indicates that patients who had undergone screening sigmoidoscopy within the previous ten years had a lower risk of dying of CRC (85). Two large uncontrolled clinical trials demonstrated a shift to lower stage at diagnosis and better survival from CRC in patients receiving periodic rigid sigmoidoscopy (86).

Since sigmoidoscopy has an important role in primary prevention of CRC by removal of premalignant polyps it remains to be determined if screening can be stopped after a period if no further polyps are identified (87). This approach would serve to maximize the potential benefits of screening and minimize the costs and discomforts of screening particularly in the older individual.

Recommendations of Other Groups

The American Cancer Society (20), American Gastroenterological Association (88) and ACOG (25) recommend annual DRE for all adults beginning at age 40, annual FOBT beginning at age 50 and sigmoidoscopy every 3–5 years. These recommendations are supported by the USPSTF (21). The American College of Physicians (22) has recommended CRC screening for patients 50–70 at 10 year intervals using sigmoidoscopy, barium enema or colonoscopy.

Summary

There is ample data to support annual FOBT and periodic sigmoidoscopy in persons over the age of 50. Annual FOBT should be done and periodic sigmoidoscopy should be recommended for patients fit enough to undergo the preparation and diagnostic study.

Cervical Cancer

There are approximately 16,000 cases of cervical cancer diagnosed in the United States each year. About 5,000 women die from cervical cancer each year (1). The incidence of this disease has decreased strikingly. There has been a 70% decrease in both the incidence of invasive disease and in mortality from 1950 to 1970. Since 1980 the rate of decrease has slowed suggesting that screening efforts have reached a plateau. Carcinoma *in situ* peaks between ages 20 and 30, while invasive cancer peaks in later years. Mortality increases with age. Older women, particularly those who have never been screened, are an important group to reach. Over 25% of invasive cancers occur in women who are over 65 years of age. More concerning is that almost half the women who die of cervical cancer are over 65 (89).

The most important causative factor related to cervical cancer risk is sexual intercourse. The agent thought to be important in causing cervical cancer is human papilloma virus (HPV) particularly subtypes 16,18,31,33 and 35 (90).

The evidence supporting the use of Pap smears is derived from observational studies (91–94). These studies provide substantial evidence that mortality can be reduced by screening. There are data from Scandinavia, Canada, the US and Iceland showing stunning decreases in mortality following the introduction of population-wide screening programs. In addition to observational studies, there are several confirmatory case control studies which demonstrate a reduction in cervical cancer mortality (95,98). Unfortunately, such observational studies cannot prove that Pap smear screening is the reason why cervical cancer mortality is reduced. Because there is such widespread acceptance of the utility of the Pap smear in reducing mortality from this disease, no randomized controlled trial is likely be done.

The accuracy of the Pap smear depends on several factors. First, is the adequacy of the specimen submitted for cytologic evaluation. For older women who have been estrogen deprived for a long period of time, the vagina becomes atrophic and it may be extremely difficult to introduce the speculum (13) making it difficult to obtain an adequate specimen (13). The adequacy of the specimen obtained is also a function of the skill of the operator in finding and sampling the squamocolumnar junction.

The ACS recommends the following technique for accurate detection of cervical cancer: The endocervical canal is aspirated with an endocervical brush, or glass pipette. The aspirate is placed on a glass slide and quickly fixed without air drying. The squamocolumnar junction on the ectocervix and the entire portio are then scraped gently with a bifid spatula and material obtained placed on another glass slide (99). Also critical is the adequacy of the facility interpreting the results of the Pap smear. Efforts are ongoing among state departments of health, the ACS and the Center for Disease Control (CDC) to ensure minimal standards for cytology laboratories. Currently, false negative rates range from 5–30% (99).

Cure of this disease is clearly related to stage at discovery. In pre-malignant, *in situ* and very localized disease, cure is the usual outcome. By contrast, cure is rarely possible, and mortality certain in the majority of cases with advanced disease. Therefore, screening to find early disease is imperative. Particularly important is the screening of older women who have never been screened or who have not had a normal Pap smear within two years. There are several studies which report that at least 17% of women over 65 and 32% of poor women 65 and older have never had a Pap smear (100,101). Remember, the burden of invasive disease and death is borne by those women 65 and over who have never been screened or who have not had consecutive normal smears.

Not every woman needs to have a Pap smear. Women who have never been sexually active (102) and those who have had hysterectomies with the cervix removed should not have Pap smears. The interval at which screening should be done is a matter of some discussion although most of the controversy pertains to younger women. For older women, most experts agree that after several annual normal smears, the interval can be lengthened to three years (103). The evidence for this is inferential, and related to the natural history of cervical cancer. Most authorities believe that there is an orderly progression from pre-neoplasia through cancer *in situ* to invasive cancer. What is not agreed upon is the time frame for progression and the extent to which retrogression occurs. Again, the general consensus is that the time frame from confirmed *in situ* to invasive disease is about 10 years. Hence, screening at intervals of 3–5 years seems appropriate after one has established several annual normal tests results. It is also well known that perhaps as many as 30% of *in situ* lesions will regress during observation.

When, if ever, should routine Pap smears be discontinued? There is some evidence that older women may not really benefit from continued screening (104,105). In modeling studies, the suggestion is that the death rate from cervical cancer in women over 73 would only be 6 per 1000 (106).

The barriers to Pap smear screening are considerable among the elderly cohort (107–110). Often mentioned are issues of modesty, particularly among women of various ethnic groups and women who have immigrated to this country. The recent rapid increase of female practitioners is helpful in this regard. Female physicians are more likely to have their patients comply with screening guidelines and this may be due to a greater ability to acknowledge patient fears and concerns. Most likely, the Pap test will be performed by the primary care physician, as few older women in this age cohort seek regular gynecologic care. Since most elderly patients will see a primary care physician at least once during the year, there will be an opportunity, at least in principle, for the primary care doctor to recommend this preventive test. Unfortunately, many of the elderly encounters with medical providers are tied to symptomatic or chronic health problems, and the preventive service may assume a low priority.

Recommendations of Other Groups

There is a general consensus that all women who have been or are sexually active should have annual Pap smears. Most organizations also allow for less frequent intervals after three or more normal annual smears. There is no consensus about when to stop. The AAFP (24) suggests that screening can be stopped at age 65 if there have been several recent normal annual smears. The ACP suggests a Pap test every 3 years until age 65, and then stopping; however for women 66–75 every 3 years if not screened in the prior 10 years before age 66 (22). The ACS (20) and the ACOG (111) do not address the issue of stopping. The American Geriatric Society (112) recommends that screening can be stopped between ages 60 and 70, as long as there have been several recent normal screens. But the AGS also notes that all previously unscreened women, no matter their age, should have at least one Pap smear since a high rate of invasive disease has been noted in the elderly who have never been screened. The Canadian Task Force (113) recommends screening every three years and stopping at age 69. The USPSTF (114) recommends Pap smears every three years, and notes no evidence to suggest an age at which to stop screening but suggests that there are other reasons to discontinue regular screening in women over the age of 65 who have had several recent normal smears.

Summary

There is excellent observational and case control data supporting the reduction in mortality from cervical cancer by the routine use of Pap smears. We recommend an interval of 3–5 years for screening, once several normal annual screens have occurred. We recommend Pap smears only in women who are or who have been sexually active. While there is no firm data regarding the appropriate time to stop doing smears, we recommend that for older women who have been screened adequately in the past and who are no longer sexually active that screening may stop at age 70. Physician judgment and patient acceptance will most likely determine the appropriate stopping point.

Cancer of the Uterus: (*corpus uteri*)

Cancer of the endometrium affects 34,000 women each year. It is a relatively indolent disease with less then 10% of patients dying from the disease (1). Peak incidence is from 50–60 years old. Unlike cervical cancer, it is more frequently found in urban white middle class populations. Major risk factors include obesity, nulliparity, chronic non-ovulation and the unopposed use of postmenopausal estrogens (115). More recently, an increased incidence has been noted in women on tamoxifen therapy for breast cancer (116). The increased risk is about the same magnitude as that for unopposed estrogen therapy.

There have been no studies evaluating screening for uterine cancer. Current clinical practice is limited to a bimanual pelvic examination. Since early endometrial cancer first affects the endometrium, it is no wonder that bimanual exam has not identified Stage 1 disease. Newer screening includes recommendations to perform endometrial biopsy. This make more intuitive sense. However, there is no evidence that endometrial biopsy results in earlier stage disease, less morbidity or decreased mortality from uterine cancer. Currently, gynecologists are of differing opinions regarding routine screening endometrial biopsies in an asymptomatic population, even in women at somewhat higher than usual risk (i.e. women on tamoxifen or estrogen therapy who have experienced no symptoms). Pap smears do not identify early endometrial cancers and are not recommended by any group.

Recommendations of Other Groups

Guidelines for the screening of uterine cancer are controversial. The only group recommending endometrial biopsy is the ACS (20) and its recommendation is for a one time endometrial biopsy at menopause only in women at higher risk for the development of the disease.

Since clinical practice is often associated with a general annual exam, many primary care physicians take the opportunity to perform preventive services at this time. It may therefore be prudent to include a bimanual exam, even though evidence for its utility in decreasing the mortality or morbidity of uterine cancer is entirely lacking. Groups recommending a bimanual annual exam for prudent reasons include the ACOG and the ACS.

Summary

We do not recommend any screening test for uterine carcinoma in asymptomatic women.

Ovarian Carcinoma

Cancer of the ovary is the fifth most common cancer in women. The incidence rises between 40 and 70, but it is most common in women over 60 (117). Of the 20,000 cases diagnosed each year, ultimately about 65% will die from this disease. The incidence is slightly higher in nulliparous women (1). Most ovarian carcinomas are epithelial (adenocarcinomas). There are rare families with an increased incidence of ovarian cancers. While very few women have the hereditary syndrome (less than 1 in 1000), those who are affected have a 40% lifetime risk of developing ovarian cancer (118).

Screening tests which are used for ovarian cancers have been: bimanual pelvic examination (119), the CA-125 blood test, (120–122) and ovarian ultrasonography (123–125). Various studies have failed to confirm that these tests provide accurate and effective screening or the discovery of early stage disease. While it is true that bimanual pelvic exam may reveal an enlarged ovary, this is only rarely associated with early stage and curable disease (119–126). In the post-menopausal woman, the ovaries should be atrophic and nonpalpable. If palpable, they are enlarged and abnormal. With regard to the CA-125 blood test, the marker may be elevated in up to 1% of healthy women, 40% of women with benign masses, and up to 30% of women with other malignancies 120,127). Thus specificity is quite poor. Regarding ovarian ultrasonography, there have been few large studies to validate its usefulness, specificity and sensitivity (123,128,129). In one such large study, the predictive value was less than 3% (130). Thus, various studies have failed to confirm that these tests are accurate and effective screening tools for the discovery of early stage disease. Unfortunately, the positive predictive value even of combining all three tests is low (131). Since only treatment of early stage disease is associated with cure, the inability to find a test or combination of tests predicts that mortality will not be affected. There is a large national study examining the benefit of rigorous screening for ovarian cancer using the above mentioned tests (132). The design includes a randomized control group. The outcome will not be ready for many years.

Recommendations of Other Groups

No group recommends routine bimanual exam as effective screening for ovarian carcinoma. An NIH Consensus Conference (133) did recommend annual pelvic exam, the CA-125 blood test, and transvaginal ultrasound but only for women with presumed hereditary ovarian cancer syndrome. Two groups recommend annual bimanual pelvic exam as a prudent measure in conjunction with the annual physical exam: the ACS, (20) and ACOG (111) The USPSTF (134) does not recommend any routine screening.

Summary

We do not recommend routine screening for ovarian cancer by bimanual pelvic exam, ultrasonography or CA-125 testing in asymptomatic older women. There is no evidence to support the usefulness of such screening.

Skin Cancer

Cancer of the skin is the commonest of human malignancies. It is estimated that there about 800,000 new cases of skin cancer diagnosed each year in the US (1). Generally these cancers are classified as either melanomatous or nonmelanoma type. Melanomas which are rare (less than 35,000 cases) account for almost all deaths from skin cancers. Nonetheless, nonmelanomatous lesions, if neglected, can be associated with significant morbidity. The non-melanomatous skin cancers are either basal cell or squamous cell cancers. Causes of these epidermoid cancers were identified as early as 1775, when the association between certain chemicals (coal tar derivatives) and epidermoid skin cancer was made in chimney sweeps. In the modern era, coal tar products are not a significant health hazard but arsenical products are. The arsenicals are thought to contribute to skin cancers in industrials workers and farmers where the use of pesticides is high (135). Other less important causes are exposure to ionizing radiation and genetic defects as in *xeroderma pigmentosum* or basal cell nevus syndrome.

Apart from these causes, the most important cause of skin cancer is exposure to ultraviolet rays combined with the inability to tan (136–139). These factors explain the high incidence of skin cancers in fair-skinned individuals as well as those chronically exposed to ultraviolet light, such as outdoor workers, people living close to the equator or at high altitudes or in areas where the ozone layer has eroded. Clearly preventive measures are feasible. There is good evidence that

sunscreens will decrease the incidence of basal and squamous cell cancers but it is unclear whether they will protect against the development of melanomas (140). Accordingly, the safest preventive measure is to decrease exposure to ultraviolet light. The ACS has launched a Skin Savers Program to educate the public about the dangers of ultraviolet light exposure.

The natural history of skin lesions differs significantly depending on histology. Basal cell and squamous cancers tend to occur on the sun-exposed head and neck area. Basal cell cancers, if ignored, tend to erode local tissue (the so-called rodent ulcer). There are fewer than 100 cases of metastatic basal cell carcinoma (141,142). Death from basal cell cancer is an extremely rare event. Thus, the goal of screening would be limited to reduction in morbidity. By contrast, squamous cell carcinomas are quite capable of metastasizing although this tends to be a late event and the metastatic site is usually regional nodes (143). Again, the proper endpoint of screening will be a decrease in morbidity and rarely a decrease in mortality.

Unlike basal and squamous cell cancers, melanoma is potentially a lethal disease. It can metastasize when the primary lesion appears quite small. Each year about 35,000 cases are diagnosed and there are 7,000 deaths (1). Of concern is the rising incidence of melanomas particularly in developed countries (144, 145). This is thought to be due to increased exposure to ultraviolet light because of our modern style of wearing less protective clothing, and because of the increased voluntary increased exposure (as in tanning). Besides the role of ultraviolet as a carcinogen, there is now clear evidence that some individuals are genetically more likely to develop melanoma. These include families with the dysplastic nevus syndrome. In this syndrome, nevi are larger than 1 cm. These premalignant lesions can look quite malignant on exam: irregular borders, irregular coloration, and nodularity. When biopsied, however, they only show atypical melanocytes. If these lesions are left untreated, the risk of subsequent melanoma is high (146,150). Risk factors for developing melanoma are increased in individuals with the following characteristics (in descending order of importance): dysplastic nevi, lentigo maligna, congenital mole, fair skin, history of prior melanoma, family history of melanoma and/or excessive sun exposure.

Early detection of malignant cutaneous melanoma appears to decrease stage at diagnosis and the possibility of death from this disease. After the introduction of population-based skin screening efforts, several national observational studies have noted a decrease in melanoma staging and mortality (151,152). Screening should include careful visual examination of the entire skin surface. The practitioner must be able to recognize changes indicative of melanoma and to discriminate these from the more common benign skin lesions (153–155). The commonest sites for melanomas are the back in men and, to a lesser extent, in women; and, in women, the lower leg.

As people age, skin exposure to damaging ultraviolet rays increase presumably accounting for the high incidence of skin cancers in the elderly. Fortunately, most of these skin cancers are the relatively benign basal cell and squamous cell carcinomas. With respect to melanoma, the commonest form found in the older population is the lentigo maligna (156). The mean age at diagnosis is 70. This lesion usually develops in sun damaged skin, especially on the face, head or neck. The lesions are flat with a highly irregular border and may have a highly variegated color pattern. Typically these lesions are present for long periods of time with a horizontal or flat growth pattern. As such they are amenable to curative excision while still thin (less then 0.85mm). As the screening test (visual inspection) is painless, patient resistance should be small.

Recommendations of Other Groups

The ACS (20) recommends annual physical skin exam in persons over 40, as does the American Academy of Dermatology (157) and an NIH consensus panel (158). The AAFP (24) recommends annual skin screening only for persons at increased risk: adults with a history of increased ultraviolet light exposure, or a personal or a family history of skin cancer. The USPSTF (159) does not recommend regular skin screening, but it does recommend consideration of referral of those patients at high risk of developing melanoma to skin cancer specialists.

Summary

A careful skin exam on a regular basis seems prudent particularly in those patients thought to be at higher risk for developing skin cancers especially melanomas. For most of these skin cancers, the outcome of interest is a decrease in mortality in melanoma and decrease in morbidity for basal cell and squamous cell carcinomas.

Stomach Cancer

Stomach cancer is the 7th most frequent cause of cancer mortality in the US, but the incidence in this country has dramatically decreased over the last 70 years (160). The reasons for this decline are not known but it is suspected that improved methods of food preservation (refrigeration) may be responsible. Risks for the development of this disease are older age, being male, atrophic gastritis, pernicious anemia and familial polyposis. Although there is good observational evidence that routine endoscopy will detect stomach cancer at an earlier stage and result in increased cures as well as decreased mortality, these studies are primarily from Japan (161,163), where the prevalence of stomach cancer is high. As stomach cancer incidence is on the decline in the US, the cost effective balance is not positive. There may be a place for screening in populations at high risk for the development of this disease such as recent older immigrants from countries where the disease is endemic (Japan, Central Europe, Scandinavia, Hong Kong, China, Korea, or the Soviet Union) (164). Nonetheless, there have been no studies to inform us of the utility of such screening in this country.

Recommendations of Other Groups

Routine gastric endoscopy in this country is not recommended.

Summary

Although there are several observational studies suggesting a decrease in gastric cancer mortality, there are too few cases in this country to warrant routine screening.

Lung Cancer

Cancer of the lung is the leading cause of death from cancer in men and women. Approximately 175,000 cases of lung cancer will be diagnosed this year and there will 155,000 lung cancer deaths (1). Risk factors include tobacco use. Tobacco use is associated with about 90% of lung cancers. Most lung cancers are advanced at the time of diagnosis but even if they are detected in early stages, are often incurable.

There are no known effective screening tests for lung cancer. Chest X-rays are not accurate or sensitive enough for routine use (165). Neither is sputum cytology (165). There have been several prospective controlled studies looking at the effect of screening chest radiographs and/or sputum cytology (165–175). While some studies have shown an increase in the diagnosis of earlier stage disease, the survival rates at 5 years are no different in the screened group compared to the controls. The reasons for this negative outcome may be related be our inability to effectively treat early stage disease, the increased occurrence of second primary lung cancers and our inability to perform further curative resections. In any case, screening for "early" disease does not appear to confer any real benefit to the patient.

Recommendations of Other Groups

No group recommends any screening measure for the detection of lung cancer.

Summary

As there are no accurate or effective tests which are available, we do not recommend routine screening chest x-ray or sputum cytology.

Testicular Cancer

This is a disease of younger men, peaking between ages 20–35 (1,176). There have been no studies to evaluate the usefulness of testicular exam in asymptomatic men (177). Tumor markers have no place in routine screening but are quite useful in following diagnosed disease (178).

Recommendations of Other Groups

The ACS (20) recommends annual testicular exam and testicular self-exam.

Summary

Given the low incidence of testicular cancer in older men and the lack of evidence that annual exam decreases morbidity or mortality, we do not recommend any screening for this cancer.

Bladder Cancer

Bladder cancer is an important cancer in the older population, particularly in older men. Over 50,000 new cases are diagnosed each year. There are about 11,000 deaths from this disease each year (1). However, the risk of developing the disease and the risk of dying from it rises sharply with age. The risk of developing cancer of the bladder after age 70 is more than 20 times the risk of developing it under age 70. Half of the deaths occur after age 70 (179,180). The incidence of bladder cancer is strongly associated with tobacco use, particularly cigarette use. More than half of bladder cancers are diagnosed in current or former smokers (179). Other carcinogens associated with bladder cancer include various industrial chemicals used in the tire, leather, rubber and dye industries (181).

The usual screening test has been urinalysis to detect occult bleeding in the urine. This may be a sign of early asymptomatic bladder cancer. Urine dipsticks can have sensitivity of 90–100% and a specificity of 65–99% (182,183). Unfortunately, these are the specificity and sensitivity rates for the detection of blood in the urine and not for the detection of bladder cancer. Several large studies have reported on the utility of repeated urine dipstick screening. The positive predictive value for bladder cancer was less than 10% (184). The result of a single urine dipstick screen in a general outpatient population were even less predictive. Only 1 asymptomatic bladder cancer was detected in 20,000 screens (185).

Urine cytology is a more specific test for bladder cancer, although cytology is much less sensitive than screening for occult blood. Cytology is also much more expensive than dipstick screening (186). Most investigators have limited its use to certain industrial workers who are at high risk. The benefits of early detection are not obvious, as there may be a significant length time bias. In other words, less aggressive tumors are more easily discovered during screening, while the more aggressive tumors present less opportunity for discovery at a curable stage. Even without screening, presentation of bladder cancer is often at a superficial stage which carries an 80% 5 year survival. In special high risk populations, screening for asymptomatic bladder cancer may be worthwhile, but it is clearly not worthwhile in the general population.

Recommendations of Other Groups

No organization recommends general screening for bladder cancer.

Summary

Although the older population is at higher risk than people under 65 years of age, we do not recommend screening for bladder cancer since there are no proven effective tests at this time.

Oral Cancer

There are approximately 30,000 new cancers of the oral cavity each year and 8,500 deaths. The disease is twice as common in men than in women (1). The older age group is at highest risk for the development of oral cavity cancers, with the median age at diagnosis of 64 years. The causes of oral cancer are tobacco use, particularly smokeless tobacco, alcohol use, and possibly poor oral hygiene (187). The screening exam consists of visual inspection of the mouth, digital palpation, and retraction of the tongue in order to see hidden areas (188). The signal abnormalities are leukoplakia and erythroplastic lesions. In screening high risk populations, such a heavy smokers and drinkers, the detection rate may be as high as 1 cancer /250 persons screened (189). At such an early stage of detection, oral cavity cancers are often curable, but there have been no controlled studies to evaluate the impact of routine screening (190). In addition to screening in order to detect early curable oral cancers, screening may also result in effective treatment of pre-cancers so that surgical intervention might be unnecessary (191,192). There are several trials now examining the usefulness of anti-oxidants and vitamins in reversing the cancer pathway (193).

Recommendations of Other Groups

The ACS (20) recommends an annual oral examination. The USPSTF (194) and the Canadian Task Force (195) conclude that there is insufficient evidence to recommend for or against screening, although both suggest that an annual oral exam should be considered in the high risk population: people over 60 who smoke and drink. The National Institutes of Health recommend annual screening of the oral cavity by dentists (188).

Summary

Given the increased incidence in older people, the increased incidence in an easily identifiable group (people who are heavy smokers and drinkers), and the increased curability and decreased morbidity of early and pre-cancerous lesions, it may be worthwhile to screen these individuals on a regular basis.

Thyroid Cancer

Thyroid cancer is fairly uncommon, occurring in 14,000 Americans each year and causing only 1000 deaths. Women are more commonly affected than men (1). The known causes of thyroid cancer include irradiation to the head and neck area, especially during infancy or early childhood (196). The usual methods for screening are palpation of the thyroid gland and thyroid ultrasonography. In trained hands, the physical exam for thyroid nodules is quite accurate with a specificity as high as 93% (197). However, the specificity for thyroid cancer is much lower, since almost all palpated nodules will represent benign disease (198). In one study, routine palpation of patients who had been exposed to childhood head and neck radiation detected thyroid cancer in 1% of this high risk population (199).

There have been no controlled studies to determine whether screening by neck palpation leads to a more favorable outcome for the screened. In uncontrolled cohort studies, there has been an improvement in survival noted in those screened. However, the screened cancers had more favorable histology than the unscreened cancers, suggesting considerable bias, both in lead time and in length time bias (198).

Recommendations by other groups

The AAFP (24) recommends neck palpation for the detection of thyroid cancer but only in persons with a history of upper body irradiation. The ACS (20) recommends annual neck exam, while Canadian Task Force (200) and the USPSTF (201) both conclude that the evidence is insufficient to recommend screening.

Summary

Given the absence of sufficient evidence to merit annual neck palpation for the detection of thyroid cancer, we do not recommend this screening exam for the early detection of thyroid carcinoma.

Annual Physical Examination

As part of the annual preventive patient encounter, a physical examination is often performed. The purpose is to discover treatable abnormalities in asymptomatic people. While this may seem to be a prudent thing to do, there is very little, if any, evidence to support the utility of this as a means of reducing cancer morbidity or death (202). Many organizations recommend examination of the thyroid, nodes, the oral cavity, the breasts and the testes as a way to detect cancers of these organs. Again the evidence that such discovery will lead to a decreased morbidity or mortality is inconclusive. Intuitively, one supposes that some individuals might profit from the annual physical examination. But, it is probably more valuable for the physician to spend time during the "annual exam" discussing life style issues and counseling about preventable diseases such as those caused by tobacco use (203). The performance of the exam may thus provide an unhurried, interrupted time that by design will not be preempted by specific complaints of acute or chronic problems. During this "quiet" time, patient and physician can explore issues of maintaining well being (204).

Other reasons for performing a complete exam may be less obvious. For some patients, a complete examination may be reassuring. This may be particularly true for the older patient who is used to this concept. The laying on of hands during the annual exam may help validate the physician's attempts to offer preventive medicine advice. On the other hand, if an annual exam is not performed, an abnormality such as a lump, an enlarged node, enlarged liver or other signs of disease may undermine patient confidence in the doctor's ability, particularly if the sign becomes a symptom for the patient in the near future. How embarrassing for

the physician when a patient returns to the office in a month with a newly self discovered 3.5cm breast lesion, a bleeding ugly mole on the back or jaundice from a liver grossly enlarged with tumor. It would be hard to imagine that a thorough exam a month earlier would have failed to detect these advanced abnormalities. It would also be hard to imagine that such discovery a month earlier would have any real impact on changing the morbidity or mortality of the disease. Nonetheless, the almost complete transferral of the opportunity and responsibility to find the signs of disease first from the physician to the patient runs counter to societal expectations. It is difficult to imagine a medical insurance policy which denies the general "laying on of hands." However, whether managed care organizations will continue to permit the luxury of the annual checkup in the absence of evidence that the annual physical exam does have a beneficial outcome remains to be seen.

Recommendations of Other Groups

Many medical organizations recommend an annual or a biannual exam at which time various screening procedures can occur. The ACS (20) recommends an annual physical exam to include assessment of breasts, testes, pelvic organs, skin, oral cavity, node areas, thyroid and rectum. Other groups specify only a few organs to be examined. For example the AAFP (24) recommends exam of the breasts, pelvic exam and digital rectal exam. The AAFP recommends exam of the thyroid, skin and oral cavity only for people at high risk. The Canadian Task Force (23,113,195,205) suggests annual or biannual breast exam, and digital rectal exam for all over 50 years, but skin and oral exam only for persons at high risk. The USPSTF takes a somewhat more conservative position. Of all possible sites to examine, it only recommends annual breast exam (21). Examination of skin (159), oral cavity (194) and thyroid (201) is suggested only for persons at high risk.

Summary

For a variety of reasons outlined above, we believe the physical exam still has a place in the practice of medicine, particularly for the current cohort of persons 65 and older. We recognize that the evidence supporting that the routine physical exam will decrease morbidity and/or mortality is limited to several sites.

Screening in the Office Setting

While most physicians report a commitment to cancer screening activities, particularly breast exams, mammography recommendations, Pap smears, and digital rectal exams, review of their actual practices reveals a somewhat less rosy picture (206). For example, the National Cancer Institute Breast Cancer Screening Consortium reported that only 25% to 41% of women visiting their primary care physicians had obtained a mammogram (207). The barriers to physician participation in screening activities are many (208). One of the commonest downfalls occurs during the episodic visit for acute or chronic problems. While attention is sharply focussed on the immediacy of the complaint, the physician misses the opportunity to perform an appropriate screening exam or to order an overdue screening test. Much of this oversight can be ascribed to the hectic pace of today's office practice. Efforts to address this problem have centered on systematic changes in office procedures. This can take the form of simple or complicated reminder systems, of using chart stickers or a computer; or of restructuring office duties (209,210). One of the simplest corrections involves the use of a preventive/screening visit which is entirely devoted to such issues. When such visits are scheduled, the rate of mammography, breast exam, Pap test, and digital rectal exam doubles compared to the rate of such testing accomplished during an episodic visit (211).

Recommendations of others

Many organizations recognize the importance of the periodic health maintenance examination. The ACS (212) is promoting the use of the "Put Prevention into Practice" kits (209). The USPSTF is committed to period health visits, even though their list of cancer screening sites that are appropriate for the physical exam (breast and cervix) is limited (213).

Summary

We recommend that primary care providers review office systems and procedures to optimize the delivery of preventive and screening services for their older patients. Given that the burden of cancer increases with age, it is important that those caring for the elderly organize their practices so that the older population are routinely included in prevention and screening care.

References

1. Wingo PA, Tong T, Bolden S. Cancer Statistics. *Ca Cancer J Clin* 1995; **45**: 8–30.
2. Silverberg E, Boring CC, Squires TS. Cancer Statistics. *Ca Cancer J Clin* 1990; **40**: 9–26.
3. Kelsey JL. A review of the epidemiology of breast cancer. *Epidemiol Review* 1979; **1**: 74–109.
4. Winawer S, Shike M. Prevention and control of colorectal cancer. In *Cancer Prevention & Control*, edited by P Greenwald, BS Kramer, DL Weed. NY: Marcel Dekker, 537–559, 1995.
5. National Cancer Institute. *Diet, nutrition, and cancer prevention: the good news.* Washington, DC: Gov Printing Office 1986; Pub#DHHS (NIH): 87-2878.
6. Nixon DW. Nutrition and cancer: American Cancer Society guidelines, programs, and initiatives. *Ca Cancer J Clin* 1990; **40**: 71–75.
7. Clark R. Principles of cancer screening. *Cancer Control* 1995; **2**: 485–492.
8. Cohen HJ. Breast cancer screening in older women: the geriatrician/internist perspective. *J of Geron* 1992; **47**: 134–136.
9. Mohr V, Pacala JT, Rakowski W. Mammography for older women: who uses, who benefits? *J of Geron* 1992; **47**: 43–49.
10. Kopans DB. Screening mammography in women over age 65. *J of Geron* 1992; **47**: 59–62.
11. Faulk RM, Sickles, Edward A, Sollitto A. Clinical efficacy of mammographic screening in the elderly. *Radiology* 1995; **194**: (1)193–196.
12. Snyder RE. Detection of breast cancer in the elderly woman. In *Perspectives in the prevention and treatment of cancer in the elderly,* edited by R Yancik. New York: Raven Press, 73–81, 1983.
13. Mandelblatt J, Gopaui I, Wistreich M. Gynecological care of elderly women: another look at Papanicolaou smear testing. *JAMA* 1986; **256**: (3)367–371.
14. Fletcher SW, Black W, Harris R, *et al.* Report of the international workshop on screening for breast cancer. *J Natl Cancer Int* 1993; **85**: 1644–1656.
15. Yancik R, Reis LG, Yates JW. Breast cancer in aging women: A population-based study of contrasts in stage, surgery and survival. *Cancer* 1989; **163**: 976–981.
16. Adami HO, Malker B, Holmberg L, *et al.* The relationship between survival and age at diagnosis in breast cancer. *N Engl J Med* 1986; **314**: 559–563.
17. Host H, Lund E. Age as a prognostic factor in breast cancer. *Cancer* 1986; **57**: 2217–2221.
18. Edwards CN, Steinthorssen E, Nicholson D, *et al.* An autopsy study of latent prostate cancer. *Cancer* 1953; **6**: 531.
19. Costanza ME. Issues in breast cancer screening in older women. *Cancer* 1994; **74**: 2009–2015.
20. American Cancer Society Guidelines for the cancer-related check up: an update. Atlanta, GA: American Cancer Society, 1993.
21. US Preventive Services Task Force. In *Guide To Clinical Preventive Services,* Anonymous 2nd Ed. Baltimore: Williams and Wilkens, 1996.
22. Hayward RS, Steinberg EP, Ford DF, *et al.* Preventive Care Guidelines: 1991. *Ann Int Med* 1991; **114**: 758–783.
23. Canadian Task Force on the Periodic Health Examination. *Canadian guide to clinical preventive health care.* Ottawa: Canada Communication Group, 797–809, 1994.
24. American Academy of Family Physicians. Age charts for periodic health examination. Kansas City, MO: American Academy of Family Physicians, 1994. Reprint no. 510.
25. American College of Obstetricians and Gynecologists. Routine cancer screening Committee Opinion no. 128. Washington D.C.: American College of Obstetrician and Gynecologist, 1993.
26. American Urological Association. *Executive Committee Report.* Baltimore: American Urological Association, 1994.
27. Ferruci JT. Screening for colon cancer. Programs of the American College of Radiology. *Am J Radiology* 1993; **160**: 999–1003.
28. Kramer BS, Brown ML, Prorok PC, *et al.* Prostate Screening: what we know and what we need to know. *Ann Int Med* 1993; **119**: 914–923.
29. US Preventive Services Task Force. *Guide to Clinical Preventive Services; 2nd ed.* Baltimore: Williams and Wilkens, xxxix–lvii, 1996.
30. National Cancer Institute. PDQ. Cancer Screening Review for Physicians: Overview, 1994.
31. Volkens N. NCI replaces guidelines with statement of evidence. *J Natl Cancer Inst* 1994; **86**: 14–15.
32. Kinsella K. The Demographic Imperative. *Cancer Control* 1995, 7–10.
33. Polednak AP. Projected Numbers of Cancers Diagnosed in the U.S. Elderly Population, 1990 through 2030. *Am J Public Health* 1994; **84**: 1313–1316.
34. Tabar L, Fagerberg G, Duffy SW, *et al.* Update on Swedish two-county program of mammographic screening for breast cancer. *Radiol Clin North Am* 1992; **30**: 187–210.
35. Chu KC, Smart CR, Tarone RE. Analysis of breast cancer mortality and stage distribution by age for the health insurance plan clinical trial. *J Natl Cancer Inst* 1988; **80**: 1125–1132.
36. Kerlikowske K, Grady D, Rubin SM, *et al.* Efficacy of screening mammography: A meta-analysis. *JAMA* 1995; **273**: 149–154.
37. Council on Scientific Affairs. Mammographic screening in asymptomatic women aged 40 years and older. *JAMA* 1989; **261**: 2535–2541.
38. Smart CR, Hendrick RE, Rutledge JHI, *et al.* Benefit of mammography screening in women aged 40 to 49: current evidence from randomized controlled trials. *Cancer* 1995; **75**: 1619–1626.
39. Allen C, Cox EB, Manton KG, *et al.* Breast cancer in the elderly: current patterns of care. *J Am Geriatric Soc* 1986; **34**: 637–642.

40. Chu J, Diehr P, Feigl P, *et al*. The effect of age on the care of women with breast cancer in community hospitals. *J Gerontol* 1987; **42**: 185–190.

41. Fisher B, Constantino J, Redmond C, *et al*. A randomized clinical trial evaluating tamoxifen in the treatment of patients with node negative breast cancer who have estrogen receptor positive tumors. *N Engl J Med* 1989; **320**: 479–484.

42. Cummings FJ, Tormey DC, Davis TE, *et al*. Adjuvant tamoxifen vs placebo in elderly women with node positive breast cancer: Long term follow-up and causes of death. *JCO* 1993; **11**: 29–35.

43. Gazet JC, Markopoulos HT, Ford RC, *et al*. Prospective randomized trial of tamoxifen versus surgery in elderly patients with breast cancer. *Lancet* 1988: 679–681.

44. Bradbeer JW, Kyngdon J. Primary treatment of breast cancer in elderly women with tamoxifen. *Clin Oncol* 1983; **9**: 531–534.

45. Mandelblatt JS, Wheat ME, Monane M, *et al*. Breast cancer screening for elderly women with and without comorbid conditions. *Ann Int Med* 1992; **116**: 722–730.

46. Mettlin C, Jones OW, Murphy OP. Trends in prostate care in the United States 1974–1990: Observations from the patient care evaluation studies of the American College of Surgeons Commission in Cancer. *CA Cancer J Clin* 1993; **43**: 83–91.

47. Cope RT, Treatment geriatric perspective in prostate cancer. In *Perspectives in prevention and treatment of cancer in the elderly*, edited by R Yancik. NY: Raven Press, 1983.

48. Breslow N, Aran CW, Dhom G, *et al*. Latent carcinoma of the prostate at autopsy in seven areas. *Int J Cancer* 1977; **20**: 680–688.

49. Baron E, Angrist A. Incidence of occult adenocarcinoma of the prostate after fifty years of age. *Arch Path* 1941; **32**: 787–793.

50. Chodak GW, Thisted RA, Gerber GS, *et al*. Results of conservative management of clinically localized prostate cancer. *N Engl J Med* 1994; **330**: 242–248.

51. Johannsson JE, Adami HO, Andersson SO, *et al*. 10 year survival rate in patients with early untreated prostatic cancer. *JAMA* 1992; **267**: 2191–2194.

52. Perrin P, Maquet JH, Devonec M. Screening for prostate cancer. Comparison of transrectal ultrasound, prostate specific antigen and rectal examination. *Brit J Urol* 1991; **68**: 263–265.

53. Mettlin C, Lee F, Drago J, *et al*. The American Cancer Society National Prostate Cancer Detection Project findings on the detection of early prostate cancer in 2,425 men. *Cancer* 1991; **67**: 2949–2958.

54. Thompson IM, Ernst JJ, Gangai MD, *et al*. Adenocarcinoma of the prostate: Results of routine urological screening. *J Urol* 1984; **132**: 690–692.

55. Mostofi FK, Murphy GP, Mettlin C, *et al*. Pathology review in an early prostate cancer detection program: results from the American Cancer Society National Prostate Cancer Detection Project. *Prostate* 1995; **27**: 7–12.

56. Stamey TA. Prostate specific antigen in the diagnosis and treatment of adenocarcinoma of the prostate. *Monogr Urol* 1989: 10–49.

57. Brawer MK, Rennels MA, Schitman RA. Significance of serum PSA in men undergoing prostate surgery for benign disease. *Am J Clin Pathol* 1988; **89**: 428

58. Oesterling JE. Prostate specific antigen: a critical assessment of the most useful tumor marker for adenocarcinoma of the prostate. *J Urol* 1991; **145**: 907–923.

59. Vihko P, Kontuyri M, Lukarinen O, *et al*. Screening for carcinoma of the prostate: Rectal examination and enzymatic and radio immunogenic measurements of serum acid phosphatase component. *Cancer* 1985; **56**: 173.

60. Catalona WJ, Smith DS, Ratliff T, *et al*. Detection of organ-confined prostate cancer is increased through prostate specific antigen based screening. *JAMA* 1993; **270**: 948.

61. Catalona WJ, Smith DS, Ratliff TL, *et al*. Measurement of prostate specific antigen in serum as a screening test for prostate cancer. *N Engl J Med* 1991; **324**: 1156–1161.

62. Brawer MK, Chetner MP, Beatie J, *et al*. Screening for prostate carcinoma with prostate specific antigen. *J Urol* 1992; **147**: 841

63. Mandelson MT, Wagner EH, Thompson RS. PSA Screening: A public health dilemma. *Annual Review of Public Health* 1995; **16**: 283–306.

64. Catalona WJ, Richie JP, Ahmam FR, *et al*. Comparison of digital rectal examination and serum prostate specific antigen in the early detection of prostate cancer: Results of a multicenter clinical trial of 6,630 men. *J Urol* 1994; **151**: 1283–1290.

65. Cooner WH, Mosky BR, Rutherford CLJ, *et al*. Prostate cancer detection in a clinical urological practice by ultrasonography, digital rectal examination, and prostate specific antigen. *J Urol* 1990; **143**: 1146.

66. Bretton PR. Prostate specific antigen and digital rectal examination in screening for prostate cancer. A community based study. *South Med J* 1994; **87**: 720–723.

67. Carter HB, Pearson HD, Melter EJ, *et al*. Longitudinal evaluation of prostate specific antigen levels in men with and without prostate disease. *JAMA* 1992; **267**: 2215–2220.

68. Bazine M, Meshref AW, Trudel C, *et al*. Prospective evaluation of prostate specific antigen density and systematic biopsies for early detection of prostate carcinoma. *Urology* 1994; **43**: 44–52.

69. Oesterling JE, Jacobsen SE, Chute CG, *et al*. Serum prostate specific antigen in a community based population of healthy men: establishment of age-specific reference range. *JAMA* 1993; **270**: 860–864.

70. el-Galley RE, Petros JA, Sanders WH, *et al*. Normal range prostate — specific antigen vs. age-specific prostate-specific antigen in screening prostate adenocarcinoma. *Urology* 1995; **46**: 200–204.

71. Krahn MD, Mahoney JE, Eckman MH, *et al*. Screening for prostate cancer. A decision analytic view. *JAMA* 1994; **272**: 773–780.

72. Mettlen C, Littrup PJ, Kane RA, *et al*. Relative sensitivity and specificity of serum prostate specific antigen (PSA) level compared with age-referenced PSA, PSA density and PSA change data from the American Cancer Society National Prostate Cancer Detection Project. *Cancer* 1994; **74**: 1615–1620.

73. Potosky AL, Miller BA, Albertson PC, *et al*. The role of increasing detection in the rising incidence of prostate cancer. *JAMA* 1995; **273**: 548–552.

74. Epstein JI, Walsh PC, Carmichael M, *et al*. Pathologic and clinical findings to predict tumor extent of nonpapable (stage TIC) prostate cancer. *JAMA* 1994; **271**: 368–374.

75. Mettlin C, Murphy GP, Lee FE. Characteristics of prostate cancer detection in the American Cancer Society National Prostate Cancer Detection Project. *J Urol* 1994; **152**: 1734–1740.

76. Brandeau ML, Eddy DM. The workup of the asymptomatic patient with a positive fecal occult blood test. *Med Decision Making* 1987; **7**: 32–46.

77. Greene FL. Distribution of colorectal neoplasms. A left-to-right shift of polyps and cancer. *Am J Surg* 1983; **49**: 62–65.

78. Winawer SJ, Schottenfield D, Flehinger BJ. Colorectal cancer screening. *J Natl Cancer Inst* 1991; **83**: 243–253.

79. Kronborg O, Fenger C, Sndergaard O, *et al*. Initial mass screening for colorectal cancer with fecal occult blood test: a prospective randomized study at Funen in Denmark. *Scan J Gastroenterol* 1987; **22**: 677–685.

80. Griffith CDM, Turner DJ, Saunders JH. False negative results of Hemoccult test in colorectal cancer. *BMJ* 1981; **283**: 472

81. Crowley ML, Freeman LD, Mottet MD, *et al*. Sensitivity of guaiac-impregnated cards for the detection of colorectal neoplasms. *J Clin Gastroenterol* 1983; **5**: 127–130.

82. Ahlquist DA, McGill DB, Fleming JL, *et al*. Patterns of occult bleeding in asymptomatic colorectal cancer. *Cancer* 1989; **63**: 1826–1830.

83. Winawer SJ, Zauber AG, Ho MN, *et al*. Prevention of colorectal cancer by colonoscopic polypectomy. *N Engl J Med* 1993; **329**: 1977–1981.

84. Newcomb PA, Norfleet RG, Storer BE, *et al*. Screening sigmoidoscopy and colorectal cancer mortality. *J Natl Cancer Inst* 1992; **84**: 1572–1575.

85. Selby JV, Friedman GD, Quesenberry CJ, *et al*. A case-control study of screening sigmoidoscopy and mortality from colorectal cancer. *N Engl J Med* 1992; **326**: 653–657.

86. Gilbertson VA, Nelms JM. The prevention of invasive carcinoma of the rectum. *Cancer* 1978; **41**: 1137–1139.

87. Winawer SJ, Zauber AG, O'Brien MJ, *et al*. Randomized comparison of surveillance intervals after colonoscopic removal of newly diagnosed adenomatous polyps. *N Engl J Med* 1993; **1328**: 901–906.

88. Fleischer DE, Goldberg SB, Browning TH, *et al*. Detection and surveillance of colorectal carcinoma. *JAMA* 1989; **261**: 580–583.

89. Remington P, Lantz P, Phillips JL. Cervical cancer deaths among older women: Implications for prevention. *Wisconsin Med J* 1990; **89**(1): (30)32–34.

90. Kataja V, Syrjanen S, Jarvi RM, *et al*. Prognostic factors in cervical human papilloma virus infections. *Sex Trans Dis* 1992; **19**: 154–160.

91. Laara E, Day NE, Hakama M. Trends in mortality from cervical cancer in the Nordic countries: Association with organized screening programmes. *Lancet* 1987; **1**: (8544)1247–1249.

92. Christopherson WM, Lundin FE, Mendez WM, *et al*. Cervical cancer control: A study of morbidity and mortality trends over a twenty-one year period. *Cancer* 1976; **38**: (3)1357–1366.

93. Miller AB, Lindsay J, Hill GB. Mortality from cancer of the uterus in Canada and its relationship to screening for cancer of the cervix. *International J of Cancer* 1976; **17**: (5)602–612.

94. Johannesson G, Geirsson G, Day N. The effect of mass screening in Ireland, 1965–1974, on the incidence and mortality of cervical carcinoma. *J of Cancer* 1978; **21**: (4)418–425.

95. Herrero R, Brinton LA, Reeves WC, *et al*. Screening for cervical cancer in Latin America: a case-control study. *Int J Epidemiol* 1992; **21**: 1050–1056.

96. Aristizabal N, Cuello C, Correa P, *et al*. The impact of vaginal cytology on cervical cancer risks in Cali, Colombia. *Int J Cancer* 1984; **34**: 5–9.

97. Clarke EA, Anderson TW. Does screening by Pap smears help prevent cervical cancer? A case-control study. *Lancet* 1979; **2**: 1–4.

98. La Vecchia C, Decarli A, Gentile A, *et al*. Pap smear and the risk of cervical neoplasia: quantitative estimates from a case-control study. Lancet 1984; **2**: 779–782.

99. Fuller AF, Young RH, Tak WK. Cancer of the cervix, vulva, and vagina. In *Cancer Manual*, 8th Ed. American Cancer Society, MA Division, Boston, 253–262, 1990.

100. Mandelblatt J, Fahs MC. The cost-effectiveness of cervical cancer screening for low-income elderly women. *JAMA* 1988; **259**: 2409–2413.

101. Mandelblatt J, Traxler M, Lakin P, *et al*. Harlem Study Team. Mammography and Papanicolaou smear use by elderly poor black women. *J Am Geriatr Soc* 1992; **40**: 1001–1007.

102. Cervical cancer screening: summary of an NIH consensus statement. *BMJ* 1980; **281**: 1264–1266.

103. International Agency for Research on Cancer Working group on evaluation of Cervical Cancer Screening Programmes. Screening for squamous cervical cancer: duration of low risk after negative results of cervical cytology and its implication for screening policies. *BMJ* 1986; **293**: 659–664.

104. Van Wijngaarden WJ, Duncan ID. Rationale for stopping cervical screening in women over 50. *BMJ* 1993; **306**: 967–971.

105. Yu S, Miller AB, Sherman GJ. Optimizing the age, number of tests, and test interval for cervical screening in Canada. *J Epidemiol Community Health*.1982; **36**: 1–10.

106. Eddy DM. Screening for cervical cancer. *Ann Intern Med* 1990; **113**: 214–226.

107. Mandelblatt J, Traxler M, Lakin P, *et al*., Harlem Study Group. Breast and cervical cancer screening of poor, elderly, black women: Clinical results and implications. *Am J Prev Med* 1993; **9**: 133–138.

108. Koss LG. The Papanicolaou test for cervical cancer detection: A triumph and a tragedy. *JAMA* 1989; **261**: 737–743.

109. Harlan LC, Bernstein AB, Kessler LG. Cervical cancer screening: Who is not screened and why? *Am J Public Health* 1991; **81**: 885–891.

110. Mayer JA, Slymen DJ, Drew JA, *et al*. Breast and cervical cancer screening in older women: the San Diego Medicare Preventive Health Project. *Prev Med* 1992; **21**: 395–404.

111. American College of Obstetricians and Gynecologists. *Recommendations on frequency of Pap test screening*. Committee opinion no. 152. American College of Obstetricians and Gynecologists, 1995.

112. American Geriatrics Society Clinical Practice Committee. Screening for breast cancer in elderly women. *Amer Geriatr Soc* 1989; **37**: 883–885.

113. Canadian Task Force on the Periodic Health Examination. *Canadian guide to clinical preventive health examination*. Ottawa: Canada Communications Group, 884–889, 1994.

114. American Geriatrics Society Clinical Practice Committee. Screening for cervical carcinoma in elderly women. *J Amer Geriatr Soc* 1989; **37**: 885–887.

115. DiSaia PJ, Creasman WT. *Clinical Gynecologic Oncology*. 3rd edition St Louis. The CV Mosby Co 1989.

116. Fisher B, Costantino JP, Redmond CK. Endometrial cancer in tamoxifen-treated breast cancer patients: findings from the National Surgical Adjuvant Breast and Bowel Project (NSABP) B-14. *J Natl Cancer Inst* 1994; **86**: 527–537.

117. Young JL, Percy CL, Asire AJ. *SEER Program: Incidence and mortality 1973–1977*. National Cancer Institute Monograph 57 Washington, DC: Government Printing Office, 75, 1981.

118. Amos CI, Struewing JP. Genetic epidemiology of epithelial ovarian cancer. *Cancer* 1993; **71**: 566–572.

119. Smith LH, Oi RH. Detection of malignant ovarian neoplasm: a review of the literature. 1. Detection of the patient at risk; clinical, radiological and cytological detection. *Obstet Gynecol Surv* 1984; **30**: 313–328.

120. Bast RC, Klug TL, St. John E, *et al*. A radioimmunoassay using a monoclinal antibody to monitor the course of epithelial ovarian carcinoma. *N Engl J Med* 1983; **309**: 883–887.

121. Patsner B, Mann WJ. The value of preoperative serum CA 125 levels in patients with a pelvic mass. *AM J Obstet Gynecol* 1988; **159**: 873–876.

122. Schilthuis M, Aalders J, Bouma J, *et al*. Serum CA 125 levels in epithelial ovarian cancer: Relation with findings at second-look operations and their role in the detection of tumor recurrence. *BR J Obstet Gynecol* 1987; **94**: 202–207.

123. Bourne TH, Campbell S, Reynolds KM, *et al*. Screening for early familial ovarian cancer with transvaginal ultrasonography and color flow imaging. *BMJ* 1993; **306**: 1025–1029.

124. Rodriguez MH, Platt LD, Medearis AL, *et al*. The use of transvaginal ultrasonography for evaluation of postmenopausal ovary size and morphology. *AM J Obstet Gynecol* 1988; **159**: 810–814.

125. Zanaboni F, Vergadero F, Presti M, Gallotti P, Lombardi F, Bolis G. Tumor antigen CA 125 as a marker of ovarian epithelial carcinoma. *Gynecol Oncol* 1987; **28**: 61–67.

126. Hall DJ, Hurt WG. The adnexal mass. *J Fam Pract* 1982; **14**: 135–140.

127. DiXia C, Schwartz P, Xinguo L, *et al*. Evaluation of CA 125 levels in differentiating malignant from benign tumors in patients with pelvic masses. *Obstet Gynecol* 1988; **72**: 23–27.

128. VanNagell JR, DePriest PD, Puls NE, *et al*. Ovarian cancer screening in asymptomatic postmenopausal women by trans-vaginal sonography. *Cancer* 1991: 458–462.

129. Andolf E, Jorgensen C, Astedt B. Ultrasound examination for detection of ovarian carcinoma in risk groups. *Obstet Gynecol* 1990; **75**: 106–109.

130. Campbell S, Bhan V, Royston J, *et al*. Screening for early ovarian cancer. *Lancet* 1988; **1**: 710–711.

131. Jacobs I, Stabile I, Bridges J, *et al*. Multi modal approach to screening for ovarian cancer. *Lancet* 1988; **1**: 268–271.

132. Kramer BS, Gohagan J, Prorok PC, Smart C. A National Cancer Institute sponsored screening trial for prostatic, lung, colorectal, and ovarian cancers. *Cancer* 1993; **71**: 589–593.

133. National Institutes of Health. *Ovarian cancer: Screening, treatment, and follow-up*. National Institutes of Health Consensus Conference Statement (April 5–7, 1994).

134. US Preventive Services Task Force. *Guide to Preventive Clinical Services*. 2nd Ed Baltimore Williams and Wilkens 1996: 159–166.

135. Wick MM, Grande DJ, Lo TCM. Cancer of the skin. In *Cancer Manual* 8th ed. American Cancer Society, MA Division, Boston 1990: 125–132.

136. Urback R. Incidence of nonmelanoma skin cancer. *Dermatol Clin* 1991; **9**: 751–755.

137. Evans RD, Kopf AW, Lew RA, *et al*. Risk factors for the development of malignant melanoma-I: review of case-control studies. *J Dermatol Surg Oncol* 1988; **14**: 393–408.

138. Dubin N, Moseson M, Pasternack BS. Sun exposure and malignant melanoma among susceptible individuals. *Environ Health Perspect* 1989; **81**: 139–151.

139. Koh HK, Kligler BE, Lew RA. Sunlight and cutaneous malignant melanoma: evidence for and against causation. *Photochem Photobiol* 1990; **51**: 765–779.

140. Drolet BA, Connor MJ. Sunscreens and the prevention of ultraviolet radiation-induced skin cancer. *Journal of Dermatologic Surgery and Oncology* 1992; **18**(7): 571–576.

141. Committee on Guidelines of Care AA. Guidelines of care for basal cell carcinoma. *J Am Acad Dermatol* 1992; **26**: 117–120.

142. Costanza ME, Dayal Y, Binder S, Nathanson L. Metastatic basal cell carcinoma: review, report of a case, and chemotherapy. *Cancer* 1974; **34**: 230–235.

143. Karagas MR, Stukel TA, Greenberg ER, *et al*. Risk of subsequent basal carcinoma and squamous cell carcinoma of the skin among patients with prior skin cancer. *JAMA* 1992; **267**: (24)3305–3310.

144. Glass AG, Hoover RN. The emerging epidemic of melanoma and squamous cell skin cancer. *JAMA* 1989; **262**: 2097–2100.

145. Morbidity and Mortality Report Centers for Disease Control, Atlanta: Death rates of malignant melanoma among white men–United States, 1973–1988. *Archives of Dermatology* 1992; **128**: (4)451–452.

146. Greene MH, Clark WH, Tucker MA, *et al*. High risk of malignant melanoma in melanoma-prone families with dysplastic nevi. *Ann Intern Med* 1985; **102**: 458–465.

147. Halpern AC, Guerry DI, Elder DE, *et al*. Dysplastic nevi as risk markers of sporadic (nonfamilial) melanoma. *Arch Dermatol* 1991; **127**: 995–999.

148. Tiersten AD, Grin CM, Kopf AW, *et al*. Prospective follow-up for malignant melanoma in patients with atypical-mole (dysplastic-nevus) syndrome. *J Dermatol Surg Oncol* 1991; **17**: 44–48.

149. Mihm MC, Barnhill RL, Sober AJ, *et al*. Precursor lesions of melanoma: Do they exist? *Seminars in Surgical Oncology* 1992; **8**: (6)358–365.

150. Rhodes AR. Melanocytic precursors of cutaneous melanoma. Estimated risks and guidelines for management. *Med Clin North Am* 1986; **70**: 3–37.

151. Holman CD, James IR, Gattey PH, *et al*. An analysis of trends in mortality from malignant melanoma of the skin in Australia. *Int J Cancer* 1980; **26**: (6)703–709.

152. Keefe M, MacKie RM. The relationship between risk of death from clinical stage I cutaneous melanoma and thickness of primary tumor: No evidence for steps in risk. *Br J Cancer* 1991; **64**: 598–602.

153. Friedman RJ, Rigel DS, Silverman MK, *et al*. Malignant melanoma in the 1990s: The continued importance of early detection and the role of the physician examination and self-examination of the skin. *Ca Cancer J Clin* 1991; **41**: 201–226.

154. Ramsey DL, Fox AB. The ability of primary care physicians to recognize the common dermatoses. *Arch Dermatol* 1981; **117**: 620–622.

155. Wagner RF, Wagner D, Tomich JM, *et al*. Diagnoses of skin diseases: Dermatologists vs. nondermatologists. *J Dermatol Surg Oncol* 1985; **11**: 476–479.

156. Smith TJ, Mihm MC, Sober AJ. Malignant melanoma. In *Cancer Manual* 8th Ed. American Cancer Society MA Division, Boston. 1990; **133**–144.

157. Committee on Guidelines of Care AA. Guidelines of care for nevi I (nevocellular nevi and seborrheic keratoses). *J Am Acad Dermatol* 1992; **26**: 629–631.

158. NIH Consensus Development Panel on Early Melanoma. Diagnosis and treatment of early melanoma. *JAMA* 1992; **268**: 1314–1319.

159. US Preventive Services Task Force. *Guide to Clinical Preventive Services*, 2nd ed. Baltimore: Williams and Wilkens, 141–152, 1996.

160. Boeing H. Epidemiological research in stomach cancer: progress over the last ten years. *J of CA Research and Clinical Oncology* 1991; **117**: (3)133–143.

161. Murakami R, Tsukuma H, Ubukata T, *et al*. Estimation of validity of mass screening program for gastric cancer in Osaka, Japan. *Cancer* 1990; **65**: (5)1255–1260.

162. Kampschoer GH, Fujii A, Mousuda Y. Gastric cancer detected by mass survey: comparison between mass survey and outpatient detection. *Scandinavian Journal of Gastroenterology* 1989; **24**: (7)813–817.

163. Hirayama T, Hisamichi S, Fujimoti I, *et al*. In *Screening for Gastric Cancer*, edited by AS Miller. Screening for Cancer. NY: Academic Press, 367–376, 1985.

164. Tytgat GN, Mathus-Vliegen EM, Offerhaus J. Value of endoscopy in the surveillance of high risk groups for gastrointestinal cancer. In *Precancerous Lesions of the Gastrointestinal Tract*, edited by P Sherlock *et al*. New York: Raven Press, 305–318, 1983.

165. National Cancer Institute. Cooperative Early Lung Cancer Detection Program. Summary and conclusions. *Am Rev Respir Dir* 1984; **130**: 565–567.

166. Brett GZ. The value of lung cancer detection by six-monthly chest radiographs. *Thorax* 1968; **23**: 414–420.

167. Weiss W. Survivorship among men with bronchogenic carcinoma: three studies in populations screened every six months. *Arch Environ Health* 1971; **22**: 168–173.

168. Ebeling K, Nischan P. Screening for lung cancer: results from a case-control study. *Int J Cancer* 1987; **40**: 141–144.

169. Sanderson DR. Lung cancer screening: the Mayo study. *Chest* 1986; **89**(suppl): 324S.

170. Melamed MR, Flehinger BJ, Zamen MB, *et al*. Screening for early lung cancer: results of the Memorial Sloan-Kettering study in New York. *Chest* 1984; **86**: 44–53.

171. Berlin NI, Buncher CR, Fontana RS, *et al*. The National Cancer Institute Cooperative Early Lung Cancer Detection Program: results of the initial screen (prevalence): introduction. *Am Rev Respir Dis* 1984; **130**: 545–549.

172. Flehinger BJ, Melamed MR, Zamen MB, *et al*. Early lung cancer detection: results of the initial (prevalence) radiologic and cytologic screening in the Memorial Sloan-Kettering study. *Am Rev Respir Dis* 1984; **130**: 555–560.

173. Frost J., Ball WCJ, Levin ML, *et al*. Early lung cancer detection; results of the initial (prevalence) radiologic and cytologic screening in the John Hopkins study. *Am Rev Respir Dis* 1984; **130**: 549–554.

174. Fontana RS, Sanderson DR, Taylor WF, *et al*. Early lung cancer detection: Results of the initial (prevalence) radiologic and cytologic screening in the Mayo Clinic study. *Am Rev Repir Dis* 1984; **130**: 561–565.

175. Kubik A, Parkin DM, Khlat M, *et al*. Lack of benefit from semi-annual screening for cancer of the lung: follow-up report of a randomized controlled trial on a population of high-risk males in Czechoslovakia. *Int J Cancer* 1990; **45**: 26–33.

176. Miller BA, Ries LA, Hankey BF, *et al*. *Cancer Statistics Review 1973–1989*. Bethesda, MD. National Cancer Institute Publication NIH 92-2789, 1992.

177. Vogt HB, McHale MS. Testicular cancer: role of primary care physicians in screening and education. *Postgrad Med* 1992; **92**: 93–101.

178. Rowland RG. Serum markers in testicular germ-cell neoplasms. *Hematol Oncol Clin North AM* 1988; **2**: 485–489.

179. National Cancer Institute. *Cancer of the bladder*. Bethesda: National Cancer Inst NIH Publ# 90-722, 1990.

180. Ries LAG, Miller BA, Hankey BR, *et al*. SEER Cancer Statistics Review 1973–1991 tables and graphs. In *Anonymous HO 94-2789*. Bethesda: National Cancer Institute NIH Publication No. 94-2789, 1994.

181. Anton-Culver H, Lee-Felstein A, Taylor TH. Occupation and bladder cancer risk. *Am J Epidemiol* 1992; **136**: 89–94.

182. Sewell DL, Burt SP, Gabbert NJ, *et al*. Evaluation of the Chemstrip 9 as a screening for urinalysis and urine culture in men. *Am J Clin Pathol* 1985; **83**: 740–743.

183. Mariani AJ, Luangphinith S, Loo S, *et al*. Dipstick chemical urinalysis: An accurate cost-effective screening test. *J Urol* 1984; **132**: 64–66.

184. Messing EM, Young TB, Hunt VB, *et al*. Home screening for hematuria: Results of a multi-clinic study. *J Urol* 1992; **148**: 289–292.

185. Hiatt RA, Ordonez JD. Dipstick urinalysis screening, asymptomatic microhematuria, and subsequent urological cancers in a population-based sample. *Cancer Epidemiol Biomarkers* 1994; **3**: 1–5.

186. Farrow GM. Pathologist's role in bladder cancer. *Semin Oncol* 1979; **6**: 198–206.

187. Vokes EE, Weichselbaum RR, Lippman SM, *et al*. Head and neck cancer. *N Engl J Med* 1993; **328**: 184–194.

188. Department of Health and Human Services NC. *Tobacco effects in the mouth*. Bethesda: Public Health Service 1992; Pub# (NCI) 92–3330.

189. Prout M. Results of screening in an inner city clinic. Personal communication, 1990.

190. Mehta FS, Bhonsle RB, Daftary DK, *et al*. Detection of oral cancer using basic health worker in an area of high oral cancer incidence in India. *Cancer Detect Prev* 1986; **9**: 219–225.

191. Hong WK, Lippman SM, Itri LM, *et al*. Prevention of second primary tumors with isotretinoin in squamous cell carcinoma of the head and neck. *N Eng J Med* 1990; **323**: 795–801.

192. Lippman SM, Batsakis JG, Toth BB, *et al*. Comparison of low dose isotretinoin with beta carotene to prevent oral carcinogenesis. *New Eng J Med* 1993; **328**: 15–20.

193. Brenner SE, Winn RJ, Lippman SM, *et al*. Regression of oral leukoplakia with alpha-tocopherol: a Community Clinical Oncology Program chemoprevention study. *J Natl Cancer Inst* 1993; **85**: 44–47.

194. US Preventive Services Task Force. *Guide to Clinical Preventive Services 2nd Ed*. Baltimore: Williams and Wilkens, 175–180, 1996.

195. Canadian Task Force on the Periodic Health Examination. *Canadian guide to clinical preventative health care*. Ottowa: Canada Communication Group, 838–847, 1994.

196. Shore RE, Hildreth N, Dvoretsky P, *et al*. Thyroid cancer among persons given x-ray treatment in infancy for an enlarged thymus gland. *Am J Epidemiol* 1993; **137**: 1068–1080.

197. Brander A, Viikinkoski P, Tuuhea J, *et al*. Clinical versus ultrasound examination of the thyroid gland in common clinical practice. *J Clin Ultrasound* 1992; **20**: 37–42.

198. Ishida T, Izuo M, Ogawa T, *et al*. Evaluation of mass screening for thyroid cancer. *Jpn J Clin Oncol* 1988; **18**: 289–295.

199. Shimaoka K, Bakri K, Sciascia M, *et al*. Thyroid screening program: Follow-up evaluation. *NY State J Med* 1982: 1184–1187.

200. Canadian Task Force on the Periodic Health Examination. *Canadian guide to clinical preventative health care*. Ottowa: Canada Communication Group, 611–618, 1994.

201. US Preventive Services Task Force. *Guide to Clinical Preventive Services*, 2nd edition. Baltimore: Williams and Wilkens, 187–191, 1996.

202. Frame PS. The complete annual physical examination refuses to die. *J of Fam Pract* 1995; **40**: 543–545.

203. McCormick WC, Inui TS. Geriatric Preventive care: Counseling techniques in practice settings. *Clinics in Geriatric Care* 1996; **8**: 215–228.

204. US Preventive Services Task Force. *Guide to Clinical Preventive Service*, 2nd Ed. Baltimore: Williams and Wilkens, lxxv–lxxxiii, 1996.

205. Canadian Task Force on the Periodic Health Examination. *Canadian guide to clinical preventative health care*. Ottowa: Canada Communication Group, 850–861, 1994.

206. Lurie N, Manning WG, Peterson C, *et al*. Preventive care: do we practice what we preach? *Am J Public Health* 1987; **77**: 801–804.

207. National Cancer Institute Breast Screening Consortium. Screening mammography: a missed clinical opportunity? *JAMA* 1990; **264**: 54–58.

208. Frame PS. Health maintenance in clinical practice: strategies and barriers. *Am Fam Physician* 1992; **45**: 1192–1200.

209. Griffith HM, Rahman MI. Implementing the Put Prevention into Practice Program. *Nurse Pract* 1994; **19**: 12–19.

210. Dietrich AJ, Woodruff CB, Carney PA. Changing office routines to enhance preventive care. *Arch Fam Med* 1994; **3**: 176–183.

211. Carney P, Dietrich A, Keller A. Tools, teamwork, and tenacity: And office system for cancer prevention. *J Fam Pract* 1992; **35**: 388–394.

212. Costanza ME, Li FP, Prout M, *et al*. Cancer prevention and detection: Strategies for practice. In *Cancer Manual*, 9th Ed. American Cancer Society, MA Division, Boston, 1996.

213. US Preventive Services Task Force. *Guide to Clinical Preventive Services*, 2nd Ed. Baltimore, Williams and Wilkens, lvii–lxxiv, 1996.

25. Barriers to Cancer Prevention in the Older Person

Sarah A. Fox, Richard G. Roetzheim and Raynard S. Kington

Introduction

Barriers to the older person using preventive services regularly or at all are numerous. Examples of types of barriers covered in this chapter are: 1) demographic barriers, such as insufficient income to purchase services or differential utilization of services by racial/ethnic groups; 2) physician-patient communication patterns which are differentially effective in improving patient compliance; 3) knowledge gaps which can effect screening compliance; 4) attitudinal barriers, such as anxiety about the outcome of screening which may impede obtaining services or a belief that a preventive procedure is ineffective; and 5) community-based barriers such as the lack of a reminder system to assist providers in maintaining patient compliance. Strategies to improve compliance with screening ideally should be multi-level and include individual-level (physician and/or patient), cohort-level (physician and patient), practice-level, and community-level efforts. Research studies currently are underway at all levels to develop, refine, and improve strategies for reducing barriers to prevention.

Much of the current research knowledge about the appropriate or inappropriate utilization of screening services is applicable only to younger persons; the older person is only recently included in or focused on in research protocols. Nevertheless, although much can be learned from the body of research that focuses on persons under age 60, this chapter is devoted to findings derived from older samples since there are unique differences between age groups.

Demographic and Socioeconomic Variation in the Use of Preventive Cancer Screening Services

The comparison of utilization rates for cancer screening procedures across demographic groups provides important information for addressing potential barriers to their use. The rates of utilization of a wide range of health care services vary across demographic groups, but most of the analyses of utilization have focused on acute care services. Analyses of utilization rates are based on theoretical behavioral or descriptive models that attempt to describe patterns of use or explain why some individuals use certain health care services and others do not. Perhaps the most widely used descriptive utilization model in health services research is the Andersen model which divides potential causal factors into three broad categories: societal, health services systems, and individual determinants. Individual determinants are in turn classified as predisposing factors such as age and sex, enabling factors such as income or health insurance, and illness level or medical need (1). Although most individual level factors are not likely to change in the short run (e.g., education levels), the finding of differences in rates across demographic groups suggests that clinical and public health interventions to promote the appropriate use of the services should take into account differences across relevant demographic and socioeconomic groups.

The interpretation of differences in the rates of utilization of preventive cancer screening services, like that of acute care services, is complex because for many cancer screening procedures there is no clear consensus on the appropriate use of the services. For example, there is wide agreement in the medical community that screening for lung cancer with chest radiographs is not an effective means for improving health (2). However, even for procedures for which there is a broad consensus, such as mammography for breast cancer, there is often significant variation in the details of screening recommendations across sets of recommendations issued by various organizations (2,3). The lack of consensus is important because identification of a demographic group with a low utilization rate may have limited policy or clinical implications if there is no agreement that the use of the procedure for screening has a positive impact on health. Nevertheless, the available evidence suggests substantial variation in the use of widely accepted preventive cancer screening services across demographic groups.

Relatively few national data sets provide information on demographic variation in the utilization of preventive cancer services, and the data that are available and analyzed focus on screening for breast and cervical cancers, two cancers for which there is considerable agreement about the effectiveness of screening in reducing mortality. The primary demographic factors for which we have good evidence on utilization rates are age, race and ethnicity, income, education, and urban versus rural residence.

Very little is known about differences between men and women in rates of utilization of cancer screening services because the majority of data focuses on breast and cervical cancer screening. The primary important cancer for which there are available screening procedures and which affects both men and women is colon cancer. A range of procedures, including digital rectal examination, fecal occult blood testing, flexible sigmoidoscopy, barium enema, and colonoscopy, have been proposed as a part of strategies to reduce mortality from colon cancer (2). However, there is no consensus yet on guidelines for screening for colon cancer (3). Although several studies of geographically limited populations have found gender differences in the population that responds to community-level interventions to promote fecal occult screening, the results have been inconsistent (4–7). Furthermore, most of the studies have been unable to calculate response rates for these interventions because the total number of women and men exposed to the interventions is not known. A recent large study of an intervention to promote fecal occult screening in a defined population found that women were more likely than men to respond to fecal occult screening (8). Nevertheless, there is insufficient evidence to draw strong conclusions regarding differences between men and women in rates of cancer screening.

An additional limitation of the available evidence on the role of demographic factors in cancer screening is the lack of detailed multivariate analyses of the comparative importance of demographic factors within the older population. For example, there are few analyses of the relative importance of demographic factors such as education and income within older populations as compared to younger populations. Although we may draw inferences from studies across the adult populations, factors such as income and education may be more, less, or as important as a determining factor and a potential barrier within the older population.

Age

Several studies of use of cancer screening services have found that older persons are less likely to be screened than younger persons. When there have been analyses of differences within the over 65 population, older persons are still less likely to be screened. Among older women in the 1992 National Health Interview Survey (NHIS), the most comprehensive on-going survey of the nation's health, the percentage of women who had completed a mammogram varied significantly by age (9). While 41% among women age 60–64 had completed a mammogram, only 28% among women age 75–79 had. These age differences have been noted since mammography utilization began being tracked in the 1987 NHIS. Additionally, Los Angeles regional data demonstrate less screening among older Hispanics when compared to blacks and Anglos (10). Older women are also significantly less likely to be compliant with recommendations for cervical cancer screening (11–13).

Race and Ethnicity

Among older women, both African-American and Hispanic women are substantially less likely than white women to have completed mammography (14,15) or pap smears. Among women above age 75 in the 1987

NHIS, 83.5% of black women and 93.2% of Hispanic women had never had a mammogram, compared to 75% of white women (16). Analysis of Medicare claims in 1986 found that the relative risk of having a mammogram for white women compared to black women was 1.76 (17). The patterns may be different for cervical cancer screening. For example, although national data from the 1973 NHIS found that white women ages 60–79 were more likely than black women to have had a Pap test within the two years prior to the survey (38.2% versus 31.2%), by 1985 black women were more likely than white women in that age group to have had a Pap test within two years (50.% versus 42.4%) (12). Little is known about details of specific relative patterns of use across racial and ethnic minorities (e.g., across specific Latino or Asian sub-populations). Differences across these sub-populations may have important implications for eliminating barriers.

Socioeconomic Status

Socioeconomic status, typically measured by education and income, is an important predictor of access to health care services in general, and as is true with many health care procedures, low income persons and those with less education are less likely to undergo cancer screening compared to high income and better educated persons. Among women in the 1992 NHIS above age 40, only 26% of those from families with income less than $20,000 had a mammogram, compared to 44% among those from families with incomes greater than $20,000 (18). After adjusting for age, 64.8% of the women in the 1987 NHIS who were in families below the poverty index ratio had completed a Pap smear within three years, compared to 75.2% for women above this level (13). The findings for persons with lower education mirror those with low income. In the 1992 NHIS, 24% of women above age 40 with less than a high school education had had a mammogram, compared to 46% for women with more than a high school education (18). A study of almost 5,000 persons in the upper Midwestern U.S. found higher education to be associated with the use of a range of screening procedures including mammography, sigmoidoscopy, Pap smears, fecal occult blood testing, and rectal exams (19).

Urban versus Rural

Residence in a rural community may present barriers to access to a range of health care services, and the available evidence suggests that persons who live in rural settings are also less likely to undergo cancer screening. Among women 40+ in the 1992 NHIS, 38% of urban women above age 40 received a mammogram compared to 33% for rural women (18). Analysis of data from a Canadian population found similar findings: in spite of comparable access to physician services, women in rural areas were less likely to report a clinical breast examination or a mammogram (20). The urban-rural difference may increase racial differences. In the analysis of 1986 Medicare, the relative risk among white versus black women for undergoing mammography increases from 1.67 to 2.64 when urban and rural populations are compared (17).

Access to Care

A number of studies have stressed the importance of access to primary care in order to accomplish cancer screening. The NHIS, for example, has consistently shown higher rates of breast cancer screening among women who report a regular source of medical care (21). Women who lack health insurance have likewise been found to have much lower rates of breast and cervical cancer screening (11,22,23) and are more likely to be diagnosed with cancer at an advanced stage (24).

Presence of health insurance may, of course, be less of a problem for older patients who are almost uniformly insured by Medicare. Medicare has only recently, however, begun to provide reimbursement for mammography and Pap smears (1992) and it still does not cover costs of other cancer screening tests. Furthermore these tests are reimbursed only after appropriate deductibles have been met, and patients are still responsible for copayments. For some elderly patients, therefore, costs of cancer screening may still be a burden.

The available literature suggests that poor insurance reimbursement for cancer screening is a barrier for some Medicare-insured patients. Patients with Medicare supplement policies, for example, have significantly higher cancer screening rates than those who can not afford them (25). Interventions that have provided first dollar Medicare coverage of cancer screening tests have also shown increased rates of cancer screening (26). Physicians frequently cite cost and lack of insurance reimbursement as a barrier to screening, and may therefore be reluctant to recommend tests such as flexible sigmoidoscopy for poor patients (27–29).

Two other points about screening costs and insurance reimbursement are apparent. First, while financial costs and poor reimbursement are certainly important barriers for some patients it is unlikely that they are the major barrier for most patients. The recently enacted Medicare benefit for mammography and Pap smears, for example, has not so far, led to increased screening rates (25,30). A number of prior studies had also hinted that cost was not the main barrier for tests such as mammography (31,32). Also, interventions directed primarily at reducing screening costs have not been particularly effective unless supplemented with patient education (33). Second, it seems clear that the poor will face barriers to screening even when provided with adequate health insurance. Cancer screening rates, for example, are considerably lower among poor people even in countries with universal health insurance (34).

The structure of primary medical care may also play an important role in cancer screening. Some studies have found that patients enrolled in managed care HMO's receive more cancer screening services and have earlier stage at diagnosis (35,37). It is not known, however, if this is due to a greater emphasis on prevention,

better reimbursement for screening procedures, or simply the result of prevention-oriented individuals self-selecting into HMO's.

Physician-Older Patient Communication's Impact on Cancer Screening

Physician-patient communication is a topic of considerable interest among those who investigate patient compliance and barriers to as well as enablers of patient compliance. What impact, if any, does communication have on an older patient's compliance with cancer screening? A recent annotated bibliography by Beisecker (38) provides a thoughtful review of the communication literature relevant to patients and their doctors and communication's possible relevance to health outcomes. Additionally, Beisecker reviewed the different components of the doctor older-patient relationship that might impact communication and compliance such as provider and patient characteristics, e.g., gender and race; the context of care, e.g., the patient's companion and the length of the encounter; the content of the encounter, e.g., what is communicated factually; the process within the encounter, e.g., patient assertiveness; and the outcomes of the encounter, e.g., patient satisfaction, recall, compliance, and health status (39). These reviews are incorporated into the below sections.

Demographic Characteristics and Communication

Patient characteristics such as race, health insurance status, and age, and physician characteristics such as race and specialty are potentially strong predictors of effective doctor-patient communication about cancer screening. Although the importance of these characteristics has been examined for younger patients, fewer studies of older patients and the influence of their characteristics on communication exist. The literature on the impact of physician characteristics on communication is even smaller (40). Nevertheless, the match of physician-patient gender has been shown to interface with preventive services in the office setting. In one study, male patients over age 70 had the highest probability of being offered rectal examinations (92%) when they were seen by male physicians; male patients seen by female physicians were offered the examination considerably less (55%) (41). Additionally, there was much less gender differentiation in the patient group aged 50–70. Beisecker's review concluded that female physicians seem to be better communicators but that it was unclear what effect, if any, communication had on health status (38).

Patient age also affects communication with physicians. Weinberger found that physicians were significantly more likely to forget to mention screening to 75 year old patients as opposed to 50 and 65 year olds (42). For example, physicians were significantly more likely to believe that a clinical breast examination alone was adequate breast cancer screening for patients 75 years and older but would more likely recommend mammography as well to their younger patients (42). These physicians cited co-morbidities and an expected shortened life expectancy as their rationale for these limited screening recommendations (42).

Patient co-morbidities often are believed to influence physician communication about screening and can contribute to fewer physician recommendations for screening in the older patient. For example, communication difficulties are inevitable and complicated when accompanied by a decline in cognitive skills that may also accompany aging (43). The older old (>75) are far more likely to have problems: a decline in cognitive skills, hearing problems, physical impairments, financial concerns, transportation restraints and mobility problems. All of these are possible contributors to increased barriers to screening which the younger old are less likely to experience.

Communication Content

Older patients appear to have a more difficult time getting their needs met at the office visit. Rost found that among diabetic patients over age 60, more than a quarter reported that their problems had not been addressed at the visit; this problem is compounded by the fact that older patients are more likely than younger ones to have multiple problems (44). In fact, over half had at least one important medical problem and one psychological problem that was never addressed (44). Adelman et al. also found that older patients had difficulty getting their concerns acknowledged and that about two-thirds of the topics were ones raised by physicians rather than patients (45). Screening may be neglected if it is not on the physician's agenda.

There also is confusion among the elderly about what occurred during the visits. Greene found significantly less concordance for the older (65 years of age and older) patient-physician dyadic interactions than for the younger dyads, especially in relation to what was discussed in general and discussed medically (46).

Finally, what is communicated and by whom makes a difference. In focus groups conducted by the National Cancer Institute, it was discovered that older patients shared a considerable anxiety about cancer and were fairly pessimistic about their ability to recover after a diagnosis (47). A physician's reassurance and support could be essential in overcoming this pessimism to allow for screening compliance. Additionally, Fox found that the physician just mentioning a mammogram to patients was the strongest predictor of patients getting one, especially for patients over age 65 (15). The communication did not need to be lengthy, persuasive, or directive — it just had to occur (15). A physician's belief in prevention — if belief was communicated — served as a strong inducement for eventual patient compliance.

Communication Process

What is said or communicated, the content of messages, is important in influencing compliance with screening, as discussed above. How the content is communicated — the process of communication — is also and, maybe, more important. Adelman and others found that audiotapes of primary care follow-up appointments showed that physicians favored younger patients (<45 vs >65 years of age) in the following ways: provided more information on physician-initiated issues, provided more support on patient-initiated issues, and were nicer (48, 49). However, younger patients asked better questions and provided better information than the older patients. Although these findings might be attributable to physician ageism, they were also a result of the more successful way in which younger patients handled their physician visits. Older patients also negatively influenced the outcomes of their visits to physicians by being more passive and giving more decision-making authority to physicians (49–52).

Finally, Fox et al. found that the enthusiasm with which physicians discussed screening mammography was the strongest predictor of patient follow-up with the referral (59). Being very or somewhat enthusiastic about discussing screening was a stronger predictor of eventual screening than the mention of screening neutrally or not enthusiastically (59). As women aged, however, past age 75, the enthusiasm for screening expressed by physicians dropped markedly which served to contribute to a lowered screening rate by this group (59).

Communication Context

The context in which physician-patient communication takes place can effect its outcome. For example, the presence of third parties at an office visit has a meaningful impact on interaction, both positive and negative. Beisecker examined audiotapes of 21 patients, aged 60–85, with their physicians; 9 visits were with solo patients and 12 included a patient companion, all family members (60). The older the patient, the more likely a companion was involved (60). Companion presence did not effect the length of the visit's length but instead took time away from patients (60). Coe found that although the presence of a third party effected communication, e.g., physicians adjusted to include the presence of a third party; it was not clear whether the effect was positive or negative for the patient (61). Both authors agreed that more research is needed on the effects that third parties bring to the older patient-physician interaction and subsequent screening rate compliance.

Knowledge-Based Barriers to Screening

Patients, and their providers, generally need a minimal knowledge base, e.g., that includes risk factors regarding disease, awareness of cancer screening procedures, and knowledge about the current guidelines for their use, for there to be patient compliance regarding utilization. Therefore, patient's lack of awareness about the risk factors for breast cancer, screening procedures, e.g., mammography, or the recommended guidelines for its use, can serve as barriers to patient screening compliance. Exceptions exist, however, especially when patients or providers resist or are unaware of current guidelines. For example, the recommended utilization of screening mammography for women age 50–74 (U.S. Preventive Task Force) is every year or two; the National Cancer Institute recommends mammography every year or two from age 50 with no upper age restrictions. Nevertheless, most women in that age group still believe that annual screening is the recommended frequency, a frequency that is now endorsed only by the American Cancer Society (53). It is unclear if providers prefer annual screening. The research base, however, regarding the impact of knowledge on screening endorsements is not as broad as the literature supporting the impact of access to care or attitudes on screening. Furthermore, most studies have focused on patient knowledge instead of provider knowledge of risk factors or screening recommendations. Exceptions are two surveys of general practitioners in Australia: one survey indicated both confusion about guidelines for prostrate and testicular cancer screening as well as an under usage of these techniques with patients (54); the other survey determined that although general practitioners had a good working knowledge regarding skin cancer, there were significant gaps that needed correction (55).

Several studies indicated a similar confusion about guidelines among patients. Older women demonstrated less awareness and use of pap smears for cervical cancer screening purposes. Mamon *et al.* found that older women (over age 45) were more likely to be under-screened as well as to not know the risk factors for cervical cancer (56). Additionally, older women were more likely to not recall being told about the guidelines by their providers and to be confused about actual guidelines (56). Mandelblatt had similar findings: older black low income women who reported low levels of knowledge about cervical and breast cancer also demonstrated low levels of utilization of screening tests (57). Other studies demonstrated a relationship between actual compliance with breast cancer screening, intended compliance, and knowledge about disease and detection. Fox and Champion found that the less compliant patient had lower levels of knowledge about breast cancer and detection issues (58,62). Richardson found, similarly, that women who intended to participate in regular breast cancer screening were more knowledgeable about breast cancer (63).

Knowledge of risks also contributed to better patient compliance with screening. Rimer offered a health education program to retirement home residents that included teaching the older women about risk factors as well as detection techniques (33). These women were more likely to subsequently get screened than women who were offered subsidized mammograms (33). Alternatively, women who assessed their risks as high (younger women) were more likely to get screened than older women whose actual risk were higher; this provides a partial explanation for the lower screening rates among older women (64).

Knowledge about risks tended to decrease with age and was related to a decrease in screening rates. Mah found that although over half of the sample in her Canadian study had had a mammogram, the proportion decreased with age after age 60 (65). Knowledge of breast cancer risk factors was generally low as was knowledge of guidelines; both decreased with age (65).

Finally, there were differences in knowledge levels by race/ethnicity. Ruiz found that Latinas needed to be reached about cancer issues through the Spanish-language media (66). However, if Latinas, especially the elderly, had acquired English and were acculturated, they were more likely to know more about cancer and to have been screened (66). Perez-Stable found that misconceptions about cancer were more prevalent among Latinos than Anglos (67).

Attitudinal Barriers to Screening

Patient Attitudes

Health beliefs and attitudes are important components of several theoretical models of health behavior that have been examined in the context of cancer screening. Models such as the Theory of Reasoned Action and Health Belief Model have been found to have reasonably good predictive value for compliance with cancer screening, suggesting that patient attitudes are important determinants of screening behavior (68–71). Empirical studies have also found correlations between general health attitudes and cancer screening (72). Attitudes may play an even more important role in screening behavior for the elderly than in younger women (73).

Poor cancer screening compliance among the elderly, therefore, may in part be the result of differing health beliefs and attitudes. Studies have shown that older patients possess a number of negative beliefs and attitudes about cancer and cancer screening. For example, despite the striking age-related increase in cancer incidence, many older persons paradoxically perceive less susceptibility to cancer, and this belief has been associated with lower levels of screening (65,70,74–78).

The elderly also generally express more fatalistic views of cancer (27,47,77). Focus groups, for instance, discovered that most older Americans viewed cancers in a worst case scenario, associated with radical and painful treatments, usually fatal, and accompanied by a greatly feared dependency on others. There was very little distinction made between early and late stage disease. Cancer cures were instead attributed more often to luck or personal character traits rather than early detection with screening.

Empiric studies have found a number of negative attitudes about cancer screening that are held more frequently by the elderly. These include greater worries about radiation/safety of mammography (73,74), a greater reliance on symptoms to find cancer rather than asymptomatic detection with screening (47,67,76, 77,79), lower perceived efficacy of screening (73), less concern about cancer prevention compared to current medical problems (47,75), and greater embarrassment with screening (80,82). Older men generally report more negative views about the role of prevention, are less likely to report symptoms, and report avoiding contact with physicians if possible (83).

Although the elderly possess a great many negative cancer screening attitudes their effects on screening compliance can be moderated by other factors. Social support, for example, has been shown to greatly limit the negative effects of fear/anxiety on cancer screening (84,85). A physician's firm recommendation for screening will also likely overcome most negative health beliefs and attitudes (86). Most studies have indeed found that the effects of patient attitudes on screening are modest when compared to physician input (68).

It is not clear why the elderly possess more negative views about cancer and screening. Some of these views may be the result of a cohort effect. Most elderly patients have lived much of their lives during a time when cancer treatments were generally unsuccessful, cancer was often fatal, and the potential for early detection with screening had not been realized. It is not surprising, therefore, that their experiences with cancer would be less positive than younger patients. The elderly's perception that they are less susceptible to cancer may be a result of the failure to target screening educational programs to the elderly. Until recently, for instance, most breast cancer media promotions typically featured young women undergoing screening, leaving the impression that they were most vulnerable (87). Finally, some waning of interest in cancer screening may be appropriate for persons with poor health status and other pressing health concerns. More research is needed into the effects of health status on cancer screening.

Physician Attitudes and Beliefs

Physician attitudes and beliefs about preventive medicine and the elderly may in part be responsible for their acknowledged underscreening of older persons. Physicians (and others) generally underestimate the life expectancy of older Americans (42). For example, the average life expectancy of a 65 year old woman is 18 years, for a 75 year old woman 12 years, and for an 85 year old woman 7 years (88). If physicians perceive a limited life expectancy with poor quality of life for their elderly patients they would understandably have less enthusiasm for preventive interventions. Although changing, medical education has also traditionally provided a strong disease orientation and has not emphasized preventive care (89). All of these factors may make prevention in general a low priority for physicians who care for older patients.

Screening is also impacted to a great extent by the uncertainty of guidelines for older Americans. In addition, physicians recognize that the elderly population is quite heterogenous with respect to health status, comorbidity, and quality of life. Patients likely differ in their preferences for screening, and their willingness to follow-up and treat abnormalities. Clearly these issues need to be discussed prior to undertaking screening interventions but unfortunately this makes screening a more time consuming and complicated endeavor. Physicians also have no simple methods to assess life expectancy and functional life expectancy to assist in these decisions (90).

Physicians' screening recommendations are also likely influenced by their perceptions of patients' attitudes and beliefs. For example, physicians report that their elderly patients are less interested in preventive care compared to care for their acute and chronic medical problems (27). During focus group discussions they also report that their patients find many screening tests unpleasant, or embarrassing (28). Physicians believe that older patients do not expect certain screening tests to be done (digital rectal examination) and are more likely to refuse cancer screening recommendations (91).

On a positive note, primary care physicians do have some very encouraging attitudes about cancer screening in general. They overwhelmingly know and support ACS guidelines, often in preference to less aggressive guidelines like the US Preventive Services Task Force (92–94). They also believe cancer screening is effective (28,91) and express strong interest in cancer screening education (95). Also, although the yield of cancer screening is generally low in a typical primary care practice its emotional impact can be substantial. During focus groups, physicians report being affected greatly by the diagnosis of an early cancer by screening and also are quite effected by caring for cancer patients with terminal disease. Diagnosing cancer is likely a critical event for physicians.

Cancer screening attitudes are not uniform among primary care physicians. Most studies, for instance, have shown less favorable attitudes about cancer screening among older physicians. It is unclear if this is the result of a cohort effect reflecting training differences of younger and older physicians. It is also possible that attitudes about the value of preventive services change as physicians age or assume care for an older patient population. Although some studies have suggested gender differences in physicians preventive care, gender differences have not been apparent for older patients.

Community-Based Barriers to Screening

Office Interventions

Even physicians with a very strong commitment to screening must overcome a number of barriers, including remembering to offer screening, finding adequate time during patient encounters, and the many logistical problems of screening. A fairly substantial gap between physicians intentions to screen and actual screening rates are usually reported (40). A large number of interventions have been conducted to improve cancer screening in the primary care setting. Interventions have been directed at primary care physicians, their patients, and their staff.

Physician-directed interventions have included health promotion checklists, flow sheets, and chart tags that serve as reminders for screening (96–101). These reminder systems increase screening rates by attempting to focus attention to selected cancer screening tests. In general such reminders are effective especially when directed at a small number of screening tests. They are less effective when directed at multiple screening tests with some studies finding that non-targeted screening tests may actually decrease. Clearly physicians cannot focus their attention on all screening interventions.

Chart audit of screening compliance with feedback of screening rates to individual physicians has also been successfully used (102,103). Finally computer-generated reminders have been studied extensively (103–109). These interventions have generally shown greater increases in screening rates than chart reminders, and when directed at multiple screening tests have produced more uniform effects. Computer reminders were more cost-effective than audit with feedback (110). Patient interventions that have been found to be effective include mailed reminder postcards/letters (101,103,106,111,112), history/risk factor questionnaires (109), and patient-held minirecords (115,116). Telephone calls have not been found to be particularly effective (106,111). Interventions targeted at both physicians and patients (physician computer reminders and patient letter or postcard) have also been effective, and have generally shown additive effects (115–117). Several interventions have been directed at office nursing staff and have been effective at increasing rates of breast and colorectal screening (119–122).

Although all of the above interventions have been successful to some extent, the long-term durability of their effects is not known. One would expect effects to wane over time as the novelty of reminder systems wears off (123).

Community Interventions

A number of community-based interventions to promote cancer screening have been conducted (124–136). Most have studied breast and cervical cancer screening. Strategies to promote screening have generally been multifaceted including efforts to educate and persuade primary care physicians to increase screening (CME, newsletters), efforts to educate/motivate women (posters, brochures, direct mailings, mass media, church/work-site programs, use of celebrities and volunteers), and efforts to overcome logistic/access barriers (mobile vans, on site nurse practitioners, reminder systems, office staff training, subsidizing screening costs). The details of NCI-funded community interventions have recently been summarized (137).

Several conclusions can be drawn from these trials. First multistrategy interventions have generally been more successful than more limited interventions. It is also clear that eliminating the costs of screening without addressing other barriers has not proven successful (33). Finally, well structured community intervention have increased screening rates in an impressive variety of patient care settings, including HMOs, public hospital clinics, community health centers, and private physicians' offices, and for patients of varied ethnicities, and socioeconomic status.

Several questions regarding community interventions remain unanswered. The cost effectiveness of community interventions in general has not been established nor have individual strategies been compared with respect to their cost-effectiveness. Although community interventions have proven their effectiveness in research settings, it is also not always clear how they can be implemented in settings where resources are more limited, and specialized personnel are lacking.

Conclusions

Following are practice-based suggestions to reduce barriers to cancer prevention in the older person.

Demographic Barriers and Suggestions for Improvement:

The following patient groups need special encouragement by clinicians if there is to be more equity in screening rates: older persons, especially over age 74; non-white patients, especially those who are non-English speaking; and poverty-level and lower-education persons. In addition:

- Opposite gender (to physicians) patients should be treated with age-appropriate screening practices, in spite of any clinician embarrassment.
- The number of quality years of life expectancy that older, still healthy, patients can expect is often underestimated; health status, instead of chronological age, should be the best indicator of whether to refer patients for prevention services.
- Older people are not homogeneous. Not only do they differ in personalities, they also differ by age groups. All 65 and over people are often viewed as similar when in fact 65 year olds are quite different in co-morbidities and other problems from 85 year olds.
- Problems with aging should not be assumed to be automatic with all aged patients even though there will often be increased medical difficulties with patient aging, which needs to be inquired about.

Communication Barriers and Suggestions for Improvement:

- Taking more initiative and asking patients about their concerns at the beginning of the visit will facilitate older patients getting their needs met. Likewise, patients should learn to be more verbally assertive about the reasons for the visit at its beginning.
- Compliance with screening guidelines is likely to suffer if their mention is not easily recalled by patients or reinforced with printed matter provided by the physician's office.
- Physicians who treat older patients would be more effective if patient fears about cancer were directly addressed by their physicians.
- Physicians have enormous influence over their older patient's behaviors, even their screening behaviors;

cancer screening compliance rates can be increased significantly through a more direct physician communication of their wants for their patients, e.g., that they want their patients to get screened for cancer.

- The way in which clinicians encourage patient behavior makes a difference in whether patients respond; physicians can enjoy an increased level of screening by their patients if physicians recommend screening with enthusiasm.

Knowledge Barriers And Suggestions For Improvement:

- Knowledge levels of risk factors, awareness of screening procedures, and knowledge of screening guidelines are all predictors of higher levels of screening compliance. These issues should be reviewed with older patients. Ideally, patients should leave each visit with printed matter that reinforces verbal instructions.

Attitudinal Barriers And Suggestions For Improvement:

- Physician's enthusiasm for screening can be very effective in overcoming the older person's pessimism regarding survival from a cancer diagnosis and accompanying pessimism regarding cancer screening.
- Survey research and focus groups suggest that older persons are generally very receptive to getting regular screening. Thus, providers should not assume that older patients will resist screening recommendations.

Community Barriers And Suggestions For Improvements:

- Physician and patient reminders regarding screening tests improve compliance.
- Multiple barriers, e.g., reduction of screening costs and anxiety about a finding, etc., to screening need attention in order to increase patient compliance with screening.

Acknowledgements

This investigation was supported in part by the National Cancer Institute (NCI#SROlCA6587 and NCI#ROlCA65880) to S.A.F, the Health Resources Services Administration (#2T32PE19001) to R.G.R., and the National Institute on Aging (NIA#SP20AG12059) to R.S.K. The authors acknowledge the assistance of Sarah Connor and Robin Grant in the preparation of this manuscript.

References

1. Andersen R, Newman JF. Societal and individual determinants of medical care utilization in the United States. *Milbank Memorial Fund Q* 1973; **51**(1): 95–124.
2. Hayward RSA, Steinberg EP, Ford DE, Roizen MF, Roach KW. Preventive care guidelines. *Ann Intern Med* 1991; **114**(9): 758–783.
3. Sox HC. Preventive health services in adults. *N Eng J Med* 1994; **330**(22): 1589–1595.
4. Glober GA, Hundahl S, Stucke J, Choy M. Fecal occult blood testing for colorectal cancer in an ethnically diverse population. *West J Med* 1994; **161**(4): 377–382.
5. Cummings MK, Michalek A, Tidings J, Herrera L, Mettlin C. Results of a public screening program for colorectal cancer. *NY State J Med* Feb 1986; **86**: 68–72.
6. McGarrity TJ, Long PA, Peiffer LP. Results of a repeat television-advertised mass screening program for colorectal cancer using fecal occult blood tests. *Am J Gastroenterology* 1990; **85**(3): 266–270.
7. Chang FC, Jackson TM, Jackson CR. Hemoccult screening for colorectal cancer. *Am J Surgery* 1988; **156**: 457–459.
8. Thomas W, White CM, Mah J, Geisser MS; Church TR, Mandel JS. Longitudinal compliance with annual screening for fecal occult blood. *Am J Epidemiology* 1995; **142**: 176–82.
9. Breen N and Kessler L. *Mortality and Morbidity Weekly Report*, [In Press], 1996.
10. Fox SA and Roetzheim RG. Screening mammography and older Hispanic women. Current status and issues. *Cancer* 1994; **74**: 2028–2033.
11. Hayward RA, Shapiro MF, Freeman HE, Corey CR. Who gets screened for cervical and breast cancer. Results from a New National Survey. *Arch Intern Med* 1988; **148**: 1177–1181.
12. Makuc DM, Fried VM, Kleinman JC. National trends in the use of preventive health care by women. *Am J Public Health* 1989; **79**(1): 21–26.
13. Harlan LC, Bernstein AB, Kessler LG. Cervical cancer screening: who is not screened and why? *Am J Public Health* 1991; **81**(7): 885–890.
14. Stein JA and Fox SA. Language preference as an indicator of mammography usage among Hispanic women. *J Natl Cancer Inst* 1990; **82**: 1715–1716.
15. Fox SA, Murata PJ, Stein JA. The impact of physician compliance on screening mammography for older women. *Arch Intern Med* 1991; **151**: 50–56.
16. Caplan LS, Wells BL, Haynes S. Breast cancer screening among older racial/ethnic minorities and whites barriers to early detection. *J Gerontolo* 1992; **47**(Special Issue): 101–110.
17. Escarce JJ Epstein KR, Colby DC, Schwartz JS. Racial differences in the elderly's use of medical procedures and diagnostic tests. *Am J Public Health* 1993; **83**(7): 948–954.
18. Breen N. Tabulations communicated to S.A.F. 1995.
19. Bostick RM, Sprafka JM, Virnig BA, Potter JD. Predictors of cancer prevention attitudes and participation in cancer screening examinations. *Prev Med* 1994; **23**: 816–826.
20. Bryant H and Mah Z. Breast cancer screening attitudes and behaviors of rural and urban women. *Prev Med* 1992; **21**: 405–418.
21. Breen N and Kessler L. Changes in the use of screening mammography. Evidence from the 1987 and 1990 National Health Interview Surveys. *Am J Public Health* 1994; **84**: 62–670.
22. Woolhandler S and Himmelstein D. Reverse targeting of preventive care due to lack of health insurance. *JAMA* 1988; **259**: 2872–2874.
23. Kirkman-Liff B and Kronenfeld J. Access to cancer screening services for women. *Am J Public Health* 1992; **82**: 733–735.
24. Ayanian J, Kohler B, Abe T, Epstein A. The relation between health insurance coverage and clinical outcomes among women with breast cancer. *N Engl J Med* 1993; **329**: 326–331.
25. Blustein J. Medicare coverage, supplemental insurance, the use of mammography by older women. *N Engl J Med* 1995; **332**: 1138–43.
26. Morrissey J, Harris R, Kincade-Norburn J, *et al.* Medicare reimbursement for preventive care. Changes in performance of services, quality of life, health care costs. *Med Care* 1995; **33**: 315–31.
27. Zapka J and Berkowitz E. A qualitative study about breast cancer screening in older women. Implications for research. *J Gerontolo* 1992; **47**(Supplement): 93–100.
28. Montano D, Manders D, Phillips W. Family physician beliefs about cancer screening. Development of a survey instrument. *J Fam Pract* 1990; **30**: 313–9.

29. Frame P. Breast cancer screening in older women. The family practice perspective. *J Gerontolo* 1992; **47**(supplement): 131–3.
30. Coleman EA, Feuer EJ, The NCI Breast Cancer Screening Consortium. Breast cancer screening among women 65–74 years of age in 1987–88 and 1991. *Ann Intern Med* 1992; **117**: 961–966.
31. Burg M and Lane D. Mammography referrals for elderly women. Is Medicare reimbursement likely to make a difference? *Health Ser Res* 1992; **27**: 505–516.
32. Urban N, erson G, Peacock S. Mammography screening. How important is cost as a barrier to use? *Am J Public Health* 1994; **84**: 50–5.
33. Rimer BK, Resch N, King E, Ross E, Lerman C, Boyce A, Kessler H, Engstrom PF. Multistrategy health education program to increase mammography use among women ages 65 and older. *Pub Health Reports* 1992; **107**(4): 369–80.
34. Katz S and Hofer T. Socioeconomic disparities in preventive care persist despite universal coverage. Breast and cervical cancer screening in Ontario and the United States. *JAMA* 1994; **272**: 530–4.
35. Bernstein A, Thompson G, Harlan L. Differences in rates of cancer screening by usual source of medical care. *Med Care* 1991; **29**: 196–209.
36. Zapka J, Hosmer D, Costanza M, Harris D, Stoddard A. Changes in mammography use. Economic, need, service factors. *Am J Public Health* 1992; **82**: 1345–1351.
37. Riley G, Potosky A, Lubitz J, Brown M. Stage of cancer at diagnosis of Medicare, HMO and fee-for-service enrollees. *Am J Public Health* 1994; **84**: 1598–1604.
38. Beisecker AE. Older patients and their doctors. University of Kansas Medical Center. Commissioned by the National Institute on Aging (Annotated bibliography); 1995.
39. Beisecker AE. Older patients and their doctors. University of Kansas Medical Center (unpublished and commissioned by the National Institute of Aging); 1995.
40. Roetzheim R, Fox S, Leake B. Physician-reported determinants of screening mammography in older women. The impact of physician and practice characteristics. *J Am Geriatr Soc* 1995; **43**: 1–5.
41. Levy S, Dowling P, Boult L, Monroe A, McQuade W. The effect of physician and patient gender on preventive medicine practices in patients older than fifty. *Fam Med* 1992; **24**: 58–61.
42. Weinberger M, Saunders AF, Samsa GP, Bearon LB, Gold GT, Brown JT, Booher P, Lowehrer PJ. Breast cancer screening in older women. Practices and barriers reported by primary care physicians. *J Am Geriatr Soc* 1991; **39**: 22–29.
43. Erber NP. Communicating with elders. Effects of amplification. *J Gerontolo Nursing* 1994; **20**: 6–10.
44. Rost K and Frankel R. The introduction of the older patient's problems in the medical visit. *J Health and Aging*, 1993.
45. Adelman RD, Greene MG, Charon R, Friedmann E. The content of physician and elderly patient interaction in the medical primary care encounter. *Comm Res* 1992; **19**: 370–380.
46. Greene MG, Adelman RD, Charon R, Friedmann E. Concordance between physicians and their older and younger patients in the primary care medical encounter. *Gerontolo Soc Am* 1989; **29**: 808–813.
47. Sutton S, Eisner E, Burklow J. Health communications to older Americans as a special population. The National Cancer Institute's consumer-based approach. *Cancer* 1994; **74**: 2194–9.
48. Adelman RD, Greene MG, Charon R. Issues in the physician-elderly patient interaction. *Aging and Society* 1991; **2**: 127–148.
49. Street RL. Information-giving in medical consultations. The influence of patients' communicative styles and personal characteristics. *Soc Sci Med* 1991; **32**: 541–548.
50. Beisecker AE. Aging and the desire for information and input in medical decisions. Patient consumerism in medical encounters. *The Gerontologist* 1988; **28**: 330–335.
51. Kreps GL. A systematic analysis of health communication with the aged. In *Communication, Health and the Elderly*, edited by H Giles, N Coupland, JM Wuemann. London: Manchester University Press, 135–154, 1990.
52. Waitzkin H. Information giving in medical care. *J Health Soc Behavior* 1985; **26**: 81–101.
53. Fox SF. unpublished, Los Angeles data, 1995.
54. Sladden MJ and Dickinson JA. General practitioners' attitudes to screening for prostate and testicular cancers. *Med J Australia* 1995; **162**(8): 410–3.
55. Paine SL, Cockburn J, Noy SM and Marks R. Early detection of skin cancer. Knowledge, perceptions and practices of general practitioners in Victoria. *Med J of Australia* 1994; **161**(3): 188–9,192–5.
56. Mamon JA, Shediac MC, Crosby CB, Sanders B, Matanoski GM, Celentano DD. Inner city women at risk for cervical cancer. behavioral and utilization factors related to inadequate screening. *Prev Med* 1990; **19**(4): 363–76.
57. Mandelblatt J, Traxler M, Lakin P, Kanetsky P and Kao R. Mammography and Papanicolaou smear use by elderly poor black women. The Harlem Study Team. *J Am Geriatri Soc* 1992; **40**(10): 1001–7.
58. Champion VL. Compliance with guidelines for mammography screening. *Cancer Detection and Prevention* 1992; **16**(4): 253–8.
59. Fox SA, Siu AL and Stein JA. The importance of physician communication on breast cancer screening of older women. *Arch Intern Med* 1994; **154**: 2058–2068.
60. Beisecker AE. The influence of a companion on the doctor-elderly patient interaction. *Health Comm* 1989; **1**: 55–70.
61. Coe RM. Communication and medical care outcomes. Analysis of conversations between doctors and elderly patients. In *Health in Aging*, edited by RA Ward, SS Tobin. New York: Springer, 1987.
62. Fox SA, Klos DS, Tsou CV and Baum JK. Breast cancer screening recommendations. Current status of women's knowledge. *Fam Comm Health* 1987; **10**(3): 39–50.
63. Richardson A. Factors likely to affect participation in mammographic screening. *New Zealand Med J* 1990; **103**(887): 155–6.
64. Harris RP, Fletcher SW, Gonzalez JJ, Lannin DR, Degnan D, Earp JA, Clark R. Mammography and age: are we targeting the wrong women? A community survey of women and physicians. *Cancer* 1991; **67**(7): 2010–4.
65. Mah Z and Bryant H. Age as a factor in breast cancer knowledge, attitudes and screening behavior. *Can Med Assoc J* 1992; **146**(12): 2167–74.
66. Ruiz MS, Marks G and Richardson JL. Language acculturation and screening practices of elderly Hispanic women. The role of exposure to health-related information from the media. *J Aging and Health* 1992; **4**(2): 268–81.
67. Perez-Stable EJ, Sabogal F, Otero-Sabogal R, Hiatt RA, McPhee SJ. Misconceptions about cancer among Latinos and Anglos. *JAMA* 1992; **268**(22): 3219–23.
68. Montano D and Taplin S. A test of an expanded theory of reasoned action predict mammography participation. *Soc Sci Med* 1991; **32**: 733–741.
69. Stein J, Fox S, Murata P, Morisky D. Mammography usage and the health belief model. *Health Educ Q* 1992; **19**: 1–16.
70. Aiken L, West S, Woodward C, Reno R. Health beliefs and compliance with mammography-screening recommendations in asymptomatic women. *Health Psychol* 1994; **12**: 122–9.
71. Hyman R, Baker S, Ephraim R, Moadel A, Philip J. Health belief model variables as predictors of screening mammography utilization. *J Beh Med* 1994; **17**: 391–406.
72. O'Connor A and Perrault D. Importance of physician's role highlighted in survey of women's breast screening practices. *Can J Public Health* 1995; **86**: 42–5.
73. Taplin S and Montano D. Attitudes, age, participation in mammographic screening. A prospective analysis. *J Am Board Fam Pract* 1993; **6**: 612–23.
74. Vernon S, Vogel V, Halabi S, Jackson G, Lundy R, Peters G. Breast cancer screening behaviors and attitudes in three racial/ethnic groups. *Cancer* 1992; **69**: 165–74.
75. Burg M, Lane D, Polednak A. Age group differences in the use of breast cancer screening tests. *J Aging Health* 1990; **2**: 514–30.
76. Costanza M, Stoddard A, Gaw V, Zapka J. The risk factors of age and family history and their relationship to screening mammography utilization. *J Am Geriatr Soc* 1992; **40**: 774–778.
77. King E, Resch N, Rimer B, Lerman C, Boyce A, McGovern-Gorchov P. Breast cancer screening practices among retirement community women. *Prev Med* 1993; **22**: 1–19.

78. Lerman C, Rimer B, Trock B, Balshem A, Engstrom P. Factors associated with repeat adherence to breast cancer screening. *Prev Med* 1990; **19**: 279–290.

79. Rimer B, Keintz M, Kessler H, Engstrom P, Rosan J. Why women resist screening mammography. Patient related barriers. *Radiology* 1989; **172**: 243–246.

80. Burack R and Liang J. The acceptance and completion of mammography by older black women. *Am J Public Health* 1989; **4**: 721–726.

81. Richardson J, Marks G, Solis J, Collins L, Birba L, Hisserich J. Frequency and adequacy of breast cancer screening among elderly Hispanic women. *Prev Med* 1987; **16**: 761–774.

82. Morisky D, Fox S, Murata P, Stein J. The role of needs assessment in designing a community-based mammography education program for urban women. *Health Educ Res* 1989; **4**: 469–478.

83. Greg G and Goys J. Men's health project focus groups reports. Washington, DC: American Association of Retired Persons, 1994.

84. Suarez L, Lloyd L, Weiss N, Rainbolt T, Pulley L. Effect of social networks on cancer screening behavior of older Mexican-American women. *J Natl Cancer Inst* 1994; **86**: 775

85. Kang S and Bloom J. Social support and cancer screening among older black Americans. *J Natl Cancer Inst* 1993; **85**: 737–742.

86. Slenker S and Grant M. Attitudes, beliefs and knowledge about mammography among women over forty years of age. *J Cancer Educ* 1989; **4**: 61–65.

87. Roetzheim R, Van DD, Brownlee H, *et al.* Reverse targeting in a media-promoted breast cancer screening project. *Cancer:* 1992; **70**: 1152–1158.

88. Costanza M. The extent of breast cancer screening in older women. *Cancer* 1994; **74**(Supplement): 2046–50.

89. Williams P and Williams M. Barriers and incentives for primary care physicians in cancer prevention and detection. *Cancer* 1988; **61**: 2382–2390.

90. Cohen H. Breast cancer screening in older women. The geriatrician/internist perspective. *J Gerontolo* 1992; **47**: 134–6.

91. Clasen C, Vernon S, Mullen P, Jackson G. A survey of physician belief and self-reported practices concerning screening for early detection of cancer. *Soc Sci Med* 1994; **39**: 841–9.

92. Czaja R, McFall S, Warnecke R, Ford L, Kaluzny A. Preferences of community physicians for cancer screening guidelines. *Ann Intern Med* 1994; **120**: 602–8.

93. Weinberger M, Saunders A, Bearon L, *et al.* Physician-related barriers to breast cancer screening in older women. *J Gerontol:* 1992; **47**: 111–117.

94. Stange K, Kelly R, Chao J, *et al.* Physician agreement with US Preventive Services Task Force recommendations. *J Fam Pract* 1992; **34**: 409–16.

95. Warner S, Worden J, Solomon L, Wadland W. Physician interest in breast cancer screening education. *J Fam Pract* 1989; **29**: 281–285.

96. Cohen D, Littenberg B, Wetzel C, Neuhauser D. Improving physician compliance with preventive medicine guidelines. *Med Care* 1982; **20**: 1040–5.

97. Prislin M, Vandenbark M, Clarkson Q. The impact of health screening flow sheet on the performance and documentation of health screening procedures. *Fam Med* 1986; **18**: 290–2.

98. Cheney C and Ramsdell J. Effect of medical records' checklists on implementation of periodic health measures. *Am J Med* 1987; **83**: 129–36.

99. Schreiner D, Petrusa E, Rettie C, Kluge R. Improving compliance with preventive medicine procedures in a housestaff training program. *South Med J* 1988; **81**: 1553–7.

100. Robie P. Improving and sustaining outpatient cancer screening by medicine residents. *South Med J* 1988; **81**: 902–5.

101. Pierce M, Lundy S, Palanisamy A, Winning S, King J. Prospective randomized controlled trials of methods of call and recall for cervical cytology screening. *Br Med J* 1989; **299**: 160–2.

102. Winickoff R, Coltin K, Morgan M, Buxbaum R, Barnett G. Improving performance through peer comparison feedback. *Med Care* 1984; **22**: 527–34.

103. McPhee S, Bird J, Jenkins C, Fordham D. Promoting cancer screening. A randomized, controlled trials of three interventions. *Arch Intern Med* 1989; **149**: 1866–1872.

104. McDonald C, Hui S, Smith D, *et al.* Reminders to physicians from an introspective computer medical record a two-year randomized trial. *Ann Intern Med* 1984; **100**: 130–8.

105. Tierney W, Hui S, McDonald C. Delayed feedback of physician performance vs. immediate reminders to perform preventive care. *Med Care* 1986; **24**: 659–66.

106. McDowell I, Newell C, Rosser N. Computerized reminders to encourage cervical screening in family practice. *J Fam Pract* 1989; **28**: 420–4.

107. Chambers C, Balaban D, Carlson B, Ungemack H, Grasberger D. Microcomputer generated reminders. Improving the compliance of primary care physicians with mammography screening guidelines. *J Fam Pract* 1989; **29**: 273–280.

108. Chodroff C. Cancer screening and immunization quality assurance using personal computer. *QRB Qual Rev Bull* 1990; **16**: 279–87.

109. Turner B, Day S, Borenstein B. A controlled trial to improve delivery of preventive care. Physician or patient reminders? *J Gen Intern Med* 1989; **4**: 403–9.

110. Bird J, McPhee S, Jenkins C, Fordham D. Three strategies to promote cancer screening. How feasible is wide-scale implementation? *Med Care* 1990; **28**: 1005–1012.

111. Petravage J and Swedberg J. Patient response to sigmoidoscopy recommendations via mailed reminders. *J Fam Pract* 1988; **27**: 387–9.

112. Wolosin R. Effect of appointment scheduling and reminder postcards on adherence to mammography recommendations. *J Fam Pract* 1990; **30**: 542–7.

113. Dioptric A and Duhamel M. Improving geriatric preventive care through a patient-held checklist. *Fam Med* 1989; **21**: 195–8.

114. Dickey L and Petitti D. A patient-held minirecord to promote adult preventive care. *J Fam Pract* 1992; **34**: 457–63.

115. Nattinger A, Panzer R, Janus J. Improving the utilization of screening mammography in primary care practices. *Arch Intern Med* 1989; **149**: 2087–2092.

116. McPhee S, Bird J, Fordham D, Rodnick J, Osborn E. Promoting cancer prevention activities by primary care physicians. *JAMA* 1991; **266**: 538–544.

117. Becker D, Gomez E, Kaiser D, Yoshihasi A, Hodge R. Improving preventive care at a medical clinic. How can the patient help? *Am J Prev Med* 1989; **5**: 353–9.

118. Ornstein S, Garr D, Jenkins R, Rust P, Arnon A. Computer-generated physician and patient reminders. Tools to improve population adherence to selected preventive services. *J Fam Pract* 1991; **32**: 82–90.

119. Davidson R, Fletcher S, Retchin S, Duh S. A nurse-initiated reminder system for the periodic health examination. Implementation and evaluation. *Arch Intern Med* 1984; **144**: 2167–70.

120. Thompson R, Michnich M, Gray J, Friedlander L, Gilson B. Maximizing compliance with Hemoccult screening for colon cancer in clinical practice. *Med Care* 1986; **24**: 904–14.

121. Belcher D. Implementing preventive services. Success and failure in an outpatient trial. *Arch Intern Med* 1990; **150**: 2533–41.

122. Foley E, D'Amico F, Merenstein J. Improving mammography recommendation. A nurse-initiated intervention. *J Am Board Fam Pract* 1990; **3**: 87–92.

123. Dioptric A, Sox C, Tosteson T, Woodruff C. Durability of improved physician early detection of cancer after conclusion of intervention support. *Cancer Epidemiol Biomarkers Prev* 1994; **3**: 335–40.

124. Suarez L, Nichols D, Brady C. Use of peer role models to increase Pap smear and mammogram screening in Mexican-American and black women. *Am J Prev Med* 1993; **9**: 290–6.

125. Herman C, Speroff T, Cebul R. Improving compliance with breast cancer screening in older women. Results of a randomized controlled trial. *Arch Intern Med* 1995; **155**: 717–22.

126. Lantz P, Stencil D, Lippert M, Beversdorf S, Jaros L. Breast and cervical cancer screening in a low-income managed care sample. The efficacy of physician letters and phone calls. *Am J Public Health* 1995; **85**: 834–6.

127. Costanza M, Zapka J, Harris D, *et al.* Impact of a physician intervention program to increase breast cancer screening. *Cancer Epidemiol Biomarkers Prev* 1992; **1**: 581–589.

128. Trock B, Rimer B, King E, Balshem A, Cristinzio C, Engstrom P. Impact of an HMO based intervention to increase mammography utilization. *Cancer Epidemiol Biomark Prev* 1993; **2**: 151–6.

129. Zapka J, Harris D, Hosmer D, Costanza M, Mas E, Barth R. Effect of a community health center intervention on breast cancer screening among Hispanic American women. *Health Ser Res* 1993; **28**: 223–235.

130. Lane D, Polednak A, Burg M. Effect of continuing medical education and cost reduction on physician compliance with mammography screening guidelines. *J Fam Pract* 1991; **33**: 359–368.

131. Mandelblatt J, Traxler M, Lakin P, *et al*. A nurse practitioner intervention to increase breast and cervical cancer screening for poor, elderly, black women. The Harlem Study Team. *J Gen Intern Med* 1993; **8**: 173–8.

132. Metcher S, Harris R, Gonzalez J, *et al*. Increasing mammography utilization. A controlled study. *J Natl Cancer Inst* 1993; **85**: 112–120.

133. Forsyth M, Fulton D, Lane D, Burg M, Krishna M. Changes in knowledge, attitudes and behavior of women participating in a community outreach education program on breast cancer screening. *Patient Education Counseling* 1992; **19**: 241–50.

134. Zapka J, Costanza M, Harris D, *et al*. Impact of a breast cancer screening community intervention. *Prev Med* 1993; **22**: 34–53.

135. Bastani R, Marcus A, Maxwell A, Das I, Yan K. Evaluation of an intervention to increase mammography screening in Los Angeles. *Prev Med* 1994; **23**: 83–90.

136. Lane D and Burg M. Strategies to increase mammography utilization among community health center visitors. Improving awareness, accessibility, affordability. *Med Care* 1993; **31**: 175–81.

137. Haynes S and Mara J. The picture of health. How to increase breast cancer screening in your community. *National Cancer Institute No. 94–3604*, 1993.

26. Management of Cancer in the Older Person

Lodovico Balducci, Charles E. Cox, Harvey Greenberg, Gary H. Lyman,
Rafael Miguel, Richard Karl and Peter J. Fabri

Introduction

The management of cancer in the older person is an increasingly common aspect of oncologic practice (1). The central questions concern effectiveness and safety of antineoplastic therapy, clinical criteria to identify patients who may benefit from treatment, and individualized management plans. To address these questions, we review the influence of age on various forms of cancer treatment, explore the basis of treatment-related decisions in older persons with cancer, and propose areas for future investigation. Age itself is not a contraindication to cancer treatment. Individualized treatment plans, based on appropriate diagnosis, staging, and comprehensive geriatric assessment, are most beneficial to the older patients.

Cancer Treatment and Aging

Surgery

The mortality and perioperative morbidity of elective surgical oncologic procedures are little affected by patient age (2). Our review of the records of 70 patients who have undergone major surgical procedures over the past five years at the Moffitt Cancer Center shows that the mortality, length of stay, length of procedure, estimated blood loss, and major complication rate for all patients undergoing Whipple operations, major liver resections, and esophagogastrectomy were similar for patients aged 70 years and over and for younger patients, with the exception of the complication rate of liver resection, which was higher among older persons (55% vs 14%). While age itself is not a risk factor, other factors of comorbidity, such as cardiopulmonary dysfunction and malnutrition, may increase with the age of the patient and may inhibit appropriate surgical treatment of cancer (3).

For a cancer patient undergoing emergency surgery, the risk of death and surgical complications increases dramatically with the patient's age (2). The major cause of mortality is sepsis. The increased risk of surgical complications is not surprising in the emergency situation as age is associated with a progressive decline in the functional reserve of major organ systems, and the ability of older persons to cope with physical stress is consequently more limited.

One may postulate that the success of cancer surgery in the older person is determined largely by the previous commitment of that person to health maintenance. In addition to regular physician visits, this commitment includes regular exercise, abstinence from smoking and drugs, adequate nutrition, avoidance of unnecessary medication, and cancer screening (4). Early diagnosis of cancer can avoid the complications of emergency surgery.

Recent innovations in anesthesia and in surgery may be particularly beneficial to older patients Cox et al. (5) confirmed that breast cancer surgery can successfully be accomplished on an outpatient basis under local anesthesia. Modified radical mastectomies or lumpectomies with complete axillary dissection to level III lymph nodes were performed in 20 patients, using local anesthetic, with monitored anesthetic techniques. The mean age of the group was 76 ± 14 years, and 15 patients were aged 65 to 95 years. Six patients had significant comorbid conditions, which either contraindicated general anesthesia or would have altered the outcome if surgery could not be done with local anesthetics. These conditions included three cases of congestive heart failure, severe pulmonary disease, recent myocardial infarction, and Alzheimer's disease. The remaining 14 patients elected local anesthesia as a personal preference. The only complication of surgery was a hematoma in one wound, requiring reoperation under local anesthesia.

Epidural anesthesia during abdominal surgery lessens the surgical stress and limits considerably the intensity and the risks of general anesthesia (6,7). Yaeger et al. (8) compared general anesthesia with and without epidural anesthesia in abdominal surgery. The rate of lethal and nonlethal complications declined with epidural anesthesia.

Important surgical advances include modification of current surgical techniques, endoscopic surgery, and stereotactic surgery. There has been a consistent trend toward limiting the extent of surgical resections. Examples of this trend include partial mastectomy for breast cancer, low anterior resection for rectal cancer, and the adoption of small (1 cm) skin margins for malignant melanoma (9,10). Endoscopic surgery can allow palliation of some tumors of the digestive tract and of the urinary bladder with minimal morbidity. In the case of small lesions, endoscopic surgery may even be curative (11). Stereotactic techniques have made possible the biopsy and the resection of small tumors in previously inaccessible regions of the brain (12). Stereotactic breast biopsy of mammographic lesions can be performed as an outpatient procedure in all ages, and this approach has reduced the need for operative management for diagnosis. Progress in endoscopic and stereotactic surgery is in part due to safer and more effective laser beams (11).

Radiation Therapy

One of the traditional roles of radiation therapy has been the management of resectable cancer in patients who have a high risk of morbidity or mortality from surgery. In some conditions, such as early prostate cancer, the outcomes of surgery and radiation therapy for local control are comparable (13). Radiation therapy may have an increased role in the management of older persons, whose comorbidity represents an elevated surgical risk. Several studies attest to the safety of radiation therapy for cancer in the aged. Wyckoff *et al.* (14) compared the total dose of radiation, the number of treatment interruptions, and the incidence of soft tissue complications among women aged 65 years and younger and among older women receiving irradiation of the breast after partial mastectomy. Radiation therapy was equally well tolerated by women of all ages. Casey *et al.* (15) studied the tolerance of radiation therapy by 44 patients aged 80 years and older receiving treatment for cancer of the upper aerodigestive tract, the chest and the pelvis. Of these, only five patients failed to complete treatment. All other patients received the planned dose of radiation, without delay and with minimal morbidity. Radiation therapy to the pelvis was tolerated less well by older patients, with the most common complications being mucositis and diarrhea.

Aging in experimental animals is associated with increased proliferation of the epithelial cells of the digestive mucosa and by depletion of the mucosal stem cells (16). These changes may make the mucosa of older individuals particularly vulnerable to cell-cycle-active treatment, such as radiation therapy and chemotherapy. The risk of mucositis may be minimized by reducing the fractional dose of radiation, while timely hospitalization and aggressive fluid resuscitation are effective in reversing the complications of mucositis. Of special interest to older individuals, Casey *et al.* (17) demonstrated that the malnutrition complicating irradiation of the upper airways and the chest may be prevented or reversed by nutrition counseling and aggressive nutrition. Important advances in radiation therapy that may avoid surgery in the aged include brachytherapy of prostate cancer and radiosurgery of intracranial malignancies (12,13).

Cytotoxic Chemotherapy

Aging may be associated with changes is pharmacokinetics and pharmacodynamics of cytotoxic agents and with increased susceptibility to the organ-related toxicity of these compounds. Most pharmacokinetic parameters may undergo age-related derangements (Table 26.1), but the most consistent and predictable physiologic change is a progressive decline of the

Table 26.1 Pharmacokinetic parameters which may be altered in the older person.

Absorption
Volume of Distribution
Decreased total body water
Increased total body fat
Reduced concentration circulating albumin
Hepatic Uptake
Reduced hepatic blood flow
Reduced hepatocyte function
Hepatic Metabolism
Type I reactions (p^{450} cytochrome mediated activating reactions)
Type II reactions (glucuronidation, deactivating reactions)
Excretion
Renal
Hepatic

glomerular filtration rate with increasing age (18). The excretion of methotrexate, carboplatin, the oxozophosphorine alkylators (cyclophophosphamide and ifosfamide), and fludarabine is consequently reduced (19). Dosing of these agents should be adjusted to the measured creatinine clearance in persons aged 65 years and older to avoid excessive toxicity (20). Inadequate renal excretion of uridine arabinoside, an intermediate metabolite of cytosine arabinoside (ARA-C), may be responsible for the age-related cerebellar toxicity from high dose ARA-C (19). This form of treatment should be closely monitored and possibly avoided for creatinine clearance < 50 mL/min.

At least two age-related physiologic changes may alter the hepatic metabolism of drugs: diminished hepatic blood flow and consequently lessened hepatic drug uptake, and reduced activity of cytochrome p^{450} dependent microsomal enzymes (19). The cytochrome p^{450} system is also a major center of drug interactions. Drug interactions are more likely in the aged, due to a high incidence of polypharmacy. The clinical relevance of age-related changes in hepatic metabolism to cancer chemotherapy has never been convincingly demonstrated.

Pharmacodynamic changes, which are at present mostly theoretical, may lead to therapeutic refractoriness (Table 26.2). This possibility is supported by experimental findings as well as clinical observations (18,21, 23). For some neoplasms, such as acute myelogenous leukemia, intermediate grade non-Hodgkin's lymphoma, and epithelial cancer of the ovary, the response rate to chemotherapy becomes lower and the

Table 26.2 Pharmacodynamic parameters which may be altered in tumors occurring in older persons.

Decreased drug uptake

    p-Glycoprotein mediated multidrug resistance (MDR)

    Abnormal transport mechanisms

Abnormal drug metabolism

    Reduced activation

    Enhanced catabolism

Decreased sensitivity to the mechanism of action of the drug

    Increased incidence of tumor cell anoxia

    Increased concentration of glutathione reductase

    Abnormal target enzymes

duration of chemotherapy-induced cancer remission becomes shorter in the older person. This poorer outcome may be due to clones of chemotherapy resistant neoplastic cells. The most likely mechanisms of drug resistance include p-glycoprotein mediated multidrug resistance (MDR), cellular anoxia, and abnormal target enzymes of chemotherapy (24). The membrane p-glycoprotein, encoded by the MDR gene, is a slow CA^{++} channel-dependent pump which extrudes naturally occurring cytotoxic agents from the cell and may be responsible for tumor refractoriness to anthracyclines, anthraquinones, alkaloids, and epipodophyllotoxins (25). The p-glycoprotein is detectable in the myeloblasts of the majority of patients with myelodysplastic syndromes, an entity which becomes more common with age (18). The incidence of tumor anoxia, which may reduce the sensitivity of neoplastic cells to alkylating agents, increases with the age of the tumor host in experimental systems. Structural abnormalities of target enzymes, such as dihydrofolate reductase, may prevent drug-effected metabolic inhibition. These aberrations may become more common with aging because the incidence of cellular protein abnormalities from anomalous synthesis increases.

Several complications of chemotherapy are more common and more severe in the aged (Table 26.3) (18,19). Age-associated restrictions in functional reserve are probably responsible for these higher complication

Table 26.3 Complications of chemotherapy whose risk increases with the age of the tumor host.

Myelosuppression

Mucositis

Peripheral neuritis

Central neurotoxicity

Cardiotoxicity

rates. Chemotherapy-induced myelotoxicity is more severe and more prolonged in older persons with hematological malignancies, such as acute leukemia or malignant lymphoma. In these conditions the neoplasm, rather than age, may cause a depletion of hemopoietic stem cells. In the case of solid tumors with marrow involvement, the tolerance of chemotherapy does not appear to be seriously compromised, at least until age 80 years.

As in the case of radiation therapy, the incidence and severity of chemotherapy-induced mucositis increases with the patient's age. This complication may be fatal to older persons unless it is promptly recognized and treated in a timely fashion. The incidence of peripheral neuropathy is more common in older patients receiving vincristine for lymphoma. In addition to an increased risk of cytosine arabinoside-induced cerebellar toxicity, age may be a risk factor for cognitive and other neurologic abnormalities following intrathecal medications or combined treatment with systemic chemotherapy and central nervous system irradiation. The incidence of congestive heart failure following treatment with anthracyclines or anthraquinones increases progressively after age 70 years. These agents cause the formation of free radicals in the myocardium and lead to a loss of myocardial fibrils. Unexpectedly, the risk of nephrotoxicity from cisplatin does not increase with patient age. The severity of chemotherapy-induced nausea and vomiting may become less intense with age, but delayed nausea (48 to 72 hours after chemotherapy) may become more common.

Despite the increased likelihood of therapeutic refractoriness and treatment complications, chemotherapy may be very beneficial to older patients. Prolonged remissions (lasting 1 year or longer) occur in 30% to 40% of patients over 60 years with acute myelogenous leukemia, and in 40% to 50% of those with Hodgkin's disease and non-Hodgkin's lymphoma, multiple myeloma, stage III ovarian cancer, and small-cell cancer of the lung (26). Chemotherapy can also afford effective palliation to persons with metastatic cancer of the breast, colorectum, prostate and bladder. Adjuvant chemotherapy reduced by 30% the risk of cancer death in patients aged 65 years and over with stage III colorectal cancer (27). In combination with radiation therapy, chemotherapy can obviate surgical resection of the larynx, the urinary bladder, the anus, and the esophagus in patients with locally advanced tumors involving these organs (27). Functional and anatomic organ preservation is particularly important to older persons for whom organ rehabilitation and colostomy management may be problematic.

Problems related to the use of chemotherapy should not dissuade the practitioner from treating older patients. Rather, awareness of these problems should allow a more rational and effective use of chemotherapy in the elderly. The treatment of persons over 65 years with chemotherapy for malignant lymphoma (22) and for breast cancer (28) at Moffitt Cancer Center has been reviewed. In our experience, chemotherapy has been highly beneficial to older persons with these malignancies and has not caused excessive therapeutic complications.

A major advance in the field of cytotoxic chemotherapy has been the development of hemopoietic growth factors for clinical use (29). In addition to the granulocyte-colony stimulating factor (G-CSF) and granulocyte macrophage-colony stimulating factor (GM-CSF) currently available, several other compounds are undergoing clinical trials. Of these, interleukin-3 (IL-3), and stem cell growth factor (SCGF) have almost completed the clinical evaluation phase and should be released soon for general use. G-CSF and GM-CSF shorten the duration of chemotherapy-induced myelosuppression and reduce the risk of neutropenic infections. IL-3 and SCGF may also shorten the duration of thrombocytopenia and reduce the risk of hemorrhage. Hemopoietic growth factors are as effective in older persons as in younger persons (30).

Hormonal Therapy

Three common neoplasms that occur more frequently in older persons — cancer of the prostate, the breast and the endometrium — may be responsive to hormonal manipulations. Endocrine agents of current use include estrogen antagonists, progesterone derivatives, LH-RH analogs, and aromatase inhibitors (19). Although the incidence of deep vein thrombosis from tamoxifen may increase after age 70 years, the tolerance of these compounds by patients of all ages is excellent overall. The incidence of tamoxifen-induced hypercalcemia in patients with bone metastasis from breast cancer is not affected by age. Whenever possible, hormonal manipulations are preferred to cytotoxic chemotherapy in the aged.

Biological Therapy

Of the agents currently available in clinical practice — recombinant alpha interferon (r-alpha IFN) and interleukin-2 (IL-2) — only r-alpha IFN has been tested extensively in the older person. At low doses (three to five million units daily or thrice weekly) r-alpha IFN is well tolerated regardless of the patient's age. At higher doses unpredictable complications, such as cerebritis, have been reported occasionally (19).

Special Issues Related to the Management of Older Persons with Cancer

The decisions involved in the management of older persons with cancer are based on assumptions underlying any type of therapeutic intervention (Figure 26.1). Briefly, treatment is indicated when (a) treatment may improve the disease outcome and (b) the likelihood of treatment-related benefits exceeds that of treatment-related risks. In the case of older persons, the assessment of benefits and risks may be problematic and may need to be individualized. The main components of this problem are definition of treatment goals and assessment of the older person for life expectancy, quality of life, and risk of treatment-related toxicity (31).

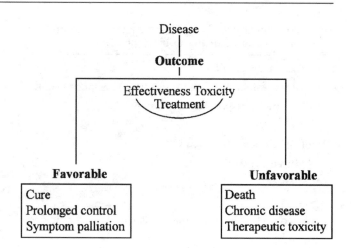

Figure 26.1 Basic assumptions of therapy of diseases: the outcome is positively weighted by treatment.

Goals of Treatment

Cure is the preferable outcome of most diseases. In older persons, however, the benefits of cure may be tempered by competitive causes of death and by the risk of therapeutic complications. This possibility is well epitomized by prostate cancer. When diagnosed in men aged 70 years and older, well-differentiated, localized (stages I and II) prostate cancer does not reduce the life expectancy of these individuals (32). Thus, the risks associated with treatment — either radical prostatectomy or external beam irradiation — may not be warranted in this population. More complex but equally instructive is the example of breast cancer. Women aged 70 years and older with early (stage I and II) breast cancer have comparable survival when treated surgically or medically (33). Surgical treatment is generally preferred in terms of quality of life because of superior cosmetic results and a lower risk of local progression.

These examples suggest that survival gain may not always represent a realistic goal of cancer treatment in all circumstances, and quality-of-life considerations may direct the management of some older persons. These suggestions should not be generalized to all cancers or to all patients. Cancer is a common cause of death for older individuals, and aggressive management of cancer may be lifesaving even in advanced ages. For example, large cell non-Hodgkin's lymphoma may be curable with chemotherapy (22). The median survival of untreated patients with large cell lymphoma is 18 months, which is shorter than the life expectancy of a 90-year-old person.

In individual clinical situations, the choice of the best course of action requires knowledge of the natural history of the disease, of the anticipated outcome of treatment, and of the life expectancy and the quality of life of each individual. A recent rewarding experience has been the aggressive management with chemotherapy of an almost moribund 82-year-old woman with bulky cell lymphoma of the stomach. She recently celebrated her 86th birthday, surrounded by an extended family and free of life-threatening or quality-of-life-compromising diseases.

Assessment of the Older Person

Aging is multidimensional and involves the functional, the cognitive, the emotional, and the socioeconomic domains (34). Alterations in any of these domains may influence the manifestations and the outcome of diseases, as well as the effects of treatment. The comprehensive geriatric assessment, discussed elsewhere in this issue (34), is most useful in evaluating the special needs and the rehabilitative potential of older persons with chronic diseases and disabilities. In oncology, the comprehensive geriatric assessment may reveal unsuspected conditions which can interfere with cancer treatment, may indicate unexpected social and rehabilitative needs, and may provide information on life expectancy, quality of life, and treatment tolerance (34). All patients referred to the geriatric service of our institution are screened with a comprehensive geriatric assessment.

A person's life expectancy is determined by age, comorbidity, and functional status (26). The importance of functional status as an independent variable has emerged only recently. In a cohort of persons aged 70 years and older, A. Siu, MD, had found that the two-year mortality varied from 8% for totally independent to 40% for institutionalized or homebound individuals (personal communication, April 1993).

Health-related quality of life may be assessed by well-validated instruments measuring one's satisfaction in the physical functional, emotional, social and spiritual domains (35). These instruments are questionnaires in which each answer is scored according to a categorical or visual analog scale. There is concern that these questionnaires may not be appropriate for older individuals for several reasons, including content, length, and complexity (35). Given the diversity of the older population, individualized instruments may be desirable. Another difficulty is the assessment of quality of life in the cognitively impaired. For this purpose, every effort should be made to obtain some type of direct and consistent information from the patient. Several studies demonstrated that the assessment of quality of life by proxy is inadequate. Psychosocial medicine and the geriatric program at our center are developing a number of projects to study the accuracy of existing instruments and to explore the generation of customized instruments for the assessment of quality of life in the older person.

A person's functional status is an important predictor of treatment tolerance and outcome. In general, functional status is measured according to the Karnofsky or the Zubrod scale. The instruments are not calibrated to persons with chronic diseases and disability, whose incidence increases with age. For many older persons, the assessment of the activities of daily living (ADL) and instrumental activities of daily living (IADL) are more informative than the Karnofsky or Zubrod performance status (3). As the functional status of the older person may decline very rapidly from serious diseases, information on premorbid functional status is paramount. We might have denied lifesaving chemotherapy to our 82-year-old woman with lymphoma of the stomach because she was bedridden if we had not known that less than a month earlier she had been fully functional. Formal decision-analysis may be extremely helpful to support difficult and controversial decisions related to the management of cancer in older persons. Lyman (36) has provided a framework of reference for the application of the principles of decision analysis to individual clinical situations involving the aged and has described a reliable instrument to predict individual outcome of treatment in terms of survival and cost.

Several other areas of geriatric oncology deserve more study. These include the natural history of cancer in the older person, the influence of chronic diseases on tumor growth and treatment tolerance, the risk of drug interactions from polypharmacy, the management and the significance of malnutrition, and the impact of depression, cognitive function, income, and social support on medical access and outcome.

We believe that the proper context to explore these issues is a longitudinal study of a large cohort of older individuals undergoing uniform evaluation and regular follow-up and receiving treatment according to flexible protocols capable of accommodating the diversity of this population. Whenever possible, these individuals should be evaluated and treated in the community in which they live, under the attention of personal physicians, to minimize discomfort and expenses related to travel. The management of such a cooperative study is a major purpose of our geriatric oncology program.

Conclusion

Antitumor treatment is beneficial to the majority of older patients with cancer, and age should not be considered a contraindication to treatment.

The management of some older individuals is best planned around a comprehensive geriatric assessment including life expectancy, functional status, and the likelihood of therapeutic complications. Quality of life represents a major endpoint of cancer treatment in older individuals: the assessment of the quality of life in the aged with cancer is a high-priority research program.

The most appropriate solution to persistent questions of cancer and aging would be a community-based clinical trial that could include the creativity of individual practitioners and accommodate the diversity of the geriatric population.

Acknowledgments

Appreciation is expressed to Susan K. Smith, manager of Moffitt Cancer Center's Tumor Registry, for her technical assistance with the information in this manuscript. "Reprinted with permission of *Cancer Control: Journal of the Moffitt Cancer Center*, H. Lee Moffitt Cancer Center and Research Institute, publisher."

References

1. Balducci L. Review: Cancer and age. *Forum* 1994; **4**(5): 554–565.
2. Donegan WL. Operative treatment of cancer in the older person by general surgeons. In *Geriatric Oncology*, edited by L Balducci, GH Lyman, WB Ershler. Philadelphia, Pa: JB Lippincott Co., 151–159, 1992.
3. Balducci L, Beghe' C, Chausmer A, *et al.* Prognostic evaluation in geriatric oncology. *Arch Gerontol Geriatr* 1991; **13**: 31–41.
4. Woolf SH, Kamerow DB, Lawrence RS, *et al.* The periodic health examination of older adults: the recommendations of the U.S. Preventive Services Task Force-Pt II. *J Am Geriatr Soc* 1990; **38**(8): 933–942.
5. Cox CE, Miguel R, Bosek V. Outpatient lumpectomy, axillary node dissection and modified radical mastectomy under local anesthesia. *15th Annual San Antonio Breast Cancer Symposium.* San Antonio, Tex, 180, 1992. Abstract.
6. Tuman KJ, McCarthy RJ, March RJ, *et al.* Effects on epidural anesthesia and analgesia on coagulation and outcome after major vascular surgery. *Anesth Analg* 1991; **73**(6): 696–704.
7. Breslow MJ, Jordan DA, Christopherson R, *et al.* Epidural morphine decreases postoperative hypertension by attenuating sympathetic nervous system hyperactivity. *JAMA* 1989; **261**(24): 3577–3581.
8. Yaeger MP, Glass DD, Neff RK, *et al.* Epidural anesthesia and analgesia in high risk surgical patients. *Anesthesiology*. 1987; **66**(6): 729–736.
9. Patterson WB. Surgical options in the treatment of cancer: how are they affected by the patient's age? In *Geriatric Oncology*, edited by L Balducci, GH Lyman, WB Ershler. Philadelphia, Pa: JB Lippincott Co., 145–150, 1992.
10. Veronesi U, Luini A, Del Vecchio M, *et al.* Radiotherapy after breast-preserving surgery in women with localized cancer of the breast. *N Engl J Med* 1993; **328**: 1587–1591.
11. Pinkas H. Gastrointestinal cancer ablation via endoscopy. In *Geriatric Oncology*, edited by L Balducci, GH Lyman, WB Ershler. Philadelphia, Pa: JB Lippincott Co., 199–207, 1992.
12. Zachariah S, Zachariah B, Wang T, *et al.* Primary brain tumors in the older patient: an annotated review. *J Am Geriatr Soc* 1992; **40**(12): 1265–1271.
13. Balducci L, Trotti A, Pow-Sang J. Advances and controversies in the prevention and treatment of prostate cancer. *L'annee' Gerontologique* 1992; **2**: 97–110.
14. Wyckoff J, Greenberg H, Sanderson R, Wallach P, Balducci L. Breast irradiation in the older woman: a toxicity study. *J Am Geriatr Soc* 1994; **42**(2): 150–152.
15. Casey L, Zachariah B, Balducci L. A profile of cancer patients aged 80 and older treated with radiation therapy: analysis of tolerance and effectiveness. *J Am Geriatr Soc* 1992; **40**: SA-43.
16. Balducci L, Phillips DM, Davis KM, *et al.* Systemic treatment of cancer in the elderly. *Arch Gerontol Geriatr* 1988; **7**(2): 119–150.
17. Casey L, Balducci L, Jensen C, *et al.* Preventing weight loss in the older man during radiation therapy for cancer. *J Am Geriatr Soc* 1992; **40**: SA-43.
18. Balducci L, Mowrey K. Pharmacology and organ toxicity of chemotherapy in older patients. *Oncology* 1992; **6**: 62–68.
19. Balducci L, Mowrey K, Parker M. Pharmacology of antineoplastic agents in older patients. In *Geriatric Oncology*, edited by L Balducci, GH Lyman, WB Ershler. Philadelphia, Pa: JB Lippincott Co., 169–180, 1992.
20. Gelman RS, Taylor SG IV. Cyclophosphamide, methotrexate and 5-fluorouracil chemotherapy in women more than 65 years old with advanced breast cancer: the elimination of age trends in toxicity by using doses based on creatinine clearance. *J Clin Oncol* 1984; **2**(12): 1404–1413.
21. Ballester OF, Moscinski LC, Morris D, *et al.* Acute myelogenous leukemia in the elderly. *J Am Geriatr Soc* 1992; **40**(3): 277–284.
22. Ballester OF, Moscinski LC, Spiers ASD, *et al.* Non-Hodgkin's lymphoma in the older person. *J Am Geriatr Soc* 1993; **41**(11): 1245–54.
23. Thigpen T, Brady MF, Omura GA, *et al.* Age as a prognostic factor in ovarian carcinoma: the gynecologic oncology group experience. *Cancer* 1993; **71**: 606–614.
24. Dietel M. Meeting report: Second international symposium on cytostatic drug resistance. *Cancer Res* 1993; **53**(11): 2683–2688.
25. Holzmayer TA, Hilsenbeck S, Von Hoff DD, *et al.* Clinical correlates of MDRI (p-glycoprotein) gene expression in ovarian and small cell lung carcinomas. *JNCI* 1992; **84**(19): 1486–1491.
26. Beghe' C, Balducci L, Geriatric oncology: perspectives from decision analysis. *Arch Gerontol Geriatr* 1990; **10**: 141–162.
27. Balducci L, Lyman GH. Adjuvant treatment of cancer in older persons. In *Geriatric Oncology*, edited by L Balducci, GH Lyman, WB Ershler. Philadelphia, Pa: JB Lippincott Co., 284–302, 1992.
28. Lyman GH, Lyman S, Balducci L, Kuderer N, Reintgen D, Harris J, Cox C, Baekey P, Greenberg H, Horton J. Age and the risk of recurrence in women with breast cancer. *Cancer Control* 1996; **3**: 421–427.
29. Shank W. Clinical use of hematopoietic growth factors in patients with cancer. In *Geriatric Oncology*, edited by L Balducci, GH Lyman, WB Ershler. Philadelphia, Pa: JB Lippincott Co., 208–20, 1992.
30. Shank W Jr, Balducci L. Recombinant hemopoietic growth factors: comparative hemopoietic response in younger and older subjects. *J Am Geriatr Soc* 1992; **40**(2): 151–154.
31. Applegate WB, Curb JD. Designing and executing randomized clinical trials involving elderly persons. *J Am Geriatr Soc* 1990; **38**(8): 943–950.
32. Chodak GW, Thiste RA, Gerber GS, *et al.* Results of conservative management of clinically localized prostate cancer. *N Engl J Med* 1994; **330**: 224–8.
33. Bates T, Riley DL, Houghton J, *et al.* Breast cancer in elderly women: a cancer research campaign trial comparing treatment with tamoxifen and optimal surgery with tamoxifen alone. The elderly breast cancer working party. *Br J Surg* 1991; **78**(5): 591–594.
34. Beghe' C, Robinson B. Comprehensive geriatric assessment: diagnostic, therapeutic, and prognostic value. *Cancer Cont: JMCC* 1994; **1**(2): 121–125.
35. Kimmick GG, Fleming R, Muss HB, Balducci L. Cancer chemotherapy in older adults: A tolerability perspective. *Drugs and Aging* 1997; **10**(1): 34–49.
36. Lyman GH. Decision analysis: a way of thinking about health care in the elderly. In *Geriatric Oncology*, edited by L Balducci, GH Lyman, WB Ershler. Philadelphia, Pa: JB Lippincott Co., 8–19, 1992.

27. Surgical Approaches to the Older Person with Cancer

Peter J. Fabri

Introduction

A surgical procedure in an elderly oncology patient must be planned with consideration of the differences in physiology of the patient, response of the patient to anesthesia and stress, and particular aspects of nutrition in surgical illness. Just as surgical procedures in neonates cannot be considered treatment of "small adults" neither can the surgical management of the elderly simply be considered treatment of "older adults." This chapter is included to provide an "overview" of the physiologic, pharmacologic, ethical, and functional issues which play an important role in the surgical treatment of the elderly. It is necessarily succinct and the interested reader is referred to the comprehensive references which address specific issues in much greater detail.

As far back as 1907, the literature suggests that the risks of surgical procedures in the elderly were high enough to warrant calling age a contraindication (1). By the late thirties, it became apparent that surgical procedures in the elderly were a necessary part of the modern therapeutic age (2), and throughout the subsequent years continued advances in our understanding of the physiology of aging (3,4) have evolved. As people have lived to older age, the surgical horizon has expanded, as described in a report on the management of patients over the age of 100 (5). As surgeons began to treat a larger number of elderly patients, interest emerged in evaluating outcome, and the result of applying objective data to improve surgical treatment was reported (6).

Effect of Age on Cancer

A quick review of the published effects of aging on the state and biologic activity of cancer yields a very complex and confusing picture, since different studies conducted at different times and at different institutions yield markedly divergent results (7,8,9,10). While it is possible that a real difference in the behavior of cancer as a direct effect of age might exist, the small size of most studies precludes the ability to confidently indicate a difference in stage or survival. It is most likely that there is a marked variation in stage at diagnosis and in biologic behavior regardless of age and that in reviews of small series, no difference will be seen in looking at different tumors. Therefore, in the absence of more convincing data it seems prudent to take each patient as a unique individual with a unique cancer and base prognosis on more objective parameters, such as traditional survival for the specific tumor, effect of associated disease, etc. In lung, breast, and colorectal cancer, however, it appears likely that a real difference exists and that elderly patients may actually have a more favorable situation than their juniors (11). Nevertheless, each patient should still be treated individually since the effects of associated illness and altered physiology are probably of greater planning significance in most patients than the effect of age on tumor biology. Epidemiologists will continue to search for relationships between age and cancer, but it is not likely that these will be of major value in decision making for an individual patient in the near future.

Many alterations in organ function have been described as a consequence of age. Significant changes in tidal volume and respiratory response (12), and a significant increase in the incidence of respiratory comorbidity (13) suggest that the elderly patient is often encumbered by pulmonary alterations which will alter the response to a surgical procedure. Changes in cardiac regulatory function (14) and response to cardiac medications (15) may have a dramatic effect on the perioperative surgical patient who develops cardiac dysfunction. Patients with acute myocardial infarction, for example, have worse prognosis as a function of age (16). This probably applies as well to postop surgical patients who have perioperative myocardial infarction and perhaps even those who have an underlying cardiac abnormality but without infarction. Alterations in thyroid function (17) can impact on the metabolic demands of a superimposed surgical procedure and the relative hypothyroidism of old age may contribute to the "euthyroid sick" syndrome which occurs in critical illness (17). Alterations in liver function (18,19) have effect not only on protein synthesis but also on the detoxification and excretion of a wide variety of pharmacologic agents. Gastrointestinal drugs for the management of peptic ulcer disease, for example, have significantly different metabolism in the elderly (20). At the same time, alteration in GI, pancreatic and hepatobiliary function with age can have a significant effect on GI motility as well as response to pharmacologic agents used in the management of abnormalities of these organs (21). It is therefore necessary to have a broad and comprehensive understanding of the pharmacotherapeutic differences of the geriatric oncology patient (22). Choice of drugs, dose of drugs, and interactions of drugs must all be considered individually.

Anesthesia in particular is a significant stress for all patients and major changes in the handling of anesthetic agents as well as the response to anesthetic agents have been described in the elderly (23). Agents such as Midazolam (24) which are often used during the conduct of outpatient procedures, should be particularly noted because of the marked increase in the frequency of outpatient and minimally invasive procedures during which such agents are likely to be a component of the conscious sedation/anesthetic plan. Accordingly, a detailed understanding of the effects of anesthesia in the elderly patient (25) is essential. Neuromuscular blocking agents (26,27), and changes in responsiveness to epidural narcotics (28) can have substantial effects on intraoperative management and, more importantly, postoperative ventilatory status. Elderly patients typically receive multiple medications for their associated medical illnesses. An understanding of the drug interactions between anesthetic agents and co-existing pharmaceutical agents should be high on the operative and postoperative lists (29). Recognized changes in autonomic responsiveness (30) may necessitate a change in the type of anesthetic agent used, as well as in postoperative pain management and sedation. Management of the elderly patient in the postoperative period (31) requires an understanding of changes in physiology, particularly of the heart, lungs, and kidney. In addition, however, alterations in drug metabolism in the liver (32) and changes in the handling of fluid and electrolytes by the kidney (33) have a substantial effect on the risk of surgical procedures in elderly patients (34). Assessment of the overall risk in the elderly patient (35) as well as an awareness of quantitative estimates of the cardiac and pulmonary risks of abdominal and thoracic procedures (36) should be used in preoperative preparation. Preparation for the co-morbid illnesses (37,33) should include recognition of the increased incidence and severity of deep vein thrombosis and pulmonary embolus (39,40) in the elderly cancer patient. Most risk classification systems for thromboembolic disease list cancer and age as independent factors for deep vein thrombosis and, therefore, all elderly surgical patients should be considered to be at high risk of deep vein thrombosis and treated with appropriate prophylactic measures. Sequential calf vein compression devices are probably indicated for all elderly patients undergoing surgical procedures for oncologic disease. In addition, certain factors (previous deep vein thrombosis, high dose estrogen use, and obesity) increase the risks independently and may justify the use of low dose subcutaneous heparin 5000 units q 8 hours in addition to calf compression.

Nutrition

Early enthusiasm for aggressive nutrition support in minimizing perioperative and postoperative risks of malnutrition may have been overly optimistic (41). Nevertheless, malnutrition is an important co-factor in postoperative morbidity and preoperative identification in the elderly patient is an important part of patient assessment. The increased incidence of malnutrition in the elderly (42,43,44) is multifactorial, probably cannot be fully addressed in the preoperative period, but can be included in peri- and postoperative planning. The preoperative serum albumin is an excellent indicator of nutrition status (45) but the increased risk associated with hypoalbuminemia cannot be remedied by the infusion of albumin. Even though elderly patients have a relative decrease in their caloric requirement (46), and while it may be appropriate to allow a week of relative starvation in postoperative patients of younger age, this may not be appropriate in the elderly patient. Early and aggressive attention to nutrition deficiencies in the postoperative period appears warranted. Alterations in wound healing are often related to diabetes (47) and are aggravated by malnutrition and other premorbid factors. The best way to avoid such problems is early identification of malnutrition and a plan to provide appropriate and safe postoperative nutrition support. Although the use of TPN has been largely supplanted in many centers by aggressive tube feeding, it should be recognized that the actual need is for nutrition and that there is currently no evidence of a superiority of route of administration in most cases. Most patients can be fed enterally using the gastrointestinal tract, thus maintaining the integrity of the GI mucosa, but careful attention must be paid to assure its safe and effective use (48). In particular, patients should be assessed for risk of aspiration which depends largely on neurologic status and degree of sedation/analgesia.

Ethics

As a larger number of elderly patients present for surgical treatment of major oncologic problems, the ethical issues associated with such treatment assume even greater significance. The perioperative responsibilities of the surgeon in geriatric oncology are more frequent (49) and more difficult but nevertheless rewarding challenges. Recent changes in our code of law have guaranteed that individuals have the right to participate in their healthcare choices. Advance directives are now offered to all patients at the time of admission to the hospital. Rather than view these advance directives as intrusions, perhaps we should accept them as a welcome way of identifying our patients' wishes before major surgical procedures. It is far easier to address these preoperatively than it is to try to deal with family members in a complicated postoperative period. The ethical associations in geriatric care (50) and some of the moral dilemmas which develop (51) pose opportunities to improve communication with patients and family and to enhance our preoperative preparation and informed consent.

A more difficult situation is the issue of resuscitation in the operating room. Often anesthesiologists are reluctant to administer care to patients with "do-not-resuscitate" orders. In the intensive care unit, where resuscitation is frequently an issue, we can usually recognize the difference between "no CPR" and "no treatment." In the operating room, however, where resuscitation is uncommon and perhaps more "threatening," the decision to treat has already been made and the individuals involved feel compelled to proceed with CPR since the success of resuscitation may be greater than in the general hospital environment (48,53). Often the solution to the dilemma is the temporary reversal of the DNR order for the time-limited perioperative period. Nevertheless, there will be a particular subgroup of patients for whom an operation is appropriate, but the patient is clearly terminal such that resuscitation would not be warranted under any circumstance. Cases such as this should be handled individually and with open communication among all members of the family and the healthcare team. The ethics committee may be helpful.

Our understanding of the management of critical surgical illness in the elderly comes largely from studies done in trauma patients and burn patients. Changes in metabolism, cytokine release, etc. in the elderly patient (54,55,56,57,58,59,60,61,62) identify the management issues associated with elderly patients with severe, acute illness. Similarly, studies in burn patients (63,64,65) identify that there is shortened length of stay and improved outcome when burns are treated aggressively with early surgical excision in the elderly to minimize the hyper metabolic risk and risk of sepsis. Information from both of these groups (trauma and burn) has provided us with an improved understanding of the management of the elderly patient who becomes acutely ill, septic, or hyper metabolic. Cytokine release (Il-l, TNF, IL-6) following acute injury produces fever, hypermetabolism, neutrophilia and a hyperdynamic state. Aggressive, early diagnosis and treatment to minimize this inflammatory response syndrome would appear to be justifiable in the management of complications in the elderly oncologic patient based on the results obtained from the treatment of elderly trauma / burn patients since patients who develop complications have a high incidence of additional complications and subsequent death. Age and co-morbid illnesses may be independent causes of decreased survival as has been reported from ARDS (66).

Critical Care

Complicated, elderly patients consequently consume a significant percentage of healthcare dollars when they require prolonged intensive care use (67). Preadmission functional status, that is the ability to perform the activities of daily living such as transfer from bed, feeding, and maintenance of bodily functions seems to predict outcome in the intensive care unit (68). With careful attention to the unique problems of the elderly, particularly postoperative pulmonary function (69), and the recognition of the impact of age on respiratory tract disease (70), it is possible to gain very acceptable results in the elderly oncology patient in the SICU (71). Even in the extreme elderly, procedures that require

surgical intensive care should not be avoided only on the basis of age (72,73). It is important to realize, however, that co-morbid illness and the adverse effect of postoperative complications lead to a significant failure rate at one year .

Although new technologic advances such as percutaneous tracheostomy (75) and changes in the management of critically ill patients (76) will continue to improve our ability to care for elderly patients in the intensive care unit, technology will not replace sound decision making, careful attention to details, and avoidance of complications.

Infections

As previously indicated, elderly patients do not tolerate complications well. In elderly patients undergoing treatment for complex oncologic disease, infection and / or sepsis often occur and can significantly influence the outcome of the procedure. Infectious diseases in the elderly require careful consideration and prompt recognition and treatment (78). Antibiotic use may require attention to drug interactions, altered organ system function, and poorly tolerated side effects (79).

Simultaneous Surgical Problems

Although the "Principle of Parsimony" states that all of a patients symptoms can usually be explained by a single disease, elderly patients not uncommonly present with more than one serious medical problem. A commonly faced dilemma, for example, is the patient who presents with an abdominal aortic aneurysm and who is found to have a colon carcinoma — or vice versa. When both problems represent as clean surgery, the option of simultaneous surgical procedures may be considered (a typical example is carotid artery disease and coronary artery disease), but in most oncologic situations, this is a less desirable or suitable option. While there is occasionally some disagreement among surgeons about the order or preference for sequential or staged procedures, most surgeons agree that the most immediately life threatening problem should be addressed first. A symptomatic aneurysm should be repaired before an "incidental" colon cancer, whereas a nearly obstructing colon carcinoma should be resected before an asymptomatic 5 cm aneurysm is addressed.

Emergency Operations and Procedures

Emergency procedures at all ages carry higher risks than the same procedure in an elective environment. In some circumstances (e.g. tracheostomy) the difference may be absolute — life or death. In others, (e.g. drainage of wound abscess) the difference is minimal. In most circumstances, however, the addition of an emergency component to an operation is of intermediate significance and results in a substantial increase in risk. Colon operations without bowel preparation, for example, carry a 3–5 fold higher risk of infection. And even surgical procedures whose excess risk would appear to be minimum (biliary obstruction), can have a 3–4 fold increase in complications and death.

Wherever possible, emergency procedures in the elderly should be avoided. Attention to fluid and electrolytes, antibiotics, hemodynamic monitoring and optimization, etc. are each contributory to improved outcome. When an emergency situation does not allow delay (e.g. biliary obstruction with suppurative cholangitis and CNS alterations), an initial non-surgical approach (percutaneous cholangiography or ERCP) is often preferable to committing the patient and surgeon to a major surgical procedure with unanticipated and avoidable hazards. Occasionally a procedure which is not usually indicated or used, such as cholecystostomy, offers an alternative to a major operation, buys time, and allows patient preparation. This is even more true when it can be done percutaneously. But when an operation cannot be postponed and a less hazardous alternative does not exist, then the surgeon and patient must be prepared for the increased risk of an operation. Very careful hemodynamic preparation with Swan Ganz catheter is often indicated. Induction of anesthesia using cardiac surgical techniques may minimize the acute physiologic stress. Efforts to do the simplest and most direct procedure which will address the problem at hand are preferable to complex and elaborate procedures which attempt to provide the most comprehensive solution.

Common Outpatient Procedures

- node biopsy
- Breast biopsy (needle localization)
- Laparoscopy
- Colonoscopy
- mastectomy, quadrantectomy
- percutaneous g-tube
- line and port placement

Minimal Invasive and Ambulatory Surgery

Healthcare changes of the past decade have led to an increased use of ambulatory surgery programs for larger surgical procedures (80). "Minimally invasive" procedures, such as laparoscopy, (81,82,83) appear to be physiologically less stressful, may require a shorter hospital stay, and may allow an earlier return to normal functional activity. It is important to realize, however, that most of these procedures require a general anesthetic (which may carry a higher risk in the elderly patient). In addition, since most elderly surgical oncology patients have several co-morbid illnesses, the co-morbidity is often the limiting factor in the length of hospitalization and the speed of recovery and therefore minimizes the effect of minimally invasive technology and length of stay, time to recovery, etc. The preparation of patients undergoing ambulatory surgery is focused on the recognition and treatment of underlying medical problems. Age alone is not a factor in deciding about the ambulatory approach. Availability of care-givers is important, as is the recognition of the physiologic effect of age on pulmonary function

(decreased) and hepatic function (decreased). A wide variety of anesthetics and sedatives is available and different authors have their own preferences. It is crucial, however, to anticipate the need to change dosing. Midazolam, a widely used benzodiazepine, is safe and effective in a small dose (lmg) either IV or IM. Adequate time must be allotted before a subsequent dose to avoid respiratory depression. The rapid onset and short duration (1 hr) together with both anterograde and retrograde amnesia make this agent quite suitable for outpatient procedures as long as subsequent redosing is avoided. Similarly, fentanyl (50–100 mg) or meperidine (10–25 mg) can be given intravenously for analgesia during monitored procedures with local or regional anesthesia. Agents which are not reversible should be avoided since wide variation in metabolic clearance is possible in the elderly because of intrinsic alterations in clearance or competition with other medications.

Wound Healing

Although surgical expertise inside a body cavity is the ultimate determinant of the success of a major surgical procedure, it is the external wound which is most noticed by patients and their families. Wound healing may be affected by factors that are common in oncologic practice and may be aggravated in the elderly. Factors such as competition of the tumor for nutrients, tumor induced malnutrition, and perhaps tumor derived wound factors may all inhibit the rate of intrinsic wound healing (84). Similarly, chemotherapy and radiation therapy are known to adversely affect wound healing and may be additive to other risk factors (85). It is possible that available nutrient supplementation, such as vitamin A, or investigational factors such as growth hormones, growth factors, etc., may restore wound healing to normal (1). In the elderly oncology patient, wounds should be closed per primum whenever possible (to minimize the metabolic stimulus) and perhaps even with subcuticular closure to allow more rapid return to normal function and to avoid the need for return for suture removal. Conversely, however, when there is a high risk for wound infection, wounds should be allowed to heal by secondary intention, because the secondary complications of inadequately treated infection are usually poorly tolerated in the elderly. Thoughtful decision making and finely honed judgment are essential in assuring an excellent outcome.

Rehabilitation

Many cancer patients have already lost function prior to surgery. Rapid recovery (86) of function may be a critical factor in patient outcome. Likewise, return to normal function has significant social as well as economic implications for many of these individuals. In the management of younger patients, discharge from the hospital usually represents a marker of the completeness of care. In the elderly, however, rehabilitation, which may be extended and multifactorial, may be an equally important phase of the total surgical process (87,88,89,90,86,91,92). For example, elderly patients recover less well from extremity amputation (92), due to loss of muscle mass, underlying osteoporosis, degenerative joint disease and vascular disease. In preoperative evaluation, it is crucial for the primary care physician and healthcare team to begin to plan for postoperative rehabilitation to allow ongoing continuity and a transition to longer term care. Surgical care is thus one phase in a continuous process of care which begins with diagnosis but ends only when the patient has been returned to a pre-illness state of function.

Advance Directives

As indicated earlier the discussion of advance directives, including intraoperative DNR, becomes an important part of the overall surgical management of the elderly cancer patient. While each institution may approach the specifics differently, all institutions should have an organized program for assuring that each elderly patient has been appropriately informed about the opportunity for an advance directive prior to a major oncologic surgical procedure (93). In many cases, the patient's wishes can be met best by the choice of a less aggressive surgical procedure than might ordinarily be recommended in a younger patient (94,95). Since elderly patients are usually very aware of issues and values that are important to them they are typically quite prepared to discuss matters related to dying and quality of life-matters which may be critical factors in the decision process and which may be pivotal if a major complication occurs. All of this is much easier to discuss and clarify with the patient himself before the patient undergoes a procedure. Once the patient develops a complication that forebodes a long phase of in hospital treatment, perhaps in an intensive care unit where social isolation is often prevalent, the decision making process becomes even more complex. Careful estimation of prognosis and frequent communication with the family greatly facilitate decisions to forego additional treatment (96,97). or to withdraw treatment when the likelihood of success seems small (95). These decision making issues in the final phase of an individual's life are important, potentially costly, and emotionally challenging (95).

Case Study #1

Advance directive and do not resuscitate. An 85 year old male is admitted to the hospital for management of a low-lying rectal carcinoma. Sigmoidoscopic examination demonstrates the lesion to be 8 cm from the anal verge. There is no evidence of metastatic disease on pre-op evaluation. The patient indicates that he will not agree to an abdominoperineal resection, no matter what. Furthermore, he has met with an attorney and has created an advance directive and has granted durable power of attorney to his son. Following a transrectal excision of the lesion, the patient has a cerebrovascular accident and requires intubation and

mechanical ventilation. The patient's wife, the stepmother to his son wants everything to be done. How should you proceed?

Case Study #2

Comorbid illness. An 80 year old woman is referred for management of a 1.5 cm pigmented lesion on the right leg. Biopsy by the dermatologist showed a melanoma, superficial spreading. Because of a prior history of myocardial infarction, the operative risk is considered to be high. The planned procedure is a local excision of the lesion, using local incision and intravenous sedation. In addition, sentinel lymph node mapping is planned to stage the patient.

Summary

Just as pediatric surgical patients are not "small adults" neither are elderly and geriatric patients "old adults." Elderly oncology patients present with a variety of unique problems that require forethought, preparation, and accuracy. The identification and management of associated health problems is paramount. The choice of an appropriate operation may be different from that used in a younger patient. Attention to the need for social considerations, such as advance directives, takes on a greater importance in the elderly patient with cancer. Similarly, postoperative recovery of function, response to complications, and the length and complexity of rehabilitation may all be markedly different in this age group. Good results often depend on thoughtfulness, attention to details, and communication skills.

References

1. Smith KP, Zardiackas LD, Didlake RH. Cortisone, vitamin A, and wound healing. The importance of measuring wound surface area. J Surg Res 1986; 40: 120–125.
2. Brooks B. Surgery in patients of advanced age. Ann Surg 1937; 105: 481–495.
3. Marshall WH, Fahey PJ. Operative complications and mortality in patients over 80 years of age. Arch Surg 1964; 88: 896–904.
4. Glenn F. Surgery in the care of the elderly. Gerontol Geriatr Educ 1980; 1(2): 107–10.
5. Katlic MR Surgery in centenarians. JAMA 1985; 253: 3139–3141.
6. Seymor DG, Pringle R. A new method of auditing surgical mortality rates. Application to a group of elderly general surgical patients. BMJ 1982; 284: 1539–1542.
7. Goodwin JS, Sarnet JM, Key CR et al. State at diagnosis of cancer varies with the age of the patient. J Am Geriatr Soc 1986; 34: 20–26.
8. Holmes FF. Clinical evidence for a change in tumor aggressiveness with age. Semin Oncol 1989; 16: 34–40.
9. Kant AK, Glover C, Horm J, et al. Does cancer survival differ for older patients? Cancer 1992; 70: 2734–2740.
10. Kennedy BJ. Aging and cancer. J Clin Onco 1988; 16: 1903–1911.
11. Mor V, Guadagnoli E, Masterson-Allen S, et al. Lung, breast and colorectal cancer: the relationship between extent of disease and age at diagnosis. J Am Geriatr Soc 1988; 36: 873–876.
12. Brandstetter RD, Kazemi H. Aging and the respiratory system. Med Clin North Am 1983; 67: 419.
13. Beernaeris A. Surgery in the aged. Associated pathologies of aged people. Acta Chir Belg 1993; 93(3): 112–4.
14. Lakatta EG. Cardiovascular regulatory mechanisms in advanced age. Physiol Rev 1993; 73: 413–467.

15. Rich MW, Imburgia M. Inotropic response to dobutamine in elderly patients with decompensated congestive heart failure. *Am J Cardiol* 1990; **65**: 519–521.

16. Sinclair D. Myocardial infarction. Consideration for geriatric patients. *Canadian Family Physician* 1994; **40**: 1172–7.

17. Burrows V, Shenkcman L. Thyroid function in the elderly. *Am J Med Sci* 1982; **283**: 8–17.

18. Kampmann JP, Sinding J, Moller-Jorgensen I. Effect of age on liver function. *Geriatrics* 1975; **30**: 91.

19. James OFW. Gastrointestinal and liver function in old age. *Clin Gastroenterol* 1983; **12**: 671.

20. Chiverton SG, Hunt RH. Pharmacokinetics and pharmaco-dynamics of treatments for peptic ulcer disease in the elderly. *Am J Gastroenterol* 1988; **83**: 211.

21. Altman DF. Changes in gastrointestinal, pancreatic, biliary and hepatic function with aging. *Gastroenterol Clin North Am* 1990; **19**: 227–234.

22. Delafuente JC. Perspectives on geriatric pharmacotherapy. *Pharmacotherapy* 1991; **11**(3): 222–4.

23. Djokovic JL, Hedley-Whyte J. Prediction of outcome of surgery and anesthesia in patients over 80. *JAMA* 1979; **242**: 2301.

24. Greenblatt DJ, Abernathy DR, Loeniskar A, *et al.* Effect of age, gender, and obesity on midazolam kinetics. *Anesthesiology* 1984; **61**: 27.

25. Kreehel SW. Anesthesia for surgical care of the elderly. In *Surgical Care of the Elderly*, edited by JL Meakins, JC McClaran. Chicago: Year Book Medical Publishers, pp. 276–287, 1988.

26. Matteo RS, Baeku WW, McDaniel DD, *et al.* Pharmacokinetics and pharmacodynamics of D tubocurarine and metoeurine in the elderly. *Anesth Analg* 1985; **64**: 23.

27. Rupp SM, Castagnoli KP, Fisher DM, *et al.* Pancuronium and vecuroniurn pharmacokinetics and pharmacodynamics in younger and elderly adults. *Anesthesiology* 1987; **67**: 45.

28. Moore AK, Vilderman S, Lubensky W, *et al.* Differences in epidural morphine requirements between elderly and young patients after abdominal surgery. *Anesth Analg* 1990; **70**: 316.

29. Mattison RA. Anesthesia drug interaction in the elderly. In *Problems in Anesthesia*. Philadelphia: JB Lippincott, pp. 589–601, 1989.

30. Taseh MD. The autonomic nervous system and geriatric anesthesia. *Intl Anesthesiol Clin* 1988; **26**(2): 143–51.

31. Watters JM, McClaran JC. The elderly surgical patient. In *Care of the Surgical Patient*, edited by DW Wilmore, MF Brennan, AH Harken. New York: Scientific American/American College of Surgeons, 1990.

32. Woodhouse KW, Mutch E, Williams FM, *et al.* The effect of age on pathways of drug metabolism in human liver. *Age Ageing* 1984; **13**: 328.

33. Zawada ET Jr, Horning JR, Salem AG. Renal, fluid, electrolyte, and acid-base problems during surgery in the elderly. In *Geriatric Surgery*, edited by MR Katlic. Baltimore: Urban & Schwarzenberg, pp. 85–96, 1990.

34. Denny JL, Denson JS. Risk of surgery in patients over 90. *Geriatrics* 1972; **27**: 115–118.

35. Johnson JC. Surgical assessment in the elderly. *Geriatrics* 1988; **43**: Suppl. 83–90.

36. Gerson MC, Hurst JM, Hertzberg VS, *et al.* Prediction of cardiac and pulmonary complications related to elective abdominal and noncardiac thoracic surgery in geriatric patients. *Am J Med* 1990; **88**: 101.

37. Kauder DR, Schwab CW. Comorbidity in geriatric patients. *Advances in Trauma* 1989; **29**: 541.

38. Ritter-Sterr C, Janssen I, List M, Lansky S, Benson A, Mullane M. Surgery in the elderly cancer patient. A descriptive analysis of patient characteristics, comorbidities and psychosocial variables (meeting abstract). *Proc Ann Meet Am Soc Clin Oncol* 1993; **12**: A1559.

39. Mereli GJ. Prophylaxis for deep vein thrombosis and pulmonary embolism in the geriatric patient undergoing surgery. *Clin Geriatr Med* 1990; **6**(3): 531–42.

40. Palmberg S, Hirsjarvi E. Mortality in geriatric surgery. With special reference to the type of surgery, anaesthesia, compli-cating diseases, and prophylaxis of thrombosis. *Gerontology* 1979; **25**(2): 103–12.

41. Buzby GP. Perioperative total parenteral nutrition in surgical patients. *NEJM* 1991; **325**: 525–532.

42. Department of Health and Social Security. A nutrition survey of the elderly. *Rep Health Soc Subj (Lond)* 1979; **16**: 1–209.

43. Morley JE. Nutrition in the elderly. *Ann Intern Med* 1988; **109**: 890–904.

44. Pinchcofsky-Devin GD, Kaminski MV. Incidence of protein calorie malnutrition in the nursing home population. *J Am Coll Nutri* 1987; **6**: 109–112.

45. Rudman D, Feller AG, Nagruj HS, *et al.* Relation of serum albumin concentration to death rate in nursing home men. *JPEN* 1987; **11**: 360–363.

46. Shizgal HM, Martin MF, Gimmon Z. The effect of age on the caloric requirement of malnourished and individuals. *Am J Clin Nutr* 1992; **55**: 783–789.

47. Gavin LA. Management of diabetes mellitus during surgery. *West J Med* 1989; **151**: 525–529.

48. Cohen CB, Cohen PJ. Do not resuscitate orders in the operating room. *NEJM* 1991; **325**: 1879–1882, *Letters* 1992; **326**: 1571–1572.

49. Cohen MM. Perioperative responsibilities of the surgeon. *Clin Geriatr Med* 1990; **6**(3): 459–67.

50. Lockwood M. Ethical dilemmas in surgery. some philosophical reflections. *J Med Ethics* 1980; **6**(2): 82–4.

51. Reiss R. Moral and ethical issues in geriatric surgery. *J Med Ethics* 1980; **6**(2): 71–7.

53. Walker RM. DNR in the OR. Resuscitation as an operative risk. *JAMA* 1991; **266**: 2407.

54. Champion HR, Copes WS, Buyer D, *et al.* Major trauma in geriatric patients. *Am J Public Health* 1989; **79**: 1278.

55. Demarest GB, Turner MO, Clevenger FW. Injuries in the elderly. Evaluation and initial response. *Geriatrics* 1990; **45**: 36.

56. Finelli FC, Jonsson J, Champion HR, *et al.* A case control study for major trauma in geriatric patients. *J Trauma* 1989; **29**: 541.

57. Grisso JA, Schwartz DF, Wishner AR, *et al.* Injuries in an elderly inner-city population. *J Am Geriatr Soc* 1990; **38**: 1326.

58. Horst HM, Obeid FN, Sorensen VJ, *et al.* Factors influencing survival of elderly trauma patients. *Crit Care Med* 1986; **14**: 681.

59. Lehman LB. Head trauma in the elderly. *Postgrad Med* 1988; **83**: 140.

60. Luna GK, Carrico VA. Trauma in the elderly. In *Surgical Medical Publishers*, edited by JL Meakins, JC McClaran, p. 473, 1988.

61. McCoy GF, Johnstone BA, Duthie RB. Injury to the elderly in road traffic accidents. *J Trauma* 1989; **29**: 494.

62. Osler T, Hales K, Baack B, *et al.* Trauma in the elderly. *Am J Surg* 1988; **156**: 537.

63. Deitch EA, Clothier J. Burns in the elderly. An early surgical approach. *J Trauma* 1983; **23**: 891.

64. Hunt JL, Purdue GF. The elderly burn patient. *Am J Surg* 1992; **164**: 472.

65. Kara M, Peters WJ, Douglas LG, *et al.* An early surgical approach to burns in the elderly. *J Trauma* 1990; **30**: 430.

66. Gee MH, Gottlieb JE, Albertine KH, *et al.* Physiology of aging related to outcome in the adult respiratory distress syndrome. *J Appl Physiol* 1990; **69**: 822–829.

67. McClish DK, Powell SH, Montenegro H, Nochomovitz M. The impact of age on the utilization of intensive care resources. *J Am Geriatr Soc* 1987; **35**: 983–988.

68. Mayer-Oakes SA, Oye RK, Leake B. Predictors of mortality in older patients following medical intensive care — the im-portance of functional status. *J Am Geriatr Soc* 1991; **39**: 862–868.

69. Craig DB. Postoperative recovery of pulmonary function. *Anesth Analg* 1981; **60**: 46.

70. Heuser MD, Case LD, Ettinger WH. Mortality in intensive care patients with respiratory disease — is age important? *Arch Intern Med* 1992; **152**: 1683–1688.

71. Kass JE, Castriotta RJ, Malakoff T. Intensive care unit outcome in the very elderly. *Crit Care Med* 1992; **20**: 1666.

72. Margulies DR, Lekawa ME, Bjerke S, *et al.* Surgical intensive care in the nonagenarian. No basis for age discrimination. *Arch Surg* 1993; **128**: 753–758.

73. Nicholas F, LeGall Jr, Alperovitch A, *et al.* Influence of patient's age on survival, level of therapy and length of stay in intensive care units. *Intensive Care Unit* 1982; **13**: 9–13.

74. Rockwood K, Noseworthy TW, Gibney RTN, *et al.* One-year outcome of elderly and young patients admitted to intensive care units. *Crit Care Med* 1993; **21**: 687–691.

75. Worthley L, Holt A. Percutaneous tracheostomy. *Intens Care World* 1992; **9**: 187–192.

76. Bowser-Wallace BH, Cone JB, Caldwell FT. Hypertonic lactated saline resuscitation of severely burned patients over 60 years of age. *J Trauma* 1985; **25**: 22.

77. Schneider EL. Infectious diseases in the elderly. *Ann Intern Med* 1983; **98**: 395–400.

78. Madden JW, Croker JR, Beynon GPJ. Septicemia in the elderly. *Postgrad Med J* 1981; **57**: 502.

79. Yoshikawa TT. Antimicrobial therapy for the elderly patient. *J Am Geriatr Soc* 1990; **38**: 1353–1372.

80. Leiber CP, Seinige UL, Sataloff DM. Choosing the site of surgery. An overview of ambulatory surgery in geriatric patients. *Clin Geriatri Med* 1990; **6**(3): 493–7.

81. Larach SW, Salomon MC, Williamson PR, *et al.* Laparoscopic assisted abdominoperineal resection. *Surgical Laparoscopy and Endoscopy* 1993; **3**: 115–118.

82. Quattlebaum JK Jr, Flanders HD, Usher CH III. Laparoscopic assisted colectomy. *Surgical Laparoscopy and Endoscopy* 1993; **3**: 81–87.

83. Shimi S, Nathanson LK, Cuschieri A. Laparoscopic cardiomyotomy for achalasia. *J R Coll Surg Edinb* 1969; **36**: 152–154.

84. Dvorak HF. Tumors. Wounds do not heal. *N Eng J Med.* **315**: 1650–1659. 1986;

85. Falcone RE, Nappa JF. Chemotherapy and wound healing. *Surg Clin North Am* 1984; **64**: 779–794.

86. Nicaise J, Jonckers J, Smeis P, Provosi J, Asiel M. Social rehabilitation of the elderly after surgical intervention. *Acta Chir Belg* 1993; **93**(3): 122–5.

87. Clark GS, Murray PK. Rehabilitation of the geriatric patient. In *Practices and Principles of Rehabilitation Medicine*, edited by JA DeLisa. Philadelphia: JB Lippincott, p. 410, 1988.

88. Delisa JA, Miller RM, Melnick RR, *et al.* Rehabilitation of the cancer patient. In *Cancer. Principles and Practices of Oncology*, 2nd ed, edited by VTG Devita, S Hellman, J Rosenberg. Philadelphia: JB Lippincott, p. 2333, 1989.

89. Felsenthal G. Rehabilitating older patients. Primary care evaluation, treatment, and resources. *Geriatrics* 1989; **44**: 81.

90. Harris KA, van Schie L, Carrole SE, *et al.* Rehabilitation potential of elderly patients with major amputations. *J Cardiovasc Surg* 1991; **32**: 463.

91. Reyes RL, Leahey EB, Leahey EB Jr. Elderly patients with lower extremity amputations: Three year study in a rehabilitation setting. *Arch Phys Med Rehabil* 1977; **58**: 116.

92. DeVivo MJ, Kartus PL, Rutt RD, *et al.* The influence of age at time of spinal cord injury on rehabilitation outcome. *Arch Neurol* 1990; **47**: 687.

93. Emanuel LL, Barry MJ, Stoeckle JD, *et al.* Advance directives for medical care. A case for greater use. *N Eng J Med* 1991; **324**: 889.

94. Ewen EF Jr, Keating HL. 3d: Alternatives to major surgery in the high-risk elderly. *Clin Geriatr Med* 1990; **6**(3): 481–92.

95. Fried TR, Gillick MR. Medical decision-making in the last six months of life. choices about limitation of care. *J Am Geriatr Soc* 1994; **42**(3): 303–7.

96. Society of Critical Care Medicine Ethics Task Force. Consensus report on the ethics of foregoing life-sustaining treatments in the critically ill. *Crit Care Med* 1990; **18**: 1435.

97. Faber-Langendoen K, Bartels DM. Process of forgoing life-sustaining treatment in a University hospital. An empirical study. *Crit Care Med* 1992; **20**: 570.

98. Smedira NG, Evans BH, Grais LH, *et al.* Withholding and withdrawal of support from the critically ill. *N Eng J Med* 1990; **322**: 309.

28. Advances in Geriatric Surgery

Peter J. Fabri

Introduction

As a larger percent of the population lives into their eighties or nineties or above, the likelihood of encountering malignancy likewise goes up. Accordingly, the incidence of most malignancies increases in the elderly. At the same time, improvements in anesthetic technique, patient preparation, and management of co-existent medical conditions now allow surgical procedures in the older cancer patient which previously might not have been considered. Concurrently, changes in the health care environment are necessitating shorter hospital stays, increasing use of ambulatory surgery, and a burgeoning use of "minimally invasive" surgical procedures (1), such as laparoscopy, thoracoscopy, interventional endoscopy, and interventional radiology. The surgical treatment of malignancies in elderly patients may translate into improved outcome (2,3,4) but also increases the risk for surgical complications, lengthy hospitalizations and dramatic costs.

In the past, upper abdominal operations (5,6,7) were often considered too risky in elderly patients, and in many institutions age limits were established for high risk procedures such as pancreaticoduodenectomies and trisegmentectomies of the liver. Recent studies, however, suggest (8,9,10) that the outcome of major surgery is comparable in the elderly if careful patient selection and appropriate attention to detail is exercised (12,13,14). In very high risk, elderly patients, the choice of a surgical procedures for specific diseases may need to be modified (15). Attention to cardiac and pulmonany risk factors in the elderly is essential (16) and the influence of co-existing disease must be anticipated (17). A careful social and functional history, in addition to past and current illnesses, is essential. If these factors have been considered, it should be possible to offer appropriate and effective surgical therapy for many malignancies in elderly patients. Surgical oncology in the elderly does not require alteration in the technical performance of a given operation; therefore, we will not "reiterate" traditional surgical atlases (18). Rather, surgical oncology in the elderly is a matter of decision making and patient management.

Esophageal Disease

Cancer of the esophagus often presents in an advanced stage. Even when it appears localized, however, submucosal spread and lymph node involvement are common. Consequently, because of the very poor response of esophageal cancer to resection, many surgeons have been reluctant to operate on elderly patients with malignancies of the esophagus. Therefore, medical evaluation and treatment of esophageal symptoms, endoscopic stenting and dilation (19) and endoscopic laser therapy (20) have been offered as alternatives. In recent years, however, it has been demonstrated that esophageal resection can be performed safely in the elderly (21,22,23) and with quite acceptable long term survival even in elderly patients (24). We are faced with the situation of a high risk operation and a patient population with multiple associated diseases. Therefore, a very careful selection process to define the optimum candidates based on each of these two groups of risk factors is essential. Patients whose risk is too high might be offered chemotherapy, radiation, and palliative laser treatment with stent placement. The chosen surgical patients, however, should undergo resection since it is the only therapeutic modality that currently offers the possibility of cure.

Blunt esophagectomy, using a transhiatal approach, has been recommended (25) as having fewer complications. While the evidence of complications has been argued, it appears clear that an anastomotic leak from a cervical esophagogastrostomy is better tolerated than a similar leak in an intrathoracic location. This favors the transhiatal approach with cervical reconstruction. One must consider, however, the risk of reflux and aspiration as well as that of postop complications.

Applying the increasing experience in blunt dissection of the lower esophagus, it has often become possible to resect lesions of the distal esophagus using a smaller procedure, and a primary transhiatal anastomosis constructed using a circular stapling device (EEA) through the abdomen. This approach avoids the need for thoracotomy with its attendant pulmonary complications, postoperative discomfort, and delayed recovery. Similarly, the introduction of thoracoscopic surgery allows careful dissection of the esophagus under direct vision with wide margins, with subsequent performance of a "controlled blunt esophagectomy" through a cervical and abdominal approach and the same cervical anastomosis where complications appear to be less.

Stomach and Duodenum

Even as the incidence of peptic ulcer disease has decreased in the United States, the incidence of gastric malignancy appears to be increasing. Similarly, there is a change in histology of distal esophageal lesions, with decreasing proportion of squamous and increasing incidence of adenocarcinoma. In a sense, gastric cancer is "migrating" proximally into the gastric fundus and GE junction. Meanwhile antral carcinoma, previously the most common gastric location, is clearly decreasing. The upper gastric lesions are more undifferentiated and less radio responsive. Consequently, a great portion of the surgical attention to esophageal and gastric neoplasms is now focused on the esophagogastric junction. It is probably not critical to distinguish between an adenocarcinoma that originates in the distal esophagus and migrates caudad versus a carcinoma in the proximal stomach that extends proximally into the esophagus. The surgical approach and the expected outcome are probably similar in both cases.

Carcinoma of the body of the stomach has been treated aggressively in many countries in the elderly patient. Experience gained in the treatment of benign diseases of the stomach in the elderly (26,27,28,29,30,31) has allowed transfer of these skills toward more aggressive gastric resections for malignancy (32,33,34, 35,36,37,38,39). An unusual variant of gastric carcinoma is that which occurs following a previous procedure for peptic ulcer disease. Recent data would suggest that a period of approximately twenty five years is required for the development of gastric malignancy following antral resection. Although there is continued debate whether the incidence of cancer in this setting is actually increased, it is clear that the entity exists and should be suspected in patients with upper GI symptoms and a remote history of gastric resection (40,41). Aggressive surgical treatment of these patients is justifiable even in advanced stage as long as appropriate patient selection and management of associated conditions are undertaken.

Endocrine Tumors

The use of screening both by imaging and by biochemical assays has identified elderly patients with previously unrecognized mass lesions in the thyroid (thyroid scans, thyroid ultrasounds, etc.), parathyroids (hypercalcemia) and adrenals (abdominal CT scan and MRI). Management of these asymptomatic "tumors" is controversial since these lesions are usually benign. Most authors would recommend that careful selection of patients for surgical treatment will result in better surgical results. Older patients tolerate total thyroidectomy or wide parathyroid exploration without much difficulty regardless of chronological age (42,43). Many patients in this age group present with vague neuromuscular symptoms and are subsequently found to be hypercalcemic by lab screening (44). If patients are selected because of acceptable risk, expectation of improvement can be anticipated. Clark, in a recent review of asymptomatic hyperparathyroidism, demonstrated that virtually all patients actually have significant preoperative symptoms which aren't actually realized until after they are eliminated by parathyroidectomy.

Introduction of a laparoscopic approach to the adrenal gland may be a major advance in managing patients with adrenal mass lesions identified on CAT scan which are smaller than 6 cm in size. Traditionally, pheochromocytoma has required laparotomy and bilateral adrenal exploration. Currently, MRI can identify pheochromocytoma with a high degree of accuracy, confirming whether it is unilateral thus allowing even a pheochromocytoma to be approached laparoscopically when the opposite adrenal gland is normal on MRI. In the case of endocrine disease of the elderly, it is more important than ever to establish an accurate diagnosis and to avoid aggressive treatment in "incidental" disease. Examples of these are lesions in the thyroid that are cystic or multilobar which are very unlikely to be malignant. Similarly, hypercalcemia should be evaluated thoroughly to exclude metastatic carcinoma or hypercalcemia associated with medical diseases such as sarcoidosis, multiple myeloma as should lesions on CT scan. This latter group has been most puzzling. Recent data from many centers suggest that patients without evidence of endocrinopathy (no high blood pressure, hypokalemia, Cushing's symptoms) and with lesions less than 4 to 5 cm can be observed with serial CT scans. Patients with lesions over 6 cm regardless of symptoms should undergo surgical exploration. The upper limit for size for safe removal laparoscopically is probably about 6 cm so that all lesions over 6 cm should probably be approached through an open surgical incision. Malignancy of the adrenal carries a very high mortality since it is identified late. Yet most small adrenal lesions are not malignant. A very cautious approach to large lesions in the elderly because of the poor prognosis is suggested.

Breast Cancer

The incidence of breast cancer continues to increase throughout life with the highest frequency in our oldest patients. As life span increases, an increasing number of patients in the latter years of life will develop breast tumors. Particularly with the increased use of screening mammography (45), many breast lesions in the elderly are being found that perhaps might not have been found before. The traditional approach to breast cancer in older women is to perform mastectomy routinely with the thought that breast conservation and cosmesis are not particularly important in the elderly female. Many recent studies, however, suggest that cosmesis and sense of self-image are probably quite important in the elderly and should be considered in the treatment planning. It is uncertain whether age affects breast cancer favorably or unfavorably since studies have been contradictory (46,47,48,49). Most authors would suggest that actuarial survival of breast cancer patients is probably not influenced by age at diagnosis. Since survival data appear favorable, women with small lesions can safely undergo lumpectomy with axillary dissection and radiation. If the size of the tumor relative to the breast would preclude an acceptable cosmetic result, mastectomy is probably warranted. Several centers are evaluating or using tamoxifen alone in the elderly patient with breast cancer, demonstrating good short term results. Long term results, however, are not yet available. Studies to date would suggest, however, that recurrence after tamoxifen therapy can still be treated surgically without apparent compromise in staging or curability of the disease. The use of chemotherapy in this age group is extremely controversial. Most studies do not show a distinct survival advantage of adjuvant use although there may be a delay in the time to recurrence of disease. Tamoxifen has been the mainstay of treatment in this age group in both the adjuvant as well as therapeutic setting. Hospital stays are becoming shorter and shorter with many breast procedures being performed on an outpatient basis. Elderly patients tolerate this outpatient management well as long as appropriate preoperative and psychosocial evaluations have been undertaken.

Colorectal Cancer

Malignancies of the colon and rectum are one of the more common lesions to be treated in the elderly. Several authors have reviewed their experience in the management of these lesions (50,51,52,53,54,55,56,57, 58,59) and studies generally suggest that appropriately selected patients can be managed using techniques traditionally used in younger patients. Several authors suggest modified surgical approaches such as perineal rectosigmoidectomy (60), subtotal colectomy with primary ileocolonic anastomosis for obstructing carcinoma (61), laparoscopy assisted resection (62), or conservative treatment with local excision (63). Patients seem to tolerate major surgical resections of the colon and rectum well but do not tolerate the infectious complications and wound problems which may result. Careful attention to preoperative bowel preparation, both mechanical and antibiotic, is essential. Careful evaluation of the heart and lungs with correction of abnormalities preop to minimize the impact of comorbid illness is also important. Sphincter-sparing operations, which avoid the need for a permanent colostomy, appear to be well tolerated in the elderly, although they often result in an increased frequency of bowel movements and/or incontinence. Overall, patients appear to tolerate large procedures on the colon quite well; the traditional concept that elderly patients should all have a colostomy to avoid the risks of surgical anastomosis does not appear to be warranted.

Traditional abdominal perineal resection can be avoided in most cases by the performance of low anterior resection or coloanal pull through. Elderly patients do not tolerate coloanal pull through procedures as well as younger patients, however, and are frequently troubled by excessive diarrhea. Careful patient selection is therefore essential. Preoperative, sandwiched radiotherapy may simplify removal of long lesions from the rectum and certainly appears to reduce the incidence of local recurrence. Neoadjuvant chemotherapy is probably of benefit in patients with large lesions and the addition of combined radiation and chemotherapy is currently being studied but seems likely to be beneficial as well in appropriately selected patients.

Recent experience confirms that local excision of rectal lesions is adequate therapy in selected patients. With or without adjuvant therapy, local recurrence rates are low and survival appears comparable to larger operations. Careful evaluation of the surgical specimen for level of penetration and lymphatic involvement is important if such minimal excision is to be recommended.

Pancreas

Many surgeons have recommended that pancreatic resection should not be accomplished in patients over the age of 65 because of the high operative risk and low survival yield. Recent studies (64,65,66), however, have documented that pancreatic resection in the elderly patient is both possible and effective. Endoscopic treatment of pancreatic cancer for palliation (67) is effective but requires frequent (every 6–12 weeks) replacement via ERCP. Renewed enthusiasm for resection of the pancreas (Whipple procedure) is found in the markedly decreased operative mortality following pancreaticoduodenectomy at Johns Hopkins (63). Pylorus preservation in this operation has rapidly become the treatment of choice because it minimizes gastric emptying disorders and does not appear to be associated with a significant incidence of marginal ulceration. The use of Octreotide in an adjuvant setting to decrease the incidence and severity of pancreatic anastomotic dehiscence appears to be justified. The postoperative recovery times and tolerance to major surgery appear to be normal in elderly patients and the stress of the initial procedure is not nearly as disadvantageous as are major surgical complications. Accordingly, the intent should be to perform the ideal operation at the first setting with perfect anastomoses and attention to all necessary details (69). Localized excision of lesions of the ampulla and duodenum may be quite suitable in elderly patients, particularly if co-morbid illness necessitates a rapid operation.

Liver

Hepatic and biliary resections have also been considered to be high risk procedures and therefore not appropriate for the elderly. In recent years, however, aggressive resections in both United States and abroad (70,71,72,73,74) confirm that operation appears possible for primary liver tumors as well as for metastatic disease from the colon. Primary liver tumors should probably be resected if they are small, not associated with advanced cirrhosis, and not involving major vascular structures such as the vena cava. CAT scans and MRI's have reached a level of sophistication which allows appropriate evaluation of the suitability of patients for resection and avoids the need for unnecessary pre-resection abdominal exploration. Many studies suggest that anatomic resection of segments of the liver is preferable to wide local excision in many cases. Patients appear to tolerate hepatic resection well if they are appropriately screened preoperatively and if particular attention is paid to preservation of adequate liver to assure adequate liver function (22).

Biliary tract tumors similarly can be resected with very acceptable results (75) in appropriately selected patients. Where preoperative imaging demonstrates unresectability due to anatomic factors or metastases, patients with advanced disease can be treated with endoscopic endoprosthesis (76). Patients who present acutely with obstruction due to malignant disease may derive benefit from temporary decompression via endoscopically placed biliary stents or by either percutaneous cholecystostomy or percutaneous transhepatic catheterization when endoscopic approaches are unsuccessful. Long term palliation with stents (77) is certainly possible; the average "survival" of a stent is about three months before replacement is necessary and therefore treatment should be carefully matched to the expected survival of the patient.

Gallbladder cancer has been a difficult problem because of the very poor prognosis. Several studies have demonstrated a place for aggressive surgical excision (78,79). Controversy continues about the role of extended surgical resection with portal lymph node dissection. At the present time, extended resection and lymph node dissections of the porta hepatis should be reserved for centers that are actively studying this problem and perform the operations frequently. Approaches to bypass both gallbladder and bile duct tumors by use of hepaticojejunostomy using segments three or four of the liver have proven useful (70,80).

Prostate

The incidence of prostate cancer increases linearly with age (81) and perhaps should be considered almost a routine diagnosis in the octogenarian. Treatment of this condition has been difficult because many patients appear to do quite well with no treatment at all. Nevertheless, many patients have a rapidly progressive and fatal course and therefore serious consideration of appropriate diagnosis, staging, and management is essential. The symptoms of urinary obstruction can now be relieved endoscopically with the use of an endoprosthesis (82) followed by treatment of obstructing prostatic lesions with laser (83). Some authors recommend deferring treatment in the elderly (86) for low grade stage T3 tumors without metastasis. Others, citing the excellent results of prostatectomy, recommend radical surgical excision in the elderly (85). Balducci (86) and Gibbons (87) discuss the relative role of the various treatment modalities in this disease. The difficulty in interpreting the literature for prostate cancer is the difference between treating an individual and a population. The results from large population studies employing radical resection suggests a benefit, although it is not clearly a large benefit. In younger, healthy patients, the risk of nerve sparing prostatectomy appear justified. In the older patient, careful decision-making is essential since many of these patients will never have clinical progression of disease. Accordingly, many authors would recommend expectant management for lesions in elderly patients, or

perhaps radiation. Additional studies are required to clarify the optimum way to treat prostate cancer in the elderly.

Bladder Cancer

Carcinoma of the bladder in the elderly patient can be managed easily by repeated transurethral resection of bladder tumors with careful restaging of the depth of penetration of the tumor at each excision. However, many of these patients will require more aggressive therapy. Even in the elderly patient, radical cystectomy appears to be a well accepted and tolerated procedure if it can be performed with minimal associated morbidity (88,89,90,91,92). Although a radical procedure may appear difficult, the mechanisms of urinary reconstruction are now sufficiently evaluated to allow even elderly patients to undergo a minimal risk procedure with suitable long term results. Urinary incontinence can be a difficult problem in this age group (93) but resection to control local disease outweighs the need to treat hemorrhage, obstruction, and necrosis at a later time.

When patients present with obstruction of the urinary tract due to cancers impinging on the ureter or ureteral orifices, percutaneous nephrostomy is a safe and effective measure for restoring excretion (94). Urologic procedures can often be performed through the tract of the percutaneous nephrostomy utilizing laser technology and flexible scopes.

Gynecologic

Gynecologic malignancies are often considered to be diseases of middle aged women. As with most malignancies, however, the actual incidence in elderly women is substantial and increases over time. Cancer in particular may be identified in elderly women long after their reproductive years (95). Radical resection of the uterus carries an increased risk in the elderly patient but this again can be managed quite suitably if associated underlying diseases can be effectively controlled (96). Elderly patients with gynecologic malignancy undergo non-operative staging including CAT scan and possible laparoscopy. In patients with a minimal number of risk factors and suitable perioperative staging and preparation, radical surgery should be recommended. Surgical stays are decreasing in length and the elderly appear to tolerate this change well. In resection of the ovaries, hormonal replacement is probably justified although debate continues about the side effects of hormonal replacement. Currently, replacement therapy for symptomatic females is being recommended as being of more benefit than risk. In the elderly woman, however, risk/benefit is an important consideration since replacement therapy may increase coronary disease, may decrease osteoporosis, and probably increases endometrial cancer. Although some clinicians feel strongly about the cardiac risks, and there is some evidence of an increased incidence of cardiovascular disease, this appears to be minimal if the patients are chosen appropriately and the dose minimized to that necessary to control symptoms.

Thoracic

Although the incidence of smoking is decreasing, the long term effects of smoking still result in a high frequency of lung cancer in elderly patients (97,98). Over the years, the relative benefit of pulmonary resection has been questioned. During the most recent decade, however, the optimism for chemotherapy and radiation alone has been tempered by a realization that surgical excision is still the best treatment for long term control of symptoms as well as the potential for cure. Pulmonary disease often has significant underlying cardiac disease which must be identified and treated. If patients can have underlying diseases adequately managed, pulmonary resection in the elderly patient appears to be a reasonable approach (99,100,101,102, 103,104,105). Patients often present with a large apical mass, may have a histologic diagnosis of adenocarcinoma on percutaneous biopsy, and may not have any evidence of metastatic disease (106,107). These patients are ideal candidates for resection if their surgical risk is otherwise reasonable. Preoperative thoracoscopy may be indicated in the marginal patients to assure that a lesion is resectable prior to making a commitment to a thoracotomy (108). Follow up of patients with non-small cell carcinoma appears to be favorable in elderly (109,101).

Head and Neck Surgery

Incidence of carcinoma of the larynx, base of the tongue, and palette increase with duration of smoking and exposure to other risk factors (102). Accordingly, elderly patients are not spared from these diseases. Since radiation therapy, chemotherapy, and surgical resection each have a role in treatment, planning for the management of these patients requires a multi modality approach which includes head and neck surgery, radiation oncology, and medical oncology. Careful staging including triple endoscopy and thin section CAT scans are essential to appropriately stage the tumor before definitive therapy is considered. Many favorable patients will benefit from a multi modality approach. Other patients with substantial risk factors may benefit from radiation alone with regular followup. If such patients develop recurrence, salvage with surgery and/ or chemotherapy is possible.

If surgical resection is chosen, careful attention to identification of risk factors allows an appropriate planned approach (113,114,115,116,117,118,119,120,121, 122,123,124,125,l26,127, 128). Many patients will present with significant malnutrition. Studies evaluating preoperative nutrition support have not shown improvement and this should be reserved for patients with marked malnutrition. Rather, consideration of nutrition requirements should include establishment of a suitable route for continued enteral nutrition in the postoperative period. Many institutions have placed percutaneous endoscopic gastrostomy tubes at the time of initial diagnosis to allow continued use of the gastrointestinal tract throughout the remainder of staging, adjuvant therapy, and postoperative recovery.

Elderly patients tolerate large, radical head and neck operations as well as multiple modality therapy well if underlying, associated illnesses are identified and treated. Accordingly, aggressive pursuit of nutrition maintenance is essential for the healing of flaps, stomas, and suture lines in radiated tissue. In many cases, hemilaryngectomy can be accomplished which preserves voice, and tracheostomy may also be avoided.

Neurosurgery

Many studies of benign and malignant disease have shown that elderly patients tolerate neurosurgical procedures quite well (128,129,130,131,132). Debulking tumor burden for malignant tumors in elderly patients may have a very limited role and therefore appropriate patient selection is warranted. In particular, removal of metastatic lesions to the brain should be limited to situations where a solitary lesion from a responsive tumor is identified on staging in a symptomatic patient whose symptoms are expected to be improved by resection (133). As more lesions are identified in patients who have imaging studies, particularly MRI, in advanced aged (134,135,136), more difficult decisions will have to be made about the appropriate surgical therapy. In particular, silent lesions in the elderly may not benefit from aggressive therapy. Again, very careful selection of patients is essential.

Development of less invasive approaches such as stereo tactic surgery (137), laparoscopic surgery via small ventriculostomy, gamma knife, neutron beam radiation, etc. may be suitable modalities in patients at higher risk. Meningiomas and acoustic neuromas appear to be identified with increasing frequency in this age group as the use of imaging modalities increases. Very careful consideration of possible benefit should be included in the preoperative evaluation of these patients since many of them are asymptomatic or minimally symptomatic and are unlikely to derive substantial benefit from surgery. On the other hand, patients with substantial symptoms that limit their ability to function can be expected to derive comparable benefits to younger patients if their associated illnesses are appropriately treated (138,138,140,141).

Skin

After many years of sun exposure, elderly patients are at high risk of developing skin cancer (142). Similarly, both unusual and common malignancies (143) occur with increased frequency. Melanoma is common, can usually be treated with local excision and follows an unpredictable course just as in younger patients. 2 cm margins seem adequate in most cases. Age is probably not a negative factor in the treatment of these lesions. Careful consideration of the total body skin coverage, however, should also be made at the time that a single lesion is excised. Careful documentation of co-existent premalignant lesions, small malignant lesions in critical areas, etc. which may alter the outcome, is important before embarking on surgical intervention. Wide excision should be limited in magnitude, particularly on the face, but function is clearly the most important factor to consider and particular attention should be paid to eye closure. Recent studies using radiolabelled vital dyes (injected around the tumor) have suggested that patients can be treated adequately without the associated morbidity by undergoing only the excision of the "sentinel node." Most data have been accumulated in patients with melanoma but recent studies have also shown an advance in carcinoma of the breast. Although short term data and actuarial evaluation of the data are too new, evaluation of the data suggests that comparable staging can be accomplished and formal lymph node dissection of the axilla, groin and neck can be avoided without apparent adverse reaction.

Orthopedics

Elderly are still at risk of developing common orthopedic problems; the most frequent problem is fracture secondary to falls (144). Patients do not tolerate long hospitalizations and so prompt medical evaluation and preparation for surgery is indicated. Although recent, larger procedures, including total hip replacement have received favorable support, it may be more prudent in elderly patients, particularly if their mobility is already severely restricted, to use limited procedures including pinning. Patients who are extremely high risk or have underlying terminal conditions may benefit from in-line traction in bed and control of pain. If patients are appropriately selected, surgical repair or replacement in the elderly patient with acute fracture can be accomplished with very acceptable morbidity and mortality. A common problem in the elderly oncology patient is lytic lesions of bone leading to instability. Successful techniques for bone repair using prosthetic devices and radiotherapy have shown improved clinical response and, more importantly, symptomatic improvement. Such a procedure does not lead to a large number of cures, but does allow patients to become ambulatory.

Summary

While surgical techniques remain much as they are described in atlases, the philosophy of surgery for cancer in the elderly has evolved in recent years in ways which influence the preparation of the patient for the surgical procedure itself.

1. Increasingly, patients are being treated in an ambulatory setting regardless of age.
2. An increased use of minimally invasive surgical procedures allows more rapid mobilization and return to normal activity and therefore better functional results.
3. Patients are being treated concurrently for other medical problems which are often factors in management decisions.
4. Limited surgical procedures may be preferable in elderly patients.

Accepted Limited Surgical Procedures

breast-lumpectomy with axillary dissection

carcinoma of the rectum transanal resection

carcinoma of the lung-thoracoscopic wide excision. (VATS)

References

1. Adkins RB, Scott HW Jr. Surgical procedures in patients aged 90 years and older. *South Med J* 77: 1357, 1984.
2. Baranofsky A, Myers M. Cancer incidence and survival in patients 65 years of age and older. *Cancer* 36: 27–41, 1986.
3. Becker TM, Goodwin JS, Hunt WC, Key CR, Samet JM. Survival after cancer surgery of elderly patients in New Mexico, 1969–1982. *J Arm Geriatr Soc* 37: 155–159, 1989.
4. Boring C, Squires T, Tong T. Cancer statistics, 1991. *Cancer* 47: 28, 1991.
5. Alexander HR, Turnbull AD, Salamone J, Keefe D, Melendez J. Upper abdominal cancer surgery in the very elderly. *J Surg Oncol* 47(2): 82–6, 1991.
6. Burns GP, Parikh SR. Abdominal surgery in the elderly patient. *Clin Geriatr Med* 6(3): 589–607, 1990.
7. Fenyo G. Acute abdominal disease in the elderly. *Am J Surg* 143: 751, 1982.
8. Donegan WL. Operative treatment of cancer in the older person by general surgeon. In *Geriatric Oncology*, edited by L Balducci, GH Lyman, WB Ershler. J.B. Lippincott, pp: 51–159, 1992.
9. Hoskin MP, Warner MA, Lobdell CM, Offord KP, Melton LJ III. Outcomes of surgery in patients 90 years of age and older *JAMA* 261: 1909–1915, 1989.
10. Koruda MJ, Sheldon GF. Surgery in the aged. *Adv Surg* 24: 293–331, 1991.
11. Morel PH, Egeli RA, Wachtl S, Rohner A. Results of operative treatment of gastrointestinal tract tumors in patients over 80 years of age. *Arch Surg* 124: 662–664, 1989.
12. Patterson WB. Surgical issues in geriatric oncology. *Semin Oncol* 16: 57–65, 1989.
13. Keating HJ 3d, Lubin MF. Perioperative responsibilities of the physician/geriatrician. *Clin Geriatr Med* 6(3): 459–67, 1990.
14. Reiss R, Deutsch AA, Eliashiv A. Decision-making process in abdominal surgery in the geriatric patient. *World J Surg* 7(4): 522–6, 1983.
15. Samet JM, Hunt WC, Key CR, *et al.* Choice of cancer therapy varies with age of patient. *JAMA* 255: 3385–3390, 1986.
16. Ziffren SE. Comparison of mortality rates for various surgical operations according to age groups, 1951 to 1977. *J Am Geriatr Soc* 27: 433, 1979.
17. Weitz HH. Noncardiac surgery in the elderly patient with cardiovascular disease. *Clin Geriatr Med* 6(3): 511–29, 1990.
18. Zollinger RM, Zollinger RM Jr. *Atlas of surgical operations*, 6th Ed. New York: MacMillan, 1988.
19. Castell DO. Esophageal disorders in the elderly. *Gastroenterol Clin North Am* 19: 235–254, 1990.
20. Siegel HI, Laskin KJ, Dabezaies MA, *et al.* The effect of endoscopic laser therapy on survival in patients with squamous-cell carcinoma of the esophagus. Further experience. *J Clin Gastroenterol* 13: 142–146, 1991.
21. Keeling P, Gillen P, Hennessy TP. Oesophageal resection in the elderly. *Ann R Coll Surg Engl* 71: 34–36, 1988.
22. Karl R, Smith S, Fabri P. Validity of major cancer operations in elderly patients. *Ann Surg Oncology* 2: 107–113, 1995.
23. Muechrcke DD, Kaplan DK, Connelly RJ. Oesophagogastrectomy in patients over 70. *Thorax* 44: 141–145, 1989.
24. Sugirnachi K, Matsuzaki K, Kuwano H, *et al.* Evaluation of surgical treatment of carcinoma of the esophagus: 20 years' experience. *Br J Surg* 72: 28–30, 1985.
25. Orringer MB, Stirling MC. Transhiatal esophagectomy for benign and malignant disease. *J Thoracic and Cardiovascular Surg* 105: 265, 1993.

26. Feliciano DV, Bitondo CG, Burch JM, et al. Emergency management of perforated peptic ulcers in the elderly patient. *Am J Surg* **148**: 764, 1984.

27. Fiser WP, Wellborn JC, Thompson BW, et al. Age and morbidity of vagotomy with antrectomy or pyloroplasty. *Am J Surg* **144**: 694, 1982.

28. Kane E, Fried G, McSherry CK. Perforated peptic ulcer in the elderly. *J Am Geriatr Soc* **29**: 224, 1981.

29. McGee GS, Sawyers JL. Perforated gastric ulcers. *Arch Surg* **122**: 555, 1987.

30. Nussbaum MS, Schusterman MA. Management of giant duodenal ulcer. *Am J Surg* **149**: 357, 1985.

31. Permutt RP, Cello JP. Duodenal ulcer disease in the hospitalized elderly patient. *Dig Dis Sci* **27**: 1, 1982.

32. Bandoh T, Isoyama T, Toyoshima H. Total gastrectomy for gastric cancer in the elderly. *Surgery* **109**(2): 136–42: 1991.

33. Coluccia C, Ricci EB, Marzola GG, Molaschi M, Nono MG. Gastric cancer in the elderly. Results of surgical treatment. *Int Surg* **72**: 4–10, 1987.

34. Edelman DS, Russin DJ, Wallack MK. Gastric cancer in the elderly. *Am Surgeon* **53**: 170–173, 1987.

35. Habu H, Endo M. Gastric cancer in elderly patients — results of surgical treatment. *Hepatogastroenterol* **36**: 71–74, 1989.

36. Saario I, Salo J, Lempinen M, et al. Total and near-total gastrectomy for gastric cancer in patients over 70 years of age. *Am J Surg* **154**: 269, 1987.

37. Svartholm E, Larsson SA, Haglund U. Total gastrectomy in the elderly patient. *Acta Chir Scand* **153**: 677–680, 1987.

38. Takeda J, Hashimoto K, Tanaka T, Koufuji K, Kodama I, Aoyagi K, Yano S, Kakegawa T. Gastric cancer surgery in the elderly. *Kurume Med J* **39**(2): 89–94, 1992.

39. Teixeira CR, Haruma K, Teshima H, Shimamoto T, Tanaka S, Yamamoto G, Sumil K, Kajiyama G. Comparative report on endoscopic and surgical treatment for early gastric cancer in elderly patients. *Arquivos de Gastroenterologia* **29**(3): 75–9, 1992.

40. Northfield TC, Hall CN. Carcinoma of the gastric stump. Risks and pathogenesis. *Gut* **31**: 1217, 1990.

41. Toftsgard C. Gastric cancer after peptic ulcer surgery. *Ann Surg* **220**: 159, 1989.

42. Whitman ED, Norton JA. Endocrine surgical diseases of elderly patients. *Surg Clin North Am* **74**: 1: 127–44, 1994.

43. Miccoli P, Iacconi P, Cecchini GM, Caldarelli F, Ricci E, Berti P, Puccini M. Thyroid surgery in patients aged over 80 years. *Acta Chir Belg* **94**(4): 222–3, 1994.

44. Delbridge LW, Marshman D, Reeve TS, et al. Neuromuscular symptoms in elderly patients with hyperparathyroidism. Improvement with parathyroid surgery. *Med J Aust* **149**: 74, 1988.

45. Mandelblatt J, Wheat M, Monane M, et al. Breast cancer screening for elderly women with and without co-morbid conditions. *Ann Intern Med* **116**: 722–730, 1992.

46. Adami H, Malker B, Holmberg L, et al. The relation between survival and age at diagnosis in breast cancer. *N Eng J Med* **315**: 559–563, 1986.

47. Adami H, Malker B, Meirik O, et al. Age as a prognostic factor in breast cancer. *Cancer* **56**: 898–902, 1985.

48. Bergman L, Dekker G, Van Leeuwen F, et al. The effect of age on treatment choice and survival in elderly breast cancer patients. *Cancer* **67**: 2227–2234, 1991.

49. Hunt K, Fry D, Bland K. Breast carcinoma in the elderly patient. An assessment of operative risk, morbidity, and mortality. *Am J Surg* **140**: 339–342, 1980.

50. Armaud JP, Schloegel M, Ollier JC, et al. Colorectal cancer in patients over 80 years of age. *Dis Colon Rectum* **34**: 896–898, 1991.

51. Fitzgerald SD, Longo WE, Daniel GL, Vernava AM. Advanced colorectal neoplasia in the high-risk elderly patient: is surgical resection justified? *Diseases of the Colon & Rectum* **36**(2): 161–6, 1993.

52. Hesterberg R, Schmidt WU, Ohmann C, et al. Risk of elective surgery of colorectal carcinoma in the elderly. *Dig Surg* **8**: 22–27, 1991.

53. Hobler KE. Colon surgery for cancer in the very elderly. Cost and 3-year survival. *Ann Surg* **203**: 129–131, 1986.

54. Lewis AAM, Khoury GA. Resection for colorectal cancer in the very old. Are the risks too high? *Br Med J* **296**: 459–461, 1988.

55. Payne JE, Chapuis PH, Pheils MT. Surgery for large bowel cancer in people aged 75 years and older. *Dis Colon & Rectum* **29**: 733–737, 1986.

56. Richards PC. Colorectal cancer in the elderly. *Front Radiat Ther Oncol* **20**: 139–142, 1986.

57. Tomoda H, Tsujitani S, Furusawa M. Surgery for colorectal cancer in elderly patients — A Comparison with younger adult patients. *Jap J Surg* **18**: 397–402, 1988.

58. Vivi AA, Lopes A, Cavalcanti S de F, Fossi BM, Marques LA. Surgical treatment of colon and rectum adenocarcinoma in elderly patients. *J Surg Oncol* **51**: 3: 203–6, 1992.

59. Whittle J, Steinberg EP, Anderson GF, Herbert R. Results of colectomy in elderly patients with colon cancer, based on Medicare claims data. *Am J Surg* **163**: 6: 572–6, 1992.

60. Johansen OB, Wexler SD, Daniel N, et al. Perineal recto sigmoidectomy in the elderly. *Dis Colon Rectum* **36**: 767–772, 1993.

61. Kluger Y, Shiloni E, Jurim O, Katz E, Rivkind A, Ayalon A, Durst A. Subtotal colectomy with primary ileocolonic anastomosis for obstructing carcinoma of the left colon. valid option for elderly high risk patients. *Israel J Med Sci* **29**: 11: 726–30, 1993.

62. Vara-Thorbeck C, Garcia-Caballero M, Salvi M, Gutstein D, Toscano R, Gomez A, Vara-Thorbeck R. Indications and advantages of laparoscopy-assisted colon resection for carcinoma in elderly patients. *Surg Laparoscopy & Endoscopy* **4**: 2: 110–8, 1994.

63. Rouanet P, Saint Aubert B, Fabre JM, Astre C, Liu JZ, Dubois JB, Joyeux H, Solassol C, Pujol H. Conservative treatment for low rectal carcinoma by local excision with or without radiotherapy. *Brit J Surg* **80**: 11: 1452–6, 1993.

64. Connolly MM, Dawson PJ, Michelassi F, et al. Survival in 1001 patients with carcinoma of the pancreas. *Ann Surg* **206**: 366–373, 1987.

65. Hannoun L, Christophe M, Ribeiro J, Nordlinger B, Elriwini M, Tiret E, Parc R. A report of forty-four instances of pancreaticduodenal resection in patients more than seventy years of age. *Surg Gynecol Obstet* **177**: 6: 556–60, 1993.

66. Sciannameo F, Ronca P, Alberti D, Uccellini R. Therapeutic strategies in the surgical management of pancreatic neoplasms in the elderly. *Panminerva Medica* **35**: 2: 93–5, 1993.

67. Huibregtse K, Katon RM, et al. Endoscopic palliative treatment in pancreatic cancer. *Gastrointest Endosc* **32**: 334, 1986.

68. Yeo CJ, Cameron JL, Maher MM, Sauter PK, Zahurak ML, Talamin MA, Lillemoe KD, Pitt HA. A prospective randomized trial of pancreaticogastrostomy versus pancreaticojejunostomy after pancreaticoduodenectomy. *Ann Surg* **222**: 4: 580–592, 1995.

69. Gadzijev E, Pegan V. Extended excision of the ampulla of Vater–a new operative technique for elderly patients. *Hepato-Gastroenterology* **39**: 5: 475–7, 1992.

70. Bismuth H, Castaing D, Traynor O. Resection or palliation. Priority of surgery in the treatment of hilar cancer. *World J Surg* **12**: 39, 1988.

71. Ezaki T, Yukaya H, Ogawa Y. Evaluation of hepatic resection for hepatocellular carcinoma of the elderly. *Br J Surg* **74**: 471, 1987.

72. Mentha G, Huber O, Robert J, Klopfenstein C, Egeli R, Rohner A. Elective hepatic resection in the elderly. *Brit J Surg* **79**: 6: 557–9, 1992.

73. Nagasue N, Chang YC, Takemoto Y, Taniura H, Kohno H, Nakamura T. Liver resection in the aged (seventy years or older) with hepatocellular carcinoma. *Surgery* **113**: 2: 148–54, 1993.

74. Takenaka K, Shimada M, Higashi H, Adachi E, Nishizaki T, Yanaga K, Matsumata T, Ikeda T, Sugimachi K. Liver resection for hepatocellular carcinoma in the elderly. *Arch Surg* **129**: 8: 846 50, 1994.

75. Saunders K, Tompkins R, Longmire W Jr, Roslyn J. Bile duct carcinoma in the elderly. A rationale for surgical management. *Arch Surg* **126**: 10: 1186–90; discussion 1190–1, 1991.

76. Shepherd HA, Royle G, et al. Endoscopic biliary endoprosthesis in the palliation of malignant obstruction of the distal common bile duct. A randomized trial. *Br J Surg* **75**: 1166, 1988.

77. Speer AG, Russell RCG, et al. Randomized trial of endoscopic versus percutaneous stent insertion in malignant obstructive jaundice. *Lancet* **2**: 57, 1987.

78. Nakamura S, Sakaguchi S, et al. Aggressive surgery for carcinoma of the gallbladder. *Surgery* **106**: 467, 1989.

79. Silk YN, Douglass HO Jr, et al. Carcinoma of the gallbladder, the Roswell experience. *Ann Surg* **210**: 751, 1989.

80. Blumgart LH, Thompson JN. The management of malignant strictures of the bile duct. Tumors of the biliary and intrahepatic bile ducts. *Current Problems in Surgery* **Vol. XXIV**(2): 81, February 1987.

81. Stamey TA, McNeal JE. Adenocarcinoma of the prostate. In *Campbell's Urology*, ed 6, edited by PC Walsh, AB Retik, TA Stamey, et al. Philadelphia: WB Saunders, pg. 2829, 1992.

82. Adam A, Jager R, McLoughlin J, et al. Wall stent endoprosthesis for the relief of prostatic urethral obstruction in high risk patients. *Clin Radiol* **42**(4): 228–32, 1990.

83. Kabalin JN. Urolase laser prostatectomy. *Monographs in Urology* **14**: 23–36, 1993.

84. Adolfsson J. Deferred treatment of low grade stage T3 prostate cancer without distant metastases. *J Urol* **149**: 326, 1993.

85. Kerr LA, Zincke H. Radical retropubic prostatectomy for prostate cancer in the elderly and the young: complications and prognosis. *Europ Urol* **25**(4): 305–11; discussion 311–2, 1994.

86. Balducci L, Trotti A, Pow-Sang J. Advances and controversies in the prevention and treatment of prostate cancer. *L'Annee' Gerontologique* **2**: 97–110, 1992.

87. Gibbons RP. Localized prostate carcinoma. Surgical Management. *Cancer.* **72**(10): 2865–12, 1993.

88. Kursh ED, Rabin R, Persky L. Is cystectomy a safe procedure in the elderly patients with carcinoma of the bladder? *J Urol* **118**: 40, 1977.

89. Skinner EC, Lieskovsky G, Skinner DG. Radical cystectomy in the elderly patient. *J Urol* **131**: 1065, 1984.

90. Tachibana M, Deguchi N, Jitsukawa S, et al. One-state total cystectomy and ileal loop diversion in patients over eighty years old with bladder carcinoma. *Urology* **22**: 512, 1983.

91. Wood DP, Montie JE, Maatman TJ, et al. Radical cystectomy for carcinoma of the bladder in the elderly patient. *J Urol* **138**: 46,1987.

92. Zincke H. Cystectomy and urinary diversion in patients eighty years or older. *Urology* **19**: 139, 1982.

93. Rousseau P, Fuenteville-Clifton A. Urinary incontinence in the aged, Part 2. Management strategies [published erratum appears in *Geriatrics* 1992 **47**(9): 87].

94. Segura JW. Percutaneous nephrostomy. Technique, indications and complications. *AUA Update Series*, **Vol 12**, Lesson 20, 1993.

95. McGonigle KF, Lagasse LD, Karlan BY. Ovarian, uterine, and cervical cancer in the elderly woman. *Clin Geriatr Med* **9**(1): 115–30, 1993.

96. Fuchtner C, Manetta A, Walker JL, Emma D, Berman M, DiSaia PJ. Radical Hysterectomy in the elderly Patient. Analysis of morbidity. *Am J Obstet & Gynec* **166**(2): 593–7, 1992.

97. Ershler WB, Socinski MA, Greene CJ. Bronchogenic carcinoma, metastases, and aging. *J Am Geriatr Soc* **31**: 673–676, 1983.

98. O'Rourke MA, Feussner JR, Fiegl P, Laszlo J. Age trends of lung cancer stage at diagnosis. *JAMA* **258**: 921–926, 1987.

99. Brucke P. Is lung cancer resection justified in patients aged beyond 70 years? *Europ J Cardio-thoracic Surg* **7**(6): 336, 1993.

100. Osaki T, Shirakusa T, Kodate M, Nakanishi R, Mitsudomi T, Ueda H. Surgical treatment of lung cancer in the octogenarian. *Ann Thorac Surg.* **57**(1): 188–92, discussion 192–3, 1994.

101. Plotrlikov VI, Kulish VL, Malaev SG. Surgery for elderly patients with cancer of the cardia. *Seminars in Surg Oncol* **8**(1): 41–5, 1992.

102. Roxburgh JC, Thompson J, Goldstraw P. Hospital mortality and long term survival after Pulmonary resection in the elderly. *Ann Thorac Surg* **51**: 800–803, 1991.

103. Sherman S, Guidot CE. The feasibility of thoracotomy for lung cancer in the elderly. *JAMA* **258**: 927–930, 1987.

104. Shiracusa T, Tsutsui M, Iriki N et al. Results of resections for bronchogenic carcinoma in patients over the age of 80. *Thorax* **44**: 189–191, 1989.

105. Thomas P, Sielezneff I, Ragni J, Giudicelli R, Fuentes P. Is lung cancer resection justified in patients aged over 70 years? *Europ J Cardiothoracic Surg* **7**(5): 246–50; discussion 250–1, 1993.

106. DeMaria LC, Cohen HJ. Characteristics of lung cancer in elderly patients. *J Gerontol* **42**: 540–545, 1987.

107. Teeter SM, Holmes FF, MacFarlane MJ. Lung cancer in the elderly population. Influence of histology on the inverse relationship of stage to age. *Cancer.* **60**: 1331–1336, 1987.

108. Reilly JJ Jr, Mentzer SJ, Sugarbaker DJ. Preoperative assessment of patients undergoing pulmonary resection. *Chest* **103**(4 Suppl): 342S–345S, 1993.

109. Gebitekin C, Gupta NK, Martin PG, Saunders NR, Walker DR. Long-term results in the elderly following pulmonary resection for non-small cell lung carcinoma. *Europ J Cardio-thoracic Surg* **7**(12): 653–6, 1993.

110. Ishida T, Yokoyama H, Kaneko S, et al. Long term results of operation for non-small cell lung cancer in the elderly. *Ann Thorac Surg* **50**: 919–922, 1990.

111. Whittel J, Steinberg EP, Anderson GF, Herbert R. Use of Medicare claims data to evaluate outcomes in elderly patients undergoing lung resection for lung cancer. *Chest* **100**(3): 729–34, 1991.

112. Barzan L, Veronesi A, Caruso G, et al. Head and neck cancer and aging. A retrospective study in 438 patients. *J Laryngol Otol* **104**: 634–640, 1990.

113. McGuirt WF, Loevy S, McCabe BF et al. The risks of head and neck surgery in the aged population. *Laryngoscope* **87**: 1378–1382, 1977.

114. Harries M, Lund VJ. Head and neck surgery in the elderly. A maturing problem. *J Laryngol Otol* **103**: 306–309, 1989.

115. John AC, Vaughan ED. Laryngeal resection in patients of seventy years and older. *J Otol* **94**: 629–635, 1980.

116. Johnson JT, Rabuzzi D, Tucker HM. Composite resection in the elderly. A well tolerated procedure. *Laryngoscope* **87**: 1509–1515, 1977.

117. Jun MY, Strong EW, Saltzman EI, et al. Head and neck cancer in the elderly. *Head Neck Surg* **5**: 376–382, 1983.

118. Kowalski LP, Alcantara PS, Magrin J, Parise Junior O. A case-control study on complications and survival in elderly patients undergoing major head and neck surgery. *Am J Surg* **168**(5): 485 90, 1994.

119. Linn BS, Robinson DS, Klimas SETTING. Effects of age and nutritional status on surgical outcomes in head and neck cancer. *Ann Surg* **207**: 267–273, 1988.

120. Loewy A, Huttner DJ. Head and neck surgery in patients past 70. *Arch Otol* **84**: 523–S26, 1984.

121. Martin H, Rasmussen LH, Perras C. Head and neck surgery in patients of the older group. *Cancer* **8**: 707–711, 1955.

122. McGuirt WF, Davis SP rd. Demographic portrayal and outcome analysis of head and neck cancer surgery in the elderly. *Arch Otolaryngol — Head & Neck Surg* **121**(2): 150–4, 1995.

123. Morgan RF, Hirata RM, Jacques DA, et al. Head and neck surgery in the aged. *Am J Surg* **144**: 449–451, 1982.

124. Morton RP, Benjamin CS. Elderly patients with head-and-neck cancer. *Lancet.* **335**: 1597, 1990.

125. Robinson DS. Head and neck considerations in the elderly patient. *Surg Clin North Am* **74**(2): 431–9, 1994.

126. Sanders AD, Blom ED, Singer MI, et al. Reconstructive and rehabilitative aspects of head and neck cancer in the elderly. *Otol Clin North Am* **23**: 1141–1156, 1990.

127. Tucker HM. Conservation laryngeal surgery in the elderly patient. *Laryngoscope* **87**: 1995–1999, 1977.

128. Amacher AL, Bybee De. Toleration of head injury by the elderly. *Neurosurgery* **20**: 954, 1987.

129. Caruso R, Salvati M, Cervoni L. Primary intracranial arachnoid cyst in the elderly. *Neurosurg Review* **17**(3): 195–8, 1994.

130. Gijtenbeek JM, Hop WC, Braakman R, Avezaat CJ. Surgery for intracranial meningiomas in elderly patients. *Clinical Neurol & Neurosurg* **95**(4): 291–5, 1993.

131. Howard MA, Gross AS, Dacey RG, et al. Acute subdural hematomas. An age-dependent clinical entity. *J Neurosurg* **71**: 858, 1989.

132. Jamjoom A, Nelson R, Stranjalis G, *et al.* Outcome following surgical evaluation of traumatic intracranial hematomas in the elderly. *Br J Neurosurg* **6**: 27, 1992.

133. Kelly PJ, Hunt C. The limited value of cytoreductive surgery in elderly patients with malignant gliomas. *Neurosurg* **34**(1): 62–6; discussion 66–7, 1994.

134. Maurice-Williams RS, Kitchen ND. Intracranial tumors in the elderly. The effect of age on the outcome of first time surgery for meningiomas. *Brit J Neurosurg* **6**(2): 131–7, 1992.

135. Maurice-Williams RS, Kitchen N. The scope of neurosurgery for elderly people. *Age & Ageing* **22**(5): 337–42, 1993.

136. Nishizaki T, Kamiryo T, Fujisawa H, Ohshita N, Ishihara H, Ito H, Aoki H. Prognostic implications of meningiomas in the elderly (over 70 years old) in the era of magnetic resonance imaging. *Acta Neurochirurgica* **126**(2–4): 59–62, 1994.

137. Popovic EA, Kelly PJ. Stereotactic procedures for lesions of the pineal region. *Mayo Clin Proc* **68**(10): 965–70, 1993.

138. Ramsay HA, Luxford WM. Treatment of acoustic tumors in elderly patients: is surgery warranted? *J Laryngol Otolog* **107**(4): 295–7, 1993.

139. Rubin G, Ben David U, Gornish M, Rappaport ZH. Meningiomas of the anterior cranial fossa floor. *Acta Neurochirurgica* **129**(1–2): 26–30, 1994.

140. Samii M, Tatgiba M, Matthies C. Acoustic neurinoma in the elderly. Factors predictive of postoperative outcome. *Neurosurg* **31**(4): 615–9; discussion 619–20, 1992.

141. Umansky F, Ashkenazi E, Gertel M, Shalit MN. Surgical outcome in an elderly population with intracranial meningioma. *J Neurol Neurosurg Psychiatry* **55**(6): 481–5, 1992.

142. Jones EW. Some special skin tumors in the elderly. *Br J Dermatol* **122** (Suppl 35): 71–75, 1990.

143. Ries WR, Aly A, Vrabec J. Common skin lesions of the elderly. *Otol Clin North Am* **23**: 1121–1139, 1990.

144. Perez ED. Hip fracture: physicians take more active role in patient care. *Geriatrics* **49**(4): 31–7, 1994.

29. Perioperative Considerations in the Geriatric Oncology Patient

Rafael Miguel

Introduction

Setting arbitrary age limits for the geriatric patient population is somewhat difficult. These limits are arbitrary in that change in the age which classifies a patient "geriatric," is continual. For example, in the early 20th Century, surgery on patients above the age of 50 was considered dangerous and not recommended (1). Indeed, in 1927 Alton Ochsner suggested that "an elective operation for inguinal hernia in a patient older than 50 years is not justified" (2). This impression has certainly changed. By 1985, Catlic (3) reported six patients over the age of 100 who underwent anesthesia and surgery. His impression at the time reflected the changing mood in society and medicine. He stated that "elective surgery should not be deferred nor emergency surgery denied, even for centenarians on the basis of chronologic age." Data from the US Census Bureau has shown changing demographics of the population (Figure 29.1). Furthermore, as the population ages, this will have a significant impact in those patients going to surgery. Since patients going to surgery tend to be older rather than young, a greater portion of patients of any hospital's operating rooms will be occupied by geriatric patients.

Common knowledge would dictate that older patients have a markedly higher incidence of perioperative complications, even death, when compared to their younger counterparts. However, little information is available that implicates age *per se* as a risk factor. The most important consideration in the elderly is to search for and identify associated abnormalities. These may occur secondary to the natural decline of basic organ function due to the aging process. For this reason, a basic understanding of the physiologic changes of aging that impact perioperative management is useful whether a patient undergoes an inpatient or an outpatient operation. The latter is important since more mandates are being received from Medicare and third party payors for outpatient and same day admit procedures, as greater emphasis is placed on decreasing costs. This emphasis needs to be directed to preoperative evaluation during clinic visits, so that associated abnormalities may be identified and optimized, if present. It is hoped that a thourough understanding of the physiologic changes commonly found in the elderly and tailoring their anesthetic techique and perioperative management would lead to improved outcomes.

Physiologic Changes of Aging and their Anesthetic Implications

General Considerations

There is a significant decrease in body mass, accounted for by a decrease in the number of functioning parenchymal cells, with an increase in interstitial substances. This accounts for a generally accepted decrease in basal metabolic rate (BMR) of 1% per year after the age of 30. There is a significant change in the composition of body fluids. Total body water decreases 10–15%. This change effects a drop from 60% in younger patients to 45% total body water found in the elderly. Since extracellular body fluid volume remains the same, the drop is primarily due to a decrease in intracellular fluid. Total plasma proteins remain unchanged, although the ratio changes significantly. Albumin concentration decreases while globulin concentration increases.

Regulation of temperature becomes more difficult as there is a decrease in the number of skin capillaries. This causes a decreased capacity for vasoconstriction and vasodilatation. Sweat gland atrophy contributes for a decrease in the capacity to sweat and release heat.

These changes in the elderly renders them unable to adapt to ambient temperature changes, making them

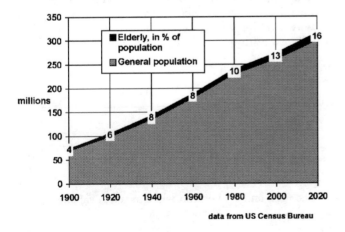

Figure 29.1 US Demographics.

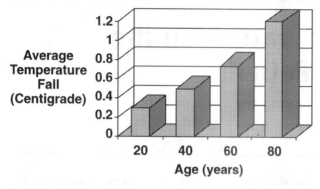

modified from McClesky C, in Clinical Anesthesia, 2nd Ed.

Figure 29.2 Age and intraoperative rectal temperature.

especially susceptible to hypo- and hyperthermia. Decreases in body temperature are routine in the anesthetized surgical patient, but that drop is accentuated in the elderly (Figure 29.2). Recent studies have demonstrated improvements in morbidity by decreasing perioperative hypothermic events. Kurz *et al.* found a decrease in surgical wound infections and shorter hospitalizations by maintaining normothermia perioperatively (4). Frank and his collaborators demonstrated that in patients with cardiac risk factors, maintenance of perioperative normothermia was associated with a lower incidence of morbid cardiac events (i.e., unstable angina/ischemia, cardiac arrest or myocardial infarction) as well as, ventricular tachycardia, when compared to hypothermic patients (5). Particular attention needs to be placed on perioperative temperature monitoring and actively warming and cooling them as necessary.

Structural Characteristics

The musculoskeletal system undergoes dramatic changes in the elderly. Some of the structural changes and their management are listed in Table 29.1. The elderly patient generally adopts a posture of generalized flexion. The thoracic spine becomes kyphotic secondary to degenerative changes in the vertebral column, intravertebral discs and paraspinal tendons and mus-

cles. The amount of osteoporosis seen is progressive and is of staggering importance. Females greater than the age of 45 demonstrate presence of osteoporosis and it is estimated that by the age of 65, 33% of all females have vertebral fractures and by the age of 81, one-third of all women and one-sixth of all men will have had a hip fracture (4). Osteoporosis becomes a problem in males above the age of 55. While the bone is qualitatively normal, whatever bone there is, is less dense and there is less of it. The patient is more susceptible to bony fractures with otherwise negligible trauma. At present, it is unknown whether this is part of the natural aging process or a disease entity in and of itself.

Osteoarthritic changes are seen throughout the body and joint changes are universal with increased aging. There is thinning of joint cartilage, a loss of joint fluid and hardening of joint capsules with proliferation of adjacent bones. This leads to osteophyte formation. Skeletal muscle wasting is seen secondary to a decrease in the number and size of individual muscle fibers. Encouraging, however, was a recent study (5) which pointed out that nonagenarians could significantly increase strength and endurance by progressive weight training. There is degradation of motor end-plates. The generalized wasting with loss of skin elasticity, vascularity and tensile strength is accompanied by a decrease in subcutaneous fat. This decrease is accentuated with age. This makes the patient particularly vulnerable to even minor trauma. Because of this loss of support structures and subcutaneous tissue, great attention to pressure points needs to be done in the perioperative period. Padding with sheep skin, foam or other suitable materials are indicated. Skin and muscular atrophy lead to problems with cannulation of veins, which are more fragile and mobile.

Changes in orofacial structures contribute to a loss of elasticity and tone over the mouth muscles. There is significant resorption of alveolar bone and weakening of support for dental structures. This is commonly accompanied by lost or loose teeth. The anesthetic implications of these structural changes are many. Airway management is primarily affected by loss of orofacial support. Difficulty maintaining a patients airway can be encountered. The question remains whether dentures should be left in or out. While den-

Table 29.1 General and structural changes in the elderly.

Changes	Implications	Management
Loss of functioning parenchymal cells, decreased # of skin capillaries, sweat gland atrophy	10–15% drop in BMR Decreased ability to vasoconstrict or vasodilate	Actively warm or cool as necessary
Osteoarthritis	Decreased mobility of joints, neck and mouth	Position while awake, evaluate airway access
Loss of muscle and subcutaneous fat, bony resorption	Ease of developing pressure trauma, facial anatomy changes	Pad pressure points, dentures/oral packs may help airway support

BMR = basal metabolic rate

Table 29.2 Cardiorespiratory changes in the elderly.

Changes	Implications	Management
Fibrosis of sinoatrial node, ventricular conduction	Arrhythmias, decreased heart rate	Continual EKG monitoring
Atherosclerotic vessel walls	Decreased BP accommodation Compensatory LVH	Avoid rapid changes in blood volume
Myocardial fiber atrophy, decrease in LV cavity, valvular calcification	Decrease in CO, increased circulation time, decreased ejection fraction	Afterload reduction, avoid cardiodepressant medication, titrate medications
Calcific, arthritic thoracic joints, bronchi and chest wall	Inefficient expiration, RV increases 50%, VC/IC decrease, dead space ventilation increases	Maximize preoperative pulmonary function, support ventilation postoperatively
CV increases, MVV decreases, chemoreceptor response decrease	Increased V/Q mismatch, resting P_aO_2 lower, less ventilatory reserve, response to P_aCO_2 increase/P_aO_2 decrease blunted	Supplemental O_2, monitor $ETCO_2$/S_pO_2, always R/O in postoperative delirium, light sedation/narcosis

EKG = Electrocardiogram, LVH = left ventricular hypertrophy, LV = left ventricle, CO = cardiac output, RV = residual volume, VC/IC = vital capacity/inspiratory capacity, CV = closing volume, MVV = maximum voluntary ventilation, V/Q = ventilation/perfusion

tures are commonly removed prior to anesthesia for fear of losing them or causing airway obstruction under anesthesia, they may improve the ability to maintain a good seal while performing bag-mask ventilation. It may be advantageous to leave dentures in place. Similarly, since elderly patients have significant resorption of their facial structures, gauze may be used under the lips to increase facial bulk and facilitate a tight fitting seal around the mask and face. Close examination of the oral cavity needs to be done to identify loose teeth and to remove any dislodged teeth. Neck and jaw mobility are restricted in the elderly and should be evaluated preoperatively. This evaluation is important as many patients will refer pain on positioning which would otherwise appear to be appropriate and indeed may reveal the presence of vascular abnormalities, such as carotid stenosis. This may manifest as lightheadedness, dizziness or even fainting when changing head position in the awake patient. Waiting until the patient is asleep to assess the position for operation, will obviously fail to reveal problems. This evaluation becomes even more important when one considers the degree of cervical osteoarthritis seen in the elderly. This results in a decrease in size of transverse process canals through which the vertebral artery passes. It can be easily understood how manipulation of the head can further impair flow leading to vertebrobasilar insufficiency and global cerebral ischemia.

Cardiovascular System

The cardiovascular system presents the most important age related physiologic changes which affect anesthetic management. While once thought to be part of the natural aging process, many of the changes seen in the cardiovascular system are now considered to be related to preexisting diseases in the patient and lifestyle changes associated with prolonged deconditioning (6).

The heart demonstrates increased amounts of subpericardial fat. There are patches of fat in the endocardium and capillary muscles with increased fibrotic thickening and rigidity of all valves. There is left atrial enlargement, an increase in left ventricular (LV) wall thickness and a decrease in LV cavity size (Table 29.2). The ventricular conduction system is invaded by fibrosis, which causes an increased frequency of arrhythmias. Vessel walls are less resilient, so therefore there is a lower capacity to accommodate for wide changes in arterial pressure. While cardiac output (CO) averages approximately 6.5 L/min at 25 years of age, there is a progressive decrease to 50% of that value by the age of 80 (7). This is primarily due to a decrease in stroke volume and heart rate. There is increasing evidence that this decrease may ocurr only in patients who have adopted a sedentary lifestyle or are affected by disease (8). Circulation time is increased by 33%, which facilitates patient overdosing especially when considered in combination with a decrease in blood flow to metabolic end-organs. There is a decrease in systolic blood pressure with an increase in diastolic pressure. Longstanding disease, such as hypertension or congestive heart failure, will greatly exacerbate all of the aforementioned cardiovascular changes. Therefore, maintaining near normal vital signs, maintaining satisfactory oxygenation and producing a favorable myocardial O_2 supply: demand ratio, is of utmost importance.

Pulmonary System

The pulmonary system is important in anesthesia because of the increased need for homeostasis and gas

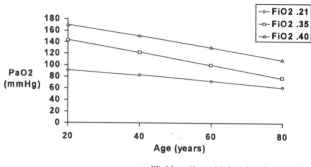

Figure 29.3 Age related decrease in P_aO_2.

exchange and the involvement of the lung with uptake and elimination of anesthetic gases. Alveoli are affected by the aging process and septal membranes weaken and are often disrupted. This causes a significant coalescence (i.e., increase in size with a decrease in number) of alveoli in the elderly. Calcific and arthritic changes are seen in cartilage and joints of the thorax and bronchi. Ventilatory muscles become weaker, so therefore, there is increased rigidity of lung parenchyma, tracheobrochial tree and thorax (Table 29.2). Inspiration becomes more inefficient, there is a decrease in chest wall mobility and muscle strength. Expiration becomes more inefficient because of a decrease in elastic recoil. All these changes significantly affect lung volumes. Total lung capacity decreases by approximately 10%. Residual volume (RV) increases approximately 50% at the expense of vital capacity (VC) and inspiratory capacity (IC). These decrease 30 and 70%, respectively. Anatomic dead space increases with age. At 20 years of age, approximately 20% dead space ventilation is seen. This doubles by the time the patient is 60. There is a decrease in tidal volume, minute ventilation and the ventilatory response to a CO_2 challenge is impaired. Closing volume (CV), the volume of lung in which airways collapse, increases (9). This may be the most important change in the pulmonary system. When closing volume is greater than functional residual capacity, the closing volume will be within normal tidal volumes, so some airways will be collapsed until inspiration. At approximately 36 years of age closing volume is greater than functional residual capacity in the supine patient. At 60, this occurs in the sitting position. Obviously, this will include essentially all positions which will lead to an increase in V/Q mismatch units and decreased P_aO_2 (Figure 29.3). The ideal P_aO_2 value can be calculated by the following formula:

$$P_aO_2 = 109 \text{ mmHg} - (0.43 \times \text{age in years}).$$

The anesthetic implication of these changes in the pulmonary system is evidenced by the increase in pulmonary problems seen perioperatively in elderly patients. While operative mortality for lobectomy in younger patients is 2–4% and up to 10% for pneumonec-

tomy, in the elderly patient with poor lung function operative mortality may exceed 15 and 30%, respectively (10). Lower postoperative P_aO_2 values are seen in these patients. In addition to all these changes in the ventilatory system, the effects of positive pressure ventilation, endotracheal intubation, decrease in mucociliary transport, central respiratory depression and residual neuromuscular blockade have to be considered. Particularly important to the respiratory system are the influence the latter two have perioperatively. The use of opioids perioperatively would be expected have a significantly more intense and long-lasting effect in elderly patients. Scott and Stanski (11) have found dose requirements of fentanyl and alfentanil to decrease by 50% from the age of 20 to 85 years. Residual neuromuscular blockade can also contribute negatively to pulmonary function. This is especially significant when older agents, such as pancuronium, metocurine, or d-tubocurarine are used. An increase in dosing intervals should be effected as 25%-75% twitch recovery time, an index of neuromuscular recovery, is considerably longer than in younger patients (12).

Nervous System

The weight of the brain decreases to 80% of peak weight secondary to neuron loss in the cerebellum, cerebral cortex and thalamus. There are chemical alterations which contribute to the decrease in CNS function. These include a decrease in the rate of conversion of tyrosine and DOPA. The activity of MAO and COMT are increased. In combination, these contribute to an overall decrease in catecholamines. Serotonin synthesis is decreased and its catabolism is increased. Cholinesterase and acetylcholine activity is decreased. With this overall decrease in CNS activity, there is a corresponding decrease in anesthetic requirements. For example, greater pain relief may be achieved from a given dose of agent and the patient will be able to tolerate a less than a perfect regional anesthetic.

Fear of developing significant confusion with supplemental sedation may steer many Anesthesiologists away from regional anesthetics. The well described "Sundowner Syndrome," which occurs when sedating elderly patients and maintaining them in poorly lit areas leading to hallucinations, is a real concern. Two avenues may be taken in treating this syndrome. Heavily sedate the patient or withdraw all sedative medications. This author favors the latter. However, one must never lose sight of supplying pain relief during the immediate postoperative period despite the desire to enhance mental clarity.

Genitourinary System

There are morphologic changes seen after the age of 40. A progressive decrease in renal mass is observed with a great loss of cortex and medulla. There are intrarenal vascular changes. There is a decrease in cortical blood flow and in the medulla there is a progressive shunt contributing to a more, non-perfused medulla. After 40 there is a 10% per decade decrease in renal blood flow. Primarily, glomerular filtration decreases progressively to 90 to 50% of what it was at 20 years of age. BUN also increases in a linear fashion. At 20, 30, and 40 years of age, it is 10, 13, and 20 mg/100 ml, respectively. Creatinine clearance decreases by 50% in patients above the age of 65, but is matched by a decrease in creatinine production, so therefore, serum creatinine remains unchanged (13). Concentrating capacity decreases, so therefore, the capacity to conserve sodium and excrete acid is diminished (14). There is difficulty compensating for acute acidosis, be it respiratory or metabolic.

The anesthetic considerations of these renal changes are that the renal excretion of medications administered perioperatively is decreased. This is another reason to decrease anesthetic medication doses. Futhermore, while renal function is generally maintained to prevent uremia, the reserve capacity to compensate for fluid overloaod or dehydration, congestive heart failure or sodium loads is impaired and can easily lead to acute renal failure. The direct effects of general anesthesia on the kidneys are relatively small when compared to the combined effects general anesthesia and surgery have in decreasing renal blood flow and glomerular filtration rate through the renin-angiotensin system (15,16). This is dependent on the type of anesthetic utilized. An inhalational anesthetic decreases renal blood flow and glomerular filtration rate > nitrous oxide : narcotic technique > regional anesthetic. Oliguria is the rule rather than the exception during anesthesia and surgery and does not necessarily imply that renal damage is ocurring, although it should not be ignored. It is imperative that brisk urine output be maintained perioperatively. Maintenance of at least 0.5 ml/kg/h urine flow is mandatory. Postoperative confusion and lethargy may be medication or hypoxemia related but could be secondary to water intoxication and should always be included in the differential diagnosis. Acute renal failure accounts for 20% of perioperative deaths among elderly surgical patients (17).

Gastrointestinal System

There is significant atrophy in the stomach accompanied by a decrease in acid secretion. The rate of gastric emptying decreases. There is progressive salivary gland atrophy. While there is no specific age attributable deterioration in liver function, there is some deterioration secondary to decrease in cardiac output.

The anesthetic implications of these changes are important. Since there is a significant decrease in gastric emptying, there is an increase in gastric residual volume in the elderly. This emphasizes the need for more consideration with time to last oral intake. It is not uncommon to have regurgitation and subclinical aspiration occur while mask ventilation is done in the elderly. A decrease in gastroesophageal sphincter tone accompanies the aging process and may contribute to this complication. The elderly patient essentially survives with a chronic xerostomia. Therefore, drying agents to decrease saliva production are much less indicated in the elderly, than in their younger counterparts.

Endocrine System

There is a 25% decrease in the weight of the pituitary gland by the age of 80, but no significant alterations of secretion is attributable to age. The ACTH response relative to stress is not affected. Adrenal function and circadian rhythm are well maintained. Thyroid function is decreased, but does not appear to require treatment. Myxedema is probably the most common thyroid disease of the elderly, but is often confused with the aging process *per se*. Hyperthyroid disease is uncommon in the elderly but accounts for 10–17% of all patients with thyrotoxicosis. Parathyroid function remains normal. Ovarian function deterioration is probably the most significant endocrine function change seen in females. Estrogen concentration is 1/3 to 1/2 of women in their 20's. Testosterone levels fall and decreased spermatogenic activity is seen in men above the age of 65. The endocrine pancreas is significantly affected. This is manifested by the fact that diabetes mellitus is present in 10% of all patients above the age of 65. The urinary threshold for glucose increases, so therefore, urinary glucose testing is not reliable. It correlates with much higher serum glucose levels then the 160 mg/dl concentration seen in younger patients.

Table 29.3 Pharmacologic changes in the elderly.

Changes	Implications	Management
Decrease in TBW and muscle mass	Higher, more prolonged blood/tissue levels	Decrease doses of medications greater than a function of body weight
Liver parenchyma and blood flow decrease	Conversion of fat soluble to water-soluble forms impaired	Some decrease in dose, caution with prolonged effects
Increase in total body fat, decrease in [albumin]	Greater accumulation of fat soluble medications, higher protein-bound [free drug], more prolonged effects	Decrease doses of fat soluble (e.g., fentanyl, inhaled agents) and highly protein-bound (e.g., thiopental, morphine) medication

TBW = total body water

Pharmacologic Changes in the Elderly

Perioperatively, a multitude of medications are given, so knowledge of the differences in behavior of commonly used drugs is indicated. Furthermore, the elderly comprise approximately 12% of the general population, yet they receive 30% of all prescriptions. Over-the-counter medications are used by almost 70% of the elderly, compared to 10% of the general adult population. Understanding the need for a specialized prescription and differences in behavior of medications is essential for successful perioperative management.

Distribution Phase

There is a decrease in total body weight and skeletal muscle mass (Table 29.3). A dose regimen based on a per kilogram basis will result in higher and more prolonged blood tissue levels, as most medications are distributed over lean body mass. For example, diazepam has a half-life of 20 hours at 20 years of age. By the time the patient is 80 it is increased to 90 hours. This accounts for an increased depressant effect for days after a single dose of diazepam. In addition to the more prolonged effects, a more intense effect from a given dose can be expected. Bell *et al.* (18) found that the dose of midazolam required to induce ptosis in a 20 year-old patient was 10 mg yet the same effect was attained with 2 mg in patients aged 85. The relative increase in total body fat will result in accumulation and prolongation of fat soluble medications and inhaled anesthetic agents. All highly protein bound medications (e.g., sodium thiopental, meperidine) will exhibit higher free drug concentrations secondary to a decrease in serum albumin, which is compounded by the smaller initial volume of distribution seen in the elderly. The decrease in cardiac output will delay delivery of drug to end-organs. This effect will also decrease the removal of medications, increasing the possibility of overdosing and prolongation of effects.

Biotransformation

The capacity to change lipid soluble medications to water soluble forms is diminished as liver mass and liver blood flow decreases, so therefore, excretion will be slower. Esterase activity is lower, so there is an increased duration of succinylcholine and ester local anesthetics (e.g., tetracaine, 2-chloroprocaine). There is a decreased number of receptors and changes in receptor states which lead to decreased responsiveness to agents such as atropine, which produces a lower tachycardic response. The need for muscle relaxation in many operations makes choosing the appropriate agent an important consideration. There is a small decrease in succinylcholine requirements secondary to a decrease in plasma cholinesterase level and a decrease in peripheral nerve axons (19). Non-depolarizing agents, however, are significantly affected. D-tubocurarine, metacurine and pancuronium have been shown to have prolonged recovery times due to prolongation of elimination half-life in the elderly. The newer agents such as vecuronium, atracurium, mivacruium, rocuronium

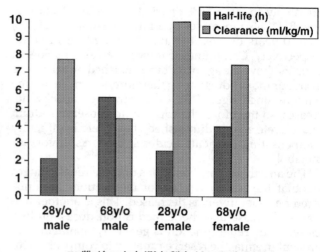

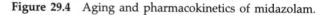
modified from Janis KM, in Clinical Anesthesia Practice

Figure 29.4   Aging and pharmacokinetics of midazolam.

and cis-atracurium are less affected by the aging process. The initial dose remains unchanged and a decrease in distribution in the elderly offsets the decrease in clearance rate, so therefore, their half-life is virtually unchanged.

Anesthetic Management

Premedication

The more elderly and ill the patient, the less sedation necessary. Often, the elderly patient will have a slightly clouded mental status which would be sufficient for preoperative sedation. This should not be further jeopardized by adding sedative or narcotic medications. Consideration should be made of the fact that elderly patients tolerate hospital experiences much better than their younger counterparts. They are accustomed to hospital visits and tend to be more tolerant to invasive procedures than younger patients. A small dose of a short acting anxiolytic (e.g., midazolam 1–2 mg IV) can produce adequate sedation and amnesia for a longer period than younger patients (Figure 29.4). Preoperative opioids should be reserved for those patients undergoing potentially painful procedures before induction (e.g., CVP/Swan-Ganz line insertion, epidural catheter placement, etc...).

In-depth inquiry should be made of the elderly patient regarding drug use, prescription and over-the-counter. Most drugs will be continued throughout the perioperative period. In general, all cardiovascular medications except diuretics, should be continued through surgery. The elderly commonly suffer from diabetes and perioperative management of their disease begins prior to arrival at the hospital (Table 29.4). While most patients receive "routine" NPO orders, these may not be appropriate in the diabetic. A glass of juice (e.g., apple, pulp-free orange) is necessary alimentation in a modified fasting preoperative state.

Table 29.4 Perioperative diabetic management.

- At home (or in hospital) AM of surgery
    - Glass of juice
    - NPO for solids/milk products
    - No regular insulin
    - 50% long–acting insulin
    - Carry hard candy
- Preoperative holding area
    - Start IV and piggyback glucose at 5–10g/h
    - Measure blood glucose, K$^+$, urine glucose/ketones
- Intraoperative
    - Draw periodic glucose (q2–4h)
    - Treat hyperglycemia with IV regular
- Postoperative
    - Draw PACU blood glucose, K$^+$, urine glucose/ketones
    - "Sliding scale"

Insulin dose is reduced. No regular insulin is given the morning of surgery and 50% of the long-acting dose is given. A supplemental D_5W infusion is started at 50–75ml/h. Serial blood sugars will be checked and treated with intravenous regular insulin aliquots as necessary. While much discussion has transpired on the long duration of some of the oral hypoglycemics and the expectation that the patient will be eating soon, it is more prudent that oral hypoglycemics be withheld.

Induction Agents

Sodium thiopental requirements are decreased 25–75%. There is an increase in onset time secondary to a decrease in cardiac output and an increase in circulation time. There is an initial higher serum concentration secondary to a decrease in volume of distribution. Elimination half-life is dramatically prolonged from 6–12 hours to 13–25 hours. Etomidate is a hemodynamically stable induction drug. Its clearance depends on hepatic blood flow which may result in an increase of its elimination half-life. While a single induction dose of sodium thiopental may have prolonged effects in the elderly, more efficient short-acting alternatives are available. Propofol has the most rapid recovery profile of the induction agents with a paucity of side effects. The dose needs to be decreased or significant cardiovascular depression is seen. The drop in blood pressure may be greater than seen with sodium thiopental secondary to its absence of a reflex tachycardia. The drop in blood pressure is primarily due to a negative inotropic effect with little change in systemic vascular resistance.

Narcotics play an important role in anesthetic and postoperative pain management. Elderly postoperative patients have an increased duration of analgesia and an increase in sensitivity as drug free-fraction (i.e., nonprotein bound) is increased. This allows a significant reduction in narcotics dose. Recent studies have shown significant pharmacokinetic changes with fentanyl (20). Beta half-lives for fentanyl and its analogues (i.e., alfentanil, sufentanil) are significantly prolonged. The 50% decrease in age related requirements are also due to increased brain sensitivity (21). Attention should be given to cardiovascular responses to intubation. Elevation of heart rate and left ventricular end-diastolic pressure are two major determinants of myocardial O_2 consumption and should be avoided, if possible. The addition of small amounts of opioids decreases the dose of induction drug and will decrease the hypertensive and tachycardic response seen with laryngoscopy and endotracheal intubation. Other agents, such as esmolol and nitroglycerin, have been used for the same effect with success.

Muscular atrophy leads to a decrease by 33% in the dose of muscle relaxants to be used. Similarly, any residual neuromuscular blockade is more significant as the remaining end-plates cannot increase whatever function needs to be compensated.

Anesthetic Technique

No specific technique has been documented to demonstrate significant superiority over another. Every technique should be considered dangerous and can be misused. Cohen *et al.* found that advanced age, males, large operations, preoperative condition, intraoperative complications and emergency surgery were major determinants of morbidity and mortality (22). They found that narcotic-based anesthetics seemed to be associated with higher mortality, however, that may be due to that technique being a more popular choice in higher risk patients. Other multicenter studies have yielded similar results (23).

Induction and maintenance doses of all analgesic and anesthetic medications should be significantly decreased in the elderly. Elderly patients tend to drop their blood pressure greater on induction and raise it greater on skin incision than their younger counterparts. This increased hemodynamic instability is secondary to a decrease in blood volume and decreased blood vessel reactivity. The decrease in efficiency of the baroflex response and increase in the adrenergic hormonal response to stimulation, makes the availability of more rapid and shorter acting agents more useful in medication titration.

Of all the anesthetic techniques, local anesthetic infiltration with a field block is the safest. Unfortunately, it's useful in very few instances. Inhalational anesthetic requirement, defined by MAC (Minimum Alveolar Concentration) is affected by the aging process and is decreased from 25–75% (24). For example, isoflurane MAC in the newborn is 1.3%, whereas, in the 70 year old patient, it is 0.9%. Desflurane, a recent introduction into the inhalation armamentarium has the lowest metabolization (0.02%) of all of the inhaled anesthetic agents. Since it undergoes less degradation than any of the other inhaled agents, produces less cardiac depression, and offers a more rapid recovery profile due to its insolubility, it is an attractive choice in the elderly.

General vs. Regional Anesthesia: Is Outcome Changed?

Shulman et al. (25) in 1984 demonstrated improvement in pulmonary function testing after thoracotomy utilizing epidural anesthesia with postoperative epidural opioids, as compared to a narcotic based general anesthetic and intravenous opioids postoperatively. This study raised the possibility that a regional anesthetic may have advantages over a general and possibly influence outcomes. This was studied by Yeager et al. (26) in 1987 in high-risk surgical patients. High-risk surgical patients were defined as patients who, because of their operation, would be expected to be admitted to the intensive care unit. They found a variety of endpoints such as heart failure, respiratory failure, infections, intubation time, hospital cost, physician cost and most importantly, mortality were improved when utilizing a regional anesthetic with postoperative spinally administered opioids. Unfortunately, Yeager et al. terminated their study early as they saw a change in mortality and felt they could not ethically continue. Why these differences were seen, is still left to question. Part of the reason may be the effect of epidural opioids in blunting the adrenergic stress hormone response to surgery. Breslow and his collaborators (27) at Johns Hopkins, published a report demonstrating epidural morphine decreases postoperative hypertension by attenuating sympathetic nervous system hyperactivity. They found decreases in plasma cortisol and norepinephrine levels when utilizing epidural morphine, but not when using intravenous opioids. These studies in the late 1980's opened the way for a variety of studies in the 90's to evaluate the influences of regional vs. general anesthesia on postoperative outcome. Some studies caused great excitement (28, 29,30) describing a potential, previously unrecognized beneficial effect of local anesthetics. By interfering with the coagulation cascade, a decreased re-operation rate of lower extremity revascularization procedures was seen with the use of epidurally administered local anesthetics. Unfortunately, no differences in outcome parameters such as, angina, myocardial infarction or mortality was seen. A recent large scale study was undertaken by Bode et al. (31) to determine whether a regional or general anesthetic influenced cardiac outcome after peripheral vascular surgery, a group of patients likely to have coronary artery disease. After evaluating 423 randomized patients receiving general, epidural, or spinal anesthetics for femoral to distal artery bypass surgery, it appeared that choice of anesthesia did not significantly influence cardiac morbidity and overall mortality.

In summary, although some early studies indicated that outcome differences may have existed between general and regional anesthetics in high-risk patients,

more recent, randomized trials aimed at identifying differences in cardiac outcome have not been able to demonstrate them due solely to the two techniques. A reasonable argument for differences found between the techniques in some studies is the change in *overall perioperative* management as put forth by Sharrock et al. (32). They found differences in mortality when comparing elderly patients receiving total hip and/or knee arthroplasty in the period from 1981–1985 as compared to those patients from 1987–1991 (0.39% vs. 0.10%, p = 0.0003). Differences in management included almost exclusive use of epidural anesthesia, decreased duration of surgery, decreased blood loss/intravenous fluid administration and increased intraarterial/CVP/Swan-Ganz line use. Non-anesthetic factors that should be considered are the introduction of new medications (e.g., antibiotics, ACE-inhibitors and ß/Ca^{++} channel blockers), use of autologous blood, improved DVT prophylaxis/suveillance and improved perioperative nursing.

Cognitive function postoperatively and long-term is a concern in older patients undergoing surgery and anesthesia. A large scale study (33) recently evaluated whether differences in these parameters existed between regional and general anesthetics in older patients. Ten tests of memory, psychomotor and language skills showed no differences 1 week and 6 months postoperatively in 262 patients with a median age of 69 (86% of all patients studied were older than 60) undergoing orthopedic operations. While there was no difference between the types of anesthetic utilized with respect to delirium, those patients that developed postoperative delirium fared worse in one test of psychomotor function one week and six months postoperatively (p < 0.003).

Perioperative Management of Chemotherapy Patients

Since the modern age of chemotherapy was instituted in the early 1940's with meclorethamine, significant developments in antineoplastic agents have been achieved. Unfortunately, some agents are associated with serious side effects that occur more frequently and at lower doses in the elderly. There is increasing popularity of multi-dose regimens which work synergistically to combat cancer. This synergism also increases the capacity to induce side effects. While a more complete review of these agents is appropriate elsewhere, basic knowledge of the complications associated with chemotherapy administration, and considerations in the surgical patient, is essential.

Pulmonary System

Bleomycin and nitrosoureas administration are associated with development of progressive pulmonary fibrosis. The threshold dose for pulmonary fibrosis after bleomycin is of the order of 450–500 mg/m^2. That toxic threshold is reduced in patients above the age of 65, in patients with pre-existing pulmonary disease and in

Table 29.5 Perioperative management of patient with pulmonary fibrosis.

- Preoperative pulmonary optimization
    - Steroids
    - Antibiotics as indicated
    - Smoking cessation
    - Light or no sedation
- Intraoperative
    - Low F_iO_2 (maintain $S_pO_2 > 90\%$)
    - Limit crystalloids to maintenance and fasting deficit replacement
    - Consider central hemodynamic monitoring
- Postoperative
    - Aggressive pulmonary toilet
    - Bronchodilators as necessary
    - Bronchodilators as indicated

patients who receive adjuvant thoracic radiotherapy. Use of combination chemotherapy, especially cyclophosphamide, further decreases the toxic threshold (34). Of perioperative significance is the controversy surrounding O_2 administration and bleomycin-induced pulmonary fibrosis (Table 29.5). While it is commonly recommended that O_2 administration be restricted in these patients,(35) as it has been implicated in the development of postoperative pulmonary failure and exacerbation of pulmonary fibrosis (36), at least one study has found no difference with its use (37). Present available information warrants caution with O_2 administration and careful titration of the lowest amount of O_2 to maintain $S_pO_2 > 90\%$ by pulse oximetry appears appropriate in any patient with a prior history of bleomycin therapy.

Another perioperative problem seen with pulmonary fibrosis is fluid overload (Table 29.5). The lungs can increase lymph drainage up to twentyfold in response to fluid overload. However, patients with pulmonary fibrosis lose lymphatics and are extremely sensitive to crystalloid administration. Strict limitation of crystalloids to replace fasting and maintenance fluid deficits is mandatory. Colloid agents (e.g., hydroxyethyl starch, albumin) are preferred for volume replacement due to their greater intravascular duration. A central venous pressure or pulmonary artery catheter are useful to titrate fluids and guide therapy to maintain hemodynamic stability.

Cardiovascular System

Elderly patients with malignancies may already have a compromised cardiovascular system. A detailed history and physical examination is essential, with attention directed to the patients exercise tolerance and change in exercise pattern. Unfortunately, in many patients, deterioration may be seen which is not solely attributable to a decrease in cardiac function but also to a generalized weakened state. Chemotherapeutic agents may contribute to this cardiac deterioration. The major drugs implicated in cardiac toxicity are doxorubicin, daunorubicin, cyclophosphamide, methotrexate, and cis-platinum. All are cardiotoxic in a dose-related fashion. Paclitaxel has also been found to cause cardiovascular/ECG disturbances but without a relation to dose. The toxic threshold for doxorubicin is 500 mg/m^2 and 900 mg/m^2 for daunorubicin. Cardiac toxicity, both acute and chronic may limit effectiveness and limit dosing. Acute cardiac toxicity may manifest during or shortly after an intravenous infusion. Acute toxicity does not appear to be dose related and does not predict who will develop a more serious cardiomyopathy. It is commonly associated with EKG changes, such as, ventricular tachycardia, heart block, supraventricular arrhythmias, PAC/PVC's, sinus tachycardia, low EKG voltage and non-specific ST-T wave changes. At low doses, a left ventricular dysfunction syndrome may occur which may not be clinically evident, if the patient does not have pre-existing decreased cardiac reserve. These patients are particularly sensitive to cardiac effects of inhalation agents and dysrhythmic effects of catecholamines. Therefore, close observation in those patients who have received cardiotoxic agents over the previous two weeks to operation is warranted. A preoperative EKG is mandatory and preoperative echocardiogram, searching for evidence of cardiomyopathy is strongly recommended. Clinical signs are not sufficient for diagnosis, as a low level asymptomatic cardiac dysfunction syndrome may exist, which may become manifest when periods of stress are encountered, such as those seen during operation. Obviously, if the patient demonstrates any sign of cardiac decompensation, such as, shortness of breath, JVD or S_3, then a full cardiac evaluation is indicated. Chronic toxicity is infrequent in young healthy patients below cumulative levels under 500 mg/m^2 doxourbicin, however, 50% of all patients will have left ventricular dysfunction and weakness reaching 500 mg/m^2, regardless of risk factors. The presence of risk factors (i.e., age > 60 years, cardiac irradiation, underlying valvular or coronary artery disease, history of hypertension, administration of single doses of doxorubicin > 50 mg/m^2, co-administration of mitomycin-C and systemic disease that can decrease myocardial reserve, such as diabetes mellitus) should all be considered when approaching the threshold. At a dose of over 600 mg/m^2 in patients received doxorubicin, overt cardiomyopathy is seen in > 40% of patients. Morphologic changes increase linearly between 100 and 600 mg/m^2. This can be seen early with electron microscopy. While endomyocardial biopsy is a sensitive method to track the progression of disease, a continuous decline in cardiac function can be followed by ejection fraction measurements with radionuclide angiography (38). MUGA is much more sensitive than clinical findings. All patients should be followed by MUGA regardless of how long ago cardiotoxic chemotherapy agents were received. Symptoms can occur weeks to years after the last dose and clinically present as congestive heart failure. Therapy would include avoiding further injury by eliminating cardiotoxic medications, maintaining contractility and reducing afterload.

As these patients may pose significant challenges in the operating room, a risk:benefit ratio needs to be established to determine the appropriate anesthetic technique and degree of invasive monitoring. A short superficial, non-bloodletting procedure in a patient with a history of mild to moderate cardiac dysfunction may be satisfactorily managed with noninvasive monitors. However, a patient undergoing a larger operation with significant fluid shifts and a potential for blood loss merits invasive monitoring, such as, intra-arterial blood pressure monitoring and Swan-Ganz catheter placement to accurately determine fluid requirements and optimize cardiovascular conditions.

Summary

As we have seen, the elderly posses organic and functional differences which must be taken into consideration when developing a perioperative plan. It is well established that age is not the major consideration in assessing risk. The single most important risk factor are associated abnormalities. Evidence of deterioration in organ function should be sought and changes in the perioperative plan made accordingly. The elderly not only may posses more organ dysfunction than their younger counterparts, but also have a greater potential for significant drug interaction. The elderly are much more likely to be taking prescription and over-the-counter medications than their younger counterparts. How these medications interact with the multitude of pharmacologic agents given perioperatively is imperative.

While average *life expectancy* continues to increase, the species-specific *life span* value continues unchanged at 115–120 years. Continued improvement in maintaining the biological machinery by leading healthier lifestyles (e.g., non-smoking, aerobic exercise, dietary intake) allows greater numbers to approach maximal life span values. Where once they were rarely seen, octa- and nonagenarians are succesfully undergoing surgery and anesthesia with increasing regularity. This trend is certain to continue.

"The straw that breaks the camel's back may be a small one, when the camel is near the end of his journey"

Harold Griffiths, M.D.

References

1. Smith OC. *Advanced age as a contraindication to operation*. Medical Record (NY). **72**: 642, 1907.
2. Oshner A. Is risk of operation to great in the elderly? *Geriatrics* **22**: 121, 1927.
3. Catlic MR. Surgery in centenarians, *JAMA* **253**: 31–39, 1985.
4. Kurz A, Sessler DI, Lenhardt R for the Study of Wound Infection and Temperature Group. Perioperative normothermia to reduce the incidence of surgical wound infection and shorten hospitalization. *NEJM* **334**: 1209–1215, May 9, 1996.
5. Frank SM, Fleisher LA, Breslow MJ, Higgins MS, Olson KF, Kelly S, Beattie C. Perioperative maintenance of normothermia reduces the incidence of morbid cardiac events. *JAMA* **277**: **14**: 1127–1134, April 9, 1997.
6. McClesky CH. Anesthesia for the Geriatric Patient. In *Clinical Anesthesia*, 2nd ed, edited by S Barash. J.B. Lippincott Company: 1353–1387, 1992.
7. Fiatarone MA, Marks EC, Ryan ND, Meredith CN, Lipsitz LA, Evans WJ. High-intensity strength training in nonagenarians. Effects on skeletal muscle. *JAMA* **263**: **22**: 3029–2034, 1990.
8. Lakatta EG, Fleg JL. Aging of the adult cardiovascular system. In *Geriatric Anesthesia Principles and Practices*, edited by CR Steven, Assafare. Boston, MA: Butterworths, p. 1, 1986.
9. Brandfonbrener M, Landowne M, Shock NW. Changes in cardiac output with age. *Circulation* **69**: 557–566, 1955.
10. Rodeheffer RJ, Gerstenblith G, Becker LC, *et al.* Exercise cardiac output is maintained with advancing age in healthy human subjects. Cardiac dilatation and increased stroke volume compensate for a diminished heart rate. *Circulation* **69**: 2: 203–213, 1984.
11. Smith TC. Respiratory effects of aging. *Seminars in Anesthesiology* **5**: 14, 1986.
12. Pontoppidan H, Geffin D, Lowenstein E. Acute respiratory failure in the adult. *New England Journal of Medicine* **287**: 690–697, 1982.
13. Scott JC, Stanski DR. Decreased fentanyl and alfentanil dose requirements with age. A simultaneous pharmacokinetic and pharmodynamic evaluation. *J PharmExp Therapeutics* **240**: 1: 159–166, 1987.
14. Matteo RS, Backus WW, McDaniel DD, Brotherton WP, Abraham R, Diaz J. Pharmacokinetics and pharmacodynamics of d-tubocurarine and metocurine in the elderly. *Anesth Analg* **64**: 23–29, 1985.
15. Rowe JW, Andres R, Tobin JD *et al.* The effect of age of creatinine clearance in man. A cross sectional and longitudinal study. *Journal of Gerontology* **31**: 2: 155–163, 1976.
16. Mirenda JV, Grissom TE. Anesthetic implications of the renin-angiotensin system and angiotensin-converting enzyme inhibitors. *Anesth Analg* **72**: 667–683, 1991.
17. Miller ED, Longnecker DE, Peach MJ. The regulatory function of the renin-angiotensin system during general anesthesia. *Anesthesiology* **48**: 399–403, 1978.
18. Sweny P. Is postoperative oliguria avoidable? *Br Journal of Anaesthesia* **67**: 137–145, 1991.
19. Muravchik S. Anesthesia for the Elderly. In *Anesthesia*, 3rd Ed, edited by RD Miller. Churchill Livingstone: 1990.
20. Bell GD, Spichett GP, Reeve PA, Morden A, Logan RF. Intravenous midazolam for upper gastrointestinal endoscopy. A study of 800 consecutive cases relating dose to age and sex of patient. *Br J Clin Pharmacol* **23**: 2: 241–243, 1987.
21. Shanor SP, Van Hees GR, Baart N, *et al.* The influence of age and sex on human plasma and red cell cholinesterase. *Am J Med Sci* **242**: 357, 1961.
22. Bently JB, Borel JE, Nenad RE, Gillespie TJ. Influence of age on the pharmacokinetics of fentanyl. *Anesth Analg* **61**: 12: 968–971,1982.
23. Scott JC, Stanski DR. Decreased fentanyl and alfentanil dose requirements with age. A simultaneous pharmacokinetic and pharmacodynamic evaluation. *J Pharmacol Exp Ther* **240**: 1: 159–166, 1987.
24. Cohen MM, Duncan PG, Tate RB. Does anesthesia contribute to operative mortality? *JAMA* **260**: 19: 2859–2863, 1988.
25. Forrest JB, Rehder K, Cahalan MK, Goldsmith CH. Multicenter study of general anesthesia. III. Predictors of severe perioperative adverse outcomes. *Anesthesiology* **76**: 3–15, 1992.
26. Munson ES, Hoffman JC, Eger EI. Use of cyclopropane to test generality of anesthetic requirement in the elderly. *Anesth Analg* **63**: 998–1000, 1984.
27. Shulman M, Sandler AN, Bradley JW, Young PS, Brebner J. Postthoracotomy pain and pulmonary function following epidural and systemic morphine. *Anesthesiology* **61**: 569–575, 1984.
28. Yeager MP, Glass DD, Neff RK, Brink-Johnsen FT. Epidural anesthesia and analgesia in high risk surgical patients. *Anesthesiology* **66**: 729–736, 1987.

29. Breslow MJ, Jordan DA, Christopherson R, Rosenfeld B, Miller CF, Hanley DF, Beattie C, Traystman RJ, Rogers MC. Epidural morphine decreases postoperative hypertension by attenuating sympathetic nervous system hyperactivity. *JAMA* **261**: 24: 3577–3581, 1989.

30. Cook PT, Davies MJ, Cronin KD, Moran T. A postoperative, randomized trial comparing spinal anesthesia using hyperbaric cinchocaine with general anesthesia for lower limb vascular surgery. *Anaesth Intensive Care* **14**: 373–380, 1986.

31. Tuman KJ, McCarthy RJ, March RJ, DeLaria GA, Patel RV, Ivankovich AD. The effects of anesthesia and analgesia on coagulation and outcome after major vascular surgery. *Anesth Analg* **73**: 696–704, 1991.

32. Christopherson R, Beattie C, Frank SM, Morris EJ, Meinert CL, Gottlieb SO, Yates H, Rock P, Parker ST, Perler BA. Perioperative morbidity in patients randomized to epidural or general anesthesia for lower extremity vascular surgery. Perioperative Ischemia Randomized Anesthesia Trial Study Group. *Anesthesiology* **79**: 422–434, 1993.

33. Bode RH, Jr., Lewis KP, Zarich SW, Pierce ET, Roberts M, Kowalchuk GJ, Satwicz PR, Gibbons GW, Hunter JA, Espanola C, Nesto RW. Cardiac outcome after peripheral vascular surgery. Comparison of general and regional anesthesia. *Anesthesiology* **84**: 3–13, 1996.

34. Sharrock NE, Cazan MG, Hargett MJL, Williams-Russo P, Wilson PD. Changes in mortality after total hip and knee arthroplast over a ten-year period. *Anesth Analg* **80**: 242–248, 1995.

35. Williams-Russo P, Sharrock NE, Mattis S, Szatrowski TP, Charlson ME. Cognitive effects after epidural vs general anesthesia in older adults. *JAMA.* **274**: 44–50, 1995.

36. Cooper JA, White DA, Matthay RA. Drug-induced pulmonary disease. *Am Rev Resp Dis* **133**: 321–340, 1986.

37. Waid-Jones MI, Coursin DB. Perioperative considerations for patients treated with bleomycin. *Chest* **99**: 4: 993–999, 1991.

38. Goldiner PL, Carlon GC, Cvitkovic E, *et al.* Factors influencing postoperative morbidity and mortality in patients treated with bleomycin. *Br Med Jour* **1**: 1664–1667, 1978.

39. LaMantia KR, Glick JH, Marshall BE. Supplemental oxygen does not cause respiratory failure in bleomycin-treated surgical patients. *Anesthesiology* **60**: 65–67, 1984.

40. Gottdiener JS, Mathisen DJ, Borer JS, *et al.* Doxorubicin cardiotoxicity. Assessment of late left ventricular dysfunction by radionuclide cineangiography. *Ann Int Med* **94**: 430–435, 1981.

30. Hemopoiesis and Aging

Lynn C. Moscinski

Introduction

The aging process is characterized by alterations in the function of many organ systems. Changes occur in the cardio-vascular, endocrine and immune systems, and have been studied extensively. Changes in bone marrow function are also evident, but the physiologic basis for these alterations is less well understood. Clearly, the bone marrow plays an important role in normal homeostasis, producing cells responsible for maintenance of oxygen delivery, hemostasis and host defense against infection. Evidence that a significant decline in bone marrow function occurs with aging is debated. Whether the observed cellular alterations are a normal physiologic response or the consequence of coexistent disease processes remains controversial. In order to place published experimental data in perspective, an understanding of the regulation of normal hematopoiesis is essential.

Normal Bone Marrow Function

The production of mature peripheral blood cells from primitive precursors within the marrow results from a complex interaction between primitive hematopoietic stem cells, the stromal microenvironment and a set of soluble regulatory cytokines produced locally. The orderly development of the hematopoietic system requires that a strict balance be maintained between cell self-renewal, cell differentiation and cell death. Continued production of terminally differentiated peripheral blood cells occurs, while maintaining a balance between amplification of immature precursors and maturation with transit into the peripheral blood compartment. Most immature precursors go unrecognized by traditional light microscopic examination. The earliest morphologically recognizable myeloid, erythroid and megakaryocytic precursors are actually relatively mature progeny of a cell found at low numbers within the marrow. This self-renewing cell is referred to as the primitive hematopoietic stem cell (Figure 30.1).

The concept of a primitive hematopoietic stem cell was introduced by Till and McCulloch in the early 1960s (1). They analyzed the number and nature of cells giving rise to trilineal spleen colonies in an irradiated mouse model, and noted that each colony was derived from a single clonogenic precursor. Furthermore, these precursors were capable of continuous repopulating ability (2,3). The cell type giving rise to the spleen colonies was termed a colony-forming unit-spleen (CFU-S). This same cell was later shown to also

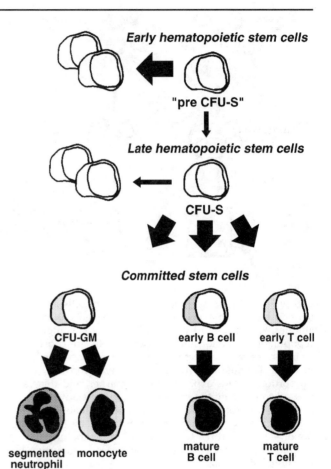

Figure 30.1 Early hematopoietic stem cells have a high proliferative potential, with more limited differentiation kinetics. Their progeny, the late stem cells, undergo preferential differentiation to form stem cells committed to the various hematopoietic lineages. These undergo terminal maturation to form the recognizable peripheral blood and lymph node elements. Each stage of stem cell differentiation is antigenically characterized by a constellation of surface antigens which can be readily measured by flow cytometry.

be capable of giving rise to peripheral blood and thymic lymphocytes (4,5), and thus became the prime candidate for the then elusive pluripotent stem cell. Since this initial description, a series of cell types has been characterized, and both early and late stages of stem cell differentiation are identified. It is now known that pluripotent stem cells are short-lived (6,7), and represent only a small fraction of cells within the bone

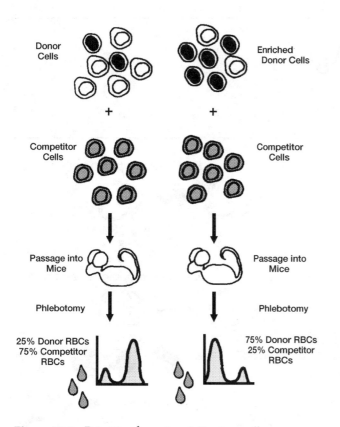

Figure 30.2 Primitive hematopoietic stem cells are defined by their maximal differentiating and repopulating abilities, as measured by a technique called "competitive repopulation." Donor and competitor cells are chosen from mouse strains to express different surface allelic markers. The mature progeny are assayed for the proportion of cells expressing each marker, and this value is used to estimate the stem cell number (relative to a standard dose of competitor cells) and evaluate for stem cell enrichment efficiency. In this example, the "enriched" donor sample is three times as efficient as the original sample, and therefore reflects an increased proportion of functional stem cells.

marrow and fetal liver. They can be defined by their maximum differentiating and repopulating ability as measured by "competitive repopulation" assays (8,9). Such assays measure the long term functional ability of stem cells (Figure 30.2). Using this methodology, competitor and donor hematopoietic populations are derived from mice that carry allelic variants of genes specifying quantifiable cellular markers. One population, termed the competitor, is an aliquot of fresh bone marrow cells that serves as an internal standard for repopulating potential. In each experiment, different donor populations containing unknown stem cell contents are measured relative to the repopulating ability of the internal standard competitor pool. Thus, various donor cell populations and bone marrow fractions can be compared (10).

Hematopoietic stem cells have been subfractionated based on size, density and the expression of cell surface

molecules (5,11,12). There is a general consensus that human stem cells are contained within the cell population expressing surface CD34 (where "CD" refers to the international nomenclature for antigens, the so-called "clusters of differentiation"). CD34 positive stem cells represent a spectrum of stages of differentiation and lineage commitment, with variable functional properties, *in vitro* laboratory properties and surface antigen expression (Table 30.1). The majority of CD34 positive bone marrow cells are "late stem cells", already committed to either the hematopoietic or stromal cell lineages (13,14). The most immature progenitors within the CD34 positive population are further fractionated by the differential expression of CD38, CD45RA, CD71, CDw90 (Thy-1), and HLA-DR (15–20).

The establishment of hematopoiesis during embryonic development, as well as the continued maturation and differentiation of bone marrow precursors *in vivo*, requires an interaction with both cellular and soluble factors. Observed changes in stem cell numbers coincide with alterations in the stromal cell content of yolk sac, liver, spleen, and bone marrow when these sites become active in hematopoiesis (21,22). In liver, spleen and bone marrow, increased numbers of fibroblastoid colony-forming units (CFU-f) precede the onset of hematopoiesis (23). When re-cultured *in vitro*, CFU-f are capable of maintaining hematopoiesis in both human and mouse long term marrow cultures (24,25). This suggests a close interaction between stem cell proliferation/maintenance and stromal cell support. CFU-f are primarily fibroblastoid stromal cell types, and are assayed by plating bone marrow in soft agar *in vitro*. However, normal hematopoietic stroma *in vivo* is heterogeneous, and in addition to CFU-f is composed of macrophages, endothelial cells and fibroblast (reticular) cells with many of the fibroblasts converting to adipocytes over time (26–31).

The mechanism for stem cell dependence on stromal cell layers is most likely an interaction of stem cell membrane proteins with adhesion molecules present on the surface of stromal cells (Figure 30.3). Such adhesion is postulated to "activate" the stromal cell components, with resultant production of cytokines (32–38).

The most primitive pluripotent stem cells do not appear to respond to any one cytokine given alone. Colony growth in soft agar can be seen when these cells are incubated with interleukin-3 (IL-3) in combination with a variety of other growth factors (39). Response of committed myelomonocytic precursors and lymphoid progenitors has been demonstrated to the early acting growth factors stem cell factor (c-kit ligand) and interleukin-1 (IL-1), as well as IL-6, G-CSF, GM-CSF, M-CSF, IL-7, and IL-5. Commitment to the erythroid lineage requires both early acting growth factors and erythropoietin. Megakaryocytic differentiation is less well understood. Many of the same early-acting growth factors are needed, although recently thrombopoietin (40,41) has been shown to play an important maturational role.

Table 30.1 Definition of hematopoietic stem cells.

	early stem cells (pre CFU-S)	late stem cells (CFU-S)	lineage-committed stem cells
A. Functional properties	Self-renewal; long-term radioprotection of the host	Production of myeloid, erythroid and lymphoid elements	Radioprotection of the host
B. Laboratory properties	CFU-S formation in secondary transplantation into lethally irradiated mice (long-term re-population) High proliferative potential	Secondary spleen colony assays (CFU-S) Long-term liquid Dexter bone marrow cultures	Methylcellulose colony formation for multi-potential lineage growth
C. Antigenic properties	Mouse — Sca-1 (stem cell antigen) positive, Thy-1.1 weak positive, LIN (lineage markers) negative Human — CD34 positive, Rh 123 (rhodamine dye) weak positive, CD38 negative, CD71 (transferrin receptor) negative, HLA-DR negative, c-kit receptor positive, CD45 RO positive, CD45 RA weak positive, Cdw90 (Thy-1.1) weak positive		Human — CD34 positive, Rh 123 (rhodamine dye) strong positive May express variable CD33 (myeloid), CD10/CD19 (B-lymphoid), CD38 and HLA-DR

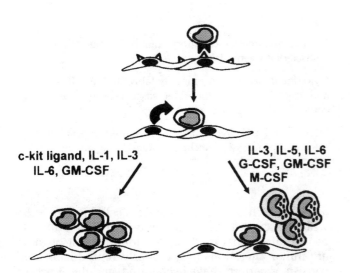

c-kit ligand, IL-1, IL-3
IL-6, GM-CSF

IL-3, IL-5, IL-6
G-CSF, GM-CSF
M-CSF

Figure 30.3 Binding of hematopoietic stem cells to stroma via surface adhesion molecules results in the release of multiple cytokines by the now "activated" stromal cells. The relative levels of these cytokines and the efficiency with which they can bind to receptors on the stem cell allows for a balance between stem cell replication and differentiation.

The Effect of Aging on Stem Cell Function

A multitude of alterations in hematopoiesis have been ascribed to the aging process, when studied in mice (Table 30.2). There is a general consensus that aging causes decrements in the proliferative potential of some cell types (42–44). There may be blunting of the proliferative response of normal marrow hematopoietic cells, resulting in inadequate amplification of myelopoiesis. This could potentially lead to neutropenia (45,46) or could be manifested as a slow recovery from myelotoxic chemotherapy (47). Age related deficits in compensatory myelopoiesis have also been ascribed to changes in the number of bone marrow progenitors, alterations in the responsiveness of these progenitors to regulatory cytokines (48), decreased production of cytokines (49–51), or defects in the bone marrow microenvironment (52).

The majority of studies to delineate the effects of aging on hematopoietic cell proliferation have been performed in rodents, predominantly mice or senescence accelerated strains of mice. Contradictory studies exist, and alterations in the function of the hematopoietic system during the aging process are not univer-

Table 30.2 The physiologic basis of "aging" in the hematopoietic system of mice.

Observed "Aging" Phenomenon	Probable Physiologic Mechanism
A. Myeloid Abnormalities	
Increased proliferative capacity of late stem cells (CFU-S)	Unknown
Increased differentiative capacity of late stem cells (CFU-S) with production of more committed stem cells	Altered stromal cell regulation and increased demand for mature cells
Decreased resynthesis of cytokine substances in bone marrow	Altered stromal cell regulation with increased fibroblast content of bone marrow
Decreased ability of early stem cells to repopulate the bone marrows of lethally irradiated mice	Decreased marrow graft content of "activated" stromal cell components capable of cytokine secretion and initiation of hematopoietic reconstitution
Decreased *in vitro* CFU-GM colony formation	Decreased sensitivity of CFU-GM to exogenous IL-3, G-CSF and GM-CSF
Reduction in hemopoietic reserve	Blunted proliferative response to stress, most likely secondary to abnormal cytokine regulation
Reduced cycling of committed stem cells (CFU-GM)	Increased demand for mature cells and increased complement of CFU-GM
Increased spontaneous chromosomal abnormalities	Decreased DNA repair mechanisms; ? altered telomerase activity
B. T-Lymphoid Abnormalities	
Blunted T cell proliferative response to mitogen	Increased content of mature T cells in bone marrow with shortened duration of response to cell activation accompanied by a decrease in bone marrow derived thymocyte progenitors; decreased local cytokine production by macrophages and stromal cells
Increased T cell content of bone marrow	Compensatory increase in infiltrating effector T cells secondary to blunted T cell proliferative response
C. B-Lymphoid Abnormalities	
Increased auto-antibody production	Cytokine dysregulation, most notably increased IL-6; restricted V_H gene usage
Decreased production of normal immunoglobulin-producing cells	Cytokine dysregulation, most notably IL-7 and IL-4; abnormal T cell regulation; decreased B-progenitor content of bone marrow
Restricted V_H gene usage	Decreased B cell precursors and increased peripheral selection; progressive decline in Rag-1 gene activity

sally accepted. It is likely that some of the confusion results from differences in experimental procedures, differences between strains of laboratory mice, or inherent differences between rodent models and normal human physiology. For example, bone marrow cellularity in rodents increases with increasing age, while cellularity in humans decreases with increasing age. Such basic differences in physiology may impact significantly on the extrapolation of results from experimental animal studies. However, despite some limitations, many lessons can be learned from *in vitro* evaluations. In the following sections, the specific effects of aging on each stage of normal stem cell differentiation will be discussed. As will become obvious, a multitude of laboratory abnormalities are found. Most of these are minor alterations or are poorly reproducible. No consistent patterns have been found, and the effects of aging on stem cell function remains a debated topic.

The Effect of Aging on Pluripotent Stem Cells (pre CFU-S and CFU-S)

A major question with regard to the aging hematopoietic system is whether or not the pluripotent stem cell has a finite replicative capacity (53). Evidence exists that stem cells are heterogeneous in self-renewal capacity; young CFU-S (pre CFU-S) show a high self-renewal capacity and give rise to older CFU-S with diminishing self-renewal and increasing differentiation potential (Figure 30.3) (54,55).

In order to understand why elderly people appear to possess less hematopoietic reserve than their youthful counterparts, early stem cell function has been evaluated in aging mice. Several studies have attempted to quantitate the number of pluripotent stem cells in the bone marrow (56,57). In the majority of cases, no differences could be detected in the absolute number of late stem cells (CFU-S) or committed multilineage stem cells (CFU-mix) when comparing bone marrows obtained from young or old mice. Marginal differences in proliferative potential, however, have been found (56). There is a suggestion that cells originating from older bone marrows proliferate to a *greater* extent and produce *more* committed stem cells than those from younger donors. This finding appears somewhat confusing, and its relevance to physiologic stem cell functioning during aging is uncertain. The basic mechanism for this observation clearly involves many factors extrinsic to the stem cell itself and appears to be a result of stromal cell dysregulation.

It is generally accepted (57) that the function of marrow stem cells, when these cells are transplanted into other animals or studied in culture, does not change significantly with age, although alterations in accessory cells occur. Resynthesis of cytokine substances appears to be slower in older mice, suggesting abnormalities in cytokine regulation or stromal cell function. However, while stromal cell dysfunction and abnormalities of stem cell proliferation can be demonstrated *in vitro*, these abnormalities do not appear capable of resulting in a significant decrement in stem cell function *in vivo*.

As an exception to these findings, a single study (58) identified a decrease in absolute CFU-S number using a novel chronobiological approach. The authors suggested that both circadian and seasonal variations in stem cell number exist. Using a calculation of mean CFU-S number, as identified by day 8 spleen colony assays, older mice appeared to have a slight decrement in absolute stem cell number. They also demonstrated less variability by season and time of day than younger littermates. The magnitude of this change, however, was quite small. It is probable that normal physiologic variations in stem cell number contributed to the difficulty in interpreting these data.

Applying these results to elderly human patients is problematic. Whether or not a small decrement in *in vitro* stem cell number leads to *in vivo* abnormalities is unclear. In order to answer this question, functional studies were attempted. Using serial transplantation to assess the replicative capacity of stem cells, conflicting data have again resulted (53). When cells are subjected to *in vivo* serial transfer in mice, by repeated injection into lethally irradiated recipients, they show a gradual loss of self-replicative ability (55). While early evidence suggested that CFU-S from young donors were better able to repopulate the marrow of irradiated mice than stem cells obtained from older donors, this difference was probably related to stromal cell content and induced cytokine secretion. Recent evidence suggests that many of the early published serial transplant studies had significant methodologic artifacts (59,60). Furthermore, as noted above, any defect in stem cell number or function is marginal. Therefore, in summary, it appears that the CFU-S has sufficient reserve capacity to produce adequate numbers of hematopoietic cells for periods that far exceed the maximum life expectancy of the host (61). Furthermore, most observed abnormalities of stem cell function are most likely secondary to alterations in stromal cells or stem cell/stromal cell interactions.

The Effect of Aging on Committed Hematopoietic Precursors

Aged people respond poorly to hematologic stress, and frequently show a blunted proliferative reaction. Such an abnormality could be caused by a decrease in basal hematopoiesis, or by end effects which inhibit late stem cells during "activation" by inflammatory stimuli. Each of these potential mechanisms has been investigated.

Studies have examined the effect of aging on the number of both committed hematopoietic stem cells (CFU-GM, CFU-E, BFU-E, etc.) and differentiated bone marrow cells (62). In mice, the results parallel those for early stem cells. Most studies show no age related reduction in the number of erythroid (BFU-E, CFU-E) or myeloid/macrophage (CFU-GM) progenitor cells. Furthermore (63), there appear to be no age related differences in the proportion of CD34 positive marrow cells or of more mature CD34 positive subsets, defined as CD34+/CD33+ cells. Maximum colony formation by primitive CD34 positive cells stimulated with combinations of cytokines, including G-CSF, GM-CSF and IL-3 is also similar in young and old subjects. Stem cell numbers, therefore, appear constant. However, similar again to early stem cells, the kinetics of the proliferative response may be altered, although no consistent pattern of abnormalities is found. Alterations appear to be growth factor specific, and thus do not represent a generalized stem cell defect. For example, dose response studies have identified a decrement in the sensitivity of cells obtained from elderly subjects to G-CSF, but not to IL-3 or GM-CSF. Similarly, the ability of early erythroid committed progenitors (CFU-E) to respond to erythropoietin and IL-3 (64) is unchanged.

As described previously for pluripotent stem cells (CFU-S), Sletvold *et al.* (65) have documented an effect of biologic rhythms on the cycling pattern and absolute numbers of CFU-GM in mice. Seasonal variations are again identified. The amplitude of the circadian variation and the mean value obtained over a 24-hour period appears to decrease slightly in older mice as opposed to younger controls. However, the significance of this variation is unclear, as the magnitude of the differences is small. When using a similar strategy to evaluate the mature progeny of committed stem cells (66), no significant decrement in mature peripheral blood neutrophils, erythroid cells or platelets can be identified.

These findings and those of others (67,68) indicate that no major change in basal hematopoiesis occurs with aging. However, the aging process is typically characterized by a reduction in functional reserve capacity. Thus, while basal function is normal, the ability to respond to increasing demand and infectious or inflammatory stress is compromised. This compromise may involve all lineages within the bone marrow, and is the most frequently cited mechanism for the anemia of aging. Older mice and humans recover hemoglobin values more slowly after phlebotomy than do their younger counterparts (69), and a less than optimum increase in hemoglobin level is noted during transitions to high altitude (70).

The fragility of the aging hematopoietic system is further highlighted by studies of mice approaching their maximal life expectancy (62). The median lifespan of the experimental mouse line C57BL/6 is 24 months and the maximum reported life expectancy is 48 months. Mice at 48 months of age have been used in experiments in which they are housed either individually or in groups of five or more animals. Under experimental conditions where crowding occurs, a significant alteration in bone marrow function results, and the majority in animals become anemic. Examination of their bone marrow shows decreases in the number of countable stem cells and morphologically recognizable mature progeny. Therefore, when viewed globally, these experiments support the clinical impression that minor stresses which may not affect hematopoiesis in younger individuals can cause significant abnormalities in aged animals. Since no abnormalities in basal hematopoiesis can be detected, it is probable that these clinically apparent effects are secondary to blunting or suppression of cell proliferation and function during inflammatory or other physiologic stresses. Cytokine mediation of this response is likely.

The Effect of Aging on Progenitor Cell Cycle Kinetics

Another explanation for the changes in marrow reserve which are noted in aging mice is an abnormality in the ability of stem cells to maintain proliferation, either temporally or in response to a stimulus. Several subtle abnormalities in both early and committed stem cell proliferation have already been discussed. Additionally, it has been reported that the cycling rate of granulocyte/macrophage colony forming cells (CFU-GM), as measured using the thymidine suicide technique (71), is lower in elderly than in young adult mice (72,73). Data suggest that the reduced cycling of CFU-GM in older mice may be due to a constant demand for mature cells and an increased complement of CFU-GM modulated by stromal regulation (74).

The Effect of Aging on Stem Cell Integrity

The proliferative lifespan of the stem cells that sustain hematopoiesis throughout life is not clearly delineated.

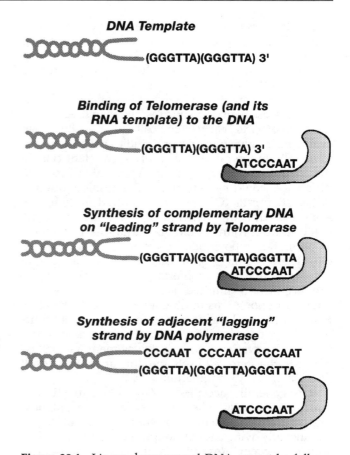

Figure 30.4 Linear chromosomal DNA cannot be fully replicated by DNA polymerase. Therefore, special DNA sequences, called telomeres, have evolved at the ends of human chromosomes. A special enzyme called telomerase contains an integral RNA template. It is capable of adding nucleotides to the replicating (leading) end of the chromosome in an attempt to extend its 3' end, allowing replication to be completed. DNA polymerase presumably fills in the adjacent (lagging) strand, but uses telomeric DNA as a site of initiation of synthesis (primer). If telomerase is not present, the chromosomal ends become progressively shortened until chromosomal replication can no longer proceed.

It has been proposed that the sequential loss of telomeric DNA from the ends of human chromosomes during cell division eventually reaches a critical point that triggers cellular senescence (75). This occurs because of the absolute requirement for DNA synthesis to begin at the binding site for the DNA replicative enzyme, DNA polymerase (a process called "priming"), and the fact that this enzyme causes unidirectional DNA synthesis only. This unidirectional process results in incomplete replication of the terminal ends of the linear chromosomes distal to the DNA polymerase binding site (76,77). In order to compensate for this replicative defect, eukaryotes have evolved a specialized rescue mechanism involving both chromosomal nucleoprotein modifications and a novel enzyme known as telomerase (Figure 30.4). Eukaryotic chromosomes end in specialized nucleoprotein structures called telomeres, which in humans contain tandem repeats of the nucleotides (TTAGGG). Telomeres are critical for chromosome stability and function, and the loss of telomeres signals cell cycle arrest and chromosomal loss in yeast (78). Shortening of telomeres during mammalian aging *in vivo* has been observed in skin dermal and epidermal cells (79), peripheral blood leukocytes (80) and colonic epithelium (81), but not in sperm DNA (79). Recent evidence (75) suggests that early (pre CFU-S) human stem cells (CD34+/CD38 dim-negative) from bone marrows of adult donors have shorter telomeres than similar cells obtained from fetal liver or umbilical cord blood. This finding suggests that the proliferative potential of hematopoietic stem cells may be limited. If proliferative potential does indeed decrease with age due to a progressive and sustained loss of telomeres, this has widespread implication for models of normal and abnormal hematopoiesis. Thus, recent molecular evidence supports the data from earlier cellular studies, and suggests that stem cells may indeed have a limited proliferative capacity *in vivo*. However, whether or not this proliferative period is less or greater than the lifespan of an individual is unknown.

The process of aging is also associated with a general loss in the biologic competence of both single cells and the individual as a whole. At the cellular level, this loss is seen as a decrease in the ability of proliferating cells to replicate and of post mitotic cells to function effectively. When cytogenetic analysis was performed on the dividing bone marrow of rats (82), the incidence of chromosomal abnormalities (predominantly hypodiploidy) increased gradually with aging. Other abnormalities, such as polyploidy or changes in mitotic index were not significant. Overall DNA content remains constant due to the small number of hypodiploid cells present (6.57% in males and 5.99% in females). When other tissues outside of bone marrow are examined for similar abnormalities, an increase in univalency and nondisjunction are found (83) in the ovaries of females. No significant alterations in sperm chromosome number or structure could be identified in even the very oldest males, although the division frequency did decline sharply at the extremes of aging (82).

Evidence for possible abnormalities of DNA repair and chromosomal dysregulation during aging was found in studies in which cytogenetic alterations were examined following exposure to mutagens (84). Older animals developed a higher frequency of micronuclei, reduced metaphase indices and lower sister chromatid exchange per cell when compared to younger counterparts. Treatment with mutagens will significantly increase micronuclei and sister chromatid exchange in most strains of mice at all ages. The important point to note, however, is that the magnitude of this change increases significantly in the older animals. When strain-dependent genetic predispositions are taken into account, sensitivity to mutagens and a decreased ability to repair abnormalities appear to characterize the aging animal.

The Effect of Aging on Bone Marrow Stroma

Age related variations in hematopoiesis are well documented, but, as noted previously, it is sometimes difficult to distinguish between the influence of extrinsic (marrow microenvironment) and intrinsic (genetic or stem cell) factors. Bone marrow stroma is an important source of extrinsic signals necessary for maintenance of both *in vitro* and *in vivo* hematopoiesis. Direct contact signaling between stem cells and stromal cells via adhesion receptors and secretion of cytokines has been documented (32–38). Serial transplantation studies in aging mice have suggested that defective secretion of cytokines and decreases in the ability of bone marrow stroma to maintain stem cell replication are the major factors responsible for the decreased cell proliferation which characterizes aging. This deficiency has been further evaluated in other experimental models (85) where a variety of latent deficiencies of the hematopoietic microenvironment have been documented. When colony formation in culture is studied during aging (86), an increase in the bone marrow content of stromal precursor cells forming fibroblast colonies (CFU-f) is noted. This increase in bone marrow stroma is not associated with changes in bone marrow stem cell content, although a relationship between stromal cell number and bone marrow cellularity is apparent. The changes in stromal cell content, cell number and cellular organization (87–89) point to an age related reorganization of the bone marrow microenvironment.

How stromal cell re-organization influences stem cell physiology is not well understood. This most likely reflects a general lack of experiments designed to evaluate the contribution of stroma on cell proliferation and function. The few functional studies which are in the literature are generally not well controlled. A single report suggests decreased neutrophil function when granulocytes are grown in long term cultures of stroma from older as opposed to younger donors (90). In this study, neutrophil function following stimulation by mitogen (PMA) was decreased in cultures initiated from the bone marrow stroma of older mice. However, neither cytokine production nor variability in culture conditions were evaluated.

The Effect of Aging on Cytokine Production and Release

While evidence exists for both alterations in cytokine secretion and cellular responses to cytokines *in vitro*, few of these proteins have been measured directly *in vivo* (Table 30.3). No published studies have identified decreases in the serum levels of cytokines necessary for myeloid proliferation or differentiation (91). An age-related decline in secretion of interleukin-3 (IL-3) has been identified in mice, but has not been directly measured in human sera.

Several studies have, however, shown age-related decreases in cytokines necessary for T-cell function (92,93). These have concentrated predominantly on the

Table 30.3 A variety of cytokine abnormalities (*in vivo* and in vitro) have been associated with aging.

	Mouse	Human
I. *In vivo* Abnormalities	Decreased serum IL-3 Decreased serum IL-2 Increased serum IL-6	Increased serum IL-6
II. *In vitro* Abnormalities A. Abnormalities in cytokine production and/or secretion	Decreased production of IL-1, IL-6 and tumor necrosis factor (TNF) by lipopolysaccharide (LPS) and thioglycolate stimulated peritoneal macrophages	Decreased production of IL-2 by anti-CD3 stimulated T cells
	Decreased production of IL-7 by long-term bone marrow cultures	Decreased production of IL-4 and interferon gamma by concanavalin A (conA) stimulated mononuclear cells
		Increased production of IL-6 by phytohemagglutinin (PHA) stimulated lymphocytes
B. Abnormalities in cellular responses to cytokines	Decreased responsiveness of B precursors to IL-7	Decreased responsiveness of marrow progenitors to G-CSF
	Decreased responsiveness of bone marrow stromal cells to platelet-derived growth factor (PDGF) and insulin-like growth factor-1 (IGF-1)	

effects of interleukin-2 (IL-2) on immune activation. A single study (94) has evaluated the contribution of interleukin-7 (IL-7) to altered B-lymphoid differentiation during aging. IL-7 is produced by bone marrow stromal cells, and is required for pre-B cell development (95). Whether alterations in cytokine secretion or production *in vitro* will translate into meaningful *in vivo* phenomena remains to be seen. Decreases in IL-2 and IL-7 production correlate with clinical data showing decreased immune function in elderly individuals.

Perhaps the most important cytokine for gerontologists is interleukin-6 (IL-6) (96). IL-6 is a multifunctional protein (Figure 30.5) produced by a wide variety of cells under varied conditions. It is the critical factor in the acute phase inflammatory response, and appears to be involved in such diverse activities as induction of B-cell proliferation and maturation, regulation of protease inhibitors such as α_1-antichymotrypsin and α_2-macroglobulin, and stimulation of bone resorption *in vitro*. Dysregulation of IL-6 expression has been implicated in the pathogenesis of a variety of neoplastic and non-neoplastic disorders including multiple myeloma (97,98), non-Hodgkin's lymphoma (99,100), rheumatoid arthritis (101,102), Castleman's disease (103,104), and cardiac myxoma (105).

The regulation of IL-6 gene expression is complex, with low to absent levels found in the serum of normal individuals. With aging, however, there is a gradual increase in the level of measurable IL-6, even in the absence of documented inflammatory stimuli (106–108). It has been postulated that changes in IL-6 regulation may constitute one of the fundamental aging processes and could conceivably contribute to a broad spectrum of age-associated diseases (96). Because of the known

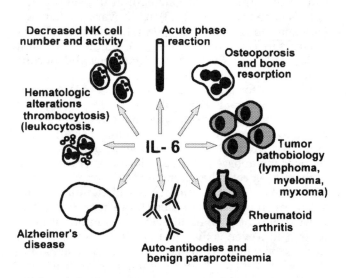

Figure 30.5 Interleukin-6 (IL-6) exerts a number of important effects on many organ systems. Increases in IL-6 during normal aging is felt to contribute to the pathogenesis of several neoplastic and non-neoplastic (predominantly inflammatory) disorders.

effects on B-cell proliferation, dysregulation of IL-6 gene expression may well be related to the appearance of autoantibodies and perhaps the benign paraproteinemias which occur in aging mice (109,110). Furthermore, since α_1-antichymotrypsin and α_2-macroglobulin may adversely alter the breakdown of amyloid precursor proteins, IL-6 induced increases in these protease inhibitors may contribute to the pathogenesis of Alzheimer's disease (111–113).

When administration of recombinant human IL-6 was tested *in vivo* in Rhesus monkeys, a number of alterations in hematologic and immune parameters were observed (114). IL-6 treated animals lost an average of 10.9% of their body weight over a 28-day period of IL-6 administration. In addition to weight loss, there was a decrease in hemoglobin and hematocrit without evidence of peripheral hemolysis or obvious bone marrow suppression. A transient leukocytosis, as well as a sustained thrombocytosis, were also noted. Decreases in natural killer (NK) activity and number were identified. Such changes are transient when normal young adult monkeys are studied, but are sustained in elderly animals. A similar dichotomy is noted when examining serum protein. In normal adult monkeys, total protein levels rise after administration of IL-6, secondary to increases in acute phase reactants and the appearance of a hypergammaglobulinemia. However, unlike the young adult animals, older subjects show a fall in serum total protein which remains depressed for up to one week after the administration of IL-6 is discontinued. Thus, IL-6 clearly has a multitude of diverse effects on metabolism and homeostasis, and these effects may be variable during aging.

Perhaps the most extensively studied effect of IL-6 on aging is that related to osteoporosis. Osteoblasts are among the many cell types that secrete IL-6, and IL-6 stimulates bone resorption *in vitro* (115). Increasing levels of IL-6 with aging may contribute to postmenopausal osteoporosis (116). The suggested mechanism is a negative influence of estrogen on IL-6 gene expression (117) with increases in bone resorption and osteoclast activation. The system is complex, however. In addition to IL-6, at least two other cytokines are implicated in the generation of osteoporosis. Both insulin-like growth factor-1 (IGF-1) (118) and platelet derived growth factor (PDGF) (119) have been identified as mitogens for marrow stromal cells. They enhance cell growth and bone turnover through actions on bone formation and bone resorption. Both of these latter cytokines are less potent when used to stimulate stromal cells obtained from older marrow donors. This lack of stimulation does not produce any observable changes in osteoblast differentiation, but may result in decreased progenitor cell proliferation and less subsequent expansion of new osteoblast cells.

The Effect of Aging on Immune Function

Bone Marrow T-Cells

The reported decline in immune responses during aging has been largely attributed to reduced functioning of

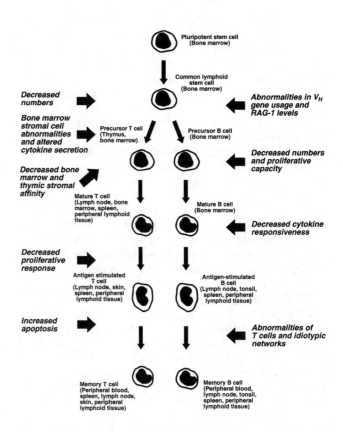

Figure 30.6 A multitude of abnormalities in both T and B cell differentiation and proliferation have been ascribed to the aging process. These defects occur at all stages of T and B lymphocyte development.

the T-cell compartment (Figure 30.6). Early evidence suggested developmental failure, since levels of immature and mature T-lymphocytes appeared to increase with aging (120–122). The majority of studies designed to investigate the biologic basis for the T-lymphocyte changes utilize mouse models. Sharp *et al.* (123) have shown an increase in the proportion of T-lymphocytes in bone marrow with age. When these cells were sorted by flow cytometry and studied for proliferative response to mitogen (concanavalin A), T-lymphocytes from bone marrows of older mice showed a significantly lower response than those obtained from younger donors. When adjusting the cultures for the presence of equal numbers of T-lymphocytes, older bone marrows appeared to initially manifest a higher level of proliferation. However, the response was maintained for a shorter duration, suggesting a functional deficit. Thus, there are greater numbers of effector T-lymphocytes in the bone marrows of older animals, but they show a proliferative response of shorter duration. Concomitant with the increase in mature T-cells, Globerson *et al.* (124) have identified a decrease in the number of bone marrow derived thymocyte progenitor cells with aging. It was suggested that this decrease may be a normal function of aging which accompanies involution of the thymus. The proportion of mature T-cell subsets (CD4/CD8 ratios) derived from bone marrows of both young and older individuals appears similar. Since these mature T-cells are long lived and can continue to proliferate in response to immunogenic stimuli, the observed decrease in thymocyte progenitors may have little functional impact.

Thymic involution, however, imparts additional functional abnormalities to T-lymphocyte proliferation and function during aging. As previously demonstrated (125), the ability of bone marrow derived prothymocytes from aged individuals to migrate in response to thymic supernatants is grossly defective. This initially suggested functional defects in the thymic stem cell. However, pre-incubation of these same bone marrow cells with neonatal thymic epithelium dramatically improved the ability of the aged bone marrow stem cells to migrate *in vitro*. It is apparent that thymic factors and bone marrow cytokines are necessary for both the function and differentiation of prothymocytes in the bone marrow.

When bone marrow derived T-lymphocytes are studied by flow cytometry (126), the majority are CD3 positive cells possessing a cytotoxic/suppressor phenotype (CD8 positive), although both CD8 and CD4 positive cells do increase numerically with aging. These T-lymphocytes are thymic derived, and are not biased for any usage of specific T-cell receptor beta chains. Their proportions differ from T-cell subsets within the spleen and peripheral blood, suggesting that this population of T-lymphocytes preferentially proliferates in the bone marrow microenvironment. Their proliferation appears to be dependent on the surrounding bone marrow non-T-cell population (126). Direct contact between bone marrow T-cells and non-T-cells leads to inhibition of T-lymphocyte proliferation after addition of exogenous mitogen. Whether or not this inhibition prevents cytotoxic T-cells from recognizing homologous bone marrow hematopoietic elements and proliferating (autoimmunity) is unknown at this time, but certainly appears feasible. Recently, Globerson (127) has identified an additional mechanism responsible for abnormal T-cell differentiation and function in aging mice. Studies involved co-culturing bone marrow cells from young and old mice with lymphoid depleted fetal thymic explants. This allowed comparison of thymocyte progenitors from young and old donors under similar experimental conditions. Although the proportion of total T-cells developing from older bone marrow donors was significantly lower than that of younger bone marrow donors, there was no difference in the proportion of T-cell subsets or reactivity to mitogen. Unlike previous studies which implicated only thymic-derived defects, this study suggested an intrinsic lesion in the donor bone marrow. Whether this reflected a lesion of differentiation or an increase in programmed cell death has not been established. It was noted that the frequency of thymocyte progenitors in older bone marrow donors was reduced by approximately 40% during aging. This decline, in of itself, would not be sufficient to account for the developmental inferiority of older bone marrow derived cells. If the older cells were

cultured in the presence of fetal thymic explants 24 hours longer than those of younger donors, the developmental inferiority was abolished. This suggests an alternate hypothesis in which the bone marrow derived cells of older donors have a decreased affinity for thymic stroma. This decreased affinity, in addition to the aforementioned decrease in sequential cell replications, can represent a major impact of aging on T-cell development.

Bone Marrow B-Cells

B-lymphocyte development is modulated by a complex network of positive and negative acting cytokines, as well as cell to cell interactions. T-lymphocyte function appears to exert a major role in B-cell development. Few abnormalities of aging have been directly attributed to defects in B-cell development or function within the bone marrow (Figure 30.6). Several authors (128,129) have found an age-related decrease in the number of pre-B lymphocytes in the bone marrow. These cells were identified by cell surface phenotyping. The decrease in early B cell precursors was accompanied by a decreased capacity to generate surface immunoglobulin positive mature B-cells. Both the numbers and proliferative capacity of these mature cells, as measured by tritiated thymidine incorporation after mitogenic stimulation are affected. In mixing experiments, it was concluded that suppressor T-cells were not the cause of these effects. Instead, it is likely that supportive cells might be missing or deficient (130). However, although less likely, a primary B-cell defect cannot be completely ruled out.

Development of B-cell precursors into mature immunoglobulin bearing B-cells depends on soluble factors such as interleukin-4 (IL-4) and IL-7, as well as cellular interactions provided by stromal cells and T-cells (131). In addition to the absolute decrease in B-cell precursors in bone marrows during senescence, data suggests a decreased overall response to cytokine induced proliferation. Johnsson *et al.* (132) identified a two to five-fold less response to IL-7 in mice over 20 weeks of age when compared to younger animals. This decrease appeared to be secondary to a reduced frequency of IL-7 responsive pro/pre-B cells in the bone marrow of the older mice, and could not be overcome by the addition of large amounts of IL-7. This observation suggested that the age associated decrease in B-cell production might result from unknown factors acting early in B-cell development.

Most of the age-related changes in B-lymphocyte immune responses appear to be reflective of aging T-lymphocytes. There is a constant decrease in the amount and the affinity of antibody produced by aged animals (133–136), accompanied by age-associated increases in autoantibody production (137). The decline in antigen responsiveness associated with aging has been characterized in both qualitative and quantitative terms (128,133–136). The magnitude of responses to both thymic independent and thymic dependent antigens are depressed. Furthermore, in the aged, the expressed antibody repertoire is principally composed of low affinity antibodies with a decrease in, or absence of, medium and high affinity antibodies. Along with this lack of maturation in antigen affinity, there occurs a concomitant change in the expressed repertoire of antibodies to a given antigen. This suggests that regulatory mechanisms involving idiotypic networks are markedly altered in the immune responses of the aged. Auto-anti-idiotypic antibodies produced during the normal immune response of the aged animal are markedly enhanced when compared to those seen in the immune responses of younger adults. This abnormality is accompanied by a rise in titers of autoantibodies and a gradual increase in total serum immunoglobulin concentration. These auto-anti-idiotypic antibodies have a potent ability to modulate the immune response, although both beneficial and detrimental effects can be observed. An increase in the amount of this antibody can assist in the downregulation of anti-self cross reactivity and potentially decrease the ability for generation of autoimmunity. However, the potential downside is that of a generalized decrease in the magnitude of antibody responses, with changes in specific immune responses to infectious and other environmental antigens.

In addition to these functional abnormalities of B-cells, molecular genetic abnormalities have also been described. Aging mice have been found to have higher frequencies of peripheral mature B-cells utilizing restricted variable gene (V_H) families. This suggests that older animals express less diversified antibody repertoires as a consequence of reduced B-cell precursors and increased peripheral selection (137). A less diversified repertoire could be related to the progressive establishment of immunodeficiency during aging, and limit the ability of aged mice to mount immune responses to microbial antigens. It is also noteworthy that restricted gene usage may contribute to the increase in autoimmunoreactivity noted during aging. Although CD5 positive B-cells have been associated with immune reactive populations, no significant differences in frequency of CD5 positive B-cells have been observed during aging. These cells do not appear to play an important role in the senescence of the immune system.

A mechanism postulated for the increase in V_H gene usage is the progressive decline in expression of recombination activating gene-1 (Rag-1). This gene is expressed in early pre-B lymphocytes, where it is involved in the process of recombination and rearrangement of immunoglobulin gene segments to produce mature immunoglobuluin. Rag-1 messenger RNA is expressed by B-cell precursors, and in mouse bone marrow increases during the first two months of life to reach a maximum level at two months of age (138). This level is maintained until adulthood where levels progressively decrease. A decrease in Rag-1 gene expression is directly correlated with a loss of antigen diversity within the immunoglobulin gene family (139). This finding may explain why, with increasing age, the antibody response becomes progressively more dominated by IgM and low affinity antibody with decreased immunoglobulin class switching and decreased somatic mutation. This abnormality is also closely related to T-cell function, as has been shown by studies in nude mice (138). Transfer of T-cells is capable of restoring full antigen diversity and Rag-1 gene expression to bone marrow cells.

Thus, despite considerable effort, it is not possible to state unequivocally that there are intrinsic changes in bone marrow B-cells with aging. The number of B-cell progenitors may be affected. However, the majority of evidence suggests that changes in regulatory mechanisms, predominantly T-cell function, are responsible for the major decline in B-cell immune response with age. The interactions of B-cell production, B-cell differentiation and thymic involution remain to be elucidated.

Conclusions

While many defects in hematopoiesis have been ascribed to the aging process, their specificity remains controversial. The difficulty in assessing functional abnormalities is in part related to the coexistence of other disease processes in the aging population. However, more importantly, it is the complex interactions between normal stem cells and their progenitors, the bone marrow stroma, the immune system (both T and B-lymphocytes), as well as the multitude of cytokines produced which contribute to a vast interactive network. While multiple studies in mice and other rodents have attempted to dissect this complex process, few human studies can be found in the literature. The importance of these studies cannot be underestimated, since an understanding of the physiology of hematopoiesis is paramount to our constructing less toxic and more effective therapies for this patient population.

References

1. Till JE, McCulloch EA. A direct measurement of the radiation sensitivity of normal mouse bone marrow cells. *Radiat Res* 1961; **14**: 213–222.
2. Becker AJ, McCulloch EA, Till JE. Cytological demonstration of the clonal nature of spleen colonies derived from transplanted mouse marrow cells. *Nature* 1963; **197**: 452–454.
3. Wu AM, Till JE, Siminovitch L, McCulloch EA. Cytological evidence for a relationship between normal hematopoietic colony-forming cells and cells of the lymphoid system. *J Exp Med* 1968; **127**: 455–464.
4. Abramson S, Miller RG, Phillips RA. The identification in adult bone marrow of pluripotent and restricted stem cells of the myeloid and lymphoid systems. *J Exp Med* 1977; **145**: 1567–1579.
5. Visser JWM, Van Bekkum DW. Purification of pluripotent hematopoietic stem cells. *Exp Hematol* 1990; **18**: 248–256.
6. Micklem HS, Lennon JE, Ansell JD, Gray RA. Numbers and dispersion of repopulating hematopoietic cell clones in radiation chimeras as functions of cell dose. *Exp Hematol* 1987; **15**: 251–257.
7. Harrison DE, Astle CM, Lerner C. Number and continuous proliferation pattern of transplanted primitive immunohematopoietic stem cells. *Proc Natl Acad Sci USA* 1988; **85**: 822–826.
8. Harrison DE. Competitive repopulation. a new assay for long-term stem cell functional capacity. *Blood* 1980; **55**: 77–81.

9. Harrison DE, Jordan CT, Zhong RK, Astle CM. Primitive hematopoietic stem cells. direct assay of most productive populations by competitive repopulation with simple binomial, correlation, and covariance calculations. *Exp Hematol* 1993; **21**: 206–219.

10. Jordan CT, Astle CM, Zawadzki J, Mackarehtschian K, Lemischka IR, Harrison DE. Long-term repopulating abilities of enriched fetal liver stem cells measured by competitive repopulation. *Exp Hematol* 1995; **23**: 1011–1015.

11. Lu L, Walker D, Broxmeyer HE, Hoffman R, Hu W, Walker E. Characterization of adult human marrow hematopoietic progenitors highly enriched by two-color cell sorting with My10 and major histocompatibility class II monoclonal antibodies. *J Immunol* 1987; **139**: 1823–1829.

12. Terstappen LWMM, Lund-Johansen F. Hematopoietic progenitors in fetal and adult tissue. *Blood Cells* 1994; **20**: 392–396.

13. Civin CI, Strauss LC, Brovall C, Fackler MJ, Schwartz JF, Shaper JH. Antigenic analysis of hematopoiesis. III. A hematopoietic progenitor cell surface antigen defined by a monoclonal antibody raised against Kg-1a cells. *J Immunol* 1984; **133**: 157–165.

14. Simmons PJ, Torok-Storb B. CD34 expression by stromal precursors in normal human adult bone marrow. *Blood* 1991; **78**: 2848–2853.

15. Terstappen LWMM, Huang S, Safford M, Lansdorp PM, Loken MR. Sequential generations of hematopoietic colonies derived from single non-lineage committed CD34+CD38-progenitor cells. *Blood* 1991; **77**: 1218–1227.

16. Huang S, Terstappen LWMM. Lymphoid and myeloid differentiation of single human CD34+, HLA-DR+, CD38-hematopoietic stem cells. *Blood* 1994; **83**: 1515–1526.

17. Baum CM, Weissman IL, Tsukamoto AS, Buckle AM, Peault B. Isolation of a candidate human hematopoietic stem-cell population. *Proc Natl Acad Sci USA*. 1992; **89**: 2804–2808.

18. Lansdorp PM, Sutherland HJ, Eaves CJ. Selective expression of CD45 isoforms on functional subpopulations of CD34+ hemopoietic cells from human bone marrow. *J Exp Med* 1990; **172**: 363–366.

19. Brandt J, Srour EF, Van Besien K, Bridell RA, Hoffman R. Cytokine-dependent long-term culture of highly enriched precursors of hematopoietic progenitor cells from human bone marrow. *J Clin Invest*. 1990; **86**: 932–948.

20. Verfaillie CM, Blakholmer K, McGlave PB. Purified primitive human hematopoietic progenitors with long term *in vitro* repopulating capacity adhere selectively to irradiated bone marrow stroma. *J Exp Med* 1990; **172**: 509–520.

21. Klein AK, Dyck JA, Stitzel KA, Shimizu J, Fox LA, Taylor N. Characterization of canine fetal lymphohematopoiesis: studies of CFU-GM, CFU-L and CFU-F. *Exp Hematol* 1983; **11**: 263–274.

22. Van Den Heuvel RL, Versele SRM, Schoeters GER, Vanderborght OLJ. Stromal stem cells (CFU-f) in yolk sac, liver, spleen and bone marrow of pre- and postnatal mice. *Br J Haematol*: 1987; **66**: 15–20.

23. Van Den Heuvel R, Schoeters G, Leppens H, Vanderborght O. Stromal cells in long-term cultures of liver, spleen, and bone marrow at different developmental ages have different capacities to maintain GM-CFC proliferation. *Exp Hematol* 1991; **19**: 115–121.

24. Van Den Heuvel RL, Schoeters GER, Vanderborght OLJ. Haemopoiesis in long-term cultures of liver, spleen and bone marrow of pre- and postnatal mice. CFU-GM production. *Br J Haematol* 1988; **70**: 273–277.

25. Cappellini MD, Potter CG, Wood WG. Long-term haemopoiesis in human fetal liver cell cultures. *Br J Haematol* 1984; **57**: 61–70.

26. Westen H, Bainton DF. Association of alkaline phosphatase-positive reticulum cells in bone marrow with granulocytic precursors. *J Exp Med* 1979; **150**: 919–937.

27. Allen TD. Haemopoietic microenvironments *in vitro*: ultrastructural aspects. *Ciba Found Symp*. 1980; **84**: 38–67.

28. Tavassoli M, Friedenstein A. Hemopoietic stromal microenvironment. *Am J Hematol* 1983; **15**: 195–203.

29. Xu CX, Hendry JH, Testa NG, Allen TD. Stromal colonies from mouse marrow. characterization of cell types, optimization of plating efficiency and its effects on radiosensitivity. *J Cell Sci.* 1983; **61**: 453–466.

30. Laver J, Ebell W, Castro-Malaspina H. Radiobiological properties of the human hematopoietic microenvironment: contrasting sensitivities of proliferative capacity and hematopoietic function to *in vitro* irradiation. *Blood* 1986; **67**: 1090–1097.

31. Wang Q-R, Wolf NS. Dissecting the hematopoietic microenvironment. VIII. Clonal isolation and identification of cell types in murine CFU-F colonies by limiting dilution. *Exp Hematol*. 1990; **18**: 355–359.

32. Wolf NS, Bertoncello I, Jiang DZ, Priestley G. Developmental hematopoiesis from prenatal to young-adult life in the mouse model. *Exp Hematol*. 1995; **23**: 142–146.

33. Wolf NS. Dissecting the hematopoietic microenvironment. III. Evidence for a positive short range stimulus for cellular proliferation. *Cell Tissue Kinetics* 1978; **11**: 335–345.

34. Ploemacher RE, Moledijk WJ, Brons NHC, de Ruiter H. Defective support of Sl/Sl^d splenic stroma for humoral regulation of stem cell proliferation. *Exp Hematol* 1986; **14**: 9–15.

35. Zsebo K, Wypych J, McNiece I, Lu H, Smith K, Karkare S, Sachdev R, Yuschenkoff V, Birkett N, Williams L, Satyagal V, Tung W, Bosselman B, Mendiaz E, Langley K. Identification, purification, and biological characterization of hematopoietic stem cell factor from buffalo rat liver conditioned medium. *Cell* 1990; **63**: 195–201.

36. Anderson DM, Lyman SD, Baird A, Wignall JM, Eisenman J,Rauch C, March CJ, Boswell HS, Gimpel SD, Cosman D, Williams DE. Molecular cloning of mast cell growth factor, a hematopoietin that is active in both membrane bound and soluble forms. *Cell* 1990; **63**: 235–243.

37. Huang E, Nocka K, Beier DR, Chu T-Y, Buck J, Lahm H-W, Wellner D, Ledner P, Besmer P. The hematopoietic growth factor KL is encoded by the Sl locus and is the ligand of the c-kit receptor, the gene product of the W locus. *Cell* 1990; **63**: 225–233.

38. Williams DE, Eisenman J, Baird A, Rauch C, van Ness K, March CJ, Park LS, Martin U, Mochizuki DY, Boswell HS, Burgess GS, Cosman D, Lyman SD. Identification of a ligand for the c-kit proto-oncogene. *Cell* 1990; **63**: 167–174.

39. Heimfeld S, Hudak S, Weissman IL, Rennick D. The *in vitro*response of phenotypically defined mouse stem cells and myeloerythroid progenitors to single or multiple growth factors. *Proc Natl Acad Sci USA* 1991; **88**: 9902–9906.

40. Bartley TD, Bogenberger J, Hunt P, Li YS, Lu HS, Martin F, Chang MS, Samal B, Nichol JL, Swift S, Johnson MJ, Hsu RY, Parker VP, Suggs S, Skrine JD, Merewether LA, Clogston C, Hsu E, Hokom MM, Hornkohl A, Choi E, Pangelinan M, Sun Y, Mar V, McNinch J, Simonet L, Jacobsen F, Xie C, Shutter J, Chute H, Basu R, Selander L, Trollinger D, Sieu L, Padilla O, Trail G, Elliott G, Izumi R, Covey T, Hu MC-T, Pacifici R, Ponting I. Saris C, Wen D, Yung YP, Lin H, Bosselman RA. Identification and cloning of a megakaryocyte growth and development factor that is a ligand for the cytokine receptor Mpl. *Cell* 1994; **77**: 1117–1124.

41. Kaushansky K, Lok S, Holly RD, Broudy VC, Lin N, Bailey MC, Forstrom JW, Buddle MM, Oort PJ, Hagen FS, Roth GJ, Papayannopoulou T, Foster DC. Promotion of megakaryocyte progenitor expansion and differentiation by the C-Mpl ligand thrombopoietin. *Nature* 1994; **369**: 568–571.

42. Hayflick L. The cell biology of human aging. *N Engl J Med* 1976; **295**: 1302–1308.

43. Norwood TH, Smith JR, Stein GH. Aging at the cellular level. the human fibroblast like cell model. In *The Handbook of the Biology of Aging*, 3rd ed., edited by EL Schneider, JW Rowe. San Diego: Academic Press, 1990; 131-154.

44. Goldstein S. Replicative senescence. the human fibroblastcomes of age. *Science* 1990; **249**: 1129–1131.

45. Finklestein M, Petkun W, Friedman M. Pneumococcal bacteremia in the elderly. *J Am Geriatr Soc* 1983; **31**: 19–27.

46. Weinstein M, Murphy J, Reller L. The clinical significance of positive blood cultures — 500 episodes of bacteremia in adults. *Rev Infect Dis* 1983; **5**: 54–70.

47. Begg C, Carbone P. Clinical trials and drug toxicity in the elderly. The experience of the Eastern Cooperative Oncology Group. *Cancer* 1983; **52**: 1986–1992.

48. Lipschitz D, Udupa K, Milton K, Thompson C. Effect of age on hematopoiesis in man. *Blood* 1984; **63**: 502–509.

49. Gillis S, Kozan R, Durante M, Weksler M. Decreased production of and response to T-cell growth factor by lymphocytes from aged humans. *J Clin Invest* 1981; **67**: 937–942.

50. Nagel J, Chopra R, Chrest F, McCoy MT, Schneider EL, Holbrook NJ, Adler WH. Decreased proliferation, IL-2 synthesis, IL-2 receptor expression are accompanied by decreased mRNA expression in PHA stimulated cells from elderly donors. *J Clin Invest* 1988; **81**: 1096–1102.

51. Buchanan J, Rothstein G. Deficient growth factor production as a cause of hematopoietic dysregulation in aged subjects. *Clin Res* 1989; **37**: 149A (abstr).

52. Lee M, Segal G, Bagby G. The hematopoietic microenvironment in the elderly: defects in IL-1 induced CSF expression *in vitro*. *Exp Hematol* 1989; **17**: 952–956.

53. Lipschitz DA, Udupa KB. Age and the hematopoietic system. *JAGS* 1986; **34**: 448–454.

54. Schofield R, Lajtha LG. Effect of isopropyl methane sulphonate (IMS) on haemopoietic colony-forming cells. *Br J Haematol* 1973; **25**: 195–202.

55. Schofield R, Lord BI, Kyffin S, Gilbert CW. Self maintenance capacity of CFU-s. *J Cell Physiol* 1980; **103**: 355–362.

56. Sharp A, Zipori D, Toledo J, Tal S, Resnitzky P, Globerson A. Age related changes in hemopoietic capacity of bone marrow cells. *Mechanisms of Ageing and Development* 1989; **48**: 91–99.

57. Schofield R, Dexter TM, Lord BI, Testa NG. Comparison of haemopoiesis in young and old mice. *Mechanisms of Ageing and Development* 1986; **34**: 1–12.

58. Sletvold O, Laerum OD. Multipotent stem cell (CFU-S) numbers and circadian variations in aging mice. *Eur J Haematol* 1988; **41**: 230–236.

59. Harrison DE, Astle CM, Delaittre JA. Loss of proliferative capacity in immunohemopoietic stem cells caused by serial transplantation rather than aging. *J Exp Med* 1978; **147**: 1526–1531.

60. Ross EAM, Anderson H, Micklem HS. Serial depletion and regeneration of the murine hematopoietic system. Implication for hematopoietic organization and the study of cellular aging. *J Exp Med* 1982; **155**: 432–444.

61. Harrison DE. Normal production of erythrocytes by mouse marrow continuous for 73 months. *Proc Natl Acad Sci USA* 1972; **70**: 3184–3188.

62. Williams LH, Udupa KB, Lipschitz DA. Evaluation of the effect of age on hematopoiesis in the C57BL/6 mouse. *Exp Hematol* 1986; **14**: 827–832.

63. Chatta GS, Andrews RG, Rodger E, Schrag M, Hammond WP, Dale DC. Hematopoietic progenitors and aging: alterations in granulocytic precursors and responsiveness to recombinant human G-CSF, GM-CSF, and IL-3. *J Gerontol* 1993; **48**: M207–M212.

64. Hirota Y, Okamura S, Kimura N, Shibuya T, Niho Y. Haematopoiesis in the aged as studied by *in vitro* colony assay. *Eur J Haematol* 1988; **40**: 83–90.

65. Sletvold O, Laerum OD, Riise T. Age-related differences and circadian and seasonal variations of myelopoietic progenitor cell (CFU-GM) numbers in mice. *Eur J Haematol* 1988; **40**: 42–49.

66. Sletvold O, Laerum OD, Riise T. Rhythmic variations of different hemopoietic cell lines and maturation stages in aging mice. *Mechanisms of Ageing and Development* 1988; **42**: 91–104.

67. Everitt AV, Webb C. The blood picture of the aging male rat. *J Gerontol* 1958; **13**: 255–260.

68. Coggle JE, Proukakis C. The effect of age on the bone marrow cellularity of the mouse. *Gerontologia* 1970; **16**: 25–29.

69. Boggs DR, Patrene KD. Hematopoiesis and aging III. Anemia and a blunted erythropoietic response to hemorrhage in aged mice. *Am J Hematol* 1985; **19**: 327–338.

70. Udupa KB, Lipschitz DA. Erythropoiesis in the aged mouse. I. Response to stimulation *in vivo*. *J Lab Clin Med* 1984; **103**: 574–580.

71. Lord BI, Schofield R. Haemopoietic spleen colony forming units. In *Cell Clones. Manual of Mammalian Cell Techniques*, edited by CS Potten, JH Hendry. Edinburgh: Churchill-Livingstone, **13**, 1985.

72. Iscove NN, Till JE, McCulloch EA. The proliferative states of mouse granulopoietic progenitor cells. *Proc Soc Exp Biol Med* 1970; **134**: 33–36.

73. Tejero C, Testa NG, Lord BI. The cellular specificity of haemopoietic stem cell proliferation regulators. *Br J Cancer.* 1984; **50**: 335–341.

74. Tejero C, Testa NG, Hendry JH. Decline in cycling of granulocyte — macrophage colony-forming cells with increasing age in mice. *Exp Hematol* 1989; **17**: 66–67.

75. Vaziri H, Dragowska W, Allsopp RC, Thomas TE, Harley CB, Lansdorp PM. Evidence for a mitotic clock in human hematopoietic stem cells: loss of telomeric DNA with age. *Proc Natl Acad Sci USA* 1994; **91**: 9857–9860.

76. Olovnikov AM. A theory of marginotomy. The incomplete copying of template margin in enzymic synthesis of polynucleotides and biological significance of the phenomenon. *J Theor Biol* 1973; **41**: 181–190.

77. Watson JD. Origin of concatemeric T7 DNA. *Nature.* (New Biol) 1972; **239**: 197–201.

78. Lundblad V, Szostak JW. A mutant with a defect in telomere elongation leads to senescence in mice. *Cell* 1989; **57**: 633–643.

79. Allsopp RC, Vaziri H, Patterson C, Goldstein S, Younglai EV, Futcher AB, Greider CW, Harley CB. Telomere length predicts replicative capacity of human fibroblasts. *Proc Natl Acad Sci USA* 1992; **89**: 10114–10118.

80. Vaziri H, Schachter F, Uchida I, Wei L, Zhu X, Effros R, Cohen D, Harley CB. Loss of telomeric DNA during aging of normal and trisomy 21 human lymphocytes. *Am J Hum Genet* 1993; **52**: 661–667.

81. Hastie ND, Dempster M, Dunlop MG, Thompson AM, Green DK, Allshire RC. Telomere reduction in human colorectal carcinoma and with ageing. *Nature* 1990; **346**: 866–868.

82. Sen S, Talukder G, Sharma A. Chromosomal alterations and DNA content in rats during ageing. *Genome* 1989; **32**: 389–392.

83. De Boer P, van der Hoeven FA. The use of translocation derived marker bivalents for studying the origin of meiotic instability in female mice. *Cytogenet Cell Genet* 1980; **26**: 49–58.

84. Singh SM, Toles JF, Reaume J. Genotype- and age-associated *in vivo* cytogenetic alterations following mutagenic exposures in mice. *Can J Genet Cytol* 1986; **28**: 286–293.

85. Boggs SS, Patrene KD, Austin CA, Vecchini F, Tollerud DJ. Latent deficiency of the hematopoietic microenvironment of aged mice as revealed in W/Wv mice given +/+ cells. *Exp Hematol* 1991; **19**: 683–687.

86. Sidorenko AV, Andrianova LF, Macsyuk TV, Butenko GM. Stromal hemopoietic microenvironment in aging. *Mechanisms of Ageing and Development* 1990; **54**: 131–142.

87. Sidorenko AV. Stromal precursor cells of hemopoietic and lymphoid organs in aged mice. *Arch Biol (Bruxelles)* 1985; **96**: 237–251.

88. Schofield R, Dexter TM, Lord BI, Testa NG. Comparison of hemopoiesis in young and old mice. *Mechanisms of Ageing and Development* 1986; **34**: 1–12.

89. Sidorenko AV, Gubrii IB, Andrianova LF, Macsijuk TV, Butenko GM. Functional rearrangement of lymphohemopoietic system in heterochronically parabiosed mice. *Mechanisms of Ageing and Development* 1986; **36**: 41–56.

90. Udupa KB, Lipschitz DA. Effect of donor and culture age on the function of neutrophils harvested from long-term bone marrow culture. *Exp Hematol* 1987; **15**: 212–216.

91. Li DD, Chien YK, Gu MZ, Richardson A, Cheung HT. The age-related decline in interleukin-3 expression in mice. *Life Sci* 1988; **43**: 1215–1222.

92. Fong TC, Makinodan T. *In situ* hybridization analysis of age associated decline in IL-2 mRNA expressing murine T cells. *Cell Immunol* 1989; **118**: 199–207.

93. Holbrook NJ, Chopra RK, McCoy MT, Nagel JE, Powers DC, Adler WH, Schneider EL. Expression of interleukin 2 and the interleukin 2 receptor in aging rats. *Cell Immunol* 1989; **120**: 1–9.

94. Updyke LW, Cocke KS, Wierda D. Age-related changes in production of interleukin-7 (IL-7) by murine long-term bone marrow cultures (LTBMC). *Mechanisms of Ageing and Development* 1993; **69**: 109–117.

95. Namen AE, Lupton S, Hjerrild K, Wignall J, Mochizuki DY, Schmierer A, Mosley B, March CJ, Urdal D, Gillis S, Cosman D, Goodwin RG. Stimulation of B-cell progenitors by cloned murine interleukin-7. *Nature* 1988; **333**: 571–573.

96. Ershler WB. Interleukin-6. A cytokine for gerontologists. *JAGS* 1993; **41**: 176–181.

97. Kawano M, Hirano T, Matsuda T, Tago T, Horii Y, Iwato K, Asaoku H, Tang B, Tanabe O, Tanaka H, Kuramoto A, Kishimoto T. Autocrine generation and requirement of BSF-2/IL-6 for human multiple myelomas. *Nature* 1988; **332**: 83–85.

98. Klein B, Zhang XG, Jourdan M, Content J, Houssiau F, Aarden L, Piechaczyk M, Bataille R. Paracrine rather than autocrine regulation of myeloma — cell growth and differentiation by IL-6. *Blood.* 1989; **73**: 517–526.

99. Nachbaur DM, Herold M, Maneschg A, Huber H. Serum levels of interleukin-6 in multiple myeloma and other hematologic disorders: correlation with disease activity and other prognostic parameters. *Ann Hematol* 1991; **62**: 54–58.

100. Merz H, Fliedner A, Orscheschek K, Binder T, Sebald W, Muller-Hermelink HK, Feller AC. Cytokine expression in T-cell lymphomas and Hodgkin's disease. Its possible implication in autocrine or paracrine production as a potential basis for neoplastic growth. *Am J Pathol* 1991; **139**: 1173–1180.

101. Ganter U, Arcone R, Toniatti C, Morrone G, Ciliberto G. Dual control of CRP gene expression by interleukin-1 and interleukin-6. *EMBO J* 1989; **8**: 3773–3779.

102. Garman RD, Jacobs KA, Clark SC, Raulet DH. B cell stimulatory factor 2 (ß2-interferon) functions as a second signal for interleukin-2 production by mature murine T cells. *Proc Natl Acad Sci USA* 1987; **84**: 7629–7633.

103. Brandt SJ, Bodine DM, Dunbar CE, Nienhuis AW. Dysregulated interleukin-6 expression produces a syndrome resembling Castleman's disease in mice. *J Clin Invest* 1990; **86**: 592–599.

104. Yoshizaki K, Matsuda T, Nishimoto N, Kuritani T, Taeho L, Aozasa K, Nakahata T, Kawai H, Tagoh H, Komori T, Kishimoto S, Hirano T, Kishimoto T. Pathogenic significance of interleukin-6 (IL-6/BSF-2) in Castleman's disease. *Blood* 1989; **74**: 1360–1367.

105. Jourdan M, Bataille R, Seguin J, Zhang XG, Chaptal PA, Klein B. Constitutive production of interleukin-6 and immunologic features in cardiac myxoma. *Arthritis Rheum* 1990; **33**: 398–403.

106. Daynes RA, Araneo BA, Ershler WB, Maloney CD, Li GZ, Ryu SY. Altered regulation of IL-6 production with normal aging. Possible linkage to the age-associated decline in dehydroepiandrosterone (DHEA) and its sulfated derivative. *J Immunol* 1993; **150**: 5219–5230.

107. Tang B, Matsuda T, Akria S, Nagata N, Ikehara S, Hirano T, Kishimoto T. Age-associated increase in interleukin-6 in MRL/lpr mice. *Int Immunol* 1991; **3**: 273–278.

108. Foster KD, Conn CA, Kluger MJ. Fever, tumor necrosis factor and interleukin-6 in young, mature and aged Fischer 344 rats. *Am J Physiol* 1992; **262**: R211.

109. Radl J. Age-related monoclonal gammopathies. clinical lessons from the aging C57BL mouse. *Immunol Today* 1990; **11**: 234–236.

110. Radl J, Sepers JM, Skvaril F, Morell A, Hijmans W. Immunoglobulin patterns in humans over 95 years of age. *Clin Exp Immunol* 1975; **22**: 84–90.

111. Abraham CR, Shirahama T, Potter H. α1–Antichymotrypsin is associated solely with amyloid deposits containing the B-protein. Amyloid and cell localization of α1-antichymotrypsin. *Neurobiol Aging* 1990; **11**: 123–129.

112. Vandenabeele P, Fiers W. Is amyloidogenesis during Alzheimer's disease due to an IL-1/IL-6-mediated "acute phase response" in the brain? *Immunol Today* 1991; **12**: 217–219.

113. Bauer J, Konig G, Strauss S, Jonas U, Ganter U, Weidemann A, Monning U, Masters CL, Volk B, Berger M, Beyreuther K. *In vitro* matured macrophages express Alzheimer's ßA4-amyloid precursor protein indicating synthesis in microglial cells. *FEBS Lett* 1991; **282**: 335–340.

114. Sun WH, Binkley N, Bidwell DW, Ershler WB. The influence of recombinant human interleukin-6 on blood and immune parameters in middle-aged and old Rhesus monkeys. *Lymphokine Cytokine Res* 1993; **12**: 449–455.

115. Ishimi Y, Miyaura C, Jin CH, Akatsu T, Abe E, Nakamura Y, Yamaguchi A, Yoshiki S, Matsuda T, Hirano T, Kishimoto T, Suda T. IL-6 is produced by osteoblasts and induces bone resorption. *J Immunol* 1990; **145**: 3297–3303.

116. Roodman GD. Interleukin-6: an osteoporotic factor? *J Bone Miner Res* 1992; **7**: 475–478.

117. Girasole G, Jilka RL, Passeri G, Boswell S, Boder B, Williams DC, Manolagas SC. 17B-Estradiol inhibits interleukin-6 production by bone marrow-derived stromal cells and osteoblasts *in vitro*: a potential mechanism for the anti-osteoporotic effect of estrogens. *J Clin Invest* 1992; **89**: 883–891.

118. Tanaka H, Quarto R, Williams S, Barnes J, Liang CT. *In vivo* and *in vitro* effects of insulin-like growth factor-I (IGF-I) on femoral mRNA expression in old rats. *Bone.* 1994; **15**: 647–653.

119. Tanaka H, Liang CT. Effect of platelet-derived growth factor on DNA synthesis and gene expression in bone marrow stromal cells derived from adult and old rats. *J Cell Physiol* 1995; **164**: 367–375.

120. Makinodan T, Adler W. Effect of aging on the differentiation and proliferation potentials of cells of the immune system. *Fed Proc* 1975; **34**: 153–158.

121. Ligthart GJ, Schuit HRE, Hijmans W. Subpopulations of mononuclear cells in ageing: expansion of the null cell compartment and decrease in the number of T and B cells in human blood. *Immunology* 1985; **55**: 15–21.

122. Jensen TL, Hallgren HM, Yasmineh WG, O'Leary JJ. Do immature T cells accumulate in advanced age? *Mechanisms of Ageing and Development.* 1986; **33**: 237–245.

123. Sharp A, Kukulansky T, Malkinson Y, Globerson A. The bone marrow as an effector T cell organ in aging. *Mechanisms of Ageing and Development* 1990; **52**: 219–233.

124. Globerson A, Sharp A, Fridkis-Hareli M, Kukulansky T, Abel L, Knyszynski A, Eren R. Aging in the T lymphocyte compartment. A developmental view. *Ann NY Acad Sci* 1992; **673**: 240–251.

125. McCormick KR, Haar JL. Bone marrow-thymus axis in senescence. *Am J Anat* 1991; **191**: 321–324.

126. Hozumi K, Masuko T, Nishimura T, Habu S, Hashimoto Y. Characterization of the T cells in aged rat bone marrow. *Immunol Lett* 1993; **36**: 137–144.

127. Globerson A. Thymocyte progenitors in ageing. *Immunol Lett* 1994; **40**: 219–224.

128. Schulze DH, Goidl EA. Age-associated changes in antibody-forming cells (B cells). *Proc Soc Exp Biol Med* 1991; **196**: 253–259.

129. Kim YT, Goidl EA, Samarut C, Weksler ME, Thorbecke GJ, Siskind GW. Bone marrow function. I. Peripheral T cells are responsible for the increased auto-anti-idiotypic response in older mice. *J Exp Med* 1985; **161**: 1237–1242.

130. Zharhary D. Age-related changes in the capability of the bone marrow to generate B cells. *J Immunol* 1988; **141**: 1863–1869.

131. Kincade PW. Experimental models for understanding B lymphocyte formation. *Adv Immunol* 1987; **41**: 181–267.

132. Jonsson JI, Phillips RA. Interleukin-7 responsiveness of B220+ B cell precursors from bone marrow decreases in aging mice. *Cell Immunol* 1993; **147**: 267–278.

133. Walford RL. *The Immunologic Theory of Aging.* Copenhagen: Munksgaard, 1969.

134. Makinodan T, Perkins EH, Chen MG. Immunologic activity of the aged. *Adv Gerontol Res* 1971; **3**: 171–198.

135. Price GB, Makinodan T. Immunologic deficiencies in senescence. I. Characterization of intrinsic deficiencies. *J Immunol* 1972; **108**: 403–412.

136. Nordin AA, Makinodan T. Humoral immunity in aging. *Fed Proc* 1974; **33**: 2033–2035.

137. Viale AC, Chies JAB, Huetz F, Malenchere E, Weksler M, Freitas AA, Coutinho A. V_H-gene family dominance in ageing mice. *Scand J Immunol* 1994; **39**: 184–188.

138. Ben-Yehuda A, Szabo P, Dyall R, Weksler ME. Bone marrow declines as a site of B-cell precursor differentiation with age: relationship to thymus involution. *Proc Natl Acad Sci USA* 1994; **91**: 11988–11992.

139. Ben-Yehuda A, Szabo P, Weksler ME. Age-associated change in the B-cell repertoire: effect of age on RAG-1 gene expression in murine bone marrow. *Immunol Lett* 1994; **40**: 287–289.

31. The Aging Bone Marrow

Lynn C. Moscinski

The bone marrow is a highly organized cellular network held together by a complex stroma and rich vascular supply. Functionally and anatomically, it is the largest organ of the body (1). Taken in aggregate, there are approximately 1,500 gm of active marrow in the adult, weighing 3,000 to 4,000 gm when including both hematopoietic and fatty components. The bone marrow is located within the cavities of the bones, surrounded by dense cortical bone and consisting of approximately 15% medullary trabecular bone and 85% cellular marrow (2). Structurally, the marrow is composed of thin walled venous blood vessels commonly referred to as sinuses and adjacent areas of hematopoiesis (Figure 31.1). Small nutrient arteries penetrate the bone shaft and branch into an extensive periosteal capillary network. This network eventually drains into central venous sinuses through fenestrations in endothelial basement membranes. Bone marrow capillaries are covered by a single layer of endothelial cells on one side and reticular or fibroblastic cells on the other side. It is these latter cells, collectively referred to as the stroma, which create the lattice work along which the

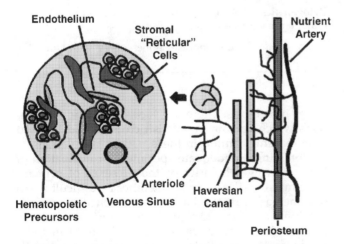

Figure 31.1 The anatomy of normal bone marrow is illustrated both macroscopically and microscopically. Nutrient arteries penetrate the periosteum where they form an extensive arborizing network which eventually fills the Haversian system and nourishes the cancellous bone. Arterioles leaving the Haversian canals penetrate the bone marrow interstitium where they eventually drain into a complex system of venous sinuses. These sinuses are lined by endothelium internally and supporting stromal "reticular" cells externally. The stroma forms a critical support matrix for the developing hematopoietic precursors.

hematopoietic cells form islands or cords between the sinuses. Stroma is heterogeneous and derived from marrow fibroblasts and progeny of the monocyte-macrophage lineage. It encompasses reticulum cells, osteoblast and osteoclast progenitors, histiocytes, adipocytes, and fibroblastic cells. Differentiation along one or more of these lineages is dependent on local production of cytokines, soluble growth factors and intercellular signals. There is a tight interaction between the stroma, bone, hematopoietic precursors, and interdigitating blood vessels. There are no lymphatics.

The bone marrow functions as both an immune and hematopoietic organ. Its role in generating the cells which populate the peripheral blood (granulocytes, monocytes, red blood cells, and platelets) is probably its best known function. It releases basal levels of these cells to maintain constant peripheral blood counts, but can increase their production to up to 10 times normal values when under stress. No less important, however, is the role of the bone marrow as a reticuloendothelial organ involved in antigen processing, production of B lymphocytes and participation in cellular immune reactions. It plays an important role in the removal and recycling of senescent and abnormal cells, including defective hematopoietic precursors.

The bone marrow is easily examined by either aspiration or biopsy (or both), typically through use of a Jamshidi needle (3). Marrow aspirate obtained by this method is placed onto glass slides where aspirate smears, containing bone marrow particles, are prepared and stained with Wright-Giemsa. A small cylinder of bone, the core biopsy, is fixed in a suitable histology fixative, decalcified and embedded in paraffin. Sections of these paraffin blocks are cut, placed onto glass slides, and stained with hematoxylin and eosin (H & E) or periodic acid-Schiff (PAS) for examination. The procedure for obtaining and evaluating bone marrow aspirate and biopsy specimens is standard in adults of all age groups, although some special considerations in interpretation are inherent in specimens from elderly patients. A good understanding of bone marrow physiology and its histologic correlates during aging is critical if one hopes to obtain meaningful data on hematopoietic reserve and the presence of bone marrow disease in this population.

Special Considerations in the Performance of Bone Marrow Examinations in the Elderly

Few modifications are needed in performing bone marrow aspirations and biopsies in elderly individu-

Table 31.1 Recommendations for obtaining diagnostic material in the evaluation of common bone marrow disorders in the elderly.

A.   Conditions in which a diagnosis is best established on bone marrow aspirate

Diagnosis	Other Diagnostic Ancillary Tests
Pernicious anemia	Serum B12 and red cell folate levels
Anemia secondary to ineffective erythropoiesis (chronic disease)	Serum and aspirate smear iron studies with clinical correlation
Acute leukemia (both myeloid and lymphoid subtypes)	Cytogenetics, flow cytometry, cytochemical stains

B.   Conditions in which a diagnosis is best established on bone marrow biopsy

Diagnosis	Other Diagnostic Ancillary Tests
Follicular lymphoma	Immunohistochemistry for bcl-2
Diffuse large cell lymphoma	Immunohistochemistry for B and T lymphocyte antigens
Hodgkin's disease	Immunohistochemistry for LeuM1, Ki-1 and common leukocyte antigens
Myelofibrosis	—
Metastatic carcinoma or other solid tumor	Immunohistochemistry for epithelial (keratin) or other tumor antigens

C.   Conditions in which aspirate smear cytology and either bone marrow biopsy or clot section histology are useful

Diagnosis	Other Diagnostic Ancillary Tests
Myelodysplasia	Cytogenetics, iron stains to evaluate for ringed sideroblasts
Chronic lymphocytic leukemia	Flow cytometry
Small lymphocytic lymphoma, marginal zone B cell lymphoma, mantle cell lymphoma	Flow cytometry
Chronic myelogenous leukemia and chronic myeloproliferative disorders without myelofibrosis	Cytogenetics, molecular studies for evaluation of a Philadelphia chromosome
Multiple myeloma	Serum protein electrophoresis, bone survey with clinical correlation

als, when compared to the younger adult population. In the absence of co-morbid conditions, which may make positioning of the patient difficult or inhibit their ability to lay flat on a firm table surface, no significant alterations in technique need be made. It is important to note, however, that the administration of local anesthetics (lidocaine and related compounds) should be carefully titered to avoid overdosage of the patient. Vascular absorption of these compounds can result in accumulation of lidocaine and its metabolites in the blood, and can result in central nervous system toxicity (anxiety, depression or restlessness), cardiac toxicity (bradycardia or hypotension) or neurologic toxicity (seizures). Since tolerance of elevated blood levels of these drugs varies with the status of the patient, it is generally recommended that debilitated, very elderly or acutely ill patients be given reduced doses commensurate with their age and physical condition. Patients with peripheral vascular disease or those with hypertensive vascular disease may exhibit exaggerated vasoconstrictor responses which could result in ischemic

injury or necrosis. Therefore, local anesthetic preparations which contain vasoconstrictors should be used with extreme caution in these patient populations.

Obtaining an adequate specimen for evaluation of bone marrow cellularity or the presence of primary bone marrow disease can sometimes be difficult when osteopenia is present. Lack of bone density can make obtaining an adequate core biopsy technically difficult, and good clinical judgement must be used in these instances. Where cellularity or primary hematopoietic disease is suspected, additional aspirate material submitted for clot section histology can often take the place of a biopsy specimen. When this is attempted, adequate care must be taken that sufficient aspirate is obtained to produce a representative sample. In conditions associated with marrow fibrosis (metastatic carcinoma, myeloproliferative disorders or multiple myeloma), aspirate clot sections may not be as helpful, and an increased effort to obtain multiple portions of core biopsy may be necessary. Sometimes obtaining a specimen with an attached portion of cortical or cancellous bone can help preserve the integrity of the biopsy and prevent severe crush artifact from occurring. In patients with a suspected diagnosis of malignant lymphoma, or in whom multiple lymphoid aggregates were demonstrated on previous biopsies, submission of additional aspirate material for either flow cytometric immunophenotyping or molecular analysis can be helpful. When the physician has knowledge of the differential diagnosis at the time of the procedure, adequate diagnostic material should be obtainable in virtually every patient, irrespective of age (Table 31.1).

Age Related Variations in the Bone Marrow: Physiologic

Generally speaking, the majority of parameters evaluated in the bone marrow aspirate and biopsy do not change with patient age. Cellular maturation, relative numbers of megakaryocytes and their precursors, and the relative ratios of myeloid and erythroid precursors remain constant throughout life. There are, however, several unique aspects to the evaluation of the aging bone marrow (Table 31.2).

Bone Density

Bone continues to undergo remodeling throughout life (4). The remodeling process involves the formation of new bone by osteoblasts, and the resorption of existing bone matrix by osteoclasts. With advancing age in humans and other vertebrate animals, the dynamics of this remodeling gradually change such that more matrix is removed than is newly formed. Thus, a subtle imbalance between formation and resorption of bone matrix occurs over time, resulting in the development of osteopenia (5). Regression of trabecular bone with age has been established in both animal and human studies (6, 7). In carefully prepared, decalcified and paraffin-embedded bone marrow biopsies from eld-

erly individuals, this process is frequently observed as thinning of the bony trabeculae with an irregularity to the bony trabecular surface. The changes observed in routine iliac crest marrow biopsies appear to parallel generalized changes throughout the body (6) as demonstrated by necropsy studies. Bone loss is most severe in areas of the skeleton containing large amounts of trabecular bone. Cancellous bony plates are resorbed and converted to slender spicules that appear split or transected. This is accompanied by thinning of the cortical bone. Osteopenic bone has a reduced overall mass, although it has the same composition as normal bone. Mineralization is appropriate, so increased amounts of osteoid or widened osteoid seams (osteomalacia) are not observed.

The precise basis for accelerated bone loss in older individuals is unclear, but is likely to be multifactorial. In women, most important appears to be estrogen deficiency; androgen deficiency has been reported to play a similar but less central role in men. How estrogen acts on bone is still under investigation, although bone cells have been shown to possess estrogen receptors *in vitro*. One theory is that estrogen binds to bone and inhibits the local synthesis of bone substance by bone cells. Estrogen-regulated promoters and other DNA sequences have been identified in many genes expressed by bone-forming cells under experimental conditions. However, more likely is the suggestion that accelerated bone loss associated with absent estrogen is secondary to heightened osteoclastic activity, especially during the immediate period post-menopausal. With time, a more gradual process of bone loss ensues which is closely associated with a decrease in the number of osteoblasts recruited for bone forming activity (8). Activation of lymphocytes, monocytes and other stromal cells which promote the release of osteoblast activating factors is probably a key-factor.

A number of these growth factors have been iden-

Table 31.2 Physiological changes in the aging bone marrow and their reflected morphologic abnormality.

Physiologic Alteration	Diagnostic Correlate
Regression of trabecular bone (osteopenia)	– Thinned bony trabeculae – Irregular trabecular surfaces with frequent "moth eaten" indentations
Decrease in tissue blood flow	– Increased marrow arterioles and small/medium size intramedullary arteries
Progressive fatty replacement of the marrow	– Decreased hematopoietic cellularity – Altered distribution of hematopoietic cellularity with subcortical hypoplasia/aplasia and increased paratrabecular fat accumulation
Immunologic stimulation	– Increased numbers of benign interstitial lymphoid aggregates
Alterations in chromosomal DNA during cell senescence	– Loss of the Y chromosome (-Y) on karyotypic analysis of bone marrow aspirate

tified, among them interleukin-6 (IL-6), interleukin-1 (IL-1), tumor necrosis factor (TNF), platelet derived growth factor (PDGF), tumor growth factor ß and insulin growth factor-I. These cytokines appear to be capable of stimulating both osteoclastic and osteoblastic activity in variable proportions, depending on the timing and the actual stimulus for secretion. While little experimental data is available in humans, several studies in mice (8, 9) suggest that osteopenia in the elderly results from a cytokine-mediated decrease in osteoblast function (4) with an increase in the progenitor pool which gives rise to monocytes, macrophages and osteoclast-like cells.

Other conditions known to affect the frequency of osteopenia in the elderly include deficiency of vitamin D and decreased levels of general physical activity.

Vascular Channels

A decrease in tissue blood flow is typical of the aging process, but the association between this process and histologic change in bone marrow biopsies is poorly understood (10). When examining specially prepared, plastic-embedded bone marrow biopsy sections (6), the presence and number of bone marrow vessels can be quantitated. During infancy and adolescence, when hematopoiesis is most active, the overall number of capillaries and sinusoids is higher than in the adult. The geriatric patient shows a slight, although not significant, increase in arterial capillaries with a marked decrease in marrow sinusoids. This is accompanied by a marked increase in marrow arterioles and small to medium sized intramedullary arteries. These vascular changes appear to correlate with osseous remodeling and the maintenance of active hematopoiesis. An interaction between the endothelial cells of paratrabecular sinusoids and bone forming cells is reported (11). Age dependent diminution of bone marrow sinusoids accompanied by osteopenia and decreasing marrow cellularity suggests an essential role of capillaries in hematopoiesis, the release of blood cells and morphogenesis of trabecular bone. This hypothesis is supported by *in vitro* studies documenting a correlation between oxygenation and both hematopoiesis and bone formation (12, 13). However, while these findings are of physiologic importance, changes in the number or size of bone marrow sinusoids is not a reproducible observation when examining routinely processed marrow specimens.

Marrow Cellularity

The percentage of cellular bone marrow (red marrow) when compared to marrow fat (yellow marrow) changes with the advancing age of the patient, but shows considerable variability within each age group in adults (14). A rough guideline for the estimation of marrow cellularity is 100% minus 1% for each year of age up to the age of 80 years. In the very elderly, marrow cellularity should not decrease below 15–20%. In iliac crest bone marrow core biopsy specimens from older individuals, it must be remembered that the immediate subcortical region is more hypocellular than deeper

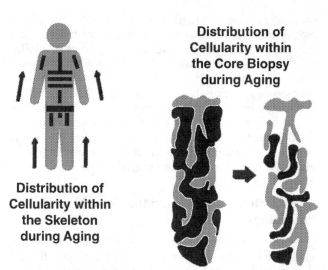

Figure 31.2 The distribution of bone marrow cellularity changes significantly with age. Conversion of cellular "red marrow" to fatty "yellow marrow" begins peripherally and progresses centrally during adulthood. In older persons, the marrow cellularity becomes limited to portions of the vertebral column and sternum, ribs, pelvis, and small segments of the proximal humerus and femur. Further changes also occur within individual bones. Bone marrow biopsy specimens show progressive subcortical hypoplasia during aging, as well as an increase in paratrabecular fat accumulation.

regions of the bone. Thus, a relatively long and adequate biopsy of at least 1 cm is important to avoid an erroneous diagnosis of marrow hypoplasia or aplasia on sampling artifact.

The anatomic characteristics of age associated marrow conversion from cellular to fatty tissue were first described in the early 1920s and 1930s (15, 16). More recently, these findings have been verified by imaging studies utilizing magnetic resonance (MRI) (17–20). The pattern of overall timing and anatomic sites of marrow conversion have been delineated as a function of age. At birth, all marrow is hematopoietic. With aging, there is progressive fatty replacement which begins in the peripheral skeleton and progresses centrally. In the long bones, this replacement starts first in the diaphyses with relative preservation of metaphyseal hematopoiesis. By the end of adolescence, active hematopoietic red marrow remains in the proximal metaphyses of the femur and humerus as well as in the vertebral bodies, sternum, ribs, and skull. With continued aging, there is progressive involution of the remaining hematopoietic tissues. No appreciable sex difference in this distribution is apparent (20). In older adults, the majority of hematopoietic bone marrow is contained within the sternum, clavicle, vertebral column, and iliac crests (Figure 31.2). This axial distribution enables routine sampling of the posterior iliac crest as representative of the overall bone marrow cellularity. Furthermore, the sites of marrow cellularity appear to parallel the sites of marrow involvement by metastatic lesions, enabling accurate staging information to be collected (21) from routine biopsy specimens.

In addition to the progressive anatomic centralization of active hematopoietic marrow, and decreases in subcortical cellularity within these central sites, changes in the distribution of hematopoietic cells and marrow fat within an individual core biopsy can also be observed. In elderly patients with osteopenia or primary bone disease, marrow fat tends to accumulate in a paratrabecular location (6) with islands of hematopoiesis confined to the central bone marrow spaces. This peculiar relationship has been ascribed to the intimate interactions between osseous remodeling and hematopoietic precursor proliferation (22), support for the theory of co-regulation of these two processes.

Lymphoid Aggregates

Benign lymphocytic aggregates are relatively common findings in the bone marrow biopsy and aspirate slides obtained from adult patients (23). They are composed of small, round mature benign lymphocytes mixed with small numbers of histiocytes, reticulum cells, plasma cells, eosinophils, and mast cells. They may occasionally be associated with germinal centers or epithelioid histiocytes. These aggregates range from 0.05 to 1 mm and are generally well delineated from the surrounding hematopoietic tissue. They are frequently referred to as lymphoid nodules or lymphoid follicles. Rarely, they may have irregular or serpentine borders, and have been referred to as lymphoid infiltrates (24). The reported incidence in autopsy material ranges from 15–42%, with vertebral bone marrow being richer in aggregates than either sternal or iliac crest marrow. They are more frequent in women, and their incidence increases with age. They are also more frequent in bone marrows of healthy individuals than those affected by chronic illnesses, cachexia or non-hematopoietic tumors (25). The incidence in normal iliac crest biopsy specimens is approximately 15% of the general adult population (26).

The presence of lymphoid aggregates is felt to be a physiologic reaction to infection and/or chronic immunologic stimulation (27). Since their incidence steadily increases with advancing age, they become a nearly ubiquitous finding in individuals over the age of 70 years. The significance of lymphoid aggregates has remained undetermined, although they do not appear to evolve into a malignant lymphoproliferative disorder. Morphologic criteria have been used to separate patients with undiagnosed bone marrow involvement by lymphoproliferative disorders from those with benign or reactive lymphoid aggregates. These criteria include the size and composition of the aggregate (benign aggregates are well circumscribed and contain a heteromorphous cellular population), the presence of well defined borders (benign lymphoid aggregates tend to be well circumscribed), and the number and size of these entities (benign aggregates are single, and generally number fewer than three per biopsy specimen).

Studies performed prior to the utilization of flow cytometry to define clonality have documented an inci-

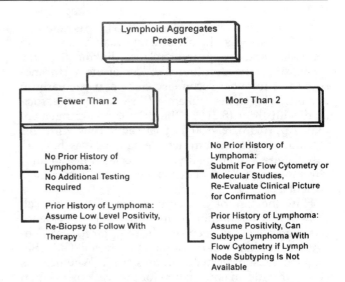

Figure 31.3 Recommendations for the evaluation of bone marrow lymphoid aggregates should take into account a knowledge of the clinical setting, patient history and physical exam. Additional diagnostic studies may be helpful if unusually large or confluent aggregates are present, or if multiple aggregates are identified.

dence between 15 and 50% (24, 28, 29). With the advent of ready access to flow cytometric immunophenotyping, a small, yet important, number of patients can be identified as having malignant lymphoproliferative disorders. While flow cytometry or molecular pathology studies (Southern blotting or polymerase chain reaction analysis for clonal immunoglobulin gene rearrangements) can be diagnostic, it is important to place these laboratory tests in the context of the patient. The expense and time needed for their evaluation must be weighed against their contributions to changing treatment decisions, especially in the very elderly. Guidelines are needed to help standardize evaluation (Figure 31.3).

Chromosomal Abnormalities

Loss of the Y chromosome (-Y) in the bone marrow cells of elderly males is relatively common, and has generally been accepted as a normal age related phenomenon. It appears to be without pathogenetic significance (30). While chromosomal instability is not generally accepted as a normal aging phenomenon, there is evidence to point to the occurrence of alterations in chromosomal DNA during the processes of cellular senescence (31, 32). Aberrations have been identified in tissue culture cells obtained from humans and other mammals, and it has been suggested that genetic factors may be related to their prevalence (31).

Although commonly noted in routine chromosomal analysis on bone marrow specimens in elderly males, the presence of –Y can occasionally be associated with neoplastic changes. Thus, identification of –Y as a karyotypic abnormality should always be evaluated in the context of the clinical scenario. Its appearance as the only karyotypic abnormality noted in acute myelogenous leukemia or myelodysplasia (33, 34) is reported. In these instances, the abnormality may disappear in remission and reappear in relapse, linking it to the neoplastic clone. Additionally, loss of the Y chromosome is a frequent secondary change, particularly in acute myelogenous leukemia (FAB M2 type) associated with the t (8;21) as the primary rearrangement (35). Approximately 50% of leukemic cells with this translocation isolated from male patients may have an associated –Y abnormality. An associated loss of an X chromosome (-X) is occasionally reported in female patients.

How the loss of a Y chromosome influences cell growth and maturation is unknown. Recent evidence has suggested that a gene for the receptor for granulocyte macrophage colony stimulating factor (GM-CSF) maps to the short arm of chromosome Y. Whether this could provide an explanation for the weak association between premature marrow aging and chromosome loss is unclear.

Common Hematopoietic Abnormalities in the Elderly: Non-Physiologic

While morphologic changes have been associated with the process of aging in normal individuals, little evidence exists for bone marrow compromise or development of cytopenias as a "normal" physiologic phenomenon. The identification of significant cellular defects (including anemia, neutropenia and abnormal infiltrates) should always be taken as a sign of disease.

Anemia in Aging Individuals

As men and women age in our population, the incidence of anemia appears to increase (36, 37) such that cross-sectional studies of healthy individuals have shown a progressive decrease in hemoglobin with age (38). When clinically stable healthy persons are studied longitudinally, rather than cross-sectionally, hemoglobin and hematocrit do not appear to fall in the absence of demonstrable disease (39). The overall incidence of anemia in the elderly has been estimated to average 20%, with a range of 2–30% reported in the literature (36, 37, 40).

When the causes of anemia can be identified in elderly patients, they are similar to those of younger patients. The presence of chronic disease and iron deficiency resulting from blood loss appear to be the most frequent contributors (41). In elderly patients living alone, vitamin deficiencies (particularly folate deficiency) may occur as a result of poor nutritional habits (42). Although the incidence of pernicious anemia also increases with age, vitamin B12 deficiency in the elderly is rare (43). Thus, while one must keep in mind that elderly individuals with pernicious anemia may have unusual presentations, such as dementia as the only obvious clinical abnormality, the rarity of this disorder makes routine supplementation with vitamin B12 of unproven value in the aging population.

Although the presence of anemia does not appear to be a normal physiologic phenomenon, several pub-

lished studies have suggested that bone marrow response to stress may be blunted in the elderly. When anemia develops in young normal individuals, the level of 2,3-diphosphoglycerate (2,3-DPG) increases, with a subsequent decrease in the oxygen affinity of hemoglobin and increase in oxygen delivery. This adaptive mechanism to anemia results in a shift of the oxygen dissociation curve to the right. It has been reported (44) that elderly individuals with anemia may have lower 2,3-DPG levels than a group of corresponding young anemic subjects. However, while these levels are indeed lower than younger individuals, they are still elevated from baseline in non-anemic elderly people. This finding suggests that the response to 2,3-DPG, while blunted, is present. Therefore, it remains doubtful that abnormalities in 2,3-DPG significantly contribute to the development of anemia or the long-term ability of older persons to produce marrow compensation to it. Results of complete hematologic workup, including iron studies, bone marrow aspirations and biopsies, hemolysis evaluation, and the concentration of erythroid stem cells (BFU) have been examined and found to be within normal limits, showing no change with aging. However, there is one abnormality which is reproducibly observed, and that is a partial defect in marrow response to erythropoietin, often accompanied by a decreased level of erythropoietin (43). This decrease in functional erythropoietin response, associated with a compromised bone marrow proliferative capacity, has been well documented (45–47), and may underlie the observation that many elderly patients have a decreased capacity to respond to hematologic stress.

Neutropenia

Generally speaking, neither total white blood cell count nor differential tends to change with advancing age (48). However, several cross-sectional studies (49, 50) have shown a fall in the absolute lymphocyte count with aging, and have suggested that this change is a possible predictor of death within three years. No decreases in peripheral neutrophil count, monocyte count or eosinophil count have been observed (5). Despite the stability of peripheral blood numerical values, it is generally felt that elderly patients are more susceptible to infections. Furthermore, when infections develop, these same individuals are more likely to be hospitalized longer and to succumb more frequently than younger patients with similar diagnoses (51, 52). While there is most likely a multifactorial etiology for the observed enhancement of susceptibility to infectious complications, impairments in neutrophil supply and/or neutrophil function are postulated (44, 53). A higher incidence of neutropenic complications of infections, autoimmune diseases and chemotherapy in the elderly also suggest the presence of disordered neutrophil production and/or regulation (43). Recent studies (54) have searched for such a defect with little success, and could identify no measurable decrement in marrow response to stimulation by either growth factor (G-CSF) or epinephrine. Thus, the supposition that neutrophil reserves are decreased in the elderly has not been substantiated by concrete experimental data (55, 56).

Since peripheral neutrophil counts do not change with aging, it should be assumed that the presence of neutropenia in elderly individuals is a sign of primary marrow dysfunction or the presence of enhanced cellular destruction. Certainly, the presence of clonal marrow disorders such as myelodysplasia must be excluded, as this disorder demonstrates a markedly increasing incidence with increasing patient age. Furthermore, although uncommon, autoimmune disorders also increase in frequency with increasing age. Autoimmune neutropenia, while rare, is important to recognize because it is treatable in the majority of patients, resulting in improvements or normalization of neutrophil count and function. Care must be taken to avoid diagnosing a "treatable" autoimmune disorder as myelodysplasia, since these two diseases can sometimes be confused when evaluating bone marrow aspirate material.

Lymphoid "Hyperplasia" and Non-Hodgkin's Lymphoma

As previously mentioned, the distinction between benign lymphoid nodules and lymphoproliferative disorders of the marrow is often difficult to discern. Generally speaking, a few well demarcated lymphoid nodules are common in the normal older adult, in contrast to larger or more numerous irregularly shaped nodules that may be present in patients with lymphomatous involvement of the marrow (57). When identified in a paratrabecular orientation, or when seen as confluent or diffuse infiltrates, these lymphoid nodules suggest the presence of a malignant lymphoproliferative disorder, rather than a benign lesion.

Occasionally, lymphoid nodules may be numerous, although they still retain their benign histologic architecture. A particularly high incidence of lymphoid nodules is found in systemic autoimmune disorders such as rheumatoid arthritis and systemic lupus erythematosus, in aplastic anemia and pure red cell aplasia, myelodysplasia or myeloproliferative disorders, idiopathic thrombocytopenia purpura or infection with human immunodeficiency virus (HIV) (23). The most significant association is with autoimmune disorders, where lymphoid infiltrates can be associated with the presence of germinal centers or a granulomatous response (58).

One must be cautious and not simply assume that all lymphoid aggregates in older persons are benign. Low grade lymphoproliferative disorders show an increasing incidence with patient age, with a documented increased prevalence over recent years. Careful evaluation for the presence of peripheral lymphadenopathy, splenomegaly or circulating abnormal lymphocytes should be performed in patients demonstrating abnormally large or frequent lymphoid infiltrates in their bone marrow specimens. If available, flow cytometric immunophenotyping or other molecular assays for demonstration of clonality are highly recommended.

Other Malignancies

When faced with an elderly patient showing selected cytopenias or pancytopenia, marrow infiltrative disorders should be ruled out. As seen in myelodysplasia, there is also an increasing incidence of the acute leukemias (predominantly acute myelogenous leukemia) with advancing patient age. The increased association of acute leukemia with myelodysplasia and marrow failure in the elderly population, make the prevalence of "aleukemic" leukemia more frequent. Bone marrow aspiration and biopsy are diagnostic.

Marrow infiltration by solid tumors, including metastatic carcinomas of the prostate, breast or gastrointestinal tract can also occur. Atypical presentations of metastatic disease with primary pancytopenia, while uncommon, are found in aged persons more frequently than younger individuals.

Conclusions

Although there are clearly age related physiologic changes noted within the bone marrows of elderly individuals, the majority of these are histologic changes without a significant impact on basal hematopoiesis. Aged individuals may show evidence of decreased marrow reserve or hematopoietic compromise when stressed by infection or other co-morbid conditions. However, the identification of cellular abnormalities in this population (anemia, neutropenia or thrombocytopenia) should be investigated, as an underlying pathologic state is likely to coexist. Aged individuals show a gradually increasing incidence of malignancies (both hematopoietic and non-hematopoietic) such that a malignant cause of marrow dysfunction is not uncommon. The performance of routine bone marrow aspiration and biopsy is not complicated by patient age alone. Thus, these procedures can be safely and effectively utilized in the elderly individual, and may contribute significant information as to the etiology of any observed peripheral blood abnormality.

References

1. Gulati GL, Ashton JK, Hyun BH. Structure and function of the bone marrow and hematopoiesis. *Hematol/Oncol Cl NA* 1988; **2**: 495–511.
2. Politis C, Karamerou A, Block. Pathophysiologic aspects of the bone/marrow/fat relationship. *Lab Management* 1983; **21**: 40–55.
3. Jamshidi K, Swain W. Bone marrow biopsy with unaltered architecture. *J Lab Clin Med* 1971; **77**: 333–342.
4. Parfitt AM. Bone remodeling and bone loss: understanding the physiology of osteoporosis. *Clin Obstet Gynecol* 1987; **30**: 789–811.
5. Smith R. Osteoporosis. Cause and management. *Br Med J* 1987; **294**: 329–332.
6. Burkhardt R, Kettner G, Bohm W, Schmidmeier M, Schlag R, Frisch B, Mallmann B, Eisenmenger W, Gilg TH. Changes in trabecular bone, hematopoiesis and bone marrow vessels in aplastic anemia, primary osteoporosis, and old age: A comparative histomorphometric study. *Bone* 1987; **8**: 157–164.
7. Whitehouse WJ. Cancellous bone in the anterior part of the iliac crest. *Calcif Tissue Res* 1977; **23**: 67–76.
8. Kahn A, Gibbons R, Perkins S, Gazit D. Age-related bone loss: A hypothesis and initial assessment in mice. *Clin Orthop Relat Res* 1995; **313**: 69–75.

9. Perkins SL, Gibbons R, Kling S, Kahn AJ. Age-related bone loss in mice is associated with an increased osteoclast progenitor pool. *Bone* 1994; **15**: 65–72.

10. Kita K, Kawai K, Hirohata K. Changes in bone marrow blood flow with aging. *J Orthop Res* 1987; **5**: 569–575.

11. Burkhardt R. Interrelations between bone marrow and bone (report). *Verh Detsch Ges Pathol* 1994; **58**: 205–218.

12. Rutishauser E, Rohner E, Held D. Experimentelle untersuchungen uber die wirkung der ischamie auf den knochen und das mark. *Virch Arch Path Anat* 1960; **333**: 101–118.

13. Rhinelander F, Stewart CL, Wilson JW Bone vascular supply. In *Skeletal Research*. New York: Academic Press, pp. 367–395, 1979.

14. Hartsock RJ, Smith EB, Petty CS. Normal variations with aging of the amount of hematopoietic tissue in bone marrow from the anterior iliac crest. *Am J Clin Pathol* 1965; **43**: 326–331.

15. Piney A The anatomy of the bone marrow. *Br Med J* 1922; **2**: 792–795.

16. Custer RP. Studies on the structure and function of bone marrow. *J Lab Clin Med* 1932; **16**: 951–962.

17. Zawin JK, Jaramillo D. Conversion of bone marrow in the humerus, sternum, and clavicle: Changes with age on MR images. *Radiology* 1993; **188**: 159–164.

18. Richardson ML, Patten RM. Age-related changes in marrow distribution in the shoulder: MR imaging findings. *Radiology* 1994; **192**: 209–215.

19. Mirowitz SA. Hematopoietic bone marrow within the proximal humeral epiphysis in normal adults: Investigation with MR imaging. *Radiology* 1993; **188**: 689–693.

20. Ricci C, Cova M, Kang YS, Yang A, Rahmouni A, Scott WW Jr, Zerhouni EA. Normal age-related patterns of cellular and fatty bone marrow distribution in the axial skeleton: MR imaging study. *Radiology* 1990; **177**: 83–88.

21. Kricun ME. Red-yellow marrow conversion: Its effect on the location of some solitary bone lesions. *Skeletal Radiol* 1985; **14**: 10–19.

22. Lips P, van Ginkel FG, Netelenbos JG. Bone marrow and bone remodeling. *Bone* 1985; **6**: 343–344.

23. Navone R, Valpreda M, Pich A. Lymphoid nodules and nodular lymphoid hyperplasia in bone marrow biopsies. *Acta Haemat* 1985; **74**: 19–22.

24. Rywlin AM. *Histopathology of the Bone Marrow*. Boston: Little, Brown Co., pp. 95–110, 1976.

25. Chomette G, Dumont J, Pinaudeau Y, Auriol M, Brocheriou C. Les ilots lymphoides dans la moelle osseuse. *Annls Anat Path* 1967; **12**: 91–100.

26. Navone R, Vigliani R, Valpreda M. Studio dei noduli linfatici del midollo osseo in una casistica autopsica. *Pathologica* 1982; **74**: 231–240.

27. Liu PI, Takanari H, Yatani R, Nelson G. Comparative studies of bone marrow from the United States and Japan. *Ann Clin Lab Sci* 1989; **19**: 345–351.

28. Maeda K, Hyun BH, Rebuck JW. Lymphoid follicles in bone marrow aspirates. *Am J Clin Pathol* 1977; **67**: 41–52.

29. Hashimoto M, Hashimoto N. The occurrence of lymph nodules in human bone marrow with particular references to their number. *Kyushu J Med Sci* 1963; **14**: 343–354.

30. United Kingdom Cancer Cytogenetics Group. Loss of the y chromosome from normal and neoplastic bone marrow. *Genes, Chrom Cancer* 1992; **5**: 83–88.

31. Nisitani S, Hosokawa M, Sasaki MS, Yasuoka K, Naiki H, Matsushita T, Takeda T: Acceleration of chromosome aberrations in senescence-accelerated strains of mice. *Mutation Res* 1990; **237**: 221–228.

32. Bergtold DS, Lett JT. Alterations in chromosomal DNA and aging: An overview. In *Molecular Biology of Aging*, edited by A Sohal, *et al*. New York: Raven, 1985.

33. Abe S, Golomb HM, Rowley JD, Mitelman F, Sandberg AA. Chromosomes and causation of human cancer and leukemia. XXXV. The missing y in acute non-lymphocytic leukemia (ANLL). *Cancer* 1980; **45**: 84–90.

34. Holmes RI, Keating MJ, Cork A, Trujillo JM, McCredie KB, Freireich E. Loss of the y chromosome in acute myelo-genous leukemia: A report of 13 patients. *Cancer Genet Cytogenet* 1985; **17**: 269–278.

35. Riske CB, Morgan R, Ondreyco S, Sandberg AA. X and Y chromosome loss as sole abnormality in acute nonlymphocytic leukemia (ANLL). *Cancer Genet Cytogenet* 1994; **72**: 44–47.

36. Parson PL, Whitney JL, Kilpatrick GS. The prevalence of anemia in the elderly. *Practitioner* 1965; **195**: 656–660.

37. Timiras ML, Brownstein H. Prevalence of anemia and correlation of hemoglobin with age in a geriatric screening clinic population. *J Am Geriatr Soc* 1987; **35**: 639–643.

38. Baldwin JG Jr: True anemia: Incidence and significance in the elderly. *Geriatrics* 1989; **44**: 33–36.

39. Baldwin JG, Lichtenstein LS, Stuart RK: Longitudinal study of hemoglobin and hematocrit in the elderly. *Blood* 1986; **68** (suppl 1): 52a.

40. Hill RD: The prevalence of anemia in the over-65s in a rural practice. *Practitioner* 1967; **217**: 963–967.

41. Lewis R: Anemia: A common but never a normal concomitant of aging. Geriatrics 1976; **31**: 53–60.

42. Lipschitz DA, Mitchell CO. The correctability of the nutritional, immune and hematopoietic manifestations of protein calorie malnutrition in the elderly. *J Am Coll Nutr* 1982; **1**: 17–25.

43. Baldwin JG Jr. Hematopoietic function in the elderly. *Arch Intern Med* 1988; **148**: 2544–2546.

44. Lipschitz DA, Udupa KB, Milton KY, Thompson CO. Effect of age on hematopoiesis in man. *Blood* 1984; **63**: 502–509.

45. Boggs DR. Hematopoiesis and aging: IV. Mass and distribution of erythroid marrow in aged mice. *Exp Hematol* 1985; **13**: 1044–1047.

46. Williams LH, Udupa KB, Lipschitz DA. Evaluation of the effect of age on hematopoiesis in the C57BL/6 mouse. *Exp Hematol* 1986; **14**: 827–832.

47. Freedman ML. Heme and iron metabolism in aging. *Blood Cells* 1987; **13**: 227–235.

48. Zauber NP, Zauber AG. Hematologic data of healthy very old people. *JAMA* 1987; **257**: 2181–2184.

49. Mackinner AA Jr. Effect of aging on the peripheral blood lymphocyte count. *J Gerontol* 1978; **33**: 213–216.

50. Bender BS, Nagel JE, Adler WH, Andres R. Absolute peripheral blood lymphocyte count and subsequent mortality of elderly men. *J Am Geriatr Soc* 1986; **34**: 649–654.

51. Berk SL, Smith JK. Infectious diseases in the elderly. *Med Clin North Am* 1983; **67**: 273–293.

52. Yoshikawa TT, Norman DC. Aging and Clinical Practice: Infectious Diseases, Diagnosis and Treatment. New York: Igaku-Shoin, 1987.

53. Corberand J, Ngyen F, Laharrague P, Fontanilles AM, Gleyzes B, Gyrard E, Senegas C. Polymorphonuclear functions and aging in humans. *J Am Geriatr Soc* 1981; **29**: 391–397.

54. Chatta GS, Price TH, Stratton JR, Dale DC. Aging and marrow neutrophil reserves. *J Am Geriatr Soc* 1994; **42**: 77–81.

55. Cream JJ. Prednisolone-induced granulocytosis. *Br J Haematol* 1968; **15**: 259–267.

56. Timaffy M. A comparative study of bone marrow function in young and old individuals. *Gerontol Clin* 1962; **4**: 113–118.

57. Rywlin AM, Ortega RS, Dominguez CJ. Lymphoid nodules of bone marrow: Normal and abnormal. *Blood* 1974; **43**: 389–400.

58. Makonidan T, Kay MMB. Age influence on the immune system. *Adv Immunol* 1980; **29**: 287–330.

32. Radiotherapy in the Elderly

Pierre Scalliet and Thierry Pignon

Introduction

In North America and Europe more than 12% of the population is over 65 years of age. All older persons are facing decisions at the end of life which will affect their families and society (1). The simple facts that this book, and this chapter have been written proceed from the belief that older individuals constitute a distinct group deserving special consideration concerning diagnosis, treatment and the general management of cancer. Epidemiological data, however, do not define a group of older persons clearly separated from younger persons. Rather, age is a continuum variable without clear cut boundaries, and the incidence of cancer increases with age.

Radiation oncology is an important form of cancer treatment which may prove particularly valuable in the older cancer patient. The main issue of radiation oncology in the elderly concerns preservation of treatment effectiveness while minimizing the risk of therapeutic complications. This goal is dictated by several considerations. Older persons may present a reduced tolerance of cytotoxic treatment, due to reduced reserve in hemopoietic and mucosal stem cells, and in the functional reserve of multiple organ systems, such as cardiovascular, pulmonary and renal function. Older patients may develop tumors with decreased aggressiveness. Also, the picture is frequently complicated by the presence of associated conditions which are known to influence the tolerance of radiotherapy. Aged patients are more exposed to co-morbidities such as diabetes, hypertension, and heart or lung insufficiency, which may complicate the clinical course of their cancer and impair their ability to sustain a long, and sometimes aggressive, curative treatment. The effects of age and the effects of chronic disease often converge, reducing the tolerance of stress by older individuals. However, because aging is highly individualized, the respective effects of age and of chronic diseases other than cancer on treatment tolerance need to be assessed separately. It is not unusual to find persons of advanced age in excellent general condition. It would be inappropriate to deny the benefits of aggressive antineoplastic treatment to these persons.

No guidelines are established for adapting treatment strategies to patient's age (except, perhaps, in hematology) yet older patients are, as already mentioned, often treated in a different, less aggressive way than younger patients. The few available studies relevant to this question do not, however, support the indiscriminate reduction of radiation dose/intensity.

Lack of Radiobiological Data

The interactions of radiobiology and age were recently reviewed (2). The data appear very scant and inconclusive. Most experimental works explore the influence of age on radiobiology by comparing the effects of irradiation in immature and in young adult animals. These investigations were designed to study the benefits and the toxicity of irradiation in children, not to obtain information about older adults. Biological as well as logistical problems impede the study of radiation in older animals. As a matter of fact, working with old mice or rats close to the end of their lifespan is quite impractical in general for all radiation effects and, in particular, for late effects. The comorbidity of older animals may cloud the investigation of acute radiation toxicity; the short life span of these animals prevents the study of late radiation effects.

Few *in vitro* data deal with the age of cell cultures. Human fibroblasts were found to have similar survival parameters independently from the donor's age (range 11 to 78 years) (3), although the proliferative potential of such cultures decreases with age (4). In contrast, the rate of DNA damage removal has been found to decrease with increasing age in the rat skin (5), but this observation has no obvious *in vivo* counterpart (6). These projects, however, did not explore skin reactions in very old animals. Last, but not least, housing of rodents for several months is very expensive.

Interesting data were very recently published, dealing with the effect of the host age on microenvironmental heterogeneity of EMT6 tumors implanted into young and aging mice. The mice had been housed 15 to 18 months before starting the experiments, and could hence be considered very old. The most conclusive result of these experiments was the finding of a much higher radiobiological hypoxic fraction in older than in younger animals (41% vs 19%), although an identical number of tumor cells had been implanted in all mice. A higher hypoxic fraction shelters the tumor from the cytotoxicity of radiation and has obvious impact on curability. Mitomycin C, an agent with selective toxicity to hypoxic cells, produced greater antineoplastic effect in tumors in aging mice and potentiated the effects of radiation in older mice more effectively than in younger animals (7). These experimental data, however, are at odds with the clinical impression that the tumor radiocurability does not change with the age of the patient. Following, we will review the effects of irradiation on most common neoplasms occurring in elderly patients.

Prostate Cancer

The controversy regarding the best treatment for localized prostate carcinoma has been raging for decades. Consensus meetings trying to resolve the issue in the absence of appropriately controlled studies, usually tend to recommend radical radiotherapy for men over 70 years of age (8). A survey of the Metropolitan Detroit Cancer Surveillance System confirmed indeed that there is an increased awareness of radiation therapy as a means of therapy in the elderly (over 75 years). This may have caused a migration to this form of therapy (9). However, this migration was not found to be age-dependent in another population-based study from The Netherlands since identical trends were identified in younger age groups (10). Yet, it is acknowledged that attitudes regarding radical treatment of prostate carcinoma widely differ between the US and Europe.

The artificial age limit of 70 in the consensus statement represents, in reality, a surrogate for a life-expectancy of, at best, 10 years. This recommendation reflects the baseless belief that radical radiotherapy is inferior to radical prostatectomy and that it can provide adequate control of the tumor only up to ten years. In addition, early recurrence and death from prostate cancer represent a smaller loss in life-expectancy for individuals aged 70 and older than for younger men.

A true comparison between surgery and radiotherapy, however, does not exist; attitudes regarding treatment are therefore rather a matter of belief than of science.

Quality of life after treatment may be affected by gastrointestinal or urologic symptoms. Gastrointestinal complications including radiation enteritis and colitis, and even small bowel obstruction are more common with radiotherapy; urologic complication, especially urinary incontinence, are more common with surgery. The risk of complications should be openly discussed with the individual patient allowing him to express his own view on which aspect of quality of life he would be more prepared to trade-off for tumor control. As far as the patient's preference is concerned, a recent Veteran Administration study revealed that older patients are more willing to accept an impotence outcome than a urinary incontinence outcome, yet older patients were less willing to accept the impotence outcome than younger patients, even though the reported incidence of impotence increased with age (11). This study underlines the importance of obtaining information related to one's quality of life directly from the patients and not to make assumptions about an individual patient's preferences. One cannot overemphasize the risk of assuming that older patients have an already

compromised quality of life and reduced interest in sexual activity.

Adequate informed consent is as important in the elderly as it is in other age groups. This is all the more true since a recent report from Karolinska Institute suggested that the incidence of impotence after radiotherapy might be far from negligible, i.e. much more than usually reported, and with a measurable negative impact on the patient's perception of his own quality of life (12).

Regarding radical radiotherapy, the Pattern of Care Study and a series by the Fox Chase Cancer Center revealed that the outcome of this form of treatment was similar in men aged 70 and over and in younger men (13). These conclusions concern all aspects of cancer control and the whole gamut of treatment-related late morbidity. Therefore, radiation treatment should not be withheld from appropriately selected elderly patients with prostate cancer because of concerns about the patient's tolerance of treatment. Also, 3D conformal irradiation reduces the incidence of acute treatment complications and appears particularly advisable in advanced ages (14).

Head and Neck Cancer

Comorbidity is very common in patients with squamous cell carcinomas of the head and neck, which are mostly due to cigarette smoking and consumption of alcoholic beverages. Locoregional spread of these neoplasms may rapidly compromise two vital functions (swallowing and breathing) and quality of life. Despite excess of comorbidity, cancer is the most common cause of death and suffering in this population. Consequently radical treatment is used even in patients with compromised function of multiple organ systems, and simple palliative procedures are seldom used. However, elderly or frail patients are less prone to be offered surgery or combined radiotherapy and surgery (or chemotherapy); they are rather referred to radiotherapy departments for radical treatment.

In a French retrospective series of 331 elderly patients, 104 had a medical contraindication to general anesthesia (15). Mean age was 75 years (range 70–95). As far as survival was concerned, performance status proved to be a much better predictor of treatment outcome than age. Psychological problems (including confusion) interfered with the treatment in 8% of cases more prominently in the subgroup aged 80 and more. Otherwise, age and general status did not appear to have influenced the mucosal tolerance to treatment.

This finding is corroborated by another series of 277 patients in which body weight loss during radical radiotherapy was prospectively recorded and analyzed according to patient's age. Mean age was 63.3 years (range 29–91); average body weight loss during irradiation was 4% (maximum 15%). If any trend was recognizable it was a slight positive effect of age on treatment tolerance. Patient's age had no influence on survival probability (16). At variance with the previous study in which 11 patients succumbed apparently from lack of recovery after radical irradiation, there were no treatment related deaths in this series which probably reflects the positive patient selection. A third retrospective study in 88 elderly patients treated in the period 1980–1985 at the Prince of Wales Hospital supported safety and effectiveness of radiotherapy (17).

A survey of the EORTC database of all head and neck patients included in 5 prospective trials between February 1980 and March 1995 has been recently carried out at the Central Office in Brussels. One thousand five hundred eighty nine subjects have been identified. Data regarding local control, survival, early and late tolerance were available in all or part of the series. Mean age was 57 (range 20–82), i.e. relatively young given the trial exclusion criteria often mentioning 70 years as the age-limit. There were still 20% of these aged 65 or more and 13% aged 70 or more. Age was not a prognostic factor for locoregional control, body weight loss, acute objective mucosal reactions or late effects. The only statistical difference was an age-related worse functional acute toxicity of radical radiotherapy (essentially pain as experienced by the patient). It was interesting to note this discrepancy between acute objective and functional side effects; it suggested that equivalent severity levels of mucositis were differently experienced by younger and older patients. Body weight loss, as mentioned above, was however similar in both groups (18).

Lung Cancer

Patients with non-small cell lung cancer that is inoperable for medical reasons (19) or simply because of age (20) are often referred to radiotherapy. Radical irradiation will improve survival in those with a small initial tumor (< 3–4 cm) achieving complete remission and will provide valuable symptom palliation in the majority of other patients. Tumor control needs advanced planning and a total dose of at least 60–65 Gy. It seems that the initial field size does not influence critically the probability of local control and survival, i.e. irradiation of the primary is sufficient, without prophylactic mediastinal lymph node irradiation. Whether this is an equivalent treatment option to surgery remains unknown since comparative data are not available, so far.

A longitudinal prospective study described functional tolerance in a sample of 45 elderly patients (range 61–86, mean 69.8) receiving radiotherapy for breast or lung cancer. The outcome variables were weight and multidimensional functional status. A great majority had at least one comorbid condition. Radiotherapy was well tolerated. The functional status of these elderly patients was overall well preserved, despite some transient limitations in the usual activities, during treatment (21).

An important observation concerns treatment variables which might have decreased the compliance of older individuals with treatment. Of these, the distance

from the treatment center appeared to have a major impact in a Dutch study, reviewing the pattern of cancer care in south-eastern Netherlands (10). A distance of 35 km or more between the residence of the patient and the radiotherapy facility did not affect use of radiotherapy as a primary treatment, except for older patients with lung cancer; the percentage of older individuals receiving radiotherapy decreased from 48% to 28%. This observation may only reflect regional conditions, but it is nonetheless important. It reveals the influence of parameters independent from the disease and the patient's physical condition on the management of older persons.

Breast Cancer

There are several reports indicating that both tumor staging and treatment choice are inadequate in older women, especially regarding the use of radiotherapy after partial mastectomy (22, 23, 24, 25). Since treatment selection chiefly depends on tumor staging, incomplete staging procedures are prone to lead to inappropriate therapeutic strategies.

In a population-based series of 2268 patients aged 55 and older, the clinical stage was twice as frequently unknown in the oldest age group (18%) than in younger patients (8%) (23). Breast cancer patients of 75 years and older were treated with adjuvant radiotherapy less often than younger patients. Instead, the oldest age group received surgery alone or surgery followed by adjuvant hormonal therapy. This was not fully explained by stage progression with age, although stage III and IV were more frequent in older patients.

Appropriateness of treatment was retrospectively investigated in a series of 492 patients from Middelheim hospital (mean age 54.1, range 24–81). Multi variate analysis revealed that, after correction for stage, younger patients were more often offered conservative surgery than older patients. Moreover, node dissection was less frequent in older patients. Elderly patients treated with breast-conservation procedures received breast boost much less frequently than younger individuals. Finally, older patients were less likely to receive axillary irradiation, even in the absence of axillary lymph node dissection (26).

Failure to use adjuvant radiotherapy appropriately may have a serious negative impact on treatment outcome as local relapse usually occurs in the first 4 postoperative years and is likely to become a problem during the patient's lifetime (25). Replacing adjuvant irradiation with adjuvant hormonotherapy in locally advanced stages should therefore be restricted to women with a short life expectancy. A recent randomized trial, in which women older than 75 received either tamoxifen alone or surgery, concluded that surgery is the appropriate treatment for elderly patients with operable breast cancer (27). Giving tamoxifen as a unique treatment only delayed the moment when surgery became necessary, which often had to be carried out in more adverse conditions. This was confirmed in another series of 85 patients aged 75 years and older with loco-regional disease (stage I and II). Complete remission lasting for their lifetime was obtained in only 12 patients (median follow-up 28 months, range 3–97). All the others were exposed to morbidity due to the cancer which was not well controlled by hormonotherapy. Another 12 died from their cancer in the follow-up period (28). In a series from Rochester, a preferential allocation of aged women to conservative breast surgery without radiotherapy was observed, a policy which can no longer be advocated since the recurrence rate exceeded 25 % vs. 7 % only if postoperative radiotherapy was given (29).

Whether adjuvant radiotherapy is required in all cases of conservative surgery has been questioned by Veronesi in the analysis of a recent Milan randomized study. Between 1987 and 1989, 567 women with small breast tumors (< 2.5 cm) were randomly assigned to quandrantectomy followed by radiotherapy vs. quadrantectomy alone. The incidences of local recurrence were 0.3% vs 8.8%. However, there was a substantial effect of age: women older than 55 years had a lower recurrence rate of 3.8% in the absence of adjuvant irradiation (30). This finding has prompted an EORTC trial, currently ongoing, aiming at assessing the value of adjuvant radiotherapy in post-menopausal women treated for a small stage I tumor.

As far as irradiation is concerned, the few available reports do not support any difference in the early or late tolerance to radiotherapy of elderly patients (24, 25). An original comparison of local outcome after free-tissue transfer procedure for various tumor sites (including breast) in elderly patients previously treated or not by radiotherapy and/or chemotherapy concluded that free-tissue transfer success rates were high in both patient categories. Previous radiotherapy did not decrease the possibility of salvage surgery (31). Van Limbergen et al. (1989) did not find any influence of age on the cosmetic outcome of conservative breast cancer treatments in a multivariate analysis of a large group of patients (32). In contrast, a small negative impact of age on cosmesis was suggested from another series, although this did not reach statistical significance and was, at least to some extent, confounded by variations in extent of surgery (33). Another paper, dealing with the risk of developing a brachial plexus injury after radiotherapy for breast cancer found no correlation with age (449 patients with age range 18–92) (34). The only predictor for plexus injury was the use of large daily radiation doses. This contrasts with the conclusions of a French trial in a series of elderly women (average 81 years) advocating the use of large single weekly doses (seven fractions of 6.5 Gy over six weeks) associated to tamoxifen (35).

Hypofractionation however increases the risk of late radiation damage unless the total dose is reduced appropriately which, in turn, decreases the effect on the tumor. Two Gy per fraction emerged through experience as the best compromise between effectiveness and morbidity of radiotherapy. Departing from this protocol requires a very careful assessment of all factors involved, in particular the life expectancy of the individual patient.

Since many older women are anxious to preserve their breasts, they should certainly be offered the conservative treatment option combining surgery and adjuvant irradiation whenever the local stage allows for it (36, 37). Tolerance of adjuvant radiotherapy should not be of a different concern than it is in any other age group. It is also important to keep in mind that a woman of 85 years can expect to live on average 7 more years, and may therefore experience local recurrence of her cancer during her lifetime (38).

Gynecological Malignancies

Women presenting with an endometrial or a cervical carcinoma inoperable for medical reasons are often referred to radiotherapy for radical irradiation. Whether radiotherapy offers an equal chance of cure than surgery is unknown because there are no randomized trials comparing surgery and irradiation. Retrospective studies are subject to selection bias, as mostly medically unfit patients are referred for primary radiotherapy. Radical irradiation however is not always possible given the high frequency of associated morbid conditions that often are the same that contraindicate surgery. Age by itself does not determine the use of palliative or radical irradiation. Patients should be allocated to palliative or radical irradiation on the basis of their performance status.

Daly et al. analyzed a series of 188 women irradiated with large pelvic fields and presenting later on with radiation ileitis (39). Age had no influence on the risk of complications, but obese women or women older than 75 years were treated systematically with 1.8 Gy instead of 2 Gy per fraction, with the same total dose. Similar findings were reported by others (40).

The feasibility of gynecological brachytherapy is sharply dependent on the individual anatomy of each patient. The size and depth of the vaginal cavity changing with age, Senkus-Konefka et al. investigated the influence of age on the size of applicators used and dose distribution, with special attention to doses to critical normal tissues (41). They concluded that, due to a reduction in the size of the vagina, there was a consistent increase in rectum and bladder doses (due to the use of smaller ovoids). This study was unfortunately not complemented with an analysis of morbidity.

Data regarding morbidity of brachytherapy are available from a prospective study of the Institute Gustave Roussy in which patients treated for cervix or endometrial carcinoma were randomized between two different brachytherapy schedules (Scalliet P, unpublished data). When adjusted for tumor size and nodal involvement, age had an unfavorable influence on overall and recurrence-free survival. On the contrary, age had no influence on the rate of overall and late complications (i.e. those developing from 6 months after treatment on).

The EORTC Experience

The entire EORTC database has been searched for identifying those patients who participated in trials including a pelvic or abdomino-pelvic irradiation (42). One thousand six hundred nineteen patients were identified out of 9 trials initiated by the radiotherapy cooperative group or the gastro-intestinal group between 1975 and 1991 (rectum, prostate, bladder, uterus, anal canal cancer). Mean age was 61 years (range 47–80). The originality of this database is that each of these patients has been followed according to strict trial criteria regarding the prospective scoring of side effects and complications.

Acute Side Effects

Nausea and vomiting occurred when the irradiated volume encompassed the upper abdomen and was more frequent in younger patients. The same trend was identified regarding severe diarrhea (grade 2 and 3). In contrast, acute effects on skin, on the urinary tract, deterioration of performance status and body weight loss were evenly distributed among all age groups investigated.

Late Effects and Complications

Eighty percent of the patients in each age group were free of late toxicity by 5 years. There was no difference in the occurrence of late diarrhea, fibrosis or rectal complications between the different age groups. Older patients seemed to have more skin effects than younger individuals but the small number of events prevented a more detailed analysis of this complication. Data about sexual function was available in patients enrolled in prostate cancer trials. Radiotherapy caused more late sexual dysfunction in aged patients than in younger ones, which was expected, as elderly patients were more frequently subject to sexual dysfunction than younger patients. Unfortunately, quality of life assessment was not incorporated in these trials and so definitive conclusions about the effects of radiotherapy on the quality of life of older individuals remain difficult to draw.

Socio-Economic Problems

The modern family is mobile and dispersed in many western countries. While family members remain well and independent this geographical separation is of limited consequence. The impact on families of prolonged illness and disability, on the contrary, can be profound and requires attention from health professionals.

The main problem for the elderly patient with radiotherapy is having to get from home to the hospital daily, 5 times a week. Having only the week-end for resting is often not sufficient because week-ends are often dedicated to visits from or to the family and other social activities, equally and sometimes more tiresome. Hospitalization is probably of no real help because deprivation of the home surroundings may give rise to even worse problems such as disorientation and depression.

Accepting one or more leisure days during radiotherapy invariably prolongs the treatment which may be detrimental to its efficacy. Alternatively, larger daily fractions are sometimes advocated in order to keep the treatment duration within acceptable limits and to offer an additional rest day during the week. Such an attitude entails a higher risk of late effects and should only be considered if a palliative treatment option has already been selected.

There is no other guideline to advocate than to appreciate, on a personal and familial basis, a solution that is adapted to each particular case. The consequences of all possible options need to be openly discussed before any treatment decision is made. It is wise to include a social worker in the radiotherapy department staff to help with all these aspects.

The Oldest Old

Nearly a third of the very elderly (85 years or older) have some degree of dementia (43). They require an active treatment of co-morbid conditions. Home care and revalidation are even more important in this age group since coping with even a minor disability can be a problem. Patient transportation can be a serious problem. It depends on family or partner support, on community support, or on availability of public transportation. As already mentioned in the section on lung cancer, a long distance between the home and the hospital has apparently prevented some very old patients from receiving appropriate radiotherapy. It is not uncommon in our practice that surgeons favor radical mastectomy in small breast tumors in order to spare the patient 5 or 6 weeks of adjuvant radiotherapy. There is of course nothing wrong with this provided the patient has been honestly offered all the possible alternatives. However this is not a universal event: in a population-based study of 2268 patients with breast cancer, no correlation between the use of adjuvant radiotherapy and the distance of the patient's home was found (22).

A central problem, with respect to treatment strategy in the oldest old, is the dilemma of palliative vs. radical treatment. A precise definition of what is a palliative treatment in this context is a challenging intellectual exercise, but it may tentatively be put in the following way: in some circumstances, a palliative treatment schedule (with lesser burden) will give sufficient tumor regression to cover the expected survival time, a more radical treatment being otherwise still theoretically possible. This means that palliation may only be offered to some patients whose life expectancy is obviously short or very short, but for non oncological reasons. Looking back at our own practice, there is less than a handful of such patients each year. They all share the same handicap, i.e. the association of advanced age and a severe degree of dementia, so that the minimum of active collaboration necessary for the treatment to be delivered in good conditions is not guaranteed. There is also a common feeling with such patients that their quality of life is already impaired to such an extent that attempts to prolong life seem meaningless. This attitude, however, is mainly related to philosophical convictions of the doctor, of the medical staff and hopefully of the patient himself, as assessed during conversations with him or with his family if the contact with the patient has been definitively lost. A very delicate matter, indeed.

Conclusions

Most frequently, tumor related factors (stage, histology, etc) will override considerations of age in the choice of treatment, if a curative option exists. As extensively discussed elsewhere in this book, there is no indication in the major oncological pathologies that age is an appropriate factor for stratification. Patients with a good performance status are likely to respond to treatment in general, and to radiotherapy in particular, independently from their chronological age. It can even be suggested that many of the retrospective series in which age had a detrimental effect on prognosis were biased in several possible ways: inappropriate staging, unconventional curative treatment, replacement of a curative treatment by a palliative approach, wait-and-see policy instead of appropriate treatment, etc.

Hodgkin's disease, for example, is considered as having a less positive prognosis in patients aged 60 and over, yet 2 reports showed that patients whose conditions were adequate enough to allow them to receive standard therapy had similar outcomes to that seen in younger patients and that the less favorable outcome in some of the older patients was very likely to result from alterations in the standard treatment schedule (44, 45).

Many patients who are not eligible for a major operation or for major chemotherapy can still tolerate the alternative of radical radiotherapy quite well, and there is no suggestion that age will have a major influence on tolerance. Indeed, a substantial proportion of patients in radiotherapy are over 70 years, and patients over 80 years are regularly seen.

Advanced follow-up during their treatment will help them to get through treatment without major acute side effects. The use of appropriate care as antiemetic, antispasmodic or anticholinergic drugs and more recently with sucralfate, for instance, has demonstrated its ability to reduce bowel discomfort (46).

The fact that older patients more often die from intercurrent disease than from their tumor does not mean that they do not suffer from the cancer-related morbidity before ultimately dying from another cause. Less aggressive strategies based on the higher incidence of intercurrent disease (47) must then be established very carefully, after a thorough appreciation of the potential cancer morbidity which will result from a less intensive therapy. Other strategies, based on the belief that cosmesis is a less prominent concern in older patients (47) are also not supported by data; there is no evidence that the body self-image is less important with advancing age.

"Reduced" treatment is never a solution, unless the life-expectancy of the patient is obviously so short that the tumor recurrence is unlikely to occur or at least to produce substantial morbidity before the patient has died from another cause.

References

1. Gordon M, Singer PA. Decisions and care at the end of life. *Lancet* 1995; **346**: 163–166.
2. Scalliet P. Radiotherapy in the elderly. *Eur J Cancer* 1991; **27**: 3–5.
3. Little JB, Nove J, Strong LC, Nichols WW. Survival of human diploid skin fibroblasts from normal individuals after X-irradiation. *Int J Rad Biol* 1988; **54**: 899–910.
4. Martin GH, Sprague CA, Epstein CJ. Replicative life span of cultivated human cells. Effects of donor's age, tissue and genotype. *Lab Invest* 1970; **23**: 86–92.
5. Sargent EV, Burns FJ. Repair of radiation-induced DNA damage in rat epidermis as a function of age. *Rad Res* 1985; **102**: 176–81.
6. Denekamp J. Residual radiation damage in mouse skin 5 to 8 months after irradiation. *Radiology* 1975; **115**: 191–5.
7. Rockwell S, Hughes CS, Kennedy KA. Effect of host age on micro environmental heterogeneity and efficacy of combined modality therapy in solid tumors. *Int J Rad Oncol Biol Phys* 1991; **20**: 259–63.
8. Denis LJ, Murphy GP, Schroder FH. Report of the consensus workshop on screening and global strategy for prostate cancer. *Cancer* 1995; **75**: 1187–1207.
9. Severson RK, Montie JE, Porter AT, Demers RY. Recent trends in incidence and treatment of prostate cancer among elderly men. *JNCI* 1995; **87**: 532–534.
10. De Jong B, Crommelin M, van der Heijden LH, Coebergh JWW. Patterns of radiotherapy for cancer patients in southeastern Netherlands: 1975–1989. *Radiother Oncol* 1994; **31**: 213–221.
11. Mazur DJ, Merz JF. Older patient's willingness to trade off urologic adverse outcomes for a better chance at five-year survival in the clinical setting of prostate cancer. *J Am Ger Soc* 1995; **43**: 979–984.
12. Helgason AR, Frederikson M, Adolfsson J, Steineck G. Decreased sexual capacity after external radiation therapy for prostate cancer impairs quality of life. *Int J Radiat Oncol Biol Phys* 1995; **32**: 33–39.
13. Hanks GE, Hanlon A, Owen JB, Schultheiss TE. Patterns of radiation treatment of elderly patients with prostate cancer. *Cancer* 1994; **74**: 2174–2177.
14. Hanks GE, Schultheiss TE, Hunt MA, Epstein B. Factors influencing incidence of acute grade 2 morbidity in conformal and standard radiation treatment of prostate cancer. *Int J Radiat Oncol Biol Phys* 1995; **31**: 25–29.
15. Lusinchi A, Bourhis J, Wibault P, *et al.* Radiation therapy for head and neck cancer in the elderly. *Int J Radiat Oncol Biol Phys* 1990; **18**: 819–823.
16. Scalliet P, Van den Weyngaert D, Van der Schueren E. Radiotherapy. In *Cancer in the Elderly. Treatment and Research*, edited by IS Fentiman, S Monfardini. Oxford: Oxford Medical Publications, 28–37, 1994.
17. Chin R, Fisher RJ, Smee RI, Barton MB. Oropharyngeal cancer in the elderly. *Int J Radiat Oncol Biol* 1995; **32**: 1007–1016.
18. Pignon T, Horiot JC, Van den Bogaert W, Van Glabbekke M, Scalliet P. 1996; No age limit for radical radiotherapy in head and neck tumors. *Eur J Cancer.*
19. Dosoretz DE, Galmarini D, Rubenstein JH, Katin MJ, Blitzer PH, Salenius SA, Dosani RA, Rashid M, Mestas G, Hannan SE. Local control in medically inoperable lung cancer: an analysis of its importance in outcome and factors determining the probability of tumor eradication. *Int J Radiother Oncol* 1993; **13**: 83–9.

20. Nordijk EM, Poest Clement Ev.d, Hermans J, Wever AMJ, Leer JWH. Radiotherapy as an alternative to surgery in elderly patients with resectable lung cancer. *Radiat Oncol Biol Phys* 1988; **27**: 507–516.

21. Lindsey AM, Larson PJ, Dodd MJ, Brecht ML, Packer A. Comorbidity, nutritional intake, social support, weight and functional status over time in older cancer patients receiving radiotherapy. *Cancer Nurs* 1995; **17**: 113–124.

22. Bergman L, Dekker G, van Leeuwen FE, Huisman SJ, van Dam FSAM, van Dongen A. The effect of age on treatment choice and survival in elderly breast cancer patients. *Cancer* 1991; **67**: 2227–34.

23. Bergman L, Kluck HM, Van Leeuwen FE, Crommelin MA, Dekker G, Hart AAM, Coebergh JWW. The influence of age on treatment choice and survival of elderly breast cancer patients in south-eastern Netherlands: a population-based study. *Eur J Cancer* 1992; **28A**: 1475–1480.

24. Martin LM, Le Pechoux C, Calitchi E, Otmezguine Y, Feuillhade F, Brun B, Piedbois P, Mazeron JJ, Julien M, Le Bourgeois JP. Management of breast cancer in the elderly. *Eur J Cancer* 1994; **30A**: 590–596.

25. Morrow M. Breast disease in elderly women. *Surg Clin North Am* 1994; **74**: 145–161.

26. De Winter K, Van den Weyngaert D, Becquart D, Scalliet P. Breast cancer: influence of age on treatment choice of surgeon and radiation oncologist. *Eur J Cancer* 1993; **29A** (Suppl 6): S73.

27. Robertson JFR, Todd JH, Ellis IO, Elston CW, Blamey RW. Comparison of mastectomy with tamoxifen for treating elderly patients with operable breast cancer. *B M J* 1988; **297**: 510–14.

28. Bergman L, van Dongen JA, van Ooijen B, van Leeuwen FE. Should tamoxifen be a primary treatment choice for elderly breast cancer patients with locoregional disease? *Breast Cancer Res Treat* 1995; **34**: 77–83.

29. Kantorowitz DA, Poulter CA, Rubin P, Patterson E, Sobel SH, Sischy B, *et al*. Treatment of breast cancer with segmental mastectomy alone or segmental mastectomy plus radiation. *Radiother Oncol* 1989; **15**: 141–50.

30. Veronesi U, Luini A, Del Vecchio M, Greco M, Galimberti V, Merson M, Rilke F, Sacchini V, Sacozzi R, Savio T. Radiotherapy after breast-preserving surgery in women with localized cancer of the breast. *N Engl J Med* 1993; **328**: 1587–1591.

31. Reece GP, Schusterman MA, Miller MJ, Kroll SS, Baldwin BJ, Wang B. Morbidity associated with free-tissue transfer after radiotherapy and chemotherapy in elderly cancer patients. *J Reconstr Microsurg* 1994; **10**: 375–82.

32. Van Limbergen E, Rijnders A, van der Schueren E, Lerut T, Christiaens R. Cosmetic evaluation of breast conserving treatment for mammary cancer. 2. A quantitative analysis of the influence of radiation dose, fractionation schedules and surgical treatment techniques on cosmetic results. *Radiother Oncol* 1989; **16**: 253–68.

33. Steeves RA, Phromratanapongse P, Wolberg WH, Tormey DC. Cosmesis and local control after irradiation in women treated conservatively for breast cancer. *Arch Surg* 1989; **124**: 1369–73.

34. Powell S, Cooke J, Parsons C. Radiation-induced brachial plexus injury: follow-up of two different fractionation schedules. *Radiother Oncol* 1990; **18**: 213–20.

35. Maher M, Campana F, Dreyfus H, Vilcoq JR, Gautier C, Mosseri V, Asselain B, Fourquet A. Breast cancer in elderly women: a retrospective analysis of combined treatment with tamoxifen and once weekly irradiation. *Int J Radiat Oncol Biol Phys* 1995; **31**: 783–789.

36. Toonkel TM, Fix I, Jacobson LH, Bamberg N. Management of elderly patients with primary breast cancer. *Int J Radiat Oncol Biol Phys* 1988; **14**: 677–681.

37. Amsterdam E, Birkenfield S, Gilad A, Krispin M. Surgery for carcinoma of the breast in women over 70 years of age. *J Surg Oncol* 1987; **35**: 180–183.

38. Bouvier-Colle MH, Vallin J, Hatton F. *Mortalite et causes de deces en France*, Ed. Inserm-DOIN, 1991.

39. Daly NJ, Izar F, Bachaud J-M, Delannes M. The incidence of severe chronic ileitis after abdominal and/or pelvic external irradiation with high energy photon beams. *Radiotherapy and Oncology* 1989; **14**: 287–95.

40. DeWinter K, Van den Weyngaert D, Becquart D, Scalliet P. Panabdominal radiotherapy in ovarian carcinoma: a retrospective analysis of survival and complications (abstract). Proceedings of the 9th Annual Meeting ESTRO, Montecattini, 157, 1990.

41. Senkus-Konefka E, Kobierska A, Jassem J, Serkies K, Badzio A. The impact of patient and disease related factors on the quality of pelvic dose distribution in cervical cancer patients. *Radiother Oncol* 1995; **35**: S4.

42. Pignon T.

43. Skoog I, Nilsson L, Palmertz B, Andreasson LA, Svanborg A. A population based study of dementia in 85-years-olds. *N Engl J Med* 1993; **328**: 153–158.

44. Zietman AL, Linggood RM, Brookes AR, Convery K, Piro A. Radiation therapy in the management of early stage Hodgkin's disease presenting in later life. *Cancer* 1991; **68**: 1869–187.

45. Diaz-Pavon JR, Cabanillas F, Majlis A, *et al*. Outcome of Hodgkin's Disease in elderly patients. *Hematol Oncol* 1995; **13**: 19–27.

46. Henriksson R, Frantzen L, Littbrand B. Prevention and therapy of radiation induced bowel discomfort. *Scand J Gastroenterol* 1992; **27** (suppl 191): 7–11.

47. Papillon J. Resent status of radiation therapy in the conservative management of rectal cancer. *Radiother Oncol* 1990; **17**: 275–84.

48. Abbatucci JS, Boulier N, Laforge T, Lozier JC. Radiation therapy of skin carcinomas: results of a hypofractionated irradiation schedule in 675 cases followed for more than 2 years. *Radiother Oncol* 1989; **14**: 113–20.

33. Cancer Chemotherapy in the Older Patient

Dario Cova, Gianni Beretta and Lodovico Balducci

Introduction

This chapter explores the effects of aging on the pharmacology of antineoplastic agents. Aging involves progressive changes in organ and cellular function and in tumor growth (1–3). These changes may alter the pharmacokinetics and the pharmacodynamics of drugs (4–5). Also, a progressive decline in the physiologic reserve of many organ systems may make older individuals more susceptible to the therapeutic complications of cytotoxic medications (4–5).

Aging is highly individualized and chronologic age is a poor predictor of the extent of physiologic changes in each individual. The practitioner managing older patients should be aware of the diversity of the older population and should tailor antineoplastic treatment to these individual variations.

Pharmacokinetics

Figure 33.1 summarizes the most important pharmacokinetic parameters. All of these may undergo age-related variations. We will discuss each parameter separately and we will highlight the implications of age-related variations.

Absorption

Drug absorption may be affected by a number of digestive changes. These include decreased gastro-intestinal motility, decreased splanchnic blood flow, decreased secretion of digestive enzymes, and mucosal

atrophy (6–8). The net result of these changes is a reduction in drug absorption rate (i.e in the amount of drug absorbed in the unit of time), rather than reduced overall absorption of drugs (6). Of special concern is the bioavailability of drugs in the oldest old, i.e. in persons over 80. The diffuse atrophy of the digestive mucosas described in persons of advanced ages may significantly impair the intestinal absorption of drugs (9). Absorption abnormalities unlikely affect cancer treatment, to a large extent because the majority of oncologic treatments are administered parenterally. The following areas deserve some special attention, however:

- Treatment involving administration of oral leucovorin, such as high dose-methotrexate with leucovorin rescue, or treatment regimens exploiting the synergy of fluorouracil and leucovorin. The absorption of oral folates, and seemingly the absorption of oral leucovorin are decreased in older patients (10).
- Management of lymphoid malignancies with oral alkylating agents and steroids. In persons over 70 it may be advisable to spread the total dose of the medications over 4–7 days, to allow more complete absorption of the drugs.
- Management of a number of tumors with daily oral etoposide (11). In these cases it may be advisable to check the serum etoposide levels periodically, especially if a therapeutic response is not observed.
- Management of nausea and vomiting with oral agents (compazine, ondansetron, granisetron, metoclopramide).
- Management of pain with oral narcotics.

Distribution

The volume of distribution (Vd) of drugs is a function of body composition, and of the concentration of circulating plasma proteins (12). With age there is a progressive decline in total body water and a progressive accumulation of total body fat, which results in decreased Vd for water-soluble agents and increased Vd for fat-soluble compounds. Also, a progressive decline in the concentration of plasma proteins may further reduce the Vd of water-soluble drugs, especially of those that are heavily protein-bound, such as the vinca alkaloids, the taxanes, the anthracyclines, and the epipodophyllotoxins. Though the AUC of drugs is

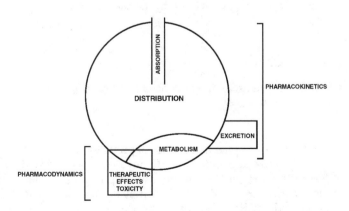

Figure 33.1 Summary of the most important pharmacokinetic parameters.

Table 33.1 Effects of hepatic metabolism on commonly used agents.

Drug	Metabolic Products	Product Activity	Dose Adjustments
A. Antimetabolites			
Methotrexate (MTX)	7-OH MTX	none	no
Fluorouracil (5FU)	CO2, NH3, F-BAL	none	no
Cytosine Arabinoside (ARA-C)	ARA-U	none	no
B. Alkylators			
Cyclophosphamide (CP)	4-OH-CP	yes*	no
Ifosfamide	Aldophosphamide	yes*	
	Phosphoramide Mustard	yes*	
	4-keto CP	no	
	Carboxyphosphamide	no	
ThioTEPA	TEPA	yes	?
BCNU	Nitrogen	no	?
	Hydroxy radical	yes	?
	Chloroethyl radical	yes	
C. Anthracyclines	Deoxyaglicones	no	
	Glucuronides	no	
Doxorubicin	Doxorubicinol	yes	yes**
Daunorubicin & Epirubicin	Daunorubicinol & Epirubicinol	yes	yes**
Idarubicin	Idarubicinol	yes	?
Mitoxantrone	Not characterized	no	yes**
D. Vinca Alkaloids			
Vincristin			
Vinblastine	4-deacetyl-derivatives	yes	yes**
Vindesine	N-Oxide-derivatives	no	
Vinorelbine	Others	no	
E. Taxanes			
Paclitaxel & Docetaxel	OH-derivatives	no	yes**
F. Epipodophyllotoxins			
Etoposide &Teniposide	Glucuronides	no	no
	Hydroxy-derivatives	no	
	Epiaglycones	yes	

ARA-U= Uridine arabinoside
F-BAL= Fluoro-beta-alanine
4-OH-CP=4-OH-cyclophosphamide
4-Keto-CP= 4-ketocyclophosphamide

* Only phosphoramide mustard acts as an alkylator. The majority of phospphoramide mustrd is formed within the tumor cell. The cytotoxic action of 4-OH-P and aldophosphamide consist mainly of transporting within the cells the precursors of phosphoramide (Figure 33.2).

** Current Recommendations are:
1/2 dose for bilirubin $\geq$ 1.5 mg
1/4 dose for bilirubin $\geq$ 3.0 mg

It should be noticed however that this recommandations are not based on extensive data: the need for dose adjustement should be left to the jaudgement of the practitioner in individual clinical situations.

unaffected by changes in Vd, the shape of the AUC may change. While water-soluble drugs may experience higher plasma levels associated with shorter half-lives, lipid-soluble agents may experience lower plasma concentrations and more prolonged half-lives.

The changes in AUC shape may influence both effectiveness and toxicity of drugs. For example, a more rapid decline in plasmatic doses of phase-specific agents (ex. methotrexate, cytarabine), may be associated with lessened therapeutic efficacy; higher plasma peak levels of cardiotoxic anthracyclines may be associated with enhanced cardiac toxicity.

Special attention should be paid to changes in the Vd of the oldest old. After ages 80–85 new changes in body composition may occur, with atrophy of many organs and depletion of total body fat (9).

Metabolism

The liver is the main site of drug metabolism. The effects of hepatic metabolism of antineoplastic drugs are described in Table 33.1. Hepatic metabolism involves two types of metabolic reactions. Type I reactions are dependent on the p450 cytocrome mixed function oxidase system (MFOS) and may lead to active as well as inactive compounds (13). One of the best known of these reactions, that are oxidative/reductive reactions, is the activation of oxaphosphorine alkylators, cyclophosphamide and ifosfamide to the active compounds phosphoramide mustard and 4-hydroxycyclophosphamide/aldophosphamide (14).

Type II reactions are conjugative reactions which may involve glucuronidation and lead to inactive compounds, excretable through the biliary system (13). This construct of drug metabolism is probably too simple. Recently it was found that some of the glucuronides, such as morphine 6-glucuronide are as active or more active than the parent compound (15).

Table 33.1 illustrates very well the complex task to predict drug effectiveness and toxicity based on hepatic function. Oxaphosphorines are both activated and deactivated by P450 microsomal reactions, and it is impossible to predict which process will be more prominent in case of liver dysfunction (14).

5-FU and ARA-C are predominately activated intracellularly and are partly catabolized by the liver: dose adjustments for these drugs are recommended only in the presence of severe liver insufficiency (16–17). In some instances (anthracyclines or vinca alkaloids, for example), both the parent compound and some hepatic metabolites are active, and it may be problematic to establish the respective contributions to the antineoplastic effect of the drug (18–19). The 13-ol derivatives of the anthracyclines provide a good example of this difficulty. Doxorubicinol and epirubicinol are formed in negligible amount, whereas daunorubicinol and especially idarubicinol are responsible for a substantial antineoplastic effect. These ol-derivatives are mostly excreted in the urine. In the case of idarubicin no dose adjustment of the drug is recommended in the presence of hyperbilibinemia, because the majority of the active drug is eliminated through the kidney.

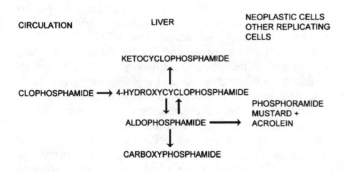

Figure 33.2 Metabolism of cyclophosphamide.

Table 33.2 Excretion of antineoplastic agents dose adjustments (% regular dose).

		Cr Cl (ml/min)		
		≤60	≤45	≤30
A.	Renal excretion			
	Bleomycin	.70	.60	NR
	Carboplatin	Calvert's Formula		
	Carmustine	.80	.75	NR
	Cisp[latin	.75	.50	NR
	2-CDA	Not established		
	Cytarabine (HD)	.60	.50	NR
	Dacarbazine	.80	.75	.70
	Fludarabine	.80	.75	.65
	Hydroxyurea	.85	.80	.75
	Idarubicin	Not established		
	Ifosfamide	.80	.75	.70
	Melphalan	.85	.75	.70
	Methotrexate	.65	.50	NR
B.	Hepatic Excretion			
	Doxorubicin			
	Daunorubicin			
	Epirubicin			
	Vinca alkaloids			
	Taxanes			
C.	Mixed excretion			
	Epipodophyllotoxins			
	Mitomycin C			

Both animal and human studies indicate that phase I reactions may become less active with age. It is not clear, however, the extent to which this reduction is a function of susceptibility to environmental factors, such as tobacco smoking, diet, and other drugs. What it is clear is that frailty is associated with decreased activity of phase I reactions (20). Also, these reactions are influenced by a number of drugs, including cimetidine, which is inhibitory, and phenobarbital, which enhance the activity of the reactions (20). Polypharmacy, a common problem in older individuals, may also affect phase I reactions. Phase II reactions appear unaffected by age.

Excretion

Urinary and biliary excretion are the main routes of drug disposal (Table 33.2). A few drugs, such as fluorouracil and cytosar, are catabolized intracellularly to inactive products (16–17). Some of these metabolic products, including carbon dioxide, are excreted though respiration. For other drugs, such as cisplatin, the final fate of the drug and its products is partly unknown (21).

A progressive decline in glomerular filtration rate (GFR) is one of the most consistent findings of normal aging (22). Controversy lingers over whether this decline is avoidable. Some investigators believe that a reduction in daily protein intake may delay or prevent the age-related reduction in GFR (22). What is clear is that comorbid conditions, including poorly controlled hypertension and diabetes, may accelerate the development of renal insufficiency and so may the chronic intake of certain drugs, such as paracetamol and non-steroidal anti-inflammatory drugs (NSAIDs) (23).

The importance of GFR impairment in the management of older persons with cancer has been highlighted by a seminal study of Gelman and Taylor (24) These authors treated metastatic breast cancer in 167 women with a combination of cyclophosphamide, methotrexate and fluorouracil. The doses of cyclophosphamide and methotrexate were adjusted to the patients' GFR, in women aged 65 and older. The therapeutic response was similar in younger and older women, but the myelotoxicity was less severe in the older women.

Kintzel and Dorr calculated the dose adjustment with declining renal function for drugs, whose parent compounds, active metabolites, or toxic metabolites are excreted through the kidneys (25) (Table 33.2). They based this calculation on the fraction of drug or drug derivative undergoing renal excretion, according to the formula:

Adjusted dose= (normal dose)X f[Kf-1]+1
where Kf = patient's CrC1/120/min
f = fraction of the parent compound, and/or active or toxic metabolite
excreted through the kidneys.

This reference might be very helpful to the busy practitioner. It should be pointed out, however, that many of these adjustments were not tested in the clinical context.

We recommend that ideally in all patients, but especially in those aged 50 and older, the creatinine clearance (CrC1) be calculated and the dosage of renally excreted medications be adjusted accordingly (25). We also recommend that the creatinine clearance be calculated with the formula of Cockcroft and Gault (26):

Males:

$$\frac{CrC1 = 1.23 \times (140\text{-age in years}) \times (\text{weight in Kg})}{\text{plasma creatinine umol}/1}$$

Females:

$$\frac{CrCL = 1.04 \times (140\text{-age in years}) \times (\text{weight in kg})}{\text{plasma creatinine umol}/1}$$

Using the plasma clearance of 99/Tc DPTA as gold standard measurement of GFR, Waller et al. (26) demonstrated that the calculation of CrCl with these formulas had smaller variation coefficients than direct measures of CrCl from 2, 4 and even 24 hours urine collection, or calculations using different formulas. Of interest, the variation coefficients were larger for GFR >50ml/ min. Thus, this formula is especially reliable in patients with reduced GFR. It is not clear how well this formula may apply to patients over 75, however, due to marked variations in body composition.

We recommend that the doses of methotrexate given iv push be adjusted according to the formula proposed by Gelman and Taylor (24), that proved adequate in the management of older individuals:

$$\text{Dose of Methotrexate} = \frac{D \times CrCl}{70}$$

Where D is the dose of methotrexate for persons with normal renal function (24).

When methotrexate is used at high doses by continuous infusion, the infusion rate may be calculated as follows (27):

$$\text{Infusion rate} = \text{plasma}\{MTX\} \times Cl\ (MTX)$$

where Cl (MTX) is the clearance of methotrexate calculated an initial push dose of 50mg/m2:

$$\frac{\text{Dose}}{\text{AUCX T}}$$

The Calvert formula allows the practitioner to calculate the dose of carboplatin for the desired AUC based on age and serum creatinine (28). For other drugs we recommend the dose adjustment proposed by Kintzel and Dorr (Table 33.2) (25).

Several drugs, such as etoposide, have a mixed hepatic and renal excretion (29). In these circumstances, a reduction of GFR up to 25 ml/minute does not seem to prevent adequate drug excretion as long as biliary obstruction is not present.

In general, biliary excretion seems to be unaffected by age. Robert and Hoerni (30) and Egorin et al. (31) have studied the $1/2$ life of doxorubicin and daunorubicin respectively in persons of different ages and were unable to demonstrate the presence of age-related changes.

Another poorly explored issue concerns the excretion of active metabolic products of active agents. For example, doxorubicin is partly transformed into an active alcohol, doxorubicinol, which is renally excreted, unlike the parent compound (19).

Of special interest is a study by Burkowski et al., who studied the pharmacokinetics of nine drugs in patients younger than 65 and aged 65 and over (32). The drugs were dichloromethotrexate, hexamethylen bisacethamide, n-methylformamide, trimetrexate, taxol, piroxantron, topotecan, bequinar and menogaril. Eighty one patients were over 65, 35 over 70 and 5 over 75; the oldest patient was 77. Fifty one percent of patients >65 and 53% of those <65 received a dose of chemotherapy equal to or higher than the maximal tolerated dose (MTD); 25.9% of the older patients and 31.7% of the younger experienced dose limiting toxicity equal to or higher than grade 3. Of special interest was the experience with dichloromethotrexate: while the renal clearance of the drug decreased with age, in accord to a decline of the creatinine clearance, the total clearance of the drug did not decrease, suggesting compensatory increased hepatic clearance. This study is very important for several reasons: first, it was the first study to include older individuals in phase I trials, second, it demonstrated that the pharmacokinetics of many drugs does not change with the age of the patient, third, it suggested the possibility of compensatory changes in drug clearance for agents at mixed excretion. The main limitation of the study was scarce representation of patients aged 75 and older. In the same line, Yamamoto et al. (33), studied the pharmacokinetics of cisplatin in lung cancer patients of different ages and found that the concentration was increased for a more prolonged period of time in older individuals, indicating a decreased rate of drug elimination.

The pharmacokinetics of the most common antineoplastic agents are summarized in Table 33.3.

Pharmacodynamics

Age-related changes in pharmacodynamics are highly speculative. This is an open and important area of research aimed at explaining age-related differences in the responsiveness of certain tumors to chemotherapy. These tumors include acute myelogenous leukemia, epithelial carcinoma of the ovaries, and possibly non-Hodgkin's lymphomas (5). We will explore three reasonable hypotheses to account for these differences:

- Age is associated with a higher prevalence of neoplastic cells with Multi Drug Resistance (MDR).
- Age is associated with abnormalities in tumor enzymes which are the target of specific agents.
- Age is associated with changes in tumor kinetics, which prevent the cytotoxic effect of cycle-active drugs.

Other important potential mechanism of drug resistance include alterations in the mechanism of intracellular transport and intracellular activation and deactivation of drugs.

Age and Multi Drug Resistance (MDR)

MDR may result from several mechanisms (34), but the best understood form of drug resistance is the expression of the MDR-1 gene. This gene encodes the P-glycoprotein 170, a membrane protein that extrudes from the cell natural antineoplastic agents, including antibiotics, vinca alkaloids, epipodophyllotoxins, taxanes. The function of this pump is related to slow Ca^{++} channels and may be reversed by Ca^{++} channel blockers and by cyclosporine (CSA) and its derivatives.

MDR-1 is expressed also in normal tissues, such as the hemopoietic stem cells and the endothelial cells lining the blood vessels of the central nervous system

and of the testicles (34–35). The relative resistance of these tissues to cancer chemotherapy may be explained in part by MDR.

The hypothesis that the prevalence of MDR-expressing leukemic blasts increases with the age of the patient was recently proved by Willman et al. (Cheryl Willman, personal communication, American Society of Hematology, Seattle, Washington, December 2,1995). These authors found the MDR1 phenotype in the blasts of 77% of patients over 55 with acute myelogenous leukemia, and in 17% of those aged 45 or less.

Several years ago Applebaum et al. also reported that the blasts of refractory anemia with excess blasts (RAEB) and refractory anemia with excess blast in transformation (RAEBT) expressed the P-glycoprotein in approximately 60% of patients (36). This is a very pertinent observation as many forms of acute myeloid leukemias in older individuals are preceded by myelodysplasia (37).

Circumstantial evidence suggests that MDR-1 may play a role in the shorter remission-duration of patients aged 60 and older with large cell lymphomas, treated with doxorubicin-containing combination chemotherapy (38) and with ovarian cancer (39).

The mechanism by which tumors of older individuals may develop MDR is not clear. The acquisition of MDR is a spontaneous mutation whose incidence is a function of the number of mitosis undergone by the tumor cell (34–35). Older organisms may not support tumor growth as well as younger organisms (40), thus the incidence of tumor cell death may be higher in older individuals and a higher number of mitosis may be required for a sizable tumor.

A second form of MDR is related to abnormalities of the enzyme topoisomerase II, which is the target of a number of agents, including the anthracyclines and the epipodophyllotoxins. Synthesis of aberrant proteins is one of the molecular abnormalities of aging (41). Thus, it is not unreasonable to hypothesize that the synthesis of topoisomerase II be abnormal in the tumors of older individuals.

A third form of MDR involves increased concentration of glutathione reductase that allows a more complete scavenging of free radicals generated by drugs and irradiation and consequent prevention of cellular damage from these compounds (42). There is no evidence that the concentration of glutathione reductase increases with age in neoplastic or in normal cells. There is evidence of higher degree of hypoxia, however, in tumors occurring in older animals, and hypoxia may prevent the formation of free radicals (43).

A fourth form of MDR concerns alterations in the mechanism of cellular death. Clearly, many drugs, including the epipodophyllotoxins and the purine analogs cause cell death by apoptosis that occurs in cells where the P53 gene is normally expressed and the Bcl-2 gene is not functional (44). When this equilibrium is altered, as it is the case of many tumors, the drugs may lose their effectiveness. The Bcl-2 is expressed in marginal zone lymphomas (maltomas), whose incidence increases in older individuals (45). The Bcl-2 product

Table 33.3 Pharmacokinetic parameters of major antineoplastic agents.

Name	Activity Parent Compound	Active Metabolitet	Elimination Active Compounds	Dose Adjustment
A. Antimetabolites				
Methotrexate (MTX)	yes	–	Renal	yes
Fluorouracil (5FU)	–	yes	cellular & hepatic metabolism	no
Cytosine Arabinoside (Cytosar)	–	yes	cellular & hepatic metabolism	no*
Fludarabine	–	yes	Renal	yes
2-chlordeoxyadenosine (Cladribine)	–	yes	Renal	?
B. Alkylating agents				
Bischloroethylamines				
Oxazaphosphorines (Cyclophos phamide & Ifosfamide)	–	yes	Hepatic metabolism; Renal	yes**
Chlorambucil	yes	–	Hepatic metabolism; Renal	?
Melphalan	yes	–	Hepatic metabolism;Renal	yes***
Aziridines				
Thiotepa	yes	yes	Hepatic Metabolism; Renal	?
Nitrosureas	yes	yes	Hepatic Metabolism	?
C. Platinum Analogues				
Cisplatin	yes	no	Inactivated intracellularly and in the circulation. Renal (minor)	no****
Carboplatin	yes	no	Renal	yes
D. Antibiotics				
Anthracycline,				
Daunorubicin & Doxorubicin	yes	yes	Biliary*****	yes
Idarubicin	yes	yes	Renal	?
Anthracendiones				
Mitoxantrone	yes	no	Biliary*****	yes
Mitomycins	yes******	no	Hepatic Metabolism; Renal	no
E. Plant derivatives				
Epipodophyllotoxins				
Etoposide	yes	no	mixed hepatic and renal for reduced CrCl	yes
Teniposide	yes	no	mixed hepatic and renal	no
Vinca Alkaloids				
Vincristine				
Vinblastine	yes	no	biliary	yes
Vinorelbine				
Taxanes				
Paclitaxel	yes	no	hepatic metabolism	?
Docetaxel	yes	no	hepatic metabolism	?
F. Hydroxyurea	yes	no	renal	?

*high doses contraindicated for Crcl<50ml/min; may also be contraindicated in patients over 60.

**especially for ifosfamide.

*** 1/2 dose for BUN>30mg/ml

**** dose adjustment should be made to prevent further renal damage

***** >50% of these drugs is tissue-bound and is not accounted for in urines or stools.

****** Spontaneously activated in hypoxic conditions and in acidic environment.

Table 33.4 Enzymes inhibited by specific chemotherapy agents.

Drug	Enzyme(s)
Methotrexate	Dihydrofolate reductase (DHFR)
Fluorouracil	Thymidylate Synthase (TS)
Cytosine Arabinoside	DNA polymerase alpha
Fludarabine	DNA polymerase alpha
	Ribonucleotide reductase
	DNA primase
	DNA Ligase 1
2-chlorodeoxyadenosine	Ribonucleotide reductase
Hydroxyurea	Ribonucleotide reductase
Anthracyclines	Topoisomerase II.

Table 33.5 Common chemotherapy related toxicity.

UNIVERSAL
Myelodepression
Mucositis
Nausea and emesis

DRUG SPECIFIC
Cardiotoxicity
Pulmonary toxicity
Central and peripheral neurotoxicity
Nephrotoxicity
Epipodophyllotoxins

was also found more frequently in the non-small cell lung cancer of older individuals (46). Thus some circumstantial evidence suggests that the prevalence of this type of MDR may increase with the age of the patient.

A fifth and only theoretical form of MDR includes enhanced repair of DNA damage caused by cytotoxic agents. In general the ability of repairing DNA appears decreased in aging tissues and this form of MDR is unlikely of interest to the older patients.

Age and Synthesis of Enzymes Target of Antimetabolites

The mechanism of action of antimetabolites involves inhibition of one or more enzymes necessary for DNA synthesis (Table 33.4). As in the case of topoisomerase II, the synthesis of these enzymes may be abnormal in tumors occurring in older individuals (41). The abnormal enzyme may escape the block effected by the drugs.

In certain circumstances drug resistance is a consequence of an amplification of the gene encoding the target enzyme (47). This mechanism of drug resistance was demonstrated "in vivo" for methotrexate. Amplification of the gene encoding the target enzyme dihydrofolate reductase followed prolonged exposure to the drug, and the excess enzyme overcame the metabolic block (47).

Age and Tumor Kinetics

The biology of some tumors may be altered in the older tumor host. These biologic alterations may include slower tumor growth from reduction of the tumor growth fraction. This possibility was demonstrated in experimental animals (3). In humans, Valentinis et al. demonstrated that the labeling index of breast cancer was significantly lower in women under 70 than in older women (48). Daidone et al. also found decreased proliferation rate of lung cancer in older individuals

(49). A reduced growth fraction may be associated with drug resistance, as the majority of antineoplastic agents are active against replicating cells.

Pharmacodynamic changes may also influence the development of drug toxicity: Rudd and all have recently reported that DNA adducts from cisplatin are completely clear in 48 hours from circulating monocytes of individuals aged 20–25 but may persist indefinitely in the monocytes of individual over 70 (50). These effects suggest inadequate ability of DNA repair in the normal tissue of older individuals which may lead to cumulative and irreversible toxicity.

Organ Specific Toxicity

In Table 33.5 the most common complications of antineoplastic treatment are listed. Some of these complications, such as myelotoxicity, nausea and vomiting, and mucositis, are almost universal; the other complications are drug-specific.

Myelotoxicity

Myelotoxicity is the most common complication of cancer chemotherapy (51). A brief review of hemopoiesis is necessary to understand the mechanisms of myelotoxicity and the treatment strategies that may minimize this complication (52).

A common view of hemopoiesis (Figure 33.3), holds that from a pluripotent hemopoietic stem cell (PHSC) hemopoietic progenitors committed to the erythroid, myeloid, megakaryocytic and lymphoid series are derived (52). From these progenitors the recognizable

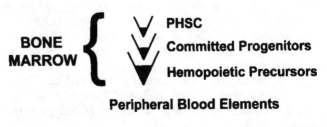

Figure 33.3 Hemopoiesis. The dark area represents the proliferative rate; the clear area, the ability for self-replication.

Table 33.6 Hemopoietic growth factors.

Granulocyte-colony stimulating factor (G-CSF)
Stimulate proliferation and maturation of granulocyte progenitors.
Synergistic withother factors in causing cycling of PHSC

Granulocyte-macrophage-colony stimualting factor (GM-CSF)
Supports proliferation of PHSC (After exiting G0)
Stimulates proliferation and maturation of granulocyte-macrophage progenitors.
Stimulates thrombopoiesis

Erythropoietin (Epo)
Stimulates proliferation and maturation of early (BFU-E) and late (CFU-E) erythropoietic progenitors. CFU-e are more
sensitive than BFU-E.

Macrophage-Colony Stimulating Factor (M-CSF)
Proliferation and differentiation of macrophage progentors
Leukemia Inhibitory Factor (LIF)

Steel Factor (SF).
Survival factor for PHSC in G0
Stimulates thrombopoiesis

Thrombopoietin (Tpo)
Stimulates thrombopoiesis

Interleukins (IL)
IL3: stimulates PHSC and early progenitors to enter cell cycle
    stimulate proliferation of PHSC and early progentors.
    survival factor for PHSC

IL5: stimulates proliferation and maturation of macrophage-monocyte progenitors
    stimulate proliferation and differentiation of eosinophi progenitor.

IL4, IL6, IL11, IL12 act synergistically with other hemopoietic factors in different hemopoietic steps.

precursors of circulating blood elements originate. The PHSC is unique in two aspects: extensive self-renewal potential and ability to become committed to different hemopoietic lines. The committed progenitors instead have limited potential of self-renewal and can differentiate only into a single hemopoietic line. The PHSC and committed progenitors can be recognized from clonal growth "in vitro" and from specific cell markers, such as the CD34 (53). The processes of proliferation, commitment, and differentiation require an intact hemopoietic stroma (54–55) and are modulated by a host of hemopoietic growth factors (Table 33.6) (54). The functions of the hemopoietic stroma include the homing of the PHSC and the production of some of the growth factors.

Any alteration in the number or function of PHSC, in the structure and the function of the stroma and in the production of growth factors may compromise hemopoiesis.

The PHSCs are largely sheltered from cytotoxic injury. Low-proliferation rate limits the proportion of

cells vulnerable to cycle-active drugs. In addition, the PHSC expresses the MDR-1 gene which encodes the P-glycoprotein, a powerful membrane pump which extrudes natural cytotoxic agents from the cell (35). Low proliferation shelters to some extent also the committed progenitors from antineoplastic agents, while highly proliferating, differentiated precursors are particularly vulnerable to these drugs. Chemotherapy-induced losses of late marrow precursors are repaired by increase differentiation of committed progenitors and enhanced commitment of PHSC.

With age, the full and timely replacement of destroyed hemopoietic elements may be hindered by three causes: exhaustion of the PHSC reserve, dysfunctional marrow stroma and decreased production of endogenous growth factors.

There is circumstantial evidence both in experimental systems and in humans, that the PHSC may become restricted with age. In a series of elegant experiments, Lipschitz et al. (56) exposed older and younger mice to crowding, which represents a hemopoietic stress in this system. Older mice experienced a rapid decline in the concentration of PHSCs not seen in younger mice. In aging humans, the incidence of aplastic anemia increases (57), the percentage of functional marrow tissue is progressively reduced (57), and the ability to cope with some forms of hemopoietic stress, such as infection and bleeding is progressively impaired. A recent study by Chatta et al. also suggests age-related depletion of PHSC reserve. These authors studied the response to G-CSF and GM-CSF in volunteers aged 20 to 30 and 70 to 80 (58). They found that comparable degrees of neutrophilia followed G-CSF administration in younger and older individuals. The concentration of PHSC in the peripheral blood following GM-CSF, however, was twofold higher in younger subjects.

The information concerning the aging hemopoietic stroma is limited (58), but indicates a progressive loss in the ability to provide homing for PHSC, which may lead to a depletion of PHSC reserve.

The endogenous production of hemopoietic growth factors may not be affected by age, but Lipschitz et al. reported a delayed and blunted response of PHSCs and early progenitors to these growth factors which suggests either a dysfunction or a reduced concentration of these elements (59).

In general, older individuals have been able to tolerate moderately toxic chemotherapy regimens without excessive complications, when the dosage of renally-excreted drugs has been properly adjusted (26). After aggressive chemotherapy, as employed in the treatment of acute leukemias and certain lymphomas, however, myelodepression has been more prolonged and more severe in older patients (37,45,60,61). Several causes might have been responsible for enhanced myelotoxicity in these conditions. These include depletion of PHSCs as a result of myelophthisis, preexisting hemopoietic insufficiency from chronic diseases and malnutrition, and interaction of chemotherapy with other myelodepressive drugs, such as sulfamethoxazole-trimetophrim or phenytoin.

In any case it is prudent to consider individuals over 65 and especially those over 80 at increased risk for chemotherapy induced myelotoxicity and its complications.

Several interventions, illustrated in more details in another chapter of this book (62), may ameliorate chemotherapy myelotoxicity in the older person. These include identification of patients at increased risk for myelotoxicity, institution of treatment regimens targeted to patients with compromised hemopoiesis, and the use of hemopoietic growth factors (62–63). Although there are no standardized tests to assess the hemopoietic reserve of individual patients, the assessment of the granulocyte reserve after hydrocortisone or after G-CSF may be helpful in individual situations, with persistent neutropenia. Effective treatment regimens with reduced myelotoxicity include combinations of low-doses of cyclophosphamide, doxorubicin, etoposide, vincristine and prednisone for the management of intermediate and high grade non-Hodgkin's lymphomas in patients aged sixty and older (61) and oral

etoposide in the management of small cell cancer of the lung (11).

Mucositis

Mucositis, caused by the destruction of rapidly proliferating gastrointestinal cells, may be particularly severe with methotrexate, fluorouracil, bleomycin, and cytarabine and the combination of fluorouracil and leucovorin. The manifestations of mucositis include inflammation of the upper digestive mucosas, with dysphagia, odynophagia and reduced oral intake of fluids, food and medications, and severe diarrhea.

Clinical evidence that older persons are at risk for severe mucositis is compelling. Gelman and Taylor could not prevent mucositis by adjusting the dose of methotrexate to the GFR in older patients and suggested that the repair of mucosal damage become compromised with aging (24). The Gastrointestinal Tumor Study Group reported ten deaths from diarrhea in patients over 65 treated with fluorouracil and leucovorin and concluded that both mucositis and dehydration are particularly severe in older persons (64). Bennett et al. also reported that only 40% of patients over 70 with colonic cancer were able to complete a full year of adjuvant treatment with fluorouracil and levamisole, and mucositis was the major dose-limiting toxicity (65). In the presence of diarrhea or impaired fluid intake, the older patient should be hospitalized and given aggressive fluid resuscitation. Prophylactic sucralfate slurs may ameliorate symptoms of mucositis and allow better fluid intake.

Nausea and Vomiting

Several forms of chemotherapy-related nausea and vomiting have been described (66). Of these, the most common form follows administration of drugs almost immediately and is due to stimulation of the chemoreceptors trigger zone of the medulla. Anticipatory nausea and vomiting is a learned reaction triggered by thoughts or sensory stimulations related to chemotherapy. Both types of nausea and vomiting seem to be less severe in older persons.

A third form of nausea and vomiting, whose pathogenesis is less well understood, is delayed nausea and vomiting (67). This includes any form of nausea and vomiting persisting 48 hours or longer after chemotherapy. Delayed nausea and vomiting are more common and more severe in the elderly and may respond to management with dexamethasone and metoclopramide. Transdermal scopolamine may also ameliorate delayed nausea and vomiting. The serotonin antagonists ondansetron and granisetron, which have been very effective in the prevention of immediate nausea and vomiting don't have any role in the management of the delayed nausea and vomiting (68).

Cardiotoxicity

Cardiotoxicity is a complication of anthracyclines, mitoxantrone, high dose cyclophosphamide, mitomycin C, and of high doses of cyclophosphamide (19). Anthracycline cardiotoxicity, the pathology of which has been best described, may be caused by an excess of free radicals in the sarcoplasm (19). Age is a risk factor for cadiotoxicity, as the myocardial reserve may be reduced in older patients. In addition, old myocardial sarcomeres may have lost the ability to scavenge free radicals. It is likely but not conclusively established that coronary artery disease, hypertension, and valvular heart disease predispose the patient to cardiac complications of chemotherapy.

Several precautionary measures may prevent heart failure in patients at risk (69). These include reduction of the total dose of anthracyclines, administration of anthracyclines by continuous infusion (70), the concomitant administration of digoxin and anthracyclines, the concomitant administration of anthracyclines and bib-piperazondione, a substance that prevents the formation of free radicals (71) or amifostine, a cytoprotective agent (72),and the use of liposomal doxorubicin (73). Of these measures, infusional doxorubicin and the concomitant administration of doxorubicin and bis-piperazondione have been best studied. It is important to underline the limitation of these studies. First, they were confined to doxorubicin, and it is not clear whether the conclusions can be extended to other anthracyclines. Second, only two diseases have been extensively studied: breast cancer and sarcomas. Third, the percentage of older individuals included in these studies was small (mean ages 55 and 57; oldest ages 75 and 77) and inadequate to draw firm conclusions about the effectiveness of these approaches in the elderly. Fourth, the main advantage of these approaches became evident for patients who received a total dose of doxorubicin >600/m2, which is seldom reached in older individuals. Fifth, the subjects of these studies were almost exclusively women. Sixth, continuous infusion of doxorubicin was associated with increased risk of mucositis, and the use of bis-piperazonedione was associated with increased risk of myelotoxicity: these complications are of particular concern in older individuals. Finally, these strategies may substantially increase the cost of treatment. A cost/effectiveness study comparing alternative strategies, such as use of mitoxantrone instead of doxorubicin, appears desirable. Serial monitoring of the cardiac ejection fraction by radionuclide angiography has been recommended in any patient receiving anthracyclines and particularly in older patients. The benefits of serial MUGA scans have recently been questioned. The main limitations of this approach are: MUGA scan do not detect diastolic dysfunctions, that may be present in as many as 30% of individuals over 65; the MUGA scans are unreliable in patients with atrial fibrillation; performance of MUGA scans is costly and time-consuming; originally, MUGA scans were used to screen patients who needed myocardial biopsy, not to dictate discontinuance of doxorubicin. Separated from myocardial biopsy, radionuclide angiography may direct discontinuance of the drug in patients who may still benefit from it (69). Also, permanent myocardial damage is very rare (<1%) prior to a total dose of doxorubicin of 300 mg/m2 (69). Our current approach, in older patients without symptoms of

congestive heart failure, is to obtain a baseline MUGA scan after a doxorubicin dose of 300mg/m2 and to repeat the test thereafter for each additional dose of 100mg/m2.

Due to a lower incidence of cardiac complications, mitoxantrone may be preferable to anthracyclines in older patients whenever the substitution is appropriate (19,74). Mitoxantrone is as effective as anthracyclines in breast cancer and acute myelocytic leukemia and may even be more effective in the blastic phase of chronic granulocytic leukemia (74).

Pulmonary Toxicity

Pulmonary toxicity is a common complication of chemotherapy, particularly when bleomycin, mitomycin C, busulfan, or nitrosureas are part of the treatment. Although decrements in vital capacity and in forced expiratory volume suggest the increased vulnerability of older patients to pulmonary injury, an excess of pulmonary toxicity with aging has not been reported (75).

Nephrotoxicity

Many chemotherapeutic agents and, in particular, cisplatin, mitomycin C, nitrosureas, ifosfamide, and fludarabine are toxic to the proximal renal tubule. Although one may expect enhanced nephrotoxicity in older patients, clinical studies with cisplatin have so far failed to demonstrate this correlation (25,76). Seemingly, the age-related reduction in the maximal reabsorptive capacity of the tubule may limit tubular exposure to nephrotoxic drugs. The cytoprotective amifostine may protect the cancer patient from cisplatin nephrotoxicity (72)

Cisplatin is contraindicated in patients of any age with renal dysfunction (creatinine clearance lower than 50mL/min). Carboplatin, a congener of cisplatin with similar antineoplastic activity but no relevant nephrotoxicity, may be substituted for cisplatin in many of these cases (77). An important caveat concerns proper adjustment of the dose of carboplatin to the creatinine clearance, as myelotoxicity may be overwhelming in renal insufficiency (28).

Peripheral Neurotoxicity

Peripheral neuropathy is a common complication of vinca alkaloids (vincristine and vinblastine), epipodophyllotoxins (etoposide and teniposide), synthetic alkaloids, such as vindesine and vinorelbine, taxanes (paclitaxel and docetaxel), and cisplatin (78).

Manifestations of neurotoxicity, which is dose limiting for vincristine, appear in a stepwise fashion and include paresthesias, abolishment of deep tendon reflexes, and weakness. Autonomic neuropathy manifested as postural hypotension, ileus, or bradycardia may also occur.

The main indication for discontinuing these drugs is progressive weakness, which is easily detectable by serial measurements of the strength of the upper extremities. Vincristine neurotoxicity is reversible, but reversal may take several months. Prevention of vincristine neurotoxicity with 1.5 g of oral glutamic acid daily is advisable for older patients who are at increased risk for this complication (79). A common manifestations of paclitaxel neurotoxicity, which is devastating for older individuals, is compromise of fine movements, such as ability to button one's shirt. Dose reductions and increased interval between consecutive administration may ameliorate this disturbing symptom.

An idiosyncratic form of neurotoxicity produced by cisplatin does not appear to be dose related and may be irreversible. Patients receiving cisplatin should undergo serial assessments of muscular strength and of touch and temperature sensitivity. Any abnormality of these parameters appearing at total doses of cisplatin lower than 300 mg/m2 mandates discontinuance of the drug (80).

A special form of neurotoxicity is dysfunction of the acoustic nerve from cisplatin. Hearing loss is caused by destruction of the outer hair cells of the organ of Corti (81). Cisplatin-related hearing impairment is seldom of clinical consequence, as it affects mainly frequencies outside the spoken language hearing range. In patients with preexisting hearing dysfunction, serial audiographic exams during cisplatin treatment and avoidance of other ototoxic drugs — furosamide, etacrinic acid, and aminoglycosides — are advisable.

Central Neurotoxicity

The central nervous system (CNS) may be affected at different levels by antineoplastic agents. Older patients may be especially vulnerable to CNS toxicity due to the age-related loss of neurons (1). Cerebellar toxicity from high-dose cytarabine is more frequent in older persons (82), but this effect may be secondary to GFR reduction (83). Neurotoxicity from 5 FU, nitrosoureas, dacarbazine, and fludarabine may also be increased. The neurotoxicity of fludarabine is of special concern as this drug is becoming the frontline treatment of chronic lymphocytic leukemia, a disease whose incidence increases with age. There are no guidelines about the prevention of this complications. Seemingly, subtle changes in cognition may herald the development of more serious dysfunctions and suggest discontinuance of the drug. Given the special vulnerability of the CNS of older patients, intracarotideal chemotherapy or concomitant administration of CNS radiotherapy and systemic chemotherapy may be ill advised.

Hormonal Agents

The hormonal agents of common use in cancer treatment include estrogens, estrogen antagonists, LH-RH analogs, progesterone derivatives, aromatase inhibitors, antiandrogens and estramustine.

The therapeutic use of estrogen has been largely discontinued both in breast cancer and in prostate cancer. These hormones were associated with congestive heart failure and deep vein thrombosis in approximately 20% to 30% of patients, and older patients were at increased risk for these complications (84–85).

Tamoxifen is an antiestrogen used almost exclusively in breast cancer. The experience with this drug is very large and involves several patients over age 80. In general, it has been remarkably safe even with prolonged administration. Its complications include thromboembolism, endometrial cancer and retinopathy (86). Of these, only thromboembolism requires treatment discontinuance. Tamoxifen-related endometrial cancer is diagnosable at an early stage with serial transvaginal ultrasounds (86). The concern that tamoxifen might enhance the rate of bone loss or the incidence of coronary events has not be substantiated (86). A new antiestrogen, toremifene, is undergoing clinical trials and may have been less side effects than tamoxifen (87). An important potential benefit of both tamoxifen and toremifene is reversal of MDR-1.

LH-RH analogues are standard treatment for metastatic prostate cancer (85) and are undergoing trials in breast and ovarian cancer. These compounds seem extremely well tolerated by persons of any age, the main complication of treatment being the development of hot flashes. The depot forms of LH-RH analogues are particularly convenient for older and confused patients for whom compliance may be a problem.

Progesterone derivatives are used in the treatment of postmenopausal breast cancer and for palliation of cancer-related cachexia (86). These compounds have been well tolerated by patients of any age, the main side effects have been increased appetite, weight gain, and fluid retention. The incidence of deep vein thrombosis may also be increased.

Aminoglutethimide, an inhibitor of adrenal desmolase and of peripheral aromatase, is very effective as front-line and salvage treatment in postmenopausal breast cancer (88). This agent may have disturbing, albeit transient, complications that include a high incidence of allergic reactions and confusion. Thus, aminoglutethimide may not be the front-line treatment of choice for older breast cancer patients. New aromatase inhibitors, including letrozole and 4-hydroxyandrostendione, may be better tolerated and more effective than aminoglutethimide. Clinical trials with these drugs are ongoing (88).

Antiandrogens include several compounds of different structures that inhibit the interaction of dihydrotestrone with cytoplasmic or nuclear receptors. Chemically, one can distinguish two main groups of antiandrogens: the steroidal antiandrogens, the prototype of which is cyproterone, and the nonsteroidal antiandrogens whose prototypes are flutamide and nilutamide (89). Cyproterone may cause deep vein thrombosis, congestive heart failure, and impotence in men. Flutamide is associated with fewer complications, of which gynecomastia is the most common (89). Although well tolerated by patients of any age, recent reports of hepatic toxicity cast some doubts on the safety of flutamide.

Estramustine, a combination of nornitrogen mustard and estradiol, is an effective front-line treatment for metastatic prostate cancer (89). This compound is associated with the complications of both chemotherapy and estrogen therapy, but has the advantage of preserving sexual functions in the majority of patients. These characteristics make estramustine the treatment of choice for sexually active patients in good general condition while contraindicating the drug in frail and debilitated patients.

Biologic Response Modifiers (BRM)

The treatment with BRM is targeted to amplify an organism's own immune defenses. This form of treatment is particularly attractive in the older aged person, in whom a progressive decline in cellular immunity and especially in the function of helper T cells may be observed (90). Biologic modulation of neoplasia has been facilitated by recombinant DNA technology, which has made effectors of immune response available in unlimited amount for clinical use. Of these, interferons (IFN) and interleukin-2 (IL-2) have been tested in several clinical trials (91–92).

Interferons (IFN)

Of the three major classes of IFNs — alpha, beta and gamma — only alpha is commercially available. The recombinant form of this compound is referred to as rIFN.

At low does (3–7 million units daily subcutaneously), IFN alpha has been very effective in some hematologic malignancies, such as hairy cell leukemia (HCL) (91), chronic granulocytic leukemia (CGL) (93–95), myeloproliferative disorders with thrombocytosis (91), and cutaneous T-cell lymphoma (91), and neuroendocrine tumors (96). In CGL, IFN alpha has shown the unique ability to eliminate the Philadelphia chromosome-bearing hemopoietic clone in some patients. Unfortunately, the majority of these patients still harbor the bcr/abl abnormality in their bone marrow, when tested with PCR. Thus, rIFN may not provide a cure of CGL. What was clearly demonstrated was the superiority of rIFN over hydroxyurea and busulfan in terms of symptom control and survival (93–95). At low doses, IFN may cause fever and malaise during the initial course of treatment, along with neutropenia, thrombocytopenia, and renal and hepatic dysfunctions, and sometimes cardiac dysfunction. These complications have not so far been more common nor more severe in older patients.

At higher doses (9–50 million units daily or thrice weekly), IFN alpha is active in a number of other malignancies, such as multiple myeloma, AIDS-related Kaposi sarcoma, malignant melanoma, renal cell carcinoma, colorectal cancer, and carcinoid tumors (91). With higher doses of IFN the risk of complications increases, and new side effects, such as peripheral and central neurotoxicity may appear. The experience with high-dose IFN in older patients has been limited. It is reasonable to assume that many of these patients may be more susceptible to treatment complications from limited functional reserve.

Interleukin-2 (IL-2)

Alone, or in combination with lymphokine-activated killer (LAK) cells, IL-2 has demonstrated activity in renal cell carcinoma and malignant melanoma (92). Although some older patients have been treated with these compounds, the numbers are not adequate to establish whether tolerance to IL-2 is a function of age.

The substantial toxicity of IL-2, which includes adult respiratory distress syndrome (ARDS) from generalized capillary leak, contraindicates this compound in debilitated patients. Of special interest, IL2 at low doses was found effective in eradicating "minimal residual leukemia." Those doses appeared well tolerated in older individuals and should be considered for the maintenance treatment of acute myelogenous leukemia in older persons and possibly for the management of myelodysplasias with excess blasts.

Age-Related Factors that May Influence Cancer Management

In the beginning of the chapter, we stated that age is associated with multidimensional changes, all of which may adversely influence cancer treatment. The focus of this review has been on physical changes. However, this discussion would not be illustrative of the complexity of aging without exploring the effects of mental, emotional, and socioeconomic conditions on antineoplastic therapy. Inadequate treatment compliance may have different causes, such as limited access to clinic and hospital care, confusing medication schedules, and lessened motivation to withstand the ordeal of aggressive treatment. Comprehensive data on the effects of age on cancer treatment are difficult to retrieve. The main sources of information — clinical trials and tumor registries — have limitations, as described in Chapter 3. Clinical trials tend to include only a small minority of older patients, who are not representative of the general population, whereas tumor registries fail to provide comprehensive patient evaluation from multiple observers due to the retrospective data collection.

We have attempted a new approach to the study of aging and cancer treatment. We have analyzed treatment-related decisions in 209 consecutive cancer patients seen at the Bay Pines Veterans Hospital over 1 year by the same consultant (Balducci, L., personal communication, 27th meeting of the American Geriatric Society, Chicago, IL, 1991). In our analysis we explored the influence of comprehensive geriatric evaluations on therapeutic decisions in patients of different ages. We found an increased incidence of cognitive and emotional disturbances, family dysfunction, poor performance status, co-morbidity and polypharmacy in patients over 65. Of these factors, poor performance status and dementia were common causes for withholding treatment in older patients. Interestingly, strong family support, represented by a caring spouse or a highly committed child, buffered the negative impact of dementias on treatment-related decisions. We are expanding our analysis to a larger number of patients. Our method appears promising for identifying age-specific problems of older patients with cancer.

References

1. Duthie E. Physiology of Aging, Relevance to Symptoms, Perceptions and Treatment Tolerance. In *Comprehensive Geriatric Oncology*, edited by L Balducci, GH Lyman, WB Ershler. Harwood Academic Press, 1997, pp.

2. Kim S, Jiang JC, Kirchman PA, *et al*. Cellular and Molecular Aging. In *Comprehensive Geriatric Oncology*, edited by L Balducci, GH Lyman, WB Ershler. Harwood Academic Press, 123–55, 1997.

3. Ershler WL. Age-related changes in tumor growth in experimental models. *Comprehensive Geriatric Oncology*.

4. Holmes FF. Clinical Course of Cancer in the Elderly. *Cancer Control* 1994; **1**: 108–114.

5. Balducci L, Cox CE, Greenberg H, *et al*. Management of Cancer in the Older Aged Person. *Cancer Control* 1994; **1**: 132–139.

6. Iber FL, Murphy PA, Connor ES. Age-related changes in the gastrointestinal system. *Drugs and Aging* 1994; **5**: 34–48.

7. Crome P, Flanagan RJ. Pharmacokinetic studies in elderly people. *Clin Pharmacokinet* 1994; **26**: 243–247.

8. Ritschel WA. Identification of populations at risk in drug testing and therapy. application to elderly patients. *Eur J Drug Met Pharmcokin* 1993; **18**: 101–111.

9. Stanta G. Morbid Anatomy of Aging. In *Comprehensive Geriatric Oncology*, edited by L Balducci, GH Lyman, WB Ershler. Harwood Academic Press, 1997, pp.

10. Johnson SL, Mayerson M, Conrad KA. Gastrointestinal absorption as a function of age: xylose absorption in healthy adults. *Clin Pharmacol Ther* 1985; **38**: 331–335.

11. Carney DN, Byrne A. Etoposide in the treatment of elderly poor prognosis patients with small cell lung cancer. *Cancer Chemother Pharmacol* 1995; **36**: 506–512

12. Montamat SC, Cusack BJ, Vestal RE. Management of Drug Therapy in the Elderly. *N Engl J Med* 1989; **321**: 303–309.

13. Moore MJ, Ehrlichman C. Therapeutic drug monitoring in oncology. Problems and potentials inantineoplastic therapy. *Clin Pharmacokin* 1987; **13**: 205–227.

14. Tew KD, Calvin M, Chabner BA. Alkylating agents. In *Cancer Chemotherapy & Biotherapy*, edited by BA Chabner, DL Longo. Lippincott-Raven, 297–332, 1996.

15. Forman W. Palliative care of the older cancer patient. *Clin Ger*, in press.

16. Grem JL. 5–Fluoropyrimidines. In *Cancer Chemotherapy & Biotherapy*, edited by BA Chabner, DL Longo. Lippincott-Raven, 149–211, 1996.

17. Chabner BA. Cytidine Analogues. *Cancer Chemotherapy and Biotherapy*. Lippincott-Raven, 213–233, 1996.

18. Rowinsky EK, Donehwer RC. Antimicrotubular agents. In *Cancer Chemotherapy & Biotherapy*, edited by BA Chabner, DL Longo. Lippincott-Raven, 263–296, 1996.

19. Doroshow JH. Anthracyclines and anthracendiones. In *Cancer Chemotherapy & Biotherapy*, edited by BA Chabner, DL Longo. Lippincott-Raven, 409–434, 1996.

20. O'Mahony MS, Woodhouse KW. Age, environmental factors, and drug metabolism. *Pharmac Ther* 1994; **61**: 279–287.

21. Reed E, Dabholkar M, Chabner BA. Platinum Analogues. In *Cancer Chemotherapy & Biotherapy*, edited by BA Chabner, DL Longo. Lippincott-Raven, 357–378, 1996.

22. Anderson S, Brenner BM. Effects of aging on the renal glomerulus. *Am J Med* 1986; **80**: 435–442.

23. Henrich WL. Analgesic Nephropathy. *Am J Med Sci* 1988; **295**: 561–568.

24. Gelman RS, Taylor SG. Cyclophosphamide, Methotrexate and 5 Fluorouracil chemotherapy in women more than 65 year old with advanced breast cancer. The elimination of age trends in toxicity by using doses based on creatinine clearance. *J Clin Oncol* 1984; **2**: 1406–1414.

25. Kintzel PE, Dorr RT. Anticancer Drug Renal Toxicity and elimination: dosing guidelines for altered renal function. *Cancer Treat Rev* 1995; **21**: 33–64.

26. Waller DG, Fleming JS, Ramsay B, *et al*. The accuracy of creatinine clearance with and without urine collection as a measure of glomerular filtration rate. *Postgrad Med J* 1991; **67**: 42–46.

27. Chu E, Allegra C. Antifolates. In *Cancer Chemotherapy & Biotherapy*, edited by BA Chabner, DL Longo. Lippincott-Raven, 109–148, 1996.

28. Calvert AH, Newell DR, Gumbrell LA, *et al*. Carboplatin dosage: prospective evaluation of a simple formula based on renal function. *J Clin Oncol* 1989; **7**: 1748–1756.

29. Pommier Y, Fesen MR, Goldwasser F. Topoisomerase II inhibitors: the epipodophyllotoxins, m-AMSA, and the ellipticine derivatives. In *Cancer Chemotherapy & Biotherapy*, edited by BA Chabner, DL Longo. Lippincott-Raven, 435–461, 1996.

30. Robert J, Hoerni B. Age dependence of the early phase pharmacokinetics of doxorubicin. *Cancer Res* 1983; **43**: 4467–4469.

31. Egorin MJ, Zuhowsky EG, Thompson B, *et al*. Age related alterations in daunorubicin pharmacokinetics. *Proc Am Soc Clin Oncol* 1987; **6**: 38.

32. Burkowski JM, Duerr M, Donehower RC, *et al*. Relation between age and clearance rate of nine investigational anticancer drugs from phase I pharmacokinetic data. *Cancer Chem Pharmacol* 1994; **33**: 493–496.

33. Yamamoto N, Tamura T, Maerla M, *et al*. The influence of aging on cisplatin pharmacokinetics in lung cancer patients with normal organ function. *Cancer Chemother Pharmacol* 1995; **36**: 102–106.

34. Moscow JA, Schneider E, Cowan KH. Multidrug resistance. In *Cancer Chemotherapy and Biological Response Modifiers*, edited by HM Pinedo, DL Longo, BA Chabner. Annual: 16, Elsevier Science BV: 111–131, 1996.

35. Murren JR, DeVita VT. another look at multidrug resistance. *PPO update* 1995; **9 (11)**: 1–12.

36. Applebaum FR, Barrall J, Storb R, *et al*. Treatment of myelodysplasia with marrow transplantation: overall results and effect of pretreatment variables on outcome. *Blood* 1989; **74 (suppl.1)**: 52:a.

37. Ballester O, Moscinski L, Morris D, *et al*. Acute leukemia in the elderly. *J Am Ger Soc* 1992; **40**: 277–284.

38. Shipp MA. Prognostic Factors in Aggressive non-Hodgkin's Lymphoma: who has "high risk" disease? *Blood* 1994: 1165–1173.

39. Thigpen T, Brady MF, Omura GA, *et al*. Age as a prognostic factor in ovarian carcinoma: the gynecologic oncology group experience. *Cancer* 1993; **71**: 606–614.

40. Ershler WB. A gerontologist's perspective on cancer biology and treatment. *Cancer Control* 1994; **1**: 103–107.

41. Balducci L, Wallace C, Khansur T, *et al*. Nutrition, cancer and aging. an annotated review. *J Am Ger Soc* 1986; **34**: 127–136.

42. O'Dwyer PJ, Hamilton TC, Yao K-S, *et al*. Modulation of glutathione and related enzymes in reversal of resistance to anticancer drugs. *Hemato/Onco Clin N America* 1995; **9**: 383–396.

43. Rockwell O , Hughes CS, Kennedy KA. Effect of host age on microenvironmental heterogeneity and efficacy of combined modality therapy in solid tumors. *Int J Rad Oncol Biol Phys* 1991; **20**: 259–263.

44. Reed JC. BCL-2. Prevention of apoptosis as a mechanism of drug resistance. *Hematol/Oncol Clin N America* 1995; **9**: 450–473.

45. Ballester O, Moscinski L, Spiers A, Balducci L. Non-Hodgkin's Lymphomas in older patients. *J Am Ger Soc* 1993.

46. Pezzella F, Turley H, Kuzu I, *et al*. bcl-2 protein in non-small cell lung carcinoma. *N Engl J Med* 1993; **329**: 690–694.

47. Ackland SP, Schilsky RL. High dose methotrexate: a critical reappraisal. *J Clin Oncol* 1987; **5**: 2017–2031.

48. Valentinis B, Silvestrini R, Daidone MG, *et al*. 3H-Thymidine labeling index, hormone receptors and ploidy in breast cancer from elderly patients. *Breast Cancer Res Treat* 1991; **20** 19–24.

49. Daidone MG, Luisi S, Silvestrini R, *et al*. Biologic Characteristics of Primary Breast Cancer in the Elderly. In *Comprehensive Geriatric Oncology*, edited by L Balducci, GH Lyman, WB Ershler. Harwood Academic Press, 197–200, 1997.

50. Rudd GN, Hartley JA, Souhani RL. Persistence of cisplatin induced DNA interstrand crosslinking in peripheral blood mononuclear cells from elderly and younger individual. *Cancer Chemother Pharmacol* 1995; **35**: 323–326.

51. Cohen HJ. Principles of treatment applied to medical oncology: an overview. *Sem Oncol* 1995 **22 (Suppl.1)**: 1–3.

52. Fraser CC, Hoffman R. Hematopoietic stem cell behavior: potential implications for gene therapy. *J Lab Clin Med* 1995; **125**.693–702.

53. Krause DS, Fackler MJ, Civin CI, *et al*. CD34: structure, biology, and clinical utility. *Blood* 1996; **87**: 1–13.

54. Ogawa M. Hematopoiesis. *J All Clin Immunol* 1994; **94**: 645–650.

55. Gordon MY. Physiology and function of the haemopoietic microenvironment. *Br J Haematol* 1994; **86**: 241–243.

56. Lipschitz DA. Age-related decline in hemopoietic reserve capacity. *Sem Oncol* 1995; **22(suppl.1)**: 3–6.

57. Rothstein G. Hematopoiesis in the aged: a model of hematopoietic dysregulation? *Blood* 1993; **82**: 2601–2604.

58. Chatta GS, Price TH, Allen RC, *et al*. Effects of "in vivo" recombinant methionyl human granulocyte colony-stimulating factor on the neutrophil response and peripheral blood colony-forming cells in healthy young and elderly adult volunteers. *Blood* 1994; **84**: 2923–2929.

59. Lipschitz DA, Udupa KB. Age and the hemopoietic system. *J Am Ger Soc* 1986; **34**: 448–454.

60. Buchner T. Treatment of Acute Leukemia in Older Patients. In *Comprehensive Geriatric Oncology*, edited by L Balducci, GH Lyman, WB Ershler. Harwood Academic Press, 1997, pp.

61. Monfardini S, *et al*. Non-Hodgkin's Lymphoma in the older patient. *Comprehensive Geriatric Oncology*.

62. Zagonel V, *et al*. *Comprehensive Geriatric Oncology*.

63. Schank W, Balducci L. Recombinant hemopoietic growth factors: comparative hemopoietic response in younger and older patients. *J Am Ger Soc* 1993.

64. Petrelli N, Douglass HO, Herrera L, *et al*. The modulation of fluorouracil with leucovorin in metastatic colorectal carcinoma: a prospective randomized phase III trial. *J Clin Oncol* 1989; **7**: 1419–1426.

65. Brower M, Asbury R, Kramer Z,, *et al*. Adjuvant chemotherapy of colorectal cancer in the elderly. Population Based Experience. *Proc Amer Soc Clin Oncol* 1993; **12** 195.

66. Diehl V, Marty M.Efficacy and safety of antiemetics. *Cancer Treat Rev* 1994; **20**: 379–392.

67. Kris MG, Gralla RJ, Tyson LB, *et al*. Controlling delayed vomiting: double blind, randomized trial comparing placebo, dexamethasone alone, and metoclopramide plus dexamethasone in patients receiving cisplatin. *J Clin Oncol* 1989; **7**: 108–114.

68. De Wit R, Schmitz PIM, Verweij J, *et al*. Analysis of cumulative probabilities shows that the efficacy of 5HT3 antagonist prophylaxis is not maintained. *J Clin Oncol* 1996; **14**: 644–651.

69. Basser RL, Green MD. Strategies for prevention of anthracycline cardiotxicity. *Cancer Treat Rev* 1993; **19**: 57–77.

70. Speyer JL, Green MD, Zeleniuch-jacquotte A, *et al*. ICRF-187 permits longer treatment wiht doxorubicin in women with breast cancer. *J Clin Oncol* 1992; **10**: 117–127.

71. Legha Ss, Benjamin RS, Mackay B, *et al*. Reduction of doxorubicin cardiotoxicity by prolonged continuous intravenous infusion. *Ann Int Med* 1982; **96**: 133–139.

72. Capizzi RL. Protection of normal tissues from the cytotoxic effects of chemotherapy by amifostine (Ethyol): clinical experiences. *Sem Oncol* 1994; **21 (supp 11)**: 8–15.

73. Uziely B, Gabizon A, Jeffers S, *et al*. Liposomal doxorubicin (doxil): antitumor activity and unique toxicities during two complementary phase I studies. *Proc Am Soc Clin Oncol* 1995; **14**: 483.

74. Balducci L. Mitoxantrone: a monography.

75. Shapiro CL, Yeap BY, Godleski J, *et al*. Drug-related pulmonary toxicity in Non-Hodgkin's Lymphoma. *Cancer* 1991; **68**: 699–705.

76. Thyss A, Saudes L, Otto J, *et al*. Renal tolerance of cisplatin in patients more than 80 years old. *J Clin Oncol* 1994; **12**: 2121–2125.

77. Muggia FM. Overview of carboplatin: replacing, complementing and expamnding the therapeutic horizon of cisplatin. *Semin Oncol* 1989; **16 (suppl 5)**: 7–18.

78. MacDonald DR. Neurotoxicity of Chemotherapeutic Agents. In *The Chemotherapy Source Book*, edited by MC Perry. Williams & Wilkins, 666–679, 1992.

79. Jackson DV, Wells HB, Atkins JN, *et al*. Amelioration of vincristine neurotoxicity by glutamic acid. *Am J Med* 1988; **84**: 1016–1022.

80. Thompson SW, Davis LE, Kornfeld M, *et al*. Cisplatin neuropathy. *Cancer* 1984; **54**: 1269–1275.

81. Shaffer SD, Post JD, Close LG. Ototoxicity of low and moderate dose cisplatin. *Cancer* 1985; **56** 1934–1939.

82. Rubin EH, Andersen JW, Berg DT, *et al*. Risk factors for high-dose cytarabine neurotoxicity: an analysis of a cancer and leukemia group B trial in patients with acute myeloid leukemia. *J Clin Oncol* 1992; **10**: 948–953.

83. Damon LE, Mass R, Linker CA. The association between high-dose cytarabine neurotoxicity and renal insufficiency. *J Clin Oncol* 1989; **7**: 1563–1568.

84. Ingle JN, Ahmann DL, Green SJ, *et al*. Randomized clinical trial of diethylstilbestrol versus tamoxifen in postmenopausal women with advanced breast cancer. *N Engl J Med* 1981; **304**: 16–21.

85. Andrejico JL, Marshall LA, Dumesic DA, *et al*. Therapeutic use of gonadotropin-releasing hormone analogs. *Obstetr Gynecol Surg* 1987; **42**: 1–21.

86. Balducci L, Baekey P, Sillimann RA. Breast Cancer in the Older woman: an oncological perspective. In *Comprehensive Geriatric Oncology*, edited by L Balducci, GH Lyman, WB Ershler. Harwood Academic Press, 1997, pp.

87. Gylling H, Pyrhonen S, Mantyla E, *et al*. Tamoxifen and toremifene lower serum cholesterol by inhibition of delta-8cholestenol conversion to lathosterol in women with breast cancer. *J Clin Oncol* 1995; **13**: 2900–2905.

88. Hoffken K. Experience with aromatase inhibitors in the treatment of advanced breast cancer. *Cancer Treatment Rev* 1993; **19 (suppl.B)**: 37–44.

89. Balducci L. Prostate Cancer in the older man. *Clin Ger*, in press.

90. Burns E, Goodwin J. Immunology of aging. In *Comprehensive Geriatric Oncology*, edited by L Balducci, GH Lyman, WB Ershler. Harwood Academic Press, 213–223, 1997.

91. Witt PL, Lindner DJ, D'Cunha J, *et al*. Pharmacology of interferons: induced proteins, cell activation and antitumor activity. In *Cancer Chemotherapy & Biotherapy*, edited by BA Chabner, DL Longo. Lippincott-Raven, 585–608, 1996.

92. Bukowski RM, Mclain D, Finke JH. Clinical pharmacokinetics of interleukin 1, interleukin 2, interleukin 4, tumor necrosis factor and macrophage colony-stimulating factor. In *Cancer Chemotherapy & Biotherapy*, edited by BA Chabner, DL Longo. Lippincott-Raven, 609–638, 1996.

93. Hehlmann R, Heimpel H, Hasford J, *et al*. Randomized comparison of interferon alpha with busulfan and hydroxyurea in chronic myelogenous leukemia. *Blood* 1994; **84**: 4064–4077.

94. The Italian Cooperative Study Group on Chronic Myeloid Leukemia. Interferon alpha 2a as compared with conventional chemotherapy for the treatment of chronic myeloid leukemia. *N Engl J Med* 1994; **330**: 820–826.

95. Ohnishi K, Ohno R, Tomonaga M, *et al*. A randomized clinical trial comparing Interferon alphawith busulfan for newly diagnosedchronic myelogenous leukemia in chronic phase. *Blood* 1995; **86**: 906–916.

96. Andreyev HJN, Scott-Mackie P, Cunningham D, *et al*. Phase II study of continuous infusion fluorouracil and interferon alfa-2b in the palliation of malignant neuroendocrine tumors. *J Clin Oncol* 1995; **13**: 1486–1492.

34. New Antineoplastic Agents of Interest to the Older Patient

John R. Eckardt and Daniel D. Von Hoff

Introduction

Recently, the combination of an increase in the number of older people in the population and increased incidence of cancer as a person ages has made the treatment of cancer in elderly patients a significant health issue. An important aspect of cancer in the elderly patient is that the most common tumor types seen are generally resistant to standard therapies when in the advanced setting. In 1995 1,252,000 cases of cancer and 547,000 deaths were estimated in the United States by the National Cancer Database (1). In 1991 approximately 87% of all cancer deaths were in patients 55 years of age or older, with 38% in patients 75 years of age or older (1). In men 75 years of age and older the five most common causes of cancer deaths are lung, prostate, colorectal, pancreas and bladder cancers, which account for 68.8% of all cancer-related deaths in that age group (1). Similarly, in women 75 years of age or older the five most common causes of cancer deaths are lung, colorectal, breast, pancreas and ovarian cancers, which account for 58.7% of all cancer-related death in that age group (1). The importance of these statistics is that the seven different tumor types listed are all generally resistant to standard chemotherapy agents with only minimal impact on survival in the advanced setting. Therefore, the development of new, more active chemotherapy agents for these tumor types is needed.

The 1990s is an exciting decade for the treatment of cancer. Technology from the 1980s and 1990s has provided new anticancer agents with unique mechanisms of action and significant clinical activity. The discovery of new chemotherapeutic agents with activity in these general tumor types is important for the elderly patient with cancer, but it is also important to address the special needs and differences of the elderly patient. The most important difference to remember is that not all elderly patients are the same. The psychosocial and physiologic changes that occur as a person ages will affect different people at different rates and at different ages. Therefore, a person at the age of 65 may have more significant changes in organ function than a person at the age of 80.

A person at the age of 85 in good physiologic condition may or may not wish the same intensity of treatment as a younger patient. Psychosocial issues, such as the prior death of a spouse or child from cancer, availability of family and friend's support, finances, and depression, may affect a person's desire for treatment. Consequently, in the development of new anticancer agents for elderly patients, all of these physiologic and psychosocial differences must be taken into account. In San Antonio, we looked at age to determine if it were a risk factor for outcome of patients treated on phase I clinical trials. The records of 601 patients treated on 26 phase I trials between 1979 and 1992 were examined. Outcomes included time to tumor progression, toxicity, and response rate. No difference in any of these outcomes was seen between patients < 65 years of age versus those ≥65. Similar results were demonstrated for all age cutoffs analyzed (2).

In this chapter we will discuss new agents which have recently been developed or are being developed which may have activity in the cancers that affect the elderly. We will also discuss the characteristics of these agents (such as pharmacokinetics, mode of excretion, toxicity profiles, and mode of delivery), which may aid in choosing one treatment over another in any individual patient. These new agents include:

- Vinorelbine with mild non-hematologic toxicities and activity in patients with non-small cell lung, breast and hormone-refractory prostate cancers;
- Docetaxel with a high level of activity in breast, non-small cell lung, bladder, pancreas and ovarian cancers;
- Topoisomerase I inhibitors (topotecan, irinotecan, etc.) with activity in small cell and non-small cell lung, colorectal and ovarian cancers;
- Gemcitabine with activity in breast, non-small cell lung, pancreas and ovarian cancers;
- Tomudex and LY231514 (second- and third-generation thymidylate synthase inhibitors) with single-dose administration schedules and activity in non-small cell lung, colorectal and pancreas cancers;
- Temozolomide which is orally administered and has activity in patients with melanomas and gliomas; and
- Losoxantrone, an anthrapyrazole with activity in breast cancer.

Vinorelbine (Navelbine)

Advantages for the Elderly Patient

- Toxicity profile

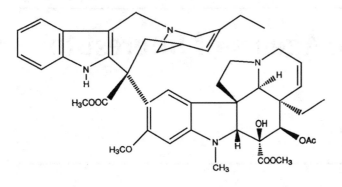

Figure 34.1   Vinorelbine: Structure.

- Administration
- Activity in patients with breast and non-small cell lung cancers
- Pharmacokinetics

Although vinorelbine is currently approved for the treatment of non-small cell lung cancer in the United States, this agent is relatively new in its development and certain characteristics make it appropriate for treatment of elderly patients with cancer. Navelbine (vinorelbine, 5'-nor-anhydrovinblastine) is a unique vinca alkaloid which is produced by semisynthesis and which differs from naturally occurring vincas in its structure and selectivity of action (Figure 34.1). Modifications have been made in the catharanthine portion of the molecule with an 8-member ring instead of the 9-member ring seen in naturally occurring vincas (3). Similar to the other vincas, navelbine's mechanism of action is the depolymerization of microtubules (4, 5).

Advantages for the Elderly Patient

Toxicity profile

Navelbine has been extensively studied in phase I, II, and III clinical trials. The most notable toxicity associated with navelbine is hematologic (Figure 34.2). Neutropenia with or without fever is the dose-limiting toxicity noted on all intravenous schedules tested (Table 34.1) (6–11). Anemia is common but rarely severe and thrombocytopenia is rare. Although age has little effect on hemoglobin and platelet toxicities, a slight increase in grade 3 and 4 neutropenia is observed in patients 65 years of age or older (Figure 34.2) (12). Although the incidence of grade 3 and 4 neutropenia is high, complications from the neutropenia are uncommon with only 7% of patients requiring hospitalization for fever or infection (12).

Non-hematologic toxicities are seen in about 85% of patients treated with navelbine and are generally mild to moderate in severity and rarely severe or life-threatening (Figure 34.3) (12). Asthenia was the most common non-digestive tract toxicity occurring in 29% of patients. The use of prophylactic antiemetics was generally not required with navelbine. Thirty-eight percent of patients developed some nausea but in only 2% was the nausea grade 3/4. A difficult toxicity for elderly patients seen with navelbine is constipation. This occurs in about 30% of patients, similar to the frequency for other vinca alkaloids. The constipation can be severe in up to 2% of patients. Preclinical studies suggest that navelbine might cause less neurotoxicity than other vinca alkaloids (5). Clinical studies have demonstrated that neuropathy, manifested as paresthesia and hypesthesia, occurs in 20% of patients but is severe in < 1% (12).

Table 34.1   Vinorelbine phase I studies.

Schedule	Route	MTD # pts	mg/m²	DLT	Antitumor Activity	Reference
Weekly	IV	34	35 .4	Leucopenia	1 PR NHL 1 PR HD	[6]
Weekly	IV	15	30	Neutropenia	1 PR breast 1 PR H&N	[7]
Weekly	IV	30	35	Leucopenia	NR	[8]
8 mg bolus plus 96 hour infusion	IV	68	10 /day	Neutropenia	5 CR breast 15 PR breast	[9]
Weekly	PO	19	160	Leucopenia	5 PR breast	[10]
Daily × 21	PO	40	40	Febrile Neutropenia	1 PR breast	[11]

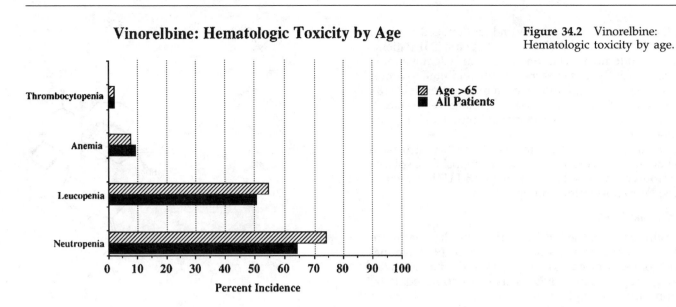

Figure 34.2 Vinorelbine: Hematologic toxicity by age.

Administration

Navelbine is given as a weekly 10-minute infusion. Studies with navelbine have demonstrated this schedule to be active in breast and non-small cell lung cancers with tolerable toxicities. Navelbine is a vesicant and needs to be administered with care. Since this agent does not cause significant nausea or vomiting, out-patient administration is feasible. This ease of administration makes navelbine appealing for the treatment of elderly patients with cancer.

Activity in patients with breast and non-small cell lung cancers

Navelbine has undergone extensive phase II and III testing in patients with breast and non-small cell lung cancers, and has demonstrated activity in both of these tumor types. In patients with metastatic breast cancer, navelbine has been evaluated as first and second-line treatment. Response rates in first-line, metastatic breast cancer have ranged from 40–52% for intravenous navelbine and 0–32% for oral navelbine (13). In patients with previous treatment, navelbine has demonstrated response rates which range from 17–46%. Multiple combination trials have looked at the activity of navelbine in combination with 5-fluorouracil, doxorubicin, epirubicin or mitoxantrone. Response rates as high as 74% have been reported (13).

Navelbine has demonstrated activity in patients with non-small cell lung cancer. Response rates of 15–40% have been reported for single-agent navelbine (14–16). In elderly patients with non-small cell lung cancer, navelbine at a dose of 25 mg/m^2 per week demonstrated a response rate of 16% in 25 patients (15). Non-hematologic toxicities were minimal. In a three-arm phase III trial of navelbine versus navelbine and cisplatin versus vindesine and cisplatin, 612 patients were randomized to one of the three arms. Response rate, median survival and one year survival were superior for the navelbine and cisplatin arm compared to the

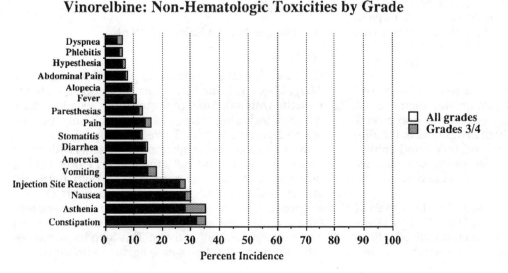

Figure 34.3 Vinorelbine: Non-hematological toxicities by grade.

other two arms (17). In a second randomized study of navelbine versus navelbine and cisplatin, 231 patients were randomized. The combination arm demonstrated a significantly higher response rate and time to tumor progression but no difference in median survival (18). Currently, a randomized trial of cisplatin versus navelbine and cisplatin has completed accrual and is being analyzed.

In addition to cisplatin, navelbine has also been evaluated in combination with etoposide/cisplatin, mitomycin-C/cisplatin, cisplatin/5-FU/leucovorin, cisplatin/ifosfamide and epirubicin.

Pharmacokinetics

Examination of the influence of age on the pharmacokinetics of navelbine has been reported (19). Examination of the pharmacokinetics of 44 cancer patients with an average age of 56 ± 7.8 years was performed. Relationships were explored by regression analysis between age and clearance, half-life, and V_{ss}. No evidence was found of an age dependency for any pharmacokinetic parameter.

Navelbine is a new vinca alkaloid well tolerated in the elderly population with activity in malignancies common to the elderly. Further evaluation of navelbine in combination with other agents and in other tumor types will better define its role in cancer of the elderly.

Docetaxel (Taxotere)

Advantages For the Elderly Patient

- High-level activity in breast, non-small cell lung, pancreas and ovarian cancers
- Pharmacokinetics: Minimal renal excretion
- Administration
- Synergistic activity with other active compounds

Disadvantage For the Elderly Patient

- Toxicity profile in patients with abnormal liver function tests

Docetaxel (N-debenzoyl-N-tert-butoxycarbonyl-10-deacytyl taxol, RP56976, taxotere) is a semisynthetic analog of paclitaxel prepared from a non-cytotoxic precursor extracted from the needles of the European yew tree *(Taxus baccata)* (Figure 34.4). Docetaxel was synthesized in 1986 and selected for clinical development in 1987, secondary to preclinical activity and a formulation which allowed for shorter infusion schedules than paclitaxel. Early preclinical testing of docetaxel demonstrated potency 2.5-fold greater than that of paclitaxel (20) The mechanism of action of docetaxel is similar to that of paclitaxel; both drugs bind to tubulin, promote the assembly of microtubules and inhibit depolymerization (20). However, the compounds are not cross resistant in many *in vitro* and *in vivo* systems (21).

In 1990 phase I dose escalation and toxicity trials of docetaxel began in Europe and the United States. Dose-limiting neutropenia has been seen on all schedules explored (Table 34.2) (22–26). Studies which have uti-

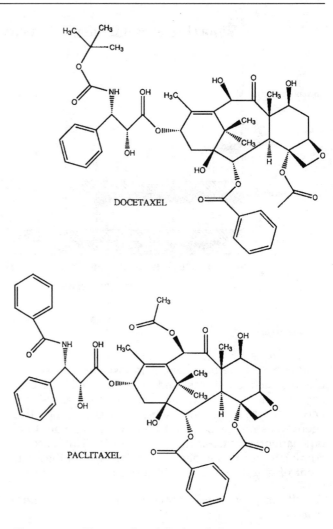

Figure 34.4   Docetaxel and Pacltaxel: Structure.

lized longer schedules or repeated-dosing schedules have found more severe mucositis along with the neutropenia. Mucositis was not found to be a significant problem on 1- and 2-hour dosing schedules. Therefore, the 1-hour infusion schedule was chosen for further clinical development.

Advantages For the Elderly Patient

High-level activity

Docetaxel has undergone broad phase II testing (Table 34.3) (27–52). Clinical activity has been documented in patients with a number of tumor types seen in elderly patients, including breast, non-small cell lung, pancreatic and ovarian cancers. There is intense interest in the activity of docetaxel for treatment of patients with breast cancer and non-small cell lung cancer. Docetaxel has demonstrated objective responses in both untreated and treated metastatic breast cancer patients (27–31). Response rates for docetaxel in untreated metastatic breast cancer are as high or higher than any other reported single-agent activity. This activity is comparable to the most active single agents in breast cancer,

Table 34.2 Docetaxel phase I studies.

Taxotere Dose/Schedule	Maximally Tolerated Dose (mg/m²)	Dose Limiting Toxicity	Recommended Phase 11 Dose (mg/m²)	Responses	References
1–2 hour infusion Q21 days	115	Neutropenia	100	1 PR Ovarian 1 PR Breast 1 PR 9CLC 1 PR Unknown Primary	[22]
24 hour infusion Q21 days	115	Neutropenia	100	2 PR NSCLC 1 PR Breast 1 PR Cholangiocarcinoma	[23]
6 hour infusion Q21 days	100	Neutropenia Mucositis	100	1 PR Breast	[23]
24 hour infusion Q21 days	90	Leucopenia Mucositis	70–90	None	[24]
1 hour daily × 5 Q21 days	80 (per cycle)	Neutropenia Mucositis	70	6 PR Ovarian 1 PR Breast	[25]
1 hour infusion Dl and D8 Q21 days	110 (per cycle)	Neutropenia	100	4 PR Breast 1 PR Unknown Primary	[26]

including doxorubicin and paclitaxel. In comparing the published response rates and survival of docetaxel to those of doxorubicin, docetaxel has similar to higher response rates and similar median survival. Although these are not randomized trials, this significant activity is encouraging. Even more encouraging is the activity of docetaxel in patients with metastatic breast cancer who have progressed after anthracycline- and/or anthracenedione-based chemotherapy. In published studies in patients resistant or refractory to anthracyclines and/or anthracenediones, docetaxel demonstrated an overall response rate of 43% with 10-month median survival (27, 28). In non-small cell lung cancer responses have been documented in patients who either are chemotherapy-naive or have progressed after a platinum-containing regimen with published response rates ranging from 21–33% (32–37). This activity in platinum-refractory patients is notable when compared to other agents in this patient population. Single-agent activity of paclitaxel, cisplatin, etoposide, epirubicin and vindesine has ranged from 2–10% when used as second-line treatment.

Single-agent activity has also been demonstrated for docetaxel in trials in patients with pancreatic and ovarian cancer. This significant activity in tumor types common in the elderly population makes docetaxel attractive for the treatment of elderly patients.

Pharmacokinetics

Population pharmacokinetics have been performed for docetaxel. Bruno *et al* (53), using a three-compartment model, found docetaxel to have a half-life of 11.1 hours with a clearance of $21.21/hr/m^2$ and a volume of distribution of 691 m². Metabolism studies have demonstrated that 80% of taxotere is recovered in the feces

over 7 days with only 5% recovered in the urine (54). Therefore, in elderly patients with decreased creatinine clearance, the elimination of docetaxel will not be affected. However, pharmacodynamic analysis of taxotere has demonstrated that patients with elevated transaminases, alkaline phosphatase, or bilirubin have a significant decreased clearance, increased AUC, and increased toxicity compared to patients with normal liver function studies. Therefore, extreme caution should be used in treating patients with abnormal liver function studies.

Administration

Docetaxl has been developed as a single 1 hour infusion every 3 weeks. Although premedication with steroids and antihistamines has been used to reduce the severity of some toxicities (see below), docetaxel has very minimal nausea and vomiting and can easily be given in the outpatient setting. This ease of administration can be an advantage for elderly patients.

Synergistic activity with other active compounds

Docetaxel with its unique mechanism of action has demonstrated synergistic activity in preclinical models when combined with cyclophospharnide, 5-fluorouracil, etoposide, vinorelbine, and methotrexate (55). Phase I combination studies are underway.

Disadvantage For the Elderly Patient

Toxicity profile

The major toxicity observed with docetaxel is neutropenia. The neutropenia is dose-dependent with a median day to nadir of 9 days and recovery by day 21. At the recommended phase II dose of docetaxel

Table 34.3 Docetaxel phase II studies.

Tumor Type	Regimen	# Evaluable Patients	Previous Chemotherapy	CR (%)	PR (%)	References
Breast Cancer	100 mg/m^2 Q21 days	24	Yes	1 (4)	13 (54)	[27]
Breast Cancer	100 mg/m^2 Q21 days	33	Yes	0	18 (55)	[28]
Breast Cancer	100 mg/m^2 Q21 days	38	No	5 (13)	12 (31)	[29]
Breast Cancer	100 mg/n^2 Q21 days	21	No	0	12 (57)	[30]
Breast Cancer	100 mg/m^2 Q21days	14	No	2 (14)	6 (43)	[31]
Non-Small Cell Lung Cancer	100 mg/m^2 Q21 days	37	No	1 (3)	7 (19)	[32]
Non-Small Cell Lung Cancer	100 mg/m^2 Q21 days	18	No	0	5 (28)	[33]
Non-Small Cell Lung Cancer	100 mg/m^2 Q21 days	11 9	Yes No	0 0	3 (27) 3 (33)	[34]
Non-Small Cell Lung Cancer	100 mg/m^2 Q21days	42	Yes	0	9 (21)	[35]
Non-Small Cell Lung Cancer	60 mg/m^2 Q21 days	84	No	0	18 (21)	[36]
Non-Small Cell Lung Cancer	100 mg/kn^2 Q21 days	39	No	0	13 (33)	[37]
Ovarian Cancer	100 mg/m^2 Q21 days	24	Yes	0	8 (33)	[38]
Ovarian Cancer	100 mg/m^2 Q21 days	52	Yes	3 (6)	18 (35)	[39]
Ovarian Cancer	100 mg/m^2 Q21 days	34	Yes	2 (6)	10 (29)	[40]
Bladder Cancer	100 mg/m^2 Q21 days	11	Yes	0	1 (9)	[41]
Melanoma	100 mg/m^2 Q21 days	13	No	1 (8)	0	[42]
Melanoma	100 mg/m^2 Q21 days	14	No	1 (7)	2 (14)	[43]
Pancreatic Cancer	100 mg/m^2 Q21 days	23	No	0	5 (22)	[44]
Renal Cell Carcinoma	100 mg/m^2 Q21days	18	No	0	0	[45]
Soft Tissue Sarcoma	100 mg/n^2 Q21 days	29	No	0	5 (17)	[46]
Head and Neck Cancer	100 mg/m^2 Q21 days	14	Yes	2 (14)	3 (21)	[47]
Head and Neck Cancer	100 mg/m^2 Q21 days	37	Yes	2 (5)	10 (27)	[48]
Colon Cancer	100 mg/m^2 Q21 days	18	No	0	0	[49]
Colon Cancer	100 mg/m^2 Q21 days	19	No	0	0	[50]
Colon Cancer	100 mg/m^2 Q21 days	33	No	1 (3)	2 (6)	[51]
Gastric Cancer	100 mg/m^2 Q21 days	33	No	0	8 (24)	[52]

(100 mg/m^2 over 1 hour), approximately 70% of patients develop grade 4 neutropenia. The neutropenia is generally of short duration and without complications, with only 18% of patients having grade 4 neutropenia lasting greater than 7 days, and 15% have fever associated with the neutropenia (22–26). Other hematologic toxicities including anemia and thrombocytopenia are generally mild ($\leq$ grade 2) and seen only in a minority of patients (< 20%).

Non-hematologic toxicities of docetaxel are shown in Figure 34.5. Non-hematologic toxicities were generally mild to moderate in severity. Treatment discontinuation was required in only 17.7% of patients for toxicity. Toxicities which caused treatment discontinuation included: febrile neutropenia, fluid retention, hypersensitivity reaction, asthenia, skin toxicity and paresthesia.

Four toxicities of docetaxel require further discussion. First is the hypersensitivity reaction. Unlike paclitaxel, docetaxel does not cause acute anaphylactic reactions. However, a unique syndrome characterized by localized or generalized flushing, rash, chest pain or heaviness, back pain, dyspnea and fever is observed in approximately 15% of patients (56). These symptoms occurred within 3 to 10 minutes of the beginning of the infusion. They resolved over a few minutes after

Docetaxel: Non-Hematologic Toxicities

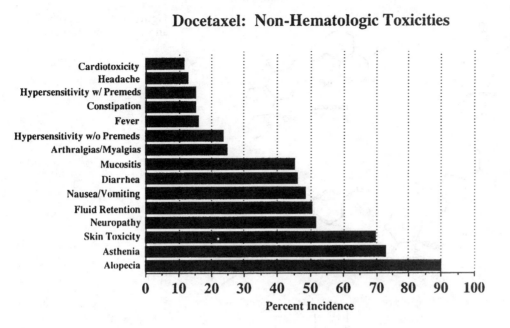

Figure 34.5 Docetaxel: Non-Hematological toxicities.

interruption of the infusion. Treatment with diphenhydramine and hydrocortisone allows the infusion to be restarted. Severe symptoms associated with hypotension and/or bradycardia were seen in only 2% of patients. Premedication with antihistamines and steroids has been found to reduce the incidence of the severe (grade 3 and 4) hypersensitivity reactions (57). Patients who develop the hypersensitivity reaction do so on the first or second cycle of therapy and rarely after the fourth cycle (56). In patients who manifest a hypersensitivity reaction on their first and/or second cycle of therapy they will rarely continue to manifest the reaction after the third cycle.

The second toxicity is fluid retention, which has been associated with the development of peripheral edema, pleural effusions and ascites. The etiology of this fluid retention syndrome is unknown but may be related to increased capillary permeability (58). The edema appears to occur after approximately 400–500 mg/m^2 total dose of docetaxel and can be minimized by premedication with steroids and the use of diuretics.

The third toxicity is a cutaneous toxicity, which is associated with a skin rash and nail changes. The skin rash is seen in greater than 50% of treatment cycles with 21% being asymptomatic and 79% being symptomatic. The most common skin reaction is characterized as discrete erythematous to violaceous patches or edematous plaques similar to acral (59). The nail changes, oncholysis, are painful in some patients. Premedication with steroids and antihistamines has been reported to reduce the severity of the local cutaneous toxicities (60).

The fourth toxicity is neuropathy that is mainly a sensory type, which is generally mild (grade 1 or 2) with symptoms of numbness and dysesthesia. The neuropathy resolves slowly when docetaxel is discontinued (61). Rarely a motor neuropathy has been re-

ported. The neuropathy is cumulative and only rarely (< 1% of patients) will require treatment to be discontinued.

Pharmacodynamic analysis of toxicity in phase II trials of docetaxel has demonstrated that patients with transaminases ≥ 1.5 × upper limits of normal and alkaline phosphatase ≥ 2.5 × upper limits of normal have increased risk of severe hematologic and non-hematologic toxicities. Extreme caution should be used in treating these patients.

Docetaxel is currently undergoing further testing including: (1) combination phase I studies with cisplatin, doxorubicin or 5-fluorouracil; (2) phase II trials in paclitaxel-resistant breast cancer, hormone-refractory prostate cancer, and cholangiocarcinoma; (3) phase III trials of both docetaxel versus best supportive care as second-line treatment for patients with non-small cell lung cancer and docetaxel versus paclitaxel in anthracycline-refractory breast cancer; (4) phase II and III trials in locally advanced breast cancer. Results of these further studies will help define docetaxel's role in the treatment of patients with cancer.

Topoisomerase I Inhibitors

Topoisomerase I inhibitors are an exciting new class of antineoplastic agents that are currently in clinical testing. This class of compounds is structurally related to the compound camptothecin, a natural product isolated from the Chinese plant, *Camptotheca acuminata* (62). Topoisomerase I is a cellular enzyme that is involved in maintaining the topographic structure of DNA during translation, transcription and mitosis (63). The double helix structure of DNA creates torsional strain in a cell that must be overcome in order for replication and translation to proceed. DNA topoisomerases are enzymes that control and modify the topological state of DNA by creating a transient break in a single strand

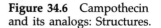

Figure 34.6 Campothecin and its analogs: Structures.

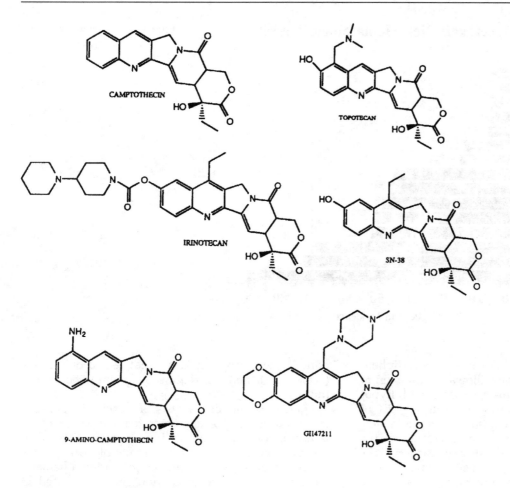

(topoisomerase I) or both complementary strands (topoisomerase II) of the DNA backbone (64). These enzymes are capable of catalyzing many types of interconversions between DNA topological isomers. Examples of interconversions include: catenation (to interlock DNA circles) and decatenation as well as knotting (passing one double strand of DNA through another strand of DNA) and unknotting (64). It is now established that the transient breakage of the DNA backbone by topoisomerases is accompanied by the formation of a covalent enzyme-DNA intermediate called the cleavable complex (65). The inhibition of topoisomerase I by camptothecin and its analogs is accomplished by stabilization of the enzyme-DNA cleavable complex. This occurs after the cleavage step and results in the trapping of the DNA and topoisomerase in the cleavable complex. When camptothecin is removed, the DNA is reannealed (the DNA backbone is resealed) and replication can proceed. This inhibition of topoisomerase I function inhibits cellular RNA and DNA synthesis. The mechanism of cell death by topoisomerase I inhibitors is presently unknown (66). Although topoisomerase inhibitors in clinical trials are all camptothecin analogs, there are significant differences in the biologic and pharmacologic properties which make each of these compounds distinctly different.

History of Topoisomerase I Inhibitors

Camptothecin

In the late 1950s, a crude extract of the oriental tree, *Camptotheca acuminata,* was found to have anticancer activity during extensive screening of random plant products by the Cancer Chemotherapy National Service Center (62). In 1966 Wall and co-workers (62) isolated camptothecin (Figure 34.6) which demonstrated significant anticancer activity in L1210 leukemia and Walker 256 carcinosarcoma (67, 68). In the preclinical studies, hemorrhagic enterocolitis was the major dose-limiting toxicity (69).

In the late 1960s and early 1970s, camptothecin underwent phase I and phase II testing. Phase I studies using single dose (69), daily (70), weekly (70) and daily × 5 (71) schedules of sodium camptothecin were performed. Although 5 of 18 patients demonstrated objective tumor responses in one phase I trial, further evaluation in phase II studies of patients with melanoma (72) and adenocarcinoma of the colon (73) were limited by severe hemorrhagic cystitis and unpredictable myelosuppression. As a result, further clinical development of camptothecin sodium was halted.

It wasn't until the 1980s, when the mechanism of action of camptothecin was identified as inhibition of

Table 34.4 Irinotecan phase II studies.

Tumor Type	Irinotecan Dose/Schedule	# Evaluable patients	Previous treatment	CR (%)	PR (%)	Reference
Non-Hodgkin's Lymphoma	40 mg/m^2/d × 5 200 mg/m^2 q 3–4 weeks, 20 mg/m^2/bid × 7, 40 mg/m^2/qd × 3 weekly	29	Yes	4 (14)	3 (10)	[79]
Non-Hodgkin's Lymphoma	40 mg/m^2/qd × 3 weekly	52	Yes	8 (15)	15 (29)	[80]
Hodgkin's Disease	40 mg/m^2/d × 5 200 mg/m^2 q 3–4 weeks 20 mg/m^2/bid × 7, 40 mg/m^2/qd × 3 weekly	3	Yes	0	1 (33)	[79]
Hodgkin's Lymphoma	40 mg/m^2/qd × 3 weekly	4	Yes	0	0	[80]
Acute Lymphoblastic Leukemia	40 mg/m^2/d × 5, 200 mg/m^2 q 3–4 weeks, 20 mg/m^2/bid × 7, 40 mg/m^2/qd × 3 weekly	11	Yes	1 (9)	1 (9)	[79]
Acute Myelocytic Leukemia	40 mg/m^2/d × 5 200 mg/m^2 q 3–4 weeks, 20 mg/m^2/bid × 7, 40 mg/m^2/qd × 3 weekly	15	Yes	0	1 (7)	[79]
Acute T-Cell Leukemia	40 mg/m^2/qd × 3 weekly	13	Yes	1 (8)	4 (31)	[81]
Colon Cancer	100 mg/m^2/w or 150 mg/m^2 qow	13	Yes	0	6 (46)	[82]
Colon Cancer	125 mg/m^2/weekly × 4 q 6 weeks	44	Yes	1 (2)	10 (23)	[83]
Colon Cancer	125 mg/m^2/weekly × 4 q 6 weeks	63	21 Yes 13 No	0 0	5 (24) 2 (15)	[84]
Colon Cancer	350 mg/m^2 Q 3 wks	85	Yes	0	12 (14)	[85]
Colon Cancer	350 mg/m^2 Q 3 wks	35	No	0	7 (20)	[86]
Colon Cancer	100 mg/m^{2}w or 150 mg/m^2 qow	63	Yes	0	17 (27)	[87]
Non-Small Cell Lung Cancer	100 mg/m^2/week	22	No	0	9 (40.9)	[88]
Non-Small Cell Lung Cancer	100 mg/m^2/week	67	No	0	23 (34)	[89]
Non-Small Cell Lung Cancer	100 mg/m^2/week	72	No	0	23 (32)	[90]
Non-Small Cell Lung Cancer	60 mg/m^{2}dl, 8,15 Cisplatin 80 mg/m^2 dl Q 28 days	69	No	1 (1)	32 (46)	[91]
Small Cell Lung Cancer	100 mg/m^2/w	35	Yes	2 (7)	7 (25)	[92]
Small Cell Lung Cancer	100 mg/m^2/week	15	Yes	0	7 (47)	[93]
Breast Cancer	350 mg/m^{2}Q 3 wks	12	Yes	1 (8)	0	[94]
Pancreas Cancer	100 mg/m^2/w or 150 mg/m^{2}qow	35	Yes	0	4 (11)	[95]
Gastric Cancer	100 mg/m^2/w or 150 mg/m^2 qow	60	Yes	0	14 (23)	[96]
Ovarian	100 mg/m^2/w, 150 mg/m^2 qow, 200 mg/m^2 q 3–4 weeks	14	Yes	1 (7)	2 (14)	[97]
Cervical	100 mg/m^2/w or 150 mg/m^2 qow	55	Yes	5 (10)	8 (15)	[98]

topoisomerase I, that interest in this class of compounds was rekindled. In addition, it was found that the lactone ring (E-ring, which is pH labile) was critical to the activity of camptothecin, and, thus, the sodium salt used in earlier trials (which mainly comprised the carboxylate (inactive) form) might have been the reason for the lack of antitumor activity observed (74). Structure-activity studies (75) were performed and it was discovered that modification of the A-ring improved water solubility and reduced protein binding. Therefore, analogues of camptothecin were developed with increased water solubility and decreased protein binding, with the anticipation of enhancing activity while decreasing the hemorrhagic cystitis and unpredictable myelosuppression. Currently, four analogues of camptothecin are in clinical development: topotecan, irinotecan (CPT-11), G1147211 and 9-aminocamptothecin (Figure 34.6).

Camptothecin is undergoing testing as an oral preparation. Giovanella and Natelson reported the preliminary results of a trial with oral camptothecin where the dose-limiting toxicity was gastrointestinal, 1 complete and 5 partial responses were noted in the 52 the patients treated (76).

Irinotecan (CPT-11)

Advantages For the Elderly Patient

- Activity in non-small cell lung and colorectal cancers
- Administration
- Synergism

Disadvantage For the Elderly Patient

- Toxicity profile

The initial preclinical and clinical development of irinotecan was in Japan. In preclinical testing, irinotecan was found to be active against a broad spectrum of tumor models (77). The decarboxylated metabolite SN-38 (7-ethyl-10-hydroxy-camptothecin) (Figure 34.6) plays the major role in the antitumor activity of irinotecan *in vivo* (78). Irinotecan was initially synthesized in 1981 and in 1986 phase I trials in Japan were initiated. Worldwide development began in France in 1990 and in the United States in 1991.

Advantages for the Elderly Patient

Activity in non-small cell lung and colorectal cancers

The single-agent activity of irinotecan has been evaluated in a number of tumor types including: non-Hodgkin's and Hodgkin's Lymphoma, acute leukemia, and colon, non-small cell and small cell lung, ovarian, cervical, breast, pancreatic, and gastric cancers (Table 34.4) (79–98). This encouraging activity seen in patients with refractory tumors, such as cervical cancer and colon cancer, has stimulated large phase II trials now being conducted in the United States and abroad.

Administration

The administration schedule has advantages for the elderly patient. Irinotecan is given intravenously over 90 minutes. The most commonly tested schedules are weekly for 4 weeks every 6 weeks and a single dose every 3 weeks. Other schedules, including an oral preparation, are being developed.

Synergism

Because of the novel mechanism of action and clinical activity, investigators have looked at combinations of irinotecan with other cytotoxic agents. *In vitro* and *in vivo* testing of camptothecin analogs has demonstrated inhibition of DNA repair as well as synergistic activity in combination with topoisomerase II inhibitors, alkylating agents, platinum compounds and radiation (99). Phase I trials of irinotecan in combination with other cytotoxic agents have been reported (Table 34.5) (100–107). Impressive activity has been demonstrated using combinations of cisplatin or etoposide with irinotecan in patients with non-small cell lung cancer, and this has prompted further development of these combinations.

Disadvantage for the Elderly Patient

Toxicity profile

The maximally-tolerated-dose (MTD) is dependent on the dose and schedule, with diarrhea and neutropenia being the major toxicities. Dosing schedules that employ a daily dose or a single dose every 3 weeks have demonstrated more neutropenia, while weekly schedules have been associated with significant diarrhea (Table 34.6) (108–116). The dose-intensity on all the schedules has remained approximately 100 mg/m²/week (Table 34.6). However, in a recently published study from France (110) escalation of the dose of irinotecan given over 90 minutes every three weeks could be accomplished with aggressive treatment of the diarrhea with antimotility agents. An MTD of 600 mg/m² every three weeks was reported with neutropenia being dose-limiting. Investigators in San Antonio are looking at age as a risk factor for the development of toxicity with irinotecan. Although neutropenia is common with irinotecan, other hematologic toxicities are generally mild with only a minority of patients developing grade 3/4 thrombocytopenia (4%) or anemia (16%).

Irinotecan is associated with two forms of diarrhea. The first type of diarrhea occurs during or just after the infusion of irinotecan and has a cholinergic mechanism. The use of atropine at the onset of this diarrhea is effective. The second type of diarrhea begins 3 to 5 days after the infusion of irinotecan and may be moderate to severe in 20% of patients. Aggressive treatment at the onset of the diarrhea with antimotility agents may obviate the severity of the diarrhea (Immodium 4 mg at the time of first loose stool then 2 mg every 2 hours until no bowel movements for 12 hours). If the diarrhea is not treated early, it usually runs a 5–7 day course. The mechanism of the diarrhea is unknown but may be secondary to the biliary excretion of the glucuronidated form of the active metabolite, SN-38 (108).

In addition to dose-limiting myelosuppression and diarrhea, other toxicities reported with irinotecan in-

Table 34.5 Irinotecan combination phase I studies.

Schedule	MTD CPT-II	MTD Other Agent	DLT	Responses (%) [tumor type]	Reference
CPT-11 dl, 8, 15, Cisplatin dl every 28 days	60	80	Neutropenia, diarrhea	13/23 (57%) [NSCLC]	[100]
CPT-11 dl, 8, 15, Cisplatin dl every 28 days ±G CSF	80	80	Diarrhea	10/20 (50%) [NSCLC]	[101]
CPT-11 dl, 8: Cisplatin dl: Vindesine dl, 8: every 28 days	37.5 with (1) or 80 with (2)	(1) Gisplatin 100 mg/m² or (2) 60 mg/m² + Vindesine 3 mg/m²	Neutropenia, diarrhea	4/9 (44%) [NSCLC]	[102]
CPT-11 dl, 8, 15, Cisplatin dl every 28 days	80	60	Diarrhea	6/14 (43%) [SCLC]	[103]
CPT-11 dl-3 Etoposide dl-3 q 28 days	60	60	Neutropenia	5/7 (71%) [NSCLC]	[104]
CPT-11 dl, 8, 15 Etoposide dl-3 q 28 days ±rhG-CSF	80	80	Neutropenia, diarrhea	2/9 (22%) [NSCLC] 7/12 (58%) [SCLC]	[105]
CPT-11 dl 5-FU Cl dl-7 q 28 days	225	400	Not reached	3/15 (20%) [Colon cancer]	[106]
CPT-11 dl Cisplatin CI dl-5 q 28 days	80	20	Neutropenia, diarrhea	9/20 (45%) [NSCLC]	[107]

Table 34.6 Irinotecan phase I studies.

Schedule	MTD (mg/m²)	Dose intensity (mg/m²/week)	Dose-limiting toxicity	Response	Reference
Single Q 21days	240	80	Neutropenia, diarrhea	1 PR colon 1 PR cervical	[108]
Single Q 21days	250	83	Neutropenia	Not reported	[109]
Single Q 21 days	600	200	Neutropenia 1 CR cervical 1 CR H & N	6 PR colon	[110]
Weekly	150	150	Neutropenia, diarrhea	2 PR NSCLC	[111]
Weekly	145	145	Neutropenia, diarrhea	1 PR	[112]
Weekly × 4 Q 6 weeks	180	120	Diarrhea	2 PR colon	[113]
Weekly × 4 Q 6 weeks	NR	NR	Diarrhea	NR	[114]
120 hour CI Q 21 days	200	67	Diarrhea	NR	[115]
QD × 3 Q 21 days	115 (QD)	115	Neutropenia 1 PR breast	1 PR mesothelioma	[116]

NR: Not Reported

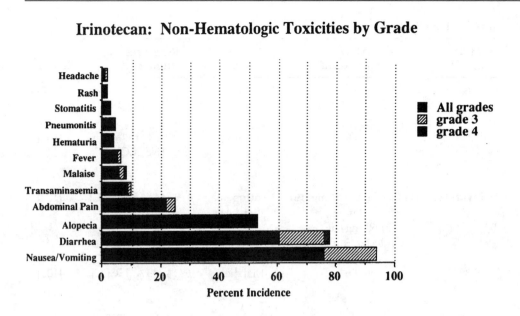

Figure 34.7 Irinotecan: Non-hematological toxicities by grade.

clude anemia, transaminasemia, anorexia, alopecia, malaise, flushing, stomatitis, pneumonitis, nausea and vomiting (Figure 34.7). These toxicities have been reported to be mild to moderate in severity and reversible with grade 3/4 toxicities reported infrequently, except for nausea/vomiting, anorexia, and the previously discussed diarrhea. Based on a retrospective analysis, it appears that age (> 65 years old) could be a risk factor for grade 3/4 diarrhea. This is now being examined in a prospective study with irinotecan in which patients are being stratified by age.

Topotecan

Advantages for the Elderly Patient

- Activity in patients with small cell lung and ovarian cancers
- Administration, oral schedule
- Synergism
- Toxicity profile

Disadvantage for the Elderly Patient

Pharamacokinetics

Topotecan is a semisynthetic analog of camptothecin that incorporates a stable basic side chain at the 9-position of the A-ring of 10-hydroxycamptothecin (Figure 34.6). The basic side chain of topotecan affords water solubility without requiring hydrolysis of the E-ring lactone.

Advantages for the Elderly Patient

Activity in small cell lung and ovarian cancers

Phase II activity of topotecan is summarized in Table 34.7 (117–126). Encouraging activity in patients with previously treated small cell lung and ovarian cancers has stimulated phase II and III trials in those patient populations. Results of these trial are expected in early 1996. Topotecan has also demonstrated activity in other tumor types seen in the elderly, including breast and non-small cell lung cancers. However, unlike irinotecan, no significant activity has been seen in patients with colorectal cancer.

Administration, oral schedule

Topotecan has minimal non-hematologic toxicities and can be given without intravenous hydration and often without antiemetic premedication. Both of these factors make topotecan appealing in the treatment of elderly patients. Topotecan has recently undergone testing as an oral preparation. The oral route has the potential advantage of ease of administration, and, in addition, the acidic pH of the stomach should maintain topotecan in the active closed lactone form. Creemers *et al.* (127) reported their experience with topotecan given orally on day one followed by an intravenous dose on day two. They found the oral form exhibited 32% bioavailability and was not affected by first-pass metabolism. Kuhn and colleagues (128) reported the use of single-dose oral topotecan compared to intravenous topotecan. They demonstrated oral bioavailability of 42% but > 100% bioequivalent toxicity. The single dose of oral topotecan of 14.0 mg/m^2 was found to have equivalent toxicities to 17.5 mg/m^2 of topotecan given intravenously. Current evaluation of topotecan orally for 5, 10 and 21 days is underway.

Synergism

Topotecan has demonstrated preclinical synergism when given in combination with topoisomerase II inhibitors, platinum compounds, alkylating agents and radiation. The role of topotecan in combination with other active antineoplastic agents is being determined. As with irinotecan, combination phase I studies with etoposide, doxorubicin, cisplatin, taxol and radiation have been reported (Table 34.8) (129–135). Encouraging responses have been reported in these combination trials.

Table 34.7 Topotecan phase II studies.

Tumor type	Regimen	# Evaluable patients	Previous Treatment	CR (%)	PR (%)	References
Small Cell Lung Caner	2.0 mg/m²/d × 5 days Q 21 days	18	No	0	7 (39)	[117]
Small Cell Lung Cancer (refractory)	1.5 mg/m²/d × 5 days Q 21 days	9	Yes	1 (11)	2 (22)	[118]
Small Cell Lung Cancer (sensitive)	1.5 mg/m²/d × 5 days Q 21 days	11	Yes	I (9)	3 (27)	[118]
Non-Small Cell Lung Cancer	1.5 mg/m²/d × 5 days Q 21 days	37	No	0	5 (14)	[119]
Non-Small Cell Lung Cancer	2.0 mg/m²/d × 5 days Q 21 days	20	No	0	0	[120]
Ovarian Cancer	1.5 mg/m²/d × 5 days Q 21 days	28	Yes	0	4 PR (14) 17 SD (61)	[121]
Head and Neck Cancer	1.5 mg/m²/d × 5 days Q 21 days	14	No	0	4 (29)	[122]
Soft Tissue Sarcoma	1.5 mg/m²/d × 5 days Q 21 days	16	No	0	2 (13)	[123]
Glioma	1.5 mg/m²/d × 5 days Q 21 days	12	Yes	1 (8)	1 (8)	[123]
Colon Cancer	1.5 mg/m²/d × 5 days Q 21 days	19	No	0	0	[124]
Pancreas Cancer	1.5 mg/m²/d × 5 days Q 21 days	15	No	0	0	[125]
Renal Cell Cancer	1.5 mg/m²/d × 5 day Q 21 days	IS	No	0	0	[126]

Table 34.8 Topotecan combination phase I studies.

Schedule	MTD Topotecan	MTD Other Agent	DLT	Responses (tumor type)	References
Topotecan QD × 5, Cisplatin dl every 21 days	0.75	50	Neutropenia Thrombocytopenia	Not reported	[129]
Topotecan QD × 5, Cisplatin d5 every 21 days	0.75	50	Neutropenia Thrombocytopenia	Not reported	[1291]
Topotecan QD × 5 wk 1 + 4 XRT 60 cGy over 6 wks	1. 0	60 cGy	Neutropenia Esophagitis	4/6 CR (67%) (NSCLC)	[130]
Topotecan 72 hr CI dl-3 Doxorubicin bolus d5	NS	NS	Not reached	1 PR SCLC 1 PR Bladder	[131]
Topotecan 72 hr CI dl-3 Etoposide d7-9 q 28 days	0.85	100	Neutropenia Thrombocytopenia	Not reported	[132]
Topotecan QD × 5 Taxol dl Q 21 days	1.0	80	Neutropenia	1 PR NSCLC	[133]
Topotecan QD × 5, Cisplatin dl every 21 days	1.0	75	Neutropenia Thrombocytopenia	2/10 (20%)	[134]
Topotecan QD × 5, Cisplatin dl every 21 days	1.0	75	Neutropenia	1 PR NSCLC	[135]

Table 34.9 Topotecan phase I studies.

Schedule	MTD (mg/m^2)	Dose Intensity (mg/m^2/week)	Dose-Limiting Toxicity	Response	Reference
Single Q 21 days	22.5	7.5	Neutropenia	1 MR NSCLC 1 MR Renal cell 1 MR Squamous cell	[136]
Single Q 21 days	22.5	7.5	Neutropenia	Not reported	[137]
Daily × 5 Q 21 days	2.5	4.2	Neutropenia	2 PR NSCLC 1 CR NSCLC 1 PR Ovarian	[1381]
Daily × 5 Q 21 d + GCSF	2.5	4.2	Neutropenia Thrombocytopenia	None	[139]
Daily × 5 Q 21 days	1.5	2.5	Neutropenia	1 PR NSCLC 1 PR SCLC	[140]
Daily × 5 Q 28 days	1.75	2.2	Neutropenia	1 PR esophageal	[141]
Daily × 5 Q 21 d + CCSF	1.5	2.5	Thrombocytopenia	None	[141]
Daily × 5 Q 21 d + CCSF (pediatric)	2.4	4.0	Neutropenia Thrombocytopenia	4 MR neuroblastoma	[142]
24 hour CI Q week	2.0	2.0	Neutropenia	1 PR colon	[143]
24 hour CI Q 21 days	8.4	2.8	Neutropenia Thrombocytopenia	None	[144]
24 hour CI Q 21 days	10	3.3	Neutropenia Thrombocytopenia	None	[145]
24 hour CI Q 21 d + CCSF	15	5.0	Thrombocytopenia	None	[145]
24 hour CI Q 21 days (pediatric)	7.5	2.5	Neutropenia Thrombocytopenia	None	[146]
72 hour CI Q 21 days (pediatrics)	1.0	1.0	Neutropenia	1 CR Neuroblastoma	[147]
72 hour CI Q week	0.7	2.0	Neutropenia	Not reported	[148]
72 hour CI Q 14 days	0.87	1.3	Neutropenia	Not reported	[148]
72 hour CI Q 21 days	1.6	1.6	Neutropenia Thrombocytopenia	1 MR NSCLC 2 MR Ovarian	[149]
120 hour CI Q 21 days	0.68	1.1	Neutropenia Thrombocytopenia	1 MR NSCLC 1 MR Ovarian	[149]
120 hour CI Q 21–28 days (leukemia)	2.1	2.6	Mucositis	1 CR AML/CML 2 PR AML	[150]
120 hour CI Q 21–28 days (leukemia)	2.1	2.6	Mucositis	1 CR CML 1 PR AML	[151]
21 day CI Q 28 days	0.53	2.8	Neutropenia Thrombocytopenia	1 PR Breast 2 PR Ovarian 1 PR Renal cell 1 PR NSCLC	[152]
24 hour CI Q 28 days (intraperitoneal)	4.0	1.0	Neutropenia	Ascites Reduction	[153]

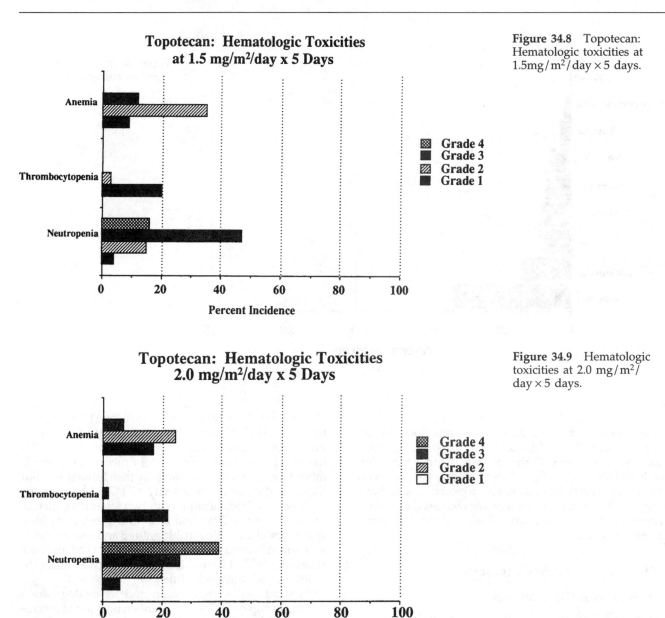

Figure 34.8 Topotecan: Hematologic toxicities at 1.5mg/m^2/day × 5 days.

Figure 34.9 Hematologic toxicities at 2.0 mg/m^2/day × 5 days.

Toxicity profile

Based on the preclinical activity seen with topotecan, a number of phase I clinical studies were initiated (Table 34.9) (136–153). To date, 18 phase I studies using 9 different schedules of topotecan have been reported. The dose-limiting toxicity observed with topotecan in all schedules (except in leukemia where mucositis was dose-limiting) has been myelosuppression, consisting of neutropenia and thrombocytopenia. The dose limiting hematologic toxicities are dose dependent (Figures 34.8 and 34.9). Neutropenia and mild thrombocytopenia were observed with the short infusion schedules, whereas schedules with longer infusion times experienced both dose-limiting neutropenia and thrombocytopenia. The neutropenia and thrombocytopenia have generally been short lived (less than 7 days) and rarely associated with fever. Non-hematologic toxicities have been mild and include nausea and vomiting, anorexia, diarrhea, alopecia, fatigue, and stomatitis (Figure 34.10). The mild non-hematologic toxicities make topotecan an attractive drug for the treatment of the elderly patients with cancer.

Because the major toxicities are hematologic, the use of G-CSF to further dose escalate topotecan has been explored (139, 141, 142, 145). Unfortunately, no significant dose escalation has been accomplished with the use of colony-stimulating factors, secondary to the development of thrombocytopenia as the dose-limiting toxicity (139).

Disadvantage for the Elderly Patient

Pharamacokinetics

Topotecan has also been evaluated in patients with hepatic or renal dysfunction. Patients with renal insuf-

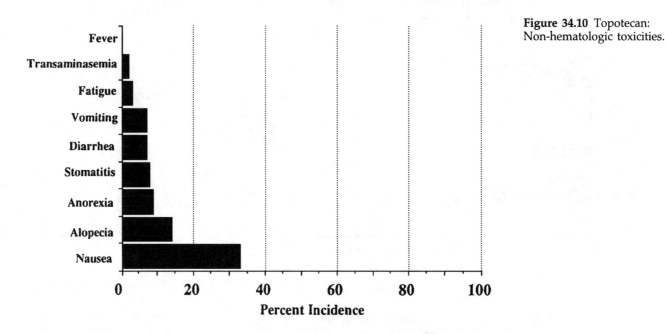

Figure 34.10 Topotecan: Non-hematologic toxicities.

ficiency had significantly decreased clearance and required dose reduction. Hepatic dysfunction did not change clearance and patients with hepatic dysfunction tolerated doses similar to those with normal hepatic function (154). Therefore in elderly patients with decreased creatinine clearance, topotecan will have decreased clearance and may have increased toxicities. These patients should have dose adjustments when given topotecan.

Other Topoisomerase I Inhibitors

9-Amino-20(S)-Camptothecin

9-amino-20(S)-camptothecin (9-AC) (Figure 34.6) has demonstrated potent preclinical activity. In potency studies conducted at the National Cancer Institute, 9-AC was found to be slightly more potent than topotecan and significantly more potent than CPT-11, but slightly less potent than SN-38 (the active metabolite of CPT-11) and camptothecin in measurements of DNA strand breaks and cytotoxicity against HT-29 cell lines. Clinical development of 9-AC has proceeded slowly due to its relative water insolubility. In a phase I study of 9-AC as a 72-hour continuous infusion in patients with solid tumors, dose-limiting neutropenia occurred at 59 mg/m^2/day (155). Other toxicities (all grade ≤ 2) included nausea, vomiting, mucositis, and diarrhea. Further dose escalation of 9-AC in combination with G-CSF is currently underway.

GI147211

GI147211 is a new water-soluble analog of camptothecin (Figure 34.6). In human tumor xenograft models, HT-29 and SW-48 (colon), PC-3 (prostate), and MX-1 (breast), GI147211 demonstrated activity 1.5–1.8 times greater than topotecan in suppressing growth. GI147211 has also been found to be 2.3–4.3 times more potent in inhibiting topoisomerase I activity than topotecan (156). Based on the preclinical activity, GI147211 has recently undergone clinical testing with two schedules, including daily for five days and a 72-hour continuous infusion every 21 days. Reversible grade 3 and 4 neutropenia and thrombocytopenia have been observed on both schedules (157). Phase II trials are underway using the daily for five days schedule.

In summary, camptothecin and its analogs are a unique group of anticancer agents with a novel mechanism of action. Encouraging phase I and II activity has stimulated further development of these agents alone and in combination with other cytotoxic agents. The ultimate role of these compounds in elderly patients is to be determined.

Gemcitabine

Advantages for the Elderly Patient

- Activity in patients with breast, non-small cell lung, pancreatic and ovarian cancers
- Administration

Disadvantage for the Elderly Patient

- Toxicity profile

Gemcitabine (2'2'-difluorodeoxycytidine; dFdC) is a synthetic pyrimidine antimetabolite structurally related to cytosine arabinoside (ara-C). It differs from the endogenous nucleoside, deoxycytidine, by the pres-

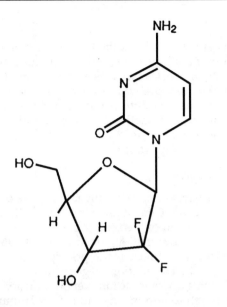

Figure 34.11 Gemicitabine: structure.

ence of two flourine atoms in its deoxyribofuranosyl ring (Figure 34.11). Gemcitabine was originally synthesized as an antiviral agent inhibiting both RNA and DNA viruses in cell culture. Its narrow therapeutic index during *in vivo* evaluation, however, precluded further development as an antiviral drug (158). It subsequently was found to have excellent *in vitro* antineoplastic activity in tumor cell lines, as well as broad-spectrum activity against a panel of murine solid tumors and human tumor xenografts (159, 160).

Gemcitabine's cytotoxic activity is due to the inhibition of DNA synthesis and repair. It is a pro-drug requiring intracellular metabolic activation to its phosphorylated forms by deoxycytidine kinase. Gemcitabine triphosphate competes with deoxycytidine triphosphate (dCTP) as a substrate for incorporation into DNA (161) Once incorporated into DNA, gemcitabine triphosphate causes a profound inhibition of DNA elongation and chain termination (162). Gemcitabine diphosphate is an inhibitory substrate for ribonucleotide reductase (RbNR) (163). This enzyme is required for the production of deoxynucleotides, which are used for DNA synthesis and repair. Cell death is a combination of these events and exhibits the morphological and biochemical characteristics of apoptosis (164).

Gemcitabine appears to have the ability to enhance its own activity (self-potentiation). Inhibition of ribonucleotide reductase causes lowering of intracellular dCTP levels. Through feedback mechanisms, low dCTP levels activate deoxycytidine kinase and inactivate dCMP deaminase, leading to increased phosphorylation (activation) and decreased deamination (elimination) of gemcitabine (165). Low intracellular levels of dCTP

Table 34.10 Phase II trials of gemcitabine.

Tumor Type	Dose (mg/m²) Schedule	Prior Chemotherapy	Response/ Evaluable Patients	Response Rate %	Reference
Non-small cell lung cancer	800–1000 weekly × 3	No	16/79	20	[167]
Non-small cell lung cancer	1000–1250 weekly × 3	No	15/76 (2 CR's)	20	[168]
Non-small cell lung cancer	1250 weekly × 3	No	19/93 (1 CR)	20	[169]
Non-small cell lung cancer	1000–1750 weekly × 3	No	4/19	21	[170]
Non-small cell lung cancer	1000–1250 weekly × 3	Not Stated	11/37	30	[171]
Non-small cell lung cancer	1000–1250 weekly × 3	Not Stated	9/37	24	[171]
Non-small cell lung cancer	90 twice weekly	No	5/40	13	[172]
Small cell lung cancer	1000–1250 weekly × 3	No	7/26 (1 CR)	27	[173]
Gastric cancer	1000 weekly × 3	No	1/26	4	[174]
Gastric cancer	800 weekly × 3	No	0/15	0	[175]
Malignant melanoma	1000 weekly × 3	No	1/33	3	[174]
Ovarian Cancer	800 weekly × 3	Yes	8/42	19	[176]
Squamous cell of head and neck	800–1250 weekly × 3	Yes	7/54	13	[177]
Breast cancer	800 weekly × 3	Yes	9/35	29	[178]
Renal cell cancer	800–1250 weekly × 3	No	1/18	6	[179]
Renal cell cancer	800 weekly × 3	No	3/30 (1 CR)	10	[180]
Pancreas	800–1250 weekly × 3	No	5/39	13	[181]
Pancreas	800–1000 weekly × 3	No	2/23	9	[182]
Colon cancer	800 weekly × 3	Not stated	0/14	0	[183]
Colon cancer	1000 weekly × 3	No	1/25	4	[184]

also enhance gemcitabine triphosphate's incorporation into DNA due to competition for DNA polymerase. These mechanisms may explain the increased cellular accumulation and increased activity seen in solid tumors with gemcitabine as compared to ara-C.

Advantages for the Elderly Patient

Activity in breast, non-small cell lung, pancreatic and ovarian cancers

Clinical activity was demonstrated in patients with non-small cell lung, pancreatic, breast, head and neck, bladder, renal cell and colon cancers. Among the several dosing schedules studied (daily times five, twice a week, weekly, and biweekly), the weekly schedule was chosen for phase II trials due to safety profile, adequate dose intensity and preclinical data suggesting schedule-related efficacy (166).

Based on the activity profile seen in phase I trials, broad phase II testing with gemcitabine is being conducted in a wide variety of malignancies. As summarized in Table 34.10 (167–184), activity has been confirmed in patients with small cell and non small cell lung, breast, ovarian, pancreatic cancers and with squamous cell carcinoma of the head and neck.

Clinical benefit as assessed by change in pain, performance status and weight is the primary objective of two ongoing trials with gemcitabine in patients with advanced pancreatic cancer (185).

Gemcitabine's favorable toxicity profile makes it an attractive candidate for combination therapy with other antineoplastic agents. Several trials utilizing gemcitabine with other agents such as cisplatin, carboplatin, taxol and hydroxyurea are currently underway.

Administration

The most commonly studied schedule of gemcitabine is a 30-minute infusion given weekly for 3 weeks followed by 1 week rest. This administration schedule does not require prehydration or anaphylactic prophylaxis. The nausea and vomiting are well controlled with routine antiemetics. This ease of administration makes gemcitabine attractive for the treatment of elderly patients with cancer.

Pharmacokinetics

The pharmacokinetics of gemcitabine have been extensively studied. Gemcitabine undergoes intracellular phosphorylation by deoxycytidine kinase to its active metabolites. Deamination to uridine metabolites (dFdU) by cytidine deaminase is the principal mechanism involved in the elimination of gemcitabine.

Following a 30-minute intravenous infusion, gemcitabine has a short terminal half-life of 4–20 minutes (186). Its deaminated metabolite (dFdU), however, has a much longer half-life ranging from 4–24 hours. Gemcitabine clearance was found to be lower in women than in men, perhaps related to differences in the activity of cytidine deaminase (187).

Disadvantage for the Elderly Patient

Toxicity profile

Results of single-agent phase I trials are summarized in Table 34.11 (188–195). Dose-limiting toxicity has been found to be particularly schedule-dependent (i.e., there is a marked difference in the maximally tolerated dose, dependent on the schedule of administration). Because

Table 34.11 Phase I trials of gemcitabine.

Schedule	Dose Range (mg/m²)	MTD (mg/m²)	Toxicity	Responses	Reference
Daily × 5 (30 min inf)	1–12	9	Flu-like symptoms, Hypotension	None	[188]
Twice weekly (30 min inf)	5–90	75	Thrombocytopenia fever	Renal cell	[189]
Twice weekly (5 min inf)	30–150	150	Thrombocytopenia fever	None	[189]
Weekly × 3 q 4wks 24 hr inf)	10–180	Not reached	Neutropenia	NSCLC	[190]
Weekly × 3 q 4wks (30 min inf)	10–1000	790	Thrombocytopenia, Anemia, granulocytopenia	Colon, NSCL C	[191]
Weekly × 3 q 4wks × (30 min inf)	300–1370	1370	Myelosuppression	Bladder	[192]
Weekly × 3 q 4wks (30 min inf)	1000–2200	1500	Myelosuppression, Reversible hepatotoxicity, flu-like symptoms	NSCLC	[193]
Weekly × 3 q 4wks (30 min inf)	1000–1750	1750	Reversible myelosuppression	NSCLC	[170]
Every other week (4 hr inf)	1000–5700	3600	Myelosuppression, rash	Breast, pancreas head and neck	[194]
Every other week (30 min inf)	40–5700	4560	Myelosuppression reversible hepatoxicity	Breast	[195]

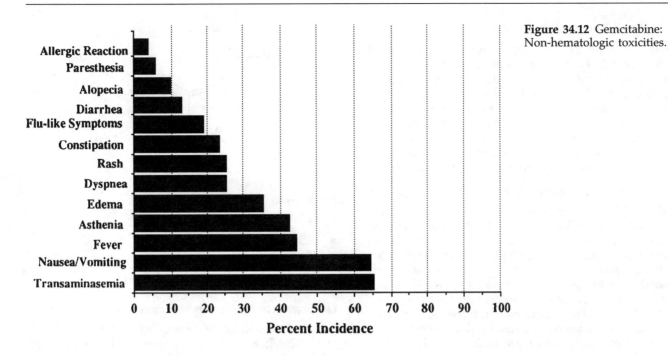

Figure 34.12 Gemcitabine: Non-hematologic toxicities.

toxicities for gemcitabine are generally mild to moderate, the elderly population generally tolerate gemcitabine well (Figure 34.12). However, the non-hematologic toxicities which can be seen with this agent may not be as well tolerated in patients who are elderly compared to those who are younger. Toxicities have included myelosuppression, reversible skin rash, fever, mild nausea and vomiting, alopecia, lethargy, a flu-like syndrome, peripheral edema and reversible elevations in liver function tests (170, 188–195). Cumulative toxicity has not been observed. Less frequent dosing schedules demonstrate more hematologic and fewer non-hematologic toxicities.

Thymidylate Synthase Inhibitors

Thymidylate synthase is an enzyme which catalyzes the conversion of DUMP by reductive methylation into deoxythymidine monophosphate (dTM) and dihydrofolate. This reaction requires the presence of a reduced folate cofactor and provides the precursor of deoxythymidine triphosphate (dTT), one of the deoxyribonucleotides necessary for DNA synthesis. Inhibition of thymidylate synthase is probably the most important mechanism of action of 5-FU and related compounds. Total thymidylate synthase activity is measured by a catalytic assay (the capacity to convert DUMP to dTM) and thymidylate synthase inhibition has been shown to correlate with response to 5-FU (196). An array of new agents has been developed to produce a more effective inhibition of this enzyme.

Tomudex

Advantages for the Elderly Patient

- Activity in non-small cell lung and colorectal cancers

- Schedule
- Toxicity profile and polyglutamation

Tomudex (ZD1694, ICI D1694) was synthesized as an alternative to the agent CB3717, a quinazoline-based thymidylate synthase inhibitor that competes with reduced folates, producing potent inhibition of the enzyme. Unfortunately, CB3717 has poor aqueous solubility and produces life-threatening nephrotoxicity and dose-independent hepatotoxicity. Tomudex, however, has the advantage of water solubility and rapid intracellular polyglutamation. The polyglutamate derivatives are more active against thymidylate synthase and are retained longer intracellularly giving this compound more efficacy *in vivo* (197).

Advantages for the Elderly Patient

Activity in non-small cell lung and colorectal cancers

Tomudex has demonstrated activity in the majority of tumors found in elderly patients. In phase II trials of tomudex using the 3 mg/m^2 dose, significant activity has been demonstrated in patients with advanced colorectal carcinoma (31/124 patients [25%] with 2 complete responses) and those with breast cancer (11/45 patients [24%] with 2 complete responses), as well as in patients with pancreatic, non-small cell lung and ovarian cancers (198). Minimal toxicity was observed on these trials. Phase III trials will randomize patients with colorectal cancer between tomudex and a standard 5-day regimen of 5-FU/leucovorin.

Schedule

Tomudex has a favorable dosing schedule of once every 21 days. No hydration or antiemetics are required for treatment with tomudex.

Toxicity profile and polyglutamation

Phase I trials in Europe with tomudex recommended a dose of 3.0 mg/m² over 15 minutes every 21 days. Dose-limiting toxicities were diarrhea, neutropenia, malaise and asthenia. Escalation of this drug up to 4.5 mg/m² has been reported, with a recommended phase II dose of 4 mg/m² (198). These higher doses of tomudex have demonstrated increased myelosuppression and hepatic transaminasemia. Because tomudex is polyglutamated, prolonged toxicities have been reported.

Other Thymidylate Synthase Inhibitors

Other folate antimetabolites undergoing clinical trials are AG-331 and LY231514. AG-331 lacks a glutamate moiety but is very lipophilic which facilitates tissue penetration. The lack of polyglutamation contributes to its favorable toxicity profile. Phase I trials with both 1- and 24-hour continuous infusions of AG-331, daily for 5 days, are currently being conducted.

LY231514 undergoes extensive intracellular polyglutamation producing a more sustained drug effect. Data from two phase I studies are available (199). In the first study the drug was administered weekly for 4 weeks every 42 days. Dose-limiting neutropenia was encountered at 40 mg/m²/week. Two minor responses in patients with colorectal cancer were documented. In the second study, the drug was administered as a single dose every 21 days. Reversible neutropenia was the dose-limiting toxicity with dose escalation up to 700 mg/m². Minor responses in 6 patients with colorectal cancer and in 1 patient with pancreatic cancer were reported.

Dipyrimidine Dehydrogenase Inhibitors

776C85

776C85 is 5-Ethynyluracil, which binds to dipyrimidine dehydrogenase and irreversibly inactivates it. This drug has been demonstrated to markedly increase the area under the concentration/time curve, oral bioavailability and therapeutic index of 5-FU in animals (200). Recent data in animals suggest that this compound is considerably more effective than high-dose uracil in sustaining plasma 5-FU generated from ftorafur (201). In addition, 776C85 has been shown in dogs to protect against 5-FU-induced neurotoxicity. This may occur through the inhibition of the formation of neurotoxic catabolites or through the protection conferred by high serum levels of uracil (202). Phase I trials testing this drug in combination with 5-FU (with or without leucovorin modulation) are currently underway in San Antonio and at the University of Chicago. To date no toxicity has been demonstrated for 776C85 alone. In combination with 5-FU at doses of 20 mg/m²/day daily × 5, grade 3 leucopenia and grade 2 mucositis have been seen (203). The study is ongoing.

Temozolomide

Advantages for the Elderly Patient

- Activity in melanoma and glioma

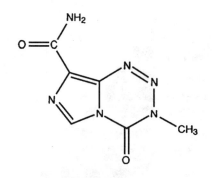

Figure 34.13 Temozolomide: Structure.

- Schedule
- Toxicity profile

Disadvantage for the elderly patient

Unknown activity in common tumors of the elderly

Temozolomide (NSC 362856; CCRG 81045; M&B 39831; SCH 52365; 8-carbamoyl-3-methyl-imidazo[5,1-d]-1,2,3,5-tetrazin-4(3H)-one) (Figure 34.13) is an analog of dacarbazine displaying similar broad spectrum activity in mouse tumors, but showing considerably less myelosuppression in the toxicology screen. Temozolomide undergoes chemical degradation to its active metabolite MTIC, whereas dacarbazine undergoes metabolic degradation to MTIC (Figure 34.14). The chemical degradation of temozolomide may decrease some of the unpredictable myelosuppression seen with dacarbazine.

Advantages for the Elderly Patient

Activity in melanoma and glioma

In phase I studies, clinical activity was observed using the 5 day schedule in 4 (2CR, 2PR; 17%) out of 23 patients with melanoma and in 1 patient with mycosis fungoides (CR lasting 7 months). Two patients with recurrent, high-grade gliomas also had partial responses.

Temozolomide has been evaluated in patients with primary brain tumors (204). Twenty-eight patients with primary brain tumors were given 150 mg/m²/day of temozolomide for 5 days. If no significant myelosuppression was noted on day 22, the dose was escalated to 200 mg/m²/day for 5 days for subsequent courses. All patients received oral ondansetron prior to dosing with temozolomide with no significant gastrointestinal toxicities noted. A major response was noted in 5 of 10 patients with astrocytomas recurrent after radiotherapy, with one further patient demonstrating a clinical response with a minor improvement on CT scan. Reduction in the size of the CT lesion was also observed in 4 of 7 patients with newly diagnosed high-grade astrocytomas given 2–3 courses of temozolomide prior to irradiation. One patient with recurrent medulloblastoma had a clinical response in bone metastases. Temozolomide was found to be well tolerated with predictable myelosuppression.

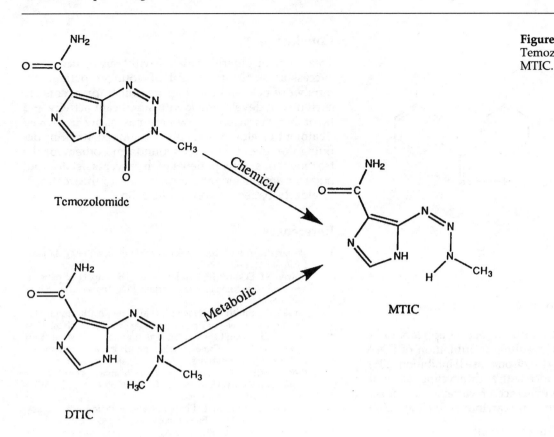

Figure 34.14 Conversion of Temozolomide and DTIC to MTIC.

Schedule

Initial phase I studies of temozolomide were performed using a single intravenous dosing schedule (205). A total of 51 patients were entered on the single dose schedule with doses of 50–1200 mg/m². Temozolomide exhibited linear pharmacokinetics with dose escalation. Myelotoxicity was dose-limiting. No antitumor activity was seen on this schedule. Secondary to the schedule dependency of temozolomide, a phase I study of the oral administration daily × 5 was initiated with dose escalation to a total dose of 750 to 1,200 mg/m² in 42 patients. The oral preparation was found to be well tolerated and myelosuppression was again dose-limiting. This oral route of administration makes temozolomide an appealing treatment for elderly patients.

Toxicity profile

In phase I studies of oral temozolomide given on a daily × 5 schedule, toxicities were mainly myelosuppression and nausea. The recommended dose for Phase II trials is 150 mg/m² oral for 5 days (total dose 750 mg/m²) for the first course, and if no major myelosuppression is detected on day 22 of the 4-week cycle, then subsequent courses can be given at 200 mg/m² for 5 days. No cumulative myelosuppression has been reported with temozolomide. Mild to moderate nausea and vomiting were dose related but readily controlled with antiemetics. This mild toxicity profile makes temozolomide an encouraging new treatment for elderly patients.

Disadvantage for the Elderly Patient

Unknown activity in common tumors of the elderly

The activity of temozolomide in other solid tumors is not known. Future plans for temozolomide include the evaluation of combination regimens with a nitrosourea secondary to the preclinical synergism seen with these two agents. Also further phase II testing in primary brain tumors and melanoma is underway. The ease of oral administration and the documented activity in tumors which are generally resistant to chemotherapy make temozolomide attractive for the treatment of elderly patients with cancer. Evaluation of temozolomide in tumor types common to the elderly is needed to better define the role of temozolomide in the treatment of this patient population.

Losoxantrone

Advantages for the Elderly Patient

- Activity in breast cancer
- Toxicity profile

Losoxantrone is a member of the anthrapyrazole family of antineoplastic agents synthesized in an attempt to retain the antitumor activity of the anthracyclines while reducing the risk for cardiotoxicity. The cardiac toxicity of the anthracyclines is believed to result from the formation of free radicals, which damage the myocardial sarcoplasmic reticulum. The anthrapyrazoles were created by modification of the chromophore ring of the anthracenedione structure in order to de-

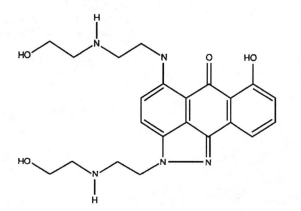

Figure 34.15 Losoxantrone: Structure.

crease the potential for free radical formation (Figure 34.15).

The mechanism of antitumor action appears to be intercalation of DNA, resulting in inhibition of DNA and RNA synthesis via topoisomerase II inhibition (206). Although cross-resistance with anthracyclines is usual, there has been some evidence of variable non-cross-resistance in some mammary carcinoma cell lines (207).

Advantages for the Elderly Patient

Activity in breast cancer

Encouraging results for losoxantrone have been seen in phase II studies. Losoxatrone has been studied as a single agent in advanced breast cancer in doses of 50 mg/m² every 3 weeks. The overall objective response rate was 63% in patients with chemotherapy-naive breast cancer, with 2 patients (7%) experiencing a complete response (208). In a second study of losoxantrone in previously treated and untreated patients with metastatic breast cancer, responses were demonstrated in 35% and 43% of the patients, respectively.

Losoxantrone has also recently been reported to have activity in patients with hormone-refractory prostate cancer. Twenty patients were treated with 50 mg/m² of losoxantrone. Sixty percent of patients with pain had improvement in symptoms, with 25% of patients demonstrating > 50% decline in PSA values (209).

Toxicity profile

The toxicity profile of losoxantrone is similar to the other anthrapyrazoles. Dose-limiting toxicity in phase I trials was myelosuppression, predominantly neutropenia. Cardiac toxicity has been reported and has consisted mainly of asymptomatic ECG changes or small declines in left ventricular ejection fraction (208). Non-hematologic toxicities are mild, consisting of nausea and vomiting, alopecia, stomatitis, diarrhea, fatigue and phlebitis.

Currently trials of losoxantrone in combination with taxol (210) and cyclophosphamide (211) are underway.

Conclusion

Treatment of elderly patients with cancer can be as successful as the treatment of younger patients. A number of new and exciting chemotherapy agents are currently in development with significant activity and favorable characteristics which may allow improved treatment of elderly patients. Continued work in defining the role of these compounds and others for the treatment of elderly patients with cancer is needed, but hope for novel chemotherapy options for the treatment of elderly patients is on the horizon.

References

1. Wingo PA, Tong T, Bolden S. Cancer Statistics, 1995. *CA Cancer J Clin* **45**(1): 8–30, 1995.
2. Bowen KJ, Eckardt JR, Clark G, et al. The impact of patients' age on the outcome of phase I trials. *Proc Am Soc Clin Onc* **12**: 184, 1993.
3. Jones AL, Smith IE. Navelbine and the Anthrapyrazoles. *Hematology/Oncology Clinics of North America* **8**(1): 141–52, 1994.
4. Benit S, Chaineau E, Fellous A, et al. Immunofluorescent study of the action of navelbine, vincristine and vinblastine on mytotic and axonal microtubules. *Int J Cancer* **46**: 262, 1990.
5. Binet S, Fellous A, Lataste H, et al. *In situ* analysis of the action of navelbine on various types of microtubles using immunofluorescence. *Semin Oncol* **16**: 5–8, 1989.
6. Mathe G, Reizenstein P. Phase I pharmacologic study of a new vinca alkaloid. Navelbine. *Cancer Let* **27**: 285–93, 1985
7. Favre R, Garnier G, Depierre A, et al. A phase I study of (nov-5'-anhydrovinblastine). *Recent Adv Chemother*, pp. 641–2, 1985.
8. Furuse K, Niitani H, Wakui A, et al. Phase I study on vinorelbine (Navelbine) by single or intermittent administration. *Invest New Drugs* **7**: 456 1989.
9. Izzo J, Toussaint C, Chabot G, et al. High activity and dose-intensity relationship in advanced breast cancer with continuous infusion of navelbine. *Proc Am Soc Clin Oncol* **11**: 71, 1992.
10. Favre R, Delgado M, Bsenval M, et al. Phase I trial of escalating doses of orally administered Navelbine (NVB). Part II—Clinical results. *Proc Am Soc Clin Oncol* **8**: 64, 1989.
11. Bowen K, Burris H, Rodriguez G, et al. A phase I trial of chronic oral Navelbine administration. *Proc Am Assoc Cancer Res* **33**: 519, 1992.
12. Hohneker JA. A summary of Vinorelbine (Navelbine) safety data from North American clinical trials. *Semin Oncol* **21**(5) suppl 10: 42–7, 1994.
13. Hortobagyi G. Future directions for vinorelbine (Navelbine). *Semin Oncol* **22**(2) suppl 5: 80–87, 1995.
14. Furuse K, Kubota K, Kawahara M, et al. A phase II study of vinorelbine, a new derivative of vinca alkaloid, for previously untreated advanced non-small cell lung cancer. Japan Vinorelbine Study Group. *Lung Cancer* **11**: 385–91, 1994.
15. Colleoni M, Gaion F, Nelli P, et al. Weekly vinorelbine in elderly patients with non-small cell lung cancer. *Tumori* **80**(6): 448–52, 1994.
16. Vokes EE, Rosenberg RK, Jahanzeb M, et al. Multicenter phase II study of weekly oral vinorelbine for stage IV non-small cell lung cancer. *J Clin Oncol* **13**(3): 637–44, 1995.
17. Le Chevalier T, Pujol JL, Douillard JY, et al. A three-arm trial of vinorelbine (navelbine) plus cisplatin, vindesine plus cisplatin and single-agent vinorelbine in the treatment of non-small cell lung cancer An expanded analysis. *Semin Oncol* **21**(5) suppl 10: 28–33, 1994.
18. Depierre A, Chastang C, Quoix E, et al. Vinorelbine versus vinorelbine plus cisplatin in advanced non-small cell lung cancer. A randomized trial. *Ann Oncol* **5**(1): 37–42, 1994.
19. Wargin WA, Lucas VS. The clinical pharmacokinetics of Vinorelbine (Navelbine). *Semin Oncol* **21**(5) suppl 10: 21–27, 1994.

20. Cassidy J, Kaye SB. New drugs in clinical development in Europe. *Hematology/Oncology Clinics of North America* 8(2): 289–303, 1994.

21. Ringel I, Horwitz SB. Studies with RP56976 (taxotere): a semi-synthetic analogue of taxol. *J Natl Cancer Inst* 83(4): 288–91, 1991.

22. Extra JM, Rousseau F, Bruno R, et al. Phase I and pharmaco-kinetic study of taxotere (RP 56976, NSC 628503) given as a short intravenous infusion. *Cancer Res* 53(5): 1037–42, 1993.

23. Burris H, Irvin R, Kuhn J, et al. Phase I clinical trial of taxotere administered as either a 2 or 6 hour intravenous infusion. *J Clin Oncol* 11(5). 950–8, 1993.

24. Bissett D, Setenoians A, Cassidy J, et al. Phase I and phar-macokinetic study of taxotere (RP 56976) administered as a 24-hour infusion. *Cancer Res* 53(3): 523–7, 1993.

25. Pazdur R, Newman RA, Newman BM, et al. Phase I trial of taxotere. Five-day schedule. *J Natl Cancer Inst* 84(23): 1781–8, 1992.

26. Tomiak E, Piccart MJ, Kerger, et al. Phase I study of docetaxel administered as a 1-hour intravenous infusion on a weekly basis. *J Clin Oncol* 12(7): 1458–67, 1994.

27. Ten Bokkel Huinink WW, Prove AM, Piccart M, et al. A phase II trial with docetaxel (taxotere) in second line treatment with chemotherapy for advanced breast cancer. A study of the EORTC Early Clinical Trials Group. *Ann Oncol* 5(6): 527–32, 1994.

28. Valero V, Walters R, Theriault R, et al. Phase II study of docetaxel (Taxotere) in anthracycline-refractory metastatic breast cancer (ARMBC). *Proc Am Soc Clin Oncol* 13: 470, 1994.

29. Dieras V, Fumoleau P, Chevallier B, et al. Second EORTC-clinical screening group (CSG) Phase II trial of Taxotere (docetaxel) as first line chemotherapy (CT) in advanced breast cancer (ABC). *Proc Am Soc Clin Oncol* 13: 78, 1994.

30. Trudeau ME, Eisenhauer E, Lofters W, et al. Phase II study of Taxotere as first line chemotherapy for metastatic breast cancer. A National Cancer Institute of Canada Clinical Trials Group (NCIC CTG) study. *Proc Am Soc Clin Oncol* 12: 64, 1993.

31. Seidman AD, Hudis C, Crown JP, et al. Phase II evaluation of Taxotere (RP56976, NSC628503) as initial chemotherapy for metastatic breast cancer. *Proc Am Soc Clin Oncol* 12: 63, 1993.

32. Cerny T, Kaplan S, Pavlidis N, et al. Docetaxel (taxotere) is active in non-small cell lung cancer. A phase II trial of the EORTC Early Clinical Trials Group (ECTG). *Br J Cancer* 70(2): 384–7, 1994.

33. Rigas JR, Francis PA, Kris MG, et al. Phase II trial of Taxotere in non-small cell lung cancer (NSCLC). *Proc Am Soc Clin Oncol* 12: 336, 1993.

34. Burris H, Eckardt J, Fields S, et al. Phase II trials of Taxotere in patients with non small cell lung cancer. *Proc Am Soc Clin Oncol* 12: 335, 1993.

35. Fossella FV, Lee JS, Shin DM, et al. Taxotere (docetaxel. DTXL), an active agent for platinum-refractory non-small cell lung cancer (NSCLC). Preliminary report of a Phase II study. *Proc Am Soc Clin Oncol.* 13: 336, 1994.

36. Watanabe K, Yokoyama A, Furuse K, et al. Phase II trial of docetaxel in previously untreated non-small cell lung cancer (NSCLC). *Proc Am Soc Clin Oncol* 13: 331, 1994.

37. Fossella FV, Lee JS, Murphy WK, et al. Phase II study of docetaxel for recurrent or metastatic non-small-cell lung cancer. *J Clin Oncol* 12(6): 1238–44, 1994.

38. Francis P, Hakes T, Schneider J, et al. Phase II study of docetaxel (Taxotere) in advanced platinum-refractory ovarian cancer (ca). *Proc Am Soc Clin Oncol* 13: 260, 1994.

39. Kavanagh J, Kudelka A, Freedman R, et al. Taxotere (docetaxel). Activity in platinum refractory ovarian cancer and amelioration of toxicity. *Proc Am Soc Clin Oncol* 13: 237, 1994.

40. Aapro M, Pujade-Lauraine E, Lhomme C, et al. Phase II study of Taxotere (T) in ovarian cancer: EORTC Clinical Screening Group (CSG). *Proc Am Soc Clin Oncol* 12: 256, 1993.

41. Sadan S, Bajorin D, Amsterdam A, et al. Docetaxel in pahents with advanced transitional cell cancer (TCC) who failed cisplatin-based chemotherapy. A Phase II trial. *Proc Am Soc Clin Oncol* 13: 244, 1994.

42. Einzig AI, Schuchter LM, Wadler S, et al. Phase II trial of Taxotere (RP 56976) in patients (pts) with metastatic melanoma previously untreated with cytotoxic chemotherapy. *Proc Am Soc Clin Oncol* 13: 395, 1994.

43. Bedikian A, Legha S, Eton O, et al. Phase II trial of docetaxel (taxotere, RP 56976) in patients with advanced cutaneous malignant melanoma (ACMM) previously untreated with chemo-Rx. *Proc Am Assoc Cancer Res* 35: 86, 1994.

44. Rougier P, De Forni M, Adenis A, et al. Phase II study of Taxotere (RP56976, docetaxel) in pancreatic adenocarcinoma (PAC). *Proc Am Soc Clin Oncol* 13: 200, 1994.

45. Mertens WC, Eisenhauer EA, Jolivet J, et al. Docetaxel in advanced renal carcinoma. A phase II trial of the National Cancer Institute of Canada Clinical Trials Group. *Ann Oncol* 5(2): 185–7, 1994.

46. Van Hoesel QG, Verweij J, Catimel G, et al. Phase II study with docetaxel (taxotere) in advanced soft tissue sarcomas. *Ann Oncol* 5(6): 539–42, 1994.

47. Dreyfuss A, Clark J, Norris C, et al. Taxotere (TXTR) for advanced, incurable squamous cell carcinoma of the head and neck (SCCHN). *Proc Am Soc Clin Oncol* 13: 287, 1994.

48. Catimel G, Verweij J, Mattijssen V, et al. Docetaxel (taxotere). An active drug for the treatment of patients with advanced squamous cell carcinoma of the head and neck. EORTC Early Clinical Trials Group. *Ann Oncol* 5(6): 533–7, 1994.

49. Clark T, Kemeny N, Conti JA, et al. Phase II trial of docetaxel (Taxotere, RP56976) in previously untreated patients (pts) with advanced colorectal cancer (CRC). *Proc Am Soc Clin Oncol* 13: 212, 1994.

50. Pazdur R, Lassere Y, Soh L, et al. Phase II trial of docetaxel (taxotere) in metastatic colorectal carcinoma. *Ann Oncol* 5(6): 468–70, 1994.

51. Sternberg CN, Ten Bokkel Huinink WW, Smyth JF, et al. Docetaxel (taxotere), a novel taxoid, in the treatment of advanced colorectal carcinoma. An EORTC Early Clinical Trials Group study. *Br J Cancer* 70(2): 376–9, 1994.

52. Sulkes A, Smyth J, Sessa C, et al. Docetaxel (taxotere) in advanced gastric cancer: results of a phase II clinical trial. EORTC Early Clinical Trials Group. *Br J Cancer* 70(2): 380–3, 1994.

53. Bruno R, Cosson V, Vergniol JC, et al. Taxotere population pharmacokinetics. *Proc Am Assoc Cancer Res* 34: 234, 1993.

54. De Valeriola D, Brassinne C, Gaillard C, et al. Study of excretion balance, metabolism, and protein binding of ¹⁴C radiolabelled taxotere (RP 56976, NSC 628503) in cancer patients. *Proc Am Assoc Cancer Res* 34: 373, 1993.

55. Lavelle F, Bissery MC, Combeau C, et al. Preclinical evaluation of docetaxel (taxotere). *Semin Oncol* 22(2) suppl 10: 3–16, 1995.

56. Wanders J, Schrijvers D, Bruntsch U, et al. The EORTC-ECTG experience with acute hypersensitivity reactions (HSR) in taxotere studies. *Proc Am Soc Clin Oncol* 12: 73, 1993.

57. Wanders J, Van Oosterom A, Gore M, et al. Taxotere toxicity effects of premedication. *Eur J Cancer* 29A(6). S206, 1993.

58. Oulid-Aissa D, Behar A, Speilmann M, et al. Management of fluid retention syndrome in patients treated with taxotere (docetaxel). Effect of premedication. *Proc Am Soc Clin Oncol.* 13: 465, 1994.

59. Zimmerman GC, Keeling JH, Burris HA, et al. Acute cutaneous reactions to docetaxel, a new chemotherapeutic agent. *Arch Dermatol* 131(2): 202–6, 1995.

60. Eisenhauer EA, Lu F, Muldal A, et al. Predictors and treatment of docetaxel toxic effects. *Ann Oncol* 5(5): 202, 1994.

61. New P. Neurotoxicity of taxotere. *Proc Am Assoc Cancer Res* 34: 233, 1993.

62. Wall ME, Wani MC, Cook CE, et al. Plant antitumor agents. 1. The isolation and structure of camptothecin, a novel alkaloidal leukemia and tumor inhibitor from Camptotheca Acuminata. *J Amer Chem Soc* 88: 3888–90, 1966.

63. Zijlstra JG, De Jong S, De Vries, et al. Topoisomerases, new targets in cancer chemotherapy. *Med Oncol Tumor Pharmacother* 7: 11–18, 1990.

64. D'Arpa P, Liu LF. Topoisomerase-targeting antitumor drugs. *Bioch Biophy Acta* 989: 163–77, 1989.

65. Wang JC. DNA Topoisomerases. *Ann Rev Biochem* 54: 665–97, 1985.

66. Hsiang YH, Lihou MG, Liu LF. Arrest of replication forks by drug-stabilized topoisomerase I-DNA cleavable complexes as a mechanism of cell killing by camptothecin analogues. *Cancer Res* **49**: 5077–82, 1989.

67. DeWys WD, Humphreys SR, Goldin A. Studies on therapeutic effectiveness of drugs with tumor weight and survival time indices of Walker 256 carcino sarcoma *Cancer Chemother Rep* **52**: 229–42, 1968.

68. Venditti JM, Abbott BJ. Studies on oncolytic agents from natural sourses. Correlations of activity against animal tumors and clinical effectiveness. *Lloydia* **30**: 332–48, 1967.

69. Gottlieb JA, Guarino AM, Call JB, et al. Preliminary pharmacologic and clinical evaluation of camptothecin sodium (NSC-100880). *Cancer Chemother Rep* **54**(6): 461–70, 1970.

70. Muggia FM, Creaven PJ, Hansen HH, et al. Phase I clinical trial of weekly and daily treatment with camptothecin (NSC-100880). Correlation with preclinical studies. *Cancer Chemother Rep* **56**(4): 515–21, 1972.

71. Creaven PJ, Allen LM, Muggia FM. Plasma camptothecin (NSC-100880) levels during a 5-day course of treatment. Relation to dose and toxicity. *Cancer Chemother Rep* **56**(5): 573–78, 1972.

72. Gottlieb JA, Luce JK. Treatment of malignant melanoma with carnptothecin (NSC-100880). *Cancer Chemother Rep* **56**(1): 103–5, 1972.

73. Moertel CG, Schutt AJ, Reitemeier RJ, et al. Phase II study of camptothecin (NSC-100880) in the treatment of advanced gastrointestinal cancer. *Cancer Chemother Rep* **56**(1): 95–101, 1972.

74. Wall ME and Wani MC. Camptothecin. In *Anticancer Agents Based on Natural Product Models*, edited by JM Cassady, JD Douros. New York: Academic Press, NY, pp. 417–36, 1980.

75. Jaxel C, Kohn KW, Wani MC, et al. Structure-activity study of the actions of camptothecin derivatives on mammalian topoisomerase I. Evidence for a specific receptor site and a relation to antitumor activity. *Cancer Res* **49**: 1465–9, 1989.

76. Giovanella BC, Natelson E. Preclinical and clinical trials of oral 20-(S)-camptothecin (CPT) and of 9-nitro-so-(S)-camptothecin (9NC). The Proceedings of the Fifth Conference on DNA Topoisomerases in Therapy 31(Abstr: 32), 1994.

77. Kunimoto T, Nitta K, Tanaka T, et al. Antitumor activity of 7-ethyl-10-[4-(1-piperidino)-1-piperidino]carbonyloxy-camptothecin, a novel water-soluble derivative of camptothecin, against murine tumors. *Cancer Res* **47**: 5944–7, 1987.

78. Kaneda N, Nagata H, Furuta T, et al. Metabolism and pharmacokinetics of the camptothecin analogue CPT-11 in the mouse. *Cancer Res* **50**: 1715–20, 1990.

79. Ohno R, Okada K, Masaoka T, et al. An early phase II study of CPT-11. A new derivative of camptothecin for the treatment of leukemia and lymphoma. *J Clin Oncol* **8**(11): 1907–12, 1990.

80. Tsuda H, Takatsuki K, Ohno R, et al. A late phase II trial of a potent topoisomerase I inhibitor, CPT-11, in malignant lymphoma. *Proc Am Soc Clin Oncol* **11**: 316, 1992.

81. Tsuda H, Takatsuki K, Ohno R, et al. Treatment of adult T-cell leukaemia lymphoma with irinotecan hydrochloride (CPT-11). CPT-11 Study Group on Hematological Malignancy. *Br J Cancer* **70**(4): 771–4, 1994.

82. Shimada Y, Yoshino M, Wakui A, et al. Phase II study of CPT-11, new camptothecin derivative, in the patients with metastatic colorectal cancer. *Proc Am Soc Clin Oncol* **10**: 135, l991.

83. Rothenberg ML, Eckardt JR, Burris HA, et al. Irinotecan (CPT-11) as second-line therapy for patients with 5-FU-refractory colorectal cancer. *Proc Am Soc Clin Oncol* **13**: 198, 1994.

84. Pitot HC, Wender D, O'Connell MJ, et al. A Phase II trial of CPT-11 (irinotecan) in patients with metastatic colorectal carcinoma. A North Central Cancer Treatment Group (NCCTG) study. *Proc Am Soc Clin Oncol* **13**: 197, 1994.

85. Bugat R, Suc E; Rougier P, et al. CPT-11 (irinotecan) as second-line therapy in advanced colorectal cancer (CRC). Preliminary results of multicentric Phase II study. *Proc Am Soc Clin Oncol* **13**: 200, 1994.

86. Rougier P, Culine S, Bugat R, et al. Multicentric Phase II study of first line CPT-11 (irinotecan) in advanced colorectal cancer (CRC). Preliminary results. *Proc Am Soc Clin Oncol* **13**: 200, 1994.

87. Shimada Y, Yoshino M, Wakui A, et al. Phase II study of CPT-11, a new camptothecin derivative, in metastatic colorectal cancer: CPT-11 Gastrointestinal Cancer Study Group. *J Clin Oncol* **11**(5): 909–13, 1993.

88. Fukuoka M, Negoro S, Niitani H, et al. Phase II study of a new camptothecin derivative, CPT-11 in previously untreated non-small cell lung cancer (NSCLC). *Proc Am Soc Clin Oncol* **9**: 226, 1990.

89. Ogawa M, Taguchi T. Clinical studies with CPT-11: the Japanese experience. *Ann Oncol* **3**(Suppl 1): 118, 1992.

90. Fukuoka M, Niitani H, Suzuki A, et al. A phase II study of CPT-11, a new derivative of camptothecin, for previously untreated non-small-cell lung cancer. *I Clin Oncol* **10**(1): 16–20, 1992.

91. Nakagawa K, Fukuoka M, Niitani H. Phase II study of irinotecan (CPT-11) and cisplatin in patients with advanced non-small cell lung cancer (NSCLC). *Proc Am Soc Clin Oncol* **12**: 332, 1993.

92. Negoro S, Fukuoka M, Niitani H, et al. Phase II study of CPT-11, new camptothecin derivative, in small cell lung cancer (SCLC). *Proc Am Soc Clin Oncol* **10**: 241, 1991.

93. Masuda N, Fukuoka M, Kusunoki Y, et al. CPT-11: A new derivative of camptothecin for the treatment of refractory or relapsed small-cell lung cancer. *J Clin Oncol* **10**(8): 1225–9, 1992.

94. Bonneterre J, Pion JM, Adenis A, et al. A Phase II study of a new camptothecin analog CPT-11 in previously treated advanced breast cancer patients. *Proc Am Soc Clin Oncol* **12**: 94, 1993.

95. Sakata Y, Wakui A, Nakao I, et al. A late Phase II study of irinotecan (CPT-11), in advanced pancreatic cancer. *Proc Am Soc Clin Oncol* **12**: 211, 1993.

96. Kambe M, Wakui A, Nakao I, et al. A late Phase II study of irinotecan (CPT-11) in patients (pts) with advanced gastric cancer. *Proc Am Soc Clin Oncol* **12**: 198, 1993.

97. Takeuchi S, Takamizawa H, Takeda Y, et al. Clinical study of CPT-11, camptothecin derivative, on gynecological malignancy. *Proc Am Soc Clin Oncol* **10**: 189, 1991.

98. Takeuchi S, Noda K, Yakushiji M. Late phase II study of CPT-11, a topoisomerase I inhibitor, in advanced cervical carcinoma. *Proc Am Soc Clin Oncol* **11**: 224, 1992.

99. Kaufmann SH. Induction of endonucleolytic DNA cleavage in human acute myelogenous leukemia cells by etoposide, camptothecin, and other cytotoxic anticancer drugs. A cautionary note. *Cancer Res* **49**: 5870–8, 1989.

100. Masuda N, Fukuoka M, Takada M, et al. CPT-11 in combination with cisplatin for advanced non-small-cell lung cancer. *Clin Oncol* **10**(11): 1775–80, 1992.

101. Masuda N, Fukuoka M, Kudoh S, et al. Phase I study of irinotecan and cisplatin with granulocyte colony-stimulating factor support for advanced non-small-cell lung cancer. *J Clin Oncol* **12**(1). 90–6, 1994.

102. Shinkai T, Arioka H, Kunikane H, et al. Phase I clinical trial of irinotecan (CPT-11), 7-ethyl-10-[4-(1-piperidino)-l-piperidino] carbonyloxy-camptothecin, and cisplatin in combination with fixed dose of vindesine in advanced non-small cell lung cancer. *Cancer Res* **54**(10): 2636–42, 1994.

103. Masuda N, Fukuoka M, Kudoh S, et al. Phase I and pharmacologic study of irinotecan in combination with cisplatin for advanced lung cancer. *Br J Cancer* **68**(4): 777–82, 1993.

104. Karato A, Sasaki Y, Shinkait I, et al. phase 1 study of CPT-11 and etoposide in patients with refractory solid tumors. *J Clin Oncol* **11**(10): 2030–5, 1993.

105. Masuda N, Fukuoka M, Kudoh S, et al. Phase I and pharmacologic study of irinotecan and etoposide with recombinant human granulocyte colony-stirnulating factor support for advanced lung cancer. *J Clin Oncol* **12**(9): 1833–41, 1994.

106. Shimada Y, Sasaki Y, Sugano K, et al. Combination Phase I study of CPT-11 (Irinotecan) combined with continuous infusion of 5-fluorouracil (5FU) in metastatic colorectal cancer. *Proc Am Soc Clin Oncol* **12**: 196, 1993.

107. Mori K, Suga U, Kishiro I, et al. A Phase I study of CPT-11 and cisplatin (5-day continuous infusion) for advanced non-small cell lung cancer. *Proc Am Soc Clin Oncol* **13**: 366, 1994.

108. Rowinsky EK, Grochow LB, Ettinger DS, *et al.* Phase I and pharmacological study of the novel topoisomerase I inhibitor 7-ethyl-10-[4-(1-piperidino)-1 piperidino]carbonyloxy campto-thecin (CPT-11) administered as a ninety-minute infusion every 3 weeks. *Cancer Res* **54**(2): 427–36, 1994.

109. Taguchi T, Wahui A, Hasegawa K, *et al.* Phase I clinical study of CPT-11. *Jap J Cancer Chemother* **17**: 115–20, 1990.

110. Abigerges D, Chabot GG, Armand JP, *et al.* Phase I and pharmacokinetic studies of the camptothecin analog irinotecan administered every 3 weeks in cancer patients. *J Clin Oncol* **13**(1): 210–21, 1995.

111. Negoro S, Fukuoka M, Masuda N, *et al.* Phase I study of weekly intravenous infusions of CPT-11, a new derivative of campto-thecin, in the treatment of advanced non-small-cell lung cancer. *J Natl Cancer Inst* **83**(16): 1164–8, 1991.

112. de Forni M, Bugat R, Chabot GG, *et al.* Phase I and pharmaco-kinetic study of the camptothecin derivative irinotecan, admi-nistered on a weekly schedule in cancer patients. *Cancer Res* **54**(16): 4347–54, 1994.

113. Rothenberg ML, Kuhn JG, Burris HA, *et al.* Phase I and pharmacokinetic trial of weekly CPT-11. *J Clin Oncol* **11**(11): 2194–204, 1993.

114. Gupta E, Lestingi TM, Mick R, *et al.* Metabolic fate of irinotecan in humans. Correlation of glucuronidation with diarrhea. *Cancer Res* **54**(14): 3723–5, 1994.

115. Ohe Y, Sasaki Y, Shinkai T, *et al.* Pharmacokinetics with a 5-day continuous infusion of a camptothecin derivative, CPT-11. *Proc Am Soc Clin Oncol* **10**: 117, 1991.

116. Clavel M, Mathieu-Boue A, Dumortier A, *et al.* Phase I study of CPT-11 administered as a daily infusion for 3 consecutive days. *Proc Am Assoc Cancer Res* **33**: 262, 1992.

117. Schiller JH, Kim K, Johnson D. Phase II study of topotecan in extensive stage small cell lung cancer. *Proc Am Soc Clin Oncol* **13**: 330, 1994.

118. Ardizzoni A, Hansen H, Dombernowsky P, *et al.* Phase II study of topotecan in pretreated small cell lung cancer (SCLC). *Proc Am Soc Clin Oncol* **13**: 336, 1994.

119. Perez-Soler R, Glisson BS, Kane J, *et al.* Phase II study of topotecan in patients with non-small-cell lung cancer (NSCLC) previously untreated. *Proc Am Soc Clin Oncol* **13**: 363, 1994.

120. Lynch TJ Jr, Kalish L, Strauss G, *et al.* Phase II study of topotecan in metastatic non-small-cell lung cancer. *J Clin Oncol* **12**(2): 347–52, 1994.

121. Kudelka A, Edwards C, Freedman R, *et al.* An open Phase II study to evaluate the efficacy and toxicity of topotecan adminis-tered iv as 5 daily infusions every 21 days to women with advanced epithelial ovarian carcinoma. *Proc Am Soc Clin Oncol* **12**: 259, 1993.

122. Robert F, Wheeler RH, Molthrop DC, *et al.* Phase II study of topotecan in advanced head and neck cancer. Identification of an active new agent. *Proc Am Soc Clin Oncol* **13**: 281, 1994.

123. Eisenhauer EA, Wainman N, Boos G, *et al.* Phase II trials of topotecan in patients (pts) with malignant glioma and soft tissue sarcoma. *Proc Am Soc Clin Oncol* **13**: 175, 1994.

124. Sugarman SM, Ajani JA, Daugherty K, *et al.* A Phase II trial of topotecan (TPT) for the treatment of advanced, measurable colorectal cancer. *Proc Am Soc Clin Oncol* **13**: 225, 1994.

125. Sugarman SM, Pazdur R, Daugherty K, *et al.* A Phase II trial of topotecan (TPT) for the treatment of unresectable pancreatic cancer (PC). *Proc Am Soc Clin Oncol* **13**: 224, 1994.

126. Ilson D, Motzer RJ, O'Moore P, *et al.* A Phase II trial of topotecan in advanced renal cell carcinoma. *Proc Am Soc Clin Oncol* **12**: 248, 1993.

127. Creemers GJ, Schellens JH, Beijnen JH, *et al.* Bioavailability of oral topotecan. A new topoisomerase I inhibitor. *Proc Am Soc Clin Oncol* **13**: 132, 1994.

128. Kuhn J, Rizzo J, Eckardt J, *et al.* Phase I bioavailability study of oral topotecan. *Proc Am Soc Clin Oncol* **14**: 474, 1995.

129. Rowinsky E, Grochow L, Kaufmann S, *et al.* Sequence-depen-dent effects of topotecan (T) and cisplatin (C) in a Phase I and pharmacokinetic (PK) study. *Proc Am Soc Clin Oncol* **13**: 142, 1994.

130. Graham MV, Jahanzeb M, Dresler C, *et al.* Preliminary results of a Phase I study of topotecan plus thoracic radiotherapy for locally advanced non-small cell lung cancer (NSCLCA). *Proc Am Soc Clin Oncol* **13**: 340, 1994.

131. Tolcher AW, O'Shaughnessy JA, Weiss RB, *et al.* A Phase I study of topotecan (a topoisomerase I inhibitor) in combination with doxorubicin (a topoisomerase II inhibitor). *Proc Am Soc Clin Oncol* **13**: 157, 1994.

132. Eckardt JR, Burris HA, Von Hoff DD, *et al.* Measurement of tumor topoisomerase I and II levels during the sequential administration of topotecan and etoposide. *Proc Am Soc Clin Oncol* **13**: 141, 1994.

133. Lilenbaum RC, Rosner GL, Ratain MJ, *et al.* Phase I study of taxol and topotecan in patients with advanced solid tumors (CALGB 9362). *Proc Am Soc Clin Oncol* **13**: 131, 1994.

134. Eckardt JR, Von Hoff DD, Rinaldi DA, *et al.* Phase I trial of cisplatin followed by topotecan in patients with untreated non-small cell lung cancer. *The Proceedings of the Fifth Conference on DNA Topoisomerases in Therapy.* **48**(Abstr: 47), 1994.

135. Miller AA, Hargis JB, Lilenbaum RC, *et al.* Phase I study of topotecan and cisplatin in patients with advanced solid tumors. A cancer and leukemia group B study. *J Clin Oncol* **12**(12): 2743–50, 1994.

136. Wall JG, Burris HA, Von Hoff DD, *et al.* A Phase I clinical and pharrnacokinetic study of the topoisomerase I inhibitor topotecan (SK&F 104864) given as an intravenous bolus every 21 days. *Anti-cancer Drugs.* **3**(4): 337–45, 1992.

137. Hasegawa K, Nishimura R, Fukuoka M, *et al.* Phase I and pharmacologic evaluation of topotecan on a 30 min infusion. *Proc Am Assoc Cancer Res* **34**: 421, 1993.

138. Rowinsky EK, Grochow LB, Hendricks CB, *et al.* Phase I and pharmacologic study of topotecan. A novel topoisomerase I inhibitor. *J Clin Oncol* **10**(4): 647–56, 1992.

139. Rowinsky E, Sartorius S, Grochow L, *et al.* Phase I and pharmacologic study of topotecan, an inhibitor of topoiso-merase I, with granulocyte colony-stimulating factor (G-CSF). Toxicologic differences between concurrent and post-treat-ment G-CSF administration. *Proc Am Soc Clin Oncol* **11**: 116, 1992.

140. Verweij J, Lund B, Beijnen J, *et al.* Phase I and pharmacokinetics study of topotecan, a new topoisomerase I inhibitor. *Ann Oncol* **4**(8): 673–8, 1993.

141. Saltz L, Sirott M, Young C, *et al.* Phase I clinical and pharma-cology study of topotecan given daily for 5 consecutive days to patients with advanced solid tumors, with attempt at dose intensification using recombinant granulocyte colony stimu-lating factor. *J Natl Cancer Inst* **85**(18): 1499–507, 1993.

142. Tubergen D, Pratt C, Stewart C, *et al.* Phase I study of topotecan in children with refractory solid tumors. A Pediatric Oncology Group study. *Proc Am Soc Clin Oncol* **13**: 167, 1994.

143. Haas NB, LaCreta FP, Walczak J, *et al.* Phase I / pharmacokinetic study of topotecan by 24-hour continuous infusion weekly. *Cancer Res* **54**(5): 1220–6, 1994.

144. ten Bokkel Huinink WW, Rodenhuis S, Beijnen J, *et al.* Phase I study of the topoisomerase I inhibitortopotecan (SK&F104864-A). *Proc Am Soc Clin Oncol* **11**: 110, 1992.

145. Abbruzzese JL, Madden T, Schmidt S, *et al.* Phase I trial of topotecan (TT) administered by 24-hr infusion without and with G-CSF. *Proc Am Assoc Cancer Res* **34**: 329, 1993.

146. Blaney SM, Balis FM, Cole DE, *et al.* Pediatric Phase I trial and pharmacokinetic study of topotecan administered as a 24-hour continuous infusion. *Cancer Res* **53**(5): 1032–6, 1993.

147. Pratt CB, Stewart C, Santana VM, *et al.* Phase I study of topotecan for pediatric patients with malignant solid tumors. *J Clin Oncol* **12**(3): 539–43, 1994.

148. Sabiers JH, Berger NA, Berger SJ, *et al.* Phase I trial of topotecan administered as a 72-hr infusion. *Proc Am Assoc Cancer Res* **34**: 426, 1993.

149. Burris HA III, Awada A, Kuhn JG, *et al.* Phase I and pharma-cokinetic studies of topotecan administered as a 72- or 120-hour continuous infusion. *Anti-Cancer Drugs* **5**(4): 394–402, 1994.

150. Kantarjian HM, Beran M, Ellis A, et al. Phase I study of topotecan, a new topoisomerase I inhibitor, in patients with refractory or relapsed acute leukemia. Blood 81(5): 1146–51, 1993.

151. Rowinsky EK, Adjei A, Donehower RC, et al. Phase I and pharrnacodynamic study of the topoisomerase I-inhibitor topotecan in patients with refractory acute leukemia. J Clin Oncol 12(10): 2193–203, 1994.

152. Hochster H, Liebes L, Speyer J, et al. Phase I trial of low-dose continuous topotecan infusion in patients with cancer: an active and well-tolerated regimen. J Clin Oncol 12(3): 553–9, 1994.

153. Plaxe S, Christen R, O'Quigley J, et al. Phase I trial of ip topotecan. Proc Am Soc Clin Oncol 12: 140, 1993.

154. Slichenmyer W, Chen TL, Donehower R, et al. Clinical pharmacology of topotecan in cancer patients with renal or hepatic dysfunction. Proc Am Soc Clin Oncol 13: 142, 1994.

155. Dahut W, Brillhart N, Takimoto C, et al. A phase I trial of 9-aminocamptothecin (9-AC) in adult patients with solid tumors. Proc Am Soc Clin Oncol 13: 138, 1994.

156. Emerson DL, Besterman JM, Brown HR, et al. In vivo antitumor activity of two new seven-substituted water-soluble campto-thecin analogues. Cancer Res 55(3): 603–609, 1995.

157. Wissel P, Verweij J, Eckardt J. On-going phase I trials on intravenous GI147211, a totally synthetic camptothecin analog, administered by the daily × 5 and 72 hour CI regimens. The Proceedings of the Fifth Conference on DNA Topoisomerases in Therapy 32 (Abstr: 33), 1994.

158. Delong DC, Hertel LW, Tang J, et al. Antiviral activity of 2',2'-difluorodeoxycytidine. Am Soc of Microbiology Abstracts 1986.

159. Grindey GB, Boder GB, Hertel LW, et al. Antitumor activity of 2'2'-difluorodeoxy-cytidine (LY188011). Proc Am Assoc Cancer Res; 27: 296, 1986.

160. Hertel LW, Boder GB, Kroin JS, et al. Evaluation of the antitumor activity of gemcitabine (2'2'-difluoro 2'-deoxycytidine). Cancer Res 50(14): 4417–22, 1990.

161. Chubb S, Heinemann V, Novotny L, et al. Metabolism and action of 2',2'-difluorodeoxycytidine (dFdC) in human leukemia cells. Proc Am Assoc Cancer Res 28: 324, 1987.

162. Cuddy DP and Ross DD. Gemcitabine (2'2' difluoro deoxycyti-dine) is not a DNA chain terminator in intact HL-60 human leukemia cells. Proc Am Assoc Cancer Res 34: 417, 1993.

163. Heinemann V, Xu YZ, Chubb S, et al: 2',2'-difluorodeoxycytidine inhibits ribonucleotide reductase in CEM cells. Proc Am Assoc Cancer Res 30: 554, 1989.

164. Bouffard DY and Momparler RL. Comparison of cytosine arabinoside and 2',2'-difluorodeoxycytidine (Gemcitabine) on the induction of apoptotic cell death in HL-60 myeloid leukemic cells. Proc Am Assoc Cancer Res 35: 317, 1994.

165. Heinemann V, Xu YZ, Chubb S. Cellular elimination of 2',2'-difluorodeoxycytidine 5'-triphosphate. A mechanism of self-potentiation. Cancer Res 52(3): 533–9, 1992.

166. Boven E, Erkelens CA, Pinedo HM, et al. The new cytidine analog gemcitabine (CEM) has schedule- rather than dose-related activity in human tumor xenografts. Proc Am Assoc Cancer Res 32: 382, 1991.

167. Anderson H, Lund B, Bach F, et al. Single-agent activity of weekly gemcitabine in advanced non-small cell lung cancer. A phase II study. J Clin Oncol 12(9): 1821–6, 1994.

168. Abratt RP, Bexwoda WR, Falkson G, et al Efficacy and saftey profile of gemcitabine in non-small-cell lung cancer. A phase II study. J Clin Oncol 12(8): 1535–40, 1994.

169. Shepherd FA, Gatzemeier U, Gotfried M, et al. An extended phase II study of gemcitabine in non-small cell lung cancer (NSCLC). Proc Am Soc Clin Oncol 12: 330, 1993.

170. Fosella FV, Lippman S, Pang A, et al. Phase 1/II study of gemcitabine (G) by 30 min weekly iv infusion × 3 wk every 4 wk for non-small cell lung cancer (NSCLC). Proc Am Soc Clin Oncol 12: 326, 1993.

171. Negoro S, Fukuoka M, Kurita Y, et al. Results of Phase II studies of gemcitabine in non-small cell lung cancer (NSCLC). Proc Am Soc Clin Oncol 13: 367, 1994.

172. Lund B, Ryberg M, Meidal P, et al. A Phase II study of gemcitabine in non-small cell lung cancer (NSCLC) using a twice-weekly schedule. Ann Oncol 3(Suppl 5): 31, 1992.

173. Cormier Y, Eisenhauer E, Muldal A, et al. Gemcitabine is an active new agent in previously untreated extensive small cell lung cancer (SCLC). A study of the National Cancer Institute of Canada Clinical Trials Group. Ann Oncol 5(3): 283–5, 1994.

174. Sessa C, Aamdal S, Wolff I, et al. Gemcitabine in patients with advanced malignant melanoma or gastric cancer. Phase II studies of the EORTC Early Clinical Trials Group. Ann Oncol 5(5): 471–2, 1994.

175. Christman K, Kelsen D, Saltz L, et al. Phase II trial of gemcitabine in patients with advanced gastric cancer. Cancer 73(1): 5–7, 1994.

176. Lund B, Hansen OP, Theilade K, et al. Phase II study of gemcitabine (2',2'-difluorodeoxycytidine) in previously treated ovarian cancer patients. J Natl Cancer Inst 86(20): 1530–3, 1994.

177. Catimel G, Vermorken JB, Clavel M, et al. A phase II study of Gemcitabine (LY188011) in patients with advanced squamous cell carcinoma of the head and neck. EORTC Early Clinical Trials Group. Ann Oncol 5(6): 543–7, 1994.

178. Carmichael J, Possinger K, Philip P, et al. Difluorodeoxycytidine (gemcitabine): a Phase II study in patients with advanced breast cancer. Proc Am Soc Clin Oncol 12: 64, 1993.

179. Mertens WC, Eisenhauer EA, Moore M, et al. Gemcitabine in advanced renal cell carcinoma. A phase II study of the National Cancer Institute of Canada Clinical Trial Group. Ann Oncol 4(4): 331–2, 1993.

180. Weissbach L, de Mulder P, Osieka R, et al. Phase II study of gemcitabine in renal cancer. Proc Am Soc Clin Oncol 11: 219, 1992.

181. Casper ES, Green MR, Brown TD, et al. Phase II trial of gemcitabine (2',2'-difluorodeoxycytidine) in patients with pancreatic cancer. Proc Am Soc Clin Oncol 10: 143, 1991.

182. Carmichael J, Jink U, Rusell RC, et al. Phase II study of gemcitabine in patients with advanced pancreatic cancer. Proc Am Soc Clin Oncol 12: 227, 1993.

183. Moore DF Jr, Pazdur R, Daugherty K, et al. Phase II study of gemcitabine in advanced colorectal adenocarcinoma. Invest New Drugs 10(4): 323–5, 1992.

184. Fink U, Molle B, Daschner H, et al. Phase II study of gemcitabine in metastahc colorectal cancer. Proc Am Soc Clin Oncol 11: 173, 1992.

185. Andersen JS, Burris HA, Casper E, et al. Development of a new system for assessing clinical benefit for patients with advanced pancreatic cancer. Proc Am Soc Clin Oncol 13: 461, 1994.

186. Peters G, Tanis B, Clavel M, et al. Pharmacokinetics of gemcitabine (LY188011) (difluoro-deoxycytidine) administered every two weeks in a Phase I study. Proc Am Assoc Cancer Res 31: 180, 1990.

187. Allerheiligen S, Johnson R, Hatcher B, et al. Gemcitabine pharmacokinetics are influenced by gender, body surface area (BSA), and duration of infusion. Proc Arn Soc Clin Oncol 13: 136, 1994.

188. O'Rourke TJ, Brown TD, Havlin K, et al. Phase I clinical trial of gemcitabine given as an intravenous bolus on 5 consecutive days. Eur J Cancer 30A(3): 417–8, 1994.

189. Poplin EA, Corbett T, Flaherty L, et al. Difluorodeoxycytidine (dFdC), gemcitabine. A Phase I study. Invest New Drugs 10(3): 165–70, 1992.

190. Anderson H, Thatcher N, Walling J, et al. A Phase I study of 24 hour infusion of gemcitabine in patients with previously untreated, locally advanced, non-small cell lung cancer. Proc Am Soc Clin Oncol 13: 348, 1994.

191. Abruzzese JL, Grunewald R, Weeks EA, et al. A Phase I clinical, plasma and cellular pharmacology study of gemcitabine. J Clin Oncol 9(33): 491–8, 1991.

192. Pollera CF, Ceribelli A, Crecco M, et al. Prolonged infusion of gemcitabine. A prelirrinary report of a Phase I study. Ann Oncol 3(Suppl 5): 52, 1992.

193. Richards F, White D, Muss H, et al. Phase I trial of gemcitabine (2',2' difluorodeoxycytidine) (G) over 30 minutes in patients (pts) with non-small cell lung cancer (NSCLC). Proc Am Soc Clin Oncol 13: 344, 1994.

194. Brown T, O'Rourke T, Burris H, et al. A Phase I trial of gemcitabine (LY188011) administered every two weeks. Proc Am Soc Clin Oncol 10: 115, 1991.

195. Tanis B, Clavel M, Guastalla I, et al. Phase I study of gemcitabine (difluorodeoxycytidine; dFdC; LY188011) administered in a two-weekly schedulG Proc Am Assoc Cancer Res 31: 207, 1990.

196. Peters GJ, van der Wilt CL, van Groeningen K, et al. Thymidylate synthase inhibition after administration of fluorouracil with or without leucovorin in colon cancer patients. Implications for treatment with fluorouracil. J Clin Oncol 12(10): 2035–42, 1994.

197. Jackman AL, Taylor GA, Gibson W, et al. ICI D1694, a quinazoline antifolate thymidylate synthase inhibitor that is a potent inhibitor of L1210 tumor cell growth in vitro and in vivo. A new agent for clinical study. Cancer Res 51: 5579–86, 1991.

198. Weiss GR, Eckardt JR, Eckhardt SG, et al. New anticancer agents. In Cancer Chemotherapy and Biological Response Modifiers Annual 16. Elsevier Science Publishers B.V., Amsterdam, 1995 (in press).

199. Rinaldi DA, Burris HA, Dorr FA, et al. A Phase I evaluation of the novel thymidylate synthase inhibitor LY231514, in patients with advanced solid tumors. Proc Am Soc Clin Oncol 13: 159, 1994.

200. Cao S, Rustum YM, Spector T. S-Ethynyluracil (776C85). Modulation of 5-fluorouracil efficacy and therapeutic index in rats bearing advanced colorectal carcinoma. Cancer Res 54: 1507–10, 1994.

201. Davis ST, Joyner SS, Baccanari DP, et al: 5-Ethynyluracil (5-EU, 776C85) irnproves the pharmacokinetics of S-fluorouracil (S-FU) in rats dosed with ftorafur (FT). Proc Am Assoc Cancer Res 35: 321, 1994.

202. Davis ST, Joyner SS, Baccanari DP, et al: 5-Ethynyluracil (776C85). Protection from S-fluorouracil-induced neurotoxicity in dogs. Biochem Pharmacol 48(2): 233–6, 1994

203. Burris H, Schilsky R, Fields S, et al. lnitial phase I trial of the dihydropyrimidine dehydrogenase inactivator 5-ethynluracil (776C85) plus 5-fluorouracil. Proc Am Soc Clin Oncol 14: 171, 1995.

204. O'Reilly SM, Newlands ES, Glaser MG, et al. Temozolomide. a new oral cytotoxic chemotherapeutic agent with promising activity against primary brain tumours. Eur J Cancer 29A(7). 940–2, 1993.

205. Newlands ES, Blackledge GR, Slack JA, et al. Phase I trial of temozolomide (CCRG 81045: M&B 39831: NSC 362856). Br J Cancer 65(2): 287–91, 1992

206. Showalter HDH, Fry DW, Leopold WR, et al. Design, biochemical pharmacology, electrochemistry and antitumor biology of anti-tumor anthrapyrazoles. Anti Cancer Drugs Des I: 73–85, 1986 .

207. Leopold WR, Nelson JM, Ploughman J, et al. Anthrapyrazoles, a new class of intercalating agents with high level, broad spectrum activity against murine tumours. Cancer Res 45: 5532, 1985.

208. Talbot DC, Smith IE, Mansi JL, et al. Anthrapyrazole CI 940. A highly active new agent in the treatment of advanced breast cancer. J Clin Oncol 9: 2141, 1991.

209. Haun SD, Natale RB, Stewart DJ, et al. A phase II multicenter trial of losoxantrone (DUP 941) in patients with metastatic hormone refractory prostate cancer (HRPC). Proc Am Soc Clin Oncol 14: 238, 1995.

210. Cobb P, Burris H, Peacock N, et al. Phase I trial of losoxantrone plus paclitaxel given every 21 days. Proc Am Soc Clin Oncol 14: 476, 1995.

211. Vokes EE, O'Brien SM, Schilsky RL, et al. A phase I study of high-dose DUP941 (losoxantrone) in combination with cyclophosphamide (CTX). Proc Am Soc Clin Oncol 14: 478, 1995.

35. Bone Marrow Transplantation in the Older Patient

Karen K. Fields, David H. Vesole, Philip A. Rowlings, Mary M. Horowitz and Gerald J. Elfenbein

Introduction

In recent years, the use of high-dose chemotherapy for the treatment of various hematologic and nonhematologic malignancies has resulted in improved response rates and improvement in overall survival for patients with refractory malignancies when compared to historical controls (1–5). Bone marrow transplantation enables the clinician to exploit the steep dose-response curves observed with many chemotherapeutic agents (6,7) by providing protection from the myeloablative effects of otherwise intolerable doses of chemotherapy. Apparent cures have been achieved in 50–60% of patients with acute myelogenous leukemia in first remission and chronic myelogenous leukemia in the chronic phase (1–3). Cure rates for patients with aplastic anemia range from 60–80% after allogeneic bone marrow transplantation (8,9).

Successful bone marrow transplantation is largely influenced by the incidence of transplant-related complications. Increasing age has been associated with an increased risk of morbidity and mortality following standard therapies, thus, limiting the application of bone marrow transplantation in older patients (10–12). Presently, many centers restrict transplantation to patients under 60 to 65 years of age.

Analysis of studies of patients older than age 60 with acute myelogenous leukemia suggests that these patients tolerate intensive doses of chemotherapy well and older patients routinely undergo induction and consolidation chemotherapy following the diagnosis of acute myelogenous leukemia (13,14). The risks and benefits of this therapy are discussed in subsequent chapters. Although response rates and long-term disease-free survival rates do not appear to be as great as in the younger age group, it does appear that those older patients who do achieve complete remission may have remission durations comparable to those of the younger group. It is, therefore, reasonable to assume that some older patients may benefit from bone marrow transplantation with potential cure of their disease. Consequently, several transplant centers have actively explored the use of allogeneic and autologous bone marrow transplantation in older patient (15–17). Recent advances in supportive care, such as the availability of hematopoietic growth factors and other manipulations to shorten the period of aplasia following myeloablation, have decreased the associated mortality and morbidity and broadened the indications for bone marrow transplantation, especially in the older patient population.

Principles of High Dose Therapy

The goal of bone marrow transplantation is the delivery of curative doses of chemotherapy with or without the addition of radiation therapy. For most tumors, the doses of therapy necessary to achieve this goal would result in lethal marrow damage. Stem cells derived from bone marrow or peripheral blood provide rescue from this dose-limiting side effect, thus enabling the clinician to escalate the doses of chemotherapy or radiation therapy beyond marrow toxicity to the next level of toxicity, the non-hematologic dose-limiting toxicity. For example, thioTEPA, a mechlorethamine-like alkylating agent, has been given in the nontransplant setting in doses up to 60 mg/m^2 with myelosuppression as the main dose-limiting side effect (18). However, when autologous bone marrow rescue is provided, the maximum tolerated dose of thioTEPA given alone or in combination has been found to be up to 1200 mg/m^2 with mucositis, protracted myelosuppression and, in some reports, central nervous system toxicity constituting the main non-hematologic dose-limiting toxicities (19,20).

Unfortunately, although the delivery of high dose therapy is possible with bone marrow transplantation, not all malignancies can be cured in this setting. Dose escalation increases the overall response rates of most hematologic and non-hematologic malignancies. However, in some diseases the doses necessary to achieve complete tumor cell kill exceed the nonmarrow lethal doses of chemotherapy or radiation therapy. Therefore, some cancers remain incurable in spite of our ability to provide maximum anticancer therapy.

Figure 35.1 illustrates this concept. Tumor type A represents tumors that are highly responsive to conventional therapy. Dose escalation beyond the marrow lethal dose results in virtually 100% cell kill and probable cure of disease. An example of this tumor type is acute and chronic leukemia. Tumor type B represents malignancies that undergo marked increases in tumor cell kill when doses are escalated beyond conventional limits. These cancers can potentially be cured if the

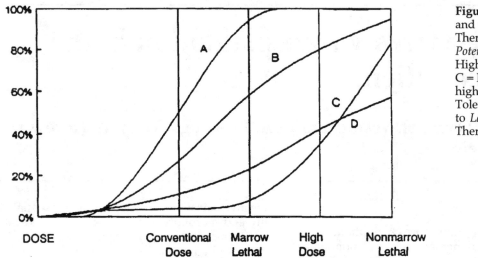

Figure 35.1 A = Sensitive and *Curable* with High Dose Therapy; B = Sensitive and *Potentially* curable with Higher Dose Therapy; C = Incurable unless *Ultra-*high Dose Therapy is Tolerable; D = Incurable due to *Lack of Sensitivity* to All Therapy.

doses of chemotherapy are elevated to the nonmarrow lethal dose. Examples of these tumor types include the lymphomas and breast cancer. Tumor type C represents tumors for which dose escalation beyond the marrow lethal dose results in only modest increases in cell kill, and unless non-hematologic, dose-limiting toxicities are survivable, these tumors are not curable with high dose therapy. With existing regimens, melanoma is an example of this tumor type. Tumors that are incurable by all types of therapy are illustrated by tumor type D. Dose escalation fails to result in adequate cell kill at any level of toxicity. Non-small cell lung cancer is one such tumor.

Tolerance of High Dose Therapy in the Older Patient

Multiple myeloma is one example of a malignancy that is very chemosensitive but seen almost exclusively in an elderly population. In recent years, high dose therapy and autologous stem cell rescue for this otherwise incurable B cell malignancy has resulted in increased response rates and improved overall survival when compared to standard therapy (21–23). Since multiple myeloma primarily affects an elderly population with a median age of onset of 65 years, high dose therapy trials directed at the treatment of this disease have provided a large body of data concerning transplant-related outcomes in the elderly patient. Until recently, patients with multiple myeloma were not considered for dose intensive regimens because of their usually advanced age and frequently incapacitating non-malignant clinical conditions. However, with the advent of peripheral blood stem cells and hematopoietic growth factors, younger age is no longer a prerequisite for consideration of myeloablative therapy with hematopoietic stem cell support.

The group of investigators at the University of Arkansas for Medical Sciences in Little Rock, Arkansas have included myeloma patients up to and, on occa-

sion with special exception, exceeding age 70 for treatment in their tandem autotransplant protocols (16). In a recent analysis of 420 patients completing autotransplant at this center, 94 patients were 60 years and older (median 63 years with a range of 60 to 76 years) (21). The myeloablative regimen consisted of high dose melphalan 200 mg/m² supported with peripheral blood stem cells with or without bone marrow for the first autotransplant. Patients achieving either a partial or complete remission received a second cycle of high dose melphalan within 3–6 months. Those patients who did not achieve at least a partial remission were offered a preparative regimen of melphalan 140 mg/m² with total body irradiation 850 to 1125 cGy.

The older patients were equally likely to complete the tandem autotransplant protocol as the younger patients (55% versus 62%, respectively) and similarly, 35% and 21%, respectively, are awaiting second transplant accounting for over 80% of the patients in each group (Table 35.1) Although there was a greater inci-

Table 35.1 Patient flow on tandem autotransplant trials for the treatment of Multiple Myloma at the University of Arkansas.

	Age	
Time of Study	<60 (n = 326)	>60 (n = 94)
Tx-1 Completed	100%	100%
Early Death	1%	6%
Died Prior to Tx-2	12%	5%
Disease Progression	1%	0
Tx-2 Declined	3%	0
Tx-2 Pending	21%	34%
Tx-2 Completed	62%	55%
Early Death	2%	6%

Tx = Transplant

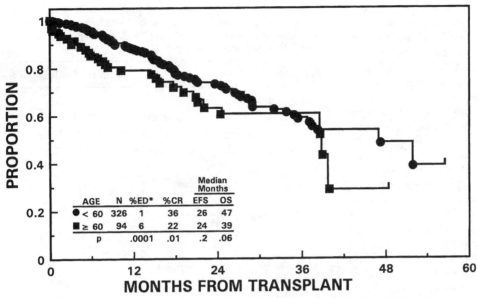

Figure 35.2 Autotransplants for multiple myeloma. Overall survival according to age in patients less than 60 years and 60 years and older (N = 420).

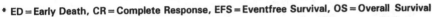

AGE	N	%ED*	%CR	Median Months EFS	OS
● < 60	326	1	36	26	47
■ ≥ 60	94	6	22	24	39
p		.0001	.01	.2	.06

MONTHS FROM TRANSPLANT

* ED = Early Death, CR = Complete Response, EFS = Eventfree Survival, OS = Overall Survival

dence of early death in the older patients (6% versus 1%), the overall survival between the two groups was comparable (Figure 35.2). Detailed analysis of prognostic factors, remission rates and survival are discussed in Chapter 44.

In these studies, stem cell reserves in younger and older patients, as determined by the number of mononuclear cells per kilogram body weight expressing CD34 antigen in apheresis products collected following high dose cyclophosphamide supported with hematopoietic growth factors were virtually identical (Figure 35.3). The major impact on stem cell reserve was the duration of prior therapy, particularly evident in patients who had received prior alkylating agents

(24). When corrected for CD34 count, post-transplant hematologic engraftment was similar in younger and older age groups for both granulocytes and platelets.

The myeloablative therapy was generally well tolerated in both age groups. Older patients demonstrated a higher incidence of World Health Organization (WHO) Grade III/IV stomatitis and diarrhea, particularly for the first autotransplant. No significant difference in nausea/vomiting and pneumonia/sepsis was observed. Although the extra-medullary toxicities were greater in the older patients, the median days of hospitalization following autotransplant for the older and younger age groups were 16 and 15 days, respectively (p = 0.09) indicating the rapid reversal of these morbi-

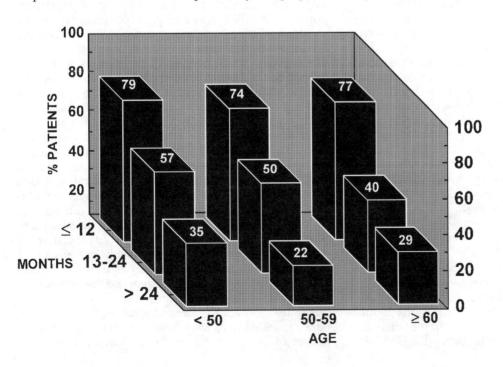

Figure 35.3 Stem cell mobilization following high dose cyclophosphamide. Shown are the percentage of patients with $>5 \times 10^6$ CD34+ cells/kg based upon age and months of prior therapy.

dities. Finally, due to the rapid hematologic recovery utilizing peripheral blood stem cells with hematopoietic growth factors and the well-tolerated extramedullary toxicities post-transplant, the Arkansas group has piloted a study to evaluate the feasibility and safety of performing autotransplantation of myeloma patients completely in the outpatient setting (25). The initial analysis indicates that older patients tolerate outpatient autotransplant as well as the younger patients.

Another study evaluating the effects of age on the tolerance of high dose therapy and autologous transplant compared 11 patients aged 55 to 59 to 157 patients aged 19 to 54 treated with high dose ifosfamide, carboplatin, and etoposide to compare transplant-related side effects and mortality (26). Patients were treated as part of a phase I/II dose escalation trial (27) with doses of ifosfamide ranging from 10,200 to 24,000 mg/m^2, carboplatin doses ranging from 1,500 to 2,100 mg/m^2, and etoposide doses ranging from 1,800 to 3,000 mg/m^2. Transplant-related morality was 9% in the younger patients compared to no transplant-related deaths in the oldest patient group (a difference that was not statistically significant). Engraftment and time to discharge following transplant did not vary by age. The risk of developing WHO grade III/IV hemorrhagic cystitis was significantly greater in the older patients despite the use of Mesna® in all patients with a trend, although not significant, toward an increased risk of WHO grade III/IV mucositis and peripheral neuropathy noted in the older patients. No other differences in specific organ toxicity were noted by age group. These data suggest that older patients tolerate high dose therapy as well as younger patients, although there may be an increased incidence of some organ specific side effects related to individual high dose regimens.

From these data, it appears that patients over the age of 60 are likely to tolerate myeloablative therapy with autotransplantation. A case in point is the oldest patient who has been reported to have completed an autotransplant, a virtually bedridden 76 year old female with advanced stage myeloma treated at the University of Arkansas, who remains in clinical remission with an excellent performance status 1 year following autotransplant. Elderly patients, with adequate stem cell reserves and physiologic organ function with the exception of renal insufficiency (28) should not be excluded from high dose therapy trials based solely upon chronological age. The increased risks of coexisting conditions, such as coronary artery disease or pulmonary disease, would be more likely to limit the use of autotransplant than age itself.

Allogeneic Transplantation

There are few reports of allogeneic transplants performed in the older patient. Therefore, available data concerning the outcome of patients in this age group are scant and it is difficult to draw conclusions about this type of therapy. The data reported to the International Bone Marrow Transplant Registry (IBMTR) be-

Table 35.2 Characteristics of patients > 50 years of age receiving HLA-identical sibling bone marrow transplants for leukemia between 1983 and 1993 and reported to the IBMTR by 75 teams worldwide.

Variable	Number Evaluable (%)
Diagnosis	
Acute lymphoblastic leukemia	9 (5%)
Acute myelogenous leukemia	48 (24%)
Chronic myelogenousis leukemia	141 (71%)
Disease State at Transplant	
Early	124 (64%)
Intermediate	32 (16%)
Advanced	38 (20%)
Karnofsky Score Pretransplant	
≥90%	154 (78%)
<90%	44 (22%)
Acute Graft Versus Host Disease	61 (34%)
Among 179 patients surviving ≥ 21 days with engraftment	
Chronic Graft Versus Host Disease	67 (46%)
Among 144 patients surviving ≥ 90 days with engraftment	

tween 1983 and 1993 includes information from 198 patients over the age of 50 receiving HLA-identical sibling bone marrow transplants for leukemia reported by 75 teams worldwide. Table 35.2 lists the characteristics of this group of patients. The oldest patient reported to the IBMTR is a 73 year old female receiving an identical twin bone marrow transplant for chronic myelogenous leukemia in 1988. As noted, the majority of allogeneic transplants in older patients were performed for a diagnosis of chronic myelogenous leukemia. Additionally, most of the patients transplanted had a good performance status and were transplanted with less advanced disease and would have, therefore, been expected to have a relatively good prognosis following transplant. The 90 day mortality for the entire group was 27%. The incidence of acute and chronic graft versus host disease, 34% and 46%, respectively, is comparable to that expected in a younger population. Table 35.3 describes transplant-related outcomes for these patients based on the status of disease at the time of transplant, i.e., early versus advanced stage leukemia. As predicted, patients with less advanced disease had a superior leukemia-free survival at 2 years compared to those with more advanced disease. Again, these data compare favorably to transplant-related outcomes in similar groups of younger patients. (The data presented here were obtained from the Statistical Center of the International Bone Marrow Transplant

Table 35.3 Transplant-related outcomes for patients >50 years of age receiving HLA-identical sibling bone marrow for leukemia between 1983 and 1993 and reported to the IBMTR by 75 teams worldwide.

Disease State	Number Evaluable	2-Year Probability (+ 95% Confidence Interval)		
		Relapse Rate	Survival	LFS*
Early	124	14 ± 8%	61 ± 9%	59 ± 9%
Not Early	70	52 ± 18%	23 ± 10%	19 ± 10%

*LFS = Leukemia-Free Survival

Registry. The analysis has not been reviewed or approved by the Advisory Committee of the IBMTR.)

The bone marrow transplant center at the University of Washington in Seattle has reported the largest number of older patients to receive allogeneic bone marrow transplantation at a single institution (15). In 1986, they reported the results of 63 patients aged 45 to 68 years who had undergone bone marrow transplantation for various hematologic disorders. Of these patients, 24 patients underwent syngeneic transplants and 39 underwent allogeneic transplant from an HLA-matched sibling or other relative. Seven patients were age 60 or older. The oldest patient in this series, age 68, successfully received a syngeneic transplant for a diagnosis of acute myelogenous leukemia dying of relapse 237 days after transplant.

In this series, the actuarial disease-free survival for patients undergoing syngeneic transplantation was 20% at 7 years. The main causes of death in this group were due to leukemic relapse and interstitial pneumonitis. For patients undergoing allogeneic transplantation, the actuarial disease-free survival at 7 years was 11%. Deaths in this group were most frequently attributed to cytomegalovirus pneumonia and septicemia. The actuarial incidence of acute graft versus host disease in patients over the age of 50 was 79%, compared to an incidence of 30% in patients aged 45 to 50 years treated at the same institution during the same time period. Analysis of those data suggested that older patients with chronic myelogenous leukemia were more likely to benefit from allogeneic transplantation than older patients with acute leukemia. This was attributed to the amount of prior therapy in patients with acute leukemia. In addition, in this series, patients with acute leukemia were more likely to have been transplanted with advanced disease. These investigators concluded that allogeneic transplants should be considered in patients over the age of 45, especially in patients with good performance status and early stage disease. Patients with chronic myelogenous leukemia and pre-leukemia were considered to be good candidates for transplant.

A recent update of patients receiving allogeneic bone marrow transplantation for the treatment of chronic myelogenous leukemia at the Fred Hutchinson Cancer Research Center in Seattle evaluated 328 patients older than age 10 treated between 1983 and 1994 which included 87 patients aged 40 to 50 and 57 patients aged 50 to 60 (29). Adverse factors associated with a significantly poorer survival in this group included age between 40 and 50 and age greater than 50 with a relative risk compared to patients less than 30 years of age of 2.84 and 2.66, respectively. An additional risk factor included the time from diagnosis to treatment; patients transplanted more than 2 years following diagnosis fared significantly worse than patients transplanted less than one year following diagnosis. However, the predicted survival of patients between the ages of 50 and 60 was not worse than patients between the ages of 40 and 50. Of note, 3 of 5 patients in the series transplanted at age 60 remained in remission between 18 and 24 months following transplant. The authors concluded that age itself is not a valid reason to deny patients curative intent therapy by bone marrow transplantation.

Few other centers report experience with allogeneic transplantation in the older patient. Beelen and coworkers (30) evaluated 20 allogeneic transplant patients with acute leukemia and chronic myeloid leukemia transplanted in the fifth decade of life compared to 32 similar patients transplanted between the ages of 30 and 39. They found that standard risk patients, defined as HLA-identical sibling donors for patients in the first chronic phase of chronic myelogenous leukemia or acute leukemia in first remission, had a higher probability of survival than poor-risk advanced stage patients in both age groups, although the differences were not statistically significant. Older patients with advanced disease at the time of transplant, however, had an actuarial survival that was statistically inferior to that of younger patients. The cumulative incidence of acute and chronic graft versus host disease was 27% in patients who received bone marrow from an HLA-identical sibling, an incidence similar to that seen in younger patients. The most frequent cause of death was interstitial pneumonitis, the incidence of which did not differ statistically from the incidence in younger patients. The authors concluded that allogeneic bone marrow transplantation could be regarded as first-line therapy for patients with acute leukemia in first remission and patients in the first chronic phase of chronic myelogenous leukemia. Transplanters at the Johns Hopkins Oncology Center in Baltimore reported 14 patients aged 50 to 55 who received allogeneic bone marrow transplants for a variety of diagnoses (31). The actuarial disease free survival at 3 years was 31% compared to an actuarial disease free survival of 48% in patients aged 20 to 49 treated concurrently on the same protocols; this difference was statistically significant (p = 0.05). Of the 14 older patients, there were 9 transplant-related deaths, including 5 deaths due to refractory graft versus host disease and 1 death due to relapse. The authors concluded that allogeneic bone marrow transplantation in the older patient is associated with a high risk of transplant-related mortality and suggested that future clinical trials in older patients should focus on the treatment or prevention of graft versus host disease.

Although several other centers have reported their experiences with allogeneic transplantation in older patients, the majority of patients transplanted in these studies are less than age 45 (32–35). Only a handful of patients reported in these studies were over the age of 50. In general, the older patients reported in these series tended to do well, a finding that was generally attributed to improved graft versus host disease prophylaxis.

In summary, there is little data available in the literature concerning the role of allogeneic bone marrow transplantation in the older patient. Data from the largest transplant registry, the IBMTR, suggests that patients over the age of 50 have similar leukemia-free survival and transplant-related outcomes as compared to younger patients. The majority of older patients reported to this registry tended to have less advanced disease, a diagnosis of chronic myelogenous leukemia, and a good performance status. Although some centers have reported an increased risk of graft versus host disease in the older patients, this is not universal. However, the problem of graft versus host disease is associated with an increased risk of transplant-related morbidity and mortality in all age groups and efforts to modulate the incidence and severity of graft versus host disease could be expected to improve treatment-related outcomes for all patients undergoing allogeneic bone marrow transplantation. The incidence of infectious complications, specifically interstitial pneumonitis, appears to be increased in older patients compared to younger patients in some series. At the present time, allogeneic transplantation should be limited to good risk patients, such as patients with aplastic anemia, acute leukemia in first remission, chronic myelogenous leukemia in the first chronic phase, or preleukemic states. Patients with a poor performance status, patients with advanced disease or heavily pretreated patients should not be considered candidates for allogeneic bone marrow transplantation. Potential candidates should be referred to centers with specific interest in allogeneic transplantation in the older patient.

Autologous Transplantation

High dose therapy and autologous stem cell transplantation using stem cells derived from the bone marrow or peripheral blood has proven to be a useful modality in the management of a variety of hematologic and non-hematologic malignancies (4,5). Its value has been demonstrated in the acute leukemias, lymphomas, and several solid tumors. One advantage of this therapy is that maximum doses of chemotherapy, doses beyond bone marrow tolerance, can be administered with subsequent increases in antitumor effects yielding potential cures in previously incurable malignancies.

At least one study has suggested, however, that event-free survival and risk of relapse may be increased in older patients following high dose therapy and autologous stem cell transplantation compared to younger patients (36). Of 458 patients receiving autotransplants for a variety of diagnoses, 45 were between the ages of 55 and 65. Several different high dose regimens were used to treat a variety of malignancies in these patients although in these series the majority of patients had a diagnosis of high risk or metastatic breast cancer (48%). Transplant-related mortality for patients aged 18 to 55 was 16% compared to a mortality rate of 24% in the older patient group (p value not significant). In patients less than 55 years of age, the event-free survival, overall survival, and risk of relapse at 2 years was 33%, 47%, and 59%, respectively. However, in patients older than age 55, the event-free survival, overall survival, and risk of relapse at 2 years was 12%, 18%, and 82%, respectively. These differences were statistically significant and suggested that older patients tolerate high dose therapy as well as younger patients but that the risk of relapse following high dose therapy may be greater in older patients following high dose therapy for the treatment of certain malignancies. Reasons for these differences still remain to be clarified but may be due to inherent differences in tumor biology or immune reconstitution following transplant in older patients compared to younger patients.

The largest body of data concerning treatment outcomes following autotransplantation is available from the Autologous Blood and Marrow Transplant Registry (ABMTR). Between 1989 and 1994, 158 teams in North and South America reported a total of 16,617 autologous transplants from all age groups to the ABMTR (data from 1994 is incomplete at this time). It is estimated that this represents about one half of all autotransplants performed in North and South America during that time period. The oldest patient in the ABMTR database is a 79 year old male who received a peripheral blood stem cell transplant in 1993 for a diagnosis of non-Hodgkin's lymphoma. (All subsequent data presented for specific diseases were obtained from the from the Statistical Center of the ABMTR. The analysis has not been reviewed or approved by the Advisory Committee of the ABMTR.)

Lymphoma

Recurrent lymphomas are among the most common malignancies to be treated with high dose therapy and autologous stem cell transplant and represent the largest number of older patients receiving autotransplants reported to the ABMTR. Table 35.4 describes the characteristics and treatment outcomes for 1298 patients over the age of 50 who received autotransplants for lymphoma between 1989 and 1994. As noted, the majority of patients had a diagnosis of non-Hodgkin's lymphoma. Two year mortality and survival rates are comparable in both Hodgkin's disease and non-Hodgkin's lymphoma and treatment outcomes are similar to outcomes reported in the literature for patients which include a majority of younger patients.

The University of Nebraska reported its experience with autotransplant in patients over the age of 60 with non-Hodgkin's lymphoma and Hodgkin's disease (17). Between 11/84 and 10/91, 7 patients 60 to 68 years of age with non-Hodgkin's lymphoma underwent high

Table 35.4 Characteristics of patients > 50 years of age receiving autotransplants for non-Hodgkins lymphoma and Hodgkins disease between 1989 and 1994 and reported to the ABMTR by 104 teams worldwide.

Variable	Number Evaluable	N (%)
Disease	1298	
Non-Hodgkins lymphoma		1191 (92%)
Hodgkins disease		107 (8%)
Type of graft	680	
Bone marrow		286 (42%)
Peripheral blood		303 (45%)
Both		91 (13%)
Interval from diagnosis to transplant median (range)	1040	22 months (range 1–474)
100-day mortality		
Non-Hodgkins lymphoma	1146	$19 \pm 2\%$*
Hodgkins disease	101	$22 \pm 8\%$*
2-year probability of survival		
Non-Hodgkins lymphoma	1146	$50 \pm 4\%$*
Hodgkins disease	101	$50 \pm 12\%$*

*95% confidence interval

dose therapy and autologous bone marrow transplantation; there were 4 transplant-related deaths and only one patient survived beyond one year. Between 3/92 and 11/93, 14 patients aged 60 to 67 with non-Hodgkin's lymphoma and 1 patient aged 63 with Hodgkin's disease underwent autotransplant. Five patients received autologous bone marrow and 10 patients received peripheral blood stem cells. Although two patients experienced significant morbidity, no transplant-related deaths were seen in this group and patients were discharged a median of 20 days post-transplant. Overall survival and progression-free survival were similar to that seen in younger patients with lymphoma transplanted at the same institution during the same interval. Hematopoietic growth factors were not routinely available for use post-transplant prior to 1992, however, following 1992, all patients received hematopoietic growth factors which was felt to have accounted for some of the differences in transplant-related mortality. The authors concluded that selected patients over the age of 60 tolerate high dose chemotherapy and, therefore, older patients should not be excluded high dose protocols.

Breast Cancer

In recent years, breast cancer has become the most frequent indication for high dose therapy and autologous stem cell rescue (37). In a recent review of transplant-related outcomes for women with breast cancer undergoing high dose therapy, 4004 women were reported to the ABMTR as having received autotransplant (38). For all patients in the registry, the three year probability of progression-free survival following high dose therapy was 62% for stage II breast cancer, 52% for stage III breast cancer, and 24% for patients with metastatic breast cancer in a complete response at the time of transplant. Patients with metastatic breast cancer achieving less than a complete response had a three year probability of progression-free survival of 4% with an overall survival of 12%.

The ABMTR reported 721 women over the age of 50 who received autotransplants for high risk stage II and III and metastatic breast cancer between 1989 and 1994. Patient characteristics, source of stem cells, early mortality and treatment-related outcomes for these patients are described in Tables 35.5 and 35.6. Patients with metastatic breast cancer comprised the majority of evaluable cases. As can be seen, there is a trend toward greater early mortality in the metastatic breast cancer group (12%) compared to the early stage patients (6%). In this series of patients over the age of 50 undergoing high dose therapy, progression-free survival and transplant-related mortality are similar to transplant-related outcomes reported in the literature for comparable groups of which include a large proportion of younger breast cancer patients.

One study suggests, however, that not all older patients with advanced breast cancer benefit in terms of progression-free survival following high dose therapy. Between 10/89 and 8/95, 219 patients with metastatic or inflammatory breast cancer undergoing high dose therapy and autologous stem cell rescue were treated at the Moffitt Cancer Center in Tampa, Florida (36). Eighteen patients in these studies were

Table 35.5 Characteristics of patients > 50 years of age receiving autotransplants for metastatic breast cancer between 1989 and 1994 and reported to the ABMTR by 72 teams worldwide.

Variable	Number Evaluable	N (%)
Number of patients	542	
Type of graft	419	
Bone marrow		153 (37%)
Peripheral blood		166 (40%)
Both		100 (23%)
Interval from diagnosis to treatment median (range)	510	37 months (range <1–301)
100-day mortality	517	$12 \pm 3\%$*
2-year probability of survival	517	$35 \pm 7\%$*
2 year probability of progression-free survival	334	$17 \pm 6\%$*

*95% confidence interval

Table 35.6 Characteristics of patients > 50 years of age receiving autotransplants for stage II and III breast cancer between 1989 and 1994 and reported to the ABMTR by 49 teams worldwide.

Variable	Number Evaluable	N (%)
Number of patients	179	
Stage II		110 (62%)
Stage III		69 (38%)
Type of graft	153	
Bone marrow		49 (32%)
Peripheral blood		57 (37%)
Both		47 (31%)
Interval from diagnosis to transplant median (range)	154	6 months (range 3–131)
100-day mortality		
Stage II	97	6 ± 5%*
Stage III	60	6 ± 6%*
2-year probability of survival		
Stage II	97	84 ± 14%*
Stage III	60	91 ± 10%*
2-year probability of progression-free survival		
Stage II	78	84 ± 14%*
Stage III	43	58 ± 34%*

*95% confidence interval

Table 35.7 Characteristics of patients > 50 years of age receiving autotransplants for acute leukemia in second remission between 1989 and 1994 and reported to the ABMTR by 36 teams worldwide.

Variable	Number Evaluable	N (%)
Disease	69	
Acute lymphoblastic leukemia		5 (7%)
Acute myelogenous leukemia		64 (93%)
Type of graft	60	
Bone marrow		48 (80%)
Peripheral blood		3 (5%)
Both		9 (15%)
Interval from diagnosis to transplant, median (range)	67	20 months (<1–92)
100-day mortality	68	32 ± 11%*
2-year probability of survival	67	25 ± 12%*
2-year probability of relapse	48	59 ± 19%*
2-year probability of progression-free survival	47	25 ± 12%*

*95% confidence interval

between the ages of 55 and 65. Patients were treated with a variety of high dose regimens; (19,27,39) 24% of all patients had refractory metastatic breast cancer with 22% of older patient group having refractory metastatic breast cancer. Event-free survival, overall survival, and risk of relapse at 2 years following high dose therapy for patients less than age 55 was 20%, 33%, and 75% compared to 0%, 11%, and 100% for patients ages 55 to 65. There were no significant differences based on the responsiveness of disease at the time of transplant or the high dose regimen used. Although the differences in event-free survival and risk of relapse were significant, the overall survival was not significantly different between age groups (two tailed p from Chi^2 was 0.25). Of note, transplant-related mortality did not differ by age. Although older women tolerated high dose therapy as well as younger women, older patients appeared to have a higher risk of relapse following autotransplant. This observation requires further evaluation to ascertain the benefits of high dose therapy for older patients with advanced breast cancer.

Acute Leukemia

Since only about 40% of patients have are expected to have an HLA-identical sibling donor and, since unre-

lated HLA-identical donors can be identified in only about 40% of the patients enrolled in various donor registries, autotransplantation represents a viable alternative in patients with acute leukemia who would not otherwise be considered for allogeneic transplant (40). Although newer potential sources of allogeneic donors such as mismatched or haploidentical family donors and placental-derived ("cord blood") stem cells are available, these therapies remain investigational and are generally only applicable in a younger population (41). The results of autologous transplantation in the acute leukemias, for example, appear to be similar to that of allogeneic transplantation, with comparable overall survival rates in some series (42–45). An absence of graft versus host disease in the autologous stem cell recipients results in similar 5 year survival rates due to less transplant-related mortality in the autotranplanted patients despite an increased risk of leukemic relapse.

The ABMTR reported 69 patients over the age of 50 who received autotransplants for acute leukemia in second remission between 1989 and 1994. As noted in Table 35.7, the majority of these patients had a diagnosis of acute myelogenous leukemia. Early mortality in this group of patients was substantial; however, a significant number of patients (25%) remain progression-free at 2 years. These data suggest that earlier use of high dose therapy and autotransplantation, i.e., in first remission, would be a reasonable approach for the treatment of acute leukemia in the older patient.

Conclusions

The available data suggest that older patients undergoing bone marrow transplantation, both allogeneic and autologous, generally tolerate therapy as well as younger patients. In many diseases, progression-free survival is comparable to younger patients following both allogeneic and autologous transplantation. There remains a paucity of data in patients undergoing transplant over the age of 60 and therefore continued evaluation of this group of patients is necessary to define the role of high dose therapy in the older patient. In the allogeneic transplant setting, recent advances in prophylaxis and treatment of graft versus host disease have allowed clinicians to consider older patients as transplant candidates. Continuing improvements in supportive care, including the development of hematologic growth factors and new antibiotics, will also enable transplanters to consider a wider variety of patients for both allogeneic and autologous transplants. The future limiting factors in determining transplant eligibility are likely to be performance status and organ function although differences in tumor biology or host immune defects associated with aging could ultimately limit the use of this type of therapy in the elderly population.

Elderly patients with a good performance status and early stage disease should be referred to transplant centers with a specific interest in transplantation in the older patient. Such centers are more likely to have access to the continuing developments in the field of supportive care and novel therapies. Careful selection of patients with diseases likely to benefit from high dose therapy (i.e., acute leukemias in first remission, the first chronic phase of chronic myelogenous leukemia, and early stage breast cancer) is essential to ensure the cost effective use of this potentially expensive therapy. Yet, as the proportion of older patients in the population continues to grow, so does the need to provide innovative approaches to their care.

References

1. Bortin MM, Horowitz MM, Gale RP. Current status of bone marrow transplantation in humans. Report from the International Bone Marrow Registry. *Nat Immunol Cell Growth Regul* 1980; **7**: 334–350.

2. Champlin R, Gale RP. Acute myelogenous leukemia. Recent advances in therapy. *Blood* 1987; **69**: 1551–1562.

3. Thomas ED. The use and potential of bone marrow allograft and whole-body irradiation in the treatment of leukemia. *Cancer* 1982; **50**: 1449–1454.

4. Dicke KA, Spitzer G, Jagannath S, Evinger-Hodges. *Autologous Bone Marrow Transplantation.* Proceedings of the Fourth International Symposium, Houston, 1989.

5. Cheson BD, Lacerna L, Leyland-Jones B, *et al.* Autologous bone marrow transplantation. Current status and future directions. *Ann Intern Med.* 1989; **110**: 51–56.

6. Frei E III, Canellos GP. Dose. A critical factor in cancer chemotherapy. *Am J Med* 1980; **69**: 585–594.

7. Frei E III, Teicher BA, Holden SA, *et al.* Effect of alkylating agent dose. Preclinical studies and clinical correlation of alkylating dose. *Cancer Res* 1988; **48**: 6417–6423.

8. Bortin MM, Gale RP, Rimm AA. Allogeneic bone marrow transplantation for 144 patients with severe aplastic anemia. *JAMA* 1981; **245**: 1132.

9. Camitta BM, Storb R, Thomas ED. Aplastic anemia. Pathogenesis, diagnosis, treatment and prognosis. *N Engl J Med* 1982; **306**: 645.

10. Applebaum FR, Dahlberg S, Thomas ED, *et al.* Bone marrow transplantation or chemotherapy after remission induction for adults with acute nonlymphoblastic leukemia. *Ann Intern Med.* 1984; **101**: 581.

11. Bross DS, Tutschka PJ, Farmer ER, *et al.* Predictive factors for acute graft-versus-host disease in patients transplanted with HLA-identical siblings. *Blood* 1984; **63**: 12–15.

12. Storb R, Prentice RL, Sullivan K, *et al.* Predictive factors in chronic graft-versus-host disease in patients with aplastic anemia treated by marrow transplantation from HLA-identical siblings. *Ann Intern Med* 1983; **98**: 461.

13. Foon KA, Sigelboim J, Yale C, Gale RP. Intensive chemotherapy is the treatment of choice from elderly patients with acute myelogenous leukemia. *Blood* 1981; **58**: 467.

14. Reiffers J, Raynal F, Broustet A. Acute myeloblastic leukemia in elderly patients. *Cancer* 1980; **45**: 2816.

15. Klingemann HG, Storb R, Fefer A, *et al.* Bone marrow transplantation in patients aged 45 years and older. *Blood* 1986; **67**: 770–776.

16. Vesole DH, Jagannath S, Tricot G, *et al.* High-dose intensive therapy with autologous transplantation (AT) in multiple myeloma (MM) patients over age 60. *Proc Ann Meet Am Soc Clin Oncol* 1995; **14**: 939a.

17. Stewart D, Bierman P, Anderson J, *et al.* High dose chemotherapy (HDC) with autologous hematopoietic rescue in patients (pts) age 60 and over. *Proc Ann Meet Am Soc Clin Oncol* 1994; **13**: 1260a.

18. Edwards MS, Levin VA, Seger ML, *et al.* Phase II evaluation of thiotepa for treatment of central nervous system tumors. *Cancer Treat Rep* 1979; **63**: 1419–1421.

19. Fields KK, Elfenbein GJ, Perkins JB, *et al.* Two novel high-dose treatment regimens for metastatic breast cancer — Ifosfamide, carboplatin, plus etoposide and mitoxantrone plus thiotepa. Outcomes and toxicities. *Sem Oncol* 1993; **20**(suppl 6): 59–66.

20. Lazarus HM, Reed MD, Spitzer TR, *et al.* High-dose IV thiotepa and cryopreserved autologous bone marrow transplantation for therapy of refractory cancer. *Cancer Treat Rep* 1987; **71**: 689–695.

21. Vesole D, Jagannath S, Tricot G, *et al.* 400 autotransplants (AT) for multiple myeloma (MM). *Blood* 1994; **84**: 535a.

22. Jagannath S, Barlogie B, Dicke K, *et al.* Autologous bone marrow transplantation in multiple myeloma. Identification of prognostic factors. *Blood* 1990; **76**: 1860–1866.

23. Barlogie B, Jagannath S, Dixon D, *et al.* High-dose melphalan and GM-CSF for refractory multiple myeloma. *Blood* 1990; **76**: 677–680.

24. Tricot G, Jagannath S, Vesole D, *et al.* Peripheral blood stem cell transplants for multiple myeloma. Identification of favorable variables for rapid engraftment in 225 patients. *Blood* 1995; **85**: 588–596.

25. Jagannath S, Vesole D, Tricot G, Barlogie B: 118 outpatient (OPT) autotransplants in multiple myeloma (MM). *Blood* 1994; **84**: 212a.

26. Partyka JS, Fields KK, Perkins JB, *et al.* The effects of age on tolerance of high dose ifosfamide, carboplatin and etoposide and autologous stem cell rescue. Morbidity and mortality. *In press.*

27. Fields KK, Elfenbein GJ, Lazarus HM, *et al.* Maximum tolerated doses of ifosfamide, carboplatin, and etoposide given over six days followed by autologous stem cell rescue. Toxicity profile. *J Clin Oncol.* **13**: 323–332, 1995.

28. Tricot G, Alberts DS, Barlogie B, *et al.* High-dose melphalan pharmacokinetics in multiple myeloma. *In press.*

29. Clift RA, Buckner CD, Storb R, *et al.* The influence of patient age on the outcome of transplantation during chronic phase (CP) of chronic myeloid leukemia (CML). *Blood* 1995; **86**: 616a.

30. Beelen DW, Quabeck K, Mahmood HK, *et al.* Allogeneic bone marrow transplantation for acute leukemia or chronic myeloid leukemia in the fifth decade of life. *Eur J Cancer Clin Oncol* 1987; **23**: 1665–1671.

31. Miller CB, Kennedy MJ, Santos GW, Jones RJ. Bone marrow transplantation (BMT) in patients over the age of fifty. *Proc Ann Meet Am Soc Clin Oncol* 1992; **11**: 1138a.

32. Copelan EA, Kapoor N, Berliner M, Tutschka PJ. Bone marrow transplantation without total-body irradiation in patients aged 40 and older. *Transplantation* 1989; **48**: 65–68.

33. Elfenbein GJ, Winton E, Lazarus H, *et al.* Improved outcome for older patients receiving allogeneic bone marrow transplants for chronic myelogenous leukemia. *Proc Ann Meet Am Soc Clin Oncol* 1989; **30**: 235.

34. Ramond E, Ash R, Doukas M, *et al.* Allogeneic bone marrow transplantation (BMT) in older patients (PTS) with Philadelphia chromosome positive (PH1+) chronic myelogenous leukemia (CML). *Proc Ann Meet Am Soc Clin Oncol* 1985; **4**: 158.

35. Blume KG, Forman SJ, Nademantee AP, *et al.* Bone marrow transplantation for hematologic malignancies in patients aged 30 years or older. *J Clin Oncol* 1986; **4**: 1489–1492.

36. Fields KK, Ballester OF, Goldstein SC, *et al.* Age effects in patients undergoing autologous bone marrow or peripheral blood stem cell transplantation. *In press.*

37. Antman K, Corringham R, de Vries E, *et al.* Dose intensive therapy in breast cancer. *Bone Marrow Transplant* 1992; **10** (suppl): 67–73.

38. Antman KH, Rowlings PA, Vaughan WP, *et al.* High dose chemotherapy with autologous hematopoietic stem cell support for breast cancer in North America. *In press.*

39. Minton SE, Fields KK, Elfenbein GJ, *et al.* High dose Taxol®, Novantrone®, and thiotepa (TNT) followed by autologous stem cell rescue (ASCR) is a very active regimen for the treatment of anthracycline refractory metastatic breast cancer. *Breast Cancer Res and Treat* 1995; **37**: 47a.

40. Bortin MM, Rimm AA. Increasing utilization of bone marrow transplantation. *Transplantation* 1986; **42**: 229–234.

41. Fleming DR, Henslee-Downey PJ, Harder EJ, *et al.* Success of partially matched related donor allogeneic bone marrow transplantation (BMT) in acute lymphoblastic leukemia (ALL). *Proc Ann Meet Am Soc Clin Oncol* 1994; **13**: 1338a.

42. Gale RP. Current status of autotransplants in acute leukemia, in Dicke KA, Spitzer G, Jagannath S, Evinger-Hodges. *Autologous Bone Marrow Transplantation.* Proceedings of the Fourth International Symposium, Houston, 1989, pp. 813–817.

43. Vellekoop L, Jagannath S, Spitzer G, *et al.* High-dose cyclophosphamide, BCNU, and etoposide followed by autologous bone marrow rescue as treatment for adult acute leukemia in relapse. *Am J Clin Oncol* 1986; **9**: 307–310.

44. Meloni G, De Fabritiis P, Pap G, *et al.* Cryopreserved autologous bone marrow infusion following high-dose chemotherapy in patients with acute myeloblastic leukemia in first relapse. *Leuk Res* 1985; **9**: 407–412.

45. Burnett AK, Tansey P, Watkins R, *et al.* Transplantation of unpurged autologous bone marrow in acute myeloid leukemia in first remission. *Lancet* 1984; **2**: 1068–1069.

36. Strategies to Prevent Chemotherapy Related Toxicity in the Older Person

Vittorina Zagonel, Antonio Pinto and Silvio Monfardini

Introduction

The use of dose-effective chemotherapy is unfortunately associated with a broad variety of unwanted side effects which are related to both the type of drug administered and to the acute or cumulative dose delivered. Anticancer agents usually exhibit a relatively narrow therapeutic index, leading to significant toxicity to normal tissues even at standard doses (1). The therapeutic index may become further restricted with the increasing age of the patient, so that many elderly patients cannot be treated as effectively as younger individuals. As a matter of fact, chemotherapy toxicity may be particularly unpleasant in the elderly, owing to the reduced physical and psychological compliance of these patients, and may often result in life-threatening complications.

On the other hand, some malignancies are highly curable with chemotherapy also in the older person and a clear-cut correlation between chemotherapy dose intensity and the probability of complete remission (CR), relapse-free survival (RFS), and overall survival (OS) has been convincingly demonstrated in the cases of aggressive lymphomas, adenocarcinoma of the breast and other chemosensitive tumors (2–5). While about 50% of cancer patients aged 65 years and over are considered able to undergo combination chemotherapy at standard doses at the time of diagnosis (6–7), only one half of these subjects actually complete the chemotherapy program fully and without significant delay (8, 9). Thus, the administration of effective and potentially curative chemotherapy to elderly subjects affected by chemosensitive tumors is a critical challenge of geriatric oncology (10, 11). As an example, it has been clearly shown by the National High Priority Lymphoma Study Group that elderly patients with intermediate and high grade non Hodgkin's lymphoma (NHL) have a survival similar to their younger counterparts if they are able to carry out full doses of second (CHOP) or third generation (m-BACOD, ProMACE-CytaBOM) chemotherapy regimens (12).

Most of the complications of chemotherapy related to age may actually reflect changes in physiologic functional parameters such as hypoalbuminemia or impaired renal function occurring in some but not all elderly subjects (13, 14). Therefore, accurate assessment of renal, hepatic, and hemopoietic function represents more reliable guide in predicting benefits and risks of chemotherapy in the elderly than chronologic age (11–16).

Based on the above considerations a number of strategies and comedications which have been developed over the last few years to make the use of appropriate doses of anticancer drugs more and more tolerable, can be now adopted in the elderly. The exact knowledge and application of these strategies may facilitate today the design of clinical protocols for older individuals and allow an increasing number of elderly cancer patients to undergo dose-effective chemotherapy. These advances include the availability of recombinant hemopoietic growth factors (HGF) and *ex vivo* manipulated stem cells progeny for ameliorating treatment-related myelotoxicity, of desrazoxane for the prevention of anthracycline cardiomyopathy (17), the availability of broad spectrum cytoprotective agents, the increased knowledge of age-related changes in pharmacokinetics (14,18) and a clearer understanding of the mechanisms of drug-related toxicity (l, 14). An accurate assessment of risks and benefits is essential to treat older patients safely and effectively. In older individuals the risk/benefit ratio of cytotoxic chemotherapy is based on the effectiveness of chemotherapy in different neoplasms (in terms of clinical responses, symptom palliation, disease-free survival and survival), the general physical conditions of each patients, comorbidity, emotional stability, cognitive ability to participate in the treatment plans, cooperation from family members, and social support (13, 14).

The Choice of Chemotherapy in the Elderly

The decision of treating elderly cancer patients with cytotoxic drugs should rely on specific reasons justifying such therapeutic approach (Table 36.1). We will herewith provide a frame of reference to answer the questions involved in this decision.

Which Kind of Tumors Should be Treated?

The use of chemotherapy, and in particular of regimens carrying a significant toxicity, should be limited to chemosensitive tumors in which the clinical efficacy of a given chemotherapy program has been clearly demonstrated in the adults. One such regimen is the combination of cyclophosphamide, doxorubicin (hydroxydaunorubicin), vincristine and prednisone (CHOP) in intermediate/high grade NHL (11–13). For other types of neoplasms, whose chemosensitivity has not been clearly demonstrated, one should consider the enrollment of elderly patients in prospective controlled phase II trials aimed at evaluating the efficacy

Table 36.1 Criteria for the choice of chemotherapy in the elderly.

1. Chemotherapy should be limited to chemosensitive tumors. Elderly could be enrolled into phase II trials, aimed at evaluating the efficacy and tolerance of newly anticancer drugs.

2. Due to the better compliance and tolerability, single agent chemotherapy must be preferred to combination chemotherapy, provided that the expected results are similar.

3. Multidimensional geriatric assessment, instead of performance status evaluation, is needed to guide clinical decision-making and therapeutic choice.

4. Informed consent is required from both patients and their relatives.

and tolerance of newly developed anticancer drugs (19). Such an approach, while allowing the short-term collection of a great amount of relevant clinical information on newer drugs, will ensure a most appropriate clinical management and follow up from qualified referral centers to a large fraction of older patients (20). Since dose-intensity is often important for therapeutic effectiveness, inclusion of older patients in phase II trials will enlarge the scope of these trials, to include the entire patient population (19, 20).

Which Kind of Chemotherapy?

When comparable clinical results are expected, single agent therapy is preferable to combination chemotherapy in terms of compliance and tolerance (13, 14, 21). As an example, there is no conclusive evidence supporting the advantage of combination vs single agent (Etoposide or Teniposide) chemotherapy for the treatment of metastatic small cell lung carcinoma (SCLC), in terms of both clinical efficacy and cost-effectiveness (based on the incidence of toxicity, overall treatment compliance, need for hospitalization, requirement of aggressive supportive therapy) (13, 21). Oral etoposide has actually provided excellent results in SCLC, leading to an OS competitive with the most effective combination chemotherapy regimens (13). Similarly, the use of single agent weekly vinorelbine may represent an effective therapeutic strategy in older patients affected by advanced non-SCLC (13) and metastatic breast cancer not responsive to hormonal therapy (22). In contrast, the need for combination chemotherapy to improve survival also in older patients is clearly established for aggressive NHL (12, 23, 24).

Another important aspect of this question concerns the choice of the route of drug administration, which may be oral or intravenous by push, by short or by continuous infusion. The oral route may be advantageous to the older subject even though it may imply some differences in treatment efficacy, related to bioavailability, pharmacology and individual compli-

ance with treatment (13, 14, 25). It is well established, for instance, that alterations in gastrointestinal absorption, quite typical in the elderly, may significantly reduce the bioavailability of orally administered anticancer drugs (25, 26).

Is Performance Status (PS) an Adequate Criteria for Treatment Choice?

PS provides a reliable prognostic parameter for the treatment of younger adults, but it may not be adequate parameter for the elderly. Other, more important, variables should be accounted for in making the therapeutic choice for older subjects. These may include: a) comorbid conditions influencing the overall physical status and causing important interactions in the pharmacologic disposition of drugs. Comorbidity may also dramatically affect *quoad vitam* prognosis in the aged cancer patient and should be therefore taken into account in the basic decision between life-prolonging treatment and pure symptom palliation; b) physical impairments which may enhance the risk of treatment complications, and mental impairments which may interfere with compliance; c) transportation and financial resources.

Seventy consecutive elderly cancer patients, observed at the Aviano Cancer Center, were enrolled into a prospective study and interviewed by means of multidimensional geriatric assessment (MGA) protocol. MGA was specifically designed to collect information, among others, on socio-demographic characteristics, economic resources, cognitive status (Mini Mental State – MMS test), emotional stability screened with the Geriatric Depression Scale (GDS) and physical activity (Physical Performance test – PPT; Activity of Daily Living – ADL – and the Instrumental Activity of Daily Living – IADL – tests). The reproducibility and validity of MGA among elderly cancer patients was preliminarily tested on a sample of our study group (27). The statistical correlation between PS (according to the Karnofsky scale) and MGA was evaluated by using the correlation coefficient (r). A correlation emerged between PS and both IADL (r = 0.55) and ADL (r = 0.50), indicating that PS may identify only about 30% of the differences measured by MGA. A less significant positive correlation was found between PS and MMS (r = 0.31) and PPT (r = 0.29), whereas an increased PS was correlated with a reduced prevalence of depressive symptoms (28). These results overall suggest that more than 70% of the variability measured by MGA could not be predicted by PS alone. They also highlight substantial limitations of the single use of PS for evaluating elderly patients, and underline the need for a multidimensional assessment approach also in the oncology setting. A more accurate evaluation of the global (physical, mental and disease-related) status of older patients, including the above described MGA approach, may facilitate the choice of the most appropriate chemotherapy strategy for each individual, and proved central to the process of clinical-decision making (28, 29).

Patient's or Relatives' Informed Consent?

It is daily clinical experience that older patients referred to specialized oncology centers, at least in Europe, represent a selected fringe of the older patient population. This selection is mainly based on social and/or mental status, education and patient's or family members' attitude toward cancer (10). For these reasons it is usually easy to communicate with the elderly and, after reassurance on his/her clinical conditions and on the possibilities of therapeutic intervention is given, to agree on an appropriate treatment plan. Unfortunately, most older subjects are strictly dependent on family member for what concerns logistic support (i.e. transportation to the care center), economic, and emotional support and for the solution of routine daily problems. Frequently, the treatment related decisions become family decisions in the management of older patients. As a matter of fact, patient willingness of being effectively treated may be frequently challenged by a negative attitude of family members, often based on economic and/or logistic issues, and by the relatives' perception that older persons are less likely to benefit from anticancer therapy or to withstand treatment-related side-effects (29). The decision of treating an older cancer patient willing to undergo an appropriate therapy program, should therefore be negotiated with family members to obtain their full agreement and cooperation (30). In such a way one may hopefully avoid patients succumbing from severe or unexpected, but clinically manageable, treatment-related toxicities because medical attention and hospital admissions were not timely pursued. Likewise, many complications of chemotherapy which are bothersome even when they are not life-threatening, may be avoided or minimized by a cooperative family and with appropriate home care. Cooperating family members can be easily educated on recognizing most common side effects and disease-related events and instructed to alert the attending physician for consultation or hospital admission.

Active Protection from Chemotherapy Toxicity

Bone Marrow Toxicity

Several recombinant HGF and cytokines (G-CSF, GM-CSF, erythropoietin, IL-3), able to temper or to prevent myelosuppression secondary to chemotherapy (17,31) have been introduced in the current clinical practice over the last few years (Tables 36.2 and 36.3). Most studies in adult patients have convincingly shown that administration of GM-CSF or G-CSF can: a) reduce both intensity and duration of granulo-monocytopenia; b) accelerate hemopoietic recovery to allow optimal timing of the administered chemotherapy; c) decrease number and severity of infectious episodes related to drug-induced neutropenia (31–33). Studies evaluating the cost-effectiveness of growth factor therapy in adult patients have concluded that prophylactic use of cytokines is cost-effective only with dose-intensive chemotherapeutic protocols (34), involving a risk of

hospitalization for neutropenic fever $\geq 40\%$. This situation may be faced more frequently in the management of older individuals. Also, the conclusion of cost/effectiveness studies were based on the assumption that the use of HGF had no effects on mortality (34). This may not be the case in older individuals, with a limited hemopoietic reserve (32, 35). In this regard most studies are concordant that elderly subjects display a higher degree of hematologic toxicity (7, 13, 14, 18), a more prolonged and severe neutropenia and a higher rate of infection-related deaths secondary to chemotherapy, as compared to younger individuals (7, 36, 37). Studies evaluating the functional activity of intermediate and mature myeloid cells, i.e. all morphologically recognizable hemopoietic precursors of the bone marrow and circulating neutrophils, have not clearly demonstrated significant differences in the aged (31, 38–40), suggesting that age-related changes primarily affect the early stages of hemopoiesis and the most immature blood cell progenitors within the bone marrow (41, 42). The physiologic basis of impaired myelopoiesis in the elderly is not completely understood even though age-associated changes in bone marrow microenvironment (43), decreased production of regulatory cytokines (44), reduced numbers of bone marrow progenitors (42) and a suboptimal response of hemopoietic precursors to specific growth factors such as G-CSF (39), or a combination of these factors (41, 45) have been proposed. As age-related hemopoietic impairment appears to affect the early hemopoietic phases, i.e. hemopoietic stem cells and early lineage progenitors (42, 45), one can expect hemopoietic growth factors in clinical use (G-CSF, GM-CSF) to prove equally effective in younger and older individuals. These cytokines may in fact recruit and expand the committed progenitors pool or the proliferating myeloid cell compartment (i.e. myeloblasts, promyelocytes and myelocytes) which are both distal to early stem cells. This expectation was supported by different investigators who demonstrated that dose- and time-dependent hematologic responses to most HGF and cytokines (G-CSF, GM-CSF, IL-3) are well maintained in patients and normal volunteers aged 65 years and more (31, 39, 40). More recently, we have shown that in patients with aggressive NHL aged 60 — 70 years and treated with a second generation combination chemotherapy (CHVmP-VB), the administration of G-CSF resulted in a significant increase in peripheral absolute neutrophils counts (ANC). This response does not fade with time, but is fully maintained throughout the eighth consecutive course of chemotherapy (33). Therapy with G-CSF facilitated the on-schedule delivery of chemotherapy, resulting in fewer and shorter delays between treatment courses. Delayed courses were observed in 19% of the patients given G-CSF and in 32.5% of the patients in the control arm. Dose reductions due to concurrent infection were also significantly less frequent in patients receiving G-CSF as compared to controls (16.6% vs 55%). The picture may however turn different in patients aged more than 70 years, at least in terms of a reduced response to repeated administration of HGFs. At our

Table 36.2 Prevention of chemotherapy toxicity.

Target Organ	Guidelines
Bone marrow	– growth factors (G-CSF, GM-CSF, IL-3, Epo, Pixy 321, stem cell factor) – transfusion support – cytoprotective agents (amifostine)
Immune system (Infections)	– antibiotic prophylaxis – antimycotic prophylaxis – immunoglobulins administration – avoidance or careful use of highly immunosuppressive drugs (i.e. purine analogues, corticosteriods)
Heart	– cytoprotective agents (ICRF-187, amifostine) – doxorubicin: continuous infusion or weekly administration; stop administration upon a more than 20% reduction of EF; a total dose of 450 mg/m2 should not be exceeded. – use of doxorubicin analogs (i.e. epirubicin) if EF < 50% – switch to mitoxantrone in breast cancer. – correct malnutrition and vitamin E deficiency
Gastro-intestinal tract	Mucositis: – GM-CSF, G-CSF = retinoic acid, oral cryotherapy (for 5-FU), KGF, IL-11. Diarrhea: – rapid correction of dehydration; i.v. fluid support and adequate liquid intake.
Liver	MEGX test in pre-treatment evaluation.
Lung	– Always perform pre-treatment PO2 and functional tests, check for anamnestic lung diseases. – Bleomycin: continuous infusion or intramuscular administration – Nitrosoureas: ambroxol
Kidney	– creatinine clearance and proteinuria evaluation. – cytoprotective agents (DDTC, sodium thiosulfate, amifostine)
Bladder	– Ifosphamide: Mesna
Nervous System	– Vincristine: do not exceed the total dose of 2 mg for each course; do not recycle before 15 days; use of continuous infusion; use of prophylactic mild laxatives; oral glutamic acid could be useful; mobilization (cyclette); light physical exercise; substitute with vindesine. – ARA-C: thetrahydrouridine. – cytoprotective agents (amifostine).

institution 20 consecutive patients older than 70 years with intermediate and high grade NHL, were treated with the VMP combination (46) and alternated G-GSF (i.e. every other course) from the 7th to the 20th day of the course (47). Therefore, the same patient was scheduled to receive consecutive courses of VMP with or without G-CSF support (47). Preliminary results of this study indicate that the number of delayed cycles after G-CSF was significantly lower. Patients receiving the first chemotherapy course without G-CSF displayed, as expected, a longer and more marked neutropenia following VMP, but also a reduced response, in terms of neutrophil increase, to G-CSF administered in subsequent courses. In patients first given VMP without growth factor, the hematologic response to G-CSF was also progressively reduced with the administration of further courses of chemotherapy. In contrast, in patients receiving G-CSF from the beginning, the magnitude of HGF-stimulated neutrophils increase was reduced to a lesser extent during subsequent courses of chemotherapy (47). The biologic mechanisms underlying the early and progressive reduction in bone marrow response to G-CSF in elderly (>70 years) NHL patients, and especially in those starting first chemotherapy without growth factor support, remain to be established. One possible explanation may be that, in these subjects, age-impaired stem cells are unable to efficiently reconstitute in a due time the intermediate pool of committed progenitors hit by the first course of chemotherapy and then exhausted by G-CSF. Alternatively, the pool of committed progenitors (i.e. CFU-GM, CFU-G) in patients older than 70 years may display a reduced sensitivity to G-CSF, as compared to more mature proliferating myelopoietic precursors (i.e. myeloblasts, promyelocytes and myelocytes). It has been suggested in fact that G-CSF- induced neutrophilia in these patients may be mainly due to increased PMN production and shortened PMN maturation time in the marrow, more than to the recruitment of early progenitors (39). This might explain the early good response to G-CSF and the progressively reduced extent of neutrophilia in subsequent administrations of the factor. Differences in bone marrow kinetic response to increasing dosages (30 and 300 µg/day) of G-CSF were explored in a very interesting randomized study by Chatta *et al.* comparing younger (aged 20 to 30 years) and older (aged 70 to 80 years) normal volunteers (39). Baseline ANCs and circulating hemopoietic progenitors (granulocyte-macrophage colony-forming units/CFU-GM) were comparable in both age groups. Similarly, the two groups had equivalent increases in ANCs after administration of both G-CSF doses. In contrast, the concentration of peripheral CFU-GM at the G-CSF dose of 30 µg were increased 2-fold in younger individuals, but were not increased in the elderly. At doses of G-CSF 300 µg a 24- and 12-fold increase in circulating CFU-GM were respectively found in younger and older subjects (39). These results confirm that while the early response to growth factors (i.e. expansion and recruitment of late myeloid precursors) is well preserved in the elderly, the population of hemopoietic stem cells and early progenitors may undergo a progressive reduction with age. This age-related hemopoietic alteration may be particularly evident with suboptimal doses of growth factors. These results suggest that long-term administration of cytokines and suboptimal growth factor dosing may have very different effects in older and younger patients (39, 47). Based on these assumptions, patients aged more than 70 years should be given full dose G-CSF since the beginning of the first chemotherapy course, especially when multiple courses (six to eight) of standard-dose combination chemotherapy have been planned. G-CSF (5 µg/kg/die subcutaneously) could be administered a few days before the expected neutrophil nadir and discontinued at least 72 hours before the next chemotherapy administration, in order to avoid exposure to cytotoxic drugs of hemopoietic progenitor cells recruited and triggered to proliferation by the growth factor (17, 48). In addition, another beneficial effect of G-CSF, i.e. protection against T-cell-mediated lethal shock triggered by bacterial superantigens, has been recently demonstrated (49). Since older patients may be particularly prone to develop infection-related fatal complications, the prompt addition of G-CSF to combination chemotherapy appears further justified.

Studies on bone marrow cell kinetics in patients receiving GM-CSF have shown that, early after growth factor suspension, the proliferative activity of the bone marrow cell progenitors quickly decreases to a level significantly lower than that observed before the administration of GM-CSF (50). Whatever the biological reason for the phenomenon, it is possible that the 48-hour to 96-hour lag phase, after GM-CSF is discontinued, may represent a period of partial refractoriness of hemopoietic progenitor cells to the action of cell-cycle-specific cytostatic drugs (49). This observation suggests that a short period of treatment with GM-CSF before chemotherapy and some days after delivering of cytotoxic drugs, might decrease the hemopoietic toxicity of antineoplastic treatments and reduce the extent and duration of drug-related neutropenia (51).

GM-CSF and G-CSF have never been directly compared in elderly cancer patients. In a randomized trial comparing G-CSF to GM-CSF in the setting of chemotherapy induced neutropenia, Miller concluded that both G-CSF and GM-CSF appear equally effective (52). GM-CSF might have an additional advantage for the elderly as it may prevent chemotherapy induced mucositis (53). Even though specific studies of elderly patients receiving standard-dose chemotherapy are relatively few, one can reasonably conclude that the use of G- or GM-CSF at a proper dosage is safe also in these patients, and results in effective early hemopoietic stimulation along with a significant reduction of neutropenia-related infections, septic deaths, and, possibly, of mucosal cell damage (32, 33, 49–53).

Management of drug-induced thrombocytopenia remains a problem since most of the widely used HGFs (i.e. G-CSF, GM-CSF) are unable to stimulate thrombopoiesis. Phase I studies in humans utilizing the stromal cell-derived cytokine IL-11, have shown however promising results for the prevention and management of drug-related thrombocytopenia. IL-11 is able to increase circulating platelet counts and to stimulate megakaryocytopoiesis in humans, along with the promotional multi lineage hematopoiesis. Preliminary studies in patients receiving myelosuppressive chemotherapy, including the strong thrombocytopenic agent carboplatin, have shown that this cytokine is able to reduce both extent and duration of thrombocytopenia, resulting in a significant reduction of the need for platelet transfusions and of hemorrhagic complications. Phase II — III studies are currently ongoing, but it appears that the concurrent use of IL-11 and/or of the recently cloned megakaryocyte growth and development factor (MGDF, c-mpl ligand) will provide an effective protection against the thrombocytopenic effects of most

Table 36.3 Hemopoietic growth factors and cytokine of current and prospective clinical use for the management of chemotherapy-induced bone marrow toxicity in elderly cancer patients.

Growth Factor/Cytokine	Main Cellular Targets	Clinical Activity	Tested in the Elderly
GM-CSF	– early CD34+ progenitors – committed progenitors (CFU-GEMM, CFU-GM, (CFU-M, CFU-MK) – proliferating myeloid cells (myeloblasts — myelocytes) – mature monocytes – mature neutrophils	– increase and activation of circulating neutrophils, monocytes and eosinophils – mobilization of CD34+ progenitors into peripheral blood	YES (active)
G-CSF	– late CD34+ progenitors – late committed progenitors (CFU-G) – proliferating myeloid cells (myeloblasts — myelocytes) – mature neutrophils	– increase and activation of circulating neutrophils – mobilization of CD34+ progenitors into peripheral blood	YES (active)
IL-3	– early CD34+ progenitors – committed progenitors (CFU-GEMM, BFU-E, CFU-GM, CFU-G, CFU-M, CFU-MK)	– increase of circulating neutrophils – increase in platelets when combined with GM-CSF? – mobilization of CD34+ progenitors into peripheral blood	YES (active)
EPO	– intermediate and committed progenitors (CFU-GEMM, CFU-E, CFU-MK)	– increase in RBC's – increase in HTC	YES (active)
M-CSF	– late CD34+ progenitors – committed progenitors (CFU-M, CFU-GM) – mature monocytes	– increase and activation of circulating monocytes – treatment of invasive fungal infections	NO
Pixy 321 (GM-CSF/IL-3 fusion protein)	– early and late CD34+ progenitors – committed progenitors (CFU-GEMM, CFU-GM, CFU-MK, BFU-E)	– increase in circulating neutrophils – increase in platelets? – mobilization of CD34+ progenitors in peripheral blood	limited experience
SCF	– early and late CD34+ progenitors – mast cells – megakaryocytes – costimulatory factor synergizing with other growth factors/cytokines	– increase in circulating CD34+ progenitors usually combined with G-CSF – increase in platelets when combined with G-CSF?	NO
IL-6	– early CD34+ progenitors – committed progenitors (CFU-GEMM, CFU-MK) – synergy factor with GM-CSF	– increase in circulating CD34+ progenitors when combined with GM-CSF – increase in platelets when combined with GM-CSF?	NO

Table 36.3 Continued.

Growth Factor/Cytokine	Main Cellular Targets	Clinical Activity	Tested in the Elderly
IL-11	– early CD34+ progenitors – committed progenitors (CFU-GEMM, CFU-GM, CFU-MK, BFU-E, CFU-M) – mesenchimal cells, preadipocytes, intestinal mucosa epithelial cells (?), stromal cells within intestinal mucosa (?) – synergy factor G-SCF, IL-3, SCF	– increase in platelets – increase in circulating CD34+ progenitors when combined with G-CSF – reduction of thrombocytopenia duration and extent in patients receiving myelo-suppressive chemotherapy – reduction of the need for platelet transfusions in the patients receiving myelosuppressive chemotherapy – protection from chemotherapy — and — radiotherapy — induced mucosal cell damage (oral and intestinal mucosa) in animal models – reduction of Gram-negative sepsis in neutropenic animals	NO
MGDF (mpl-ligand)	– early CD34+ progenitors – committed progenitors (CFU-GEMM, CFU-MK) – megakaryocyte	– increase in platelets – increase in circulating CD34+ progenitors – reduction of thrombocytopenia duration and extent in patients receiving myelosuppressive chemotherapy – reduction of the need for platelet trans-fusions in patients receiving chemotherapy – stimulation of platelet production for autologous collection (platelet autotransfusion) – *ex-vivo* expansion of CD34+ progenitors	NO

anticancer drugs, including organoplatinum compounds.

The issues of hemopoietic exhaustion and suboptimal response over prolonged HGF administration, remain to be fully addressed in the elderly and appropriate studying is required. Current treatment protocols for a number of malignancies, i.e. NHLs, involve the administration of repeated courses of combination chemotherapy and the risk of neutropenic deaths may therefore increase in the elderly (> 70 years) during later chemotherapy courses despite the use of growth factors. Since the hemopoietic deficit in the elderly mainly resides on stem cells and/or early multipotent progenitors (39, 41, 42, 45), the prospective use of newly developed cytokines (i.e. stem cell factor, Pixy 321, IL-1, IL-6, IL-11, MGDF) acting on these earlier hemopoietic precursors (48) (Table 36.3), may provide a further tool for improving hemopoietic functions in aged individuals. The recent identification and cloning of c-mpl ligand as a prospective megakaryocyte growth factor (54, 55), and of a specific ligand (FLT 3-ligand) for the stem cell associated tyrosine kinase-l (56, 57), a growth factor receptor expressed by earliest progenitors, may also represent an important advance for the prevention and management of myelosuppression in the elderly.

Owing to the redundancy of growth factor receptors on hemopoietic stem cells (58), it appears however probable that a combination of appropriate cytokines (i.e. SCF, FLT3-Ligand, MGDF) will provide the most effective tool for circumventing the impairment in early-stage hemopoiesis typical of the elderly. Specific studies on the phenotype and biology of CD34+ progenitors in older individuals are lacking. Dissecting the functional heterogeneity of these progenitors and establishing their growth factor receptors repertoire appear as promising research areas. New insights in these areas my direct new cytokine combinations for elderly individuals.

The possible use of peripheral blood progenitor cells (PBPC), mobilized by growth factors may also be explored in older individuals as a means to rescue drug-induced myelotoxicity. Preliminary data from our group indicates that adequate numbers of CD34+ progenitors can be obtained in elderly NHL patients treated either with standard dose CHVmP-VB (60–70 years) or a specifically devised chemotherapy combination (VMP; patients aged 70 or more) plus G-CSF, provided that the harvest is made early in the treatment. In our experience, harvests performed after the second course of chemotherapy have been consistently unproductive. PBPC preparations may be employed in elderly patients affected by tumors, such as NHL, in which the probability of increased survival is strictly associated with the on-time delivery of full-dose conventional chemotherapy.

Newer developments in the field of stem cell biology and *ex vivo* expansion of targeted populations of intermediate hemopoietic cells, i.e. neutrophils and platelet progenitors, may turn out to be of even greater relevance for the treatment of elderly patients. As an example, it appears now possible to drive purified CD34+ cells toward becoming neutrophils precursors still capable of some division. Therefore, while with peripheral blood stem cells an average of about ten days is required for neutrophil recovery, the use of *ex vivo* expanded neutrophil progenitors should be able to reduce neutrophil recovery to five days or less. Owing to the higher rate of neutropenia-related deaths in older subjects (7, 36, 37), any strategy taking down neutropenic periods to less than a few days would result in a dramatic advantage for such patients. Similarly, attempts to drive CD34+ cells into megakaryocyte progenitors are being developed which may allow to significantly shorten or prevent thrombocytopenia and avoid older patient problems related to frequent platelet transfusions.

In conclusion, cytokines, recombinant HGF and *ex vivo* expanded targeted hemopoietic cell fractions should be used in older patients to support standard-dose chemotherapy regimens in chemosensitive tumors, and appear safe and cost-effective. The purpose of growth factor therapy should be to allow the timely administration of full dose chemotherapy, to decrease chemotherapy-related morbidity and mortality and subsequently, to reduce hospitalization rate.

Anemia

A large number of cancer patients are anemic, and up to 19% of patients receiving chemotherapy require blood transfusions (59). Recently, a recombinant form of human erythropoietin (Epo) has become available for clinical use. In a randomized trial of 413 patients Abels *et al.* have reported an increase in hematocrit (HCT) levels from 27.6% to 29.3%, following Epo administration (60). When given at a dose of either 100 U/kg three times weekly, in patients not receiving chemotherapy, or at a dose of 150 U/kg three times weekly, in patients undergoing chemotherapy, Epo can significantly reduce transfusion requirements and increase HCT, although at least one month of therapy may be necessary before the results are observed (61). Therapeutic benefits are maximal after three months of continued therapy. Patients responding to Epo also show a significant improvement in overall performance, and Epo administration appears overall safe and well tolerated in anemic patients with cancer (61). No differences in hemoglobin levels increase among subjects older and younger than 65 years were noted following Epo administration (31), indicating that this cytokine is equally effective in older patients (31, 32). However, in elderly patients developing chemotherapy-related acute anemia, transfusion therapy remains the most appropriate choice due to the more rapid correction of hemoglobin levels and HCT and to its minor cost (62). Additional studies are warranted to better define the subsets of older patients who may obtain the greatest therapeutic benefit from Epo.

Cytotoxic Drug-Related Immunodeficiency

While it is well known that several anticancer agents can severely impair the immune system, aging-associated changes in immune cell functions and decreased immune competence have been emphasized by several studies (63). Older patients may present hypogamma-globulinemia, lymphopenia and a specific decrease of CD4+ T-cells levels and function (63, 64). Decreased T-cell function and the resulting impairment in cellular immunity in healthy elderly individuals appear also correlated with an increased likelihood of death (65). In addition, aging is associated with a shift toward a grater proportion of CD4+ T-cells of memory (CD45R0+) phenotype and a consensual reduction of cells showing a naive (CD45RA+) phenotype (66, 67). It has been suggested that a number of T-cell alterations (i.e. decreased mitogen- and antigen-driven proliferation, reduced response to T cell receptor mediated and co-stimulatory molecules-dependent activation, alterations in the profile of cytokine production) noted in the elderly (63) may be the result of the aging-associated shift from naive to memory T-cell predominance. More recently, an age-dependent deficiency in CD4+/CD45RA+ T-cell recovery has been demonstrated in cancer patients undergoing cytotoxic therapy (68). Thus chemotherapy-induced worsening of the age-associated physiologic impairment in CD4+/CD45RA+ T-cell generation, may make elderly cancer patients most vulnerable to life-threatening complications of T-lymphocyte malfunction, including infections by intracellular organisms. One should therefore pay a special attention in evaluating and preventing lymphopenia-related complications of chemotherapy, since any cytotoxic drugs that depletes CD4+ T-cells may have a more profound effect in older patients that in younger adults. Such may be the case of recently developed purine analogs (37). Purine analogs such as fludarabine, cladribine (2-chloro-deoxyadenosine) and pentostatine (deoxyco-formycin), represent very active agents for the treatment of indolent lymphoid malignancies (i.e. chronic lymphocytic leukemia, low grade NHL, hairy cell leukemia), which are particularly frequent in the elderly population. Each of these analogs has been shown to induce a profound lymphocytopenia and a drug-related marked decrease in CD4+ T-cells, which may persist for several years after the recovery of other mononuclear blood cell populations (37). The incidence of infections in patients treated with purine analogs has been shown to be age-related and their spectrum includes a wide range of opportunistic organisms. Because of the high risk of life-threatening infections by unusual pathogens in elderly patients (37), the use of purine analogs should be limited, in the elderly, to subjects without other immunologic deficiencies and not receiving concurrent corticosteroid therapy (Table 36.2). Whenever feasible, avoidance of chronic steroid therapy in these patients may prevent both infectious complications related to administration of purine analogs and metabolic alterations (i.e. diabetes) due to corticosteroid treatment. In addition, it is advisable to deliver the lowest possible number of courses of purine analogs (37).

Immunoglobulin prophylaxis appears indicated in older patients with a circulating IgG level of less than 600 mg/mL (Table 36.2). The prophylactic use of cotrimoxazole reduces the risk of lymphopenia-related lung infections, especially pneumocystis carinii pneumonia, but may worsen bone marrow damage from chemotherapy.

Cardiac Toxicity

Cardiovascular disease is a major cause of comorbidity and mortality in older patients with cancer (69). Cardiotoxic potential of the various chemotherapeutic agents is critical in defining the maximum dose that older patients may tolerate (1, 29, 70). Doxorubicin and other anthracyclines represent very active anticancer drugs and are therefore frequently employed for treatment of a wide variety of chemosensitive tumors (1). Anthracycline cardiotoxicity is primarily related to cumulative dose, even though these drugs may also cause acute cardiac disfunction (70, 71). Aging of the cardiovascular system and the frequent conmitance of cardiac diseases renders the older patient very susceptible to anthracycline cardiotoxicity (1, 29, 70). The elderly are likely to experience cardiac toxicity at lower cumulative doses of doxorubicin than adults. Specific strategies should therefore be adopted for preventing and reducing anthracycline cardiac toxicity in these patients (Table 36.2). As reported several years ago, it is possible to reduce anthracycline cardiotoxicity using continuous infusion (24–48 hours) instead of pulse administration of the drugs (72). Cardiotoxicity may also be reduced with repeated small weekly doses of the drugs (73) to maintain the same dose intensity. Clinical studies using these approaches have shown significantly less cardiotoxicity while maintaining comparable antitumor effects. Current recommendations advise, however, that patients over the age of 70, should not exceed a total doxorubicin dosage of 450 mg/m^2, and that anthracycline administration should be avoided for reductions $\geq$ 20% of left ventricular Ejection Fraction (LVEF), regardless of coexisting heart disease and of schedule or administration route (1, 25, 70). Furthermore, a number of doxorubicin analogues, such as 4'-epidoxorubicin and more recently idarubicin, have been developed which possess comparable anti-tumor activity in breast cancer (74) and hematological malignancies (74, 75) of the elderly, but carry a reduced risk of causing cardiac damage. These analogues should be considered for substituting doxorubicin in combination chemotherapy program for elderly subjects with anthracycline-responsive tumors. Due to its favorable toxicity profile, mitoxantrone has been recently explored as a possible replacement for doxorubicin (76). In several trials comparing mitoxantrone and doxorubicin in patients with metastatic breast cancer, mitoxantrone was better tolerated than doxorubicin, and caused a lesser overall toxicity including cardiac damage. In two of three randomized studies of doxorubicin and mitoxantrone in breast cancer, antitumor efficacy of the two drugs was comparable, both showing a response rate within the range of 20% to 30% (77, 78). One study however demonstrated a slightly higher response rate for doxorubicin when compared with mitoxantrone (79). Results obtained in older patients with NHL are more controversial since in some randomized studies the clinical activity of the CHOP combination has been demonstrated to be statistically superior to mitoxantrone containing regimes. The Dutch Cooperative Group recently completed a prospective randomized trial of CHOP versus CNOP in patients 60 years old or more affected by aggressive NHL (80). Treatment with CHOP resulted in a higher CR rate (49% vs 31% P = .03) and OS (P = .03) as compared to CNOP (80). Results of a randomized study from the EORTC lymphoma group also showed the superiority of the CHOP regimen as compared to VMP in terms of CR, RFS, and OS (81) in patients aged 70 years and more. These results suggest that anthracylines should be maintained in chemotherapy regimes for elderly patients with aggressive NHL showing a LVEF > 50%, also by taking into account the higher costs of mitoxantrone.

Recently, the iron chelator ICRF-187 (desrazoxane) has been shown to be an effective cardioprotector (82). Laboratory studies and randomized clinical trials with ICRF-187, support the concept that anthracycline-related cardiotoxicity can be circumvented without diminishing the antitumor activity of the drugs (83, 84). In a randomized trial enrolling more than 100 women with advanced breast cancer, Speyer et al. compared treatment with 5 Fluorouracil (5-FU), doxorubicin, and cyclophosphamide, given every 21 days, with the same regime preceded by administration of ICRF-187 (85). Cardiac toxicity was evaluated by clinical examination, determination of the left ventricular ejection fraction (LVEF) by multigated nuclear scans (MUGA), and endomyocardial biopsy. The authors concluded that ICRF-187 offers substantial protection against doxorubicin-induced cardiac toxicity along with a reduced incidence of non-cardiac toxic reactions (85). These results were confirmed by other studies (86, 87). IRCF-187 may prevent cardiomyopathy in elderly cancer patients who are particularly susceptible to the cardiotoxicity of anthracyclines. In particular, the use of ICRF-187 appears indicated for treatment regimens implying prolonged administration of doxorubicin, or combination of doxorubicin and chest irradiation. It should be underlined, however, that desrazoxane may worsen chemotherapy induced myelotoxicity.

The recent introduction in clinical practice of cytoprotective agents, such as amifostine (see below), may probably offer an alternative approach to prevent anthracycline cardiotoxicity in older patients.

In addition, a number of factors which have been shown to increase the risk of anthracycline-related cardiomyopathy should be especially accounted for in older patients. These include malnutrition, with a special regard to vitamin E deficiency, and the concomitant administration of drugs (i.e. cyclophosphamide, etoposide, vincristine, melphalan, bleomycin) which may impair the elimination and/or inactivation of anthraycyclines (70). Correction of malnutrition, the use of vitamin supplements, including tocopherol 2g/day starting one week before anthracyclines, accounting for pharmacologic interactions among anthracyclines and other drugs, along with a careful assessment of concomitant cardiovascular diseases (i.e. long standing hypertension and arrhythmias) may represent additional tools to prevent or reduce anthracycline-related cardiotoxicity in the elderly.

Finally, one should also bear in mind that a number of other anticancer drugs have sometimes induced cardiotoxic effects, even though the information has appeared in the literature in the form of case reports or small series (70). These include bleomycin, cyclophosphamide, taxol, 5-FU, methotrexate, busulfan and plant alkaloids (70). Even though of intermediate or little clinical significance in younger subjects, cardiac alterations induced by non-anthracycline drugs (myo/pericarditis, angina, bradycardia, ECG alterations, ventricular dysrhythmia, hypotension) may turn relevant in older patients with coexisting cardiovascular disorders.

Gastro-Intestinal Toxicity

The most common chemotherapy-induced gastrointestinal complication is nausea and vomiting (l, 26, 88). Clearly, the incidence and the severity of nausea and vomiting decrease with the patient age (88). This decline has never been satisfactorily explained. The sensitivity of vomiting centers and/or of the chemoreceptor trigger zone of the central nervous system may decline with age (29), but this is a hypothesis wanting experimental proof.

Mucositis, manifested primarily as stomatitis or severe diarrhea, appears to be more frequent and more severe in the elderly, although no conclusive studies are available. Mucosal damage may be particularly severe in the older patient due to the concurrent deficiency of vitamin B 12 and folates and to the age-related depletion of mucosal stem cells accompanied by increased epithelial cell proliferation (14). In addition, mechanisms regulating the repair of mucosal damage may be compromised in the aged (26). During periods of mucosal inflammation and damage, the barrier function of mucosa may be severely impaired so that the risk of serious infection should be also accounted for. Treatment of mucositis in the elderly is usually conservative and symptomatic, and includes warm saline mouth rinses, local antimicrobial agents (i.e. chlorhexidine), topical anesthetics such as viscous xylocaine given before fluid and food ingestion, topical nystatin to prevent mycotic over infection, and topical carafate. Ongoing studies of special interest to older patients, explore the possibility to prevent stomatitis with carafate. Fluid intake may be facilitated with a straw; timely administration of intravenous fluids and nutrition may be indicated in patients with severe mucositis (Table 36.2). Oral cryotherapy may ameliorate 5-FU induced mucositis (89). A prompt treatment with Aciclovir or Foscarnet may be also required in patients with concurrent mucositis and chemotherapy-related Herpes simplex virus reactivations. In this way one may avoid the worsening and complication of mucositis by viral-induced oral lesions. The concurrent use of GM-CSF, in addition to the effects on the hemopoietic system, may reduce mucosal cells damage (53). Similarly, a 75% decrease in the incidence of moderate to severe mucositis has been reported in bladder cancer patients when G-CSF was added to the M-VAC regime and to high-dose chemotherapy in patients undergoing autologous bone marrow transplantation (90, 91). More recently, the association of 13-cis-retinoic acid in patients receiving anthracyclines, has been suggested as an effective tool for reducing anthracycline-related mucosal damage (92). Oral 1 3-cis-retinoic acid is currently being tested also to reduce and prevent mucositis in elderly patients with acute myeloid leukemia undergoing dose-intense aggressive chemotherapy. A promising way to prevent or to manage severe mucositis may be the administration of recombinant Keratinocyte growth factor (KGF). KGF has been recently cloned (93) and showed to enhance survival and stimulate proliferation and differentiation of cultured keratinocytes and epithelial cells. In addition, a great amount of KGF is secreted in the dermis during wound healing processes (94). Pre-clinical testing on animal models suggests that this cytokine is effective in protecting the intestinal mucosas from the injury of cytotoxic agents, including anthracyclines (94). Recombinant human IL-11 may also be used for prevention and management of mucositis. Experimental studies have convincingly shown that recombinant IL-11 is able to stimulate recovery of intestinal and oral mucosal cells following myeloblative chemo-radio-therapy. Other investigators have also shown that IL-11 is able to induce the proliferative arrest of mucosal epithelial cells during the administration of chemotherapy. This antiproliferative effect may protect epithelia from cicle-active drugs. Phase I trials in humans are currently ongoing.

The risk of dehydration from reduced fluid intake and diarrhea should be always considered in older patients (25). Dehydration must be rapidly and effectively corrected in the elderly to avoid more severe complications such as renal insufficiency or failure and hypovolemic shock. In a trial from Petrelli et al. 20% of patients older than 65 years of age treated with 5-FU and high dose leucovorin for metastatic colorectal cancer died from dehydration due to diarrhea (95). However, it appears probable that in these patients preceding colon surgery might have caused malabsorption, which lead to weight loss and malnutrition, which made the mucosas particularly vulnerable to the treatment with 5FU/Leucovorin (96). Bloody diarrhea in the presence of mucositis may be particularly frequent following the administration of drugs such as 5-FU and Citosine-arabinoside (ARA-C) (1, 25, 26, 95, 96). Should the 5FU-related diarrhea be particularly severe and life-threatening, as frequently may occur in the elderly, the somatostatin-like octapeptide, octreotide may be used when other drugs (i.e. Loperamide, Diphenoxylate) have failed. In contrast, profuse diarrhea is an uncommon event in patients receiving methotrexate, hydroxyurea, nitrosoureas, and alkylating agents (26).

Attempts have been made to ameliorate the gastro-intestinal side effects of chemotherapeutic agents by supplemental nutritional sources (97). Enhancement of the caloric intake may lessen the malnutrition associated with neoplasia and/or anticancer treatments but does not eliminate the cause of malnutrition (98). It is likely that leucovorin worsens the 5FU related mucositis. Protracted infusions of 5FU at low daily doses may be effective in chemoresponsive tumors even without the addition of leucovorin, and may involve minimal mucositis.

Gastro-intestinal candidiasis is a common problem following chemotherapy, particularly in elderly patients with lymphoma and leukemia undergoing long term contricosteroid therapy. Treatment of oral candidiasis involves nystatin suspension or miconazole troches. Esophageal candidiasis requires systemic antifungal treatment with oral ketoconazol or fluconazol. The intestinal tract represents the main entry for gram (–) pathogens during neutropenia, which may be more prolonged in older individuals. Whenever neutropenia is expected to last one week or longer, prophylaxis with bactrim or quinolones is indicated. These antibiotics favor the overgrowth of anaerobic micro-organisms, which prevent the growth of gram (–) gastrointestinal bacteria.

Hepatic Toxicity

Assessment of liver function in cancer patients is essential for planning appropriate therapy (1,13). Hepatic function is known to decline with advancing age (99). Liver blood flow, liver mass, enzymatic activity of liver cells and the capability to replace damaged hepatocytes can be all strikingly reduced or impaired in the elderly, although the extent and severity of such changes is often unpredictable and extremely variable among different individuals (13–16, 25). On the other hand, since a large number of anticancer agents are actively metabolized by the liver, the therapeutic index of these drugs may be dramatically restricted by alterations in the hepatic function (25). In addition, while acetylation and conjugation are not usually affected by age, the activity of oxidative microsomal enzymes is greatly reduced in the aged. Hepatic oxidation is essential for the activation of certain antineoplastic agents including cyclophosphamide or ifosphamide. Age-related impairment of the oxidative hepatic functions may imply the reduction of the therapeutic activity of some anticancer agents given at a standard dosage (25). The accurate evaluation of liver function is mandatory in elderly cancer patients undergoing cytotoxic chemotherapy and should guide the clinician in determining proper dosage adjustments (25, 26). Unfortunately, the determination of circulating liver enzymes concentration bears no significant relationship to the oxidative function of the liver. No well established endogenous markers are available to monitor changes in hepatic function. A strategy is to encourage the adoption of "bio-dynamic" techniques based on the administration of model substrates followed by the subsequent detection of their specific metabolites (25). Lidocaine, a drug routinely employed for the treatment of ventricular arrhythmias, is characterized by hepatic metabolism and its main metabolite, monoethylglycinxilidide (MEGX), is the product of an oxidative N-dealkylation by cytochrome P450 system (100). MEGX concentrations are measurable in serum of patients receiving lidocaine, and correlate positively with liver function. In a study by Schinella *et al.*, performing MEGX tests in 49 elderly patients, the mean serum level of MEGX was markedly lower than that reported for younger adults and children (99). The measurement of blood MEGX may be useful for studying the declining hepatic function in elderly patients (100) (Table 36.2). MEGX determination is a safe, fast and reliable quantitative test that seems to play a key role in assessing not only the extent of hepatic impairment, but also in selecting optimal dosing and combination of anticancer drugs (101).

Pulmonary Toxicity

A higher prevalence of lung fibrosis following bleomycin treatment in patients over the age of 70 has been reported (102). The morbidity of pneumotoxicity may be enhanced in older patients due to aging-associated loss of pulmonary elasticity and higher prevalence of chronic obstructive lung disease (103). The higher risk of drug-related pulmonary fibrosis in the elderly is also probably related to a longer exposure to pre existing environmental conditions (air pollution, workplace, hygiene) or to different life-styles (smoking habits) among patients (103, 104). Recently, the mechanisms underlying drug-related pulmonary fibrosis in subjects receiving cytotoxic chemotherapy (in particular bleomycin, cyclophosphamide, nitrosoureas), have been explored. Several cytokines including transforming growth factor β1 (TGF-β1), tumor necrosis factor (TNF) and IL-1 have been shown to be involved in drug-stimulated intra alveolar collagen deposition (105). Biologic response modulation aimed at inhibiting the activity of such cytokines including receptor blockade through agents such IL-1 receptorial antagonists, may be entertained. More recently, the protective effect of recombinant KGF against bleomycin-induced lung fibrosis has been described in the rat (106). Whether KGF may be used in humans for lung protection from bleomycin damages remains to be established. A randomized, double-blind, controlled study was designed to verify whether ambroxol (Mucosolvan), a drug enhancing alveolar surfactant synthesis and modulating inflammatory cells afflux to alveo-capillary structures, can play a role in the prevention of nitrosoureas-induced pulmonary toxicity in patients with brain tumors (107). No cases of pulmonary fibrosis were shown, either in the placebo group, nor in the ambroxol-treated arm. In this latter group however there were no significant variations in functional ventilatory parameters (107). The authors anticipated a role for ambroxol in preventing pulmonary changes induced by long-term administration of nitrosourea derivatives. A reduction of bleomycin lung toxicity may also be achieved by administering the drug as a continuous infusion or via the intramuscular route (1, 25) (Table 36.2).

The lung represents also a major site of infectious complications in elderly patients undergoing combination chemotherapy.

Renal Toxicity

It does not appear that elderly patients are at increased risk for chemotherapy-induced nephrotoxicity (108). This may reflect the fact that toxicity from renally excreted drugs, including nephrotoxicity, is more likely a function of creatinine levels than of age itself (109). Studies of one of the most nephrotoxic anticancer agents, cisplatin, have confirmed this lack of age-enhanced nephrotoxicity (110–112). A retrospective study on 34 patients over the age of 70 receiving cisplatin in combination with other agents was reported by Lichtman *et al.* (111). Results show that 76% of patients completed therapy without significant cisplatin related kidney toxicity and the Authors emphasized that non-renal toxicity plaid a more important role in the management of patients receiving this drug. In addition, cisplatin at moderated doses (60 to 100 mg/m2) can be reasonably administered to patients aged more than 80 years who may benefit from such antineoplastic chemotherapy (112). Sodium thiosulfate is a neutralizing agent for cisplatin that protects against drug-induced renal damage (113). Several studies have demonstrated how the concurrent administration of thiosulfate can allow at least a twofold increase in dose and total exposure to cisplatin (112). Diethyldithiocarbamate (DDTC), a metabolite of disulfiran, has been employed as a heavy metal-chelating agent for treatment of nickel poisoning (114). Berry *et al.* demonstrated that DDTC can protect against cisplatin nephrotoxicity and suggested that ototoxicity remains the main dose limiting toxicity in patients given DDTC and platinum compounds (115). As discussed in another section of this chapter, the introduction of the cytoprotective agent Amifostine may represent a new effective tool to prevent platinum compounds-related nephrotoxicity (116, 117). As for cisplatin, elderly patients aged up to 80 years affected by rheumatoid arthritis do not appear to be at higher risk of developing toxicity from methotrexate (118). However, the risk of overall toxicity increases along with the decline in renal function, and the concurrent administration of nephrotoxic antibiotics, *i.e.* aminoglycosides, may significantly worsen kidney damage from anticancer drugs such as cisplatin (l 19).

Paradoxically, in some cases, the age-associated reduction in renal tubular reabsorption of drugs may also contribute a protective effect towards cytotoxic agents (25).

Neurologic Toxicity

Common manifestations of chemotherapy-induced neurotoxicity include peripheral neuropathies with parethesias and weakness, autonomic disfunction, mental disturbance, and neurologic ototoxicity (120). Though physiologic changes associated with aging (decreased peripheral nerve conduction, progressive autonomic dysfunctions, and age-related hearing loss) would predict a predisposition to neurologic toxicity for the elderly, conclusive data is lacking (1, 13, 120). Autonomic nerve dysfunction manifested as colicky abdominal pain, constipation, and adynamic ileus is frequently reported in patients, especially the older ones, receiving vincristine (26, 120). Constipation may be treated prophylactically with mild laxatives and stool softeners. In this regard, the administration of lactulose three times a day may prove very effective. Should an ileus nevertheless occur, the use of parasympathomimetic agents such as neostigmin is indicated. Avoidance of serious vincristine-related toxicity in the elderly requires careful attention to both total drug dose and bowel function. Currently, there are no effective tools for preventing or decreasing neurotoxicity associated with the use of vinca alkaloid, except for drug discontinuation, dose modification or changing from a push to a continuous intravenous administration (120) (Table 36.2). While vincristine neurotoxicity appears to be fully reversible in the younger adult, clinical experience suggest that such may not be the case in the elderly. In these patients vincristine may be administered as a continuous infusion at the maximal dose of 2 mg/course, and at intervals not shorter than two weeks. Folinic acid and pyridoxine have been tested as possible antidotes for vincristine associated neurotoxicity, but no clear protective effect was demonstrated (1). Recently, oral glutamic acid (at a dose of 1.5 grams daily) has been employed with more encouraging results (121). Since various vinca derivatives seem to show quantitative differences in the degree of neurotoxic potential (i.e. vincristine > vindesine > vinblastine), the less neurotoxic synthetic alkaloid vindesine may be substituted for vincristine, to prevent peripheral neuropathy (25, 120, 122).

Finally, minimizing the duration of bed confinement and prescription of light but regular physical activity, *i.e.* cyclette or short in and outside walks, may represent additional strategies to prevent or ameliorate vincristine-induced neuropathy in older patients.

In addition to vinca alkaloids, the taxanes (i.e. Paclitaxel) may induce a peripheral neuropathy which appears to be dose-dependent and more severe in patients previously treated with organo-platinum drugs.

A clear cut correlation between doses of cytarabine (ARA-C), age of patients and cerebellar toxicity has been observed (123). A major limit to the cytotoxic efficacy of ARA-C is its rapid deamination to uracil arabinoside (ARA-U). The use of high doses (up to 2–3 gr/m2) of ARA-C (HiDA) has emerged as an effective tool to circumvent ARA-C deamination and enhance the intracellular concentration of the drug. HiDA has produced definite benefits in patients with acute myelogenous leukemia (AML) resistant or refractory to conventional doses of ARA-C, but is associated with a severe extra hematological toxicity, mainly neurotoxicity (124). HiDA-induced neurotoxicity is related to the accumulation of high ARA-U levels in the central nervous system (CNS) and is particularly severe in elderly patients who display a prolonged CNS clearance of ARA-U (124). The use of non toxic

inhibitors of the cytidine deaminase enzyme might represent a strategy to reduce toxicity and to exploit the whole potential clinical efficacy of ARA-C in elderly AML patients (125) (Table 36.2). The clinical use of one of such inhibitors, the thetrahydrouridine (THU) has been recently proposed in cancer patients who were treated with conventional dose ARA-C plus THU coinfusion (126). This combination therapy resulted in plasma ARA-C levels comparable to those achieved with HiDA and concomitant reduction of ARA-U levels. The incidence of cerebellar toxicity or other forms of neurotoxicity was negligible with this combination (126). These results, if confirmed in a large series of patients, might represent an interesting example of biochemical modulation of drug efficacy/toxicity to be applied in elderly cancer patients with ARA-C responsive tumors.

Other Toxicities and Special Problems

Owing to a deteriorated cognitive function and a reduced self-awareness, in addition to a common "better-not-disturb" attitude, the older patients may be particularly prone to suffer from the worsening of apparently "minor" side effects of chemotherapy. These side effects may be particularly unpleasant for the elderly and, if unattended by the caring team, may drastically affect the overall quality of life and worsen the depression which, albeit latent, is commonly experienced by older individuals. Furthermore, due to age-associated changes in the pharmacologic disposition of some anticancer agents, these infrequent side effects may unexpectedly occur at dosages lower than usual. As an example, the keratoconjunctivitis associated with the use of methotrexate, high- and intermediate-dose ARA-C, chlorambucil and pentostatin therapy may be extremely painful and discomforting (127). Mild to moderate conjunctivitis has been also noted in patients receiving doxorubicin, 5-FU and interferon (127). Therefore, a regular prophylaxis with frequent eye-washes of normal saline and the use of steroid-containing eye drops should be carefully pursued in these patients. These measures along with the use of darkened sunglasses to manage the increased photosensitivity, may help to reduce discomfort, allow the patient to continue at their best daily activities such as walking, reading and watching television, and avoid further isolating the older subjects from the environment, due to the worsening of pre-existing visual problems. A number of anticancer agents have shown to induce endothelial cell damage, a broad array of miscellaneous vascular toxicities and cerebrovascular accidents (128). While it is not always clear whether these disorders are related to drugs themselves, the underlying malignancy or a combination of both, these events may have a particular clinical relevance in older patients given the age-reduced compliance of the vascular system, and to the frequently concomitant vascular disorders. Deep venous thrombosis, pulmonary embolism and cerebrovascular accidents have been recorded in patients treated with cisplatin/bleomycin plus etoposide or vinblastine (128). Arterial and venous thrombosis have been reported in breast cancer patients undergoing chemotherapy including cyclophosphamide, methotrexate and 5-FU plus vincristine, tamoxifen or doxorubicin (128). In addition, the administration of cisplatin, bleomycin and vinblastine has been related to the development of Raynaud's phenomenon in some patients, and thrombosis or thromboembolisms have been reported in patients undergoing chemotherapy for lymphomas and advanced prostate cancer (128). Finally, the development of leukocytoclastic vasculitis, Sweet and Sweet-like syndromes have been noted upon administration of drugs such as hydroxyurea, methotrexate, busulfan, HMBA and, more recently, following the use of the cytidine analog 5-aza-2'-deoxycytidine or HGF's such as GM-CSF and G-CSF.

Broad Spectrum Active Cytoprotection

The recent availability of the broad-spectrum cytoprotective agent Amifostine has provided the "dreamed" opportunity of utilizing a single drug which appears theoretically able to protect normal tissues from most of the toxicities elicited by different classes of anticancer agents.

Amifostine (WR-2721, Ethyol), was selected as the most promising compound among a number of drugs developed by the United States Army to protect tissues from radiation-related injuries. It is an organic thiophosphate compound that is dephosphorylated by membrane-bound alkaline phosphatase to an active thiol form, the free thiol WR-1065. This latter metabolite has been shown to provide effective cellular protection against oxygen-derived free-radicals and electrophilic compounds such as alkylating drugs and organoplatinum agents (129). More importantly, a preferential uptake (up to 100 times greater) of Amifostine by normal cells as compared to tumor cells has been shown, being partly related to the higher activity of membrane alkaline phosphatase and higher pH of normal vs tumor tissues (129). Normal cells and tissues in which amifostine has been shown to induce a transient period of "acquired chemoresistance" include bone marrow, kidney, cardiac myocytes, lung, and peripheral nervous tissues (Table 36.2). In contrast, brain and spinal cord are not adequately protected by amifostine. Results from different clinical studies have indicated that amifostine may effectively protect healthy tissues from hematologic and extrahematologic toxicity of several anticancer drugs including alkylators, mitomycin C, platinum compounds and anthracyclines, without causing a significant loss of their antitumor activity (130–133) (Table 36.4). This could allow the safe administration of chemotherapy doses higher than those usually employed in the clinical setting to increase specific tumor cytotoxicity (112, 113, 130–133). The use of Amifostine may appear of particular relevance in the prevention of cisplatin-induced nephrotoxicity. Due to its cumulative nature, cisplatin-related renal toxicity may not only limit the appropriate dosing of initial chemotherapy but may also hamper the proper administration of further courses of platinum-based chemotherapy and/or of other drugs (amino-

glycosides, cephalosporins, amphotericin B, loop diuretics, H_2 receptor antagonists, non-steriodal anti-inflammatory drugs, etc.) (134), which frequently need to be utilized in the elderly for the management of comorbid conditions and cancer-related complications. Therefore the preservation of renal function, as achieved by Amifostine pretreatment, may turn out to be of a relevant clinical benefit in older patients to ensure both appropriate dosing and tolerance of initial platinum-based chemotherapy and the proper administration of subsequent therapies (135). Preliminary studies on fetal heart myocytes have also indicated that both amifostine and its metabolite WR-1065 can protect cardiac myocytes from doxorubicin-induced damage (135–136). The broad spectrum of normal tissues protection offered by amifostine suggests that it may represent an important addition to the oncologist's armamentarium especially for the management of elderly cancer patients. Maximal tissue protection can be obtained when amifostine is given shortly (15–30 minutes) before the administration of cytotoxic therapy at doses usually ranging from 740 to 910 mg/m2 (130, 135, 136). These doses have been found to be relatively nontoxic in most patients, although a transient hypotension may occur in about 50% of patients and a few episodes of hypocalcemia were observed (130, 135). This should be considered when administering amofostine to elderly patients, who may often be dehydrated and hypotensive and frequently receive antihypertensive therapy as a part of their routine clinical management. Moderate nausea and vomiting have been also reported in patients given amifostine. Controlled clinical studies on patients with NHL, non SCLC, head and neck tumors, ovarian cancer and metastatic melanoma have shown that amifostine may effectively protect against both hematologic and non-hematologic toxicities (i.e. nephrotoxicity, cardiotoxicity, and neurotoxicity) induced by cisplatin, carboplatin, cyclophosphamide, ifosphamide, vinblastine. Interestingly, in several of these trials a significant protection against chemotherapy-(carboplatin, mitomycin C, cyclophosphamide) induced thrombocytopenia was noted (135, 136). This aspect may be particularly relevant since most of the currently adopted hemopoietic growth factors (i.e. G-CSF, GM-CSF) are unable to prevent or ameliorate chemotherapy-related thrombocytopenia (48). In a randomized trial by Glick et al., women with stage III/IV ovarian cancer were treated with cyclophosphamide 1 g/m2 plus cisplatin 100 mg/m2 with or without amifostine (133, 135). This study showed that amifostine effected a significant reduction in the frequency of hospitalization for neutropenic fever (28% vs 8%; P = .004), duration of hospitalization, and number of days spent on antibiotic therapy (133). The response rate (pathologically confirmed in all cases) and survival were similar in both arms of the study, indicating that a selective bone marrow and renal protection was achieved while the antitumor effects of the drug combination were preserved (133). Other studies on cisplatin-induced neurotoxicity and ototoxicity have shown that amifostine pretreatment reduced the frequency of neuropathy and allowed higher cumulative dose of cisplatin to be

Table 36.4 Amifostine: a broad-spectrum cytoprotective agent for elderly persons.

Advantages:

1. Prevention of multiorgan toxicity.

   (bone marrow, kidney, heart, peripheral nervous system, lung).

2. No loss in antitumour activity of cytotoxic drugs.

3. Reduced risk for genotoxicity and carcinogenicity.

4. Well tolerated (no studies available in elderly patients).

Side Effects:

1. Usually well tolerated. A transient hypothension may occur in 50% of subjects. No specific studies have been performed in elderly patients.

2. Modest nausea and vomiting.

Problems:

1. High cost.

delivered (114, 115). More recent studies by Gorin *et al.* have also indicated that amifostine is able to protect human normal progenitor cells from the toxicity of cyclophosphamide-derivatives (i.e. mafosfamide), while the cytotoxic effects of these compounds on leukemic progenitors were fully preserved (131, 136, 137). The therapeutic advantage of an agent offering the protective ability of amifostine on hemopoietic progenitors is obvious in the setting of autologous bone marrow transplantation, *ex-vivo* purging and in the clinical management of elderly patients, whose bone marrow function is compromised by aging (40–42, 44, 135). Other studies have demonstrated that G-CSF accelerates hemopoietic reconstitution from amifostine-protected stem and progenitor cells, by increasing the survival-enhancing effects of amifostine (135, 138). This finding demonstrates that radioprotective drugs and recombinant HGF can be used in combination with amifostine to reduce risks associated with severe myelosuppression (138). Owing to the capacity of amifostine to provide a multi-organ protection, this drug appears promising in the prevention of chemotherapy side effects in older patients (Tables 36.2 and 36.4). Prospective controlled clinical trials of amifostine plus chemotherapy in the elderly are lacking and should be rapidly designed to evaluate the actual impact of the "cytoprotection strategy" in such patients' population. Given the radioprotective effects of amifostine, a special emphasis should also be given in studying its efficacy for the prevention of radiation-induced damage in older patients with head and neck cancer, lung or esophageal carcinoma. Since radiation therapy remains an effective and frequently adopted option for older patients with solid tumors (10, 15, 21), finding a way to circumvent its toxic effects may have a significant impact in the overall management of these patients.

Conclusions: A Voyage Across the "Conventional"

Recent progress in strategies aimed at preventing or ameliorating hematopoietic and extrahemopoietic toxicity of chemotherapy have led to a significant enhancement in the therapeutic index of several anticancer drugs (139–140). The use of HGFs with or without autologous progenitor cell support, the design of less organotoxic drug-analogs and the introduction of organ- or cyto-protective agents (ICRF- 187, sodium thiosulphate, amifostine, retinoids) represent strategies mainly developed to increase dose-intensity and dose-size of aggressive chemotherapy regimes. These efforts have led to the concept of a "unconventionally high" dose of chemotherapy for circumventing drug resistance and increasing the cure rate of chemosensitive tumors in adult patients (141). Oncologists involved in the management of elderly cancer patients may exploit such achievements under a different perspective. Despite the evidence that cancers in the elderly are not primarily more resistant to chemotherapy and that disappointing clinical results (*i.e.* in aggressive NHL) are mainly due to the inappropriate delivery of standard dose chemotherapy (12), several older patients with chemosensitive tumors are still excluded from conventional chemotherapy protocols adopted for younger adults. While a number of chronologically older patients, whose biologic status allows the use of proper chemotherapy, may happen to be excluded on a mistaken attitude from both clinicians and family members, other patients may need special strategies to be effectively treated (10, 11, 142, 143). Unfortunately, no specific treatment regimes devised for elderly patients have been shown to be superior to those currently used in the adults (24, 81). The main goal of the geriatric oncologist must remain therefore to increase, whenever possible, the fraction of elderly cancer patients receiving conventional dose chemotherapy under the same standard dosage and timing currently adopted for adult patients. A fine-tuning of the strategies developed to deliver "unconventionally high" doses of chemotherapy in the adults may help to achieve this difficult task. Turning the "unconventional" into "conventional" is the challenge of geriatric oncology for the years to come.

Acknowledgments

This work was supported by a grant of the National Research Council (C.N.R.), contract no. 9500520, PF ACRO, 39 and by Associazione Italiana per la Ricerca sul Cancro (AIRC).

References

1. Schwartsmann G, Dekker AW, Verhoff J. Complications of cytotoxic therapy. In *Oxford Textbook of Oncology*, edited by M Peckham, H Pinedo, U Veronesi. Oxford: Oxford University Press, pp. 2307–3227, 1995.

2. Hryniuk WM. The importance of dose intensity in the outcome of chemotherapy. In *Important Advances in Oncology*, edited by VT De Vita, S Hellman, SA Rosenberg. J.B. Lippincott Company, pp. 121–42, 1988.

3. Kwak LW, Halper J, Olshen RA, Horning SJ. Prognostic significance of actual dose intensity in diffuse large-cell lymphoma. Results of a tree structured survival analysis. *J Clin Oncol* 1990; **8**: 963–977.

4. Epelbaum R, Faraggi D, Ben-Arie Y, Ben-Shahar M, Haim N, Ron Y, Robonson E, Cohen Y. Survival of diffuse large cell lymphoma. A multivariate analysis including dose intensity variables. *Cancer* 1990; **66**: 1124–1129.

5. Bonadonna G, Valagussa P. Dose-response effect of adjuvant chemotherapy in breast cancer. *N Engl J Med* 1981; **304**: 10–15.

6. O'Reilly SE, Connors JM, Howdle S, Hoskins P, Klasa R, Klimo P, Stuart DS. In search of an optimal regimen for elderly patients with advanced-stage diffuse large-cell lymphoma. Results of a phase II study of P/DOCE chemotherapy. *J Clin Oncol* 1993; **11**: 2250–2257.

7. Tirelli U, Zagonel V, Serrino D, Thomas J, Hoerni B, Tangury A, Ruhl U, Bey P, Tubiana N, Breed WPM, Roozendaal KJ, Hagenbeek A, Hupperts PS, Somers R. Non-Hodgkin's lymphomas in 137 patients aged 70 years or older. A retrospective European Organization for Research and Treatment of Cancer Lymphoma Group study. *J Clin Oncol* 1988; **6**: 1708–1713.

8. Dixon DO, Neilan B, Jones SE, Lipschitz DA, Miller TP, Grozea PN, Wilson HE. Effect of age on therapeutic outcome in advanced diffuse histocytic lymphoma. The Southwest Oncology Group experience. *J Clin Oncol* 1986; **4**: 295–305.

9. Vose JM, Armitage JO, Weisenburger DD, Bierman PJ, Sorensen S, Hutchins M, Moravec DF, Howe D, Dowling MD, Mailliard J, Johnson PS, Pevnick W, Packard WM, Okerbloom J, Thompson RF, Langdon RM, Soori G, Peterson C. The importance of age in survival of patients treated with chemotherapy for aggressive non-Hodgkin's lymphoma. *J Clin Oncol* 1988; **6**: 1838–1844.

10. Monfardini S, Aapro M, Ferucci L, Zagonel V, Scalliet P, Fentiman I. Commission of the European Communities "Europe Against Cancer" programme. European School of Oncology advisory report. Cancer treatment in the elderly. *Eur J Cancer* 1993, **29A**: 2325–2330.

11. Kennedy BJ. Needed clinical trials for older patients. (Editorial) *J Clin Oncol* 1991; **9**: 718–720.

12. Gaynor ER, Dahlberg S, Fisher RI. Factors affecting reduced survival of the elderly with intermediate and high grade lymphoma. An analysis of SWOG-8516 (INT 0067). The national high priority lymphoma study. A randomized comparison of CHOP vs m-BACOD vs ProMACE-Cyta BOM vs MACOP-B. *Proc Am Soc Clin Oncol* 1994; **13**: 370 (abstr).

13. Einhorn LH. Approaches to drug therapy in older cancer patients. *Oncology* 1992; **6**: 69–73.

14. Balducci L, Mowry K. Pharmacology and organ toxicity of chemotherapy in older patients. *Oncology* 1992; **6**: 62–68.

15. Raghavan D, Findlay MPN, McNeil EB. Cancer in the elderly. In *Oxford Textbook of Oncology*, edited by M Peckham, H Pinedo, U Veronesi. Oxford: Oxford University Press, pp. 2169–2189, 1995.

16. Conti JA, Christman K. Cancer chemotherapy in the elderly. *J Clin Gastroenterol* 1995; **21**: 65–71.

17. Lieschke GJ, Burgess AW. Granulocyte colony stimulating factor and granulocyte-macrophage colony stimulating factor. *New Engl J Med* 1992; **327**: 28–35, 99–106.

18. Begg CB, Carbone PP. Clinical trials and drug toxicity in the elderly. The experience of the Eastern Cooperative Oncology Group. *Cancer* 1983; **52**: 1986–1992.

19. Giovanazzi-Bannon S, Rademaker A, Lai G, Benson AB. Treatment tolerance of elderly cancer patients entered onto phase II clinical trials. An Illinois Cancer Center study. *J Clin Oncol* 1994; **12**: 2447–2452.

20. Monfardini S, Sorio R, Renard J, Kaye S, van Glabbeke M. Entry of elderly patients in EORTC new drug development studies. *Proc Am Soc Clin Oncol* 1993; **12**: 132 (abstr).

21. Zagonel V, Pinto A, Serraino D, Babare R, Sacco C, Merola MC, Trovo MG, Tirelli U, Monfardini S. Lung cancer in the elderly. *Cancer Treat Rev* 1994; **20**: 315–329.

22. Winer EP, Chu L, Spicer DV. Oral vinorelbine (navelbine) in the treatment of advanced breast cancer. *Semin Oncol* 1995; **22**: 72–79.

23. Armitage JO. Treatment of non-Hodgkin's lymphoma. *New Engl J Med* 1993; **328**: 1023–1030.

24. Coiffier B. What treatment for elderly patients with aggressive lymphoma? (editorial). *Ann Oncol* 1994; **5**: 873–875.

25. Fleming RA, Capizzi RL. General aspects of cancer chemotherapy in the aged. In *The Underlying Molecular, Cellular, and Immunological Factors in Cancer and Aging*, edited by SS Yang, HR Wamer. New York: Plenum Press, pp. 271–286, 1993.

26. Mitchell EP. Gastrointestinal toxicity of chemotherapeutic agents. *Semin Oncol* 1992; **19**: 566–579.

27. Monfardini S, Ferrucci L, Fratino L, Del Lungo I, Serraino, Zagonel V. Validation of a multidimensional evaluation scale for use in elderly cancer patients. *Cancer* 1996; **77**: 395–401.

28. Monfardini S, Fratino L, Zagonel V, Serraino D. How much does performance status correlate with multidimensional geriatric assessment in elderly patients with cancer (EPC)? *Eur J Cancer* 1995, **31A (Suppl 5)**: 255 (abstr).

29. Balducci L, Mowrey K, Parker M. Pharmacology of antineoplastic agents in older patients. In *Geriatric Oncology*, edited by L Balducci, GH Lyman, WB Ershler. Philadelphia: J.B. Lippincott Company, pp. 169–180, 1992.

30. Monfardini S. What do we know on variables influencing clinical decision-making in elderly cancer patients? *Eur J Cancer* 1996; in press.

31. Shank WA Jr, Balducci L. Recombinant hemopoietic growth factors. Comparative response in younger and older subjects. *J Am Geriatr Soc* 1992; **40**: 151–154.

32. Vose JM. Cytokine use in the older patient. *Semin Oncol* 1995; **22 (Suppl 1)**: 6–8.

33. Zagonel V, Babare R, Merola MC, Talamini R, Lazzarini R, Tirelli U, Carbone A, Monfardini S. Cost-benefit of granulocyte colony-stimulating factor administration in older patients with non-Hodgkin's lymphoma treated with combination chemotherapy. *Ann Oncol* 1994; **5 (Suppl 2)**: 127–132.

34. American Society of Clinical Oncology recommendations for the use of hematopoietic colony-stimulating factors. Evidence-based, clinical practice guidelines. *J Clin Onc.ol* 1994; **12**: 2471–2508.

35. Lyman GH, Lyman CG, Sanderson RA, Balducci L. Decision analysis of hematopoietic growth factor use in patients receiving cancer chemotherapy. *J Natl Cancer Inst* 1993; **85**: 488–493.

36. Armitage JO, Potter JF. Aggressive chemotherapy for diffuse histocytic lymphoma in the elderly. Increased complications of advancing age. *J Am Geriatr Soc* 1984; **32**: 269–273.

37. Cheson BD. Infectious and immunosuppressive complications of purine analog therapy. *J Clin Oncol 5*, **13**: 2431–2448.

38. Chatta GS, Andrews RG, Rodger E, Shragg M, Hammond WP, Dale DC. Hematopoietic progenitors and aging. Alternations in granulocytic precursors and responsiveness to recombinant human G-CSF, GM-CSF, and IL-3. *J Gerontol* 1993; **48**: M207 (abstr).

39. Chatta GS, Price TH, Allen RC, Dale DC. Effets of *in vivo* recombinant methionyl human granulocyte colony-stimulating factor on the neutrophil response and peripheral blood colony-forming cells in healthy young and elderly adult volunteers. *Blood* 1994; **84**: 2923–2929.

40. Chatta GS, Price TH, Stratton JR, Dale DC. Aging and marrow neutrophil reserves. *J Am Geriatr Soc* 1994; **42**: 77–81.

41. Lipschitz D, Udupa K, Milton K, Thompson C. Effect of age on hematopoiesis in man. *Blood* 1984; **63**: 502–509.

42. Mori M, Tanaka A, Sato N. Hematopoietic stem cells in elderly people. *Mech Aging Dev* 1986; **37**: 41–47.

43. Lee M, Segal G, Bagby G. The hematopoietic microenvironment in the elderly. defects in IL-I induced CSF expression *in vitro*. *Exp Hematol* 1989; **17**: 952–956.

44. Buchanan J, Rothstein G. Deficient growth factor production as a cause of hematopoietic dysregulation in aged subjects. *Clin Res* 1989; **37**: 149A (abstr).

45. Baldwin J. Hematopoietic function in the elderly. *Arch Intern Med* 1988; **148**: 2544.

46. Tirelli U, Zagonel V, Errante D, Serraino D, Talamini R, De Cicco M, Carbone A, Monfardini S. A prospective study of a new combination chemotherapy regimen in patients older than 70 years with unfavourable non-Hodgkin's lymphoma. *J Clin Oncol* 1992; **10**: 228–236.

47. Monfardini S, Sacco C, Babare R, Merola MC, Carbone A, Zagonel V. VP-16, mitoxantrone and prednimustine (VMP) with or without G-CSF in patients (PTS) with non-Hodgkin's lymphomas (NHL) older than 70 years (YRS). *Proc Am Soc Clin Oncol* 1994; **13**: 377 (abstr).

48. Vose JM, Armitage JO. Clinical applications of hematopoietic growth factors. *J ClinOncol* 1995; **13**: 1023–1035.

49. Aoki Y, Hiromatsu K, Kobayashi N, Hotta T, Saito H, Igarashi H, Niho Y, Yoshikai Y. Protective effect of granulocyte colony-stimulating factor against T-cell-mediated lethal shock triggered by superantigens. *Blood* 1995; **86**: 1420–1427.

50. Aglietta M, Piacibello W, Sanavio F, Stacchini A, Apra F, Schena M, Mossetti C, Carnino F, Caligaris-Cappio F, Gavosto F. Kinetics of human hemopoietic cells after *in vivo* administration of granulocyte-macrophage colony stimulating factor. *J Clin Invest* 1989; **83**: 551–557.

51. Tafuto S, Abate G, D'Andrea P, Silvestri I, Marcolin P, Volta C, Monteverde A, Colombi S, Andorno S, Aglietta M. A comparison of two GM-CSF schedules to counteract the granulomonocytopenia of carboplatin-etoposide chemotherapy. *Eur J Cancer* 1995; **31A**: 46–49.

52. Miller JA, Beveridge RA. A comparison of efficacy of GM-CSF and G CSF in the therapeutic setting of chemotherapy induced neutropenia. *Blood* 1994; **84**: 78a (Suppl), (abstr).

53. Chi KH, Chen ChH, Chan WK, Chow KCh, Chen SY, Yen SH, Chao JY, Chang ChY, Chen KY. Effect of granulocyte-macrophage colony stimulaying factor on oral mucositis in head and neck cancer patients after cisplatin, fluorouracil, and leucovorin chemotherapy. *J Clin Oncol* 1995; **13**: 2620–2628.

54. Bartley TD, Bogenberger J, Hunt P, Li YS, Lu HS, Martin F, Chang MS, Samal B, Nichol JL, Swift S, Johnson MJ, Hsu RY, Parker VP, Suggs S, Skrine JD, Merewether LA, Cloyston C, Hsu E, Hokom MM, Hornkohl A, Choi E, Pangelinan M, Sun Y, Mar V, McNinch J, Somonet L, Jacosen F, Xie C, Shutter J, Chute H, Basu R, Selander L, Trollinger D, Sieu L, Padilla D, Trail G, Elliot G, Izumi R, Covey T, Crouse J, Garcia A, Xu W, Del Castillo J, Biron J, Cole S, Hu CT, Pacifici R, Ponting I, Saris C, Wen D, Yung YP, Lin H, Bosselman RA. Identification and cloning of a megakaryocyte growth and development factor that is a ligand for the cytokine receptor Mpl. *Cell* 1994; **77**: 1117–1124.

55. de Sauvage FJ, Hass PE, Spencer SD, Malloy BE, Gurney AL, Spencer SA, Darbonne WC, Henzel WJ, Wong SC, Kuang W-J, Oles KJ, Hultgren B, Solberg LA Jr, Goeddel DV, Eaton DL. Stimulation of megakaryocytopoiesis and thrombopoiesis by the c-Mpl ligand. *Nature* 1994; **369**: 533–538.

56. Small D, Levenstein M, Kim E, Carow C, Amin S, Rockwell P, Witte L, Burrow C, Ratajczak MZ, Gewirtz AM, Civin CI. STK-1, the human homolog of the flk-2/flt-3, is selectively expressed in CD34+ human bone marrow cells and is involved in the proliferation of early progenitor/stem cells. *Proc Natl Acad Sci USA* 1994; **91**: 459–463.

57. Hannum C, Culpepper J, Campbell D, McClanahan T, Zurawski S, Bazan JF, Kastelein R, Hudak S, Wagner J, Mattson J, Luh J, Duda G, Martina N, Peterson D, Menon S, Shanafelt A, Muench M, Kelner G, Namikawa R, Rennick D, Roncarolo M, Zlotnik A, Rosnet O, Dubreuil P, Birnbaum D, Lee F. Ligand for flt-3/flt-2 receptor tyrosine kinase regulates growth of hematopoietic stem cells and is encoded by variant RNAs. *Nature* 1994; **368**: 643–648.

58. Metcalf D. Hematopoietic regulators: redundancy or subtlety? *Blood* 1993; **12**: 3515–3523.

59. Skilings JR, Sridhar FG, Wong C, Paddock L. The frequency of red cell transfusion for anemia in patients receiving chemotherapy. A retrospective cohort study. *Am J Clin Oncol* 1993; **16**: 22–25.

60. Abels RI. Use of recombinant human erythropoietin in the treatment of anemia in patients who have cancer. *Semin Oncol* 1992; **19 (Suppl 8)**: 29–35.

61. Henry DH, Abels RI. Recombinant human erythropoietin in the treatment of cancer and chemotherapy-induced anemia. Results of double-blind and open-label follow-up studies. *Semin Oncol* 1994; **21 (Suppl 3)**: 21–28.

62. Denton TA, Diamond GA, Matloff JM, Gray RJ. Anemia therapy. Individual benefit and social cost. *Semin Oncol* 1994; **21 (Suppl 3)**: 29–35.

63. Hodes RJ. Molecular alterations in the aging immune system. *J Exp Med* 1995; **182**: 1–3.

64. Kaiser FE, Morley JE. Idiopathic CD4+ Iymphopenia in older persons. *J Am Geriatr Soc* 1994; **42**: 1291–1294.

65. Roberts-Thomson IC, Whittingham S, Youngchaiyud U, Mackay IR. Ageing, immune response, and mortality. *Lancet* 1974; **2**: 368–370.

66. Nagelkeren L, Hertogh-Huijbregts A, Dobber R, Drager A. Age-related changes in lymphokine production related to a decreased number of CD45RBhi CD4+ T cells. *Eur J Immunol* 1991; **21**: 273–281.

67. Gabriel H, Smidt B, Kindermann W. Age-related increase of CD45RO+ lymphocytes in phisically active adults. *Eur J Immunol* 1993; **23**: 2704 2706.

68. Mackall CL, Fleisher TA, Brown MR, Andrich MP, Chen CC, Feuerstein IM, Horovitz ME, Magrath IT, Shad AT, Steinberg SM, Wexler LH, Gress RE. Age, thymopoiesis, and CD4+ T-lymphocyte regeneration after intensive chemotherapy. *New Engl J Med* 1995; **332**: 143–149.

69. Wei JY. Cardiovascular comorbidity in the older cancer patient. *Semin Oncol* 1995; **22 (Suppl 1)**: 9–10.

70. Allen A. The cardiotoxicity of chemotherapeutic drugs. *Semin Oncol* 1992; **19**: 529–542.

71. Buzdar AV, Marcus C, Smith TL, Blumenschien GR. Early and delayed clinical cardiotoxicity of doxorubicin. *Cancer* 1985; **55**: 2761–2765.

72. Hortobagyi GN, Frye D, Buzdar AU, Ewer MS, Fraschini G, Hug V, Ames F, Montague E, Carrasco CH, MacKay B, Benjamin RS. Decreased cardiac toxicity of doxorubicin administered by continous intravenous infusion in combination chemotherapy for metastatic breast carcinoma. *Cancer* 1989; **3**: 37–45.

73. Weiss AJ, Metter GE, Flztcher WS, Wilson WL, Grage TB, Ramirez G. Studies on andriamycin using a weekly regimen demonstrating its clinical effectiveness and lack of cardiac toxicity. *Cancer Treat Rep* 1976; **60**: 813–822.

74. Bonadonna G, Gianni L, Santoro A, Bonfante V, Bidoli P, Casali P, Demicheli R, Valagussa P. Drugs ten years later. Epirubicin. *Ann Oncol* 1993; **4**: 359–369.

75. Petti MC, Mandelli F. Idarubicin in acute leukemias. Experience of the Italian Cooperative Group GIMEMA. *Semin Oncol* 1989; **16**: 10–15.

76. Benjamin RS. Rationale for the use of mitoxantrone in the older patient. Cardiac toxicity. *Semin Oncol* 1995; **22 (Suppl 1)**: 11–13.

77. Henderson IC, Allegra JC, Woodcock Wolff S, Bryan S, Cartwright K, Dukart G, Henry DT. Randomized clinical trial comparing mitoxantrone with doxorubicin in previously treated patients with metastatic breast cancer. *J Clin Oncol* 1989; **7**: 560–571.

78. Neithart JA, Gochnour D, Roach R, Hoth D, Young D. A comparison of mitoxantrone and doxorubicin in breast cancer. *Clin Oncol* 1986; **4**: 672–677.

79. Covan JD, Neidhart J, McClure S, Coltman CA, Gumbart C, Martino S, Hutchins LF, Stephens RL, Vaughan CB, Osborne CK. Randomized trial of doxorubicin, bisantrene, and mitoxantrone in advanced breast cancer. A Southwest Oncology Group study. *J Natl Cancer Inst* 1991; **83**: 1077 1084.

80. Sonneveld P, de Ridder M, van der Leile H, Nieuwenhuis K, Schouten H, Mulder A, van Reiswoud I, Hop V, Lovenberg B. Comparison of doxorubicin and mitoxantrone in the treatment of elderly patients with advanced diffuse non-Hodgkin's lymphoma using CHOP vs CNOP chemotherapy. *J Clin Oncol* 1995; **13**: 2530–2539.

81. Tirelli U, Errante D, Van Glabbeke M, Teodorovic I, Kluin-Nelemans JC, Thomas J, Bron D, Rosti G, Somers R, Zagonel V, Noordijk EM. CHOP is the standard regimen in patients of 70 years of age or more with intermediate and high grade non-Hodgkin's lymphoma: results of a randomized study of the EORTC lymphoma cooperative study group. *J Clin Oncol*, (in press).

82. Speyer JL, Green MD, Kramer E, Rey M, Sanger J, Ward C, Dubin N, Ferrans V, Stecy P, Zeleniuch-Jacquotte A, Wemz J, Feit F, Slater W, Blum R, Muggia F. Protective effect of the bispiperazinedione ICRF-187 against doxorubicin-induced cardiac toxicity in women with advanced breast cancer. *N Engl J Med* 1988; **319**: 745–752.

83. Koning J, Palmer P, Franks CR, Mulder DE, Speyer JL, Green MD, Hellmann K. Cardioxane — ICRF-187. Towards anticancer drug specificity through selective toxicity reduction. *Cancer TreatRev* 1991; **18**: 1–19.

84. Hershko C, Link G, Tzahor M, Pinson A. The role of iron and iron chelators in anthracycline cardiotoxicity. *Leukemia and Lymphoma* 1993; **11**: 207–214.

85. Speyer JL, Green MD, Zeleniuch-Jacquotte A, Wernz JC, Rey M, Sanger J, Kramer E, Ferrans V, Hochster H, Meyers M, Blum RH, Feit F, Attubato M, Burrows W, Muggia F. ICRF-187 permits longer treatment with doxorubicin in women with breast cancer. *J Clin Oncol* 1992; **10**: 117–127.

86. Michelotti A, Venturini M, Conte PF, Carnino F, Gallo L, Pronzato P, Tibaldi C, Del Mastro L, Garrone O, Boni G, Mammoliti S, Fuda GC, Da Prato M, Testore F, Bruzi P, Cyrus P, Rosso R. Cardioxane (ICRF-187) protects against epirubicin (EPI) induced cardiomyopathy in advanced breast cancer (ABC) patients. A phase III study. *Proc Am Soc Clin Oncol* 1995, **14**: 98 (abstr).

87. Vici P, Di Lauro L, Ferraironi A, Carpano S, Serrone L, Conti F, Della Bitta R, Lopez M. A randomized trial of dexrazoxane (DEX) cardioprotection in patients (PTS) with metastatic breast cancer (MBC) and advanced soft tissue sarcoma (ASTS) treated with high-dose epirubicin (EPI). *Proc Anl Soc Clin Oncol* 1994; **13**: 94 (abstr).

88. McMillan S. Intensity of pain, nausea, and vomiting in relationship to age in persons with cancer. In *Geriatric Oncology*, edited by L Balducci, GH Lyman, WB Ershler. Philadelphia: J.B. Lippincott Company, pp. 326–331, 1992.

89. Mahood DJ, Dose AM, Loprinzi CL, Veeder MH, Athmann LM, Themeau TM, Sorensen JM, Gainey DK, Milliard JA, Gusa NL, Finck GK, Johnson C, Goldberg RM. Inhibition of fluorouracil-induced stomatitis by oral cryotherapy. *J Clin Oncol* 1991; **9**: 449–452.

90. Gabrilove JL, Jakubowsky A, Scher H, Sternberg C, Wong G, Grous J, Yagoda A, Fain K, Moore MAS, Clarkson B, Oettgen HF, Alton K, Welte K, Souza L. Effect of granulocyte colony-stimulating factor on neutropenia and associated morbidity due to chemotherapy for transitional cell carcinoma of the urothelium. *New Engl J Med* 1988; **318**: 1414–1422.

91. Sheridan WP, Wolf M, Lusk J, Layton JE, Souza L, Morstyn G, Dodds A, Maher D, Green MD, Fox RM. Granulocyte colony-stimulating factor and neutrophil recovery after high-dose chemotherapy and autologous bone marrow transplantation. *Lancet* 1989; **ii**: 891–895.

92. Mandelli F, personal communication.

93. Finch PW, Rubin JS, Miki T, Ron D, Aaronson SA. Human KGF is FGF related with properties of a paracrine effector of epithelial cell growth. *Science* 1989; **245**: 752–755.

94. Wemer S, Peters KG, Longaker MT, Fuller-Pace F, Banda MJ, Williams LT. Large induction of keratinocyte growth factor expression in the dermis during wound healing. *Proc Natl Acad Sci USA* 1992; **89**: 6896–6900.

95. Petrelli N, Douglass HO, Herrera L, Russell D, Stablein DM, Brucker HW, Mayer RJ, Schinella R, Green MD, Muggia FM, Megibow A, Greenwald ES, Bukowski RM, Harris J, Levin B, Gaynor E, Loutfi A, Kalser MH, Barkin JS, Benedetto P, Wooley PV, Nauta R, Weaver DW, Leichman LP. The modulation of fluorouracil with leucovorin in metastatic colorectal carcinoma. A prospective randomized phase III trial. *J Clin Oncol* 1989; **7**: 1419–1426.

96. Stein BN, Ptrelli NJ, Douglass HO, Driscoll DL, Arcangeli G, Meropol NJ. Age and sex are independent predictors of S-fluorouracil toxicity. Analysis of a large scale phase III trial. *Cancer* 1995; **75**: 11–17.

97. Morley JE. Nutritional status of the elderly. *Am J Med* 1986; **81**: 679–698.

98. De Cicco M, Panarello G, Fantin D, Veronesi A, Pinto A, Zagonel V, Monfardini S, Testa V. Parenteral nutrition in cancer patients receiving chemotherapy. Effects on toxicity and nutritional status. *J Parenter Enteral Nutr* 1993; **17**: 513–518.

99. Popper H. Aging and the liver. *Prog Liver Dis* 1986; **8**: 659–683.

100. Schinella M, Tellini U, Pravadelli B, Caputo M. Monoethyl-glycine xylilide. Levels in elderly patients. *Eur J Lab Med* 1994; **2**: 108–111.

101. Cannizzaro R, Robieux I, Valentini M, Sorio R, Amoroso B, Tumolo, Campagnutta E. Liver function assessment by MEGX. Application to oncology. *Ann New York AC Science* 1996; **784**: 486–490.

102. Ginsberg SL, Comis RL. The pulmonary toxicity of antineoplastic agents. *Semin Oncol* 1982; **9**: 34–51.

103. Mahler DA, Rosiello RA, Lorie J. The aging lung. *Geriatr Clin North Am* 1986; **2**: 216–225.

104. Sostman HD, Matthay RA, Putnam CE. Cytotoxic induced lung disease. *Am JMed* 1977; **62**: 608–615.

105. Lazo JS, Dale GH. The molecular basis of interstitial pulmonary fibrosis caused by antineoplastic agents. *Canc Treat Rev* 1990; **17**: 165–167.

106. Sugahara K, Iyama K, Sakanashi Y, Sano K. Keratinocyte growth factor (KGF) prevents bleomycin-induced lung fibrosis in rats. *Mol Biol Cell* 199S; **6**: 203a (Suppl), (abstr).

107. Gaetani P, Silvani V, Butti G, Spanu G, Rossi A, Knerich R. Nitrosourea derivatives-induced pulmonary toxicity in patients treated for malignant brain tumors. Early subclinical detection and its prevention. *Eur l Cancer Clin Oncol* 1987; **23**: 267–271.

108. Patterson WP, Reams GP. Renal toxicities of chemotherapy. *Semin Oncol* 1992; **19**: 521–522S.

109. Kintzel PE, Dorr RT. Anticancer drug renal toxicity and elimination. Dosing guidelines for altered renal function. *Cancer Treat Rev* 1995; **21**: 33–64.

110. Hrushesky WJM, Shimp W, Kennedy BJ. Lack of age-dependant cisplatin nephrotoxicity. *Am J Med* 1984; **75**: 578–586.

111. Lichtman SM, Buchholtz M, Marino J, Schulman P, Allen SL, Weiselberg L, Budman D, DeMarco L, Schuster M, Lovecchio J, Boothby R, Vinciguerra V. Use of cisplatin for elderly patients. *Age and Ageing* 1992; **21**: 202–204.

112. Thyss A, Saudes L, Otto J, Creisson A, Gaspard MH, Dassonville O, Schneider M. Renal tolerance of cisplatin in patients more than 80 years old. *J Clin Oncol* 1994; **12**: 2121–2125.

113. Pfeifle CE, Howell SB, Felthouse RD, Woliver TBS, Andrews PA, Markman M, Murphy MP. High-dose cisplatin with sodium thiosulfate protection. *J Clin Oncol* 1985; **3**: 237–244.

114. Quazi R, Chang AYC, Borch RF, Montine T, Dedon P, Loughner J, Bennett JM. Phase I clinical and pharmacokinetic study of diethyldithiocarbamate as a chemoprotector from toxic effects of cisplatin. *J Natl Cancer Inst* 1988; **80**: 1486–1488.

115. Berry JM, Jacobs Ch, Sikic B, Halsey J, Borch RF. Modification of cisplatin toxicity with diethyldithiocarbamate. *J Clin Oncol* 1990; 1585–1590.

116. Glover DJ, Glick JH, Weiler C, Fox K, Guerry D. WR-2721 and high dose cisplatin. An active combination in the treatment of metastatic melanoma. *J Clin Oncol* 1987; **5**: 574–578.

117. Treskes M, van der Vijgh WJF. WR-2721 as a modulator of cisplatin- and carboplatin-induced side effects in comparison with other chemoprotective agents: a molecular approach. *Cancer Chemother Pharmacol* 1993; **33**: 93–106.

118. Rheumatoid Arthritis Clinical Trial Archive Group. The effect of age and renal function on the efficacy and toxicity of methotrexate in rheumatoid arthritis. *J Rheumatol* 1995; **22**: 218–223.

119. Christensen ML, Stewart CF. Evaluation of aminoglycoside disposition in patients previously treated with cisplatin. *Ther Drug Monit* 1989; **11**: 631–636.

120. Tuxen MK, Hansen SW. Neurotoxicity secondary to antineoplastic drugs. *Cancer Treat Rev* 1994; **20**: 191–214.

121. Jackson DV, Wells HB, Atkins JN, Zekan PJ, White DR, Richards F, Cruz JM, Muss HB. Amelioration of vincristine neurotoxicity by glutamic acid. *Am J Med* 1988; **84**: 1016–1022.

122. Babare R, Zagonel V, Ferrara F, Merola MC, Bordonaro R, Pinto A, Cimino R, Monfardini S. Cost-benefit of chemotherapy on refractory resistant multiple myeloma (MM). VAD vs VID combination. *Ann Oncol* 1994; **5 (Suppl 8)**: 125 (abstr).

123. Gottlieb D, Bradstock K, Koutts J, Robertson T, Lee Ch, Castaldi P. The neurotoxicity of high-dose cytosine arabinoside is age-related. *Cancer* 1987; **60**: 1439–1441.

124. Lopez JA, Agarwal RP. Acute cerebellar toxicity after high dose cytarabine associated with CNS accumulation of its metabolite, uracil arabinoside. *Cancer Treat Rep* 1984; **68**: 1309–1310.

125. Feldman EJ. Acute myelogenous leukemia in the older patient. *Semin Oncol* 1995; **22**: 21–24.

126. Kreis W, Chan K, Budman DR, Schulman P, Allen S, Woiselberg L, LIchtman S, Henderson V, Freeman J, Deere M, Andreeff M, Vinciguerra V. Effect of tetrahydrouridine on the clinical pharmacology of 1-3-D arabinofuranosylcytosine when both drugs are coinfused over three hours. *Cancer Res* 1988; **48**: 1337–1342.

127. Burns LJ. Ocular toxicities of Chemotherapy. *Semin Oncol* 1992; **19**: 492–500.

128. Doll DC, Yarbow JW. Vascular toxicity associated with antineoplastic agents. *Semin Oncol* 1992; **19**: 580–596.

129. Yuhas JM. Active versus passive absorption kinetics as the basis for selective protection of normal tissues by S-2-(3-aminopropylamino) ethylphosphorothioic acid. *Cancer Res* 1980; **40**: 1519–1524.

130. Capizzi RL. Protection of normal tissues from the cytotoxic effects of chemotherapy by amifostine (Ethyol). Clinical experiences. *Semin Oncol* 1994; **21 (Suppl 11)**: 8–15.

131. Capizzi RL, Scheffler BJ, Schein PS. Amifostine-mediated protection of normal marrow from cytotoxic chemotherapy. *Cancer* 1993; **72**: 3495 3501.

132. van der Vijgh WJF, Peters GJ. Protection of normal tissues from the cytotoxic effects of chemotherapy and radiation by amifostine (Ethyol). Preclinical aspects. *Semin Oncol* 1994; **21 (Suppl 11)**: 2–7.

133. Glick J, Kemp G, Rose P, McCulloch W, Scheffler B, Schein P. A randomized trial of cyclophosphamide and cisplatin + WR-2721 in the treatment of advanced epithelial ovarian cancer. *Proc Am Soc Clin Oncol* 1992; **11**: 109 (abstr).

134. Walker EM Jr, Fazekas-May MA, Bowen WR. Nephrotoxic and ototoxic agents. *Clin Lab Med* 1990; **10**: 323–354.

135. Spencer CM, Goa KL. Amifostine. A review of its pharmacodynamic and pharmacokinetic properties, and therapeutic potential as a radioprotector and cytoxic chemoprotector. *Drug Evaluation* 1995; **50**: 1001–1031.

136. Bukowski RM, Capizzi RL, Alberts DS, Vermorken JB, van der Vijgh WJF, Dorr T, Douay L, Facchini T, Budd GT, Schuchter LM, Gorin NC, Coiffier B, Schiller JH, Thatcher N, Wasserman TH. Ethyol: Current and future applications in cytoprotection. International Congress Abstract Booklet 1995, Monte Carlo 28 September–1 October.

137. Dounay L, Hu Ch, Giarratana MC, Gorin NC. Comparative effects of amifostine (ethyol) on normal hematopoietic stem cells versus human leukemic cells during *ex vivo* purging in autologous bone marrow transplants. *Semin Oncol* 1994; **21 (Suppl 11)**: 16–20.

138. Patchen ML, MacVittle TJ. Granulocyte Colony-stimulating factor and amifostine (ethyol) synergize to enhance hemopoietic reconstruction and increase survival in irradiated animals. *Semin Oncol* 1994; **21 (Suppl 11)**: 26–32.

139. Gianni AM, Siena S, Bregni M, Lombardi F, Gandola L, Valagussa P, Bonadonna G. Prolonged disease-free survival after high-dose sequential chemoradiotherapy and hemopoietic autologous transplataton in poor prognosis Hodgkin's disease. *Ann Oncol* 1991; **2**: 645–653.

140. Coiffier B, Philip T, Bumett AK, Symann ML. Consensus Conference on intensive chemotherapy plus hematopoietic stem cell transplantation in malignancies. *J Clin Oncol* 1993; **12**: 266–331.

141. Armitage JO. Bone marrow transplantation. *N Engl J Med* 1994; **330**: 827–838.

142. Shipp MA. Prognostic factors in aggressive non-Hodgkin's lymphoma: who has "high-risk" disease? *Blood* 1994; **83**: 1165–1173.

143. Monfardini S, Yancik R. Cancer in the elderly. Meeting the challenge of an aging population. *J Natl Cancer Inst* 1993; **85**: 532–538.

37. The Role of Endoscopy in the Management of Gastrointestinal Cancers

Haim Pinkas, Dobromir Pencev and Patrick G. Brady

Introduction

Endoscopic management of gastrointestinal (GI) malignancies provides safe and effective palliation. The curability of localized GI cancer by endoscopic ablation, used alone or in combination with other treatment modalities, is now being explored actively. In this chapter, alternative forms of endoscopic cancer treatment are reviewed.

Upper Gastrointestinal Neoplasia

Esophageal Cancer Palliation by Dilation and Prosthesis

Most esophageal cancers diagnosed in the Western world are in advanced stage and need some palliation of dysphagia. Peroral dilation using different dilators is possible in most patients and can be safely performed before, during and after radiation therapy. Mercury-filled rubber dilators with a tapered tip (Maloney) are used under fluoroscopic control when the lumen diameter is not too small or angulated and tortuous.

For most malignant esophageal strictures dilation we use the over the wire technique with the Savary tapered tip dilators. This technique involves placement of the scope on the proximal end of the tumor and insertion of a steel guidewire, with both direct endoscopic and fluoroscopic guidance through the narrow lumen and positioning of the tip of the guidewire in the antrum of the stomach. The scope is pulled away and under fluoroscopic control progressively increasing size thermoplastic non-compressible dilators are passed through the stenosis. Three dilators are passed per sitting that require moderate or severe resistance. Dilations are performed every two to four days and most malignant strictures require three to five sessions with about 90% initial success (1).

Esophageal prosthesis

Prosthesis insertion is indicated when dilation becomes ineffective, or too frequent and difficult for the patient. This occurs in about 15% of the patients who have completed radiation/chemotherapy with recurrence of the cancer and post radiation fibrosis causing circumferential malignant stricture. The second indication is malignant tracheo-esophageal fistula resulting in aspiration pneumonia and constant coughing.

Relative contraindications to prosthesis placement include (2):

- Short life expectancy without prospect of improving the patient's quality of life.
- Airway compromise by tumor invasion or incasement, determined by bronchscopy.
- Location of the lesion within 2 cm of the upper esophageal sphincter; prosthesis in this location is not well tolerated by the patient.
- Tracheoesophageal fistula without luminal narrowing to anchor the prosthesis.
- Non-circumferential tumor growth.
- Alteration in the axis at the lumen interfering with gravity emptying of the prosthesis.

Two types of prosthesis are available: non-expandable and expandable. The non expandable prosthesis are made out of different plastic-rubber materials such as polyvinyl (tygon), silicone, latex and rubber with or without metal spiral reinforcement. They come in 14–16 mm outside diameter and 11–12 mm inside lumen with a variable length adapted to the tumor measurements and with an upper funnel to prevent leakage around the prosthesis.

The placement of a non-expandable prosthesis require prior progressive dilation of the stenosed lumen to a 50–52 French size over 5–10 days. Under fluoroscopic control the prosthesis is forced into the lumen over a guidewire using an appropriate placement apparatus. Tube position is difficult and may require the use of a repositioning device.

A special "fistula prosthesis" was designed by "Wilson-Cook," adding a soft air cuff containing a sponge to the silicone prosthesis. After insertion of the prosthesis the cuff fills with air, expanding the sponge and gently occluding a large fistula.

Expandable prosthesis

The self expandable prosthesis are made of different metal materials such as stainless alloy or mercury metal coil. They are inserted in a compressed state requiring a small caliber lumen (18 French) and in the majority of patients prior dilation is not needed. Placed over a guide wire, once in position, under fluoroscopic control the compressing mechanism is released and the prosthesis is allowed to expand by gaining in diameter and losing in length. Fully expanded, the stent outer diameter is about 20 mm (60 Fr) and the inner diameter

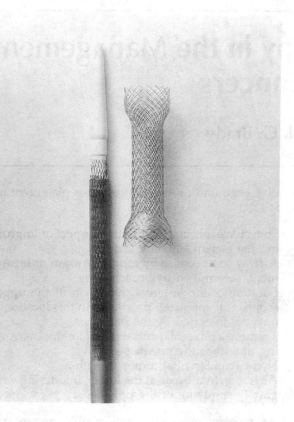

Figure 37.1 The expandable esophageal stent.
• A delivery catheter with constrained stretched stent.
• Fully expanded metal mesh stent with silicone layer covering

is 18 mm (much larger than the non expandable prosthesis diameter). Tumor ingrowing has been a problem with the early metal mesh stents and it has led to recent introduction of silicone or urethane coating (Figure 37.1).

Complications of endoprosthesis placement include perforation, migration, food impaction, tumor in-overgrowth, pressure necrosis and persistent retrosternal pain.

Perforation is a major complication occurring in about 10% of non-expandable stent insertions. A small perforation is usually managed conservatively with nasoesophageal suction and antibiotics for 7–10 days while a large perforation may require surgery on rare occasions. Massive perforation through a tumor carries a poor prognosis. The perforation rate during insertion of self-expandable prosthesis is significantly lower, below 5%.

Displacement/migration has been reported in 10–20% of the non expandable prosthesis and retainer rings on the tube itself have been used to promote anchoring. In theory the expandable metal prosthesis should hold better by constant appositional pressure but about 10% migration have been reported (3).

Tumor ingrowth, a frequent event in wire mesh biliary stents has been overcome by the use of a silicone

Table 37.1 Palliation of malignant dysphagia with prosthesis (modified from ref. 2).

Prosthesis Type	Non-Expandable	Self-Expandable
Ease of Insertion	Difficult	Easy
Degree of mural injury	Traumatic	Non-traumatic
Need for prior dilation	Always	Usually not
Perforation Risk	High	Low
Migration Risk	High	Low
Mostly solid diet	15% of patients	88% of patients
Cost	Moderate	Very High

sheath but tumor overgrowth above or below the prosthesis is seen in both non-expandable and expandable stents. The problem may be corrected by insertion of a longer expandable prosthesis, or by use of injectable ethanol or by Nd:YAG laser destruction.

The first randomized trial comparing non expandable to metal expandable stents showed a superiority of the metal stent for palliation of malignant dysphagia (4). 39 patient with esophageal carcinoma and 3 patients with malignant extrinsic obstruction were randomized to either a plastic prosthesis (16 mm outer diameter) or a metal mesh expandable stent (16 mm maximally opened diameter). The dysphagia and the Karnofsky scores improved significantly and to a similar degree in both groups. Complications were 9 in the plastic stents versus none in the metal prosthesis group. All the perforations in the study were in the plastic stent group. The most common causes of recurring dysphagia were migration of the plastic prosthesis (5 patients) and tumor in-overgrowth of the metal stent (5 patients). The rates of reintervention were similar in both groups as were the 30-day mortality rates. Despite the high cost, the metal stents appear cost effective because of the absence of complications and much shorter hospital stay. The authors concluded that metal expandable stents are a safe and cost effective alternative to conventional plastic prosthesis. Even after a successful placement of an esophageal prosthesis with good palliation of high grade dysphagia, patient's oral intake is usually not fully adequate. We place a Percutaneous Endoscopic Gastrostomy in most of our patients before the placement of the esophageal stent to assure adequate nutrition. A comparison between the two different prosthesis types is summarized in Table 37.1.

Percutaneous endoscopic gastrostomy

Percutaneous endoscopic gastrostomy (PEG) has been developed as an alternative to surgical gastrostomy in the early eighties and found world wide spread since (5). Thousands of endoscopic gastrostomies are performed yearly with high degree of safety and effectiveness. PEG is indicated in patients with functional gastrointestinal tract to maintain adequate nutrition. Patients with neuropsychiatric disorders and tumors of the oropharynx are typical candidates for this procedure. Also patients with unresectable esophageal tumors may benefit from PEG. Percutaneous gastrostomy has also been used for gastric decompression in patients with severe gastroparesis, for bile recirculation in patients with biliary fistulas and for placement of feeding jejunostomy in patients with severe gastroduodenal reflux (6,7,8). Four recent studies addressed indications, success and complications of PEG in the elderly patient (9,10,11,12). Four-hundred and seventy-three procedures in all 4 studies combined were performed. Majority of patients received gastrostomy for progressive dysphagia due to neurologic disorders but in 4% of patients for malignancy. The immediate procedure related death rate ranged from 0–3% and 30 day mortality from 14–20%. Major complications included sepsis, aspiration pneumonia and ARDS. Minor complications were encountered in 14% of patients and included mainly local wound infection and aspiration. These results compare favorably to results in younger patients except for 30 day mortality. Perhaps more vigorous patient selection and careful reflection about benefits in this specific group is needed (6,13).

Endoscopic Ultra Sonography (EUS)

EUS is an endoscopic positioning of a high resolution ultrasonographic transducer close to the GI tract wall.

The most widely used instrument is a radial scanning ultrasound endoscope with a distal tip diameter of 13 mm (The standards diagnostic upper endoscope is about 9mm wide). It uses a transducer that rotates 6.8 revolutions per second and provides a 360 degrees radial sector scan. Interface between the transducer and the gut wall is provided by a water filled latex balloon or direct instillation of water into the lumen. Frequencies of 7.5 MHZ and 12 MHZ are utilized. The EUS image of the gastrointestinal wall consists of five layers: the first layer is nearest the transducer and the fifth layer is farthest from the transducer. The first, hypoechoic layer corresponds to the superficial mucosa. The second, hypoechoic layer represents the deep mucosa and the third, hyperechoic layer corresponds to the submucosa. The fourth, hypoechoic layer represents the muscularis propria and is very important for cancer staging. The outmost, hypoechoic layer corresponds to the serosa or adventitia (see Figure 37.2).

EUS is exceptionally well suited for GI cancer staging by the TNM systems. The most recent development of EUS-guided fine needle aspiration biopsy (FNAB) adds a new dimension beyond imaging to the locoregional tumor staging of gastrointestinal tumors.

EUS staging of esophageal cancer

In a recent literature review Rosch (14) reported the combined results of 21 studies; overall accuracy of endosonographic T and N staging in patients who underwent surgery is 84% (69–102) for T staging and 77% (60–100) for N staging. EUS roles in M staging is limited to the left lobe of the liver and the celiac axis and CT evaluation is complementary for accurate M staging.

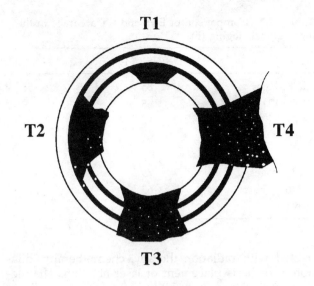

Figure 37.2 Tumor invasion staging by EUS.

Misstaging on EUS ranges between 11 to 27% and can result form microscopic infiltration (understaging) or from peritumorous inflammatory changes (overstaging). Malignant esophageal strictures represent a common dilemma in staging. The EUS scope can traverse 37% to 94% of stenosing esophageal cancers with accuracy rates of 92% for easily traversable strictures, 46% for difficult to pass strictures and 87% for non-traversable tumor. The severe strictures are almost always due to advanced tumors with higher percentage of T3 and T4 staging.

Dilation of tumor strictures before EUS examination may lead to 24% perforations and has been challenged by Catalano et al. (15). A stepwise dilation over few session could probably be done but since most of the patients with a high grade malignant stenosis have advanced disease, advanced EUS T stage is associated with a higher incidence of N-1 disease, lower rate of resectability and a poorer outcome. In a recent editorial Rubain (16) suggested to pursue dilation with EUS staging in patients with high grade malignant stricture for stage-dependent protocols and to use combined CT-EUS staging without dilation for off-protocol treatments.

The locoregional staging is of extreme importance since early T1/T2 cancers are usually completely resectable and the resectability of advanced T3/T4 tumors is dependent upon the localization above or below the tracheal bifurcation. Unlike T4 tumors, stage T3 carcinomas below the bifurcation can be resected away from the aorta and pericardium. Above the bifurcation both T3 and T4 tumors are firmly connected to the trachea/bronchi and neoadjuvent chemo/radiation therapy is being used. Therefore differentiation between stage T2 and T3 is important in choosing the appropriate treatment protocol.

In a recent retrospective cohort study Chak et al. (17) compared two groups of patients with T4 EUS staging. 42 patients underwent surgery and 37 patients were

Table 37.2 Comparison of EUS and CT accuracy in the locoregional staging (5).

Stage	EUS (%)	CT (%)
All T stages	85	58
T1/T2	65	29
T3	92	71
T4	91	41
All N stages	75	54
N0	63	77
N1	89	47

treated with radiation therapy, chemotherapy, dilation, prosthesis placement or laser ablation. The median survival times were 5.2 and 7.0 months respectively with overlapping survival curves. They concluded that EUS accurately identifies patients with invasive T4 tumors who have poor prognosis independently of the mode of therapy. Age, tumor histology and location, nodal status or resectability did not significantly affect survival of patients with advanced disease. Because surgery is associated with high cost, mortality rate of 4% to 15%, morbidity rate of 25% to 70% and prolonged recovery it seems reasonable to consider non surgical palliative therapy in patients who have regionally invasive disease identified by EUS.

EUS staging in gastric cancer

The overall staging accuracy is worse than in esophageal carcinoma, especially in detection of lymph node metastasis (18). T staging is 78% accurate and N stage is about 70% accurate. The accuracy is only 64% for T2 stage due to inflammatory and fibrous changes in the gastric mucosa surrounding the tumor. Ulcerated gastric cancers are misstaged in 4% to 21% of cases. Accuracy in detecting organ infiltration (Stage 4) varies between 64% and 100% while the accuracy in detecting distant lymph node metastasis (Stage N2) varies between 52% and 93%. Comparison with CT staging is favorable with T staging of 82% to 92% by EUS and only 25% to 43% by CT; N staging of 74% to 78% by EUS and 33% to 51% by CT (14). It is not entirely clear to which degree EUS is useful for selecting patients for different forms of treatment.

Restaging after chemo/radiation therapy

Neoadjuvant therapy is increasingly used to improve on surgical results in patients with advanced U.G.I. cancers in the Western world. In a recent review article Hordijk (19) summarized the few published studies on the use of EUS for follow-up staging. In three studies of patients with esophageal carcinoma undergoing nonsurgical treatment EUS T-overstaging was seen in 40% of cases with 3 months of radiation therapy and within few weeks of Nd:YAG laser or photo dynamic therapy. The sonographic findings are due to inflammatory changes, fibroblasts and collagen deposition.

In gastric lymphomas EUS is highly sensitive and accurate for observing the response to chemotherapy or radiation therapy with disappearance of both mural and nodal abnormalities.

New endoscopic ultrasonic miniprobes are currently being tested. These probes do not require a dedicated EUS scope but are placed through the working channel of regular scopes. They appear to be most suitable for small luminal structures such as malignant bile duct strictures. Their use in larger organ tumors is currently being studied.

Laser Tumor Ablation (ELT)

The laser's ability to recanalize obstructing esophageal cancer was demonstrated by the innovative work of Fleischer *et al.* (20). Over the last 10 years, thousands of patients with advanced gastrointestinal (GI) cancers have been treated with Nd: YAG laser, mainly to esophageal and low colorectal sites. The results of the enormous clinical experience by multiple investigators are discussed and updated in this section.

The most commonly treated UGI lesions are tumors of the esophagus and the cardia. The main indications for endoscopic laser therapy (ELT) are obstruction and/or bleeding. In general, relief of obstruction does not palliate mediastinal posterior chest pain, which continue to require analgesic treatment after ELT.

Prognostic factors for the outcome of ELT in UGI tumors were derived from the experience of 36 investigators with 1,098 patients (21–23). Most patients had undergone surgery or radiation therapy before ELT. While recurrence after esophagogastrostomy involved a short segment and quick relief was experienced with ELT (14), recurrence of proximal lesions after radiation therapy however presented a frustrating problem for the endoscopist. Radiation-induced pharyngeal mus-

Table 37.3 Prognostic factors of ELT outcome in esophagogastric cancer.

Predictors of good outcome
  Good performance status
  No anorexia
  Mid-esophageal tumor
  Involvement of a straight esophageal segment
  Tumor <5cm
  Exophytic lesion
  Mucosal involvement seen at endoscopy

Predictors of poor outcome
  Poor performance status
  Anorexia
  Tumor location in the cervical esophagus
  Fixed horizontal segment at the gastroesophageal junction
  Tumor length >8cm
  Submucosal involvement at endoscopy/extrinsic compression

cle dysfunction was discovered at videoesophagoscopy only after painstaking deobstruction by ELT (23).

The treatment of determinants described in Table 37.3 represent broad guidelines for individualized management of patients with UGI tumors rather than specific indications or contraindications to ELT. In the presence of a tracheoesophageal (TE) fistula, the procedure may be highly beneficial, albeit risky. In this case carefully performed ELT may establish sufficient esophageal lumen for the placement of a prosthesis, without enlargement of the fistula. Likewise, ELT - induced esophageal patency may permit additional nourishment through a periesophageal percutaneous endoscopic gastrostomy (PEG) placement in patients with persistent anorexia (23).

Technique

The aim of ELT is to vaporize or coagulate the intra-luminal tumor. We pass a guidewire through the narrow lumen and with the aid of fluoroscopy perform esophageal polyvinyl bougienage over the guidewire. With the scope inserted through the tumor we start the treatment distally and advance toward the proximal margin of the tumor. Treatment is applied circumferentially using laser settings of 70 to 90 W for 1 to 2 sec to vaporize the most exophytic intra-luminal parts of the tumor and settings of 40 to 60 W for 0.5 sec to induce coagulative necrosis of the flat tumor areas. In the case of endoscopically impassible stenosis we use the antegrade technique (20) and some investigators use a laser-resistant guide probe to facilitate the aiming of the laser beam (24).

Repeated sessions are carried out at 48–72 hour intervals starting with tapered polyvinyl dilators that push the necrotic debris distally and proceeding with retrograde ELT. Usually two to three treatment sessions in a outpatient setting are required to establish an 11 to 13 luminal diameter. To keep the patient dysphagia free, we repeat the laser session on a monthly basis or sooner if obstruction recurs. The results of ELT in unselected patients are summarized in Table 37.4. ELT is more effective in palliating obstruction than bleeding. We stress the difference between technical and functional success (23).

After relief of obstruction (Figure 37.3), the performance status of the majority of patients improves. These patients experience a prolongation of survival in com-

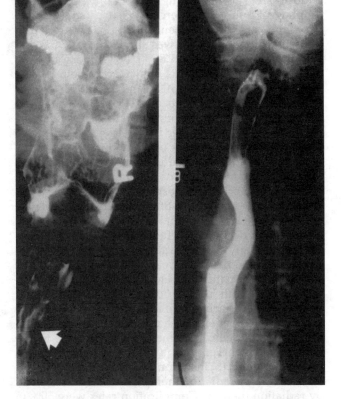

Figure 37.3 Obstructing esophageal lesion prior to (A) and after (B) ELT.

parison to historical controls (25). Karlin et al. (26) and Chatlani et al. (27) found similar impact on survival. The University of South Florida endoscopy team reported the only prospective and randomized study comparing ELT and peroral dilation in the palliation of obstructive esophageal cancer patients undergoing radiation therapy (28). The 1-year survival was 60% for ELT and 20% for peroral dilation (Brady PG, personal communication, 1988). The cost effectiveness of the two treatment modalities expressed as cost per month of survival was comparable. Siegel et al. (29) compared the survival of 36 patients with squamous cell carcinoma of the esophagus treated with ELT and 20 historical controls. The medium survival was 38% in ELT patients compared with 20% in controls. The most frequent complications of ELT are perforation and bacteremia. Perforation rates are usually 5% to 10% (21), while induced bleeding is rarely seen. Kohler et al. (30) reported bacteremia in 33% and sepsis in 10% of patients undergoing ELT. They recommend antibiotic prophylaxis in patients with valvular heart disease or artificial heart valves. Broad-heart spectrum antibiotics should be administered should a fever develop post-ELT to prevent sepsis.

Loizou et al. (31) compared ELT with intubation for palliation of malignant dysphagia. Forty-three patients

Table 37.4 Results of ELT in UGI tumors (13, 14, 16).

Indication for the procedure	End Point	Occurrence (%)
Obstruction	Luminal patency	97
	Improved dysphagia	83
	Adequate caloric intake	73
	Discharge from hospital	70
Bleeding	Decreased requirement for transfusion	53

treated with Nd: YAG laser in London were prospectively compared to 30 patients treated with Atkinson endoprosthesis in Nottingham. For those thoracic esophageal tumors, the percentage of patients achieving significant improvement in dysphagia grade initially over the long term was similar (laser, 95% and 77% intubation, 100% and 86%). For tumors crossing the cardia, intubation was significantly better (laser 59% and 50%: intubation 100% and 92%). Thirty-three percent of the ELT patients and 11% of the prosthesis patients were able to eat most or all solid foods. The perforation rate was lower in the laser treated group (2% vs. 13%). The authors concluded that both forms of therapy need to be used in complementary fashion tailored to the individual needs of each patient. If the patient was anorectic, endoscopic intubation was preferable with speedy and lasting palliation obviating the need to repeat treatments. If the patient was reasonably healthy with need for near-normal swallowing ability, the laser therapy should be attempted first. If the initial response is good, further treatment sessions should be arranged. If the patient developed only partial or short-term benefit from ELT, endoscopic intubation should be considered early in follow-up. Reed et al. (32) randomized 27 patients with unresectable and obstructing squamous cell carcinoma of the esophagus to one of three treatments groups: (a) insertions of an Atkinson prosthesis alone, (b) insertion of and Atkinson prosthesis followed by radiation therapy, and © ELT followed by radiation therapy. Complication rates were 50% in the first group (20% perforations), 38% in the second group, and none in the third group. The quality of palliation was similar in the three small groups and the authors recommend using ELT first, and using stent placement for patients with fistulae on those extrinsic compression by the tumor.

Sander et al. (33) compared laser alone with laser plus afterloading with iridium-192 for palliation in patients with malignant stenosis of the esophagus. In this prospective randomized study afterloading prolonged the first dysphagia-free time and patient survivals were similar. This combination of two local methods of palliation does not offer a significant advantage. Most authors recommend radiation therapy following local palliation. The average period of survival is expected to be twice as long when radiation therapy is combined with a local palliation such as laser or after loading therapy (34).

The combination of ELT with chemotherapy and radiation therapy promises to increase patient survival in selected cases. In 1985, Pinkas et al. (35) reported a case of squamous cell carcinoma of the esophagus that achieved complete radiologic, endoscopic, and histologic remission after combined treatment by ELT, chemotherapy, (5-FU / cisplatin), and radiation therapy. Many other investigators reported similar anecdotal cases (36). Most recently Lambert (37) reported an overall 5-year survival rate of 9% in 293 patients treated with a multimodality protocol for cancer of the esophagus that involves one ELT session, three radiotherapy courses, and up to 12 chemotherapy courses. He uses ELT at the end of the first chemotherapy course

when the tumor sensitivity to thermal injury is the highest. Further dysphagia palliation is achieved by dilation as necessary.

Other Forms of Endoscopic Tumor Ablation

The widest experience of thermal tumor ablation has been obtained with BICAP tumor probes, which were developed as an alternative to ELT (38–45). These probes resemble Eder-Peustow dilator olives with bipolar circular coagulation stripes and come in 6, 9, 12 and 15mm diameters. The coagulation stripes are 15mm long in the smallest diameter probes and 7.5 mm long in the 15mm diameter probe. The probes are passed over a standard guidewire and consist of a flexible tip and a 60 cm long shaft with centimeter markings. The power generator is a standard 50-watt ACMI / Circon system. In general, this system increases the contact in tissue asymmetric tumors and different probes capable of increasing the tissue temperature to 180°C may be used. The depth of coagulation from heating is 1–2mm; greater depth is obtainable with opposition pressure. Pulse duration varies between 6–16 seconds according to the length and diameter of the probe.

BICAP tumor probes provide effective palliation of obstructing esophageal tumors. This technique is indicated in long tumors. In all these circumstances the effectiveness of ELT is limited. Submucosal lesions may be treated with BICAP probes, but caution should be exercised to avoid the development of strictures. When treating tumors that are noncircumferential, damage of the noninvolved esophageal wall may occur. This complication may be minimized with the 180°C probe, which is more difficult to use and has not been studied adequately. The experience with BICAP probes in obstructing rectal cancer is extremely limited.

Treatment with BICAP probes is preceded by esophagoscopy for the identification of proximal and distal tumor margins, which are marked on the skin with radiopaque markers. A guidewire is placed before withdrawing the endoscope. A probe appropriate for the tumor diameter is then inserted over the guidewire. The distance of the tumor from the incisor teeth and the proximal and distal margins of the tumor are recorded and the probe is passed beyond the distal tumor and is directed by palpation, radiopaque markers, and shaft measurements. The treatment is delivered in an overlapping fashion, moving the probe cephalad until the proximal tumor edge is reached. Proximal treatment is monitored using a small-caliber endoscope passed along the shaft of the probe. When the treatment is completed, the whole apparatus is withdrawn, and the overall results are assessed endoscopically. Gray-white coagulation or, in the case of friable bleeding tumors, a black brown color is noted. A second treatment may be required after a 2-day interval. Necrotic material is pushed into the stomach with the endoscope or a dilator or may be suctioned. Follow-up endoscopic monitoring is scheduled at monthly intervals.

The use of a BICAP probe appears safe and effective, but the experience with this treatment modality is limited when compared to ELT. So far, more than 2,000 patients have been treated with ELT and probably no more than 200 with BICAP probe. Potential therapeutic complications include T-E fistulas and stricture formation, which is more likely in the proximal esophagus. Advantages of BICAP probe include its low cost, portable equipment, short treatment sessions, rapid treatment of long and submucosal lesions, and simple handling. Disadvantages are its limited experience, long pulse duration and "blind" treatment, with little room for individual dosing of energy. Also, normal tissue damage may follow the treatment of asymmetric tumors. It is hoped that ELT and BICAP will emerge as complementary treatment modalities capable together of expanding the indications for endoscopic tumor ablation.

Other forms of thermal treatment include heater probes, radar and microwaves that propagate through flexible cylindric metal wave guides (38,39)

Injectional Therapy

Local injections of substances causing tumor necrosis is another alternative to ELT, although the experience is limited with this form of therapy.

Peterlini *et al.* (40) achieved satisfactory recanalization

of the proximal and distal esophagus with intratumoral injections of concentrated polidocanol. Using 3% polidocanol Bulighin *et al.* (41) caused regression of exophytic neoplasms. Treatment of infiltrative lesions, however, resulted in stenosis and fistulas.

Payne James *et al.* (46) improved dysphagia caused by inoperable or recurrent esophagogastric cancer with intratumoral injections of ethylic alcohol. The volume of injected ethanol ranged from 1.5 to 22 ml, and there were no complications.

Wright and co-workers (47) injected a combination of 5-fluorouracil and sodium mirrhuate 2.5% into advanced squamous cell carcinoma of the esophagus, but failed to obtain appreciable tumor regression. In two cases of cancers recurring after radiotherapy, hardened tumor surface prevented adequate injection.

The injection of sclerosants in high concentration has the potential for being very damaging and should be discouraged outside clinical trials.

Photodynamic Therapy (PDT)

PDT is the destructive action of light irradiation on neoplastic tissue that contains a previously administered photosensitizer (Figure 37.4). The photosensitizer

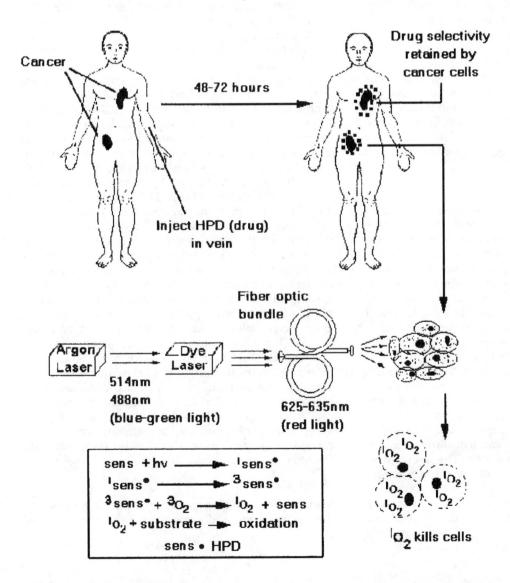

Figure 37.4 Mechanisms of action of photodynamic therapy. (From Berns MW: Hematoporphyrin derivative photoradiation therapy. *Lasers Med Surg* 1984; **4**: 3, with permission of the author and publisher.)

is initially distributed in all the tissues but is retained for a longer time by the tumor stroma, reaching a larger than 2:1 ratio 40 to 50 hours post administration (48). This difference in photosensitizer concentration enables selective destruction of tumors, since a photodynamic light dose can achieve PDT effect on the tumor while remaining below PDT threshold for the surrounding tissue. The photochemical reaction causes tissue damage by the he production of singled oxygen, the cytotoxic agent (49). Tissue studies demonstrate PDT-induced vascular damage with subsequent tumor ischemia and cirrhosis (50). An important observation was made by Barr et. al. (51) about the collagen damage by PDT versus thermal injury. In the normal colon, full thickness PDT damage spares the submucosal collagen, producing no increase in full risk of perforation. Only transmural invasion by the neoplasm itself can cause PDT-induced perforation.

The photosensitizers used in clinical trials, hemotoporphyrins, derive from our knowledge about photosensitivity disease processes like porphyria. Lipson *et al.* (52) isolated a hematoporphyrin derivative (HpD) with tumor localizing and photosensitizing properties that was used in the 1960s for endoscopic detection of carcinomas of the lung, esophagus, and gastric cardia (53). The photodynamically active ingredient of HpD was identified by Dougherty (54) as dihematoporphyrin ether/ester (DHE) and is now produced as Porfimer Sodium (Quadra Logic Technologies, Inc.). It has a major absorption peak (350–450 mm) close to the peak of a solar radiation (>400–500 mm) and a minor absorption peak at 630 mm, which is used in clinical PDT.

The light source for PDT at wavelength of 630 mm is usually a dye laser optically pumped by an argon or a copper vapor laser, while a gold vapor laser can emit this wavelength directly.

Technique

We use PDT for cancer of the esophagus as part of a multicenter cooperative study. Eligible patients receive 2mg/kg Porfimer Sodium by intravenous injection over 3 to 5 min. They become immediately photosensitive to sunlight and follow strict avoidance precautions. Endoscopically delivered red laser light treatments is performed 40 to 50 hours later and can be repeated at a similar time interval, if necessary. The light treatment is performed with a tunable argon-dye laser and is transmitted by a flexible glass fiber that is passed via the endoscope under direct visual control. If the tumor is completely obstructing, the tip of the fiber with a diffuser configuration can be inserted into the tumor central areas for interstitial treatments. For small, non-obstructing lesions a microlens is attached to the fiber tip with light focused on the lesion. The majority of the cases are done with a cylindrical diffuser that is placed in the stenotic tumor lumen. The laser power is 400 mW for each centimeter of the diffuser length and the light dose is 300 J/cm, which is translated into treatment time of 12.5 minutes at each treatment level. The diffuser is kept in place under direct fiberoptic

endoscopic control and is repositioned after each treatments interval.

The patients are endoscoped for debridement in 2 to 3 days and can be retreated with the laser while still photosensitive. The patients are shielded from sunlight for 1 month and then can carefully expose their skin to sunlight for 5 to 15 min intervals. If no sunburn occurs, sunlight is permitted and the patient is ready for a second cycle of PDT.

Results

Likier *et al.* (55) followed this protocol and reported on two patients with a completely obstructing cervical esophageal cancer, just below the cricopharyngeus muscle, in whom the guidewire would not pass to permit dilation. In this desperate setting, they were able to establish a lumen with the first cycle of PDT, avoiding potentially more dangerous antegrade Nd: YAG ELT.

Heier *et al.* (56) reported interim results of a randomized trial of PDT with DHE versus Nd: YAG. ELT using the same protocol for obstructing esophageal carcinoma. There was no difference in symptomatic improvement, esophageal patency, or survival. The complication rate was similar for both techniques. The main disadvantage of PDT was difficulty in maintaining the argon-dye laser.

Lightdale *et al.* (57) reported the results of the multi-center randomized trail of PDT versus Nd: YAG ELT for palliation of esophageal cancer, a trial in which we participated. Two hundred thirty six patients were randomized and 218 treated (PDT, 110, Nd: YAG 108). Improvement in dysphagia was equal between the two treatment modalities and about 25% of patients in both groups showed no response. Objective tumor response was equivalent at week one after treatment, about half the patients, but at month 1 the response rate was statistically higher for PDT at 32% than for Nd:YAG at 20%. Nine complete tumor responses occurred after PDT and two after Nd:YAG. Trends for improved response for PDT were seen in tumors located in the upper and lower third of the esophagus, in long tumors and in patients who had prior surgery. More mild to moderate complications followed PDT treatment including sunburn in 19% of patients, nausea, fever and plural effusion. Perforations from laser treatments or associated dilations occurred after PDT in 1% and after Nd: YAG in 7% of patients. The median survival was 123 days for PDT and 140 days for Nd: YAG.

In conclusion of the study PDT with Porfimer sodium has overall equal efficacy to Nd: YAG laser thermal ablation for palliation of dysphagia in esophageal cancer, and equal or better objective tumor response. Temporary photosensitivity is a limitation but PDT is carried out the with greater ease and is associated with fewer acute perforations.

Complication of PDT

Some patients may experience a burning sensation during treatment and some degree of chest pain and discomfort may persist. Transient dysphagia is common and esophageal strictures may occur later. Sloughing and necrosis of large lesions may cause fever, perforation, and hemorrhage.

Wooten et al. (58) reported cutaneous phototoxicity in 74% of 23 patients treated with HpD. Blisters lasting 5 to 23 weeks occurred in 18% of cases. This high complication rate was ascribed to a lack of compliance with light-avoiding precautions and was deemed a major disadvantage of PDT with HpD. The incidence of cutaneous complications may have been lessened substantially by the use of DHE. Dougherty et al. (59) reviewed the cutaneous phototoxic occurrences in patients receiving DHE. All 180 patients receiving a total of 266 injections of the photosensitizer at doses ranging from 0.5 to 2.0 mg/kg were photosensitive following the injection, but up to 40% of the patients reported some type of phototoxic response presumably due to noncompliance. Some 12% to 14% of the patients reported blistering without apparent relationship to the drug dose. Based on the data, the investigators recommend that patients receiving DHE be cautioned to avoid bright sunlight and other bright lights for at least 6 weeks following injection. Regular UV sunscreen is ineffective and only opaque cream (zinc oxide) provides protection, but it is not often cosmetically acceptable. In a pilot study of 12 PDT patients and 12 controls, treated with oral activated charcoal, Lowdell et al. (60) attempted to reduce the skin photosensitivity but failed to demonstrate a significant pharmacological or clinical difference.

Additional Treatment Reports

McCaughan et al. (61) treated 40 patients with advanced cancer of the esophagus including 19 squamous cell carcinomas, 19 adenocarcinoma, and two melanomas. They used a wide range of power settings and added Nd:YAG laser therapy, chemotherapy, and radiation therapy as well as dilation. The average luminal diameter increased form 6 to 9 mm and most patients tolerated soft diet after treatment. Probably part of the tumors treated, received a combination of PDT and interstitial hyperthermia when the fiber tip was inserted and the laser power was 1W. Complications included four perforations, six strictures, nine pleural effusions and five sunburns.

Thomas et al. (62) treated 15 patients with inoperable esophageal carcinomas, which required a total of 26 treatments with HpD at high light doses. They attempted to increase the treatment area by placing the fiber in the center of a balloon filled with intralipid to scatter the light (similar to urologic PDT in the urinary bladder filled with intralipid). Procedures lasted as long as 70 minutes and general anesthesia was used. All the patients experienced symptomatic improvement, but with the power above 1.5 W the complication rate was high. Complications included fever in seven cases, fistulas in two, mediastinitis in two, and cutaneous photosensitivity in four. The in-hospital mortality was 14%.

Of 20 patients with cancer of the esophagus, stomach, and rectum treated by Jin et al. (63), 73% experienced some type of therapeutic response, which was complete in 10% of cases.

Krasner et al. (64) treated 21 patients with GI neoplasia with PDT. Twelve rectal carcinomas, three esophageal carcinoma, one gastric cancer, and five colorectal sessile bilious adenomas were treated with curative/palliative intent. Interstitial PDT of 50 joules at four to seven treatment sites was applied. In some rectal cancers, endoscopic ultrasound was used to assess the depth of tumor invasion and the treatment response. The mean depth of tumor removed was 6 + 4 mm. Overall, 2 out of the 16 carcinomas and three out of the five adenomas were eradicated. In one case a major hemorrhage complicated the treatment of a large rectal cancer.

Like many other new cancer treatments, PDT was first tried on patients for whom all else has failed. It is clear that PDT can be used successfully for palliation in desperate cases of complete luminal obstruction but its most promising application should be in the early stage of GI cancer with primary or combined curative intent. In two international surveys of PDT, Spinelli (65) found a worldwide trend toward the treatment of early tumors and preneoplastic lesions.

Sabben et al. (66) treated 43 patients, half of whom were asymptomatic, with superficial esophageal cancer. Complete tumor destruction was obtained in 37 patients, 9 of whom experienced recurrence. Survival was 73% at least 1 year and 44% at 2 years.

Lambert (37) achieved complete destruction in 46 of 65 T1N0 or small T2.N0 esophagogastric tumors treated with PDT, chemotherapy, and radiotherapy. The five year survival rate was 26% for all cases and 37% for newly diagnosed cases. In 60% of cases, the cause of death was not related to the esophageal cancer.

Patrice et al. (67) used PDT with curative intent in 54 inoperable patients with lesions less than 4 cm in their largest diameter. Twenty-four esophageal squamous cell carcinomas, 14 gastroesophageal adenocarcinoma, and 16 rectosigmoid carcinomas were treated with 33% partial response and 44% complete response. The mean recurrence-free period varied form 13.8 to 17.4 months and 50% of the successfully treated patients were alive at 24 month. This study suggests a potential efficacy of PDT as curative treatment. Endoscopic ultrasonography staging and better dosimetry could create extension of the PDT indication from palliative to adjuvant or curative.

Karanov et al. (68) used PDT in six patients with early stage cancers of the esophagus, stomach, colon and rectum. T1, N0, M0 stage was established by computed tomography (CT) scan or endocavitary ultrasound. One to four laser sessions were required to achieve complete response in all the cases. No recurrence was observed over 7 to 16 months of follow-up.

Overholt (69) treated three patients with early esophageal cancer, achieving complete histologic and endoscopic ultrasonographic response. In one patient with adenocarcinoma in Barrett's esophagus, a reduction in the volume of Barrett's mucosa was noted.

Monnier et al. (70) treat 15 cases of "early" esophageal cancer and achieved complete response in 12. After a long theoretical review of PDT, they concluded that after 10 years of clinical trials little progress has been achieved in tumor selectivity. Partial destruction of large tumors is presumed selective because the normal mucosa gets reduced irradiation by red light while we may lose selectivity in small early cancer causing 13% of complications, such as transmural effect with fistulae and stenosis. They developed a transparent light diffusing cylinder, fixed on a Savary-Gilliard dilation bougie that permits homogenous light distribution over the whole length of the cylinder. A similar centering balloon was developed by Panjehpour et al. (71) with uniform light intensities around the lumen. The balloon increases the area illuminated by a 2.5 cm diffuser to 4.0 cm and eliminates the mucosal folds that contribute to uneven light dosimetry, Fleischer et al. (72) developed a similar dilating transparent balloon that is placed over a guidewire and contains a laser fiber for precise dosimetry.

New photosensitizers

Considerable progress has been made in the search for better sensitizers. Phtalocyanines are porphyrinlike industrial dyes with significant advantages over HpD and DHE, which are an ill-defined mixture of porphyrins with relatively weak tumor selectivity and only a weak absorption peak in the red when tissue penetration by light is the deepest. Phyalocyanines are stable compounds with known structure, easy to synthesize, and with strong absorption peaks at 600 to 750 mm when light penetration in tissue is still good. Their low absorption at wavelengths shorter than 600 mm will potentially reduce the cutaneous photosensitivity. The most promising agent appears to be aluminum chlorosulfontaed phtalocyanine (AlSPc) but animal studies (73) demonstrate a similar pattern of uptake by induced colonic and pancreatic cancer with a low therapeutic ratio to normal tissue that is unlikely to result in significant selective destruction.

When a new photosensitizer, 5-aminolevulinic acid (ALA) was compared to AIS Pc by Loh et al. (74) a new promising mechanism of action was discovered. Exogenous ALA lead to accumulation of protoporphyrin IX (PPG), producing photosensitization of the gastric mucosa (ratio 10:1) PDT with red light which resulted in marked mucosal necrosis and sparing of the underlying layers. The mechanism of cell death resulted from direct cellular photodestruction and not from damage to the microvasculature, leading to better healing without scarring. This type of PDT carries application potential for areas with severe mucosal dysplasia such as Barrett's esophagus. ALA causes only short-lived photosensitization and cutaneous side effects are unlikely after 24 hours (75).

The first study of PDT with ALA is the human gastrointestinal tract was reported by Regula et al. (76). Ten patients with eleven colorectal, duodenal and esophageal tumors were treated six hours after the first of six fractionated oral doses of ALA 30–60 mg/kg. Nine out of eleven lesions showed superficial mucosal necrosis in the areas exposed to light. Six patients had transit rises in serum aspartate aminotransferases, two had mild skin photosensitivity reactions for 48 hours only and five had mild nausea and vomiting. Gossner et al. (77) reported on two patients with small adenocarcinoma of the esophagus and stomach treated with PDT 6 to 8 hours after a oral ingestion of ALA at a dose of 60 mg/kg. Both tumors became edematous and ulcerated early after the light application and became covered with fibrin for the next few days. The patients did not exhibit prolonged photosensitivity but a transit increase of AST (x5N) was noted for 72 hours. ALA holds a greater promise for clinical use in superficial lesions such as high grade dysplasia in Barrett's epithelium.

Lower Gastrointestinal Neoplasia

Colorectal carcinoma and colon polyps

Introduction

Lower GI endoscopy of the colon developed over the last 20 years into a very effective and safe tool in the diagnosis and treatment of colonic neoplasia. With growth of elderly population the number of procedures performed in the elderly is increasing. Endoscopy not only offers cure of certain colonic polyps and cancers, but presents a variety of palliative options. In this chapter endoscopic forms of treatment will be reviewed with particular emphasis on endoscopic polypectomy, endoscopic laser and photodynamic therapy.

Endoscopic polypectomy

Recent advances in understanding of genetics of colonic carcinogenesis strongly supports a gradual development of colon cancer from adenomatous polyps often described as the adenoma — carcinoma sequence (78,79). This theory is further supported by a number of clinical retrospective studies and recent data coming out of a multi-center prospective study — The National Polyp Study. (80,81,82). Fourteen-hundred and eighteen patients compared to three historical control groups showed 76–90% lower than expected incidence of colorectal carcinoma after endoscopic polypectomy (79). The prevalence of adenomatous polyps increases with age. Presently it is unclear at what age polypectomy no longer influence overall survival. The simplicity and high degree of safety of current techniques favors removal at any age. The screening and polyp surveillance guidelines have been released through the Practice Parameters Committee of the American College of Gastroenterology and most recently summarized in the Annals of Internal Medicine and WHO Bulletin (84,85).

Most polyps up to 5 cm in size can be removed endoscopically. Several techniques have been developed according to form and size of the polyp. Description of specifics of each individual technique is beyond the scope of this revue and is referred to elsewhere (83). Small polyps (< 5 mm in diameter) should initially be removed entirely using biopsy forceps with or without electric current coagulation. The occurrence of malignancy within a small tubular adenoma is less than 5% and it remains unclear at what age further surveillance is beneficial. Patients with a single small polyp and no other risk factors for colon cancer are not at increased risk for colon carcinoma and probably do not need further colonoscopic surveillance (80). The incidence of carcinoma within a large villous adenoma is up to 40% and endoscopic polypectomy is curative for focal carcinomas within muscularis mucosa or for carcinomas without evidence of vascular or lymphatic invasion (84). The majority of large polyps are removed with snare and electrocautery. Sessile lesions may require piecemeal removal. Piecemeal removal requires repeat endoscopy and inspection of polypectomy site in 3–6 months to ensure entire removal. Multiple biopsies of the polyp base should be obtained to rule out invasive carcinoma. Once the colon has been cleared of all polyps a repeat colonoscopy in 3 and if negative for neoplasia in 5 years is sufficient. Sometimes large sessile polyps can be removed easier by injecting the base of the polyp with normal saline or 1/10000 epinephrine injection. This will raise the polyp more in to the lumen of the colon allowing removal of larger pieces. This technique appears to be safe, possibly decreases the risk of perforation and full thickness coagulation injury but may increase the risk of delayed bleeding (83,86,91). This has been reported to be close to 10% as compared to 1.7% of standard polypectomies of large polyps.

Some polyps are not amenable to endoscopic treatment and will require surgical approach. Large polyps located in the right colon particularly if sessile or extending over two folds, involving 2/3 of luminal circumference and polyps with evidence of vascular or lymphatic malignant invasion should be removed surgically. Invasive cancers within a polyp place the endoscopists in a therapeutic dilemma. The average risk of metastasis from a polyp containing poorly differentiated carcinoma is 8.5%–15% and can be as high as 50% when evidence of vascular or lymphatic invasion is present (87,88). When malignant sessile polyps are removed endoscopically the incidence of cancer detected during surgery or at follow up ranges between 4.1% for favorable histology and 20.6% for polyps with unfavorable features (89). Surgical removal however carries significant mortality which can be as high as 10% in patients over the age of 75 (90). This rate will hopefully continue to decrease with further improvement of laparoscopic colectomies. Possibly combined endoscopic and laparoscopic approach will be seen in the future.

Endoscopic laser treatment

There is a vast experience with endoscopic laser treatment successfully applied in palliation and eradication of colonic neoplasia. In more than 35 studies published just within recent 5 years endoscopic laser therapy using predominantly Nd:YAG (neodymium:yttrium aluminum garnet) laser proved to be very effective in eradication of colonic polyps (92–97) ablation and cure of certain colorectal carcinomas (98–101). It also allows recanalization of obstructing tumors (104,105) reduces the rate of bleeding, mucous discharge, diarrhea and improves incontinence (104–114).

Entire eradication of colorectal polyps can be achieved with ELT. Typically lesions located in the rectosigmoid area, non-obstructing and noncircumferential lesions are amenable to this type of therapy. Several groups reported complete ablation in 70%–92% (82,83,84). The recurrence rate was between 13–20% and about half of all polyps could be removed with subsequent treatments. In one study carcinoma was detected in 7% of biopsy specimens obtained during treatment (93). Mathus-Vliegen and Tytgat reported polyp ablation in 241 patients. Complete removal was achieved in 93% of small lesions, in 85 % of intermediate sized lesions and 56% in lesions involving 2/3 of luminal circumference (95). Seven percent of treated patients experienced complications in form of bleeding and stenosis which could be managed by conservative and endoscopic means. There were no treatment associated mortality. ELT combined with electrocautery snare debulking reduces the number of treatment sessions without concomitant increase in complications (93,94,97).

The treatment of choice of colorectal carcinoma is surgery, however in nonsurgical candidates ELT of T1 and T2 lesions may achieve cure. Mathus-Vliegen reported their experience in 35 elderly medically compromised patients (mean age 75) with evidence of invasive adenocarcinoma not beyond the submucosal layer and without evidence of lymph node involvement (98). Results were evaluable in 30 patients and complete eradication was achieved in 28 patients in follow up period of 3 years. Similar results were achieved by Brunetaud, Escourrou and Dittrich in three separate studies showing tumor free interval from 13–37 months in up to 90% of patients with early rectosigmoid tumors who were unfit for surgery (99,100,101). Endoscopic ultrasonography has been used to improve staging prior to laser treatment in some of above mentioned studies. Treatment success can be evaluated with endosonography as well, however a minimum of 6 weeks interval should be observed to avoid overstaging (102,103).

ELT plays a special role in recanalization of obstructing or near obstructing lesions. Eckhauser achieved recanalization in 31 of 55 treated patients thus allowing full peroral lavage and one stage resection (104). Interestingly in this study the majority of treated lesions were above the peritoneal deflection. In an another study Mathus-Vliegen reported 94% success in obtaining luminal patency in 31 obstructed patients. One patient died due to pararectal abscess (95). Collective experience of 7 laser centers showed 89% success rate in achieving luminal patency (105). The complication rate in this high risk patients was 11% with no treatment associated death.

Probably the most frequent application of ELT today in colonic neoplasia is to improve quality of life in nonsurgical patients by controlling symptoms of bleeding, diarrhea and pain (104–114). Hemostasis of particularly shorter and less extensive lesions is excellent and can be accomplished up to 90% of cases. The same is true for diarrhea which can be controlled in up to 90% of patients. More extensive lesions (2/3 of luminal circumference) and lesions involving the anal sphincter are much more difficult to treat (113–114) and may require alternative therapy. Brunetaud uses argon laser in lesions close to the anal sphincter which allows complete evaporation of the tumor without deep tissue injury (113). Alternatively combination therapy of ELT, chemotherapy and radiation may decrease the number of laser treatment sessions, decrease damage to the surrounding uninvolved tissue and ultimately improve palliation (115, 116).

When considering treatment of colorectal carcinoma in the elderly, overall risks and benefits of surgical endoscopic interventions have to be highly individualized. Operative mortality after abdominoperineal resection in this patient population can be as high as 10% and may be higher for rectal resection (117,118). Also significant perioperative morbidity (53%) plays a major role in the decision process and influence significantly the overall costs of surgical therapy ($22,900–23,156 versus $2,263–12,154) (119). On the other hand endoscopic treatment of extensive lesions is successful in maintenance of good palliation over extended time only in half of treated patients (113). The new trends will most certainly include direct tissue contact tips with low power lasers, photodynamic therapy and possibly combination therapies with chemo, radiation and surgery (119,120).

Photodynamic therapy

The principal of photodynamic therapy (PDT) is to potentiate laser energy by incorporation of photosensitizer in the tumor tissue. For detailed description of mechanism and techniques it is referred to previous chapter. Presently the largest experience in clinical studies is with dihematoporphyrin ether ester (DHE), systemically injected photosensitizer and argon pumped dye laser. The photosesensitizer is absorbed initially by all the tissue but slower eliminated by the neoplastic tissue reaching 2:1 distribution 40–50 hours after injection. This difference in concentration between normal and neoplastic tissue allows for cancer destruction and relative sparing of the healthy tissue. The absorption spectrum of DHE is close to that of solar radiation which explains why skin sunburn is the most common complication of this therapy. Five-amino-laevulinic acid (ALA) is a new orally administered substance which is significantly less associated with skin photosensitivity and .is overall better tolerated. It induces endogenous production of protoporphyrin IX which is differentially expressed in certain tissues such as cancer and dysplastic cells (122,75). The laser induced tumor necrosis is achieved through ischemia from destruction of blood vessel walls and also through direct tumor cell death (123).

Clinical studies

Today, it is apparent that the most beneficial role of PDT is eradication of early or preneoplastic lesions although the majority of the initial studies were done in patients who failed all other available therapies (126). Loh *et al.* treated 8 patients with 9 colosigmoid villous adenomas with PDT who previously were treated with Nd:YAG laser. Seven adenomas were entirely eradicated (median follow up of 12 months). Substantial necrosis was found in the other two polyps. There were no major complications (124). Similar results were reported by the same group in earlier studies (125). Karanov *et al.* showed complete cure of early rectal cancers (T1,No,Mo) in a small number of patients followed over a 7–16 month period (126). Interestingly, one patient with Familial Polyposis in his remaining rectum experienced complete disappearance of all polyps. In unresectable advanced cancer which previously failed other therapy, PDT offered significant improvement in luminal diameter and surrounding tissue invasion as assessed by endoscopic ultrasound (127). Again in this particular study the most benefit of PDT was seen in 2 patients with small lesions with tumor free interval of 20 and 28 months respectively. One patient experienced hemodynamically significant hemorrhage from a large rectal ulcer (127). In further studies good palliation has been achieved in more than 80% of patients with massive advanced rectal cancer (128–131). Photodynamic therapy is a relatively young technique and rapid progress is being made in improving the delivery and selectivity of new sensitizers (e.g. 5-ALA, conjugation of hematoporphyrin with albumin and transferrin) and introduction of new laser dyes such as carbocyanine and copper metal vapor (130,131).Another promising approach appears to be adjuvant intraoperative PDT which helps to control the extraluminal tumor growth (132,133).

Endoscopic Treatment of Radiation Procto — and Colopathy

Radiation therapy plays a major role of many cancer treatment programs and it is estimated that up to 50% of all cancer patients will receive radiation treatment. With development of new supervoltage techniques which decreases skin injury we are seeing more damage to the deeper tissue level including the gastrointestinal tract. The prevalence of radiation injury to the GI-tract varies between 1–25% and the incidence can be as high as 75% after pelvic irradiation (134–137). The most common colon areas affected are rectum and sigmoid colon probably due to the relative immobility of these anatomical structures and high doses of radiation used in this area. The damage to the colonic tissue follows linear relation; 16% incidence in patients receiving 3000 Gy and 37% receiving 6000 (138). Patients with radiation injury to the distal colon and rectum may present with diarrhea, tenesmus and bleeding during or within 6 weeks of completion of therapy (137,138). This is considered the acute phase (acute proctitis) and most patients will recover spontaneously (139). Endoscopy during this phase is virtually normal

Table 37.5 Success and complication rates of endoscopic polypectomy of large sessile polyps (2–5 cm in diameter) with and without invasive carcinoma.

	Number of Polyps	Complete Removal of Polyps	Complete Removal of Invasive CA	Complication Rate
Nivatvongs *et al.* 1984	28	82%	62%	4%
Bedogni *et al.* 1986	66	100%	83.5%	4.5%
Karita *et al.* 1991	71	95%	100%	0.01%
Walsh 1992	132	72%	41%	3%

showing some mild erythema. Patient who develop or progress to chronic phase will present with diarrhea, proctalgia and hematochezia typically around 9–24 months after radiation (140). It appears that chronic radiation proctosigmoiditis follows two clinical courses:patients with minimal intestinal symptoms, no transfusion requirements and high spontaneous remission (70%) and patients requiring transfusions who will develop significant morbidity and mortality. In this study the spontaneous remission rate was less than 20% in the latter group. Fifty percent required surgery and radiation associated injuries were directly responsible for 40% of death (140). Endoscopic examination reveals pale mucosa and multiple characteristic telangiectatic lesions. Also extensive areas of friable mucosa can be found in a significant number of patients whereas frank ulceration's are rather rare. It is this particular proctitis population that is difficult to treat. Many conservative attempts with 5-amino salicylic acid, sucralfate enema and hyperbaric oxygen have been made with some albeit limited success (141,142). Recent reports indicate that endoluminal formalin therapy may be more successful, reducing bleeding in 85% of treated patients and eliminates further need for transfusions (143).

The most consistent results in the control of hematochezia from chronic radiation proctitis have been achieved with endoscopic coagulation. Initial studies using endoscopic Nd:YAG laser therapy showed 80% decrease in transfusion requirements and subsequent hospital admissions (144). Subsequent series using endoscopic argon laser therapy reported similar success (145). Two groups presented their experience in two separate but comparable studies with Nd:YAG and argon laser (146,147). Patients in both studies had persistent bleeding refractory to other treatment modalities including surgical bypass colostomy. Both the Nd:YAG and argon therapies appeared to be equally effective in reduction of initial bleeding (YAG 89%, argon 100%), transfusion requirements and improving hematocrits. In inaccessible areas contact coagulation with heater probe and bipolar coagulation probe was used in the Nd:YAG study. Long-term follow up was addressed in the argon study (mean of 35 month) demonstrating the need of maintenance therapy in 71% of patients. The average symptom-free interval in these patients was 7 months. There were no complications in the argon treated patients but 6% in the Nd:YAG

group. Four percent in the Nd:YAG group required rectosigmoid resection and colostomy.

Current experience with endoscopic coagulation indicates that it is effective and safe therapy for persistent and significant bleeding associated with chronic radiation proctitis. It offers an attractive alternative to surgery which has high morbidity and mortality. Additionally, endoscopy allows dilation of colonic strictures fortunately less common radiation induced injury of the gastrointestinal tract.

Biliary and Pancreatic Neoplasia

Despite advances in diagnosis, and surgical management pancreatic carcinoma continues to have a poor prognosis. Only 20% of patients with this disease are candidates for curative resection, and of those resected the five year survival nationally is only 9% (150). The outlook is somewhat better for cholangiocarcinoma. The overall five year survival in a group of 171 patients with cholangiocarcinoma undergoing operative intervention was 16% (151). A curative resection was performed in 29% of patients and their overall five year survival was 44%. The role of endoscopy in patients with malignant pancreatic and biliary tract disease is to assist in establishing a diagnosis, to provide accurate staging, and to provide palliative therapy in patients who are poor operative candidates or who have disease which is not resectable for cure.

Diagnosis and Staging

Computed tomography (CT) is the initial test of choice for the diagnosis and staging of pancreatic and bile duct tumors. Spiral CT with oral and intravenous contrast is the preferred technique. Transabdominal ultrasound and MRI have no advantages as compared with CT and should be used selectively to answer specific questions.

Endoscopic retrograde cholangiopancreatography (ERCP) is very sensitive in the detection of ductal adenocarcinoma. The sensitivity of ERCP was 98% for pancreatic carcinomas < 2 cm in diameter in one study (152), and 97.2% for all pancreatic carcinomas in a second study (153). Biliary or pancreatic ductal cytology can be obtained at the time of ERCP and is positive in approximately 50% of cases. ERCP is the procedure of choice for the diagnosis of ampullary and duodenal carcinomas since the procedure allows direct visuali-

Table 37. 6 Indications for diagnostic ERCP.

- To evaluate equivocal findings on imaging studies.

- Suspicion of malignancy with negative imaging studies

  Unexplained pancreatitis in the elderly

  Unexplained cholestasis

  Pancreatic pain and elevated CA 19-9

- To provide an outline of ductal anatomy for preoperative planning

- For diagnosis of ampullary and duodenal carcinoma

- To establish a tissue diagnosis with cytology or biopsy if required for prognosis or to initiate therapy

Table 37.7 Staging of pancreatic and cholangiocarcinoma.

- CT — Spiral CT with IV and oral contrast the initial procedure of choice.

- Laparoscopy — Accurately detects small liver and peritoneal metastases. Recommended prior to attempted curative resection of pancreatic carcinoma.

- Endoscopic Ultrasound — Most accurate method for assessing regional lymph node involvement. Procedure of choice for staging ampullary carcinoma.

- ERCP — Demonstrates ductal anatomy. Important in determining resectability of proximal cholangiocarcinoma

- Transabdominal Ultrasound, MRI, Angiography — Not routinely indicated. Use in selected cases to answer specific questions.

zation and biopsy of these lesions which have a more favorable prognosis. Diagnostic ERCP is indicated if a diagnosis of pancreatic or biliary malignancy is suspected and CT is negative or equivocal, to outline ductal anatomy prior to surgery, and when ampullary or duodenal carcinoma is suspected. The indications for diagnostic ERCP are summarized in Table 37.6. The endoscopist performing diagnostic ERCP should be capable of inserting biliary stents, since injection of contrast beyond a partially obstructing biliary stenosis demands drainage to prevent subsequent cholangitis.

The purpose of staging is to determine prognosis and to facilitate selection of therapy. CT is the initial staging procedure of choice. However, CT is insensitive in detecting small (<1 cm in diameter) liver metastases, and peritoneal malignancies which are frequent findings in pancreatic carcinoma. These smaller lesions are detectable only by direct visualization at the time of laparoscopy or laparotomy. In one study of 88 patients with pancreatic carcinoma, 40% in whom no metastases were demonstrable by CT or angiography had small metastases on laparoscopy (154). Laparoscopy is recommended as a preoperative staging procedure in all patients with pancreatic carcinoma in whom CT shows localized disease, and who are being considered for surgical resection. An additional advantage of laparoscopy is the ability to proceed with palliative laparoscopic surgery if evidence of unresectability for cure is found. Laparoscopic cholecystojejunostomy as a palliative procedure has been reported with satisfactory results and prompt patient recovery (155).

A promising staging technique is endoscopic ultrasound. Endoscopic ultrasound has been found to be highly accurate in assessing the size, and extent of pancreatic and ampullary carcinoma. In one study, endoscopic ultrasound had an overall TNM staging accuracy of 92%, and an accuracy of 91% in the assessment of regional lymph node metastases (156). Endoscopic ultrasound can also be used to guide aspiration biopsies of pancreatic lesions with improved results (157). Newer catheter echoprobes can be inserted through the biopsy channel of ERCP endoscopes and into the pancreatic and biliary ductal systems. These

probes can supplement ERCP when the diagnosis is questionable, or when additional staging information is needed. The use of endoscopic ultrasound as a staging modality is likely to grow in the future.

Angiography has frequently been used in the past to determine resectability of pancreatic carcinoma based on major vessel involvement. CT with intravenous contrast, and endoscopic ultrasound both provide similar information. Therefore angiography should be used selectively. Staging modalities are summarized in Table 37.7.

Palliative Therapy

The majority of patients with pancreatic and biliary malignancy will be found to have unresectable disease and will require palliative therapy. A number of methods are available to achieve relief of malignant obstructive jaundice and these are summarized in Table 37.8. Palliative surgery is the traditional modality for therapy of these advanced malignancies. However, palliative surgery has a high morbidity and mortality, as well as a prolonged convalescence (158). In a prospective,

Table 37.8 Alternatives for treatment of malignant biliary obstruction.

- Palliative surgery

- Percutaneous transhepatic drainage.

  External

  Internal — External

  Endoprosthesis

- Endoscopic drainage

  Sphincterotomy (ampullary tumors)

  Conventional plasic stent

  Self expanding metal stent

- Combined percutaneous endoscopic drainage

randomized study of endoscopic biliary endoprosthesis versus surgical bypass for palliation of malignant biliary obstruction involving the distal bile duct, overall survival was found to be similar in the two groups, but initial hospital stay and overall hospitalization was shorter in the endoscopically treated group (159). The only situations favoring palliative surgery are duodenal obstruction combined with biliary obstruction, and discovery of advanced disease at the time of surgery undertaken with curative intent. Radiotherapy and chemotherapy have not been found to benefit the majority of patients with malignant biliary obstruction, the exception being the patient with lymphoma. This leaves stents placed either endoscopically or percutaneously as the major modality of palliative therapy.

Percutaneous Drainage

Several percutaneous, transhepatic biliary drainage methods have been described. Initially, external drainage by means of a catheter placed percutaneously but not advanced beyond the point of obstruction was advocated. Subsequently, techniques which involved manipulation of a guidewire and catheter through the obstructing lesion allowed both internal and external drainage (160). These techniques have the disadvantages of requiring percutaneous, transhepatic puncture with its inherent risks of bleeding and bile peritonitis as well as the external loss of fluids, electrolytes, and bile salts.

Internal biliary drainage via the percutaneous route was described by Pereras, *et al.* in 1978 (161). This technique avoids the discomfort of an external catheter, and the external loss of bile. However, it has the disadvantage of loss of access to the indwelling stent making stent exchange difficult. This becomes a problem in patients who have a longer life expectancy since these stents may occlude and require replacement. For this reason, completely internalized, percutaneously placed plastic stents have never been widely used, and internal-external drainage catheters have remained the most commonly employed percutaneous method of drainage.

The most recent development in percutaneous transhepatic stent placement has been the use of self expanding metal stents (162, 163). These stents achieve a diameter of 1cm, provide internal drainage, and occlude less frequently then conventional plastic stents. The stents consist of a stainless steel, wire mesh and may become obstructed due to tumor in-growth through the interstices of the stent. They cannot be removed, and occlusion is usually treated by placing a second stent through the occluded stent. These stents are not suitable for use in benign strictures since they are not removable.

There is one randomized trial of endoscopic versus percutaneously stent insertion in malignant obstructive jaundice (164). In this study, 75 patients were randomized to treatment with either a 12F percutaneously placed plastic stent, or a 10F endoscopically placed stent. The endoscopic method has a higher success rate for the relief of jaundice (81% versus 61%), and a sig-

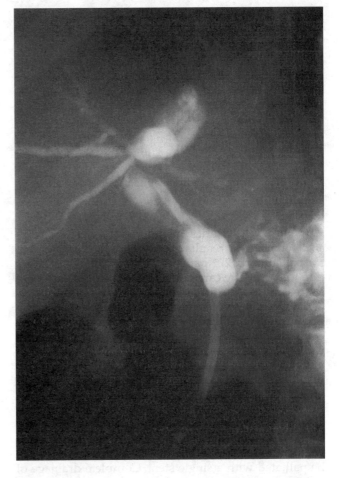

Figure 37.5 Conventional plastic stent in proper position across a malignant stricture due to pancreatic carcinoma.

nificantly lower 30 day mortality (15% versus 33%). The higher mortality after percutaneous stent placement was due to complications associated with liver puncture, namely hemorrhage and bile leaks. Based on this study, it is recommended that endoscopic stent placement be used for biliary drainage of malignant strictures. Transhepatic, percutaneous stent insertion has a role as a backup method when the endoscopic method fails. A combined technique may also be employed and is discussed below.

Endoscopic Stents

Endoscopic stent placement was first described in 1980 (165). The technique involves initial performance of a diagnostic ERCP to outline the biliary anatomy and define the extent and location of the malignant stricture. A guidewire and guide catheter are then threaded through the stricture using fluoroscopic control, and the stent is pushed into place over the guide catheter (Figure 37.5). Conventional plastic stents are held in place by side flaps. One side flap is placed just above the stenosis, and the second at the level of the ampulla. A small papillotomy can be made to facilitate stent placement, but long papillotomies are unnecessary.

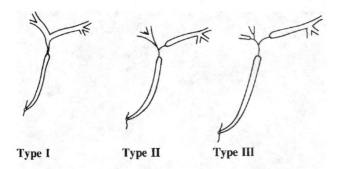

Type I   Type II   Type III

Figure 37.6 Types of malignant hilar biliary strictures.

In the largest series in the literature, Huibregtse, *et al.* reported the results of endoscopic stent placement for palliation in 221 patients with obstructive jaundice due to pancreatic carcinoma (166). The procedure was successful in 90% of patients with a morbidity of 2% and a 30 day mortality of 10%. The serum bilirubin normalized in 92% of those who survived. The major complications occurring in these patients were early cholangitis (8%) and late clogging (21%).

Hilar strictures are more difficult to palliate then distal bile duct strictures. Hilar strictures can be divided into three types (167) (Figure 37.6). Type I strictures involve the common hepatic duct just below the bifurcation. Type II hilar strictures involve the bifurcation, and type III strictures involve the bifurcation as well as the segmental bile ducts. Type I strictures can be palliated with a single stent. Complete drainage of type II strictures requires placement of two stents, one into each main hepatic duct. If it proves impossible to place two stents, it is acceptable to provide drainage with one stent (168). However, if sepsis subsequently develops it is essential to drain the remaining obstructed portion of the biliary tract (169). If this cannot be done endoscopically, combined or percutaneous drainage should be attempted. Most patients with type III hilar strictures have short life expectancies, symptoms which are difficult if not impossible to palliate, and do not develop cholangitis unless they are instrumented (169). The majority of patients with type III hilar strictures are best served by symptomatic therapy without drainage procedures. In one series of 103 patients with hilar strictures, successful drainage was achieved in only 15% of patients with a type III hilar stricture as opposed to 86% of patients with a type I stenosis (169).

Pancreatic stents can also be placed utilizing the endoscopic retrograde route. They have a minor role in palliation but may be useful in the occasional patient who has continued pain secondary to obstructive pancreatitis. Relieving pancreatic ductal obstruction with a stent relieves pain in these patients (Figure 37.7).

Complications of endoscopic biliary stents

Early complications are those occurring within seven days of stent placement. They include complications related to the initial diagnostic ERCP, endoscopic papillotomy, bile duct perforation, and cholangitis.

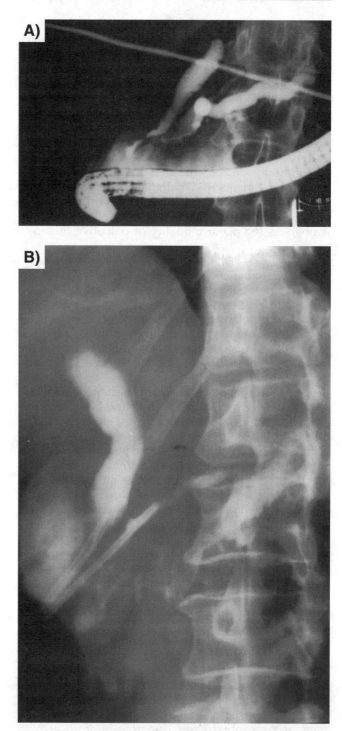

Figure 37.7 Patient with pancreatic carcinoma and recurrent episodes of pancreatitis.
A) ERCP shows a double duct sign with strictures of both pancreatic and common bile ducts.
B) Stents have been placed in both duct systems.

Attention to the details of the endoscopic procedure, and avoiding or limiting the length of the papillotomy will minimize these complications.

Early cholangitis occurs at a rate of approximately 8% (166). It is increased in frequency if more than one attempt is necessary to place a stent, if drainage is incomplete, or if contaminated instruments are used for the procedure (170). Pure diagnostic ERCP should be avoided in obstructed patients since it increases the risk of subsequent cholangitis by introducing bacteria into an undrained biliary tract. Cholangitis can be minimized by using properly disinfected instruments, using sterile water in the endoscope water reservoir, making drainage as complete as possible, and utilizing prophylactic antibiotics prior to endoscopic drainage. Antibiotic coverage should be directed at E. coli, Klebsiella, and enterococcus which are the most frequent organisms implicated in cholangitis. If a prior ERCP or drainage procedure has been attempted, antibiotic coverage should include Pseudomonas which is frequently present after failed attempts at drainage.

The most frequent late complication of endoscopic biliary stents is also cholangitis. Stents which cross the sphincter of Oddi allow access of bacteria from the upper gastrointestinal tract to the biliary tract. These bacteria adhere to conventional plastic stents and build up a bacterial biofilm ultimately leading to stent occlusion and subsequent cholangitis (171). Regardless of their caliber, plastic stents will eventually occlude. Smaller caliber stents, 8 F or less, occlude more rapidly than large caliber stents, 10 or 12F (172). Therefore only large caliber stents should be used to palliate malignant stenoses.

Potential solutions to the problem of stent occlusion include the use of oral antibiotics, the development of new polymers that do not allow bacterial adherence, and the use of self expanding metal stents. The use of oral antibiotics, and stents impregnated with antibacterial agents are ineffective in preventing stent occlusion. Expandable metal stents do not allow bacterial adherence, have better patency rates than plastic stents, but may be occluded by tumor in-growth or overgrowth. New polymers are a promising area of research. Recently a novel polymer, Vivathane, has been developed at the University of South Florida. This polymer has an ultra smooth surface that does not allow bacterial adherence (173). When perfused with infected human bile, Vivathane stents remain patent. Clinical trials will be necessary to determine if Vivathane stents are superior to conventional plastic stents in terms of stent longevity and the development of late complications.

Other late complications include duodenal stenosis due to tumor progression and acute cholecystitis. Duodenal obstruction requiring surgical therapy occurs in approximately 7% of patients with pancreatic cancer initially treated with stents. Any patient with duodenal tumor involvement should initially be treated with palliative surgery, including gastrojejunostomy as well as a biliary drainage procedure, even if it is technically feasible to place a biliary stent since surgery will eventually be required.

Acute cholecystitis is a rare complication of stent placement (174). It occurs in patients with tumor partially occluding or in close proximity to the cystic duct. Stent placement completes cystic duct occlusion and eventually results in acute cholecystitis. These patients respond well to percutaneous cholecystostomy and rarely require surgical therapy (174).

Stent replacement

Since all plastic stents will eventually occlude if the patient survives long enough, close patient follow up is necessary. Stent occlusion may be heralded by an asymptomatic rise in bilirubin or liver enzymes, by a non-specific flu like illness, or by frank cholangitis. It is important to make the patient aware of the early symptoms of stent occlusion including low grade fever, malaise, change in urine or stool color, and pruritus. Preferably stents should be replaced before cholangitis occurs. In the face of a rising bilirubin, a CT or HIDA scan may be helpful in distinguishing progressive liver metastases from stent occlusion. The patent stent will be associated with air in the biliary tract on CT, and passage of radionucleotide into the duodenum on HIDA scan. However, it should be recognized that partial stent occlusion may result in sufficient stasis to give rise to cholangitis while giving the appearance of patency on imaging studies. When doubt exists as to the adequacy of biliary drainage or the presence of cholangitis, the stent should be replaced. When cholangitis occurs, antibiotics are a necessary part of therapy, but without stent replacement to reestablish good biliary drainage they are not sufficient to effect a good outcome.

Currently the life expectancy of initial 10–12 F plastic biliary stents is 4–6 months (175). In patients with malignant biliary obstruction who remain fit, it is recommended that plastic stents be changed prophylactically at 4 month intervals. Elective stent replacement can be done on an outpatient basis, and avoids long and costly hospitalizations for treatment of cholangitis. Since many patients with malignant biliary obstruction have short life expectancies, only 25–35% will eventually require stent replacement (176).

Self expanding metal stents

Self expanding metal stents remain patent longer than conventional metal stents and partially solve the problem of stent occlusion. Metal stents are mounted on a delivery device in a collapsed state. The delivery device is then passed over a guidewire and positioned so that the stent bridges the malignant stricture. The stent is then released and allowed to expand to its full diameter, and the delivery device is then withdrawn leaving the stent in position. Currently metal stents are available in 8 and 10 mm diameters.

The most widely used metal stent is the Wallstent (Schneider, Plymouth, Mn). There have been several trials comparing Wallstents to conventional plastic stents. Davids et al. randomly assigned 105 patients with distal malignant biliary obstruction to receive either a metal or a straight 10 F polyethylene stent (177). Median patency of the metal stent was significantly longer than that of plastic stents, 273 vs. 126 days. Initial placement of a metal stent resulted in a 28% decrease in the number of endoscopic procedures.

The major cause of stent occlusion was tumor in-growth in the metal stent group, and sludge deposition in the plastic stent group. Length of patient survival was not different in the two groups. A second study in patients with hilar obstruction gave similar results (178).

A nonrandomized study of 103 patients in whom a Wallstent was inserted for mid or distal malignant common bile duct obstruction showed a 97% success rate for stent positioning, and an 18% rate of late cholangitis after a median interval of 125 days (179). Most occlusions were again due to tumor in-growth. Occlusion of metal stents can be treated by placement of a plastic stent through the metal stent to re-establish patency (Figure 37.8) (180). Following plastic stent placement, stent obstruction rarely recurs (177–180), possibly because friction between the two stents tends to erode ingrowing tumor maintaining patency of the metal stent. A second alternative is to place a second metal stent within the first.

The advantages of metallic stents are their longer patency rates, and the decreased requirements for additional endoscopic procedures. Their disadvantages include a high initial cost, and the inability to reposition or remove these stents. Currently metal self expanding stents are the palliative treatment of choice in patients with malignant biliary obstruction who have life expectancies longer than 6 months. Plastic stents remain useful in patients with shorter life expectancies, and are the stent of choice for benign strictures.

Combined Percutaneous Endoscopic Drainage

Combined percutaneous endoscopic biliary stent placement is an alternative method for placing a large caliber stent when endoscopic placement is not feasible or has failed (181). This method involves performance of a standard percutaneous transhepatic cholangiogram followed by passage of a guidewire through the obstructed duct and into the duodenum. The guidewire is then grasped by a snare and pulled through the biopsy channel of a side viewing duodenoscope by the endoscopist. The opposite end of the guidewire is secured at the skin level in the right midaxillary line and a small caliber 7F catheter is placed over it and into the biliary tract. This catheter protects the liver from the potential cutting effect of the guidewire. A stent can then be placed in a retrograde fashion over the guidewire using conventional endoscopic techniques. Securing the wire at both ends lends additional stability and allows stent passage through tight strictures which might otherwise be impossible to negotiate. Once the stent is in place, the guidewire and external catheter can be removed. Since large caliber stents are not passed through the liver, the risks of intraductal bleeding and bile leakage are minimized. In most cases, the stent placement can be accomplished in a single session without having to dilate the liver tract in stages. This procedure is a good alternative to standard PTC with drainage when endoscopic methods fail. It requires a close working relationship between the endoscopist and the radiologist if optimal results are to be achieved.

A)

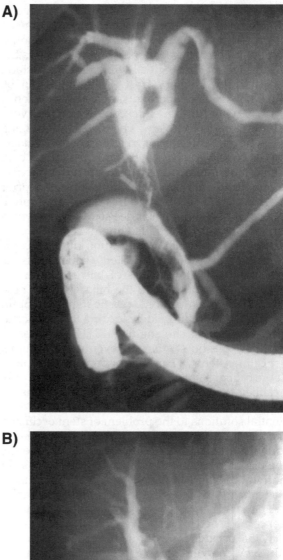

B)

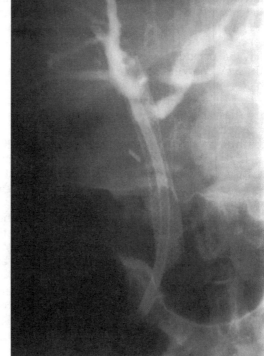

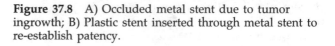

Figure 37.8 A) Occluded metal stent due to tumor ingrowth; B) Plastic stent inserted through metal stent to re-establish patency.

Intracavitary Irradiation

Intracavitary irradiation with iridium-192 wire is feasible using an endoscopic approach (182). The technique involves placement of a 7F nasobiliary drain through the malignant biliary obstruction followed by insertion of the iridium-192 wire through the nasobiliary drain and across the stricture. The iridium-192 wire is left in place until the desired dose of radiation is delivered. The nasobiliary drain containing the iridium wire is then withdrawn and replaced with a 10 or 12F stent.

Only a few non-controlled studies using iridium-192 via the endoscopic route have been published. In one study, 24 patients were studied with successful placement of iridium in 23 patients (182). The only major complication was cholangitis in 30%, and the 30 day mortality rate was 4.2%. This represents an increased risk of early cholangitis compared to stent placement alone. Survival was not significantly greater for iridium treated patients compared to historical controls treated with drainage only. Based on current information, intraluminal irradiation cannot be recommended for treatment of malignant biliary obstruction.

Ampullary Neoplasms

Carcinoma of the ampulla

Carcinoma of the ampulla of Vater is less common than pancreatic and cholangiocarcinoma, but has a much higher 5 year survival of approximately 30–40% (183, 184). Therefore every effort should be made to identify this malignancy and excise it. Since surgical excision usually requires a pancreaticoduodenectomy with its associated morbidity and mortality, the decision to proceed with surgery will depend on the stage of the tumor and the patients' comorbid conditions.

Endoscopy utilizing a side viewing duodenoscope allows optimal visualization of the ampulla of Vater. Most ampullary carcinomas will be grossly recognizable, and endoscopic biopsy will provide a tissue diagnosis. However, 20% of these malignancies are intraluminal with the papilla covered by a normal overlying mucosa (185). These cases can be accurately diagnosed with biopsy following endoscopic sphincterotomy (186). Endoscopy allows not only biopsy to establish a tissue diagnosis, but also initiation of therapy with sphincterotomy and/or stent placement to relieve obstructive jaundice.

Accurate staging of ampullary neoplasms is best accomplished with endoscopic ultrasound. Endoscopic ultrasound is the only imaging modality which can demonstrate the normal 5 layer structure of the duodenal wall. It can detect masses within the papilla as small as 8 mm in diameter (187), and invasion of the pancreatic parenchyma.

In patients with advanced lesions and in those who are poor operative candidates, palliative therapy of ampullary carcinoma is best achieved by endoscopic measures which are directed at relieving biliary obstruction. These include sphincterotomy, biliary stent placement, or a combination of the two (183, 188, 190).

Sphincterotomy relieves jaundice in most cases, 77–100% of the time (183, 190). However, if the tumor extends beyond the intramural segment of the common bile duct, stent placement will be necessary. Laser therapy with the Nd:YAG laser has also been used as an adjunct to sphincterotomy for ampullary carcinoma, however, it is not effective for complete tumor destruction and has no effect on overall survival (191). Laser therapy may be useful to treat partial duodenal obstruction secondary to primary duodenal or ampullary carcinoma (192).

Benign ampullary tumors

Adenomas of the ampulla of Vater are rare pre-malignant tumors that occur either sporadically of in association with familial polyposis. If they do not extend up the biliary or pancreatic ductal systems, they may be treated endoscopically. Lambert, et al. treated 8 patients with Nd:YAG laser therapy with successful ablation of the adenoma in 7 (88%), and recurrence in only one patient at 24 months (191).

Binmoeller et al. treated 25 patients with benign adenomas of the ampulla by endoscopic snare excision (192). Initial successful ablation was achieved in 92%. Six patients had a recurrence at a mean of 37 months, and four were again successfully treated with endoscopic methods. 16% of patients in this series eventually required surgery. The only major complication of endoscopic snare resection was pancreatitis which occurred in 12% of patients.

Both laser therapy and snare excision work well for endoscopic ablation of benign ampullary adenomas. The choice of therapy will be determined by the expertise and preference of the endoscopist.

References

1. Boyce GA. Palliation of Malignant Esophageal Obstruction *Dysphagia* 1990; **5**: 220–226.
2. Tytgat GNJ. *Endoprosthesis palliation of esophagogastric malignancy.* Practice of Therapeutic Endoscopy, edited by Tytgat and Classen. Churchill Livingston; 1994; 67–86.
3. Ell C, May A, Hahn EG. Gianturco — Z stents in palliative treatment of malignant esophageal obstruction and endotracheal fistulas. *Endoscopy* 1995; **27**: 495–500.
4. Knyrim K, Wagner NJ, Bethge N, *et al.* A controlled trial of expensible metal stent for palliation of esophageal obstruction due to inoperable cancer. *N Eng CL Med* 1993; **18**: 1302–1307.
5. Gauderer MWL, Ponsky JL, Izant RJ, Jr. Gastrostomy without laparotomy. A percutaneous endoscopic technique. *J Pediatr Surg* 1980; **15**: 872.
6. Stuart SP, Tiley EH, Boland JP. Feeding gastrostomy: a critical review of its indications and mortality rate. *South Med J* 1993; **86**(2): 169–172.
7. Ponsky JL, Aszodi A. External biliary gastric fistula: a single method for recycling bile. *Am J Gastrointest* 1985; **80**: 438.
8. Pamos MZ, Reilly H, Moran A, *et al.* Percutaneous endoscopic gastrostomy in a general hospital: prospective evaluation of indications, outcome and randomized comparison of two tube designs. *Gut* 1989; **35**(11): 1551–1556.
9. Bussone M, Lalo M, Piette F, *et al.* Percutaneous endoscopic gastrostomy: its value in assisted alimentation in malnourished elderly. Apropos of 101 consecutive cases in patients over 70 years of age. *Annales de Chirurgie* 1992; **66**(1): 59–66.
10. Raha SK, Woodhouse K. The use of percutaneous endoscopic gastrostomy (PEG) in 161 consecutive elderly patients. *Age & Aging* 1999; **23**: 162–163.

11. Finucane P, Aslan SM, Duncan D. Percutaneous endoscopic gastrostomy in elderly patients. *Postgrad Med J* 1991; **67**: 371–373.

12. Meier R, Bauerfeind P, Gyr K. Die Perkutaune Endoskopische Gastrostomy in Der Langzeiterna"hrung. *Schweiz Med Wochenschr* 1994; **124**: 655–659.

13. Taylor CM, Larson DJ, Ballard LR, *et al*. Who should receive placement of percutaneous endoscopic gastrostomy (PEG) feeding tubes? *Gastroenterology* 1991; **100**: A12.

14. Rosch T. *Endosonographic Staging of Esophageal Cancer: A review of literature results*. Gastrointestinal Endoscopy Clinics of North America. 1995; **5**(3): 537–547.

15. Catalano MF, Van Dam J, Sivak MV. Malignant Esophageal Strictures; staging accuracy of Endosonography. *Gastrointestinal Endoscopy* 1995; **41**: 535–539.

16. Roubein LD. Endoscopic Ultrasonography and the malignant esophageal stricture: implications and complications. *Gastrointestinal Endoscopy* 1995; **41**: 613–615.

17. Chak A, Canto M, Gerdes M, Lightdale CJ, Hawes RH, Weissman MJ, Kelimanis G, Tio L. Rice, TW, Boyce HW, Sivak MV. Prognosis of Esophageal Cancers Preoperatively Staged to be locally invasive (T4) by E.U.S: a multicenter retrospective cohort study. *Gastrointestinal Endoscopy* 1995; **42**: 501–506.

18. Rosch T. Endoscopic staging of gastric cancer: A review of literature results. *Gastrointestinal Endoscopy Clinics of North America* 1995; **5**(3): 549–557.

19. Hordijk ML. Restaging after radiotherapy and chemotherapy: value of Endoscopic Ultrasonography. *Gastrointestinal Endoscopy Clinics of North America* 1995; **5**(3): 601–608.

20. Fleisher D, Kessler F, Haye O. Endoscopic Nd: YAG laser therapy for carcinoma of the esophagus: a new palliative approach. *Am J Surg* 1982; **143**: 280–283.

21. Fleischer D. The Washington Symposium on Endoscopic Laser Therapy. *Gastrointest Endosc* 1985; **31**: 397–400.

22. Flesicher D, Sivak MV. Endoscopic Nd: YAG therapy as palliation for esphagogastric cancer. Parameters effecting initial outcome. *Gastroenterology* 1985; **89**: 827–831.

23. Mellow MH, Pinkas H. Endoscopic laser therapy for malignancies affecting the esophagus and the gastroesophageal junction: analysis of technical and functional efficacy. *Arch Intern Med* 1985; **145**: 1443–1446.

24. Ell CH, Reiman JF, Lux G. Denmling L. Palliative laser treatments of malignant stenosis in the upper gastrointestinal tract. *Endoscopy* 1986; **18**: (1): 21–26.

25. Mellow MH, Pinkas H. Endoscopic therapy for esophageal cancer with Nd: YAG laser: prospective evaluation of efficacy, complications and survival. *Gastrointest Endosc* 1984; **30**: 334–339.

26. Karlin PA, Fisher RS, Krevsky B. Prolonged survival and effective palliation in patients with squamous all cell carcinoma of the esophagus following E.L.T. *Cancer* 1987; **59**: 1969–1972.

27. Chatlani PT, Barr H, Krasner N. Long term survivors of Nd: YAG laser therapy for upper gastrointestinal carcinoma. *Gut* 1989; **30**: A1475.

28. Goldschmidt S, Boyce HW, Nord HJ, Brady PG. Nd: YAG laser vaporization versus peroral dilation and or prosthesis in the palliative management of obstructing squamous cell carcinoma.

29. Siegel HL, Laskin HJ, Dabezies MA, Fisher RS, Krevsky B. The effect of endoscopic laser therapy on survival in patients with squamous cell carcinoma of the esophagus — further experience, *J Clin Gastroenterol* 1991; **13**: 142–146.

30. Kohler B, Ginsbach CH, Riemann JF. Bacteremia after endoscopic laser therapy of the upper gastrointestinal tract. *Lasers Med Sci* 1988; **3**: 13–15.

31. Loizou L.A, Grigg D, Atkinson M, Robertson C, Bown SG. A prospective comparison of laser therapy and intubation in endoscopic palliation for malignant dysphagia. *Gastroenterology* 1991; **100**: 1303–1310.

32. Reed CE, Marsh WH, Carlson LS, *et al*. Palliation of advanced esophageal cancer: a (laser) light in the end of the tunnel. *Arch Thorac Surg* 1991; **51**: 522–556.

33. Sander R, Hagenmuller F, Sander C, Riess G, Classen M. Laser versus laser plus afterloading with iridium-192 in the palliative treatment of malignant stenosis of the esophagus: a prospective randomized and controlled study. *Gastrointest Endosc* 1991; **37** 433–445.

34. Bown SG. Palliation of malignant dysphagia: surgery, radiotherapy, laser, intubation alone or in combination? *Gut* 1991; **32**: 841–844.

35. Pinkas H, Cash DK, Neilan BA, Prabhu HR, Shah DE. Endoscopic Nd: YAG laser therapy followed by chemotherapy and radiation therapy for squamous cell carcinoma of the esophagus-case report of complete remission. *Gastrointest Endosc* 1985; **31**(2): 134.

36. Mellow MH. Nd: YAG laser therapy prior to radiation and chemotherapy for the primary "curative" treatment of squamous-cell carcinoma of the esophagus. *Lasers Med Sci* 1988; **80**: 392.

37. Lambert R. Endoscopic therapy of esophago-gastric tumors. *Endoscopy* 1992; **24**: 24–33.

38. Oguro Y. Laser vs heater probe and microwave treatments in endoscopic treatment for GI cancer. *Endoscopy* 1980; **20**: 5.

39. Swain CP. Laser, P.D.T. BICAP and microwaves in U.G.I. malignancy. *Endoscopy* 1988; **20**: 7.

40. Peterlini A, *et al*. An alternative to the laser in the palliative treatment of GI tract malignancy. *Endoscopy* 1987; **19**: 255.

41. Bulighin G, *et al*. Palliative treatments of upper digestive tract malignancies through sclerotherapy. *Endoscopy* 1980; **20**: 55.

42. Johnston JH, Quint R, Petruzzi C, Namihira Y. Development and testing of a large BICAP probe for palliative treatment of obstructing esophageal and rectal malignancy, abstracted. *Gastrointest Endosc* 1985; **31**: 156.

43. Johnston JH, Fleischer D, Petrini J, Nord HJ. Palliative bipolar electrocoagulation therapy for obstructing esophageal cancer. *Gastrointest Endosc* 1987; **33**: 349–353.

44. Jensen DM, Machiacado GA, Randall GM. Palliation of obstructing esophageal cancer with BICAP tumor probe of YAG laser, abstracted, *Gastrointest Endosc* 1987; **33**: 173.

45. Fleischer D, Ranard R, Kamath R, Bitterman P, Benjamin S. Stricture formation following BICAP tumor probe therapy for esophageal cancer. Clinical observations and experimental studies, abstracted. *Gastrointest Endosc* 1987; **33**: 183.

46. Payne-James II, *et al*. Use of ethanol-induced tumor necrosis to palliate dysphagia patients with esophogastric cancer. *Gastrointes Endosc* 1990; **36**: 43.

47. Wright RA, *et al*. A pilot study of endoscopic injection chemosclerotherapy of esophageal carcinoma. *Gastrointest Endosc* 1990; **36**: 47.

48. Bugelski PJ, Porter CW, Dougherty TJ. Autoradiographic distribution in malignant and normal tissue. *Cancer Res* 1979; **39**: 146–151.

49. Weishaupt KP, Gomer CJ, Dougherty TJ. Identification of singlet oxygen as the cytotoxic agent in the photoactivation of a murine tumor. *Cancer Res* 1976; **36**: 2326–2329.

50. Star WM, Marihnissen HPA, Evaunden A. Destruction of rat mammary tumor and normal tissue microcirculation by photoradiation observed vivo in sandwich observation chambers. *Cancer Res* 1987; **46**: 795–800.

51. Barr H, Tralau CJ, Boulous PB. The contrasting mechanism of colonic collagen damage between photodynamic therapy and thermal injury. *Photochem Photobiol* 1987; **46**: 795–800.

52. Lipson RL, Blades EJ, Olsen AM. Hematoporphyrin-derivative: a new aid for endoscopic detection of malignant disease. *Chest* 1964; **46**: 676–679.

53. Lipson RL, Baldes EJ, Olsen AM. Hematoporphyrin-derivative as new aid for the endoscopic detection of malignant disease. *Chest* 1964; **46**: 676–679.

54. Dougherty TJ. PDT: present and future. *Lasers Med Sci* 1988; **3**: 8.

55. Likier HM, Levine JG, Lightdale CJ. Photodynamic therapy for completely obstructing esophageal carcinoma. *Gastrointest Endosc* 1991; **37**(1): 75–78.

56. Heier SK, Rothnan K, Rosenthal WS, Heier LM. Randomized trial of photodynamic therapy vs Nd: YAG laser therapy for obstructing esophageal tumors: interim results. *Gastrointest Endosc* 1991; **37**(2): 278.

57. Lightdale CJ, Heier SK, Marcon NE. Photodynamic therapy with potrfimer sodium versus thermal ablation therapy with Nd: YAG laser for palliation of esophageal cancer: a multicenter randomized trial. *Gastrointestinal Endoscopy* 1995; **42**: 507–512.

58. Wooten RS, Smith KC, Ahlquist DA, Muller SA, Balm BK. Prospective study of cutaneous phototoxicity after systematic HpD. *Lasers Surg Med* 1988; **8**: 294–300.

59. Dougherty TJH, Cooper MT, Mang TS. Cutaneous phototoxicity occurrences in patients receiving Photofrin. *Lasers Surg Med* 1990; **10**: 485–488.

60. Lowdell CP, Gilso D, Ash DV, Holroyd JA, Vernon D, Brown SB. An attempt to reduce skin photosensitivity in clinical photodynamic therapy using oral activated charcoal. *Lasers Med Sci* 1992; **7**: 351–356.

61. McCaughan JS, Nims TA, Guy JT, Hicks WJ, Williams TE, Laufman LR. Photodynamic therapy for esophageal tumors. *Arch Surg* 1989; **124**: 74–80.

62. Thomas RJS, Abbott M, Bhothal PS. High dose photoradiation of esophageal cancer. *Ann Surg* 1987; **206**: 193–199.

63. Jin ML, Yang BQ, Zhang W, Ren P. Photodynamic therapy for the treatment of advanced gastrointestinal tumors. *Lasers Med Sci* 1989; **4**: 183–186.

64. Krasner H, Chatlani PT, Barr H. Photodynamic therapy of tumors in gastroenterology — a review. *Lasers Med Sci* 1990; **5**: 233–239.

65. Spinelli P, Dal Fonte M. PDT — state of the art. In *Laser optoelectronics in medicine 1987*, edited by W Waidelich. New York: Springer-Verlag, 609–618, 1988.

66. Sabben G, Souquet JC, Lambert R. PDT in superficial types of esophageal cancer at endoscopy. *Lasers Med Sci* 1988; **11**.

67. Patrice T, Foultier MT, Yactao S, Adam F, Galmiche JP, Douet MC, LeBodic, L. Endoscopic photodynamic therapy with hematoporphyrin derivative for primary treatment of gastrointestinal neoplasms inoperable patients. *Dig Dis Sci* 1990; **35**: (5): (233–239).

68. Karanov S, Shopova M, Getov H. Photodynamic therapy in gastrointestinal cancer. *Lasers Surg Med* 1991; **11**: 395–398.

69. Overholt BF. Photodynamic therapy and thermal treatment of esophageal cancer. *Gastrointest Endosc Clin North Am* 1992; **2**(3): 433–455.

70. Monnier PH, Savary M, Fontolliet CH, Wagineres G, Chatelain A, Cornaz P, Depeursinge CH, Van Den Bergh H. Photodetection and photodynamic therapy in "early" squamous cell carcinoma of the pharynx. esophagus and tracheo-bronchial tree. *Lasers Med Sci* 1990; **5**: 149–169.

71. Panjepour M, Overholt BF, De Novo RC, Sneed RE, Peterson MG. Centering balloon to improve esophageal photodynamic therapy. *Lasers Surg Med* 1992; **12**: 631–638.

72. Fleischer D, Cattau E Jr, Dinofsky E, Newsome J, Lack E, Andreiuk A. Benjamin S. Development of a laser balloon for the treatment of gastrointestinal obstruction. *Endoscopy* 1989; **21**: 81–85.

73. Barr H. PDT experimental studies. In *Lasers in gastroenterology*, edited by N Krasner. New York: Wiley-Liss, 233–250, 1991.

74. Loh CS, Bedwell J, MacRobert AJ, Krasner H, Phillips D, Bown SG. Photodynamic therapy of normal rat stomach: a comparative study between di-sulfonated aluminum phtalocyanine and 5-aminolevulinic acid. *Br J Cancer* 1992; **66**: 452–462.

75. Divaris XG, Kennedy Pottier RH. Phototoxic damage to sebaceous glands and hair follicles of mice after systemic administration of 5-aminolevulinic acid correlates with localized protoporphyrin IX fluorescence. *Am J Pathol* 1990: **136**: 891–897.

76. Regula J, MacRobert AJ, Gorcheim A, Buonccorsi GA, Thorpe SM, Spencer GM, Hartfield ARW Bown SG. Photosensitization and photodynamic therapy of esophageal, duodenal and colorectal tumors using 5 amino laevulinic acid induced protoporphyrin IX — pilot study. *Gut* 1995; **36**: 67–75.

77. Gossner L, Sroka R, Hahn EG, Ell C. Photodynamic therapy: successful destruction of gastrointestinal cancer after oral administration of amino levulinic acid. *Gastrointestinal Endoscopy* 1995; **41**: 55–57.

78. Peltomaki P. Aaltonen LA, Listonen P, *et al*. Genetic mapping of a locus predisposing to human colorectal cancer. *Science* 1993; 260–810.

79. Fearon ER, Vogelstein B. A genetic model of colorectal tumorigenesis. *Cell* 1990; **61**: 759.

80. Winawer SJ, Zauber AG, HO MN, O'Brien MJ, Gottlieb LS. Sternberg SS, *et al*. Prevention of colorectal cancer by colonoscopic polypectomy. *N Engl J. Med* 1993; **329**: 1977–81.

81. Morson BC. Evolution of cancer of the colon and rectum. *Cancer* 1974; **34**: 845–849.

82. O'Brien NJ, Winawer SJ, Zauber AG, *et al*. The National Polyp Study: patient and polyp characteristics associated with high grade dysplasia in colorectal adenomas. *Gastroenterology* 1990; **98**: 371–379.

83. Wayne JD. *Polypectomy Techniques in Colonoscopy: Principles and Techniques*, edited by JB Raskin and HJ Nord. Igaku-Shoin, 1995.

84. Bond JH. Polyp Guideline: diagnosis, treatment and surveillance for patients with nonfamilial colorectal polyps. *Ann Intern Med* 1993; **119**: 836–843.

85. Winawer SJ, St. John DJ, Bond JH, *et al*. Prevention of colorectal cancer: guidelines based on new data. *WHO Bulletin OMS* 1995; **Vol 73**: 7–10.

86. DePalma GD. Endoscopic treatment of sessile rectal adenoma: comparison of Nd: YAG laser therapy and injection-assisted piecemeal polypectomy. *Gastrointestinal Endosc.* 1995; **41**: 553–556.

87. Coverlizza S, Rise M, Ferrari A, *et al*. Colorectal cancers containing invasive carcinoma: pathologic assessment of lymph node, metastatic potential. *Cancer* 1989; **64**: 1937–1941.

88. Russell I, Chu D, Russell M, *et al*. When polypectomy is sufficient treatment for colorectal cancer in a polyp? *Am J Surg* 1990; **160**: 665.

89. Cranley J. Proper management of the patient with malignant colorectal polyps. *Gastrointest Endosc Clin North Am* 1993; **3**(4): 661.

90. Greenbury A, Saik R, Coyle J, *et al*. Mortality and gastrointestinal surgery in the elderly. *Arch Surg* 1981; **116**: 788.

91. Karita M, Tada M, Okita K, Kodama T. Endoscopic therapy for early colon cancer. The strip biopsy resection technique. *Gastrointest Endos* 1991; **37**: 128.

92. Brunetaud JM, Mosquet L, Houcke M, *et al*. Villous adenoma of the rectum: results of endoscopic treatment with argon and Nd: YAG lasers. *Gastroenterology* 1985; **89**: 832.

93. Brunetaud JM, Maunoury V, Cochelard D, *et al*. Endoscopic laser treatment for rectosigmoid villous adenoma: factors affecting the results. *Gastroenterology* 1989; **97**: 272.

94. Spinelli P, Dal Fante M, Mancini A. Current role of laser and photodynamic therapy in gastrointestinal tumors and analysis of a 10 year experience. *Seminars in Surg Onc* 1992; **8**(4): 204–213.

95. Mathus — Vliegen EM, Tytgat GN. The potential and limitations of laser photoablation of colorectal adenomas. *Gastrointest Endosc* 1991 **37**(1): 9–17.

96. Low D, Kozarek R. Snare cautery debridement prior to Nd: YAG photoablation improves treatment efficacy of broad-based adenomas of the colorectum. *Gastrointest Endosc* 1989; **35**; 288.

97. Aubert A, Meduri B, Fritsch J, *et al*. Endoscopic treatment of snare electrocoagulation prior to Nd: YAG laser photocoagulation in 85 voluminous colorectal villous adenomas. *Disease of the Colon & Rectum* 1991; **34**(5): 372–377.

98. Mathus — Vliegen EM. Laser ablation of early colorectal malignancy. *Endoscopy* 1993; **25**(7): 462–468.

99. Escourrou J, Delvaux T, De Bellison, *et al*. Laser for curative treatment of rectal cancer: indications and follow up. *Gastrointest Endosc* 1988; **34**: 195.

100. Brunetaud J, Maunoury V, Cochelard, *et al*. Laser palliation for rectosigmoid cancers. *Int J Colorect Dis* 1989; **4**: 6.

101. Dittrich K, Armbruster C, Hoffer, *et al*. Nd: YAG laser treatment of colorectal malignancies: an experience of $4\frac{1}{2}$ years. *Lasers in Surgery & Medicine* 1992; **12**(2): 199–203.

102. Cho E, Nakajima M, Yasuda K, Ashikara T, Kawai K. Endoscopic ultrasonography of colorectal cancer invasion. *Gastrointest Endosc* 1993; **39**: 54.

103. Hulsmans FJ, Mathus-Vliegen LM, Bosma S, Bosma A, Tygat GN. Colorectal adenomas: inflammatory changes that stimulate malignancy after laser coagulation; evaluation with tranrectal US. *Radiology* 1993; **187**: 367–371.

104. Eckhauser ML. Laser therapy of gastrointestinal tumors. *World J Surg* 1992; **16**(6): 1056–1059.

105. Eckhauser ML, Mansour EG. Endoscopic laser therapy for obstructing and / or bleeding colorectal carcinoma. *Amer Surgeon* 1992; **58**: 358–363.

106. Mlkvy P, Vrablik V, Kralik G, Laborecky M. Endoscopic Nd: YAG laser treatment of rectal sigmoidal cancer. *Neoplasma* 1994; **44**: 285–289.

107. Mesko TW, Petrelli NJ, Rodriguez-Bigas M, Nava H. Endoscopic laser treatment for palliation of colorectal carcinoma. *Surg Oncol* 1993; **2**: 25–30.

108. Escudero — Fabre A, Sack J. Endoscopic laser therapy for neoplastic lesion of the colorectum. *Amer J Surg* 1992; **163**: 260–262.

109. Tranberg KG. Moller PH. Palliation of colorectal carcinoma with the Nd: YAG laser. *Europ J Surg* 1991; **157**: 57–60.

110. Schulze S. Lyng KM. Palliation of rectosigmoid neoplasms with Nd: YAG laser treatment. *Diseases Colon & Rectum* 1994; **37**: 882–889.

111. Faintuch JS. Better palliation of colorectal carcinoma with laser therapy. *Oncology* 1988; **2**: 33–38.

112. Mandova N, Petrelli N, Herrera L, Nava H. Laser palliation for colorectal carcinoma. *Am J Surg* 1991; **162**: 212–219.

113. Van Cutsem E, Boonen A, Geboes H, *et al*. Risk factors which determine the long term outcome of Nd: YAG laser palliation of colorectal carcinoma. *Int J Colorectal Dis* 1989; **4**: 9–11.

114. Bright N, Hale P, Maso R. Poor palliation of colorectal malignancy with the Nd: YAG laser. *Brit J Surg* 1992; **79**: 308–309.

115. Daneker GW, Jr., Carlson GW, Hohn DC, *et al*. Endoscopic laser recanalization is effective for prevention and treatment of obstruction in sigmoid and rectal cancer. *Arch of Surg* 1991; **126**: 1348–52.

116. Sargeant IR, Tobias JS, Blackman G, *et al*. Radiation enhancement of laser palliation of advanced and rectosigmoid cancer: a pilot study. *Gut* 1993; **34**: 958–960.

117. Said S, Huber P, Pichlmaier H. Technique and clinical results of endorectal surgery. *Surgery* 1993; **113**: 65–69.

118. Grahm R, Garnsey L, Jessup J. Local excision of rectal carcinoma. *Am J. Surg* 1990; **160**: 306.

119. Mellow MH. Endoscopic laser therapy as an alternative to palliative surgery for adenocarcinoma of the rectum. Comparison of costs and complications. *Gastrointest Endosc* 1989; **36**: 283–287.

120. Faintuch JS. Endoscopic therapy of the totally obstructed colon. *Gastrointest Endosc* 1988; **34**(2): 196–198.

121. Harlow SP, Rodriguez-Bigas M, Mang T, Petrelli NJ. Intraoperative PDT as an adjunct to surgery for recurrent rectal cancer. *Ann Surg Onc* 1992(12): 228–232.

122. Loh CS, Mac Robert AJ, Bedwell J, *et al*. Oral versus intravenous administration of 5-amino laevulinic acid for photodynamic therapy. *Brit J Cancer* 1993; **68**(1): 41–51.

123. Foultier MT, Vonarx-Coinsman V, de Brito LX, *et al*. DNA and cell kinetics flow cytometry analysis of 33 small gastrointestinal cancers treated by PDT. *Cancer* 1994; **73**(6): 1595–607.

124. Loh CS, Bliss P, Bown SG, Krasner N. Photodynamic therapy for villous adenomas of the colon and rectum. *Endoscopy* 1994; **26**(2): 243–246.

125. Krasner N. Laser therapy in the management of benign and malignant tumours in the colon and rectum. *Internat J Colorectal Disease* 1989; **4**(1): 2–5.

126. Spinelli P. PDT state of the art. *Proceedings of the VIIth International Laser in Medicine Congress*. Munich, 1987.

127. Barr H, Krasner N, Boulos PB, Chatlani P, Bown SG. Photodynamic therapy of colorectal cancer: a quantative pilot study. *Brit J Surg* 1990; **77**(1): 93–96.

128. Kashtan H, Papa MZ, Wilson BC, Deutch AA, Stern HS. Use of photodynamic therapy in the palliation of massive advanced rectal cancer. Phase I/II study. *Dis Colon Rect* 1991; **34**(7): 600–604.

129. Patrice T, Foultier Mt, Yactao S, Douet MC, Maloisel F, LeBodic L. Endoscopic PDT with hematoporphyrin derivative in gastroenterology. *Photochem & Photobiol* 1990; **6**(1,2): 157–165.

130. Hamblin MR, Newman EL. Photosensitizer targeting in photodynamic therapy. Conjugates of hematoporphyrin with albumin and transferrin. *Photochem & Photobiol* 1994; **26**(1): 45–46.

131. Lipschutz GS. Evaluation of four new carbocyanine dyes for photodynamic therapy with lasers. *Laryngoscope* 1994; **104**: 996–1002.

132. Harlow SP, Rodriguez-Bigas T, Mang T, Petrelli NJ. Intraoperative photodynamic therapy as adjunct to surgery for recurrent rectal cancer. *Ann Surg Onc*. 1995; **2**(3): 228–232.

133. Lantz JM, Meyer C, Saussine C, *et al*. Experimental photodynamic therapy with a copper metal vapor laser in colorectal cancer. *Inter J Cancer* 1992; **52**(3): 491–498.

134. Kimose HH, Fischer L, Spjelenaes N, *et al*. Late radiation injury of the colon and rectum: Surgical management and outcome. *Dis Colon Rectum* 1989; **32**: 689.

135. Dietel M, To TB. Major intestinal complication of radiotherapy management and nutrition. *Arch Surg* 1987; **122**: 1421.

136. Decosse JJ, Rhodes RS, Wentz, *et al*. The natural history and management of radiation injury of the gastrointestinal tract. *Ann Surg* 1969; **170**: 369.

137. Perez CA, Breaux S, Bedwineic JM, *et al*. Radiation therapy alone in the treatment of carcinoma of the uterine cervix. *Cancer* 1984; **54**: 235.

138. Earnest DL. Radiation proctitis. *Practical Gastroenterol* 1991; **15**(1): 5.

139. Danielsson A, Nhylin H, Persson, *et al*. Chronic diarrhea after radiotherapy for gynecological cancer: occurrence and cytology. *Gut* 1991; **33**: 1180.

140. Gilinsky NH, Burns DG, Barbezat GO, *et al*. The natural history of radiation induced proctosigmoiditis: an analysis of 88 patients. *Q J Med* 1983; **205**: 240.

141. Kochhar R, Patel F, Dhar A, *et al*. Radiation induced proctosigmoiditis: randomized trial of oral sulfasalazine and rectal steroids versus rectal sucralfate. *Dig Dis Sci* 1991; **36**: 103.

142. Charreau J, Bouachour G, Perso B, *et al*. Severe hemorrhagic radiation proctitis advancing to gradual cessation with hyperbaric oxygen. *Dig Dis Sci* 1991; **36**(3): 373–375.

143. Mathai V, Seow-Choen F. Endoluminal formalin therapy for hemorrhagic radiation proctitis. *Brit J Surg* 1995; **8292**): 190.

144. Alexander TJ, Dwyer RM. Endoscopic Nd: YAG laser treatment of severe radiation injury of the lower GI tract: long term follow up. *Gastrointest Endosc* 1988; **34**(5)407–411.

145. O'Connor JJ. Argon laser treatment of radiation proctitis. *Arch Surg* 1989; **124**(6): 749.

146. Viggiano TR, Zieghelboim J, Ahlquist DA, *et al*. Endoscopic Nd: YAG laser coagulation of bleeding from radiation proctopathy. *Gastrointest Endsoc* 1993; **39**: 513.

147. Taylor JG, Di Sario JA, Buchi KN. Argon laser therapy for hemorrhagic radiation proctitis; long term results. *Gastrointest Endoscopy* 1993; **39**(5): 641–644.

148. Livingston EH, Welton ML. Reber HA. Surgical treatment of pancreatic cancer. The United States experience. *Int J Pancreatology* 1991; **9**: 153–157.

149. Nagorney DM, Donahue JH, Farell MB, *et al*. Outcomes after curative resection of cholangiocarcinoma. *Arch Surg* 1993; **9**: 871–879.

150. Tsuchiya a R, Noda T, Harada N, *et al*. Collective review of small carcinomas of the pancreas. *Ann Surg* 1986; **203**: 77–81.

151. Freeny PC. Radiology of the pancreas: two decades of progress in imaging and intervention. *AJR* 1988; **150**: 975–981.

152. Warshaw AL, Zhuo-Yun G, Wittenberg J, *et al*. Preoperative staging and assessment of resectability of pancreatic cancer. *Arch Surg* 1990; **125**: 230–233.

153. Shimi S, Banting S, Cushchieri A. Laparoscopy in the management of pancreatic cancer: Endoscopic cholecystojejunostomy for advanced disease. *Br J Surg* 1992; **79**: 317–319.

154. Tio TL, Tygat GNJ. Ampullopancreatic carcinoma: Preoperative TNM classification with endosonography. *Radiology* 1990; **775**: 455–461.

155. Vilmann P, Jacobsen GK, Henriksen FW, *et al*. Endoscopic ultrasonography with guided fine needle aspiration biopsy in pancreatic disease. *Gastrointest Endosc* 1992; **38**: 172–173.

156. Pretre R, Huber O, Robert J, *et al*. Results of surgical palliation for cancer of the head of the pancreas. *Br J Surg* 1992; **79**: 795–798.

157. Shepherd HA, Royle G, Ross APR, *et al*. Endoscopic biliary endoprosthesis in the palliation of malignant obstruction of the distal common bile duct: a randomized trial. *Br J Surg* 1988; **75**: 1166–1168.

158. Nakayama T, Idela A, Okuda K. Percutaneous transhepatic drainage of the biliary tract: Techniques and results in 104 cases. *Gastroenterology* 1978; **73**: 554–559.

159. Pereiras RV, Rheingold OJ, Hutson D, *et al.* Relief of malignant obstructive jaundice by percutaneous insertion of a permanent prosthesis in the biliary tree. *Ann Intern Med* 1978; **89**: 589–593.

160. Coons HG. Self expanding stainless steal biliary stents. *Radiology* 1989; **170**: 979–983.

161. Gillams A, Dick R, Dooley JS, *et al.* Self expandable stainless steal braided endoprosthesis for biliary strictures. *Radiology* 1990; **174**: 137–140.

162. Speer AG, Cotton PB, Russell RC, *et al.* Randomized trial of endoscopic versus percutaneous stent insertion in malignant obstructive jaundice. *Lancet* 1987; **2**: 57–62.

163. Sohendra N, Reijinders-Frederik V. Palliative bile duct drainage. A new endoscopic method of introducing a transpapillary drain. *Endoscopy* 1980; **12**: 8–11.

164. Huibregtse K, Katon RM, Coene PP, Tygat GNJ. Endoscopic palliative treatment in pancreatic cancer. *Gastrointest Endosc* 1986; **32**: 334–338.

165. Bismuth H, Corlette MB. Intrahepatic cholangioenteric anastomosis in carcinoma of the hilus of the liver. *Surg Gynecol Obstet* 1975; **140**: 170–178.

166. Polydorou AA, Chisholm EM, Romanos AA, *et al.* A comparison of right versus left hepatic duct endoprosthesis insertion in malignant hilar biliary obstruction. *Endoscopy* 1989; **21**: 266–271.

167. Ducreux M, Liquory CI, Lefebvre JF, *et al.* Management of malignant hilar biliary obstruction by endoscopy. Results and prognostic factors. *Dig Dis Sci* 1992; **37**: 778–783.

168. Motte S, Deviere J, Dumonceau JM, *et al.* Risk factors for septicemia following endoscopic biliary stenting. *Gastroenterology* 1991; **101**: 1374–1381.

169. Leung JWC, Ling TKW, Kung JLS, *et al.* The role of bacteria in the blockage of biliary stents. *Gastrointest Endosc* 1988; **34**: 19–22.

170. Speer AG, Cotton PB, Mac Rae KD. Endoscopic management of malignant biliary obstruction: Stents of 10 French gauge are preferable to stents of 8 French gauge. *Gastrointest Endosc* 1988; **34**: 412–417.

171. McAllister EW, Carey LC, Brady PG, *et al.* A new ultra smooth polymer that reduces bacterial biofilm deposition and clogging of biliary stents. *Gastrointest Endosc* 1993; **39**: 422–425.

172. Dolan R., Pinkas H, Brady PG, Acute cholecystitis after palliative stenting for malignant obstruction of the biliary tree. *Gastrointest Endosc* 1993; **39**: 447–449.

173. Matsuda Y, Katsuhide S, Akamatsu T. Factors affecting the patency of stents in malignant biliary obstructive disease. *Am J Gastroenterol* 1991; **86**: 843–849.

174. ASGE Technology Assessment Committee. *Status evaluation: Biliary stents.* ASGE. Boston, Ma, 1991.

175. Davids PHP, Groen AK, Rauws EA, *et al.* Randomized trial of self-expanding metal stents versus polyethylene stents for distal malignant biliary obstruction. *Lancet* 1992; **340**: 1488–1492.

176. Wagner HJ, Knyrim K, Vakil N, Klose KJ, *et al.* Plastic endoprothesis versus metal stents in the palliative treatment of malignant hilar biliary obstruction. A prospective and randomized trial. *Endoscopy* 1993; **25**: 213–218.

177. Huibregtse K, Carr-Locke DL, Cremer M, *et al.* Biliary stent occlusion-a problem solved with self expanding metal stents? European Wallstent Study Group. *Endoscopy* 1992; **24**: 391–394.

178. Mixon T, Goldschmids S, Brady PG, Boulay J. Endoscopic management of expandable metal biliary stent occlusion. *Gastrointest Endosc* 1993; **39**: 82–84.

179. Tsang TK, Crampton AR, Berstein JR, *et al.* Percutaneous-endoscopic biliary stent placement. A preliminary report. *Ann Intern Med* 1987; **106**: 389–392.

180. Levitt MD, Laurence BH, Cameron F, Klemp PFB. Transpapillary iridium-192 wire in the treatment of malignant bile duct obstruction. *Gut* 1988; **29**: 149–152.

181. Neoptolemos JP, Talbot IC, Carr-Locke DL, *et al.* Treatment and outcome in 52 consecutive cases of ampullary carcinoma. *Br J Surg* 1987; **74**: 957–961.

182. Michelassi F, Erroi F, Dawson PJ, *et al.* Experience with 647 consecutive tumors of the duodenum, ampulla, head of the pancreas, and distal common bile duct. *Ann Surg* 1989; **210**: 544–556.

183. Yamaguchi K, Enjoji M. Carcinoma of the ampulla of Vater. A clinicopathologic study and pathologic staging of 104 cases of carcinoma and 5 cases of adenoma. *Cancer* 1987; **59**: 506–515.

184. Nakao NL, Siegel JH, Stenger RJ, *et al.* Tumors of the ampulla of Vater: early diagnosis by intraampullary biopsy during endoscopic cannulation. *Gastroenterology* 1982; **83**: 459–464.

185. Yasuda K, Mukail E, Cho M, *et al.* The use of endoscopic ultrasound in diagnosis and staging of carcinoma of the papilla of Vater. *Endoscopy* 1988; **20**: 218–222.

186. Safrany L. Palliative endoscopic therapy of ampullary carcinoma. *Gastrointest Endosc* 1980; **26**: 77: (abstract).

187. Bickerstaff KI, Berry AR, Chapman RW, *et al.* Endoscopic sphincterotomy for palliation of ampullary carcinoma. *Br J Surg* 1990; **77**: 160–162.

188. Lambert R, Ponchon T, Chavaillon A, *et al.* Laser treatment of tumors of the papilla of Vater. *Endoscopy* 1988; **20**: 227–231.

189. Binmoeller KF, Boaventura S, Ramsperger K, Soehendra N. Endoscopic snare excision of benign adenomas of the papilla of Vater. *Gastrointest Endosc* 1993; **39**: 127–131.

38. Polypharmacy in the Older Patient

Mary E. Corcoran

Introduction

In the past, when an apothecary compounded medications, polypharmacy referred to the mixing of many drugs in one prescription (1, 2). Today, polypharmacy is predominantly defined as the concurrent use of several different medications, including more than one medication from the same drug classification. There are situations in which multiple drug regimens are justified. For example, congestive heart failure and hypertension are situations which frequently affect the older adult (>65 years of age), and commonly involve a multitude of medications. However, there are many instances where excessive and unnecessary medications are used.

The senior adult population comprises approximately 12% of the total population (3). The number of senior adults is projected to reach 39.3 million by the year 2010 (4). Approximately 30% of all prescription medications are utilized by the senior adult, with an unknown percentage of nonprescription medications taken (3). As the number of senior adults increases, and researchers discover and test new medications to prevent and treat medical problems, polypharmacy will continue to flourish. A risk is involved with the administration of any medication and that risk may be heightened when the patient is a senior adult. The usefulness of a drug, its side effects and any potential interactions need to be clearly defined before addition into a medication regimen.

In 1984, Simonson suggested that *polymedicine* was a more appropriate term than *polypharmacy* for the excessive and unnecessary use of medications. Seven features are noted:

- use of medications that have no apparent indication
- use of duplicate medications
- concurrent use of interacting medication
- use of contraindicated medication
- use of inappropriate dosage
- use of drug therapy to treat adverse reactions
- improvement following discontinuation of medications (5)

The Healthy People 2000 conference identified polypharmacy by older people with chronic health problems as the principal safety issue in the coming years (4).

Table 38.1 Development of polypharmacy.

number of chronic illnesses increases with age

multiple medications

a "pill for every ill"

advertisement industry

non-prescription drug availability

self-treatment

hoarding of old medications

cost of prescription products

multiple prescribers

multiple sources for medication

lack of knowledge about own medications and medical condition

Development of Polypharmacy

Four out of five elderly patients have at least one chronic illness and experience a vast array of symptoms (6). The likelihood of an elder adult experiencing a chronic illness increases rapidly with age. Elderly (>65 years old) patients are prescribed twice as many medications as are younger patients (7). The trend for multiple medications continues through 80 years of age (8). There seems to be sex specificity as the mean number of medications taken by an older woman is higher than that taken by an elder man (9).

Polypharmacy may also be attributed to the fact that senior adults seek medical advice more often than young adults. The senior adult's perception is that medication is the answer to alleviating symptoms and/or disease states. Nolan and O'Malley noticed that 35% of office visits by those more than 85 years of age resulted in a prescription of three or more medications (8). The senior adult is often targeted by the mass media in the promotion of new medications and those medications which are given over-the-counter status.

The phenomenon of treating with 'natural products' advocated and sold by health food stores and the advertisement of such products may unintentionally harm the senior adult. These products which are advertised as 'natural,' can often interact with prescribed medications and exacerbate existing health conditions.

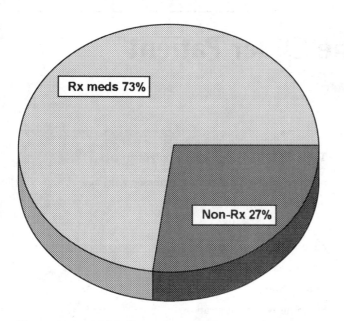

Figure 38.1 4.4 Medications per patient.

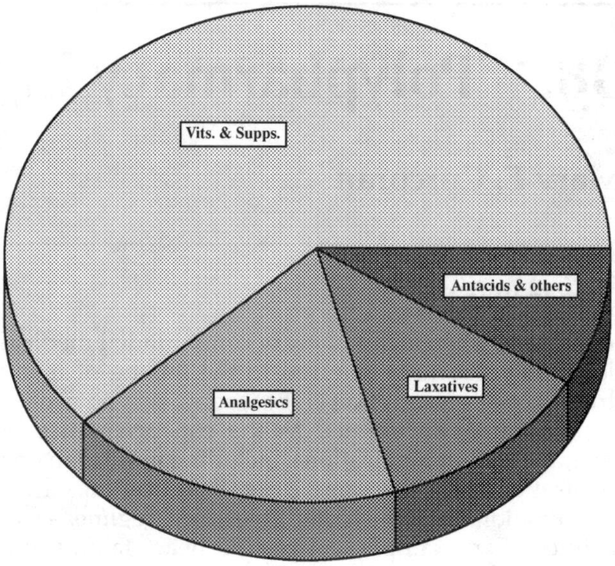

Figure 38.2 Non-prescription medications.

For example, iron products inhibit the absorption of tetracyclines, quinolones, and anti-hypertensive agents. When iron is given with thyroxine replacement therapy, it increases the serum concentration of thyrotropin (thyroid-stimulating hormone, or TSH) and thereby increases the signs and symptoms of hypothyroidism (10). Calcium products inactivate tetracycline, and should not be given with antibiotics. Calcium should be used cautiously in those seniors receiving cardiac glycosides due to the interaction between these two drug classifications. Arrhythmias may occur if these agents are given together. The term 'natural product' may tend to imply 'safe product' to the senior adult when in fact it may not be safe, depending on the overall (11) condition of the elder individual.

The danger in the use of 'natural' products by the senior adult lies in the lack of information disclosed to the health professional. When medical histories are taken, side-effects, interactions, and exacerbations of already apparent disease processes may be attributed to other causes.

The senior adult may or may not perceive the use of non-prescription products as medication and take these products without knowledge of the possibility of interactions with prescribed medications. With the volume of medications formerly obtained via prescription being given non-prescription status, the potential for polypharmacy increases. Home remedies, nutritional supplements, vitamins and alcohol have the potential for interactions; not only with prescribed medications, but also each other (12). At least one-half of the most commonly prescribed medications for the elderly have the potential to interact with alcohol (13). Forty-two percent of the 79 initial patients interviewed by the Senior Adult Oncology Program at Moffitt Cancer Center and Research Center in Tampa, Fla., were tak-

ing non-prescription items, but did not report these products as medication on their three-day medication history. An average of 4.4 medications per patient was reported; 3.2 were via prescription, and 1.2 were non-prescription items taken on a daily basis. Of the daily non-prescription items, 62% were classified as vitamins and nutritional supplements, 18% analgesics, 12% laxatives and 8% antacids and other.

Cough and cold remedies may also cause problems for seniors with high blood pressure, diabetes, and/or coronary artery disease. The recent approval of cimetidine as a non-prescription item should warrant an element of caution to the senior adult. Cimetidine reduces the hepatic metabolism of some prescription items: warfarin, phenytoin, propranolol, theophylline, terfenadine, some tri-cyclic antidepressants, and some benzodiazepines. By reducing hepatic metabolism, cimetidine decreases elimination and increases blood concentrations of the above mentioned medication. Clinically important effects that are considered to be adverse events occur. For example, the concomitant administration of cimetidine with phenytoin and theophylline leads to increased side-effects from these medications (14) that may lead to decreased dosages. Once the cimetidine is discontinued or if it is taken on a irregular basis, subtherapeutic levels may result.

The hoarding of old medications poses a potential for polypharmacy with seniors (15). 'Saving medication for later use' seems to be a common explanation given by individuals questioned as to why they did not take all their medication as prescribed (16). The fixed income of many senior adults is an issue which cannot be ignored and may potentiate an elder adults "need" to hoard medications. These situations are also compounded by the sharing of medications among friends and family members. Unfortunately, the doctor's visit may be the result of the inability of the senior adult to treat symptoms himself by using 'hoarded' medication or the medications of family members.

With the increase in number of chronic illnesses reported with advancing age, the number of physicians seen by the senior adult may increase (17). This may lead to many physicians prescribing a multitude of medications in order to achieve the same therapeutic endpoint. If these physicians do not have access to the primary medical record, therapy may be initiated without the full scope of a patient's medication history. With each additional physician seen by the senior adult, the probability of duplicate medication and other polypharmacy issues increases exponentially The lack of a "primary care" physician with the ability to orchestrate all physicians seen by one patient increases the possibility of polypharmacy.

Multiple prescribers for the senior adult are not limited to physicians. Health food store personnel, pharmacists, dieticians, nurses, friends and family members all may influence the medication practices of the elder adult. Recommendations may be made without full knowledge of the disease process, symptoms, or concomitant illness that the elder person is experiencing.

Another component that adds to the development of polypharmacy is the practice of multiple sources of prescription medications. The senior adult may go from pharmacy to pharmacy looking for the best price on a medication and not transfer all medications to that particular store. The development of the linking of pharmacies via a common computer is utilized in several of the large drug store chains. This linkage is beneficial to the senior adult who travels from one pharmacy in a chain to another pharmacy in that chain. Each pharmacy within that particular chain has access to a complete record of all prescriptions filled by that chain for the particular senior. However, this system breaks down when the senior adult uses several different chains or sources for medication that do not have a common computer source.

The lack of knowledge about medications and the corresponding medical condition for the medication may also lead to polypharmacy. Psycho-social aspects of an elder adult's ability to learn about medications has been documented (18).

The education of a patient is vital to the treatment of their medical condition. Lack of knowledge may or may not be attributed to the information resources available to the senior adult. Presentation of information must correspond to the physical limitations of patients and their education level. Beyond age 65, one in four people is affected by hearing loss or significant tinnitus (19, 20). Medication information is often presented in small print, making it difficult to read. A slowing of the cognitive process occurs with age , thereby corresponding to a decline in memory and learning procedures (21). The level of education may be such that the patient does not understand what the therapeutic endpoint in their therapy is, or why the medication is being given.

Table 38.2 Similarities in rankings of the most common prescription and non-prescription medication use by the senior adult in two studies.

Hale et al.[1]	Vener et al.[2]
1. multi-vitamins	1. Vitamins
2. antihypertensives	2. analgesics
3. non-narcotic analgesics	3. cardiovascular medications
4. antirheumatics	4. antihypertensives
5. laxatives	5. antiinflammatories
6. coronary vasodilators	6. asthma/bronchitis medications
7. diuretics	7. sedative/hypnotics
8. cardiovascular medications	8. thyroid hormones
9. anticoagulants	9. diabetic medications
10. antacids	10. laxatives

Arenas of Polypharmacy

There are three major arenas in which polypharmacy has been documented: community settings, extended care facilities, and hospital settings. Each arena has it's own special characteristics which add to the incidence of polypharmacy. Research is on-going in each particular area and is currently being reported in a number of venues.

The rate of prescribing in the ambulatory community setting is lower than in either the extended care facility or the institutionalized setting (22). Ambulatory patients are healthier than institutionalized patients. Research done in this arena in specific populations dealing with specific disease states or medication groups, has shown a lower rate of prescribing. Two studies involving the use of prescription and non-prescription drugs are presented in Table 38.2. These studies show that irregardless of study parameters, the categories of medications most frequently used in the senior population are very similar.

Shimp et al. (17) studied potential medication-related problems in non-institutionalized elderly and concluded that the total number of medications, the number of those prescribed, and the number of medical problems experienced had relationships with the number of potential drug-related problems experienced. Patients experiencing frequent changes in medication regimens may become unclear about which medication to continue or discontinue. The change from brand name to generic carries the potential of both medications taken concurrently. The change from one generic product to another may also compound the issue by changing of color or appearance. These alterations may cause confusion for senior adults who frequently identify their medications by color, shape and size of the tablet or capsule.

Approximately three quarters of ambulatory seniors take at least one prescription medication. The number of over-the-counter medications is not well documented.

Table 38.3 Medications that cause adverse drug reactions in the senior population. Similarities of different settings.

Carbonin et al. (29) (hospital)	Chrischilles et al. (32) (ambulatory)	Gerety et al. (33) (nursing home)	Burke et al. (34) (US population)
ampicillin	aspirin	analgesics	antidepressants
captopril	digoxin	cardiac meds	antihypertensives
furosemide	ibuprofen	CNS meds	antilipemics
nifedipine	prednisone	gastrointestinal	antineoplastics
nitroglycerin	propranolol		gastrointestinal

Extended care facilities have a higher number of medications used than the community setting. This may be due to more accurate records and accountability for medication use which first became mandated by federal legislation in the early 1970s (25). This legislation required a pharmacist to perform a drug regimen review in those nursing home facilities receiving Medicare or Medicaid reimbursement. The consultant pharmacist must complete a Drug Regimen Review (DRR) on each patient monthly in a skilled nursing facility or nursing facility and quarterly in an intermediate care facility or mentally retarded care facility. Each patient chart must contain documentation of the date of the review and the consultant's signature. Documentation of any medication problems and/or pertinent findings must be provided in writing to the director of nursing and the attending physician. This legislation gave rise to the multitude of studies conducted regarding the use and misuse of medication in the nursing home environment. A recent study by Beers et al. (26) found that in twelve nursing homes studied, physicians prescribed an average of 7.2 medications per patient, with 14% of those patients prescribed 10 or more medications.

The higher number of medications prescribed to the senior adult in the nursing home setting has led to more recent federal regulation (27). It is mandated that senior nursing home residents be free of unnecessary or inappropriately prescribed drugs. Unnecessary drugs are defined as any medication: given in excessive doses, for an excessive length of time, without adequate monitoring or indication, and given irregardless of adverse reactions or consequences (27). This recent legislation builds on previous legislation that impacts the consultant pharmacist (25). Legislation is aimed specifically at decreasing the use of long-acting benzodiazepines and psychotropic agents in the skilled nursing home setting. It has been reported that 44.9% of patients over the age of sixty-five in the nursing home setting have five or more medications prescribed (28). Seventy percent of the medications taken in long-term care facilities can be grouped into six categories: psychotropic agents, cardiovascular agents, laxatives, analgesics, diuretics, and vitamins.

A 1988 study by Carbonin et al. (29) studied drug use and adverse reactions in 41 medical and geriatric wards. An average of 5.1 medications was taken per patient, and this number increased with advancing age. The most common medications given during hospitalization were cardiac glycosides, loop diuretics, cardiac medications, and anti-ulcer medications. Interestingly, these medications are also reported on the top ten medications in the ambulatory setting (see Table 38.2).

Differences in study design and samples make it difficult to draw conclusions from the reporting of adverse drug reactions (ADR) in the senior hospitalized population. Drug interactions are thought to be a leading cause of ADRs (30). With the multitude of medications prescribed to the senior adult upon hospitalization, the potential for drug interactions to occur may increase. This may explain the assumption that ADRs are related to the age of the individual, when it may be due to the severity of the reason for admission (i.e. congestive heart failure, an infectious process, or respiratory difficulties).

As in the long-term care facility, several parameters for the reporting of adverse or possible adverse events are suggested. The Joint Commission on Accreditation of Healthcare Organizations (JCAHO) suggests several avenues to report these events and examines the methods for reporting upon inspection of the hospital. These requirements for ADRs have allowed for many research opportunities in the field of ADRs as well as reporting the number of medications taken by hospitalized patients.

Consequences of Polypharmacy

Adverse Drug Reactions

Adverse drug reactions can be caused by a variety of factors: drug-drug interactions, inappropriate prescribing, changes in pharmacokinetics and pharmacodynamics, multiple prescribers and sources of medication, and non-compliance. Drug-drug interactions are thought to be the leading cause of ADRs. An exponential, rather than linear, increase in the incidence of ADRs is observed with the addition of each drugs to an existing regimen (1). The potential for drug-drug interactions to be clinically significant was studied by Lipton et al. (31). This study reported 48 percent of 236 ambulatory patients experienced a drug-interaction. Only 2 percent of those reactions were determined to be clinically significant.

Several reports dealing with the common medications prescribed to the elderly have been previously listed (see Table 38.2). It is important to note that those are also the medications that most commonly cause adverse drug reactions in the senior population.

The inappropriate prescribing of medications for the elderly may also potentiate the ocurrance of adverse drug reactions. Nonpharmacologic therapy such as alterations in diet, exercise, sleeping patterns, and daily activities are not as tangible as a prescription.

Changes in the pharmacodynamics and pharmacokinetics of the senior adult may cause ADRs to occur. These include: decreased absorption (35), declining renal function (36), reduced liver mass and metabolic clearance of medications (37).

Intentional and non-intentional compliance has been studied. If information on non-compliance is not reported by the patient to the prescriber, increases or decreases in dosages of medications may result. The ramifications are multiple. The patient may be hospitalized with an ADR secondary to the dosage of the medication, not to the medication itself. Sub-therapeutic or super-therapeutic drug levels may result.

Medication Side-effects

Most side effects experienced by senior adults can be uncomfortable but usually do not warrant discontinuation of the medication. However, the consequences of treating these side-effects may themselves lead to polypharmacy. If another medication is prescribed to negate the side-effect, the potential for side-effects from the new medication is possible. This stacking of medications can become quite cumbersome, not only to the patient taking the medication, but also to the individual attempting to discover the use for those medications.

It is difficult to decide which medication is causing which problem when some medications have the same indications and side-effects. For example, narcotics and tri-cyclic antidepressants are both used in pain control and both have the potential to cause constipation. An overlapping of effects may occur with the concomitant administration of medication.

The perception that an occurrence is a side-effect may in fact be a misnomer. The patient may be experiencing a disease state that has not been diagnosed. Upon an accurate diagnosis, the addition of more medication may result. This would also increase to patient's chance for more side-effects due to polypharmacy. Some side-effects to medication subside with time, but the urgency to alleviate any unwanted symptoms is strong.

Cost

The cost of the medication as well as the cost of hospitalization due to medication is of great concern to the elder adult. Fixed incomes of the senior population may prohibit the purchasing of essential medications. The economic losses experienced by the senior adult due to the inaffordability of medication and subsequent hospitalization can be devastating. Higher medication costs have been linked to an increase in noncompliance. Medications which are not essential may take priority over essential medications because the cost versus benefit ratio is not discussed with the elder adult. Also, the cost of seeing a physician leads seniors to accept recommendation from individuals not actively involved in treatment. Friends, family, salespeople, etc. have an influence on the elder adult. Recommendations from these individuals is usually free, but the potential cost of taking those recommendations may be very high.

The senior adult may or may not be facing the financial burden alone. Insurance companies and the health care system's resources are also responsible for paying the mounting costs of addition to drug therapy.

Drug-Drug Interactions

The opportunity for drug-drug interactions increases with the addition of each medication to the drug regimen. Publicized drug interactions usually reference only one other drug and do not look at the ability of several medications potentiating one medication. It is difficult to separate which medication is causing the interaction when this occurs. There is a potential for polypharmacy to continue when the interaction is not identified. Another medication may be added to the regimen if the drug-drug interaction causes a decrease in response for the patient. An increase in response may also occur and lead the patient to describe exacerbated side-effects to medication which may result in hospitalization or an addition of medication to the therapy. This addition may include not only prescription medications but the self-treatment by the senior adult with non-prescription products.

Non-Compliance

Noncompliance is the main reason for most out-patient treatment failure, as well as a cause of serious medical complications. Rates of noncompliance have been estimated as 25 to 59 percent in the elderly (35). An average of 50 percent non-compliance has been reported in those individuals with chronic diseases (1). Noncompliance with medications has been correlated more strongly with the number of medications given than with the age of the patient. Difficulty in interpreting the importance of a medication or the directions for that medication may lead the senior adult to noncompliance.

The senior adult's knowledge base, cognition, hearing acuity, vision, memory, and physical condition may affect compliance. These may be single or additive in nature. If the senior cannot physically open the bottle of medication, or drive to get the medication, he may be viewed as noncompliant. If the elder adult does not understand the directions given to him regarding the medication, due to hearing loss or educational level, the chances for compliance are decreased. When a patient cannot take a medication as prescribed, he/she is often labeled as non-compliant. This may lead to the prescribing of more medication to the senior adult, due to the fact that the patient is embarrassed to tell the physician about their difficulties in taking medication. Confusion about therapy may increase the patient's noncompliance. Medication scheduling may be a causative factor in the development of non-compliance. An increased number of medications dispersed throughout the day may be so time consuming that the senior adult has difficulty in remembering when each medication is to be taken. The amount of time spent taking medications may actually decrease the quality of life of the senior adult. For example, diuretic use may prevent the senior adult from enjoying outdoor daily activities or traveling due to the frequency of urination which often accompanies these products. Dosages may be missed and taken at a later date or time which may result in medical problems in the future. Seniors may also play "catch-up" — taking two doses of a medication to make up for the one that was missed. This may be described as non-compliance and cause serious problems that may lead to hospitalization. Gebhardt et al. (36) reported that sixty percent of senior adults interviewed would discontinue a prescription drug without speaking to a physician if the medication did not appear to be working. Approximately one-half of those seniors interviewed thought that there were risks involved in taking medications.

Prevention of Polypharmacy

The identification of polypharmacy is the first step towards prevention. The recognition of polypharmacy can be performed in numerous ways. A comprehensive baseline assessment of the senior adult is essential to aid in the recognition of situations where polypharmacy may occur (37). All aspects of the senior adult's daily life are reviewed and may provide insight into the physical, emotional, or educational situations that may lead to the determination that polypharmacy has occurred. The possibility of illiteracy and the subsequent psychological embarrassment of the individual may lead to polypharmacy.

The medication history is another valuable tool in this determination. However, a tool is only as good as the questions asked of the senior adult. It is important to phrase questions about medication use that will allow the senior adult to expound on their experience. Open-ended questions are a very valuable tool. They allow insight into the medication habits of the senior adult and grant information that a yes/no answer will not provide. An effective evaluation allows the health care provider to learn from the patient. The medication history should include any past adverse reactions to medication as well as allergies.

The "brown bag" approach employed by Colt and Schapiro (38) is a useful and valuable tool in identification and prevention of polypharmacy. The information extracted from this approach is invaluable to the health care practitioner. This is dependant on the instructions given to the senior about the brown bag. The elder adult needs to be informed that all products, prescription and non-prescription, need to be brought to the office visit. The amount of medications remaining in a vial and calculations as to what should be remaining is available and therefore a measure of compliance can be discovered. Multiple physician use and multiple pharmacy use can be determined by the labels on the prescription. Non-prescription medication use may be available. This will provide the health care practitioner with information about possible drug interactions, actual prescribed dosages of medications, and duplications of medications.

Another valuable tool in the prevention of polypharmacy is the three day medication history. With this tool, the senior adult provides information on daily medication use (dosage and scheduling) for a three day period. The three day history, in combination with the brown bag, provide another measure of medication compliance in the senior adult.

The education of the patient concerning medication use is one of the most important tools the health care provider can use to prevent the occurrence of polypharmacy. Medication information at a level suited to the individual senior is imperative. The involvement of the senior adult in treatment options not only allows the patient some control in his/her treatment plan but also prevents possible polypharmacy occurrences. The patient needs to be an active partner in his care, and will then understand the possible ramifications of noncompliance. As an active partner, the senior adult can aid the physician in the choice of medication for the disease process. For example, if fixed income is a concern for the patient, communication with the physician will allow a possible therapeutic alternative at a lower cost. This will promote compliance in the patient, as well as make the physician aware of possible problems in the future.

Simplification of drug regimens is another means by which the health care provider can prevent polypharmacy. Single day dosing is available for many medications and may improve quality of life of the senior adult by decreasing the number of medications taken on a given day (39). One medication may have many therapeutic indications and can therefore be utilized for a number of disease states.

The utilization of a pharmacotherapy consultant can aid the physician in the prevention of polypharmacy. Lipton et al. studied the utilization of clinical pharmacists in the prescribing of medications in a geriatric population. Results indicated that clinical pharmacists can improve geriatric prescribing by physicians in the outpatient setting.

The best way to prevent polypharmacy is to change prescription habits. Prescribing medications without a diagnosis only adds to the problem of polypharmacy. The benefit of the addition of a medication to a therapeutic regimen must be weighed against the possible problems which may occur from this addition. The patient should be aware of the benefit-risk ratio of each medication addition.

Multiple sources of prescribing and providing of medications will increase the number of medications per patient unless communication among those sources occurs. A responsible party should be designated to review all medications prescribed for the senior patient and distinguish necessary and unnecessary medications. This responsible party must also maintain accurate records of non-prescription product use. A primary file or record of all medication use should be available to all practitioners as a part of the detailed history of the senior adult.

The use of 'as needed' medication should be kept to a minimum to prevent polypharmacy, as antagonism or synergism of daily medications can occur. The frequency of use of the PRN medications must be reviewed in order to prevent the misuse or overuse of these agents. The term "essential" is the key to the simplification of medications taken by the senior adult.

The outcome of drug therapy must be reviewed and medications discontinued if they are not accomplishing the therapeutic endpoint. Also, once that therapeutic endpoint is met, medications must be discontinued. This information should be shared with the senior adult upon addition to the therapeutic regimen. This will prevent the continuance of medications past their usefulness.

The use of non-medication strategies may be effective in the treatment of symptoms experienced by the senior adult. Education of the senior adult concerning non-drug treatment is a step towards the prevention of polypharmacy. Health promotion for the senior adult is an important asset to the senior adult's quality of life. Exercise, nutrition and a healthy life-style all add to a decrease in the need for medications to treat symptoms. For example, "stiffness" due to arthritis may be treated with increased exercise with or without the addition of medication.

Summary

Polypharmacy is defined as the concurrent use of several different medications, including more than one medication from the same drug classification. Unnecessary and excessive medication use is present in the senior adult population. Polypharmacy occurs in several settings including: hospital, community, and nursing facilities. The development of polypharmacy is enhanced by many factors including: multiple disease states, multiple medications, multiple prescribers, multiple sources for medication, lack of education about medication, and self-treatment. These factors may build upon each other and become additive in nature. The consequences of polypharmacy involve adverse drug reactions, drug interactions, cost to the senior adult, and noncompliance. Polypharmacy is often recognized after it has occurred.

The key to prevention of polypharmacy is the utilization of different prevention methods and the addition of these together to form a plan of action prior to the ocurrance. Education of the medical community as well as the senior adult is essential to the prevention of polypharmacy. The use of the "essential medication only" premise to medication treatment in the elderly will aid in the prevention of polypharmacy. Cost factors, therapeutic endpoints, non-drug therapy through

health promotion, education, and communication between the senior adult and all prescribers involved in medical care, are all vital components to the main goal of decreased medication use in the senior population.

References

1. Colley CA, Lucas LM. Polypharmacy: the cure becomes to disease. *Journal of General Internal Medicine* 1993; **8**: 278–283.
2. *Stedman's medical dictionary*, 24th ed. Baltimore: Williams and Wilkins, 1984.
3. Baum C, Kennedy DL, Forbes MB, *et al.* Drug use in the United States in 1981. *J am Med Assoc* 1984; **251**: 1293.
4. *Healthy People 2000: National health promotion and disease prevention objectives.* Washington DC: US Dept of Health and Human Services, 1990.
5. Simonson W. Medications and the Elderly: A Guide for Promoting Proper Use. *Aspen Systems Corporation.* Rockville, MD, p. 33,1984.
6. Kovar M. Health of the elderly and use of health services. *Public Health Rep* 1977; **92**: 9–19.
7. Colt HG, Shapiro AP. Drug-induced illness as a cause for admission to a community hospital. *J Am Geriat Soc.* 1989; **37**: 323–6.
8. Nolan L, O'Malley K. Prescribing for the elderly: part I. Sensitivity of the elderly to adverse drug reactions. *J Am Geriatr Soc.* 1989; **36**: 142–9.
9. Guttman D. Patterns of legal drug use of older Americans. *Addict Dis* 1978; **3**: 337–56.
10. *AHFS drug information 95.* Bethesda, MD, p. 922, 1995.
11. *AHFS drug information 95.* Bethesda, MD, p. 1745, 1995.
12. Ellor JR, Kurz DJ. Misuse and abuse of prescription and nonprescription drugs by the elderly. *Nurs Clin North Am* 1982; **17**: 319.
13. Atkinson RM. Alcoholism in the elderly population. *Mayo Clin Proc* 1988; **63**: 825.
14. *AHFS drug information 95.* Bethesda, MD, p. 2025, 1995.
15. Law R, Chalmers C. Medicines and elderly people: A general practice survey. *Br Med J* 1976; **1**: 565.
16. Ostrom JR, Hammerlund ER, Christiansen DB, *et al.* Medication usuage in the elderly population. *Med Care* 1985; **23**: 157.
17. Shrimp LA, Ascione FJ, Glazer HM, Atwood BF. Potential medication-related problems in non-institutionalized elderly. *Drug Intell Clin Pharm.* 1985; **19**: 766–72.
18. Back KW, Sullivan DA. Self-image, medicine and drug use. *Addict Dis* 1978; **3**: 373–82.
19. National Health Review Survey. Hyattsville, MD: US National Center for Health Statistics, 1981.
20. Oyer HJ, Oyer EJ. Social consequences of hearing loss for the elderly. *Allied Health Behav Sci* 1979; **2**: 123–38.
21. Arenberg D. Memory and learning do decline late in life. In *Aging: A Challenge to Science and Society*, 3rd ed, edited by JE Birren, JMA Munnichs, H Thomas, M Marois. Oxford: Oxford University Press, 312–22, 1983.
22. Nolan L. Prescribing for the elderly, II. Prescribing patterns: difference due to age. *J Am Geriatr Soc* 1988; **36**: 245.
23. Hale WE, May FE, Marks RG, Stewart RB. Drug use in an ambulitory elderly population: a five year update. *Drug Intell Clin Pharm* 1987; **21**: 530–5.
24. Vener AM, Krupla LR, Climo JJ. Drug usage and health characteristics in non-institutionalized retired persons. *J Am Geriatr Soc* 1979; **27**: 83–90.
25. US Federal Register. January 17, 1974; **39**: 2238–57.
26. Beers MH, Fingold SF, Ouslander JG, *et al.* Characteristics and quality of prescribing by doctors practicing in nursing homes. *J Am Geriatr Soc* 1993; **41**: 802–07.
27. Elon R, Pawlson G. The impact of OBRA on medical practice within nursing facilities. *J Am Geriatr Soc* 1992; **40**: 958–963.
28. Lamy PP, Michocki RJ: Medication management. *Clin Geriatr Med* 1988; **4**: 623.
29. Carbonin P, Pahor M, Bernabei R, Sgadari A. Is age an independent risk factor for adverse drug reactions in hospitalized medical patients? *J Am Geriatr Soc* 1991; **39**: 1093–9.

30. Lamy PP. The elderly and drug interactions. *J Am Geriatr Soc* 1986; **34**: 586–92.

31. Lipton HL, Bero LA, Bird JA, McPhee SJ. The impact of clinical pharmacist's consultations on physicans' geriatric drug prescribing. *Med Care* 1992; **30**: 646–58.

32. Chrischilles EA, Segar ET, Wallace RB. Self-reported adverse drug reactions and related resource use. *Annals of Internal Medicine* 1992; **117**: 634–640.

33. Gerety M, Cornell JE, Plichta D, Eimer M. Adverse events related to drugs and drug withdrawal in nursing home residents. *J Am Geriatr Soc* 1993; **41**: 1326–32.

34. Burke LB, Jolson HM, Goetsch RA, Ahronheim JC. Geriatric drug use and adverse event reporting in 1990. *Annu Rev Gerontol Geriatr* 1992, **12**: 1–28.

35. Col N, Fanale JE, Kronholm P. The role of medication non-compliance and adverse drug reactions in hospitalizations of the elderly. *Arch Intern Med*. 1990; **150**: 841–5.

36. Gebhardt MW, Governali JF, Hart EJ. Drug related behavior, knowledge and misconceptions among a selected group of senior citizens. *J Drug Educ* 1978; **8**: 85–92.

37. Schlarach AE, Mor-Barak ME, Katz A, *et al*. Generation: a corporate-sponsored retiree health care program. *Gerontologists* 1992; **32**: 265–269.

38. Colt HG, Shapiro AP. Drug-reduced illness as a cause for admission to a community hospital. *J Am Geriatr Soc* 1989; **37**: 323–326.

39. Stewart RB. Noncompliance in the elderly: is there a cure? *Drugs & Aging* 1991; **1**: 163–167.

39. The Diagnosis and Treatment of Cancer in the Elderly: Cost Effectiveness Considerations

Gary H. Lyman and Nicole M. Kuderer

Introduction

The resources available and permitted by society for medical care are finite. Modern medical care is costly and with the introduction of new and more expensive technologies, the demands on these resources are increasing rapidly. Many clinical decisions involve trade-offs between what is best for the individual (most effective) and what is best for society (least costly). A systematic method is needed to appropriately evaluate medical care and health care technology that carries significant risk or cost to either the patient or society. Hopefully, such evaluation methods will not only reduce cost, but also improve health care resulting in a more rational approach to the utilization of health care resources. Physicians and other health care professionals should play a leadership role in the evaluation and appropriate use of health care resources.

The cancer problem has devastating effects upon the world's population both clinically and economically. The impact of cancer and cancer treatment upon the population can be measured both clinically and economically. It is impossible to fully understand and measure the effect of this disease on the population, including the elderly, without measures of both its clinical and economic impact. As illustrated in Table 39.1, both intermediate measures and ultimate or long-term measures are utilized.

Clinical outcome may be measured in terms of both the desired effectiveness or benefit and any associated toxicity or harm which results. The favorable effect of cancer treatment is conventionally measured in terms of response and ultimately survival or life expectancy. The adverse effect of cancer treatment is conventionally measured in terms of toxicity and ultimately the effect on quality of life. Increasingly, measures which combine the positive and negative effects of cancer and cancer treatment are being utilized. The economic outcomes of cancer are generally measured as either charges or ultimately expenditures or costs. Outcome measures which combine the clinical and the economic features of cancer are available. Such measures are particularly useful for comparing the value of different diagnostic and treatment strategies. Such measures are vulnerable to misinterpretation, however, and must be fully understood. This chapter will focus on the utilization of outcome measures and their application to the elderly population with cancer.

Cancer in the Elderly

Nearly 1.4 million Americans will be diagnosed with invasive cancer in 1996 and more than 550,000 will die of the disease (1). It is estimated that nearly one-half of men and more than one-third of women will develop invasive cancer at some time during their lives. Cancer clearly is a disease of aging as age-specific incidence rates increase with increasing age. Cancer is the second leading cause of death among the elderly, accounting for nearly one-fourth of all deaths in the United States (2). Approximately 58% of all malignancies and over two-thirds of all deaths from cancer occur in individuals age 65 and over. The median age of cancer patients at the time of diagnosis is 67 years and at the time of death is 70 years. Cancer incidence rates have increased 26% over the past two decades among those 65 and over compared to only 10% among younger patients (2). Similarly, cancer mortality rates have increased 15% among individuals 65 years of age and over compared to a decrease of nearly 5% among younger individuals during the same time period. Table 39.2 summarizes the incidence and mortality trends of selected cancers among the elderly with notable increases over the past two decades. Lung cancer represents the leading cause of cancer-related mortality among the elderly and has increased three-fold during this time period among women age 65 and older (2).

Table 39.1 Cancer outcome measures.

Outcomes	Clinical		Economic
	Quantity	Quality	
Intermediate	Response	Toxicity	Charges
Ultimate	Survival	Quality of life	Direct costs
	Life expectancy	Qaly+	Indirect costs
Combined	Cost-effectiveness	Cost-utility	Cost-benefit

+Quality-adjusted life years

Table 39.2 Trends in cancer rates by selected cancer site among those age 65 and over+. Percent increase (1973–1990) (%).

Primary site	Incidence	Mortality
Female lung	182	201
Melanoma	120	65
Prostate	80	21
Non-hodgkin's lymphoma	62	49
Brain	58	67
Kidney	39	25
Liver/bilary	37	22
Breast	37	15
Esophagus	21	25
Male lung	19	34
Ovary	19	19
Bladder	14	–21
Larynx	13	1
Multiple myeloma	12	37

+SEER (2)

Table 39.3 Major quality of life dimensions*.

1. Physical concerns (symptoms)
2. Functional ability
3. Family well-being
4. Emotional well-being
5. Treatment satisfaction
6. Sexuality/intimacy
7. Social functioning

*A Global Evaluation of QOL or total score are also given Cella, 1995 (3)

There are considerable differences in both the potential for response and the risk of toxicity between older and younger individuals. The distribution of malignancies most commonly seen among the elderly are less responsive to systemic therapies while the frequency of comorbid illnesses which may complicate treatment is greater. Likewise, the potential benefit of treatment in terms of improved life expectancy becomes less with increasing age. Therefore, the importance of carefully balancing benefits and risks in the overall clinical outcome as well as considering costs is most readily apparent in clinical decision making in the elderly cancer patient. Issues related to the quality of life and the utilization of limited resources, while always of importance, are perhaps of greatest importance when considering cancer in the elderly.

Clinical Outcomes of Cancer Care

The clinical outcomes of cancer care can be measured either quantitatively or qualitatively. Effectiveness is the measurement of the clinical outcome of cancer management in the population. This must be distinguished from efficacy which represents the outcome apparent in a sample of the population in this framework of a clinical trial. Intermediate clinical outcomes are frequently utilized because they are available earlier and are often predictive of the ultimate outcome of interest. Response measured as a decrease in tumor size or a reduction in biological markers of disease activity represents an intermediate marker of effect. More powerful intermediate measures include the time

to relapse, time to recurrence or time to progression of disease. Ultimately, the benefit of cancer treatment is most frequently measured in terms of overall survival or life expectancy. Survival may be presented as actual survival where all deaths are considered or relative survival where only deaths from the disease of interest are considered. Disease-free or progression-free survival, on the other hand, consider disease recurrence or progression as well as death as adverse outcomes. In seriously ill patients such as cancer patients with limited life expectancy, the mortality rate may be considered as nearly constant. When the mortality rate is constant, the relationship between survival and time is described by a declining exponential function. Such a Declining Exponential Approximation of Life Expectancy (DEALE) is generally close enough for most clinical applications. Appendix 1 provides a brief overview of the assumptions and methods associated with utilization of the DEALE.

Organ-specific toxicity can be measured along scales which are difficult to summarize satisfactorily. Ultimately, treatment-related toxicity and symptoms related to the malignancy can be measured in terms of quality of life. Treatment and disease-related symptoms may be alleviated by supportive care measures which have little or no direct effect on the patient's malignancy. Just as survival and life expectancy measure the quantity of clinical outcome, a measure of quality of life is often sought. Quality-of-Life, unfortunately, is an outcome for which there is not complete agreement on measurement or application. As shown in Table 39.3, Quality-of-Life may be evaluated along several specific dimensions thought to measure the various aspects of life of importance to its quality (3).

Numerous instruments designed to measure quality of life are available including generic health status measures, several cancer-specific measures and cancer-site-specific measures for specific types of cancer (4). Alternatively, quality of life may be measured as a utility in terms of quantitative measures of patient preference for a certain outcome. This may provide for a combined outcome measure incorporating both the quantity and quality of life. Patient preferences may be assessed monetarily as a willingness-to-pay to achieve or avoid certain outcomes. More commonly, patient preferences are assessed as an adjustment of the effectiveness of the clinical outcome measure such as survival time or life expectancy. Such preferences may be assessed along a linear scale from 0 to 1. Alternatively, preferences can be assessed by a time trade-off method utilizing a standard reference gamble. The time in full health considered equivalent to the actual time in the diseased state is a measure of quality of life or quality adjusted life years (QALYs). Patient outcomes can be divided into a finite number of health care states with defined length and with an associated utility weight (Figure 39.1).

The sum over all health states of the product of the time spent in each state and the utility of each state will yield a summary measure termed quality-adjusted time without symptoms of disease or toxicity of treatment (Q-TWIST) (5). This provides for both a more accurate outcome measure as well as an empiric measurement of quality-adjusted survival in actual clinical settings (6). Clearly, more information is needed about the best

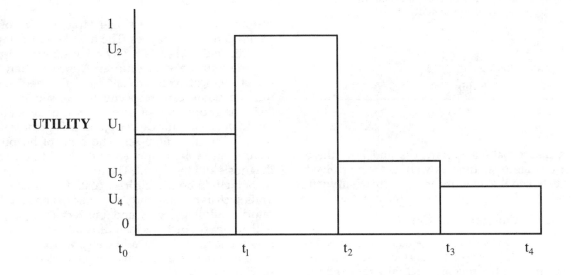

Event	Time Period	X	Utility		Product
Diagnosis	t_0		—		—
Initial Treatment	t_0 to t_1		U_1	=	$U_1 (t_1 - t_0)$
Followup	t_1 to t_2		U_2	=	$U_2 (t_2 - t_1)$
Treatment of Recurrence	t_2 to t_3		U_3	=	$U_3 (t_3 - t_2)$
Palliative Care	t_3 to t_4		U_4	=	$U_4 (t_4 - t_3)$
Death	t_4		O	=	0

Q-TWIST = $U_1 (t_1 - t_0) + U_2 (t_2 - t_1) + U_3 (t_3 - t_2) + U_4 (t_4 - t_3)$

*Gelber, 1991 (5)

Figure 39.1 Quality-adjusted time without symptoms of disease or toxicity of treatment (Q-TWIST) Schematic depiction of changes in outcome utility over time for various events from the time of diagnosis through death. Q-TWIST represents the sum over all time intervals of the product of the duration of the interval and the measured utility of the interval.

Table 39.4 Health care costs.

Direct:

- Medical: costs of medical services for prevention diagnosis and treatment of disease.

- Non-medical: costs incurred while receiving medical care; e.g., transportation.

Indirect:

- Morbidity costs: economic value of days of work lose due to illness.

- Mortality costs: value of economic output lost from premature death of workers due to disease.

Intangible:

- Pain and suffering
- Loss of companionship

Table 39.5 U.S. direct health care expenditures 1990.

	Cancer	All health care
Hospital care	65%	49%
Physician services	24%	25%
Drugs	4%	10%
Nursing home care	5%	11%
Other professional services	2%	5%

Source: National Center for Health Statistics

way to measure patient preferences and how these measures change over time as well as the perceived tradeoffs between the quantity and quality of survival.

The Economic Outcomes of Cancer

Measures utilized in evaluating the economic outcome of disease include charges for services, the cost of delivering care and the revenues actually received for services. Charges are sometimes utilized as an intermediate measure of economic outcome. Although the ratio of costs to charges may be relatively constant in certain settings, charges often have an inconsistent relationship to the actual costs of care.

There are many components to health care costs which vary greatly in measurability and accessibility (Table 39.4). As a result, there is often little uniformity in the reporting of health care costs in different studies (7,8). Direct costs include both the medical and non-medical expenses associated with the diagnosis, treatment and followup of patients. Indirect costs represent the monetary losses to the patient and family due to time lost from work and disability or due to premature death from disease. Intangible costs include the social and emotional costs of illness to the patient and family. Since these are difficult to measure objectively, economic analyses seldom consider the intangible costs of disease. In addition, most economic analyses do not consider the indirect costs of illness because of the effort required to extract and evaluate such information. In fact, most economic analyses are restricted to measures of the direct medical costs of disease ignoring any additional expenses of medical care to the patient and family (9).

Direct medical costs include several component costs, the proportion of which will vary with the type of illness. As shown in Table 39.5, hospital care represents approximately 50% of all direct medical costs in this

country making it the single largest share of direct health care expenditures. The next largest component of direct medical costs is physician services representing one-fourth of expenditures. Approximately 10% of direct medical costs are allocated for medicines and nursing home care respectively. As shown in Table 39.5, the proportion of direct medical costs allocated for hospital care for cancer patients is greater than for those with other illnesses. The costs of hospital care include multiple components which will vary with the diagnosis and treatment. The total hospital operational costs include both the direct costs for specific service units such as nursing care, pharmacy, blood bank, laboratory, radiology, etc., and indirect costs associated with support functions including administration, engineering, janitorial, education, etc., which must be allocated in some fashion to charges generated by the direct service units.

The cost of health care estimated will depend upon the ability to measure the effects of illness and the perspective from which costs are viewed. The perspectives on health care costs will vary greatly between the hospital, the physician and other professional providers, the payor, the patient and family and society as a whole. It is, perhaps, only from the global perspective of society as well as the intimate perspective of the patient and family that the true total costs of illness can be understood. From a narrow perspective, the lowest cost will be associated with minimal diagnostic and therapeutic intervention. However, from a more global perspective, the importance of new effective therapeutic strategies, early detection with screening programs and disease prevention or eradication through health education cannot be overemphasized. These will represent the ultimate answer to reducing health care costs while at the same time improving clinical outcomes.

The Cost of Cancer in the Elderly

Health care expenditures in the United States are now estimated to exceed one trillion dollars annually (10). Approximately 10% of health care costs are attributable to cancer care totaling approximately $100 billion annually. Of direct medical costs for malignancy, more than 90% is accounted for by five diagnoses: breast cancer (24%), colorectal cancer (24%), lung cancer (18%), prostate cancer (17%), and bladder cancer (8%) (10).

Approximately one-half of health care expenditures for cancer care are for patients age 65 and over.

Perhaps the most readily available information on health care costs associated with cancer in the elderly is based on Medicare coverage of cancer patients age 65 and over (11). There are several limitations to this data, however. Billed charges to Medicare generally exceed actual costs. In addition, Medicare payments do not necessarily reflect actual costs for cancer care which include nursing home costs and self-administered prescription medications. In a study from the Health Care Financing Administration (HCFA), Medicare payments for all covered services by site and stage over the first 17 years after diagnosis were studied for patients age 65 and over with cancer of the lung, breast, prostate, colon and bladder (12). This study demonstrated that Medicare payments for cancer were not uniform, but varied by site, age at diagnosis and time throughout the natural history of the disease. Medicare payments from diagnosis to death generally correlated with the duration of patient survival and were highest among those with bladder cancer ($57,629) and lowest for lung cancer ($29,184). Although higher total payments were seen among those diagnosed at an early stage, the highest average annual payment was observed in those diagnosed at later stages of disease. The highest average Medicare payments were seen during the initial six months following diagnosis and during the final six months before death. The lowest average payments were found during the interval of continuing care and monitoring. Efforts to diagnose disease early through cancer screening may increase total lifetime Medicare costs by increasing survival. Thus screening and prevention strategies must be evaluated by virtue of their ability to improve the duration and quality of life at an acceptable cost. Similar changes in cancer care costs in those age 65 and over have been reported for members of a health maintenance organization diagnosed with colon, prostate and breast cancer (13). The greatest average cost was found during the final six months of life followed by the initial six months following diagnosis. The costs of initial and terminal care were generally somewhat less among the elderly than among younger individuals. While the total costs of continuing care were higher among the elderly, the net cost of cancer care after deducting the age and sex specific costs observed for non-cancer care was actually lower among the elderly.

Economic Analyses

Economic analyses must consider both the clinical outcome as well as the economic outcome or cost (14). Economic analyses are seldom needed or of value when both an improved clinical outcome and reduced cost are found or when both a worse clinical outcome and increased cost are found. Economic analyses are called for and of greatest value when the clinical outcome is improved but the cost is greatly increased. The most efficient program will be the one with the lowest cost per unit of benefit. Economic analyses are also of value when the cost is greatly reduced, but the clinical outcome is not as good. The most efficient program would be the one with the greatest benefit per unit cost.

There are different types of economic analyses based on the available data and the purpose to which the analysis will be applied. Perhaps the most common type of economic study involves an analysis of administrative data bases collected on the basis of health care payor. Economic studies may also involve retrospective analyses of specific population cohorts based on disease or other criteria. Increasing interest has developed over the past several years in either retrospective or prospective economic analyses of cancer clinical trials. One of the most valuable types of economic analysis utilized in evaluating cancer care involves decision analytic models.

Decision analytic models require the specification of a model structure where decision points represent the focus of analysis (15). Modeling requires the explicit consideration of all decision points as well as their relationship to chance events and outcomes. This is generally schematized in the form of a decision tree where each branching point represents a chance or decision point and the leaves represent end points or outcomes. Analysis of such models also requires the explicit specification of initial estimates for the probability of each event and the value of each outcome. These estimates may be based on experience, expert opinion or data available from the clinical literature.

Decision models can be analyzed in a variety of ways. The simplest analysis involves calculating the expected value of each choice at a decision point by a process of folding back the tree. Folding back involves multiplying the assigned outcome values of each branch by the probability of that outcome and summing over all of the branches of the immediately preceding chance event. This sum represents the expected value of that event. The expected value now becomes the outcome value and the process is continued by multiplying this value by its probability. When a decision point is reached, the choice associated with the greatest expected value is the preferred choice.

One of the greatest strengths of decision analysis is the ability to vary any of the assumed probabilities and outcome values over a range of reasonable estimates in order to determine how it effects the expected value of the choices and the optimal decision. In such a sensitivity analysis, a threshold value of the variable may be found at which the expected value of two choices are exactly equal. Threshold analysis can be further elaborated by varying two or more variables simultaneously in order to define a threshold function or family of threshold functions.

Decision models are particularly suited to economic analyses by permitting the simultaneously consideration of more than one type of outcome measure; e.g., clinical outcomes and economic outcomes. In addition, costs and benefits can be modified by procedures to incorporate considerations of quality of life. Such procedures permit economic analyses based on cost-benefit, cost-effectiveness and cost-utility functions.

In the most fundamental scenario involving one disease and one treatment, there are four possible outcomes. Ideally, one would initiate treatment when the disease is present and withhold treatment when the disease is absent. Under realistic clinical conditions of uncertainty, however, treatment may be initiated when the disease is not present and treatment may be withheld when the disease is present. The expected value of each treatment strategy depends upon both the disease prevalence and the utility of each possible outcome. Clearly, the decision choice associated with the greatest expected value is the preferred one. The threshold prevalence of disease for choosing the optimal treatment strategy relates to the ratio of benefits and costs reflected in the utilities incorporated into the model. As the ratio of benefits to costs increases, the threshold changes so as to increase the indications for treatment (Appendix 2).

Cost Effectiveness Analysis

The majority of clinical investigations report outcome measured in terms of clinical benefit or quality-adjusted benefit. When clinical effectiveness is not an issue, an economic outcome such as cost may be the preferred measure of interest. However, a more accurate and complete clinical or economic analysis often requires measurement of both types of outcomes presented separately or combined. There are a variety of economic analyses that combine measures of clinical and economic outcome together into a single measure of benefit and cost (16). These measures differ substantially from one another in makeup and application and are sometimes confused with one another (17). There is increasing concern for an improved understanding of these methods including the proper utilization and reporting of such economic analyses (18).

Cost-benefit analysis is conducted by converting clinical benefits into the same economic measure as costs in order to combine them in a single term. This approach requires placing an economic value on the clinical outcome measure such as survival or life expectancy. Obviously, the measure of value for life or the willingness to pay to avoid certain events will vary with ability to pay among different socioeconomic groups. The most commonly utilized combined measure of clinical and economic outcome is that of cost-effectiveness. This approach measures the added clinical benefit of one approach over another (marginal benefit) and the added cost of that strategy over the other (marginal cost). Cost effectiveness combines these two measures into a summary measure which can be either cost-based or effectiveness based. The cost-based measure is most commonly utilized and calculates the cost per unit of clinical benefit; e.g., cost in dollars per year of life gained (marginal cost effectiveness). The effectiveness-based measure calculates the amount of added benefit per unit of economic outcome; e.g., years of life gained per dollar. Cost effectiveness is most often utilized to compare management strategies based on a common measure. Quality of life may be included as an important dimension of clinical outcome. The measures of clinical outcome can be adjusted for quality of life by assigning a utility value to different health outcome states. A cost-utility analysis can be conducted in the same fashion as a cost-effectiveness analysis by utilizing a quality-adjusted outcome measure such as quality-adjusted life years (QALYs) as the clinical outcome of interest. By measuring the added quality-adjusted benefit (marginal benefit) and the added cost of a clinical strategy (marginal cost), the cost per unit of quality-adjusted clinical benefit can be calculated; e.g., cost in dollars per QALY gained (marginal cost utility).

It is often necessary and appropriate to adjust changes in the cost or benefit measures for factors related to time or other criteria. The most common adjustment considered is related to cost discounting due to the frequent preference for delaying present costs to the future. Appendix 3 provides a brief description of cost discounting between present and future costs. In a similar fashion, future benefits can be adjusted to the present for comparison purposes based on the usual preference for immediate benefit.

It is important to note that summary measures of cost effectiveness and cost utility are marginal measures and do not provide information on the absolute amount of benefit or cost. Therefore, a strategy can potentially appear superior in terms of cost effectiveness or cost utility and yet have substantially lower absolute effectiveness or utility. In other words, a strategy may have substantially lower cost and appear more cost effective, even though it may have substantially lower clinical benefit. It is important, therefore, to measure both the absolute as well as the marginal measures of benefit and cost in such analyses. When properly estimated and presented, such methods are of value in objectively comparing strategies competing for limited resources.

Cost-Effectiveness Studies in Elderly Cancer Patients

A limited number of studies of the cost-effectiveness of cancer care in the elderly have been reported. These include studies of cancer screening efforts, early (adjuvant) treatment, the treatment of advanced (metastatic) disease and palliative care at the end of life. Each of these areas raises unique issues related to the care of the elderly and the risks and benefits of specific interventions.

Cancer Screening and Early Diagnosis

Economic analyses of cancer screening programs for several malignancies have been conducted. Decision analytic models have proven to be efficient and effective methods of economic analysis in order to develop guidelines for screening programs. These models are generally based on available incidence data, knowledge of the natural history of the disease and available information on test performance and cost. The elderly present both unique opportunities as well as important obstacles to the application of currently available screening methods (19–24). The increasing prevalence of most cancers among the elderly increases the predictive value of positive screening tests in this population. Many of the malignancies affecting the elderly are asymptomatic in their earliest phases and often present with advanced disease when symptoms bring the patient to medical attention. Early diagnosis by effective screening methods may permit treatment when curative potential is reasonably high. Alternatively, the limited life expectancy of the elderly and the frequency of comorbid conditions complicate and limit the value of effective treatment. It is precisely this type of complex trade-off of benefits and risks which calls for the application of cost effectiveness analysis in clinical and public health decision making.

The relative five-year survival for cervical cancer in women age 65 and over is approximately 50% compared to 65% in women under age 65 (2). Despite marked reductions in mortality from cervical cancer in younger patients, there has been no decrease in mortality in women over 70 years of age (25). The high frequency of abnormal smears and the high incidence of invasive cervical cancer among elderly women appears to relate to a lack of screening in this population. Compliance with recommended screening practice in women over 70 years of age has been found to be only about one-half of that among younger women. In 1990, Papanicolau smear screening for cervical cancer was adopted as a preventive health service covered by Medicare. While the evidence that cervical cancer screening is effective is substantial, few studies have included sufficient elderly women to draw definitive conclusions. A study by the Office of Technology Assessment of the cost-effectiveness of cervical cancer screening concluded that screening the elderly will not save money, but the cost per additional year of life saved is quite low (26). Utilizing a decision analysis format based on a Markov model, the impact of screening women ages 65 to 109 years of age was studied (27). Triennial screening was found to reduce mortality from cervical cancer by 75% at a cost of $2254 per year of life saved. Annual screening resulted in an increased cost to $7345 per year of life saved. These results were critically dependent upon the quality of the Papanicolau smear. Screening was seen to be most efficiently applied to women who have not had regular screening and was least efficient in those who had demonstrated consistently negative cervical cytologies. While limiting the analysis to women up to age 75 years, Eddy demonstrated that there was little difference in clinical outcome, but large increases in cost as the frequency of cervical screening changes from every four years to every year (28). This led to screening guidelines calling for a reduced frequency of screening if several annual screens were negative. The potential for more cost-effective methods for cervical cancer screening in the elderly appear promising with emerging technologies (29).

The incidence of colorectal cancer increases dramatically with increasing age although age-specific survival with this disease has remained relatively constant. The early stages of the disease may be entirely asymptomatic resulting in the majority of patients having advanced disease at presentation. When diagnosed at an early, asymptomatic stage of disease, the vast majority of patients may be cured with available treatments. Screening for occult blood has been shown to reduce mortality from colorectal cancer in a population age 50–80 years (30). However, other investigators have questioned these conclusions (31). Screening for occult blood has low sensitivity and low specificity. Sigmoidoscopy has been shown to increase the likelihood of detecting early stage disease (32). Screening colonoscopy is highly sensitive and specific, but very expensive. A cost effectiveness model developed by the Office of Technology Assessment found that annual occult blood testing would detect 17% of cancers at a cost of $35,000 per year of life saved (33). Screening schedules that included periodic sigmoidoscopy would prevent a greater proportion of cancers, but would cost between $43,000 and $47,000 per year of life saved. Although costly, colorectal cancer screening with periodic sigmoidoscopy appears to be a reasonably cost-effective preventive strategy in the elderly (34). Colonoscopy every three to five years for high risk individuals based on personal and family histories may be the most effective and cost effective screening method.

The risk of breast cancer increases rapidly with increasing age with more than 75% of breast cancers occuring in women 50 years of age and over. While previous studies suggested that elderly women with breast cancer fared poorly because of less aggressive management, several recent studies have demonstrated that elderly women actually experience a greater survival than younger women when treated in a similar fashion (35). The majority of breast cancers are found initially by the patient or the physician. Breast cancer screening incorporating breast self-examination, physical examination and periodic mammography have been shown effective at diagnosing patients at an earlier stage of disease resulting in a greater potential for curability (36). There remain many unresolved issues related to the cost-effectiveness of breast cancer screening among the elderly including the frequency of screening, type of screening, and the value of screening in the very elderly. There are also many barriers to the universal utilization of breast cancer screening among the elderly including cost, education, anxiety, and physician compliance. Currently, the American Cancer Society and the National Cancer Institute recommend monthly breast self-examination, yearly physician examination and annual mammography over the age of 50. Randomized trials provide greater evidence for the effectiveness of breast cancer screening than for screening of any other cancer. Over the past three decades, eight major randomized trials of breast cancer screening with mammography have been analyzed (37). These studies have demonstrated a mortality reduction in women age 50–69 of approximately 30%. A meta-analysis of screening mammography concluded that screening mammography of women age 50–74 years of age reduced the risk of mortality by more than 25% (38). Numerous cost-effectiveness studies of breast cancer screening have been conducted (39–41). The estimated cost-effectiveness of breast cancer screening has varied between $20,000 and $50,000 per year of life gained (42). The cost-effectiveness of breast cancer screening recruitment strategies has also been evaluated revealing that personal strategies were more cost-effective than public strategies (43). Decision analysis models have shown that the cost per year of life saved by breast cancer screening decreases with increasing age to somewhat less than $30,000 per year of life saved in the 65–70 year age group after which it increases with increasing age approaching $50,000 per year of life saved in the 80–85 year age group (44). A decision analysis model generated to look at the effects of co-morbid conditions found net benefits from breast cancer screening after adjustment for changes in long-term quality of life in elderly women of all ages (45). However, data on the effectiveness of breast cancer screening remains very limited in women age 75 and over. There are many outstanding questions concerning the application of breast cancer screening in very elderly women (46,47).

Prostate cancer is the most frequently diagnosed cancer in men in the United States and the second leading cause of cancer mortality after lung cancer (2). Prostate cancer is primarily a disease of older men with a median age at diagnosis of 77 years and an age-specific incidence of over 1% annually over the age of 75. Prostate cancer often is asymptomatic unless advanced disease is present. An analysis of benefit and risk is complicated by two clinical features of prostate cancer. First, while the prevalence of prostate cancer is extremely high in elderly men, many cases do not metastasize and cause life-threatening symptoms. Second, the therapeutic options for localized prostate cancer including surgical resection and radiation therapy are not completely effective and have considerable morbidity associated with them. Utilizing generous assumptions about the effectiveness of primary therapy, a cost-effectiveness analysis based on data from the American Cancer Society-National Prostate Cancer Detection Project concluded that the combination of digital rectal exam (DRE) and prostate specific antigen (PSA) represents an economical and ethical screening method for prostate cancer (48). In other studies utilizing a decision analytic model, DRE alone was not found to reduce mortality at any age. Screening with either PSA or transrectal ultrasound (TRUS) was found to increase life expectancy, but actually decreased quality-adjusted life expectancy (49). All strategies were found to increase costs and selecting only high prevalence subpopulations did not improve the benefit of screening. Debate continues over the value and cost effectiveness of prostate cancer screening in elderly men (50).

Cancer Treatment and Supportive Care

The cost effectiveness of treatment strategies for cancer

has only received attention over the past few years. Smith, et al., have presented an excellent review of cost-effectiveness studies of cancer treatment based on decision analysis models (51). Relatively few studies have specifically addressed the cost-effectiveness of cancer treatment in elderly patients. Without consideration of age, breast conserving surgery has been shown to yield better quality-adjusted survival than mastectomy (52). Adjunctive chemotherapy in pre-menopausal women has been shown to add benefit for all women at acceptable costs of from $4500 to $22,000 per quality-adjusted life year gained (53,54). Adjuvant chemotherapy appears to prolong the survival of older women to a lesser extent than younger women. A cost-effectiveness analysis of adjuvant chemotherapy in women age 60 to 80 years of age with lymph node positive breast cancer estimated costs per quality-adjusted year of life gained that ranged from $28,200 for a 60 year old to $57,100 for an 80 year old (55). A study of the cost-effectiveness of adjuvant therapy for stage III colorectal cancer without regard to age estimated costs per year of life saved between $2000 and $5000 (56). Several cost-effectiveness studies of first-line leukemia and lymphoma therapy have also been presented, but with little direct attention to the elderly population (57–59). There have been several cost-effectiveness analyses of treatment for advanced cancer. Few of these, however, have specifically addressed the elderly population. Cost-effectiveness in terms of incremental costs per year of life gained have generally been estimated in the range of $20,000 to $50,000 for standard dose therapy (60–65). Similarly, cost-effectiveness studies of high dose therapy with autologous bone marrow support have yielded cost estimates of $25,000 to $100,000 per year of life gained (66–67). Decision analysis methods have also been utilized to address the costs associated with the use of supportive care technologies in patients undergoing cancer treatment (68–70). There has been little systematic appraisal of the cost-effectiveness of palliative care for patients near the end of life regardless of age (71–73). There is now great interest in incorporating not only quality of life measures, but economic outcome measures into prospective randomized clinical trials (74,75). Several trials are underway which hopefully will improve our understanding of the cost-effectiveness of cancer care at all ages (5,76).

Conclusions

Cancer care is associated with both clinical and economic outcomes of interest. There is increasing interest in measuring the impact of cancer and cancer treatment on both the quantity and quality of survival. Methods are available to evaluate management strategies based on both the clinical and economic outcomes of cancer. These methods have only recently been introduced into the study of cancer care in the elderly. Over the next decade, we can anticipate a great increase in our understanding of the effectiveness and costs of cancer screening, treatment and supportive care among the elderly. This should greatly aid both clinical and health planning to provide optimal quality and cost-effective care to the elderly patient with cancer.

References

1. Parker SL, Tong T, Bolden S, Wingo PA. Cancer Statistics, 1996. *CA Cancer J Clin* 1996; **65**: 5–27.
2. Miller BA, Ries LAG, Hankey BF, Kosary CL, Harras A, Devesa SS, Edwards BK. SEER Cancer Statistics Review: 1973–1990, National Cancer Institute. NIH Pub. No. 93–2789, 1993.
3. Cella DF, Bonomi AE. Measuring Quality of Life: 1995 Update. *Oncology* 1995; **9**: 47–60.
4. Ganz PA. Impact of Quality of Life Outcomes on Clinical Practice. *Oncology* 1995; **9**: 61–65.
5. Gelber RD, Goldhirsch A, Cavelli F. Quality-of-Life-Adjusted Evaluation of Adjuvant Therapy for Operable Breast Cancer. *Ann Int Med* 1991; **114**: 621–628.
6. Weeks J. Measurement of Utilities and Quality-Adjusted Survival. *Oncology* 1995; **9**: 67–70.
7. Brown ML. The National Economic Burden of Cancer: An Update. *J Natl Cancer Inst* 1990; **82**: 1811–1814.
8. Schuette HL, Tucker TC, Brown ML, Potosky AL, Samuel T. The costs of cancer care in the United States: Implications for Action. *Oncology* 1995; **9**: 19–22.
9. Vincenzino JV. Health Care Costs: Market Forces and Reform. *Oncology* 1995; **9**: 367–372.
10. Brown ML, Fintor L. The Economic Burden of Cancer, in Cancer Prevention and Control. New York: Marcel Dekker, 1995.
11. Baker MS, Kessler LC, et al: Site-specific Treatment Costs in Cancer in Cancer Care and Cost. *Health Administration Press* 1989.
12. Riley GF, Potosky AL, Lubitz JD, Kessler LG. Medicare Payments from Diagnosis to Death for Elderly Cancer Patients by Stage at Diagnosis. *Medical Care* 1995; **33**: 828–841.
13. Taplin SH, Barlow W, Urban N, Mandelson MT, Timlin DJ, Ichikawa L, Nefcy P. Stage, Age, Comorbidity and Direct Costs of Colon, Prostate and Breast Cancer Care. *J Nat Cancer Inst* 1995; **87**: 417–426.
14. Schulman KA, Yabroff KR. Measuring the Cost-Effectiveness of Cancer Care. *Oncology* 1995; **9**: 523–533.
15. Parker SG, Kassirer JP. Decision Analysis. *N Engl J Med* 1987; **316**: 250–258.
16. Detsky AS, Naglie IG. A Clinician's Guide to Cost-Effectiveness Analysis. *Ann Int Med* 1990; **113**: 147–154.
17. Udvarhelyi IS, Colditz GA, Rai A, Epstein AM. Cost-Effectiveness and Cost Benefit Analyses in the Medical Literature: Are the Methods being used correctly? *Ann Int Med* 1992; **116**: 238–244.
18. Task Force in Principles for Economic Analysis of Health Care Technology. Economic Analysis of Health Care Technology. *Ann Intern Med* 1995; **122**: 61–70.
19. Freer CB. Screening the Elderly. *Brit Med J* 1990; **300**: 1447–1448.
20. Oddone EZ, Feussner JR, Cohen HS. Cancer Screening Older Patients for Cancer Save Lives. *Clinics in Geriatric Medicine* 1992; **8**: 51–67.
21. List ND. Problems in Cancer Screening in the Older Patient. *Oncology* 1992; **6**: 25–30.
22. Samet JM, Hunt WC, Lerchen ML, Goodwin JS. Delay in Seeking Care for Cancer Symptoms: A Population-Based Study of Elderly New Mexicans. *J Natl Cancer Inst* 1988; **80**: 432–438.
23. Suarez L, Lloyd L, Weiss N, Rainbolt T, Pulley L. Effect of Social Networks on Cancer-Screening Behavior of Older Mexican-American Women. *J Natl Cancer Inst* 1994; **86**: 775–779.
24. List ND, Kucuk O. Approaches to and Effectivenss of Current Cancer Interventions in the Elderly. *Oncology* 1992; **6**: 31–38.
25. Power EJ. Pap Smears, Elderly Women and Medicare. *Cancer Investigation* 1993; **11**: 164–168.
26. Muller C, Mandelblatt J, Schacter CJ, et al: Costs and Effectiveness of Cervical Cancer Screening in Elderly Women. *Office of Technology Assessment*. Washington, DC, 1990.
27. Fahs MC, Mandelblatt J, Schechter C, Muller C. Cost Effectiveness of Cervical Cancer Screening for the Elderly. *Ann Int Med* 1992; **117**: 520–527.
28. Eddy DM. Screening for Cervical Cancer. *Ann Int Med* 1990; **113**: 214–216.
29. Solomon D. Screening for Cervical Cancer: Prospects for the Future. *J Natl Cancer Inst* 1993; **85**: 1018–1019.
30. Mandel JS, Bond JH, Church TR, Snover DC, Bradley GM, Schuman LM, Ederer F. Reducing Mortality from Colorectal Cancer by Screening for Fecal Occult Blood. *N Engl J Med* 1993; **328**: 1365–1371.
31. Lang CA, Ransohoff DF. Fecal Occult Blood Screening for Colorectal Cancer: Is Mortality Reduced by Chance Selection for Screening Colonoscopy. *J Am Med Assoc* 1994; **271**: 1011–1013.
32. Winawer SJ, Flehinger BJ, Schottenfeld D, Miller DG. Screening for Colorectal Cancer with Fecal Occult Blood Testing and Sigmoidoscopy. *J Natl Cancer Inst* 1993; **85**: 1311–1318.
33. Wagner JL, Herdman RC, Wadha S. Cost-Effectiveness of Colorectal Cancer Screening in the Elderly. *Ann Int Med* 1991; **115**: 807–817.
34. Eddy DM. Screening for Colorectal Cancer. *Ann Int Med* 1990; **113**: 373–384.
35. Lyman GH, Lyman S, Balducci L, Kuderer N, Reintgen D, Cox C, Backey P, Greenberg H, Horton J. Age and the Risk of Breast Cancer Recurrence. *Cancer Control* 1996; **3**: 421–427.
36. Sharpiro S, Venet W, Strax P, et al: Ten-to–14-year effect of screening on breast cancer mortality. *J Natl Cancer Inst* 1982; **69**: 349–355.
37. Fletcher SW, Black W, Harris R, Rimer BK, Shapiro S. Report of the International Workshop on Screening for Breast Cancer. *J Natl Cancer Inst* 1993; **85**: 1644–1656.
38. Kerlikowski K, Grady D, Rubin SM, Sandrock C, Ernster VL. Efficacy of Screening Mammography: A Meta-analysis. *J Am Med Assoc* 1995; **273**: 149–154.
39. Eddy DM. Screening for Breast Cancer. *Ann Int Med* 1989; **111**: 389–399.
40. Okubo I, Glick H, Frankin H, et al: Cost-Effectiveness analysis of mass screening for breast cancer in Japan. *Cancer* 1991; **67**: 2021–2019.
41. Brown ML. Sensitivity Analysis in the Cost-Effectiveness of Breast Cancer Screening. *Cancer* 1992; **69**: 1963–1967.
42. Mushlin AI, Fintor L. Is screening for breast cancer cost-effective? *Cancer* 1992; **69**: 1957–1962.
43. Hurley SF, Jolley DJ, Livingston PM, Reading D, Cockburn J, Flint-Richter D. Effectiveness, Cost and Cost-Effectiveness of Recruitment Strategies for a Mammography Screening Program to Detect Breast Cancer. *J Natl Cancer Inst* 1992; **84**: 855–863.
44. Brown ML. Economic Considerations in Breast Cancer Screening of Older Women. *The Journal of Gerontology* 1992; **47**: 51–58.
45. Mandelblatt JS, Wheat ME, Manane R, Moshief RD, Hollenberg JP, Tang J. Breast Cancer Screening for Elderly Women with and without comorbid conditions: A Decision Analysis Model. *Ann Int Med* 1992; **116**: 722–730.
46. Constanza ME. Issues in Breast Cancer Screening in Older Women. *Cancer* 1994; **74**: 2009–2015.
47. Nattinger AB, Goodwin JS. Screening Mammography for Older Women: A Case of Mixed Messages. *Arch Intern Med* 1992; **152**: 922–925.
48. Lettrup PJ, Goodman AC, Mettlin CJ. The Benefit and Cost of Prostate Cancer Early Detection. *Cancer J Clin* 1993; **43**: 134–149.
49. Krahn MD, Mahoney JE, Eckman MH, Trachtenberg J, Pauker SG, Detsky AS. Screening for Prostate Cancer: A Decision Analytic View. *J Am Med Assoc* 1994; **272**: 773–780.
50. Chodak GW. Screening for Prostate Cancer: The Debate Continues. *J Am Med Assoc* 1994; **272**: 813–814.
51. Smith TJ, Hillner BE, Desch CE. Efficacy and Cost-Effectiveness of Cancer Treatment: Rational Allocation of Resources Based on Decision Analysis. *J Natl Cancer Inst* 1993; **85**: 1460–1474.
52. Verhoef LC, Stalpers LJ, Verbeck AL, et al: Breast-conserving Treatment or Mastectomy in Early Breast Cancer: a Clinical Decision Analysis with Special Reference to the Risk of Local Recurrence. *Eur J Cancer* 1991; **27**: 1132–1137.

53. Beck JR, Pauker SG. The Markov Process in Medical Prognosis. *Med Decis Making* 1983; **3**: 419–458.

54. Smith, TJ, Hillner BE. The Efficacy and Cost-Effectiveness of Adjuvant Therapy of Early Breast Cancer in Pre-menopausal Women. *J Clin Oncol* 1993; **11**: 771–776.

55. Desch CE, Hillner BE, Smith TJ, Retchin SM. Should the Elderly Receive Chemotherapy for Node-Positive Breast Cancer? A Cost-Effectiveness Analysis Examining Total and Active Life-Expectancy Outcomes. *J Clin Oncol* 1993; **11**: 777–782.

56. Brown ML, Nayfield SG, Shibley LM. Adjuvant Therapy for Stage III Colon Cancer: Economics Returns to Research and Cost-Effectiveness of Treatment. *J Natl Cancer Inst* 1994; **86**: 424–430.

57. Djulbegovic B, Hollenberg J, Woodcock TM, *et al*: Comparison of Different Treatment Strategies for Diffuse Large Cell Lymphomas: a Decision Analysis. *Med Decis Making* 1991; **11**: 1–8.

58. Rutherford CJ, Deforges JF, Barnett HI, *et al*: The Decision Between Single-and Combined-Modality Therapy in Hodgkin's Disease. *Am J Med* 1982; **72**: 63–70.

59. Lobo PJ, Powles RL, Hanrahan A, *et al*. Acute Myeloblastic Leukemia — a Model for Assessing Value for Money for new treatment programs. *Brit Med J* 1991; **302**: 323–326.

60. Rees GJG. Cost Effectiveness in Oncology. *The Lancet* 1985; **2**: 1405–1408.

61. Glimelius B, Hoffman K, Graf W, Haglund U, Nyren O, Pahlman L, Sjöden PO. Cost Effectiveness of palliative chemotherapy in advanced gastrointestinal cancer. *Ann Oncol* 1995; **6**: 267–274.

62. Goodwin PJ, Feld R, Evans WK, Pater J. Cost-Effectiveness of Cancer Chemotherapy: An Economic Evaluation of a Randomized Trial in Small-cell Lung Cancer. *J Clin Oncol* 1988; **6**: 1537–1547.

63. Smith TJ, Hillner BE, Neighbors DM, McSorley PA, LeChevalier T: Economic Evaluation of a Randomized Clinical Trial Comparing Vinorelbine, Vinorelbine Plus Cisplatin, and Vindesine Plus Cisplatin for non-small cell Lung Cancer. *J Clin Oncol* 1995; **13**: 2166–2173.

64. Hillner BE, McLeod DG, Crawford ED, Bennett CL. Estimating the Cost-Effectiveness of Total Androgen Blockade with Flutamide in M1 Prostate Cancer. *Urology* 1995: 633–640.

65. Jaakkimainen L, Goodman PJ, Pater J, *et al*. Counting the Costs of Chemotherapy in a National Cancer Institute of Canada Randomized Trial of non-small cell Lung Cancer. *J Clin Oncol* 1990; **8**: 1301–1309.

66. Hillner BE, Smith TJ, Desch CE. Efficacy and Cost-Effectiveness of Autologous Bone Marrow Transplantation in Metastatic Breast Cancer: Estimates Using Decision Analysis While Awaiting Clinical Trial Results. *J Am Med Assoc* 1992; **267**: 2055–2061.

67. Desch CE, Lasala MR, Smith TJ, *et al*: The optimal timing of autologous bone marrow transplantation in Hodgkin's disease patients following a chemotherapy relapse. *J Clin Oncol* 1992; **10**: 200–209.

68. Lyman GH, Lyman CG, Sanders RA, Balducci L. Decision Analysis of hematopoietic growth factor use in patients receiving cancer chemotherapy. *J Natl Cancer Inst* 1993; **85**: 488–493.

69. Glaspy JA, Bleecker G, Crawford J, Stoller R, Strauss M. The Impact of Therapy with Filgrastin (Recombinant Granulocyte Colony-Stimulating Factor) on the Health Care Costs Associated with Cancer Chemotherapy. *Eur J Cancer* 1993; **29A**: S23–S30.

70. Lyman GH, Kuderer NM. Incorporating Quality of Life Considerations into Decision Models for the use of colony-stimulating factors in chemotherapy patients at risk for Febrile Neutropenia. In *Febrile Neutropenia*, edited by JA Klastersky. Heidelberg: Springer-Verlag, pp. 17–22, 1997.

71. Emanuel EJ, Emanuel LL. The Economics of Dying: The Illusion of Cost Savings at the End of Life. *N Engl J Med* 1994; **330**: 540–544.

72. Bailes JS. Cost Aspects of Palliative Cancer Care. *Seminars in Oncology* 1995; **22**: 64–66.

73. Portenoy RK. Issues in the Economic Analysis of Therapies for Cancer Pain. *Oncology* 1995; **9**: 71–77.

74. Bennett CL, Armitage JL, Buchner D, Gulati S. Economic Analysis in Phase III Clinical Cancer Trials. *Cancer Invest* 1994; **12**: 336–342.

75. Simes RJ: Risk Benefit Relationships in Cancer Clinical Trials: The ECOG Experience in Non-Small-Cell Lung Cancer. *J Clin Oncol* 1985; **3**: 462–472.

76. Bennett CL, Westerman IL. Economic Analysis During Phase III Clinical Trials: Who, What, When Where, and Why? *Oncology* 1995; **9**: 169–175.

Appendix 39.1

The declining exponential approximation of life expectancy (DEALE).

When the mortality rate is constant, the relationship between time and survival can be described as a declining exponential function. If S_o is the number of patients alive at diagnosis ($t = O$), S is the number of patients alive at some time T in the future ($t = T$) and m is the mortality rate, then this relationship can be described as:

$$S/S_o = e^{-mt}$$
$$\ln(S/S_o) = -mt$$
$$m = -1/t \ln(S/S_o)$$

This model has two major advantages over other models in terms of computational simplicity. First, the life expectancy, which is the average number of years of life remaining, is $1/m$ and therefore $m = 1/\text{Life Expectancy}$. If t is the median survival time, then $m = .693/t$. Second, an individual's total mortality rate is the sum of an individual's age-specific (AS) mortality rate and the mortality rate due to disease (D). Therefore,

$$m_{total} = m_{AS} + m_D$$
or
$$m_D = m_{total} - m_{AS}$$

If the mortality rate associated with a certain cancer is known, this information can be utilized to estimate the total life expectancy of an individual even if direct observational data is not available. In addition, if the patient has more than one disease impacting on longevity, the contributions of co-morbid conditions may be incorporated into the estimate of overall life expectancy.

For example, if we need to know the life expectancy (LE) of 65 year olds with a certain cancer (CA), but only have information on 50 year olds with the same cancer that 25% survive to five years,

For 50 year olds with cancer: $m_{total} = -1/5 \ln(.25) = .277$

If the LE of 50 year olds without disease is 30 years, then $m_{50} = .033$

Therefore, $m_{CA} = .277 - .033 = .244$

If the LE for 65 year olds without cancer is 20 years, then $m_{65} = .05$

We can then calculate results for the 65 year old with cancer as:

$$m_{total} = m_{65} + m_{CA}$$

$= .05 + .244 = .294$

Life expectancy $= 1 / .294 = 3.40$ years

If the patient also has coronary artery disease (CAD) with a mortality rate of .10, then the result for a 65 year old with cancer and coronary artery disease is:

$$m_{total} = m_{65} + m_{CA} + m_{CAD}$$
$$= .05 + .244 + .10 = .394$$

Life Expectancy $= 1 / .394 = 2.54$ years.

Appendix 39.2

Decision model threshold analysis based on benefits and costs

Each possible outcome in a realistic clinical situation can be considered to have a certain value or utility (U) and a certain probability of disease (p). The expected value of the treatment and no treatment strategies is therefore:

$$EV_{treatment} = p \cdot U_{treat/disease} + (1-p) \cdot U_{treat/no\ disease}$$

$$EV_{no\ treatment} = p \cdot U_{no\ treat/disease} + (1-p) \cdot U_{no\ treat/no\ disease}$$

The treatment strategy associated with the greatest expected value should be chosen in order to optimize the likelihood of the best result. The benefits and costs can be derived from utility estimates as shown:

Benefit of treatment $= U_{treat/disease} - U_{no\ treat/disease}$

Cost of treatment $= U_{no\ treat/no\ disease} - U_{treat/no\ disease}$

A sensitivity analysis can be conducted comparing the expected value functions as the probability of disease is varied. Most often, however, we are interested in determining the threshold probability at which point the expected value of the treatment strategies are equal, i.e.,

$$EV_{treatment} = EV_{no\ treatment}$$

or

$$p \cdot U_{treat/disease} + (1-p) \cdot U_{treat/no\ disease}$$
$$= p \cdot U_{no\ treat/disease} + (1-p) \cdot U_{no\ treat/no\ disease}$$

Solving for p,

$$P_{threshold} = \frac{U_{no\ treat/no\ disease} - U_{treat/no\ disease}}{U_{treat/disease} - U_{no\ treat/disease} + U_{no\ treat/no\ disease} - U_{treat/no\ disease}}$$

$$= Cost / (Benefit + Cost) = 1 / \{(Benefit / Cost) + 1\}$$

From such a relationship, it is evident that as the ratio of benefit to cost increases the threshold probability of disease decreases. Above the threshold probability of disease, treatment will be associated with a greater expected value and will therefore be the favored strategy. The indications for treatment therefore broaden as the ratio of benefit to cost increases.

Appendix 39.3

Cost discounting based on future and present cost.

Cost discounting is based on the preference to delay present costs to some future time. The cost discount is the difference between future cost and present cost. The cost discount rate (CDR) is the cost discount as a proportion of the present cost.

$$CDR = \frac{future\ cost - present\ cost}{present\ cost}$$

If the CDR is known, then future costs can be converted into costs referable to the present as:

$$CDR = \frac{future\ cost}{present\ cost} - 1$$

$$\frac{future\ cost}{present\ cost} = CDR + 1$$

$$present\ cost = \frac{future\ cost}{CDR + 1}$$

If the discounting is conducted over several (n) years, the present value is represented by:

$$Present\ value = \frac{future\ value}{(CDR + 1)^n}$$

40. Treatment of Acute Myeloid Leukemia in Older Patients

Thomas Büchner

Introduction

Acute myeloid leukemia (AML) in older patients appears as a particular disease as does the host in whom it occurs. When compared with AML in younger patients the disease more often emerges secondary to myelodysplasia (1) or treatment of a previous cancer (2), and even without such a history, karyotype changes associated with secondary AML (3–5) occur more frequently in the older patients (6–9). The observed abnormalities of chromosomes 5 and 7 and complex abnormalities are known to predict an unfavorable prognosis (6–10). In older patients with AML different from younger patients clonality markers of the leukemic cells were also positive in all hematopoietic cells (11). It has been suggested that neutropenia after chemotherapy lasts longer in older patients (12) and a defective pool of hematopoietic stem cells could prolong myelosuppression (13). This explains in part why patients 60 years of age and older treated in multicenter randomized trials did not achieve the same remission rates (14–17) and remission duration (14,16,17) as younger patients. However, all of these trials used reduced intensity chemotherapy in the higher age group so that an inadequate antileukemic treatment might have contributed to the inferior results. Since the optimum treatment of AML in older patients and the impact of their particular disease biology have remained open we present here an analysis of published data from major multicenter randomized clinical trials, including our own data. By using this approach we can address questions about differences in patient outcome according to higher age, the effects of treatment variables, the role of full dose chemotherapy in older patients, the potential benefit of hematopoietic growth factors and differences in the disease biology between older and younger patients.

General Trends in Chemotherapy for AML

The trends in modern chemotherapy for AML in patients of all ages are best exemplified by the multicenter randomized trials and their results published since 1981 (14–32). In those trials a total of 7.545 patients were treated. The overall complete remission rate is 63% and the probability to remain free from relapse after 4–5 years is 21%. These representative average results can serve as a standard in order to judge a specific result and its relative ranking. A cer-tain chronological trend can be seen in that five year remission rates in excess of 25% are only found in publications from the 1990s. The same, however, is true for the mortality in remission exceeding 10% thus indicating the limits of the generally increasing treatment intensity.

Table 40.1

Reference No.	Age	No. of Patients	% CR	% CCR at 4–5 Y
18	<55	448	68	24
19	<60	247	36–59 [1]	no age specific data [2]
20	<60	427	57–72 [3]	not given
21	<60	255	68	8–24 [4]
22	<60	257	66	no age specific data
16	<60	740	73	18
14	<60	564	65	17
23	<60	135	60	34
15	<60	226	69	no age specific data
24	<60	449	71	no age specific data
17	<60	742	71	24–44 [5]
25	<60	707	68	33
22	60–65	30	47	no age specific data
23	60–65	39	46	30
24	60–65	73	52	no age specific data
26	55–70	117	61	not given
19	>60	105	16–45 [6]	no age specific data [7]
20	>60	226	31–47 [8]	not given
21	>60	79	39	0–28 [9]
16	>60	305	48	9
14	>60	104	41	17
15	>60	100	41	no age specific data
17	>60	346	47	15
25	>60	340	42–54 [10]	22
13	>60	388	53	not given
27	>65	172	47–70 [11]	not given

[1] Cytarabine infusion better than bolus (p < .05) and 7 + 3 better than 5 + 2 (p < .01)
[2] Cytarabine in maintenance s.c. better than i.v. (p < .01)
[3] DNR 45 better than DNR 30 or ADR 30 (p < .05)
[4] Maintenance better than no maintenance (p < .001)
[5] DFS positively correlated to post-remission cytarabine dosage (p = .002)
[6] 7 + 3 better than 5 + 2 (p?)
[7] Cytarabine in maintenance better s.c. than i.v. (p < .01)
[8] DNR 30 better than DNR 45 or ADR 30 (p < .05)
[9] Maintenance better than no maintenance (p = .002)
[10] DNR 60 better than DNR 30 (p = .026)
[11] G-CSF better than no G-CSF (p = .002)

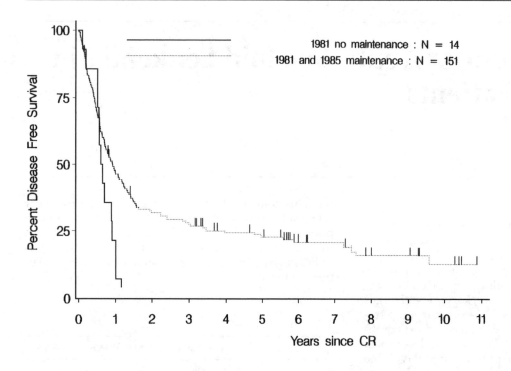

Figure 40.1 The role of prolonged maintenance in patients over age 60 demonstrated by the disease free survival in two trials of the AML-Cooperative Group. In the 1981 trial patients were randomized between maintenance and no maintenance. The identical maintenance was also used in all patients treated in the 1981 trial. Therefore, all maintenance patients in both trials are included in one combined result.

Treatment Outcome and Age

Table 40.1 represents complete remission rates and 4–5 year probabilities of continuous complete remission resulting from major multicenter randomized trials as far as age specific results have been reported. The data are listed in the order of increasing age of the groups of patients treated. Some of the reports presented significances of inferior results in older when compared with younger patients for complete remissions (14–16) and disease free survival (16). Table 40.1 reflects remission rates in excess of the multicenter trial average of 63% found in most patient groups under age 60 whereas with one exception (27) remission rates in older patients are below this average. The same is true for the average of 21% long term remissions which is exceeded by most of the results from younger patients (up to 65 years of age) and in only two results from older patients produced by the same study group and possibly reflecting a specific treatment effect (21, 25).

Therapeutic Outcome and Treatment Variables

Table 40.1 footnotes also indicate differences in treatment associated with significant differences in therapeutic outcome. When focusing on patients over age 60 the remission rates were significantly superior from daunorubicin 30 mg/m^2 than daunorubicin 45 mg/m^2 (20). In contrast, the more intensive induction regimen 7+3 was superior to 5+2 (19) and similarly daunorubicin 60 mg/m^2 was better than 30 mg/m^2 (25). G-CSF following induction treatment also significantly increased complete remissions in patients over age 65 (27). Regarding long term remissions, the only two results exceeding the average are from the administration of prolonged monthly myelosuppressive maintenance chemotherapy (21, 25).

The effect of prolonged maintenance is also demonstrated by Figure 40.1 for the disease free survival. The effects of full dose compared with reduced dose induction treatment (25) and prolonged maintenance versus no maintenance (21) in patients over age 60 strongly suggest that this strategy increases the response rates and provides long term disease free survival comparable to that from most study results in younger patients. Since the more intensive induction treatment also significantly reduced the rate of early and hypoplastic death (25) it may represent the treatment of choice for AML in older patients.

Recommended Standard Chemotherapy

Figure 40.2 presents the regimens used by the AML-Cooperative Group in their 1981 and 1985 trials referenced in Table 40.1 (21, 25). In addition, the combination of high dose cytarabine with mitoxantrone (HAM) as second induction course has also been used in patients over age 60 in the most recent 1992 trial. Among 80 older patients 59% went into complete remission with an adequate tolerability of this kind of escalation.

The Potential of Growth Factors

More than ten clinical trials have been investigating the therapeutic effect of hematopoietic growth factors administered after induction and/or consolidation chemotherapy. Those studies involving older patients with AML and their results are listed in Table 40.2 with five studies using GM-CSF and one using G-CSF. A significant reduction of neutropenia was achieved in all six studies which, in part, translated into a reduction in mortality (33), higher grade infections (26), higher remission rate (27), longer survival (26) and even disease free survival (34). Toxicity like fever and fluid

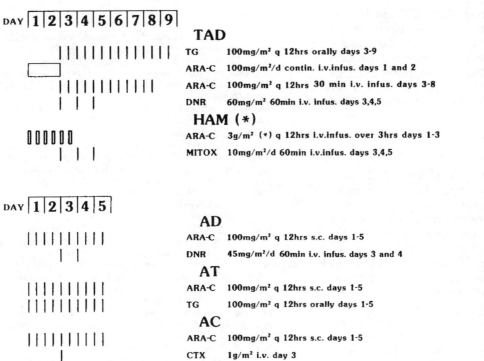

TAD

TG	100mg/m² q 12hrs orally days 3-9
ARA-C	100mg/m²/d contin. i.v.infus. days 1 and 2
ARA-C	100mg/m² q 12hrs 30 min i.v. infus. days 3-8
DNR	60mg/m² 60min i.v. infus. days 3,4,5

HAM (*)

| ARA-C | 3g/m² (*) q 12hrs i.v.infus. over 3hrs days 1-3 |
| MITOX | 10mg/m²/d 60min i.v.infus. days 3,4,5 |

AD

| ARA-C | 100mg/m² q 12hrs s.c. days 1-5 |
| DNR | 45mg/m²/d 60min i.v. infus. days 3 and 4 |

AT

| ARA-C | 100mg/m² q 12hrs s.c. days 1-5 |
| TG | 100mg/m² q 12hrs orally days 1-5 |

AC

| ARA-C | 100mg/m² q 12hrs s.c. days 1-5 |
| CTX | 1g/m² i.v. day 3 |

TG = 6-thioguanine, ARA-C = cytosine arabinoside, DNR = daunorubicin,
MITOX = mitoxantrone, CTX = cytoxan

* in patients of 60 years ARA-C 1 instead of 3g/m²

Figure 40.2 Therapeutic regimens used by the AML-Cooperative Group. In the 1981 trial patients of all ages received one to two courses of TAD for induction and were then randomized to one TAD for consolidation with or without subsequent monthly maintenance by alternating courses of AD or AT or AC for three years. Since significantly superior the same consolidation and maintenance was given to all patients in the 1985 trial. In this trial all patients under age 60 received a second induction course in any case and were randomized to the sequence TAD TAD or TAD HAM. Patients over age 60 in the 1985 trial received TAD as second induction but only in case of residual blasts and were randomized to DNR in TAD either 60 or 30 mg/m². In the 1992 trial patients over age 60 all receive full dose TAD as first induction and, if required, second induction by HAM.

Table 40.2 Supportive use of growth factors in older patients with AML: Synopsis of clinical studies.

Reference No.	Special Risk	Product	Growth Factor Daily Dose	Start	Controls	Chemotherapy Dose	No. Patients	GF Benefit	No Difference	GF Worse
33	early/mult. relapse or age 65+	GM-CSF (yeast)	250 μg/m²	day four after chemo	historic	relapses high-dose age 65+ standard	112	– neutropenia (p = .02) – mortality (p = .009)	– disease-free-survival – leukemic regrowth	
26	age 55–70	GM-CSF (yeast)	250 μg/m²	day four after chemo	placebo	standard	124	– neutropenia (p = .001) – grade 4/5 infections (p = .002) – survival (p = .048)	– disease-free survival	
13	age 60+	GM-CSF (E. coli)	5 μg/kg	day one after chemo	placebo	standard	388	– neutropenia (p = .02)	– mortality – remissions – leukemic regrowth – survival – hospitalization	
34	age 55–75	GM-CSF (E. coli)	5 μg/kg	with start of chemo	placebo	standard	209	– neutropenia (p = .002) – disease-free survival (p = .024)	– mortality – remissions – infections – survival – hospitalization	
35	age 60+	GM-CSF (E. coli)	5 μg/kg	day one before chemo	random	standard	326	– neutropenia (p = .001)	– remissions – infections – survival – disease-free survival	– fever – fluid retention
27	age 65+	G-CSF	5 μg/kg	day two after chemo	placebo	standard	172	– neutropenia (p < .001) – remissions (p = .002)	– mortality at 8 weeks – infections – leukemic regrowth – survival	

retention was only found in one study (35) and, importantly, adverse affects on the course of leukemia were not observed in any study. Although the study results leave questions about the definite clinical benefit open there are good evidences that the supportive use of growth factors in high risk populations like older patients may facilitate a full dose and even intensified chemotherapy in this age group.

AML Biology and Age

There are some features that characterize AML as a rather unfavorable disease category when compared with AML occurring in younger patients. Thus, a history of myelodysplasia (1) or treatment of a previous cancer (2) or abnormalities of chromosomes 5 and 7 and complex abnormalities associated with secondary AML (3–5) are more frequent in higher age. The AML-Cooperative Group compared among some 1000 patients with newly diagnosed AML those over 60 years of age with those under 60 (25). There was no major difference in prognostic factors like morphological subtype, white blood cell count or LDH in serum. Cytogenetics, however, disclosed significant differences in that the favorable translocations t (15; 17), t (8; 21) and inversion 16 almost did not occur and the unfavorable abnormalities of chromosomes 5 and 7 and complex karyotypes occurred three times as frequent in the older age group. Thus, the karyotype differences in favor of the younger patients amounted to 42% of patients. No difference, however, was found in the recovery time of neutrophils and platelets according to age (unpublished data).

Summary and Perspectives

Results from multicenter trials treating AML in older patients has remained disappointing. This is explained, in part, by the frequent comorbidity that makes chemotherapy less tolerable. It is also explained by the less favorable disease biology of AML in higher age, especially reflected by unfavorable chromosome abnormalities supposed to cause chemoresistance. While full dosage or even intensified chemotherapy would be required to overcome the increased chemoresistance in older patients most of the trials used reduced dosage in this age group. However, full versus reduced dose induction treatment and prolonged maintenance versus no maintenance proved significantly superior in complete remission rates, tolerability of chemotherapy and long term disease free survival approaching that published from younger patients. Thus, instead of attenuating chemotherapy, full dosage or even further intensification (see Figure 40.2) appears more promising for improving the results. A more effective antimicrobial strategy including support by hematopoietic growth factors can provide a basis for further developing the antileukemic strategy in older patients.

References

1. Hamblin TJ. The treatment of acute myeloid leukaemia preceded by the myelodysplastic syndrome. *Leuk Res* 1992: **16**: 4101–8.
2. Hoyle CF, de Bastos M, Wheatley K, et al. AML associated with previous cytotoxic therapy. MDS or myelo-proliferative disorders: results from the MRC's 9th AML trial. *Br J Haematol* 1989; **72**: 45–53.
3. Second International Workshop on Chromosomes in Leukemia. *Cancer Genet Cytogenet* 1980; **2**: 89–113.
4. Rowley J. Annotation: Chromosome changes in acute leukaemia. *Br J Haematol* 1980; **44**: 339–346.
5. Yunis JJ, Lobell M, Arnesen MA, et al. Refined chromosome study helps define prognostic subgroups in most patients with primary myelodysplastic syndrome and acute myelogenous leukaemia. *Br J Haematol* 1988; **68**: 189–194.
6. Fourth International Workshop on Chromosomes in Leukemia. *Cancer Genet Cytogenet* 1984; **11**: 332–350.
7. Keating MJ, Smith TL, Kantarjian H, et al. Cytogenetic pattern in acute myelogenous leukemia: a major reproducible determinant of outcome. *Leukemia* 1988; **2**: 403–412.
8. Schiffer CA, Lee EJ, Tomiyasu T, et al. Prognostic impact of cytogenetic abnormalities in patients with de novo acute nonlymphocytic leukemia. *Blood* 1989; **73**: 263–270.
9. Swansbury GJ, Lawler SD, Alimena G, et al. Long-term survival in acute myelogenous leukemia: A second follow up of the Fourth International Workshop on chromosomes in leukemia. *Cancer Genet Cytogenet* 1994; **73**: 1–7.
10. Yunis JJ, Brunninng RD, Howe RB, et al. High-resolution chromosomes as an independent prognostic indicator in adult acute nonlymphocytic leukemia. *N Engl J Med* 1984; **311**: 812–818.
11. Fialkow PJ, Singer JW, Raskind WH, et al. Clonal development, stem-cell differentiation, and clinical remissions in acute nonlymphocytic leukemia. *N Engl J Med* 1987; **317**: 468–73.
12. Hamblin TJ. Meeting report: 1st International Conference on reversal of multidrug resistance in cancer. *Leuk Res* 1995; **19**: 509–14.
13. Stone RM, Berg TB, George SL, et al. Granulocyte macrophage colony-stimulating factor after initial chemotherapy for elderly patients with primary acute myelogenous leukemia. *N Engl J Med* 1995; **332**: 1671–1677.
14. Preisler H, Davis RB, Kirshner J, et al. Comparison of three remission induction regimens and two postinduction strategies for the treatment of acute nonlymphocytic leukemia: A Cancer and Leukemia Group B Study. *Blood* 1987; **69**: 1441–1449.
15. Dillman RO, Davis RB, Green MR, et al. A comparative study of two different doses of cytarabine for acute myeloid leukemia: A phase III trial of Cancer and Leukemia Group B. *Blood* 1991; **78**: 2520–2526.
16. Rees JKH, Gray RG, Swirsky D, Hayhoe FGJ. Principal results of the Medical Research Council's 8th acute myeloid leukaemia trial. *The Lancet* 1986; **332**: 1236.
17. Mayer RJ, Davis RB, Schiffer CA, et al. Intensive postremission chemotherapy in adults with acute myeloid leukemia. *New Engl J Med* 1994; **6**: 896–942.
18. Mandelli F, Vegna ML, Avvisati G, et al. A randomized study of the efficacy of postconsolidation therapy in adult acute nonlymphocytic leukemia: a report of the Italian Cooperative Group GIMEMA. *Ann Hematol* 1992; **64**: 166–172.
19. Rai KR, Hollannd JF, Glidewell OJ, et al. Treatment of acute myeloid leukemia: A study by Cancer and Leukemia Group B. *Blood* 1981; **58**: 1203–1212.
20. Yates J, Glidewell O, Wiernik P, et al. Cytosine arabinoside with daunorubicin or adriamycin for therapy of acute myelocytic leukemia: A CALGB study. *Blood* 1982; **60**: 454–462.
21. Büchner T, Urbanitz D, Hiddemann W, et al. Intensified induction and consolidation with or without maintenance chemotherapy for acute myeloid leukemia (AML): Two multicenter studies of the German AML Cooperative Group. *J Clin Oncol* 1985; **3**: 1583–1589.

22. Hayat M, Jehn U, Willemze R, *et al.* A randomized comparison of maintenance treatment with androgens, immunotherapy, and chemotherapy in adult acute myelogenous leukemia. *Cancer* 1986; **58**: 617–623.

23. Hansen OP, Pedersen-Bjergaard J, Ellegaard J, *et al.* Aclarubicin plus cytosine arabinoside versus daunorubicin plus cytosine arabinoside in previously untreated patients with acute myeloid leukemia: a Danish National Phase III Trial. *Leukemia* 1991; **5**: 510–516.

24. Cassileth PA, Lynch E, Hines JD, *et al.* Varying intensity of postremission therapy in acute myeloid leukemia. *Blood* 1992; **79**: 1924–1930.

25. Büchner T, Hiddemann W, Loffler H, *et al.* Treatment of AML in the elderly: Full-dose versus reduced dose induction treatment. *Blood* 1995; **86** (1): 434 a.

26. Rowe JM, Andersen JW, Mazza JJ, *et al.* A randomized placebo-controlled phase III study of granulocyte macrophage colony-stimulating factor in adult patients (>55 to 70 years of age) with acute myelogenous leukemia: A study of the Eastern Cooperative Oncology Group (E1490). *Blood* 1995; **86**: 457–462.

27. Dombret H, Chastang C, Fenaux P, *et al.* A controlled study of recombinant human granulocyte colony-stimulating factor in elderly patients after treatment for acute myelogenous leukemia. *N Engl J Med* 1995; **332**: 1678–1683.

28. Vogler WR, Winton EF, Gordon DS, *et al.* A randomized comparison of postremission therapy in acute myelogenous leukemia. A Southeastern Cancer Study Group trial. *Blood* 1984; **63**: 1039–1045.

29. Zittoun RA, Mandelli F, Willemze R, *et al.* Autologous or allogeneic bone marrow transplantation compared with intensive chemotherapy in acute myelogenous leukemia. *N Engl J Med* 1995; **332**: 217–223.

30. Vogler WR, Velez-Garcia E, Weiner S, *et al.* A phase III trial comparing idarubicin and daunorubicin in combination with cytarabine in acute myelogenous leukemia: A Southeastern Cancer Study Group Study. *J Clin Oncol* 1992; **10**: 1103–1111.

31. Zittoun R, Jehn U, Fiere D, *et al.* Alternating v repeated postremission treatment in adult acute myelogenous leukemia: A randomized phase III study (AML6) of the EORTC Leukemia Cooperative Group. *Blood* 1989; **73**: 896–906.

32. Büchner T, Hiddemann W, Schaefer UW, *et al.* Combined effect of very early intensification and prolonged postremission chemotherapy in patients with AML. *Leukemia* 1992; **5** (suppl 4): 68–70.

33. Büchner T, Hiddemann W, Koenigsmann M, *et al.* Recombinant human granulocyte-macrophage colony stimulating factor after chemotherapy in patients with acute myeloid leukemia at higher age or after relapse. *Blood* 1991; **78**: 1190–1197.

34. Witz F, Harousseau JL, Cahn JY, *et al.* GM-CSF during and after remission induction treatment for elderly patients with acute myeloid leukemia (AML). *Ann Hematol* 1995; **70** (Suppl II): 163: A135.

35. Lowenberg B, Suciu S, Zittoun R, *et al.* GM-CSF during as well as after induction chemotherapy (CT) in elderly patients with acute myeloid leukemia (AML). The EORTC/HOVON Phase III trial (AML 11). *Blood* 1995; **86** Suppl II: 433.

41. Chronic Lymphoid Leukemias

Alexander Spiers

Introduction

This chapter will consider the diagnosis, clinical features, and management of a group of disorders that are characterized by the neoplastic proliferation of relatively mature (i.e. not blastic) lymphocytes, with involvement of the peripheral blood and the bone marrow. There are numerous subvarieties of chronic lymphoid leukemia (Table 41.1), but the T cell varieties are all so uncommon as to be of lesser importance clinically. Of the B cell leukemias, chronic lymphocytic leukemia (B-CLL or simply CLL) is by far the most frequent and the most important and will be the principal subject of discussion. For many years a relatively neglected disease, CLL has in the last decade been the focus of much important research that has increased our understanding of its biology and significantly improved its management, to the benefit of many older patients.

Terminology and Classification

The terminology outlined in Table 41.1 is widely accepted, although some variations are encountered. For example, some authors have reclassified many cases of T cell chronic lymphocytic leukemia (T-CLL) as a subacute, not a chronic, process (1), while others flatly deny the existence of T-CLL as a disease entity. The

Table 41.1 Chronic leukemias that are encountered in the older person.

Chronic myeloid leukemias

    chronic granulocytic leukemia (cgl)

    chronic myelomonocytic leukemia (cmml)

    rare subvarieties of chronic myeloid neoplasia

Chronic lymphoid leukemias

    B cell chronic lymphocytic leukemia (B-CLL)

    B cell prolymphocytic leukemia (B-PLL)

    B cell hairy cell leukemia (B-HCL)

    B cell lymphomas with blood involvement

    T cell variants of the above disorders (uncommon)

    Unique T cell disorders:

        Sezary syndrome

        Adult T cell leukemia/lymphoma (ATLL)

        Large granular lymphocytic (LGL) leukemia

nomenclature of the chronic lymphoid leukemias was until recently based mainly on morphologic considerations; descriptions of cells as "mature" or "differentiated" were based on their appearance. The ability to characterize cells by *surface markers*, antigenic determinants that are located on the cell membrane, led to major conceptual changes, the first and greatest of which was the recognition of T and B cells. With the advent of automated *flow cytometry* and the ability to study the surface markers of thousands of cells in every patient, subtle differences that are undetectable by morphologic methods alone are emerging. For example, the cells of B-CLL, despite their mature appearance, turn out to be more primitive than previously suspected. With the widespread application of flow cytometry, more accurate diagnoses of lymphoid neoplasms are now made, and revisions to current terminology can be anticipated. It remains to be seen to what extent these fine distinctions will be clinically important in selecting the most appropriate management for each patient.

B Cell Chronic Lymphocytic Leukemia (B-CLL or CLL)

Definition

CLL is a neoplastic disease of unknown etiology characterized by an absolute lymphocytosis in the bone marrow and peripheral blood. There is a usually leisurely proliferation but remorselessly progressive accumulation of monoclonal, long-lived, mature-appearing B lymphocytes that are immunoincompetent and indeed produce immunosuppression. Whereas many other clinical features are regularly encountered in CLL, for example lymphadenopathy, splenomegaly, hepatomegaly, hematopoietic failure, hypogammaglobulinemia, and autoimmune phenomena, none is constant or essential to the diagnosis.

Presentation

CLL is the leukemia *par excellence* of the older person (Table 41.2). It is rarely seen in patients aged less than 40 years, and its incidence increases steadily with advancing age, apparently without limit as it continues to rise in the ninth and tenth decades of life. The incidence of CLL increases 350-fold when ages 25 to 29 are compared with ages 80 to 84 (2). A high *incidence* of CLL (approximately one-third of all new cases of leukemia) combines with a lengthy *survival* to produce a high *prevalence* of the condition; CLL comprises

Table 41.2 Concurrent medical problems that affect the management of chronic leukemia in the older person.

Problem	Consequences
Intellectual impairment	Problems with adherence to treatment
Chronic lung disease	Mortality from intercurrent infection; problems with some cytotoxic drugs
Hypertension	Cerebral hemorrhage when thrombocytopenic
Angina	Poor tolerance of anemia
Cardiac failure	Poor tolerance of transfusion
Atherosclerosis	Poor tolerance of anemia and leukocytosis
Arthritis	Medications promote GI hemorrhage
Diabetes mellitus	Exacerbations with corticosteroid therapy
Liver disease	Altered drug metabolism
Diverticulosis	Infection, perforation, sepsis
Renal impairment	Poor tolerance of hyperuricemia; problems with antibiotic therapy
Uterine prolapse	Urinary tract infections
Prostatomegaly	Urinary tract infections
Incontinence	Decubitus ulcers
Other primary cancers	Multiple complications, depending on the primary site

This list is not exhaustive. Consideration must also be given to the psychological, social, environmental and economic problems that have a profound impact on the practice of geriatric oncology.

approximately half of all cases of leukemia in Western populations. It is safe to say that almost every geriatric practice or long term care facility will have one or more patients with CLL, and physicians in every medical specialty will regularly encounter patients with this important disease. There is a *male predominance* that appears to have decreased with time; early in this century the male-to-female ratios for CLL in Western countries ranged from 2.5 to 3.0, whereas in more recent studies they are between 1.6 and 1.9 (2). There are rare *families* that show clustering of cases of CLL, sometimes in association with cases of lymphoma or of immunological diseases. *Geographic* and *ethnic* variation in rates is greater for CLL than for any other type of leukemia (3). The highest incidences of CLL are observed in whites in North America and in northern and eastern Europe, lower rates are reported from South America and the Caribbean, and exceptionally low rates are found in India, Japan, China, and other areas of Asia, where CLL is a truly rare disease. The reason for these fascinating variations that are peculiar to CLL is unknown. The geriatric oncologist who practises in North America is in an area where the incidence of CLL is very high, and continues to increase as the population ages.

Symptoms

More than any other leukemia, CLL is apt to be diagnosed when it is still asymptomatic. A common scenario is the senior citizen who requires a surgical procedure for one of the conditions that are frequent in older age, for example inguinal hernia, uterine prolapse, or prostatomegaly. A routine preoperative blood count shows a marked absolute lymphocytosis, a follow-up bone marrow examination shows infiltration with mature-appearing lymphocytes, and flow cytometry shows the circulating lymphocytes to be positive for surface membrane immunoglobulin (sIg) and the CD5 and CD21 antigens, findings typical for B-CLL. At one time, establishing the diagnosis of CLL would have led to the immediate cancellation of surgery, which would have been appropriate if *acute* leukemia had been diagnosed, but quite unnecessary for most patients with asymptomatic CLL. It is now widely recognized that the diagnosis of uncomplicated CLL does not preclude the provision of necessary surgery or other treatment, and indeed may not alter the patient's lifestyle or longevity in any way.

Because routine physical examinations and blood tests in the absence of symptoms are becoming a regular feature of modern health care, increasing numbers of patients are being diagnosed with early CLL. Furthermore, flow cytometry has conferred the ability to diagnose CLL at a particularly early stage, when an absolute lymphocytosis has not been established, but a *monoclonal* lymphocytosis is unequivocally demonstrable. As a result of these advances, the survival of patients with CLL is likely to increase significantly, but it should be remembered that much of this "improvement" will be factitious and due to the statistical phenomenon of *lead time bias*.

Some patients with CLL present with symptoms that are often associated with malignancy and with immunodeficiency disorders: malaise, weakness, night sweats, fever without apparent infection, and weight loss. Such constitutional symptoms are less frequent in CLL than they are in Hodgkin's disease.

Other patients with CLL may present with symptoms of *anemia* - loss of energy, fatigue, dyspnea, anorexia, weight loss and pallor. In the older person with cardiac disease or peripheral vascular disease, the symptoms of anemia may be angina, cardiac failure, or intermittent claudication. In the older person with CLL, the anemia may be exacerbated — or be entirely due to — intercurrent unrelated problems, for example gastrointestinal bleeding or vitamin B_{12} or folate deficiency. A less frequent presentation of CLL is with symptoms attributable to *thrombocytopenia*: bruising, purpura, or hemorrhage. Presentation with *infection* is more common; patients with CLL are prone to infection by reason of hypogammaglobulinemia, decreased T cell function, neutropenia or combinations of these defects. Respiratory tract infections, particularly bronchitis and bronchopneumonia, may be the precipitating problem that leads to the diagnosis of CLL. Some patients present with the symptoms of one of the *autoimmune* disorders that are frequent in patients with CLL: immune thrombocytopenic purpura, autoimmune hemolytic anemia, or connective tissue disease.

Some patients with CLL initially present with symptoms of organomegaly. *Lymphadenopathy* in the neck, axilla, or groin may become quite severe before it is symptomatic. In CLL, *splenomegaly* is less frequent and usually much less marked than it is in chronic granulocytic leukemia, and symptomatic enlargement of the spleen is rarely a cause of initial presentation. Similarly, *splenic infarction* is rare in CLL.

Although *leukocytosis* greater than $200 \times 10^9/l$ is common in untreated CLL, it is almost never symptomatic. Hyperviscosity of the blood and leukostatic lesions in the lungs and brain, frequent in AML with a high blast cell count, have been reported in CLL (4) but are very rare, even when the leukocyte count exceeds one million per microliter. This is because the lymphocyte of CLL, unlike the myeloblast, is small, readily deformable, relatively nonadherent, and does not invade blood vessel walls. Thus emergency treatment for hyperleukocytosis is rarely required in CLL, and the height of the leukocyte count *per se* is seldom an indication for treatment. Most patients, and not a few physicians, are difficult to convince that this is so.

Physical Signs

The patient with CLL may not only be asymptomatic but also may have no physical signs that are referable to the disease. When abnormal findings are present, *pallor* and *lymphadenopathy* are the most frequent. Lymphadenopathy may be found in a single area or in multiple lymph node fields. The nodes are typically soft, mobile, nontender, and not matted together, and generally they are small, in the 1–2 cm range. Massive lymphadenopathy, with a bull neck or a severely distorted axilla, occurs but is uncommon. Lymphedema is rarely associated with the lymphadenopathy of CLL.

Clinically, the enlarged lymph nodes of CLL are quite different from nodes that are involved by carcinoma. *Splenomegaly* is frequently absent, and when present is rarely massive; splenic enlargement that extends below the umbilicus or across the midline is more suggestive of chronic granulocytic leukemia, prolymphocytic leukemia, or hairy cell leukemia. *Hepatomegaly*, if present at diagnosis, is usually mild. *Bruises* and *purpura* are not frequent features of newly diagnosed CLL, but both conditions may be observed in the older person in the absence of any hematologic disease, as a consequence of decreased elasticity of the skin. *Cutaneous infiltrates* may occur in B-CLL but are more frequent in the rare T cell variant of the disease. Lesions of *herpes zoster* are not uncommon in CLL and are sometimes a presenting feature. Presentation with meningeal involvement (5) or with neurologic problems suggestive of progressive multifocal leukoencephalopathy (6) is rare but important to bear in mind, particularly in the older patient in whom central nervous system disorders of diverse etiology are relatively frequent.

Laboratory Findings

CLL is characterized by an absolute and sustained lymphocytosis in the peripheral blood, with predominantly mature-appearing lymphocytes, although some atypical forms can be detected in most cases and in a few instances 50% or more of the cells possess atypical morphologic features. There is an accompanying lymphocytosis in the bone marrow but evidence of bone marrow failure — anemia, neutropenia, or thrombocytopenia — is frequently absent.

A Working Group sponsored by the National Cancer Institute has further specified typical cases of B-CLL that can be considered for protocol studies (7). Marker studies should show sIg+, CD19+, CD20+, or CD24+. The cells must be CD5+ but negative for other pan-T markers, express either kappa *or* lambda light chains, and sIg must be present at low density. The minimum threshold for blood lymphocytes is $5 \times 10^9/l$ and the blood lymphocytosis must be sustained over a period of at least 4 weeks upon repeated examinations. The lymphocytes must appear mature and no more than 55% may be atypical prolymphocytes or lymphoblasts. Patients with 11%–55% prolymphocytes — so-called prolymphocytic/CLL — should be considered for special studies because the prognostic significance of their high incidence of cellular atypia is not well-defined. The *bone marrow aspirate* must contain ≥30% lymphoid cells. The bone marrow *biopsy* may show diffuse or nodular lymphocytic infiltration and the marrow must be normocellular or hypercellular.

The above specification is not universally accepted. Some hematologists will diagnose CLL when the lymphocytosis is less than $5 \times 10^9/l$ if a B cell monoclone with the appropriate surface markers is demonstrable. While such cases may indeed have CLL at an early stage, their inclusion in clinical studies may affect survival data by the mechanism of lead time bias referred to earlier.

Cytogenetic Findings in CLL

This topic has recently been reviewed in depth (8) and only a few salient features will be considered here. Most types of chromosomal analysis require dividing cells that are in metaphase. Whereas this is no great problem in the acute leukemias or in CGL, it is a major obstacle in CLL, since the tumor cells have a very low mitotic index and must be activated in vitro with mitogens that are effective for B cells (e.g. *E. coli* lipopolysaccharide, Epstein-Barr virus). Cells from some patients with CLL do not respond to mitogens and evaluable metaphases cannot be obtained; it is not known if such unresponsive cells harbor any chromosomal anomalies.

Cytogenetic techniques in CLL cells have shown two major chromosomal abnormalities with a probable pathogenetic role: trisomy-12 and deletions of the long arm of chromosome #13 (13q14). No relevant gene on chromosome #12, and no pathogenetic mechanism by which the occurrence of trisomy-12 may lead to the development of CLL, has been documented. Terminal deletions of the long arm of chromosomes #6 and #11 might also be significant in CLL. Additional material on the long arm of chromosome #14 (14q+) to form a marker chromosome is a common additional abnormality that does not appear to be of prognostic significance. Trisomy-12 has been associated with a poor survival, whereas 13q deletions or a normal karyotype indicate a good prognosis. Complex abnormal karyotypes in the CLL cells are more commonly found at diagnosis than developing during the course of the disease, and are adverse prognostic signs.

Despite their undoubted interest and prognostic significance, it has not been convincingly shown that cytogenetic studies in CLL provide information beyond that which is obtainable from clinically staging the disease (see below).

Natural History and Prognosis of CLL

General

While it is true that CLL may run a very long and extremely indolent course, there has been a strong tendency to overemphasize the supposedly benign nature of the disease and to use this as a pretext for undertreatment. While some patients with CLL may live for more than 20 years, never require treatment for leukemia, and die from unrelated causes, most patients do far less well than this. The fact that most patients with CLL are elderly and many suffer from multiple medical problems (Table 41.2) means that in some instances the leukemia will not be the limiting factor in their survival and will not require treatment. However, many elderly people with CLL will die from the disease and effective treatment for CLL can be expected to improve both the quality and the duration of life. This is especially so now that life expectancy in the elderly has improved significantly. A 75-year-old woman has a life expectancy of 12 years; a new diagnosis of CLL with a six-year prognosis is certainly *not* a benign event.

Table 41.3 Transformations and complications in chronic lymphocytic leukemia.

acceleration without morphologic change

prolymphocytoid acceleration

Richter's syndrome: non-Hodgkin's lymphoma

Richter's syndrome: Hodgkin's disease

multiple myeloma

acute lymphocytic leukemia

acute myeloid leukemia

additional primary cancers

The Progression of CLL

Although the *rate* at which progression occurs is very variable, in almost every case of CLL there is ongoing replication of leukemia cells and the progressive accumulation of long-lived, immunoincompetent CLL cells. This increasing leukemic cell mass can induce *hematopoietic failure* with consequent anemia, thrombocytopenia, neutropenia and their complications. There is also progressive *immunologic failure*, with deficient humoral and cellular immunity, and *immune dysregulation* with the onset of autoimmune diseases. In very advanced CLL, the *leukemic cell mass* causes problems directly: hypersplenism, compression of vital structures, hypermetabolism, and cachexia. Unless death occurs from an unrelated intercurrent disease, untreated CLL progresses inexorably to a fatal termination, whether this be in 12 months or 20 years.

Transformations of CLL

During its usually lengthy course, CLL may undergo a distinct transformation to a more adverse process; this is much less frequent than the evolution that is seen in almost every case of CGL. Transformations of CLL and some neoplastic complications of the disease are listed in Table 41.3.

Acceleration of the disease to a more aggressive phase is relatively common and its time of onset is unpredictable. The blood lymphocytosis increases rapidly and the lymph nodes, liver and spleen enlarge progressively. The patient may develop constitutional symptoms and hematopoietic failure and immunodeficiency appear or worsen. Although matters may be improved with treatment, resistance to previously effective drug therapy usually appears and the patient dies from progressive and refractory CLL. In some patients, acceleration of CLL is accompanied by increasing numbers of prolymphocytoid cells in the peripheral blood and this is termed *prolymphocytoid acceleration* (9). Although the cells resemble prolymphocytes, their surface immunoglobulin density is low, like that of CLL cells, and not high as in *de novo* prolymphocytic leukemia. The immunoglobulin type is the same as that of the original CLL cells, from which the prolymphocytoid cells are apparently evolved. Once prolymphocytoid acceleration has occurred, responsiveness to therapy declines and progressive clinical deterioration is the rule. The evolution of a large cell lymphoma in a patient with CLL was first described in 1928 and bears the eponym *Richter's syndrome* (10). The literature relating to this development of CLL has recently been reviewed (11). The clinical features of Richter's syndrome include fever, weight loss, increasing lymphadenopathy, splenomegaly, hepatomegaly, lymphocytopenia, and resistance to both chemotherapy and radiation therapy. Rapid clinical deterioration is the rule; many cases of Richter's syndrome have been diagnosed at autopsy. This transformation occurs in less than 10% of patients with CLL; it appears to be more frequent in patients with multiple chromosome abnormalities in the CLL cells and a monoclonal gammopathy in the peripheral blood. In the older patient, Richter's syndrome is difficult to treat because aggressive therapies are apt to be poorly tolerated. Although Richter's syndrome usually involves a non-Hodgkin's lymphoma, cases of *Hodgkin's disease* have been reported. A very rare *myelomatous transformation* of CLL has been reported, with the heavy and light chains of the myeloma cells identical to those of the original CLL cells (12). After this transformation survival is reported as short. Whereas transformation to a picture resembling acute myeloid leukemia occurs in over 75% of patients with CGL, transformation to *acute lymphocytic leukemia* is seen in less than 1% of patients with CLL (13). In most cases the lymphoblasts are of L2 morphology. *Acute myeloid leukemia* appears to occur with increased frequency in patients with CLL, even after adjusting for their older age. It is not thought that the AML is a direct development from the CLL cells. The reason for the association is unclear; whereas treatment of the CLL with the leukemogenic alkylating agent chlorambucil may account for some cases of AML, the two diseases have been observed concurrently in patients with CLL who have never received any treatment. Reports on the occurrence of *additional primary cancers* in patients with CLL are conflicting (11), although Whipham (14) first reported the association in 1878. Gunz and Angus (15) reported that, except for an increased number of skin cancers, the incidence of other malignant diseases in CLL was not significantly higher. A later study at Roswell Park Memorial Institute (16) indicated an increased incidence of second cancers in patients with CLL; after skin cancers, lung cancer was the most frequent (14/191 patients). The confounding effects of age and smoking make firm interpretation of the data difficult, but it seems reasonable to recommend that the physician caring for a patient with CLL should always be attentive to symptoms that might indicate a lung cancer.

Immunological Complications of CLL

The immunological complications of CLL are outlined in Table 41.4.

The *immunosuppression* that is characteristic of this disease is of great clinical importance. Patients with CLL are prone to infections with tuberculosis, yeasts, and other vegetative organisms because of defective

Table 41.4 Immunological complications of chronic lymphocytic leukemia.

Immunosuppression

    hypogammaglobulinemia

    decreased cellular immunity

Immune dysregulation

    immune hemolytic anemia

    immune thrombocytopenic purpura

    immune neutropenia

    pure red cell aplasia

    connective tissue diseases

cellular immunity and are also liable to respiratory and other mucosal infections because of defective antibody production. In the older patient with CLL, opportunistic infections are productive of much morbidity and mortality. The immunosuppression of CLL is very rarely improved by treatment of the leukemia and may be made worse by it, particularly if severe neutropenia is induced by cytotoxic agents, impairing yet another of the body's defenses. *Immune dysregulation* in CLL may be the result of attempts by the immune system to control the neoplastic production of B cells, with resultant exhaustion of the system of regulatory T cells. Immune cytopenias are frequent in CLL and should always be sought when the blood count deteriorates, as they generally respond well to treatment with glucocorticoid drugs. *Pure red cell aplasia* is characterized by severe and progressive anemia with reticulocytopenia, a negative Coombs test, and severe hypoplasia or complete absence of red cell precursors in the bone marrow. This condition usually responds very well to immunosuppressive therapy; it is therefore important to distinguish it from the anemia that results when erythropoiesis is compromised by progression of the CLL itself.

Prognosis of CLL

The survival from diagnosis of CLL varies from a few months to over 20 years. For a lengthy period the survival of individual patients appeared to be unpredictable, and this made treatment decisions difficult: to treat a patient who is destined to live for years without significant progression of the disease is clearly inappropriate, while to withhold therapy until deterioration is obvious is probably leaving things too late. In the absence of reliable indicators of prognosis, recommendations regarding the timing of treatment for CLL were based largely on personal opinions. There existed both "interventionist" and "watch and wait" schools of thought and the overall results of these approaches were not very different, except that the interventionists treated many patients who would have done as well (or better) had they been left alone. Many studies iden-

Table 41.5 Proposed prognostic factors in chronic lymphocytic leukemia.

older age	multivariate analysis shows no effect (17)
sex	multivariate analysis shows no effect (17)
performance status	poor PS associated with poor survival (18)
neutropenia at dx.	does not correlate with prognosis (17)
gammaglobulin	low IgA associated with poor prognosis (19)
anemia at dx.	strong association with poor prognosis (20)
Coombs test +	no prognostic effect (21)
lymphocyte count	poor prognosis over $50 \times 10^9/1$ (11)
lymphocyte doubling	short doubling time is adverse (22, 23)
lymphocyte atypia	controversial; atypia possibly adverse (11)
marrow histology	diffuse lymphocytic infiltrate adverse (11, 24)
high serum LDH	not significant if corrected for stage (11)
cell phenotype	sIg phenotype lacks prognostic value (11, 25)
b-2-microglobulin	high serum b2M in advanced stage CLL (26, 27)
^{3}H-thymidine uptake	high uptake indicates early progression (28)
dO-thymidine kinase	elevated serum levels in progressive CLL (29)
total body K$^+$	increases with advancing stage of CLL (30)
cytogenetics	poor prognosis if complex abnormalities (8)

tified factors that were thought to possess some prognostic significance, and these are summarized in Table 41.5.

Careful study of these factors indicates that some are without prognostic value (e.g. age or sex), while others (e.g. beta-2-microglobulin, total body potassium) do not provide any information beyond that provided by the clinical stage. Certain other observations (e.g. lymphocyte doubling time, cytogenetics, tritiated thymidine uptake) may provide information that is of independent prognostic value after correction for the stage of disease, but this remains to be proved by a multivariate analysis of a large patient database. The most significant advance in assigning prognoses to patients with CLL was the development of a useful staging system.

Clinical Staging of CLL

Endeavors to identify groups of patients with CLL and different prognoses were made in the 1960's by Galton (22), Boggs and his colleagues (31) and Dameshek (32). Rai and his colleagues devised a five-stage system in 1968 and tested it retrospectively on a series of their own patients and on two published series; they then tested the system prospectively on another group of patients who were at that time undergoing therapy or

Table 41.6 The RAI system for clinical staging of CLL.

Stage	Extent of disease
0	lymphocytosis in blood and bone marrow
I	lymphocytosis plus lymphadenopathy (local or generalized, small nodes or bulky)
II	lymphocytosis plus enlarged spleen and/or liver (nodes may or may not be enlarged)
III	lymphocytosis plus anemia (Hb < 11gm/dl; enlarged nodes, spleen, or liver may or may not be present)
IV	lymphocytosis plus thrombocytopenia (< $100 \times 10^9/1$; anemia and enlarged nodes, spleen, and liver may or may not be present)

observation. In all these analyses the Rai staging system proved to be simple and easy to use and accurately predicted the survival time of patients with CLL. The system was published in 1975 (33) and is set out in Table 41.6.

The survival times that were reported in the original series (33) are shown in Table 41.7; more recent series have shown broadly similar results although in some the survivals in Stage III and Stage IV are somewhat longer. From inspection of Table 41.7 it is at once apparent that Stage 0 or I CLL is a relatively benign disease and Stage III or IV CLL is a life-threatening disease with a prognosis that is little better than that of acute leukemia in an adult. Perhaps most importantly, it is seen that *Stage II* CLL — the largest category — has a median survival of under 6 years and should not be considered in any sense a "benign" disease. This is particularly so in patients whose age and overall health would confer a prognosis of 12, 18, or more years if they did not suffer from CLL.

Other staging systems have been formulated by Binet and his colleagues (34) and by the International Workshop on CLL (35); they differ from the Rai system in detail but not in principle and they produce similar clinical results. In North America the Rai system is the most widely used.

Table 41.7 Median survival time according to RAI stage (33).

Clinical stage	Median survival in months
0	>150
I	101
II	71
III	19
IV	19
All patients	71

Table 41.8 Follow-up of an untreated patient with CLL.

Symptoms:	night sweats, fever, weight loss, malaise, infections, declining performance status.
Signs:	development of, or change in, enlarged lymph nodes, liver, or spleen.
Laboratory:	hemoglobin, platelet count, neutrophil count, lymphocyte doubling time, serum immunoglobulin level, Coombs test, bone marrow biopsy.
Note:	the above represents the desirable minimum; other investigations are done as indicated.

Table 41.9 Indications for active treatment in CLL

1) significant disease-related symptoms.

2) anemia or thrombocytopenia due to progressive leukemia (Stage III or IV CLL).

3) autoimmune hemolysis or thrombocytopenia.

4) progressive massive splenomegaly, with or without hypersplenism.

5) progressive bulky lymphadenopathy, with or without pressure effects or cosmetic problems.

6) increased susceptibility to bacterial infections.

Management of the Older Patient with CLL

General Principles

The approach to therapy of CLL varies considerably between different centers and also between individual physicians and there is no standardized policy, although advances in clinical staging and thus in assessing each patient's prognosis should now make it possible to formulate one.

Younger patients (40 to 60 years old) with CLL are a special problem because (a) they will almost certainly die of the disease, and (b) they will suffer a major loss of life expectancy because they have developed CLL. In these patients, trials of innovative and aggressive therapies, in the setting of a formal clinical study, should always be considered.

The geriatric oncologist can and should be more conservative for the following reasons. Many patients are asymptomatic at the time of diagnosis, in many the disease will pursue an indolent course for long periods, and the available treatment is palliative rather than curative and there is no demonstrated advantage to the early, as opposed to the later, exhibition of antileukemic drugs in CLL. In very elderly or infirm patients, the diagnosis of CLL may not affect the life expectancy and treatment for CLL could not be expected to produce benefit. In asymptomatic patients, who usually will have Stage 0, I, or II CLL, it is good practice to observe without treatment, whereas in Stage III or IV disease treatment is generally begun at once. Patients who are observed without treatment may be seen every 6 to 12 weeks; the features that are followed are indicated in Table 41.8.

An extremely important factor in the care of the elderly patient with CLL is the provision of a high standard of *general medical care* for any coexisting diseases; the geriatric oncologist is thoroughly familiar with this special aspect of his field. Put simply, patients with CLL who receive excellent general care will have a longer duration and a better quality of life than those who do not.

Indications for Active Treatment

The indications for the institution of active therapy in CLL have been widely discussed (11, 36, 37). They are summarized in Table 41.9.

Most oncologists would concur with these recommendations, although the threshold for considering that splenomegaly is massive or that lymphadenopathy is bulky must be subject to individual variation. Some oncologists would add other indications, for example a *short lymphocyte doubling time*, usually taken as under 6 months. This indicates progressive disease and the likelihood that the patient's disease will shortly progress to a higher Rai stage. Treatment as soon as rapid doubling of the lymphocyte count is documented may prevent this occurrence, but no formal study has been reported that tests this hypothesis. Han and Rai (11) have recommended active treatment for progressive hyperlymphocytosis, basing their recommendation on three reports of hyperleukocytosis-associated hyperviscosity syndrome in patients with CLL. They suggest instituting therapy when the total leukocyte count is between 100 and $150 \times 10^9/1$. This threshold was set empirically and it seems unlikely that the recommendation will be widely accepted unless a clinical study is done that supports it, since problems with hyperviscosity are rare and treatment for CLL is far from innocuous, particularly in the older person.

Available Treatments for CLL

Over the past half-century, many agents and very numerous schedules of administration have been employed in the management of CLL: these have been extensively reviewed (11,36,38,39). Some regimens are now of mainly historical interest and only the treatments that are most important in current clinical practice will be considered here. Aggressive therapies that are not appropriate for the older patient — for example allogeneic bone marrow transplantation — will not be discussed.

Radiation therapy

Since the advent of cytotoxic chemotherapy, radiation therapy has had only a restricted role in the management of CLL. It is no longer employed for the systemic treatment of the disease, but it is of value in the control of local problems (40). When a patient with CLL has a dominant lymph node mass that is symptomatic, local irradiation is the palliative treatment of choice. Response rates to modest doses of radiation approach 100% and local and systemic toxic effects are generally minimal. Usually the dose of radiation administered is much smaller than the doses that are administered when a lymphoma is treated with curative intent, and the same area can be irradiated again at a later date should a lymph node mass recur. If a patient is receiving chemotherapy but there is a large mass-lymph node, tonsil, or spleen- that is not responding satisfactorily to the chemotherapy, the addition of local irradiation improves the response without significant toxicity. Irradiation of the *spleen* in CLL usually reduces splenomegaly and sometimes there is an improvement in lymphocytosis, anemia, and thrombocytopenia. However, in many patients the hemoglobin level and platelet count decline significantly, and splenic irradiation must be administered with caution, particularly in patients who have received much chemotherapy.

Allopurinol

The xanthine oxidase inhibitor allopurinol prevents the conversion of xanthine to the less soluble uric acid. When lymphoid malignancies are treated with effective chemotherapy or radiation, massive lysis of tumor tissue sometimes takes place in a very short period, resulting in the production of large amounts of urate. This may lead to renal calculi, or more seriously to urate nephropathy with renal tubular obstruction and renal failure which is sometimes fatal. When treatment for CLL is begun, good hydration of the patient must be ensured, and consideration should be given to concurrent therapy with allopurinol, 300 mg daily for 21 days, to prevent hyperuricemia and the resultant hyperuricosuria. This is particularly important in the elderly, who are more likely to have reduced renal function. It is also advisable in the presence of bulky disease, or a uric acid level that is elevated *before* therapy, or if there is a history of renal disease or gout. Treatment with allopurinol is generally well tolerated but occasional patients develop drug sensitivity rashes.

Adrenal corticosteroids

The adrenal corticosteroids, usually in the form of prednisone, prednisolone, or dexamethasone, are used extensively in the treatment of CLL. They are modestly immunosuppressive and also are potent lympholytic agents, occasionally producing a response so brisk that hyperuricemia results (see above). Unfortunately, steroids produce a galaxy of adverse effects, listed in Table 41.10.

Many of these unwanted effects — for example diabetes mellitus, osteoporosis, and hypertension — are particularly serious in older people, who are prone to these conditions even without receiving corticosteroid therapy. *Single-agent* treatment with a corticosteroid is indicated when CLL is complicated by autoimmune hemolytic anemia or ITP, or when the disease has become unresponsive to other agents. In a previously untreated patient with severe hematopoietic failure, it is common practice to begin therapy with a corticosteroid alone, because these agents can bring about improvement *without* further myelosuppression. Corticosteroids are frequently administered *in combination*

Table 41.10   The side effects of adrenal corticosteroids.

General	Particularly important in the elderly
psychosis	hypertension
acne	sodium and water retention
excessive appetite	dependent edema
cutaneous striae	cardiac failure
hirsutism	osteoporosis
liability to infection	reactivation of tuberculosis
obesity	hyperglycemia, diabetes
masking of infection	peptic ulceration
	hypokalemia
	hyperuricemia

with an alkylating agent in the management of CLL, although it may be questioned if the addition of a steroid actually improves the results when the alkylating agent is administered intensively. *Long-term* therapy with corticosteroids should be avoided, because the adverse effects (Table 41.10) are much more frequent and more severe when treatment is given for an extended period. *Intermittent pulses* of a corticosteroid, for example 5–7 days per month, even in substantial doses, are better tolerated.

Androgens and estrogens

Androgens and other anabolic steroids have occasionally been used in CLL when there is bone marrow failure that has not responded to prednisone with or without an alkylating agent. Improvements in anemia and thrombocytopenia have been reported (41–43), but these agents should be used with caution because most of them are hepatotoxic and they may exacerbate preexisting prostatic hypertrophy. It is possible that erythropoietin may prove to be more effective than anabolic steroids for improving bone marrow failure in CLL; clinical studies are currently addressing this question. It is of considerable interest that some patients with CLL and carcinoma of the prostate, treated for the latter condition with diethylstilbestrol showed rapid reductions in their peripheral blood lymphocytosis (44, 45). Unfortunately, the severe cardiovascular side effects of estrogens are a contraindication to their use in an elderly patient with CLL.

Alkylating agents

Many alkylating agents, including nitrogen mustard, triethylenemelamine, busulfan, chlorambucil, and cyclophosphamide have been used in the treatment of CLL, but only chlorambucil and cyclophosphamide have remained in regular, widespread use (39). *Chlorambucil* (22, 36, 46, 47) is reliably absorbed from the gastrointestinal tract, has some selective cytotoxicity for lymphoid cells, and is relatively free of side effects such as nausea, vomiting, alopecia, and cystitis. However, it should not be forgotten that chlorambucil is mutagenic, leukemogenic, and a potent stem cell poison that can permanently impair the function of the bone marrow. Long-term myelosuppression is particularly likely to occur when low doses of chlorambucil are administered every day for many weeks or months; this is probably also the best way to induce resistance to the drug and perhaps the mode of administration that is most likely to induce AML. Fortunately, in recent years most physicians have adopted a high-dose intermittent schedule for the administration of chlorambucil (48–50). This schedule is at least as effective as low-dose daily chlorambucil, patient compliance is excellent, and the hematologic toxicity is less, dose reductions are required less frequently than with a daily dosing regimen. This suggests that the dose of chlorambucil on an intermittent regimen could be *escalated* and a higher response rate might be obtained. My practice is to administer chlorambucil at night, in a dose of 20 mg, for 4 to 7 consecutive nights, at an interval of 28 days. Nausea and vomiting are very rare and progressive hematologic toxicity is avoided because the substantial interval enables the full effects of each course to be seen before another course is prescribed. A practical point worth noting is that chlorambucil should *not* be taken with orange juice or other vitamin-C-containing vehicle, as the ascorbic acid can inactivate the alkylating agent.

Cyclophosphamide is also widely used in the treatment of CLL. Unlike chlorambucil, cyclophosphamide is available in an intravenous as well as an oral form. It has the disadvantages that it causes alopecia and also hemorrhagic cystitis. This complication, well recognized with high-dose parenteral cyclophosphamide, can also occur with chronic low doses given by mouth.[51] The principal indications for the use of cyclophosphamide in CLL are when chlorambucil is not well tolerated or when a multiple-agent chemotherapeutic regimen is administered.

Multiple-agent regimens

Several multidrug regimens have been employed in the treatment of CLL. The most frequently used are CVP (cyclophosphamide + vincristine + prednisone) (52), CHOP (cyclophosphamide + doxorubicin + vincristine + prednisone) (52), M-2 (vincristine + carmustine + cyclophosphamide + melphalan) (53), and POACH (prednisone + vincristine + cytarabine + cyclophosphamide + doxorubicin) (54). All of these regimens were originally devised for the treatment of non-Hodgkin's lymphoma or myeloma and they all contain vincristine, a drug that has *not* shown any single-agent activity in CLL. Since vincristine causes both constipation and peripheral neuropathy, both of which are frequent problems in older people without drug therapy, it should be *omitted* from these regimens as a toxic agent of unproved value. The value of multiple-drug regimens in CLL is controversial. A large French study (52) showed that CVP was more toxic, but no more effective, than single-agent chlorambucil.

The same group found that in advanced CLL, the survival of patients who were treated with CHOP was markedly superior to CVP (and possibly to chlorambucil, although this was not tested). The anthracycline antibiotics have not been particularly active as single agents in CLL, and this apparent superior survival with CHOP has not always been confirmed by other workers (39). In a study of the POACH regimen at the M.D. Anderson Cancer Center (55), 19 of 34 (56%) previously untreated patients responded, with a 21% complete remission rate, while 8 of 31 (26%) previously treated patients responded, with a complete remission rate of 7%. Mortality was very much higher in the previously treated patients. As this was a single arm study, it is not possible to assess the merits of the POACH regimen relative to other therapies. It does not appear to be very effective for previously treated patients with CLL.

Splenectomy

Although splenectomy has been widely studied in CLL (56–60), there have been no formal studies to compare it with systemic chemotherapy or with splenic irradiation. The usual indications for splenectomy are autoimmune hemolysis or autoimmune thrombocytopenia that have responded inadequately to corticosteroids or immunosuppressive drugs, and hypersplenism. Splenectomy has occasionally been performed for the relief of massive, symptomatic splenomegaly. In the older patient a careful evaluation must be made to determine their suitability for general anesthesia and surgery. As with other elective splenectomies, pneumococcal vaccine may be administered before surgery, but the patient with CLL may fail to mount a satisfactory antibody response, and long-term penicillin prophylaxis after splenectomy may be a more effective preventive measure.

Evaluation of Response to Therapy

Definitions of response to therapy in CLL have been proposed in two sets of guidelines (7, 61). Both require normalization of the peripheral blood and the bone marrow, together with disappearance of symptoms and physical signs of the disease. One group (61) recommends determining by further tests if the complete remission is a "clonal" one, by demonstrating normalization of the T:B cell ratio in the blood and normalization of the kappa:lambda light chain ratio among B cells, and decrease of CD5-positive B cells to less than 25%. The completeness of remission can be tested even further by demonstrating the resolution of markers of the neoplastic clone — idiotype, immunoglobulin gene rearrangement, and chromosomal abnormalities. From the viewpoint of the clinician, the most important criteria of response are the relief of symptoms, the correction of physical and hematologic abnormalities, the resolution of any transfusion needs, and freedom from infections. Most important, the patient's *performance status* should improve and be brought as close to normal as the patient's age and the presence of other abnormalities permit. In the case of a *partial response*, the *stage of disease* should improve — for example from Stage III to Stage 0. It seems probable that a patient who is Stage 0 by virtue of treatment may not have the excellent prognosis of an untreated Stage 0 patient: this is a subject for further study.

Fludarabine

Fludarabine monophosphate is the most recent drug to find a role in the treatment of CLL and is the most effective agent ever to be tested in that disease. It is a purine analogue with a substituted fluorine atom that confers resistance to deamination and inactivation by the cellular enzyme adenosine deaminase (62). Following injection it is dephosphorylated in plasma to form arabinosyl-2-fluoroadenine (63, 64). It is actively taken up by cells and phosphorylated to its 5'-triphosphate, F-ara-ATP, which is the active form of the drug. F-ara-ATP inhibits DNA synthesis by competing with deoxy-ATP for incorporation into DNA, and also by inhibiting ribonucleotide reductase. F-ara-ATP is also incorporated into RNA and is an inhibitor of DNA repair. The major toxicity of fludarabine is myelosuppression; it is well tolerated subjectively, with little nausea or vomiting and almost no alopecia (65). In early studies, significant neurotoxicity was encountered, but this occurred at doses approximately fourfold greater than are now employed (66). Fludarabine was first evaluated in CLL by Grever and his colleagues (67). Of 22 previously treated patients, 19 showed some response, with 1 complete remission and 3 excellent partial remissions. A study by Keating and his colleagues (68) in 68 previously treated patients with CLL showed complete remission in 15% and a partial response in 44%. These are astonishingly good results, particularly for previously treated patients, when it is recalled that in previously *untreated* patients who receive chlorambucil and corticosteroids, complete remissions are seen in perhaps 5–10% of patients at best. The major toxic effects associated with fludarabine therapy were myelosuppression and episodes of fever and infection. Ten patients died during the study, seven of them during the first three courses of treatment, and it was clear that this potent agent must be handled with caution.

When a drug performs well in patients with a previously treated neoplastic disease, results are usually even better when the drug is administered to previously untreated patients. Keating and his colleagues treated 33 previously untreated patients with advanced or progressive CLL with fludarabine, 30 mg/m^2/day intravenously for 5 days every 4 weeks (69). The complete remission rate using the NCI guidelines, which permit the presence of residual lymphoid nodules in the bone marrow, was 75%. Six of the 33 patients (18%) failed to respond and three died of infection during the first three cycles of treatment. It is very important to note that all three patients were aged over 75 years and all had Rai Stage III-IV disease. In a three-year follow-up of this study (70), there were 35 previously untreated patients with a complete remission rate of 74% and partial remissions in 6% of patients for an overall response rate of 80%. The median duration of response was 33 months. These results are far superior to any

that have been reported for alkylating agents, with or without corticosteroids or additional cytotoxic drugs.

In another study, previously treated patients with CLL received fludarabine combined with prednisone (71). The results of treatment were not better than those obtained with fludarabine alone, but as all the patients had received prednisone previously, this study does not completely rule out any synergistic effect of the drug combination if used in untreated patients.

Two other purine analogues, pentostatin and cladribine, have demonstrable activity in CLL, including refractory cases, but neither appears to be as active as fludarabine (39).

Currently the NCI is sponsoring a randomized controlled trial of fludarabine vs. chlorambucil vs fludarabine with chlorambucil in previously untreated patients with CLL. Preliminary results suggest that single-agent fludarabine is superior to single-agent chlorambucil, while the combination of the two drugs is not superior to fludarabine alone and is more toxic. This study is at too early a stage to determine effects on remission duration and survival.

If a patient cannot be entered into a formal therapeutic study, should fludarabine be used as first-line therapy in previously untreated CLL? Although all the evidence is not yet to hand, I believe the answer is "yes". This opinion is based on the high response rate (80%) and the extremely high incidence of complete remission (75%), together with preliminary evidence of a remission duration that approaches three years. These results so far exceed those that are obtained with chlorambucil, with or without prednisone, or the more toxic anthracycline-containing regimens, that it may be a disservice to the patient *not* to administer fludarabine. My policy is to administer 25 mg/m^2/day as a 30-minute intravenous infusion, daily for *three* days on the first occasion, and to repeat the treatment every four weeks, increasing its duration to four or five days if it is well-tolerated. This cautious approach is appropriate for the elderly patient, particularly if comorbid conditions are present or if there is a history of opportunistic infections.

Drug Resistance in CLL

Like many other neoplastic diseases that respond well to initial chemotherapy, CLL frequently demonstrates the phenomenon of the development of secondary resistance to previously effective drugs, evidenced by a failure of clinical and hematologic response. Although the patient whose disease has become refractory to alkylating agents and corticosteroids may in the short term do well with fludarabine as salvage therapy, the onset of drug resistance is always an ominous event that indicates a deteriorating prognosis. Further, CLL shows *primary* resistance to many drugs that are valuable in the chemotherapy of other diseases, for example methotrexate, vincristine, etoposide, and doxorubicin. The mechanisms of drug resistance in CLL have recently been reviewed (72). Resistance to methotrexate and several other antimetabolite drugs that are specifically active in the s-phase of the cell cycle appears to be attributable to the very low proliferative fraction in populations of CLL cells. Resistance to fludarabine, an antimetabolite drug that for unknown reasons is active in CLL despite the low mitotic index, is mediated by loss of enzymes that activate the drug. Resistance to chlorambucil and other alkylating agents appears to be due to enhanced mechanisms for repair of DNA and for the intracellular neutralization of alkylating molecules, while refractoriness to adrenal corticosteroids is associated with loss of the cellular receptors for these agents. Resistance to etoposide and doxorubicin may be due to the low expression of topoisomerase II, a major target of these drugs, in CLL cells (73) and/or to overexpression of the multidrug resistance gene, mdr1 (74). Activation of mdr1 leads to synthesis of the glycoprotein gp-170, which acts as an efflux pump, removing the drugs from the intracellular environment. Studies of compounds — e.g. cyclosporine analogues — that may reverse multiple drug resistance are in progress but these agents have not yet had a significant impact on clinical practice. Numerous other measures to circumvent drug resistance in CLL have been proposed (72) but have not yet entered the clinical arena.

Management of Autoimmune Complications of CLL

Anemia in CLL always requires careful evaluation. It may be due to bone marrow compromise induced by the disease, in which case the patient has Stage III disease and a median survival of less than two years. The anemia may also be due to coexisting unrelated conditions, for example deficiencies of iron, vitamin B$_{12}$, or folate, gastrointestinal bleeding, or chronic diseases such as rheumatoid arthritis. All of these conditions are more frequent in the older patient. Finally, anemia may be due to autoimmune hemolytic anemia (AIHA); this is associated with the leukemia but does not make the patient's disease Stage III. In such cases the direct antiglobulin (Coombs) test is usually positive and there is a reticulocytosis. It is not uncommon for active hemolysis to be complicated by folate deficiency because of increased folate consumption, in which case macrocytosis may be observed and reticulocytosis may be suppressed. Immune thrombocytopenic purpura (ITP) also occurs in CLL and is less serious than the thrombocytopenia of bone marrow failure; it does not make the patient's disease Stage IV. The demonstration of antiplatelet antibodies is not a well-standardized test and at many centers the diagnosis of ITP depends upon the finding of thrombocytopenia with adequate or increased megakaryocytes in the bone marrow (but this may not be the case if there is heavy marrow infiltration with CLL), and a response to corticosteroid therapy. AIHA and ITP may occur together (Evans syndrome). AIHA and ITP are usually treated with prednisone (100 mg/day) or dexamethasone (16 mg/day); these high doses can be tapered as soon as a response is seen. In the older patient it is wise to administer an H2 blocking drug (e.g. ranitidine) concurrently with the corticosteroid, and many would add anticandida prophylaxis with fluconazole. In the patient with AIHA, folate supplementation is recom-

mended while there is active hemolysis. If the response to steroid therapy is inadequate, or only occurs at an unacceptably high dose that cannot be continued long-term, high-dose intravenous immune globulin should be added: 400 mg/kg/day for 5 days and then maintenance with the same daily dose administered once every 21 days. In occasional patients, splenectomy is necessary for the control of AIHA or ITP, and this operation carries increased risks in the older patient. Overall, the prognosis of patients with AIHA or ITP who respond to prednisone therapy is better than that of patients with anemia or thrombocytopenia that are due to Stage III and Stage IV CLL respectively. Many patients may also require chemotherapy for active CLL in addition to treatment for AIHA or ITP. It should be remembered that the administration of chlorambucil or fludarabine may exacerbate the anemia of AIHA because any compensatory increase in erythropoiesis may be suppressed. The rare autoimmune condition of pure red cell aplasia (PRCA) may be treated with corticosteroid, with or without the addition of cyclosporine.

Supportive care in CLL

Anemia in a patient with CLL, if due to the leukemia itself and not to hematinic factor deficiencies, blood loss, or chronic disease, is best treated by controlling the CLL and improving the function of the bone marrow. The *transfusion* of packed red blood cells is valuable during initial therapy and also for patients whose erythrocyte production is not restored by treating the leukemia. Treatment with *erythropoietin* improves hemoglobin levels in some patients with CLL but it is not certain that this treatment is cost-effective when compared to transfusion, and in some patients it fails outright. *Platelet transfusion* in CLL is indicated only for hemorrhage, as it is in any chronic thrombocytopenic state.

For many years *immunoglobulin replacement therapy* has been employed empirically in patients with CLL for the prevention of infection, but it was only recently that a randomized, placebo-controlled study demonstrated conclusively that this therapy provides highly effective prophylaxis (75). The recommended dose is 400 mg/kg, administered intravenously once every 21 days. This treatment is very expensive and should only be administered to a patient with CLL if there is hypogammaglobulinemia *and* a history of repeated infections. As patients with CLL frequently suffer from neutropenia, an excess of suppressor T cells over T helper cells, and deficient natural killer cells, immunoglobulin replacement is unlikely to fully restore immunocompetence. Infections in patients with CLL should be investigated aggressively and treated vigorously, and their physician must be alert to the possibility of infection with unusual organisms, particularly yeasts and fungi (76).

Innovative Treatment Strategies for CLL

The introduction of fludarabine is the most significant advance in the management of CLL in four decades. Although fludarabine induces a high proportion of complete remissions in previously untreated patients with CLL, it has not been proved to have the potential for curing the disease. When patients with CLL become refractory to fludarabine, there is no alternative therapy of comparable effectiveness, so there is a pressing need for further advances in treatment. Several innovative treatment strategies are under investigation (77). Allogeneic or autologous *bone marrow transplantation* are currently considered too hazardous for the older patient with CLL and will not be discussed here. Treatment with *monoclonal antibodies* (MoAbs) has been extensively studied in patients with CLL. Passive immunotherapy with *unconjugated* MoAbs turns out to be relatively safe but the clinical responses are minor in degree and usually transient, so this cannot be considered an effective treatment. A logical extension of MoAb therapy was to give the antibodies a warhead by conjugating them with *immunotoxins* before their administration. Studies have been carried out with single-chain immunotoxins — usually the A chain of ricin — and with two-chain immunotoxins consisting of ricin A and B chains but with the nonspecific galactose-binding sites of ricin blocked. These compounds have shown major activity against CLL cells *in vitro*, but clinical experience thus far is limited and responses have been relatively minor. Clinical studies are in progress with a *fusion protein* that has been produced by recombinant DNA technology, in which the receptor-binding domain of diphtheria toxin is replaced by the sequences of human interleukin-2 (77). These compounds have significant antitumor activity but also significant toxicity, including elevated hepatic transaminases, hypoalbuminemia, fever, chest tightness, rashes, increased serum creatinine and thrombocytopenia, and clearly would have to be administered with great caution in the older patient. Studies have also been done with *radioimmunoconjugates*, in which a MoAb is coupled to a radionuclide, ^{32}P or ^{131}I. By binding to CLL cells in the bone marrow as well as the peripheral blood, these compounds deliver radiation not only to their intended targets, but also to *normal* cells in the bone marrow, and myelosuppression results. Overall, MoAbs that are armed with immunotoxins or radionuclides do possess significant activity against CLL cells but their place — if any — in therapy is undetermined. Possibly they may be of value for the eradication of minimal residual disease — for example after a complete remission has been obtained with fludarabine.

Conclusion

Chronic leukemias in the older person present the geriatric hematologist-oncologist with many problems. Curative therapy with bone marrow transplantation is not at present an option for these patients, who cannot tolerate the severe morbidity of such intensive treatment. Similarly, intensive chemotherapy at levels below those used for transplantation is hazardous in the older patient and the risk increases with advancing age. Tolerance to many drugs, particularly interferon and corticosteroids, is poor in many older patients. The presence of multiple medical problems, particularly chronic degenerative diseases, complicates the care of many patients.

The correct approach is that which prevails in all of geriatric medicine — a detailed *global* assessment of each patient, careful attention to *all* of the patient's problems, and the assignment of a *priority* to the chronic leukemia in terms of its importance in the *overall* picture of performance status and life expectancy for that individual. That done, the individual and the leukemia are treated with the best skills, compassion, and insight that can be marshalled by the physician for the patient's benefit.

References

1. Spiers ASD, Davis MP, Levine M, Li CY, Mangan KF, Mazza JJ, Neu LT, O'Brien J, Rauch AE, Wiltsie JC, Bieler L, Lorch CA. T-cell chronic lymphocytic leukaemia: Anomalous cell markers, variable morphology, and marked responsiveness to pentostatin (2'-deoxycoformycin). *Scandinavian Journal of Haematology* 1985; **34**: 57–67.
2. Linet MS, Devesa SS. Descriptive epidemiology of the leukemias. In *Leukemia*, 5th. edn, edited by ES Henderson, TA Lister. Philadelphia: Saunders, pp. 207–224, 1990.
3. Linet MS. The Leukemias: Epidemiologic Aspects. New York: Oxford University Press, 1985.
4. Baer MR, Stein RS, Dessypris EN. Chronic lymphocytic leukemia with hyperleukocytosis. The hyperviscosity syndrome. *Cancer* 1985; **56**: 2865.
5. Cash J, Fehir KM, Pollack MS. Meningeal involvement in early stage chronic lymphocytic leukemia. *Cancer* 1987; **59**: 798.
6. Case Records of the Massachusetts General Hospital (Case 45-1988). *New England Journal of Medicine* 1988; **319**: 1268.
7. Cheson BD, Bennett JM, Rai KR, *et al.* Guidelines for clinical protocols for chronic lymphocytic leukemia (CLL). Recommendations of the NCI-Sponsored Working Group. *American Journal of Hematology* 1988; **29**: 152.
8. Juliusson G, Gahrton G. Chromosome abnormalities in B-cell chronic lymphocytic leukemia. In *Chronic Lymphocytic Leukemia*, edited by RD Cheson. New York: Dekker, pp. 83–103, 1993.
9. Enno A, Catovsky D, O'Brien M, *et al.* "Prolymphocytoid" transformation of chronic lymphocytic leukemia. *British Journal of Hematology* 1979; **41**: 9.
10. Richter MN. Generalized reticular cell sarcoma of lymph nodes associated with lymphatic leukemia. *American Journal of Pathology* 1928; **4**: 285.
11. Han T, Rai KR. Chronic lymphocytic leukemia. In *Leukemia*, 5th. edn, edited by ES Henderson, TA Lister. Philadelphia: Saunders, pp. 565–611, 1990.
12. Fermand JP, James JM, Herait P, *et al.* Associated chronic lymphocytic leukemia and multiple myeloma: origin from a single clone. *Blood* 1985; **66**: 291.
13. Laurent G, Gourdin MF, Flandrin G, *et al.* Acute blast crisis in a patient with chronic lymphocytic leukemia: immunoperoxidase study. *Acta Haematologica* 1981; **65**: 60.
14. Whipham T Splenic leukemia with carcinoma. *Transactions of the Pathological Society of London* 1878; **29**: 313.
15. Gunz FW, Angus HB. Leukemia and cancer in the same patient. *Cancer* 1965; **18**: 145.
16. Moayeri H, Han T, Stutzman L, *et al.* Second neoplasms with chronic lymphocytic leukemia. *New York State Journal of Medicine* 1976; **76**: 378.
17. Binet JL, Auquier A, Dighiero G, *et al.* A new prognostic classification of chronic lymphocytic leukemia derived from a multivariate survival analysis. *Cancer* 1981; **48**: 198.
18. Zippin C, Cutler SJ, Reeves WJ, Lum D. Survival in chronic lymphocytic leukemia. *Blood* 1973; **42**: 367.
19. Rozman C, Montserrat E, Vinolas N. Serum immunoglobulins in B-chronic lymphocytic leukemia. Natural history and prognostic significance. *Cancer* 1988; **61**: 279.

20. Rundles RW, Moore JO. Chronic lymphocytic leukemia. *Cancer* 1978; **42**: 941.

21. Hansen MM. Chronic lymphocytic leukemia clinical studies based on 189 cases followed for a long time. *Scandinavian Journal of Haematology* 1973; **18 Suppl.**: 3.

22. Galton DAG. The pathogenesis of chronic lymphocytic leukemia. *Canadian Medical Association Journal* 1966; **94**: 1005.

23. Vinolas N, Reverter JC, Urbano-Ispizua A, *et al*. Lymphocyte doubling time in chronic lymphocytic leukemia: an update of its prognostic significance. *Blood Cells* 1987; **12**: 457.

24. Han T, Barcos M, Emrich L, *et al*. Bone marrow infiltration patterns and their prognostic significance in chronic lymphocytic leukemia: correlations with clinical, immunologic, phenotypic, and cytogenetic data. *Journal of Clinical Oncology* 1984; **6**: 562.

25. Baldini L, Mozzana R, Cortelezzi A, *et al*. Prognostic significance of immunoglobulin phenotype in B cell chronic lymphocytic leukemia. *Blood* 1985; **65**: 340.

26. Shatt B, Child JA, Karrgish SM, Cooper EH. Behaviour of serum beta 2-microglobulin and acute phase reactant proteins in chronic lymphocytic leukaemia. *Acta Haematologica* 1980; **64**: 73.

27. Simonsson B, Wiw L, Nilsson K. Beta 2-microglobulin in chronic lymphocytic leukaemia. *Scandinavian Journal of Haematology* 1980; **24**: 174.

28. Juliusson G, Karl-Henrik R, Nilsson B, Gahrton G. Prognostic value of B-cell mitogen-induced and spontaneous thymidine uptake *in vitro* in chronic B-lymphocytic leukaemia cells. *British Journal of Haematology* 1985; **60**: 429.

29. Kallander CFR, Simonsson B, Hagberg H, Gronowitz JS. Serum deoxythymidine kinase gives prognostic information in chronic lymphocytic leukemia. *Cancer* 1984; **54**: 2450.

30. Chandra P, Sawitsky A, Chanana AD, *et al*. Correlation of total body potassium and leukemic cell mass in patients with chronic lymphocytic leukemia. *Blood* 1979; **53**: 594.

31. Boggs DR, Sofferman SA, Wintrobe MM, *et al*. Factors influencing the duration of survival of patients with chronic lymphocytic leukemia. *American Journal of Medicine* 1966; **40**: 243.

32. Dameshek W. Chronic lymphocytic leukemia — an accumulatice disease of immunologically incompetent lymphocytes. *Blood* 1967; **29**: 566.

33. Rai KR, Sawitsky A, Cronkite EP, *et al*. Clinical staging of chronic lymphocytic leukemia. *Blood* 1975; **46**: 219.

34. Binet JL, Auquier A, Dighiero G, *et al*. A new prognostic classification of chronic lymphocytic leukemia derived from a multivariate survival analysis. *Cancer* 1981; **48**: 198.

35. International Workshop on CLL. Proposal for a revised prognostic staging system. *British Journal of Haematology* 1981; **48**: 365.

36. Spiers ASD. Chronic lymphocytic leukemia. In *Leukemia*, 4th. edn, edited by FW Gunz, ES Henderson. New York: Grune & Stratton, pp. 709–740, 1983.

37. Rai KR, Sawitsky A, Jagathambal K, *et al*. Chronic lymphocytic leukemia. *Medical Clinics of North America* 1984; **68**: 697.

38. Rai KR. An outline of clinical management of chronic lymphocytic leukemia. In *Chronic Lymphocytic Leukemia*, edited by BD Cheson. New York: Dekker, pp. 241–251, 1993.

39. Keating MJ. Chemotherapy of chronic lymphocytic leukemia. In *Chronic Lymphocytic Leukemia*, edited by BD Cheson. New York: Marcel Dekker, pp. 297–336, 1993.

40. Kempin S, Shank B. Radiation in chronic lymphocytic leukemia. In *Chronic Lymphocytic Leukemia: Recent Progress and Future Direction*, edited by RP Gale, KR Rai. UCLA Symposia on Molecular and Cellular Biology 1987, New Series, Vol. 59. New York: Alan R Liss, p. 337.

41. Kennedy BJ. Androgenic hormone therapy in lymphatic leukemia. *Journal of the American Medical Association* 1964; **190**: 1130.

42. Presant CA, Safdar SH. Oxymethalone in myelofibrosis and chronic lymphocytic leukemia. *Archives of Internal Medicine* 1973; **132**: 175.

43. West WO. The treatment of bone marrow failure with massive androgen therapy. *Ohio State Medical Journal* 1965; **61**: 347.

44. Narasimhan P, Amaral L. Lymphopenic response of patients presenting with chronic lymphocytic leukemia associated with carcinoma of the prostate to diethylstilbestrol: correlation of response to the *in vitro* synthesis of RNA by patient lymphocytes and its relationship to transcortin. *American Journal of Hematology* 1980; **8**: 369.

45. Narasimhan P, Glasberg S. Responses to diethylstilbestrol in a patient with refractory chronic lymphatic leukemia associated with non-Hodgkin's lymphoma (Richter's syndrome). *Proceedings of the Second International Congress on Hormones and Cancer* 1983. New York: Pergamon Press, (Abstr).

46. Galton DAG, Israel LG, Nabarro JDN, *et al*. Clinical trials of p(di-2-chloroethylamino)-phenylbutyric acid (CB1348) in malignant lymphoma. *British Medical Journal* 1955; **2**: 1172.

47. Han T, Ezdinli EZ, Shimaoka K, Desai DV. Chlorambucil vs. combined chlorambucil-corticosteroid therapy in chronic lymphocytic leukemia. *Cancer* 1973; **31**: 502.

48. Huguley CM Jr. Treatment of chronic lymphocytic leukemia. *Cancer Treatment Reviews* 1977; **4**: 261.

49. Knospe WH, Loeb V Jr, Huguley CM Jr. Biweekly chlorambucil treatment of chronic lymphocytic leukemia. *Cancer* 1974; **33**: 555.

50. Sawitsky A, Rai KR, Glidewell O, Silver RT, CALGB members. Comparison of daily versus intermittent chlorambucil and prednisone therapy in the treatment of patients with chronic lymphocytic leukemia. *Blood* 1977; **50**: 1049.

51. Spiers ASD, Chikkappa G, Wilbur HJ. Haemorrhagic cystitis after low-dose cyclophosphamide. *Lancet* 1983; **i**: 1213.

52. French Cooperative Group on Chronic Lymphocytic Leukaemia. Effectiveness of "CHOP" regimen in advanced untreated chronic lymphocytic leukaemia. *Lancet* 1986; **i**: 1346.

53. Kempin S, Lee BJ, Thaler HT, *et al*. Combination chemotherapy of advanced chronic lymphocytic leukemia: the M-2 protocol (vincristine, BCNU, cyclophosphamide, melphalan and prednisone). *Blood* 1982; **60**: 1110.

54. Keating MJ, Scouros M, Murphy M, *et al*. Multiple agent chemotherapy (POACH) in previously treated and untreated patients with chronic lymphocytic leukemia. *Leukemia* 1988; **2**: 157.

55. Keating MJ, Scouros M, Murphy S, *et al*. Multiple agent chemotheapy (POACH) in previously treated and untreated patients with chronic lymphocytic leukemia. *Leukemia* 1988; **2**: 157.

56. Delpero JR, Gastout JA, Letreut YP, *et al*. The value of splenectomy in chronic lymphocytic leukemia. *Cancer* 1987; **59**: 340.

57. Ferrant A, Michaux JL, Sokal G. Splenectomy in advanced chronic lymphocytic leukemia. *Cancer* 1986; **58**: 2130.

58. Merl SA, Theodarakis ME, Goldberg J, Gottlieb AJ. Splenectomy for thrombocytopenia in chronic lymphocytic leukemia. *American Journal of Hematology* 1983; **15**: 253.

59. Pegourie B, Sotto J-J., Hollard D, *et al*. Splenectomy during chronic lymphocytic leukemia. *Cancer* 1987; **59**: 1626.

60. Stein RS, Weikert D, Reynolds V, *et al*. Splenectomy for endstage chronic lymphocytic leukemia. *Cancer* 1987; **59**: 1815.

61. Binet JL, Catovsky D, Dighiero G, *et al*. Chronic lymphocytic leukemia: recommendations for diagnosis, staging and response criteria. *Annals of Internal Medicine* 1989; **110**: 236.

62. Frederickson S. Specificity of adenosine deaminase toward adenosine and 2'-deoxyadenosine analogues. *Archives of Biochemistry and Biophysics* 1966; **113**: 383.

63. Malspeis L, Grever MR, Staubus AE, Young D. Pharmacokinetics of 2-F-ara-A (9-beta-D-arabinofuranosyl-2-fluoroadenine) in cancer patients during the Phase I clinical investigation of fludarabine phosphate. *Seminars in Oncology* 1990; **17**: 18.

64. Plunkett W, Huang P, Gandhi V. Metabolism and action of fludarabine phosphate. *Seminars in Oncology* 1990; **17**: 3.

65. Von Hoff DD. Phase I clinical trials with fludarabine phosphate. *Seminars in Oncology* 1990; **17**: 33.

66. Chun HG, Leyland-Jones B, Caryk SM, Hoth DF. Central nervous system toxicity of fludarabine phosphate. *Cancer Treatment Reports* 1986; **70**: 1225.

67. Grever MR, Kopecky KJ, Coltman CA, *et al*. Fludarabine monophosphate: A potentially useful agent in chronic lymphocytic leukemia. *Nouvelle Revue Francais Hematologie* 1988; **30**: 457.

68. Keating MJ, Kantarjian H, Talpaz M, *et al*. Fludarabine: A new agent with major activity against chronic lymphocytic leukemia. *Blood* 1989, **74**: 19.

69. Keating MJ, Kantarjian H, O'Brien S, *et al*. Fludarabine: A new agent with marked cytoreductive activity in untreated chronic lymphocytic leukemia. *Journal of Clinical Oncology* 1991; **9**: 44.

70. Keating MJ, O'Brien S, Kantarjian H, *et al*. Long-term follow-up of patients with chronic lymphocytic leukemia treated with fludarabine as a single agent. *Blood* 1993; **81**: 2878.

71. Keating MJ, Kantarjian H, O'Brien S, *et al*. Fludarabine (FLU)-Prednisone (PRED): A safe, effective combination in refractory chronic lymphocytic leukemia. *Proceedings of the American Society of Clinical Oncology* 1989; 201 (abstract).

72. Silber R, Potmesil M. Drug resistance in chronic lymphocytic leukemia. In *Chronic Lymphocytic Leukemia*, edited by BD Cheson. New York: Dekker, pp. 221–239, 1993.

73. Potmesil M, Bank B, Grossberg H, *et al*. Resistance of human leukemic and normal lymphocytes to DNA cleavage by drugs correlates with low levels of DNA topoisomerase. *Cancer Research* 1988; **49**: 4385.

74. Holmes JA, Jacobs A, Carter G, *et al*. Is the mdr 1 gene relevant in chronic lymphocytic leukemia? *Leukemia* 1990; **4**: 216.

75. Cooperative Group for the Study of Immunoglobulin in Chronic Lymphocytic Leukemia. Intravenous immunoglobulin for the prevention of infection in chronic lymphocytic leukemia. A randomized, controlled clinical trial. *New England Journal of Medicine* 1988; **319**: 902.

76. Kontoyianis DP, Anaissie EJ, Bodey GP. Infection in chronic lymphocytic leukemia: A reappraisal. In *Chronic Lymphocytic Leukemia*, edited by BD Cheson. New York: Dekker, pp. 399–417, 1993.

77. Rabinowe SN, Grossbard ML, Nadler LM. Innovative treatment strategies for chronic lymphocytic leukemia: monoclonal antibodies, immunoconjugates, and bone marrow transplantation. In *Chronic Lymphocytic Leukemia*, edited by BD Cheson. New York: Dekker, pp. 337–367, 1993.

42.   Hodgkin's Disease

Paul Kaesberg

Introduction

Hodgkin's disease is an infrequent malignancy, but heavily studied as a model for the cure of advanced malignancies. In younger persons, Hodgkin's disease is notable for being among only a handful of tumors that is curable even in its most advanced stages and curable by salvage chemotherapy once relapse has occurred. In older patients, while the responsiveness to chemotherapy still is common, curability and tolerance to therapy take a sharp decline. Histologic subtype distribution alters with age toward more aggressive subtypes, and stage at presentation appears to be more advanced in older patients. The bimodal age distribution suggests different etiologies in different age groups. The combination of immune suppression that occurs with Hodgkin's disease, with treatment and with immunesenescence causes a high susceptibility to opportunistic infections, making curative treatment more problematic. Despite this, clinical remissions, relief of symptoms and prolongation of life can be achieved with treatment tailored toward the patient's age and physical condition.

Epidemiology of Hodgkin's in the Elderly

Hodgkin's disease in the United States has a bimodal age distribution (1,2). The early peak is between ages 20 and 30, while the later peak is between ages 60 and 80, with the incidence starting to increase at about age 50. The epidemiology is different in developed versus underdeveloped countries, with the early peak being smaller to absent in underdeveloped countries (3). In the younger age group, the epidemiology is similar to that of paralytic polio (higher socioeconomic class, first child in the family and fewer siblings). Based on these pieces of evidence, McMahon proposed the possibility of a viral etiology with Hodgkin's disease more likely to occur (but still very rare) if the viral infection occurs later in childhood (4). No specific virus has been proposed to date, however, Epstein-Barr virus may be associated with Hodgkin's disease. There is an increased risk of Hodgkin's disease in patients with a history of mononucleosis (5,6) and Epstein-Barr virus is present in some cases of Hodgkin's disease (7). This epidemiologic finding continues in age groups 40–54 but not in older age groups. Thus it would appear that different etiologic factors are at work in older and younger age groups. With the obvious immunologic reaction that

occurs against the malignant cell, combined with the senescence of the immune system, the increased incidence may be due to decreased immune surveillance, though there is no experimental evidence to support this theory. In the older age group, men far out number women, while women are slightly more frequent in the lower age groups. Clustering of Hodgkin's disease, suggesting the disease might be contagious, has now been discarded as a concern (8).

Biology of Hodgkin's

The cellular origin of the Reed-Sternberg Cell remains unclear. Various studies have suggested that T (9–13) or B(14,15) lymphocytes, monocytes(16,17), or reticulum cells (18–20) may be the cell of origin. However other studies can be used to attempt to dismiss each of these possibilities (10,14,15,20–23). It may be that the cell of origin is different in different types of Hodgkin's disease. T and B cell gene rearrangement studies are occasionally positive, but the data has been hard to interpret (24–31). Many times, the immunoglobulin heavy chain gene is rearranged in Reed-Sternberg cells. It is was found to be polyclonal in four patients with lymphocyte predominant disease (32), and monoclonal in some, polyclonal in other patients with nodular sclerosing and mixed cellularity disease (33). Reed-Sternberg cells from twelve patients with nodular sclerosing and mixed cellularity Hodgkin's disease showed identical immunoglobulin heavy chain gene rearrangements in three, unrelated rearrangements in six and both identical and unrelated rearrangements in three, suggesting that these cells can be derived from B cell precursors or from memory cells (34). The polyclonal nature of Hodgkin's disease derived Reed-Sternberg cells could have several explanations, as outlined by Hummel et al. (34) including continued recruitment of new cells, genetic instability, immune system abnormalities that prevent the destruction of abnormal cells, and viral or chemical transformation. B-cell specific J-chain rearrangements have been limited to the nodular variant of lymphocyte predominant Hodgkin's disease, which is now largely accepted as a separate B-cell malignancy (21). Reed-Sternberg cells from this entity uniformly express CD20 (35). Light chain genes may also be rearranged (28). Reed-Sternberg rich cell populations also have been found to be negative for immunoglobulin gene rearrangements, which appears to be a true heterogeneity, rather than a tech-

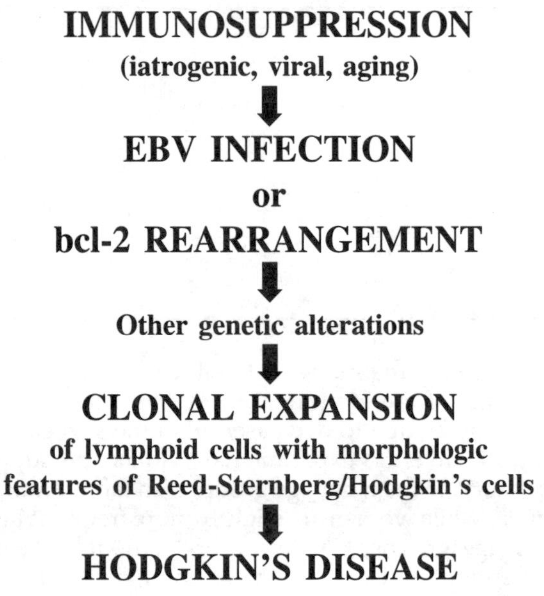

IMMUNOSUPPRESSION
(iatrogenic, viral, aging)

↓

EBV INFECTION

or

bcl-2 REARRANGEMENT

↓

Other genetic alterations

↓

CLONAL EXPANSION
of lymphoid cells with morphologic
features of Reed-Sternberg/Hodgkin's cells

↓

HODGKIN'S DISEASE

Figure 42.1 (adapted from 136).

nical problem (30). There have been inconsistent reports of rearrangements at the sites of oncogenes, especially bcl-2 (36–40), but also c-myc (41), ras (41,42) and p53 (43,44).

Cell surface marker studies have been somewhat confusing, as uniform expression of markers has not been generally found, even within subclasses of Hodgkin's disease. Some consistency has been seen. T-cell markers (CD1,CD2,CD3, and CD4) have been found frequently on Reed-Sternberg cells (31). It had been hoped that the Leu-M1 antibody, which recognizes CD15, would be a sensitive and specific marker for Reed-Sternberg cells. Reed-Sternberg are generally positive for CD15 (9,45), suggesting a monocyte origin of the Reed-Sternberg cell. T-cell non-Hodgkin's lymphomas have now been commonly identified to express CD15 (46–48). The Ki-1 antibody, raised against a Reed-Sternberg cell line, and recognizing antigen CD30, again was thought to be specific for Hodgkin's disease (49), but now is found on peripheral T-cell lymphomas (50), lymphomatoid papulosis (50–52) and anaplastic large cell lymphoma (50,53–55), which can be difficult to distinguish from Hodgkin's disease.

The most likely consideration at this time is that Reed-Sternberg and Hodgkin's cells arise from lymphocyte precursors, but they may not all arise from the same precursor. Progressive growth of Reed-Sternberg cells has been thought to be related to EBV infection (28). Figure 42.1 represents a possible pathogenesis of Hodgkin's disease.

Reed-Sternberg cells are nearly always aneuploid (56), and generally contain 4 to 8 times the normal amount of DNA (18). Chromosomal abnormalities are numerous and varied, however gains or other abnormalities in chromosomes 1,2,5,8,11,12,14, and 21 are most common. (18,25,57–60). Abnormalities involving 8q22-24, 11q23, and 14q32, which are associated with

other lymphoid malignancies, have been frequently found (58–60). At this time, these abnormalities have not been correlated with Hodgkin's disease subtypes.

Diagnosis of Hodgkin's in the Elderly

Lymphadenopathy

Hodgkin's disease frequently presents with lymphadenopathy, often rubbery and fixed to underlying tissue. Because of the myriad causes of lymphadenopathy, deciding when to biopsy a lymph node can cause a considerable dilemma. The risk of a neoplastic etiology for lymphadenopathy increases progressively with age. The incidence of most viral infections leading to lymphadenopathy declines with age, and the incidence of malignancy increases. Lymph nodes greater than 2 cm. in diameter, progressively enlarging nodes, lymph nodes found in the absence of acute infectious symptoms, lymphadenopathy found in the presence of night sweats or weight loss, and supraclavicular lymph nodes are most likely to lead to neoplastic diagnoses (61–63). Solitary enlarged nodes, fixed or matted nodes, and supraclavicular nodes should almost always be biopsied. Inguinal lymph nodes frequently do not yield a diagnosis. Adenopathy in other areas should be sought, or if the risk is high, multiple biopsies may be necessary. Sequential node biopsies often yield a diagnosis, when an initial biopsy is benign (64). In a study by Stanford (65), unexplained adenopathy was the presentation in 65% of patients with Hodgkin's disease over the age of 60, while 29% presented with B symptoms. Diagnosis requires examination of the architecture of lymph nodes as well as the cytology. For that reason, needle biopsy is not adequate for diagnosis.

Hodgkin's disease frequently involves cervical, supraclavicular, axillary, mediastinal, hilar, splenic, para-aortic, iliac and inguinal lymph nodes. It rarely involves Waldeyer's ring, mesenteric, epitrochlear and popliteal lymph nodes, suggesting that the initial site of Hodgkin's disease is in central lymph node regions and that retrograde spread through the lymphatic system is rare. Pulmonary involvement is almost always related to hilar or mediastinal involvement, and hepatic involvement almost always related to extensive splenic involvement.

Other Presentations of Hodgkin's Disease

While peripheral lymphadenopathy is the most common initial presentation of Hodgkin's disease, it certainly is not the only one. Especially in older patients, unusual presentations are possible. Older patients are more likely to have abdominal masses as their only site of disease, and initial presentations in the bone marrow, spleen, or lung can be seen. B symptoms as an initial presentation are common in older patients, and somewhat less common in younger patients.

In older patients, significant intercurrent illness is of major concern. In the Stanford study (65), 42% of patients over 60 had significant coronary artery disease, COPD, diabetes mellitus, hypertension or other illnesses that interfered with evaluation and management of the Hodgkin's disease. They considered 75% of older patients to have been adequately staged, and they were able to perform staging laparotomies in 45% of patients with significant intercurrent disease.

Histology of Hodgkin's Disease

The diagnostic cell for Hodgkin's disease is the Reed-Sternberg cell, which is a large binucleate cell with prominent nucleoli. Current understanding of the Reed-Sternberg cell is that it is of pleomorphic origin, with cell surface markings of CD30 (Ki-1), CD15 (Leu M1), HLA-DR, and CD25 (IL-2 receptor) positive (15,31,50, 66–69). These markers are not conserved across all variants of Hodgkin's disease or even within a single variant, possibly indicating differing etiologies of the disease. It is now considered the malignant cell in Hodgkin's disease, despite the fact that it may make up less than 1% of the total cells in an involved node or organ. This has been a topic of debate for many years. The diagnosis of Hodgkin's disease is still made on histologic examination of sections of lymph node tissue. While surface markings and genetic studies may serve to "rule in" diagnoses other than Hodgkin's disease, there are no unique markers for Hodgkin's disease allowing a biochemical or cytogenetic diagnosis. Strict criteria require identification of an Reed-Sternberg cell to make the diagnosis of Hodgkin's disease. On occasion, the mononuclear form — the "Hodgkin cell" — is more prominent, or multilobed variants of the Reed-Sternberg cell are found, and these may be used to make the diagnosis of Hodgkin's disease. The Reed-Sternberg cell may be present as a reactive cell in other disorders, so its presence, while considered necessary for the diagnosis of Hodgkin's disease, is not sufficient. The neoplastic cell must be observed in the appropriate background setting. (70,71).

The Rye modification of the Lukes and Butler classification divides Hodgkin's disease into four histologic categories: lymphocyte predominant, nodular sclerosis, mixed cellularity and lymphocyte depletion (71,72). Lymphocyte predominant Hodgkin's disease is characterized by an abundance of small round lymphocytes, and a small number of Reed-Sternberg cells. The nodular variant of this is considered by many to be a follicular low grade lymphoma, with an indolent and relapsing course. It may be difficult to distinguish from benign expansion of lymphoid follicles (73). The diffuse form may be difficult to distinguish from well-differentiated lymphocytic lymphoma (74). Lymphocyte depletion Hodgkin's disease is generally distinguished by the relative paucity of reactive cells and prominence of the malignant Reed-Sternberg cells. While different subgroups have been identified, most contain an amorphous background of fibrosis. In the differential diagnosis again are non-Hodgkin's lymphomas, as well as a lymphocyte depletion form of nodular sclerosing Hodgkin's disease. Mixed cellularity is often considered a midway point between Lymphocyte predominant and lymphocyte depletion Hodgkin's

disease, and contains a background of lymphocytes, plasma cells, eosinophils and fibroblasts. Differentiation from a peripheral T-cell lymphoma may be difficult. Nodular sclerosis is typified by wide bands of fibrous material separating lymph nodes into nodules. Along with this, Reed-Sternberg cells, lacunar cells and a background of lymphocytes and other cells are found. Multiple subvariants have been identified but it is unclear whether any prognostic significance can be attached to them (71,75,76).

Distribution of Hodgkin's Disease Histologies Across Age

The distribution of histologic subclasses of Hodgkin's disease varies with age. In general, it is thought that lymphocyte predominant and nodular sclerosis Hodgkin's disease are more common in younger patients while mixed cellularity and lymphocyte depletion variants are more common in older patients. Nodular sclerosing Hodgkin's disease is generally thought to be a disease of young women (76). According to Hellman et al., it is unusual in patients over the age of 50 (77). Decreased eosinophil infiltration occurs in Hodgkin's disease in older age groups (78). Again, this may be due to differing cellular reactions, or differing etiologies.

The Finsen Institute in Copenhagen examined the distribution of histologic subtypes in 506 unselected patients with Hodgkin's disease (about one-third of the cases of Hodgkin's disease in Denmark from the years 1969–1983), finding that while nodular sclerosing Hodgkin's disease was more common in younger patients, it still represented the most common subtype in patients over the age of 60 (79). The frequency of Lymphocyte predominant disease remained stable, while the frequency of mixed cellularity increased with age. The notable rarity of lymphocyte depletion Hodgkin's disease and the potential difficulty in distinguishing lymphocyte depletion Hodgkin's disease from a lymphocyte depletion subvariant of nodular sclerosing Hodgkin's disease may in part explain the discrepancy between this and other studies.

Stanford University investigators found that 64% of their "older patients" had nodular sclerosis subtype (80). Only 52 of 1,169 patients were over the age of 60. It is possible that there was a referral bias in older patients toward healthier and lower stage patients, who would be thought more to benefit from aggressive management. This selected population may have a higher proportion of better histologies such as nodular sclerosis.

The Cancer and Leukemia Group B reported on 73 patients over the age of 60 on protocol therapy for advance Hodgkin's disease (65). Seven percent of these patients had nodular sclerosing Hodgkin's disease compared to 30% of patients under the age of 40. The lower percentage of nodular sclerosing Hodgkin's disease in this study is explained by the selection of patients with advanced disease, unusual for nodular sclerosing Hodgkin's disease.

Our own tumor registry had similar distributions. Sixty-four percent of patients were under the age of 51.

Table 42.1 Staging classification of Hodgkin's disease.

Stage	Definition
I	Involvement single lymph node group (or spleen) on one side of the diaphragm
II	Involvement of more than one lymph node group (or spleen) on one side of the diaphragm)
III	Involvement of lymph node groups (or spleen) on both sides of the diaphragm
IV	Involvement of parenchymal organs (bone marrow, liver, lung, bone)
Subset E	Involvement of a single extranodal site (the differentiation between stage E and stage IV can be difficult)
Subset A	No constitutional symptoms
Subset B	Constitutional symptoms (drenching night sweats, fever >101 deg. F, weight loss greater than 10% of body weight, some investigators consider pruritis a symptom)

Stage III disease can be divided into subsets 1 (involvement of only splenic hilar, celiac or portal nodes) and 2 (involvement of para-aortic, iliac or mesenteric nodes)

Ten percent were unclassified, while 3% had lymphocyte predominant, 67% nodular sclerosing, 15% mixed cellularity and 5% lymphocyte depleted. Of those over 50 (24 patients), 42% had nodular sclerosing, 33% mixed cellularity, 8% lymphocyte predominant and 17% were unclassified (Meriter Hospital Tumor Registry, unpublished data).

These studies suggest a shift from nodular sclerosing Hodgkin's disease in younger patients to mixed cellularity and lymphocyte depletion in older patients. The cause for this is unknown. The background cellularity is vital in distinguishing histologic types, such that the differences may be in the way older patients form a reaction to Hodgkin's disease. This may be related to cellular immune senescence. It is notable that more aggressive forms of Hodgkin's disease occur in older persons, at odds with other cancers, where often less aggressive forms predominate. The strong immune reaction in younger patients to Hodgkin's disease and the well defined senescence of the immune system may explain the differing histologies with advancing age as well as the worsening stage and prognosis. Another possible explanation of differing histologies can be derived from the bimodal age distribution of Hodgkin's disease. The etiology may be different in older people, leading to differing cellular reactions and histologies.

Immunology of Hodgkin's

Cellular immunity is depressed in all patients with Hodgkin's disease, prior to the onset of treatment (81). Humoral immunity remains relatively intact. In patients with B symptoms, there is a reduction in circulating T lymphocytes (82) while it is normal in patients with stage A disease. Helper and suppressor T cell subsets remain normal in all stages of Hodgkin's disease. There is also to be an abnormality in T cell function in patients with B symptoms, while it is normal in patients without B symptoms (83). Increased T cell susceptibility to suppression by normal monocyte interactions (84) and suppressor T cells (85) occurs in all

stages of Hodgkin's disease. Interleukin 2 production also is decreased (86). It is unknown whether the immune suppression is a result of the disease or whether the immune suppression is a predecessor of the Hodgkin's disease. Older patients with Hodgkin's disease are frequently anergic, as are younger patients with stage B disease (87). These immune defects are the cause of the increase susceptibility to opportunistic organisms such as tuberculosis and fungal infections.

Staging

Hodgkin's disease is staged according to the Ann Arbor classification (88), developed in 1971 (Table 42.1). This system has both prognostic (89) and therapeutic value. Precise staging of Hodgkin's disease has importance not seen in other lymphomas. Since Hodgkin's disease spreads in an orderly manner (as opposed to many non-Hodgkin's lymphomas), precise staging allows careful tailoring of therapy to a particular pattern of involvement. Treatment of stage III Hodgkin's by radiation therapy is only possible because of precise staging, and because of the orderly manner of progression. Also, precise staging has allowed the comparison of results between studies to be much more reliable in this heavily investigated model disease.

Extranodal Hodgkin's disease comes in two forms. First is direct extension of disease from a nodal site. This is probably similar in prognosis and progression to nodal disease. Second is true non-contiguous extranodal disease. True extranodal disease represents a poorer prognosis than local extension from a nodal site into a single extranodal site (90). It is sometimes difficult to distinguish extranodal disease (what might be staged IIE, or IIIE) from stage IV disease. There can be marked disagreement among experienced clinicians given identical scenarios as to what is E disease and what is stage IV disease (91). This is of significant import for therapy, as much more intensive therapy is needed for stage IV disease, at the expense of side effects.

Table 42.2 Suggested staging plan for Hodgkin's Disease.

1. History, with emphasis on "B" symptoms: weight loss, fever, sweats

2. Physical exam, with emphasis on nodal areas, liver, spleen and skin

3. Laboratory studies to include CBC, differential, platelet count, erthrocyte sedimentation rate, creatinine, liver function studies, albumin, and total protein

4. Radiologic studies to include chest x-ray, with chest CT scan if any abnormality, CT of abdomen and pelvis, lymphangiogram (bipedal), and consideration of galllium 67 scan

5. Percutaneous bone marrow biopsy, bilateral

6. Percutaneous or laparoscopic liver biopsy

7 In select patients, exploratory laparotomy with splenectomy, wedge liver biopsy, and sampling of nodes from para-aortic, mesenteric, portal, and splenic hilar nodes

Stages are subclassified A or B. The stage is subclass B if the patient has one or more of the following: unexplained weight loss of more than 10% of body weight over the last 6 months, unexplained fever of above 38 deg. Centigrade, or drenching night sweats. The stage is subclass A if these are absent. Pruritus has been considered by some as a B symptom. In the Ann Arbor staging system, it is not considered a B symptom, however, recurrent generalized pruritus that ebbs and flows with the disease may be considered a B symptom.

It is important to note whether a given stage is based on pathologic or clinical information. Enlarged lymph nodes are assumed to be involved, but if therapeutic options would change, they should be biopsied. The spleen is often the first site of involvement in the abdomen of Hodgkin's disease arising above the diaphragm. Despite this, a homogenous, enlarged spleen on CT scan is often negative for involvement if there is no other evidence of disease below the diaphragm.

Basic Staging Procedures

A suggested plan for staging Hodgkin's disease is found in Table 42.2. History, in addition to looking for B symptoms, should concern unusual extranodal sites such as bone or gastrointestinal tract. Physical exam should include an assessment of Waldeyer's ring and skin as well as nodal sites, liver and spleen. Evaluation of thoracic disease is often accomplished with only a chest x-ray. If no abnormalities are seen, it is likely that the chest is grossly negative. If mediastinal disease obscures pulmonary parenchyma or if treatment will be altered by minimal findings in the chest, a CT of the chest is necessary. Equivocal cases may benefit from Gallium scanning (92,93). Complete evaluation of abdominal disease requires at least CT of the abdomen to evaluate the upper abdomen and lymphangiography to evaluate the lower abdomen and pelvis.

Staging Laparotomy

In the past, staging laparotomy was almost universally used in the staging of Hodgkin's disease, including many patients who were already known to be stage IV.

The technique of staging laparotomy is well described in many texts, however basically a careful abdominal exploration with routine biopsies of para-aortic, celiac and splenic hilar nodes, as well as biopsies of apparently involved mesenteric, portal and iliac nodes, splenectomy, wedge liver biopsy and two to three core liver biopsies are standard. Optionally, a large anterior iliac crest marrow biopsy is performed, however, frequently extensive bone marrow biopsies are done as a prelude to laparotomy. Staging laparotomy has been shown to upstage about 35% of patients and downstage about 15% of patients (94).

As the patterns of progression and treatment have become better understood, staging laparotomy has been needed less and less. There are several advantages to staging laparotomy: accurate mapping of lymph node involvement can guide radiation fields, or convert recommended treatment to chemotherapy or combined modality; downstaging of patients with intraabdominal node enlargement can occur; the spleen is removed which decreases side effects of radiation to the left kidney and the bowel; and, for research protocols, it is assured that patients are assigned to the appropriate stage groups for more precise evaluation of treatment efficacy.

Staging laparotomy is major abdominal surgery. Morbidity and mortality are of significant concern, especially in debilitated patients. Recent improvements in risk assessment and treatment have obviated the need for laparotomy in many cases. The use of erythrocyte sedimentation rate and C-reactive protein to estimate risk of abdominal disease is widely used in Europe and is becoming more common in the United States. Treatment protocols with short course chemotherapy, followed by consolidative radiation, can cure minimal disease in the abdomen. Thus, if gross disease is not seen on other staging studies, a laparotomy can often be avoided. It must be remembered that the elderly patient, in whom we wish to keep morbid procedures to a minimum, has the highest risk of abdominal disease (see below). The Stanford study (65) had 5 of 13 older patients with "early stage" Hodgkin's disease, not staged by laparotomy, that died of progressive Hodgkin's disease.

Staging laparotomy has allowed the subclassification of stage III abdominal disease. Stage III 1A is disease limited to the upper abdomen, the spleen as well as nodes in the celiac, splenic and hepatic portal areas, while stage III 2A is disease that has progressed to para-aortic, iliac or mesenteric nodes. When radiation is used as the sole treatment, relapse free survival is much better in patients with III 1A disease than III 2A disease, whereas this difference disappears when chemotherapy is used (95). Thus to treat stage III disease with radiation only requires staging by laparotomy, unless more extensive radiation techniques, such as prophylactic hepatic radiation, are used.

Alterations in the Elderly

Older patients have a higher likelihood of more advanced Hodgkin's disease. The Finsen Institute study (79)had stage distributions as follows: Age less than 41; stage I, 19%; stage II, 35%; stage III, 28%; stage IV 17%; Age greater than 60; stage I, 22%; stage II, 28%; stage III, 29%, stage IV, 21%. While these differences certainly would not achieve statistical significance, these distributions were noted with 60% of younger patients being staged with laparotomy, while only 18% of older patients were staged with laparotomy. Also, B symptoms were found in 54% of older patients, and only 37% of younger patients. There was a trend towards more extensive peripheral nodal and intrathoracic tumor burdens in younger patients and more extensive abdominal tumor burdens in older patients. While this would be expected with the differences in histologic distribution and the predilection of nodular sclerosing Hodgkin's disease for the mediastinum, this finding was actually independent of histologic subtype. Lokich *et al.* (96) found similar alterations in distribution with more peripheral adenopathy in younger patients and more abdominal disease in older patients, as well as 25% B symptoms in older patients and only 2% in younger patients.

Treatment

Treatment Based on Stage

The treatment of Hodgkin's disease has become better defined by clinical trials. Early stage disease (IA or IB, or IIA, especially when staged by laparotomy), are highly curable with appropriate fields of radiation. Experience with mantle and para-aortic field irradiation at the Harvard Joint Center (97) and Stanford (98) show an 85–95% five year disease free survival with radiation therapy alone, and no improvement with the addition of chemotherapy, in the absence of a large mediastinal mass. Number of involved sites appears not to have prognostic significance in stage II disease. For stage IA disease, surgically staged, mantle and para-aortic fields can be used. The mantle field includes cervical, supraclavicular, infraclavicular, axillary, mediastinal and pulmonary hilar nodes. Some evidence suggests that, with adequate surgical staging and exceptionally good risk factors, a mantle field only can

be used. Doses of radiation usually range form 3,500 to 4,400 cGy. Risk of cardiac and pulmonary complications are small with adequate blocking techniques, if a large mediastinal mass is not present (99,100). There is a somewhat higher relapse rate in pelvic nodes with mixed cellularity histology (11%) than with nodular sclerosing or lymphocyte predominant disease (5%) (101,102). Some patients with exceptionally good risk factors can be treated with mantle field alone, but one of the necessary factors is age under 40. In clinically staged IA patients, the use of subtotal lymphoid irradiation is feasible. It must include the spleen. Older patients, with greater risk of intraabdominal disease, may be less desirable candidates for this approach, but is can be considered when the risks of laparotomy and of chemotherapy appear to be excessive. Combined modality therapy reduces the risk of relapse, but has not been shown to improve survival in early stage patients (103,104).

Stage IB disease should be treated with radiation therapy as a single modality only if the patient has been surgically staged. Chemotherapy, either as a single modality, or as short course with radiation should be used for clinically staged patients (105,106).

Stage IIB disease is often treated with short course chemotherapy and radiation. Surgically staged IIB patients are curable with radiation, and may be cured with salvage chemotherapy if relapse occurs. The increased incidence of abdominal disease in clinical stage IIB disease places this in the gray zone of whether to proceed with laparotomy in hopes of avoiding chemotherapy, or to give chemotherapy to avoid laparotomy. Stage I and IIA disease below the diaphragm is uncommon, and therefore more difficult to manage precisely. Stage IA disease appears to be reasonably managed by inverted Y treatment, while stage IIA probably requires total lymphoid irradiation (complete inverted Y and upper mantle radiation) (107).

Stage III disease must be surgically staged before consideration of treatment with radiation alone. Stage IIIa1 disease is curable with total lymphoid irradiation. This is considered by most to be a reasonable treatment if there are less than five splenic nodules. Low dose radiation therapy to the liver is an option with this treatment. A recent retrospective suggests improved survival with the addition of chemotherapy but this has not been tested in randomized trials (108). Full dose chemotherapy is recommended for stage IIIa2 disease. Again, in patients where surgical staging is undesirable, short course chemotherapy plus radiation is a reasonable alternative, if gross disease within the abdomen is not found. Stage IIIB and stage IV disease is treated with full course chemotherapy.

Stage II disease with bulky mediastinal disease do poorly with radiation alone and should be treated with combined modality therapy (109). Controversy exists as to what constitutes bulky a mediastinal mass. The most common practice is to measure the maximum diameter of the mass, and maximum diameter of the pleural cavity, and calculate the ratio. Ratios greater than 1/3 are considered bulky mediastinal disease

Table 42.3 Chemotherapy for Hodgkin's disease.

MOPP:	Nitrogen Mustard 6 mg/M2 IV day 1 and 8
	Vincristine 1.4 mg/M2 IV day 1 and 8*
	Procarbazine 100 mg/M2 po day 1–14
	Prednisone 40 mg/M2 po day 1–14*
	Repeat every 28 days
	*Vincristine is often limited to 2 mg maximum dose
	Prednisone was originally given on cycles 1 and 4 only
ABVD:	Adriamycin 25 mg/M2 IV day 1 and 15
	Bleomycin 10 Units/M2 IV day 1 and 15
	Vinblastine 6 mg/M2 IV day 1 and 15
	Dacarbazine 375 mg/M2 IV day 1 and 15
	Repeat every 28 days
BCVPP:	BCNU 100 mg/M2 IV day 1
	Cyclophosphamide 600 mg/M2 IV day 1
	Vinblastine 5 mg/M2 IV day 1
	Procarbazine 100 mg/M2 po day 1–10
	Prednisone 60 mg/M2 po day 1–10
	Repeat every 28 days

(2,80,110). Some systems use absolute diameter of the mass, placing the cutoff at 6 cm (111), 10 cm (112) or 5 cm from the midline (113). Others use total tumor volume (114). These systems do not take into account the amount of lung field that may be subjected to radiation, and therefore may increase risk of serious side effects.

Multiple chemotherapy programs have been studied in Hodgkin's disease. A recently completed study showed that ABVD chemotherapy (see Table 42.3) is as or more effective than MOPP/ABV hybrid, which is more effective than MOPP alone. ABVD has some disadvantages in the elderly population. First, cardiac and pulmonary reserve must be acceptable because of the significant dosages of doxorubicin and bleomycin. Second, somewhat slower recovery of the marrow, which, in my experience, is more common in the elderly, makes treatment every 14 days difficult. BCVPP chemotherapy has a favorable acute toxicity profile, making it desirable in the debilitated or frail elderly. Here the higher risk of acute leukemia may be less of an issue than in younger patients. Full course chemotherapy is generally now given for a minimum of eight cycles or 4 cycles past complete remission, with a maximum of 12 cycles.

Complications of Therapy

Long term side effects of treatment for Hodgkin's disease are not uncommon. Acute myelogenous leukemia may occur with combined modality therapy or with combination chemotherapy, especially when alkylating agents are used. The risk is minimal but not non-existent with radiation therapy alone. MOPP chemotherapy results in about a 3% risk of AML in the first 10 years after therapy, with the peak at 5–9 years (115–117). ABVD chemotherapy appears to cause AML in somewhat less than 1% of patients (115). As mentioned above, BCVPP chemotherapy has a reputation for excess cases of leukemia. At 15 years, the risk of second malignancies in total is about 13% (115,116). Common sites of increased risk are lung and breast cancer, especially in those individuals with substantial radiation exposure at a young age to these organs (118–120). The combination of bleomycin chemotherapy and mantle radiation may result in severe pulmonary toxicity (121). Hypothyroidism is a common complication of radiation therapy to the upper mantle, even when the thyroid is blocked (122). Radiation pneumonitis, pericarditis and coronary disease may occur as complications of radiation therapy.

Recurrent Disease

Recurrent Hodgkin's disease remains a disease treatable for cure if radiation therapy was the only prior treatment, with 10 year survivals in the range of 57–80% (123–125). Relapse after chemotherapy is occasionally treatable for cure with chemotherapy. This is rarely successful if relapse has occurred within one year of completing chemotherapy, but is more likely in patients who relapse late (126,127). In eligible patients, who have been shown to have chemotherapy responsive disease, bone marrow transplantation probably offers the best chance of long term survival (128,129). Since this is rarely applicable to the elderly population, goals of therapy must be changed. Palliative care with radiation therapy to symptomatic sites, weekly injections of vinblastine, or daily oral alkylating agents may be well tolerated therapies with effective palliation.

Prognosis

Several reports outline the prognosis of older adults with Hodgkin's disease. Guinee *et al.* compared prognosis of Hodgkin's disease in 136 patients age patients age 60–79 with 223 patients aged 40–59 (130). The older group experienced twice the risk of dying from Hodgkin's disease and four times the risk of dying from other causes. Stages were similar, although increased numbers had stage I disease in the older age group. Data on frequency of staging procedures was not given. As expected, the histologies leaned toward nodular sclerosing in the younger vs older (56% vs 39%) and away from mixed cellularity in younger vs older (32% vs 50%). Complete remission rates were similar in younger and older groups (88% for younger, 84% for older), but patients aged 70–79 had a 41% relapse rate compared to less than 20% for younger patients. Looking only at deaths from Hodgkin's disease, 50% of older patients had died at 5 years, while only 20% of younger patients had.

Patients treated on CALGB protocols for advanced Hodgkin's disease had a significantly poorer prognosis if aged 60 or older compared to age less than 60 (131). Five year survival was 79% for ages less than 40, 63% for ages 40–59, and 31% for ages 60 and older. Median survival was 1.5 years for ages 60 and over, and had not been reached for younger patients. Stage was similar, although disease in the abdomen was more frequent in older patients.

Age is also an adverse factor after first relapse from Hodgkin's disease (132). Ten year freedom from second relapse was 61% for ages less than 40 and 40% for ages 40 and over. Ten year overall survival was 67% and 23% respectively, reflecting deaths from other causes. A letter by Guinee (referencing his above work) regarding this suggested that the adverse prognosis begins at about age 60 (133).

Zietman et al. studied 29 early stage patients with Hodgkin's disease over the age of 60 (134). They found that if they were able to tolerate staging and radiation therapy as would be recommended for younger patients, their prognosis was quite good (no relapses in 14 so managed patients). Patients managed suboptimally had 5 year survival and 5 year disease free survival of only 61 and 6% respectively.

Multiple other studies relating to prognosis of Hodgkin's disease show advancing age to be a poor prognostic factor (79,135–138).

Conclusions

Hodgkin's disease presents in the elderly with a differing distribution of histologies, and probably with a different etiology. While a viral etiology seems likely in younger patients, it probably is not the cause of Hodgkin's disease in a significant number of older patients. Older patients are more likely to present with intra-abdominal disease, and more advanced stage, despite less aggressive staging studies. Tolerance to treatment is decreased in the elderly, but the principles of treatment are the same as for younger patients, with some adjustments needed for the frail elderly, and those with certain co-morbid conditions. Prognosis is worse in the elderly, probably for several reasons, including higher risk histologies, more advanced stage, poorer tolerance to treatment, co-morbid conditions, and immune senescence.

References

1. MacMahon B. Epidemiologic considerations in staging of Hodgkin's disease. Cancer 1983; 31:1854–1857.
2. Young J, Percy C, Asire A, et al. Surveillance, Epidemiology and End Result: Incidence and Mortality. Bethesda, MD: National Cancer Institute, 1981.
3. Correa P, O'Conor GT, Berard CW, et al. International comparability and reproducibility in histologic subclassification of Hodgkin's disease. J Natl Cancer Inst 1973; 50: 1429–1435.
4. MacMahon B. Epidemiology of Hodgkin's disease. Cancer Res 1966; 26: 1189–1200.
5. Rosdahl N, Larsen SO, Clemmensen J. Hodgkin's disease in patients with previous mononucleosis, 30 years experience. Br Med J 1974; 2: 253–256.
6. Munoz N, Davidson RJ, Withoff B, et al. Infectious mononucleosis and Hodgkin's disease. Int J Cancer 1978; 22: 10–13.
7. Nonoyama M, Kawai Y, Huang CH, et al. Epstein-Barr virus DNA in Hodgkin's disease, American Burkitt's lymphoma and other human tumors. Cancer Res 1974; 34: 1228–1231.
8. Mueller NE. Hodgkin's disease. In Cancer epidemiology and prevention, 2nd ed., edited by D Schottenfeld, J Fraumeni. New York: Oxford University Press, 1992.
9. Pinkus G, Thomas P, Said JW. Leu-M1 — a marker for Reed Sternberg cells in Hodgkin's disease. Am J. Pathol 1985; 119: 244–252.
10. Schwarrting R, Gerdes J, Ziegler A, et al. Immunoprecipitation of the interleukin-2 receptor from Hodgkin's disease derived cell lines by monoclonal antibodies. Hematol Oncol 1987; 5: 57–64.
11. Pizzola G, Chilosi M, Sementzato G, et al. Immunohistological analysis of Tac antigen expression in tissues involved by Hodgkin's disease. Br J Cancer 1984; 50: 415–417.
12. Diehl V, Kirchner HH, Burricher H, et al. Characteristics of Hodgkin's disease derived cell lines. Cancer Treat Rep 1982; 66: 615–632.
13. Drexler HG, Gaedicke g, Lok MS, et al. Hodgkin's disease derived cell lines HDLM-2 and L428: Comparison of morphology, immunological and isoenzyme profiles. Cancer Res 1986; 10: 487–500.
14. Dorreen MS, Habeshaw JA, Stansfield AG, et al. Characterization of Sternberg-Reed and related cells in Hodgkin's disease: An immunohistological study. Br J Cancer 1984; 49: 465–476.
15. Strauchen JA, Dimitriu-Bona A. Immunopathology of Hodgkin's disease: Characterization of Reed-Sternberg cells with monoclonal antibodies. Am J Pathol 1986; 123: 293–300.
16. Foon KA, and Todd RF. Immunologic classification of leukemia and lymphoma. Blood 1986; 68: 1–31.
17. Payne SV, Wright DH, Jones KJM, et al. Macrophage origin of Reed-Sternberg cells: An immunohistochemical study. J Clin Pathol 1982; 35: 159–166.
18. Hansmann ML, Kaiserling E. The lacunar cell and its relationship to interdigitating reticulum cells. Virchows Arch 1982; 39: 323–332.
19. Kadin M. Possible origin of the Reed-Sternberg cell from an interdigitating reticulum cell. Cancer Treat Rep 1982; 66: 601–608.
20. Stein H, Gerdes J, Schwab U, et al. Identification of Hodgkin and Sternberg-Reed cells as a unique cell type derived from a newly detected small-cell population. Int. J Cancer 1982; 30: 445–459.
21. Stein H, Hansmann ML, Lennert K, et al. Reed-Sternberg and Hodgkin's cells in lymphocyte-predominant Hodgkin's disease of nodular subtype contain J chain. Am J Clin Pathol 1986; 86: 292–297.
22. Stein H, Gerdes J, Kirchner H, et al. Hodgkin and Sternberg-Reed cell antigen(s) detected by an antiserum to a cell line (L428) derived from Hodgkin's disease. Int J Cancer 1981; 28: 425–429.
23. Stein H, Gerdes J, Ulrich S, et al. Evidence for the detection of the normal counterpart of the Hodgkin and Sternberg-Reed cells. Hematol Oncol 1983; 1: 21–29.
24. Brinker MG, Poppema S, Buys CH, et al. Clonal immunoglobulin gene rearrangements in tissues involved by Hodgkin's disease. Blood 1987; 70: 186–191.
25. Griesser H, Mak TW. Immunophenotyping in Hodgkin's disease. Hematol Oncol 1988; 6: 239–245.
26. Knowles DM, Neri A, Pelicci PG, et al. Immunoglobulin and T-cell receptor B-chain gene rearrangement analysis of Hodgkin's disease: Implications for lineage rearrangement analysis of Hodgkin's disease: Implications for lineage determination and differential diagnosis. Proc Natl Acad Sci USA 1986; 83: 7942–7946.
27. Raghavachar A, Binder T, Bartram CR. Immunoglobulin and T-cell receptor gene rearrangements in Hodgkin's disease. Cancer Res 1988; 48: 3591–3594.
28. Weiss LM, Warnke RA, Sklar J. Clonal antigen receptor gene rearrangements and Epstein-Barr viral DNA in tissues of Hodgkin's disease. Hematol Oncol 1988; 6: 233–238.

29. Cossman J, Sundeen J, Uppenkamp M, *et al*. Rearranging antigen-receptor genes in enriched Reed-Sternberg cell fractions of Hodgkin's disease. *Hematol Oncol* 1988; **6**: 205–211.

30. Sundeen J, Lipford E, Uppenkamp M, *et al*. Rearranged antigen receptor genes in Hodgkin's disease. *Blood* 1987; **70**: 96–103.

31. Kadin ME Muramoto L, Said J. Expression of T-cell antigens on Reed-Sternberg cells in a subset of patients with nodular sclerosing and mixed cellularity Hodgkin's disease. *Am J Pathol* 1988; **130**: 345–353.

32. Delabie J, Tierens A, Wu G, *et al*. Lymphocyte predominance Hodgkin's disease: lineage and clonality determination using a single-cell assay. *Blood* 1994; **84**: 3291–3298.

33. Kuppers R, Rajewsky K, Zhao M, *et al*. Hodgkin disease: Hodgkin and Reed-Sternberg cells picked from histological sections show clonal immunoglobulin gene rearrangements and appear to be derived from B cells at various stages of development. *Proc Natl Acad Sci USA* 1994; **91**: 10962–10966.

34. Hummel M, Ziemann K, Lammert H, *et al*. Hodgkin's disease with monoclonal and polyclonal populations of Reed-Sternberg cells. *NEJM* 1995; **333**: 901–906.

35. Pinkus, G, Said J. Hodgkin's disease, lymphocyte predominance type, nodular — further evidence of a B-cell derivation. *Am J Pathol* 1988; **133**: 211.

36. Shibata D, Hu E, Weiss LM, *et al*. Detection of specific t(14:18) chromosomal translocations in fixed tissues. *Hum Pathol* 1990; **21**: 199–203.

37. Said H, Sassoon A, Sintaku I, *et al*. Absence of bcl-2 major breakpoint region and JH gene rearrangement in lymphocyte predominance Hodgkin's disease: Results of Southern blot analysis and polymerase chain reaction. *Am J Pathol* 1991; **138**: 261–264.

38. Louie DC, Kant JA, Brooks JJ, Reed JC. Absence of t(14:18) major and minor breakpoints and of bcl-2 protein over-production in Reed-Sternberg cells of Hodgkin's disease. *Am J Pathol* 1991; **139**: 1231–1237.

39. Athan E, Chadburn A, Knowles DM. The bcl-2 gene translocation is undetectable in Hodgkin's disease by Southern blot hybridization and polymerase chain reaction. *Am J Pathol* 1992; **141**: 193–201.

40. Poppema S, Kaleta J, Hepperle B. Chromosomal abnormalities in patients with Hodgkin's disease: Evidence for frequent involvement of the 14q chromosomal region but infrequent bcl-2 gene rearrangement in Reed-Sternberg cells. *J Natl Cancer Inst* 1992; **84**: 1789.

41. Mitani S, Sugawara I, Shiku H, Mori S. Expression of c-myc oncogene product and ras family oncogene products in various human malignant lymphomas defined by immunohisto-chemical techniques. *Cancer* 1988; **62**: 2085–2093.

42. Steenvoorden A, Janssen J, Drexler H, *et al*. Ras mutations in Hodgkin's disease. *Leukemia* 1988; **2**: 325–326.

43. Gupta RK, Norton AJ, Thompson IW, *et al*. p53 expression in Reed-Sternberg cells of Hodgkin's disease. *Br J Cancer* 1992; **66**: 649–652.

44. Gupta RK, Patel K, Bodmer WF, Bodmer JG. Mutation of p53 in primary biopsy material and cell lines from Hodgkin disease. *Proc Natl Acad Sci USA* 1993; **90**: 2817–2821.

45. Hsu G, Jaffe E. Leu M1 and peanut agglutinin stain the neoplastic cells of Hodgkin's disease. *Am J Clin Pathol* 1984; 82: **29**.

46. Strauchen J, Breakstone B. Leu-M1 antigen: Comparative expression in Hodgkin's disease and T-cell lymphoma. *Hematol Oncol* 1987; 5: **107**.

47. Wieczorek R, Burke J, Knowles D III. Leu-M1 antigen expression in T-cell neoplasia. *Am J Pathol* 1985; **212**: 374–380.

48. Sheibani K, Battifora H, Burke J, Rappaport H. Leu-M1 antigen in human neoplasms: An immunohistologic study of 400 cases. *Am J Surg Pathol* 1986; **10**: 227–236.

49. Schwab U, Stein H, Gerdes J, *et al*. Production of a monoclonal antibody specific for Hodgkin and Reed-Sternberg cells in Hodgkin's disease. *Am J Pathol* 1985; **118**: 209.

50. Stein H, Mason DY, Gerdes J, *et al*. The expression of the Hodgkin's disease associated antigen Ki-1 in reactive and neoplastic lymphoid tissue: Evidence that Reed-Sternberg cells and histiocytic malignancies are derived from activated lymphoid cells. *Blood* 1985; **66**: 848–858.

51. Kadin M. Histogenesis of Hodgkin's disease: Possible insights from a comparison with lymphomatoid papulosis. *Hum Pathol* 1987; **18**: 1085–1088.

52. Davis TH, Morton CC, Miller-Cassman R, *et al*. Hodgkin's disease, lymhomatoid papulosis, and cutaneous T-cell lymphoma derived from a common T-cell clone. *N Eng J Med* 1992; **326**: 1115–1122.

53. Kadin M, Sako D, Berliner N, *et al*. Childhood Ki-1 lymphoma presenting with skin lesions and peripheral adenopathy. *Blood* 1986; **68**: 1042–1049.

54. Kadin M. Ki-1 positive anaplastic large cell lymphoma: A clinicopathologic entity? *J Clin Oncol* 1991; **9**: 533–536.

55. Greer J, Kinney M, Collins R, *et al*. Clinical features of 31 patients with Ki-1 anaplastic large cell lymphoma. *J Clin Oncol* 1991; **9**: 533–536.

56. Andreesen R, Oslerholz J, Lohv GW, *et al*. A Hodgkin cell-specific antigen is expressed on a subset of auto- and allo-activated T(helper) lymphoblasts. *Blood* 1984; **63**: 1299–1302.

57. Fisher RI, Bates SE, Bostick-Bruton F, *et al*. Neoplastic cells obtained from Hodgkin's disease are potent stimulators of human primary mixed lymphocyte cultures. *J Immunol* **130**: 2666–2670.

58. Cabanillas F, Pathak S, Trujillo J, *et al*. Cytogenetic features of Hodgkin's disease suggest a possible origin from a lymphocyte. *Blood* 1991; **71**: 1615–1617.

59. Tilly H, Bastard C, Delastre T *et al*. Cytogenetic studies in untreated Hodgkin's disease. *Blood* 1991; **77**: 1298–1304.

60. Cabanillas F. A review and interpretation of cytogenetic abnormalities identified in Hodgkin's disease. *Hematol Oncol* 1988; **6**: 271–274.

61. Lee Y-TN, Terry R, Lukes. Lymph node biopsy for diagnosis: A statistical study. *J Surg 1 Oncol* 1980; **14**: 53–60.

62. Sinclair S, Beckman E, Ellman S. Biopsy of enlarged, superficial lymph nodes. *JAMA* 1974; **228**: 602–603.

63. Greenfield S, Jordan C. The clinical investigation of lymphadenopathy in primary care practice. *JAMA* 1978; **240**: 1388–1393.

64. Saltzman SL. The fate of patients with nondiagnostic lymph node biopsies. *Surgery* 1965; **58**: 659.

65. Peterson B, Pajak T, Cooper MR, *et al*. Effect of age on therapeutic response and survival in advanced Hodgkin's disease. *Cancer Treat Rep* 1982; **66**: 889–898.

66. Strauchen JA, Breakstone BA. IL-2 receptor expression in human lymphoid lesions. Immunohistochemical study of 166 cases. *Am J Pathol* 1987; **126**: 506–512.

67. Angel CA, Warford A, Campbell AC, *et al*. The immuno-histology of Hodgkin's disease Reed-Sternberg cells and their variants. *J Pathol* 1987; **153**: 21–30.

68. Diehl V, Pfreundschul M, Fonatsch C, *et al*. Phenotypic and genotypic analysis of Hodgkin's disease derived cell lines: Histopathological and clinical implications. *Cancer Surveys* 1985; **4**: 399–419.

69. Hansmann ML, Radzun HJ, Nebendahl C, *et al*. Immuno-electronmicroscopic investigation of Hodgkin's disease with monoclonal antibodies against histiocytes. *Eur J Haematol* 1988; **40**:25–30.

70. Lukes RJ. Criteria for involvement of lymph node, bone marrow, spleen and liver in Hodgkin's disease. *Cancer Res* 1971; **31**: 1755–1767.

71. Lukes RJ, Butler JJ. the pathology and nomenclature of Hodgkin's disease. *Cancer Res* 1966; **26**: 1063–1081.

72. Lukes RJ, Craver LF, Hall TC, *et al*. Report of the nomenclature committee. *Cancer Res* 1966; **26**: 1311.

73. Poppema S, Kaiserling E, Lennert K. Hodgkin's disease with lymphocyte predominance, nodular type (nodular paragranu-loma) and progressively transformed germinal centers — a cytohistological study. *Histopathology* 1979; **3**: 295–308.

74. Schnitzer B. Reed-Sternberg-like cells in lymphocytic lymphoma and chronic lymphocyte leukemia. *Lancet* 1970; **1**: 1399–1400.

75. Bennett MH, MacLennan, Easterling MJ, *et al*. Analysis of histological subtypes in Hodgkin's disease in relation to prognosis and survival. In *The Cytology of Leukaemias and Lymphomas*, edited by D Quaglino, FGJ Hayhoe. New York: Raven Press, pp. 15–32, 1985.

76. Keller AR, Kaplan HS, Lukes RJ, *et al*. Correlation of histopathology with other prognostic indicators in Hodgkin's disease. *Cancer* 1968; **22**: 487–499.

77. Hellman S, Jaffe E, DeVita V. Hodgkin's disease. In *Cancer: Principles and Practice of Oncology*, edited by V DeVita, S Hellman, S Rosenberg. Philadelphia: JB Lippincott Co., pp. 1698–1740, 1989.

78. Newell Gr, Cole SR, Miettnen OS, MacMahon B. Age differences in the histology of Hodgkin's disease. *J Natl Cancer Inst.* 1970; **45**: 311.

79. Specht L, Nissen NI. Hodgkin's disease and age. *Eur J Haematol* 1989; **43**: 127–135.

80. Austin-Seymour M, Hoppe R, Cox R, *et al*. Hodgkin's disease in patients over 60 years old. *Ann Intern Med* 1984; **100**: 13–16.

81. Twomey JJ, Rice L. Impact of Hodgkin's disease upon the immune system. *Semin Oncol* 1980; **7**: 114–125.

82. Posner MR, Reinherz EL, Breard J, *et al*. Lymphoid subpopulations of peripheral blood and spleen in untreated Hodgkin's disease. *Cancer* 1981; **48**: 1170–1176.

83. Fisher RI, Bates SE, Bostick-Bruton F, *et al*. Neoplastic cells obtained from Hodgkin's disease are potent stimulators of human primary mixed lymphocyte cultures. *J Immunol* 1983; **130**: 2666–2670.

84. Fisher RI, Vanhaelen CP, Bostick F. Increased sensitivity to normal adherent suppressor cells in untreated advanced Hodgkin's disease. *Blood* 1981; **57**: 830–835.

85. Vanhaelen CP, Fisher RI. Increased sensitivity of lymphocytes from patients with Hodgkin's disease to concanavalin A induced suppressor cells. *J Immunol* 1981; **127**: 1216–1220.

86. Ford RJ, Tsao J, Kouttab NM, *et al*. Association of an interleukin abnormality with the T cell defect in Hodgkin's disease. *Blood* 1984; **64**: 386–392.

87. Slivnick DJ, Ellis TM, Nawrocki JF, Fisher RI. The impact of Hodgkin's disease on the immune system. *Semin Oncol* 1996; **17**: 673–682.

88. Carbone PP, Kaplan HS, Musshoff K, *et al*. Report of the Committee on Hodgkin's Disease Staging. *Cancer Res* 1971; **31**: 1860–1861.

89. Kaplan HS. Hodgkin's Disease. Edition 2. Cambridge, Massachusetts: Harvard University Press, 1980.

90. Musshoff K. Prognostic and therapeutic implications of staging in extranodal Hodgkin's disease. *Cancer Res* 1971; **31**: 1814–1827.

91. Connors JM, Klimo P. Is it an E lesion or stage IV? An unsettled issue in Hodgkin's disease staging. *J Clin Oncol* 1984; **2**: 1421–1423.

92. Johnston GS, Go MF, Benua RS, *et al*. Gallium-67 citrate imaging in Hodgkin's disease. Final report of cooperative group. *J Nucl Med* 1977; **18**: 692–698.

93. Horn NL, Ray GR, Kriss JP. Gallium-67 citrate scanning in Hodgkin's disease and non-Hodgkin's lymphoma. *Cancer* 1976; **37**: 250–257.

94. Taylor MA, Kaplan HS, Nelson TS. Staging laparotomy with splenectomy for Hodgkin's disease. The Stanford experience. *World J Surg* 1985; **9**: 449–460.

95. Stein RS, Golomb HM, Wiernik PH, *et al*. Anatomic substages of stage IIIA Hodgkin's disease. Followup of a collaborative study. *Cancer Treat Rep* 1982; **66**: 733–741.

96. Lokich JJ, Pinkus GS, Maloney WC. Hodgkin's disease in the elderly. *Oncology* 1974; **29**: 484–500.

97. Goodman RL, Piro AJ, Hellman S. Can pelvic irradiation be omitted in patients with pathologic stages IA and IIA Hodgkin's disease? *Cancer* 1976; **37**: 2834–2839.

98. Hoppe RT, Coleman CN, Cox RS, *et al*. The management of stage I-II Hodgkin's disease with radiation alone or combined modality therapy: The Stanford experience. *Blood* 1982; **59**: 455–465.

99. Tarbell NJ, Thompson L, Mauch P: Thoracic irradiation in Hodgkin's disease. Disease control and long-term complications. *International J Rad Oncol Biol Phys* 1990; **18**: 275–281.

100. Marcus KC, Svensson G, Rhodes LP, *et al*. Mantle irradiation in the upright position. A technique to reduce the volume of lung irradiated in patients with bulky mediastinal Hodgkin's disease. *Int J Rad Oncol Biol Phys* 1992; **23**: 443–447.

101. Mauch PM: Controversies in the management of early stage Hodgkin's disease. *Blood* 1994; **83**: 318–329.

102. Zanni M, Viviani S, Santoro A, *et al*. Extended-field radiotherapy in favorable stage IA-IIA Hodgkin's disease (prognostic role of stage). *Int J Rad Oncol Biol Phys* 1994; **30**: 813–819.

103. Koziner B, Myers J, Cirrincione C, *et al*. Treatment of stages I and II Hodgkin's disease with three different therapeutic modalities. *Am J Med.* 1986; **80**: 1067–1078.

104. Longo DL, Glatstein E, Duffy PL, *et al*. Radiation therapy versus combination chemotherapy in the treatment of early stage Hodgkin's disease: Seven year results of a prospective clinical trial. *J Clin Oncol* 1991; **9**: 906–917.

105. Carde P, Hagenbeek A, Hayat M, *et al*. Clinical staging versus laparotomy and combined modality with MOPP versus ABVD in early-stage Hodgkin's disease: the H6 twin randomized trials from the European Organization for Research and Treatment of Cancer Lymphoma Cooperative Group. *J Clin Oncol* 1993; **11**: 2258–2272.

106. Crnkovich MJ, Leopold K, Hoppe RT, *et al*. Stage I to IIB Hodgkin's disease: the combined experience at Stanford University and the Joint Center for Radiation Therapy. *J Clin Oncol* 1987; **5**: 1041–1049.

107. Krikorian JG, Portlock CS, Mauch PM. Hodgkin's disease presenting below the diaphragm: A review. *J Clin Oncol* 1986; **4**: 1551–1562.

108. Marcus KC, Kalish LA, Coleman CN, *et al*. Improved survival in patients with limited stage IIIA Hodgkin's disease treated with combined radiation therapy and chemotherapy. *J Clin Oncol* 1994; **12**: 2567–2572.

109. Behar RA, Horning SJ, Hoppe RT: Hodgkin's disease with bulky mediastinal involvement: effective management with combined modality therapy. *Int J Rad Oncol Biol Phys* 1993; **25**: 771–776.

110. Rappaport H. Tumors of the hematopoietic system. In Atlas of Tumor Pathology, section III, fasc 8. Washington D.C., Armed Forces Institute of Pathology, 1966.

111. Bonnadonna G, Valagussa P, Santoro A. Prognosis of bulky Hodgkin's disease treated with chemotherapy alone or combined with radiotherapy. *Cancer Surv* 1985; **4**: 437–458.

112. Sutcliffe SB, Gospodarowicz MK, Bergsagel DE, *et al*. Prognostic groups for management of localized Hodgkin's disease. *J Clin Oncol* 1985; **3**: 393–401.

113. Mill WB, Lee FA. Prognostic parameters in early stage Hodgkin's disease. *Int J Radiat Oncol Biol Phys* 1982; **8**: 837–841.

114. Willet CG, Linggod RM, Leong JC, *et al*. Stage IA to IIB mediastinal Hodgkin's disease: Three-dimensional volumetric assessment of response to treatment. *J Clin Oncol* 1988; **6**: 819–824.

115. Valagussa P, Santoro A, Fossati-Bellani F, *et al*. Second acute leukemia and other malignancies following treatment for Hodgkin's disease. *J Clin Oncol* 1986; **4**: 830–837.

116. Tucker MA, Coleman CN, Cox RS, *et al*. Risk of second cancers after treatment for Hodgkin's disease. *N Eng J Med* 1988; **318**: 76–81.

117. van Leeuwen FE, Chorus AM, van den Belt-Dusebout AW, *et al*. Leukemia risk following Hodgkin's disease: Relation to cumulative dose of alkylating agents, treatment with teniposide combinations, number of episodes of chemotherapy and bone marrow damage. *J Clin Oncol* 1994; **12**: 1063–1073.

118. Swerdlow AJ, Douglas AJ, Hudson GV, *et al*. Risk of second primary cancers after Hodgkin's disease by type of treatment: analysis of 2846 patients in the British National Lymphoma Investigation. *Br Med J* 1992; **304**: 1137–1143.

119. Yahalom J, Petrek JA, Biddinger PW, *et al*. Breast cancer in patients irradiated for Hodgkin's disease: A clinical and pathologic analysis of 45 events in 37 patients. *J Clin Oncol* 1994; **12**: 312–325.

120. Hancock SL, Tucker MA, Hoppe RT: Breast cancer after treatment of Hodgkin's disease. *J Natl Cancer Inst* 1993; **85(1)**: 25–31.

121. Bates NP, Williams MV, Bessel EM *et al*. Efficacy and toxicity of vinblastine, bleomycin and methotrexate with involved-field radiotherapy in clinical stage IA and IIA Hodgkin's disease: A British National Lymphoma Investigation pilot study. *J Clin Oncol* 1994; **12**: 288–296.

122. Schimpff SC, Diggs CJ, Wiswell JG, *et al.* Radiation-related thyroid dysfunction: implications for the treatment of Hodgkin's disease. *Annals of Internal Medicine* 1980; **92**: 91–98.

123. Roach M, Brophy N, Cox R *et al.* Prognostic factors for patients relapsing after radiotherapy for early stage Hodgkin's disease. *J Clin Oncol* 1990; **8**: 623–629.

124. Specht L, Horwich A, Ashley S, *et al.* Salvage of relapse of patients with Hodgkin's disease in clinical stages I or II who were staged with laparotomy and initially treated with radiotherapy alone: a report from the International Database on Hodgkin's Disease. *Int J Rad Oncol Biol Phys* 1994; **30**: 805–811.

125. Healey EA, Tarbell NJ, Kalish LA *et al.* Prognostic factors for patients with Hodgkin's disease in first relapse. *Cancer* 1993; **71(8)**: 2613–2620.

126. Harker WG, Kushlan P, Rosenberg SA: Combination chemotherapy for advanced Hodgkin's disease after failure of MOPP: ABVD and B-CAVe. *Annals of Int Med* 1984; **101**: 440–446.

126a. Walker A, Schoenfild Er, Lowman JT, *et al.* Survival of the older patient compared with the younger patient with Hodgkin's disease. *Cancer* 1990; **65**: 1635–1640.

127. Canellos GP, Petroni GR, Barcos M *et al.* Etoposide, vinblastine and doxorubicin: an active regimen for the treatment of Hodgkin's disease in relapse following MOPP. *J Clin Oncol* 1995; **13(8)**: 2005–2011.

128. Bierman PJ, Bagin RG, Jagannath S *et al.* High dose chemotherapy followed by autologous hematopoietic rescue in Hodgkin's disease: long term follow-up in 128 patients. *Annals Oncol* 1993; **4**: 767–773.

129. Reece DE Barnett MJ, Connors JM *et al.* Intensive chemotherapy with cyclophosphamide, carmustine, and etoposide followed by autologous bone marrow transplantation for relapsed Hodgkin's disease. *J Clin Oncol* 1991; **9**: 1871–1879.

130. Guinee VF, Giacco GG, Durand M. *et al.* The prognosis of Hodgkin's disease in older adults. *J Clin Oncol* 1991; **9**: 947–953.

131. Mir R, Anderson J, Strauchen J *et al.* Hodgkin disease in patients 60 years of age and older. *Cancer* 1993; **71**: 1857–1866.

132. Healey EA, Tarbell NJ, Kalish LA, *et al.* Prognostic factors for patients with Hodgkin's disease in first relapse. *Cancer* 1993; **71**: 2613–2620.

133. Guinee VF. Prognostic factors for patients with Hodgkin disease in relapse (letter). *Cancer* 1993; **72**: 2290.

134. Zietman AL, Linggod RM, Brookes AR, *et al.* Radiation therapy in the management of early stage Hodgkin's disease presenting later in life. *Cancer* 1991; **68**: 1869–1871.

135. Enblad G, Glimelius B, Sundstrom C. Treatment outcome in Hodgkin's disease in patients above the age of 60: a population based study. *Ann Oncol* 1991; **2**: 297–302.

136. Haluska FG, Brufsky AM, Canellos GP. The Cellular Biology of the Reed-Sternberg Cell. *Blood* 1994; **84**: 1005–1019.

137. Terblanche AP, Falkson G, Matzner L. The prognostic significance of age in patients with advanced Hodgkin's disease. *Eur J Cancer Clin Oncol* 1988; **24**: 1805–1809.

138. Davis S, Dahlberg S, Myers MH, *et al.* Hodgkin's disease in the United States: a comparison of patients characteristics and survival in the Centralized Cancer Patient Data System and The Surveillance, Epidemiology, and End Results Program. *J Natl Cancer Inst* 1987; **78**: 471–478.

43.   Non-Hodgkin's Lymphomas

Silvio Monfardini and Antonino Carbone

Epidemiology

In Western countries, elderly individuals (aged >65 years) constitute the most rapidly growing section of the population and the group at highest risk for cancer (1–3). It has been calculated that at the turn of the century approximately 1 in 5 of the population of the industrialized countries will be over 65 (1–3). The extent to which cancer affects the elderly population is well-illustrated by the fact that in the United States from 1973 to 1981 59% of all cancers diagnosed in males, and 52% in females, occurred in persons older than 65 years (4). The absolute number and the prevalence of malignancies in older individuals is expected to increase in Western countries in the next decades as the population grows older. At the same time, the proportion of patients with cancer who are older than 65 will also increase.

The incidence of non-Hodgkin's lymphomas (NHL) has rapidly increased in recent years in the USA and Europe (5–7). Intriguingly, different published series reported a significant proportion (18–38%) of all patients as being elderly at diagnosis (8–13), although they were heterogeneously defined by different age cut-points, i.e. 60, 65 or 70 years (14). Whatever the definition of elderly patients, the incidence of lymphoma increases exponentially with age between 20 and 79 (Figure 43.1) (7,15). This increased incidence is specific for non-Hodgkin's Lymphomas (NHL) and was not observed for other hematologic neoplasias such as acute leukemia or Hodgkin's disease (16).

Causes of Increased Incidence of Lymphoma in Older Individuals

Changing trends in lymphoma incidence and mortality, whether geographical or temporal, may provide important insights into the etiology and the value of new treatments of these malignancies. In the United States the incidence of NHL increased more than 100% from the late 1940s to early 1980s (5, 17). These increases are larger than those observed in the mortality rates. Increases in age-adjusted incidence are due primarily to increases among persons aged 65 and over (5, 18). Increases in mortality rates also were greater in the oldest age groups. The pronounced increases in incidence and mortality rates among the older age groups suggest an effect of improved diagnosis among the elderly. Conversely, increments in mortality rates are probably due to several reasons (19–21): less aggressive treatment or, in some instances, over treatment; limitations to surgery, chemotherapy and radiotherapy in advanced age; the substantial lack of knowledge about the pharmacokinetics of antitumor drugs in the elderly; and the psychological attitude of such patients and their physicians toward a malignant disease, and possibly, higher prevalence of chemoresistant lymphomas.

Although more accurate diagnosis may be partly responsible for the upward trend, it is likely that risk factors are playing an important part. However, the only well-identified risk factor for NHL is the presence of a severe impairment of the immunological system, either spontaneous or acquired (22). In this regard, age-dependent alterations in immune function and host defense, in concert with rearrangements of genomes, may help to explain the increased risk of NHL in aged persons (23), although the role of the immunity for the age-related increase in tumor frequency still remains poorly understood (24). The function as well as the structure of the immune system changes with age. Even

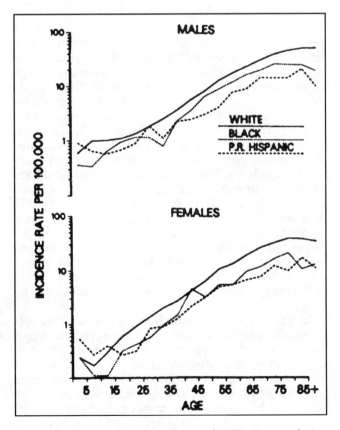

Figure 43.1 Age-related incidence of NHL. From ref 18 with permission.

Table 43.1 Lukes and Collins classification.

Undefined Cell Types

T-cell Types

    Small lymphocytic

    Mycosis fungoides/Sézary syndrome (cerebriform)

    Convoluted lymphocytic

    Immunoblastic sarcoma (T-cell)

B-cell Types

    Small lymphocytic

    Plasmacytoid lymphocytic

    Follicular center cell (follicular, diffuse, follicular and diffuse, and sclerotic)

        Small cleaved

        Large cleaved

        Small noncleaved

        Large noncleaved

    Immunoblastic sarcoma (B-cell)

Histiocytic

Unclassified

Table 43.2 Updated Kiel classification.

B	T
Low-grade	Low-grade
Lymphocytic-chronic lymphocytic and prolymphocytic leukemia; hairy-cell leukemia	Lymphocytic-chronic lymphocytic and prolymphocytic leukemia
	Small, cerebriform cell-mycosis fungoides, Sézary syndrome
Lymphoplasmacytic/cytoid (LP immunocytoma)	Lymphoepithelioid (Lennert's lymphoma)
Plasmacytic	Angioimmunoblastic (AILD; LgX)
Centroblastic/centrocytic	
– follicular ± diffuse	T zone
– diffuse	
	Pleomorphic, small cell (HTLV-I ±)
High-grade	High-grade
Centroblastic	Pleomorphic, medium/large cell (HTLV-I ±)
Immunoblastic	Immunoblastic (HTLV-I ±)
Large cell anaplastic (Ki-1+)	Large cell anaplastic (Ki-1 +)
Burkitt lymphoma	
Lymphoblastic	Lymphoblastic
Rare types	Rare types

if the total number of T-lymphocytes does not change with age (23, 24), not only are the numbers of immature T-cells in the blood increased, but the distribution of T-cell subpopulations is altered. In fact, the percentage of CD4 + T-cells increases with age and the percentage of CD8 + T-cells falls (23). Aging is associated with a disordered humoral immune system, as also revealed by the increased incidence of benign monoclonal gammopathy with age (23). Cell-mediated immune function also undergoes senescence (23, 24). One-half of healthy persons over age 60 have impaired delayed cutaneous hypersensitivity (23). The reduced cell-mediated immunity is partly a result of the thymic involution of aging (23).

Another possible etiology of NHL in the elderly is represented by 2–4 phenoxy pesticides (18). Several studies found that the relative risk of NHL increased with prolonged and intensive exposure to these substances. The mechanism of the association is completely obscure.

Pathology and Classification of Non-Hodgkin's Lymphomas

In this chapter, pathologic features of NHL in old age are discussed. Initially, a brief summary of the current NHL classifications is given for the benefit of those who are not pathologists.

Lukes and Collins (25) in the USA first proposed a classification of lymphoid tumors based on whether the tumor cell was of B-cell or T-cell origin (Table 43.1).

Lennert and Colleagues (26) in Europe proposed a classification of these neoplasms based on the cytomorphology, grade of malignancy and the functional lineage of the tumor cells. They used a terminology quite different from that used in prior classifications (Table 43.2). In 1982, the report derived from an extensive clinicopathologic study sponsored by the National Cancer Institute led to a proposal of a "working formulation for international use," which was very helpful in resolving controversies and allowed better translation among the various classifications being used (Table 43.3) (27). The "Working Formulation" (WF) was not based on immune phenotypes. It was purely a morphologic classification closely paralleling the Rappaport classification. The WF became widely accepted, especially in North America, because it was very useful in predicting survival and curability of different lymphomas and was easily understood by clinicians.

In the 16 years since the National Cancer Institute-sponsored study was initiated there have been major advances in the classification of different groups of lymphocytes, thanks to flow cytometry, which allowed recognition of different subsets of lymphocytes based on immune phenotype, and to cytogenetics which has allowed the recognition of specific chromosomal changes in different malignancies. PCR, of recent acquisition, has allowed in some cases to recognize molecular genetic changes specific of certain diseases. This

Table 43.3 Working Formulation.

Low-grade
    A. Malignant lymphoma
        Small lymphocytic
            consistent with CLL
            plasmacytoid
    B. Malignant lymphoma, follicular
        Predominantly small cleaved cell
            diffuse areas
            sclerosis
    C. Malignant lymphoma, follicular
        Mixed, small cleaved and large cell
            diffuse areas
            sclerosis

Intermediate-grade
    D. Malignant lymphoma, follicular
        Predominantly large cell
            diffuse areas
            sclerosis
    E. Malignant lymphoma, diffuse
        Small cleaved cell
            sclerosis
    F. Malignant lymphoma, diffuse
        Mixed, small and large cell
            sclerosis
            epithelioid cell component
    G. Malignant lymphoma, diffuse
        large cell
            cleaved cell
            noncleaved cell
            sclerosis

High-grade
    H. Malignant lymphoma
        Large cell, immunoblastic
            plasmacytoid
            clear cell
            polymorphous
            epithelioid cell component
    I. Malignant lymphoma
        Lymphoblastic
            convoluted cell
            nonconvoluted cell
    J. Malignant lymphoma
        Small noncleaved cell
            Burkitt's
            follicular areas

Miscellaneous
    Composite
    Mycosis Fungoides
    Histiocytic
    Extramedullary plasmacytoma
    Unclassified
    Others

new accuracy in the definition of different phenotypes, and the new advances in cytogenetics and molecular genetics, has led to a better definition of lymphoid malignancies. New clinicopathologic entities are emerging as distinctive disease with their own prognostic significance: low-grade B-cell lymphoma of MALT type, enteropathy associated T-cell lymphoma, monocytoid B-cell lymphoma, CD30 positive anaplastic large cell lymphomas (ALCL), mediastinal B large cell lymphoma, angiocentric immunoblastic lymphoma, and lethal midline granuloma. Most of these lymphomas do not fit easily into any of the current classifications of NHL. Furthermore, these classifications do not cover newly recognized entities and do not consider the refinement or redefinition of old entities. An additional problem is that these classifications ignore the methodological progress made in the field of molecular biology that provides important distinctions and relationships among the lymphoid cells and tumors derived from them. The International Lymphoma Group has recently provided an excellent review of the development in this field and, reviewing also several clinical entities recognized in recent years, has proposed a new classification of NHL (Table 43.4). The so-called R.E.A.L. classification (28) comprises nodal and extranodal lymphomas and lists seven provisional entities. The Authors of the R.E.A.L. classification devised three collective groups of lymphomas that represent separate entities in the Kiel classification: 1) in the group of follicle center lymphomas, follicular, the rare follicular centroblastic lymphoma is listed as grade III; 2) the category diffuse large B-cell lymphomas comprises centroblastic lymphoma with its subtypes, B-immunoblastic lymphoma and B-ALCL; 3) the group "peripheral T-cell lymphomas, unspecified" combines five different entities from the Kiel classification, three of which belong to the low-grade category and two to the high-grade. Its proponents have termed the Revised European American Lymphoma (REAL) Classification a "proposal" and "temporary": clinicopathologic studies should be carried out to test the clinical significance of this new classification.

Differences in Lymphoma Histology and Biology Between Younger and Older Persons

Few studies have compared the characteristics of young and elderly patients with NHL, but the initial picture of lymphoma in elderly patients did not seem very different from what was observed in younger patients. However, an increase in diffuse versus follicular histologic patterns, and in extranodal versus nodal disease was observed with advancing age (15, 29). On the other hand, little attention has been directed to the distribution of newly described entities such as CD30 positive ALCL (30), mantle cell lymphomas (MCL) (31) or low-grade B-cell lymphoma of MALT type (32) in this particular group of patients. Furthermore, it is unclear whether biologically different diseases as revealed by lymphoma immunophenotypes may develop in elderly patients when compared to younger people.

Table 43.4 Comparison of the R.E.A.L. classification and the Working Formulation for clinical usage.

Kiel Classification	Revised European American Lymphoma Classification	Working Formulation
B-lymphoblastic	Precursor B-lymphoblastic lymphoma/leukemia	Lymphoblastic
B-Lymphocytic, CLL	B-cell chronic lymphocytic leukemia/prolymphocytic leukemia/small lymphocytic lymphoma	**Small lymphocytic, consistent with CLL**
B-Lymphocytic, prolymphocytic leukemia		
Lymphoplasmacytoid immunocytoma		Small lymphocytic, plasmacytoid
Lymphoplasmacytic immunocytoma	Lymphoplasmacytoid lymphoma	**Small lymphocytic, plasmacytoid**
		Diffuse, mixed, small and large cell
Centrocytic	Mantle cell lymphoma	Small lymphocytic
Centroblastic, centrocytoid subtype		**Diffuse, small cleaved cell**
		Follicular, small cleaved cell
		Diffuse, mixed, small and large cell
		Diffuse, large cleaved cell
Centroblastic-centrocytoid subtype	Follicular center cell lymphoma, follicular	
	– Grade I	**Follicular, predominantly small cleaved cell**
	– Grade II	**Follicular, mixed small and large cell**
Centroblastic, follicular	– Grade III	Follicular, predominantly large cell
Centroblastic-centrocytic, diffuse	Follicular center cell lymphoma, diffuse, small cell (provisional)	**Diffuse, small cleaved cell**
		Diffuse, mixed small and large cell
–	Extranodal marginal zone B-cell lymphoma (low-grade B-cell lymphoma of MALT type)	**Small lymphocytic**
		Diffuse, small cleaved cell
		Diffuse, mixed, small and large cell
	Nodal marginal zone B-cell lymphoma	**Small lymphocytic**
	Diffuse, small cleaved cell (provisional)	
		Diffuse, mixed, small and large cell
		Unclassifiable
–	Splenic marginal zone B-cell lymphoma (provisional)	**Small lymphocytic**
		Diffuse, small cleaved cell
Hairy cell leukemia	Hairy cell leukemia	–
Plasmacytic	Plasmacytoma/myeloma	Extramedullary plasmacytoma
Centroblastic (monomorphic, polymorphic and multilobated subtypes)	Diffuse large B-cell lymphoma	**Diffuse, large cell**
		Large cell immunoblastic
B-immunoblastic		Diffuse, mixed small and large cell
B-cell large cell anaplastic (Ki-1 +)		
–*	Primary mediastinal large B-cell lymphoma	**Diffuse large cell**
		Large cell immunoblastic
Burkitt's lymphoma	Burkitt's lymphoma	Small noncleaved, Burkitt's
	High-grade B-cell, Burkitt-like (provisional)	**Small noncleaved, non-Burkitt's**
T-lymphoblastic	Precursor T-lymphoblastic lymphoma/leukemia	Lymphoblastic
T-lymphocytic, CLL type	T-cell chronic lymphocytic leukemia/prolymphocytic leukemia	**Small lymphocytic**
T-lymphocytic, prolymphocytic leukemia		Diffuse small cleaved cell
T-lymphocytic, CLL type	Large granular lymphocytic leukemia	**Small lymphocytic**
		Diffuse small cleaved cell
Small cell cerebriform (mycosis, fungoides, Sézary syndrome)	Mycosis fungoides/Sézary syndrome	Mycosis fungoides
T-zone	Peripheral T-cell lymphomas, unspecified	Diffuse, small cleaved cell
Lymphoepithelioid	(including provisional subtype: subcutaneous	**Diffuse, mixed small and large cell**
Pleomorphic, small T-cell	panniculitic T-cell lymphoma)	Diffuse, large cell
Pleomorphic, medium-sized and large T-cell		Large cell immunoblastic
T-immunoblastic		
–	Hepatosplenic g-d T-cell lymphoma (provisional)	–
Angioimmunoblastic (AILD, LgX)	Angioimmunoblastic T-cell lymphoma	**Diffuse, mixed small and large cell**
		Diffuse, large cell
		Large cell immunoblastic
–*	Angiocentric T-cell lymphoma	Diffuse, small cleaved cell
		Diffuse, mixed small and large cell
		Diffuse, large cell
		Large cell immunoblastic
–	Intestinal T-cell lymphoma	Diffuse, small cleaved cell
		Diffuse, mixed small and large cell
		Diffuse, large cell
		Large cell immunoblastic
Pleomorphic, small T-cell, HTLVI+	Adult T-cell lymphoma/leukemia	Diffuse, small cleaved cell
Pleomorphic, medium-sized and large T-cell HTLVI+		**Diffuse, mixed small and large cell**
		Diffuse, large cell
		Large cell immunoblastic
T-large cell anaplastic (Ki-1+)	Anaplastic large cell lymphoma, T- and null-cell types	Large cell immunoblastic

When more than one Kiel or Working Formulation category is listed, those in boldface type comprise the major of the cases.
* Not listed in classification, but discussed as rare or ambiguous type.
(Modified from Harris *et al.* (28))

The analysis of the frequency and distribution of the histologic types of NHL in old age is hampered by classification difficulties, and the lack of concordance between these systems. Since elderly patients were usually excluded from clinical trials, pathologic data concerning NHL of the elderly are fragmentary and also usually reported in one of the main classifications without mentioning the equivalent terms of the WF (27). Furthermore, newer classifications have not been incorporated in these studies.

Some clinicopathologic studies on large series of cases have provided information on the proportion of elderly patients affected by NHL. One hundred eighteen elderly (>70 years) patients formed 27.2% of all the cases of NHL seen over a 5-year period at a single institution where no particular bias in the admission of these patients has been present (29). These data are in agreement with the results of a European Organization for Research and Treatment of Cancer (EORTC) retrospective study on NHL in elderly patients (>70 years of age) seen in 13 European institutes (33). The study revealed that 137 cases of NHL were observed in the elderly during 1984, making up 28% of the total number of NHLs seen in those institutes (33). Moreover, in a population based registry it has been found that one third (38%) of the NHL patients were aged 70 or older (15). It is noteworthy that in the series of Carbone and Colleagues (29), 232 (53.6%) of the 433 patients were aged 60 years or older. By analyzing some of the major published series which contain data concerning the frequency of NHLs in old age it can be drawn that 19.8 to 38.5% of all NHL cases were found in people aged 60 years or older (9–11, 15, 29). These conflicting results are principally based on the fact that most published clinic-pathologic series are actually made up of selected elderly patients, mostly aged <70 years.

In most of the above studies "diffuse histiocytic" appeared to be the most frequent histologic type according to the Rappaport system in elderly patients. This is in agreement with the data of Carbone and Colleagues (29) which showed that 36.8% of cases were of the G (diffuse large cell) + H (large cell, immunoblastic) categories according to the WF. Equivalent of both these categories for the Rappaport classification is the "diffuse histiocytic" histologic type.

Four studies reporting pathologic data on elderly patients according to the terminology of the WF (12, 15, 33, 34) showed that most NHL cases were of intermediate — or high-grade malignancy. To the contrary, in the series of Carbone and Colleagues (29) elderly patients showed a rather similar percentage for the low (29%) and high grade (28%) NHL cases. It is of note that in the latter series no significant difference in the prevalence of low-, intermediate and high-grade subtypes was observed among patients younger or older than 70 years, although follicular growth pattern (B-follicular small cleaved cell- + C-follicular mixed cell- + D-follicular large cell-categories according to the WF) was less frequently found in the elderly group. Accordingly, Barnes and Colleagues (35) have shown a marked

trend of increasing "diffuse" vs follicular histology with advancing age. Moreover, Otter and Colleagues (36), reviewing NHL in a population-based registry reported that low malignancy grade NHLs and nodular histotypes were less frequent in the elderly (>70 years) group of patients when compared with the younger group.

In the series of Carbone and Colleagues (29), 62 NHLs (52.6%) were extranodal at presentation, the gastrointestinal tract being the most frequently involved site (47.3%). D'Amore and Colleagues (15) found out that localized cases with extranodal manifestations were more frequent among elderly (>70 years) than younger patients. The most common sites of extranodal involvement were the stomach (21% of all extranodal cases) and the bone marrow (16%). Hancock and Colleagues (37) reported that localized extranodal disease occurred more commonly in patients older than 65 years. Finally, extranodal disease was found in 27 (39%) of 70 NHL patients older than age 80 years observed over a 15-year period at two institutions (38). The fact that extranodal presentation is relatively frequent in elderly patients with NHL should be emphasized because of its prognostic implications. It has been demonstrated that patients with disseminated high grade extranodal NHL had the worst prognosis of all (39).

Recently, we have analyzed seven years of pathologic data collected in a single oncologic institution on all lymphoma patients to determine the pathologic features at presentation including histologic subtypes and cell lineage. To this end, three groups of patients were defined according to the age: >70 years, <55 years, between 55 and 69. The terminology of the WF of NHLs for clinical usage (27) was used as a means of translation among widely acknowledged classification systems for NHL. Newly described entities which are not incorporated in the WF were also included and classified according to diagnostic criteria reported by the REAL Classification (28).

Over the seven-year period from July 1988 to June 1995, 950 consecutive NHL cases have been diagnosed at the Division of Pathology of the Centro di Riferimento Oncologico, Aviano, Italy. AIDS-related lymphomas and cases diagnosed on primary or secondary lymphomatous effusions were excluded. Cases with overt chronic lymphocytic leukemia, multiple myeloma and acute leukemia diagnosed by hematologic criteria were also excluded. Elderly (>70 years) patients formed 28.5% (271/950) of all the cases of NHL. Among the 277 miscellaneous cases there were six main pathologic entities. Three of them, i.e. mycosis fungoides, extramedullary plasmacytoma and low-grade lymphoma of MALT-type were equally distributed in the three age groups. On the other hand, CD30 positive ALCL cases, which were also diagnosed in patients belonging to all three groups, were mostly seen in the group of younger patients. Finally, MCL cases were restricted to the two older groups of patients, they being absent in patients younger than 55 years, whereas mediastinal large cell lymphomas clustered in the latter group. Immunophenotypically, 739 (85.9%) of the 860 tested NHL cases expressed B-cell markers, whereas 77 (9%) expressed

T-cell markers. In the remaining 44 cases neoplastic cells did not show neither B or T-cell phenotypes. A statistically significant prevalence of T-cell marker expression was noted in the cases tested among patients younger than 55 years. In this group B-cell NHLS constitute 78% of cases, whereas T-cell NHLS appear to have a non negligible incidence, representing 12.3% of all tested cases. T-cell NHL constituted 6.9% and 8% of all tested cases in patients between 55–69 and older than 70 years, respectively.

Clinical Diagnosis and Staging

Diagnostic delay in elderly patients has been reported for some solid tumors (40) but it has not been determined if this also occurs for NHL in older persons. However, the diagnosis may be more difficult in the patient with subtle symptoms against a background of intercurrent disease, as usually occurs in older people (41).

The current clinic-pathologic staging examinations in use for NHL should be in principle the same in the elderly as well as in adults. Biochemistry and radiological examinations are easily performed in elderly cancer patients while, especially in the very old, bone marrow biopsy may encounter resistance in patients and relatives and even avert patients from treatment. Gastroscopy can be performed in most instances without any problem.

Staging procedures are probably less extensively carried out for elderly with NHL both outside specialized cancer centers and medical oncology divisions but, again, no data are available on the percentages of elderly patients referred to a specialized environment and undergoing then a correct diagnostic approach.

Combination Chemotherapy for Lymphomas of Intermediate and High Grade

Aggressive NHL can be potentially cured by intensive cytotoxic chemotherapy, if a complete remission (CR) of the disease is achieved. However this chemotherapy may cause severe and even life threatening toxicity, in older individuals. The application of chemotherapy at a high-dose intensity is believed to be the key to successful treatment. From such premises, it is easy to understand how delivery of full-dose aggressive combination chemotherapy may lead to some problems in elderly with NHL. In fact, it is well known that the treatment of elderly patients with antineoplastic agents can be complicated by many host-related factors, such as diminished bone marrow capacity of regeneration and higher likelihood of cardiac and lung toxicities (42). The pharmacokinetics processes of absorption, distribution, metabolism and elimination of drugs (and their metabolites) may be changed in the older person. In particular, the renal excretion is generally decreased, and hepatic drug metabolism may be altered (43). In addition, concomitant chronic illnesses and consequent polypharmacy may enhance the risk of drug interactions and adverse drug reactions (44).

This explains why the concern about increased risk and severity of therapeutic toxicity has led to the exclusion of older patients from most studies on NHL in Europe (33).

Combination chemotherapy in elderly with NHL has consisted, initially, in the use of the same regimens employed in younger adults and, more recently, in the development of regimens specifically designed to decrease toxicity without losing therapeutic activity. As already attempted by us (45, 46), the main retrospective studies, single arm prospective and randomized clinical trials mainly referring to NHL of intermediate-high grade in elderly patients in the English literature will be considered here, since some useful suggestions for the management can be derived from the results of this wide and various therapeutic experience.

Retrospective Studies

The main retrospective studies of the past ten years have been summarized in Table 43.5.

Armitage et al. (47) reported in 1984 the results obtained with standard CHOP without dose-adjustment for age in 20 patients aged 70 years or older who belonged to a larger group of 75 patients with aggressive NHL. The complete response (CR) rate in elderly patients (45%) did not differ from younger patients (53%) with a median overall survival of 13 months in the elderly. Considerable toxicity was seen in the aged group with a toxic death rate of 25%. Two years later, Dixon et al. (48) reviewed all clinical trials of the South-West Oncology Group from 1974 to 1982 where 307 patients with advanced diffuse large-cell lymphoma had been treated with CHOP-based regimens. CR rate was 65% in patients under 40 years but only 37% in patients 65 or older. Survival decreased from a median period of 101 months in the younger group (less than 40 years) to a median time of 16 months in patients older than 65 years. Although three fourths of patients were treated with a 50% dose reduction, one fourth received initial full dose chemotherapy. Therapy at full dose produced a better outcome but the CR rate was lower in elderly patients. In the same period, O'Connell et al. (49) presented the results of the Eastern Cooperative Oncology Group on 141 patients aged over 60 years treated with COPA (cyclophosphamide, vincristine, prednisone and doxorubicin). This study demonstrated that patients treated with full chemotherapy dose achieved a better CR rate (49%) than patients who had a 50% dose reduction (33%). The conclusion was that full-dose chemotherapy should be administered also in the elderly with NHL. Only one drug-related death occurred in one patient receiving full dose treatment.

In a following study Solal-Celigny et al. (50) treated 73 patients with an adriamycin-containing regimen (doxorubicin, etoposide, cyclophosphamide, and prednisone) and age was found to be an important prognostic factor related to survival both in a univariate and a multivariate analysis. In fact, patients under 60 years had a median survival of 48 months and survival rate was 47%.

Table 43.5 Retrospective studies in elderly patients wtih aggressive NHL.

Author, Year (reference)	# Patients	Age (Range)	Therapy	CR (%)	Overall Survival	Treatment-Related Deaths (%)
Armitage, et al. 1984 (47)	20	≥70*	CHOP	45	13 mo.	25
Dixon, et al. 1986 (48)	81	≥65*	CHOP	37	12 mo.	4
O'Connell, et al. 1986 (49)	99	≥60*	COPA	49	36 mo.	1
	48	≥60*	COPA 50%	33	20 mo.	0
Solal-Celigny, et al. 1987 (50)	34	71 (60–88)	AVmCP	56	18 mo.	0
Vose, et al. 1988 (51)	112	≥60*	CAP/BOP	61	15 mo.	7
Orlandi, et al. 1991 (52)	61	71 (65–84)	CVP 75% or CHOP 75%	42	22 mo.	0
Bruno, et al. 1992 (53)	174	≥65*	GATLA's Protocols	51	20% at 10 yrs	14
D'Amore et al. 1994 (15)	39	≥70*	CHOP CVBP	58 55	nr	nr
Grogan et al. 1994 (54)	60	71 (65–85)	CHOP m-BACOD	65	58% at 3 yrs	0

* Median not reported

In older patients (over 60 years) median survival and 5-year survival rate were 18 months and 18% respectively. CR at 5 years was seen in 72% of younger patients and in 24% of older patients. At the end of the eighties another regimen, the CAP/BOP combination (cytoxan, adriamycin, procarbazine, bleomycin, oncovin and prednisone) was used by Vose et al. of the Nebraska Lymphoma Study Group (51) to treat 112 patients older than 40 years. Forty-five other patients were younger than 60 years. Chemotherapy was administered at full dose in patients under 70 years and at two thirds of the dose in patients older than 70 years. No significant difference in CR was found in patients older and younger than 60 years, but a notable difference on 5-year survival was observed in the two groups: 62% in younger and 34% in older than 60 years. Treatment toxicity was superimposable but deaths due to other causes not obviously related to the lymphoma or its therapy occurred in 22% of patients over 60 years and in 2% of those younger (p = 0.005). CR duration was similar in the two groups of patients.

Other retrospective studies have been carried out in this first half of the nineties. Orlandi et al. (52) reviewed the results achieved in 61 patients aged 65 or older with intermediate NHL (36 cases) or high grade NHL (25 cases). Of 56 patients with stage II-IV, 14 received single-agent therapy and 32 were given attenuated CVP (25% drug dose reduction); only 10 patients were considered suitable for the CHOP or CHOP-like program with a 25% reduction of the calculated dose. Overall CR rate was 50% for intermediate- and 32% for high-grade NHL. Median survival was 33 months and 10 months respectively. The achievement of CR influenced

positively survival. Few deaths were due to treatment-related complications.

Bruno et al. (53) reported the experience of 6 consecutive GATLA's studies from 1968 to 1992 in intermediate/high-grade NHL. Details on regimens employed were not reported. Of 801 patients, 627 were younger than 65 years and 174 older. Stage, B-symptoms, PS, mediastinal involvement, bulky disease and bone marrow involvement were comparable. CR rate was higher in younger (59%) than in older patients (51%) (p = 0.0241) whereas toxic deaths were more common in the older (14%) than in the younger group (5%) (p = 0.0002). At 10-year follow-up event-free survival rate was 26% in younger patients and 16% in older patients (p = 0.0034). Overall survival was 35% in younger subjects and 20% (p = 0.0009) in the older group; no difference in CR duration was observed between the two groups. The authors concluded that such a difference in survival could be related to higher treatment toxicity and NHL-unrelated deaths in the elderly group.

In the study of D'Amore et al. (15) the large majority of non-randomized patients was treated following common general guidelines resulting in a rather homogenous therapeutic background. CHOP or CHOP-like regimens were used. The doses of cyclophosphamide, doxorubicin or other anthracyclines, and vincristine was reduced by 25% and doxorubicin was either avoided or substituted with epirubicine or mitoxantrone in patients with a left ventricular ejection fraction (LVEF) of 50% or less.

Results on response to treatment were available only in 39 patients entered in a trial for intermediate/high-grade NHL comparing standard CHOP with CVBP (cisplatin, VP16, bleomycin and prednisone). The overall results showed that CHOP was not superior to CVBP, since CR rates for CHOP and CVBP were 58% and 55%, whereas overall response rates were 74% vs 80% respectively. The median response duration was also similar. No data on survival were reported. Despite the low number of patients, overall analysis allowed the identification of some pretreatment clinical characteristics that were important, independent predictors of outcome for elderly patients, such as indicators of tumor burden (hepatic involvement, B-symptoms and elevated LDH) and tumor-cell type (high-grade histology).

Another retrospective analysis was conducted by L. Grogan et al. (54) who reviewed the clinical characteristics and outcome of 192 patients diagnosed for NHL intermediate- and high-grade seen at the Dublin Hospital between June 1984 and January 1991. Sixty out of 192 patients had a median age of 71 years and were treated with CHOP or m-BACOD according to the standard dose and schedules. This group of patients was compared with younger patients receiving the same treatment. Both age groups had similar clinic-pathological prognostic features at diagnosis. The overall response rate for patients over 65 years was 95% with 65% achieving a CR. In comparison, in the younger patients overall response rate was 92% with a higher CR rate (76%). The differences in response rates between the groups were not statistically significant (p: 0.17). The 3-year overall survival of patients >65 years (58%) was not significantly different from the survival of patients <65 years (65%) treated with the same regimen as the 3-year disease-free survival. There were no toxic deaths in elderly patients treated with CHOP or m-BACOD. The hospital admission rate was less than 10% for complications of CHOP or m-BACOD chemotherapy and was similar for younger and older patients. The results of this retrospective study indicated that it had been possible to administer full standard-dose CHOP or m-BACOD chemotherapy to the majority of elderly patients. The major prognostic factors known to affect survival in NHL could not be correlated with chronological age and there was no difference in survival between patients either younger or older than 65 years when all patients diagnosed with NHL, either pretreated or previously untreated were included in the analysis. With the exception of this last study, where probably only selected elderly patients with NHL were entered, in all the aforementioned retrospective studies advanced age was associated with a worse prognosis after combination chemotherapy.

Single Arm Prospective Studies

A summary of available results from prospective studies is presented in chronologic order in Table 43.6.

Specifically designed prospective studies on elderly patients with NHL have been performed since 1980 at the Centro di Riferimento Oncologico of Aviano — Italy. Tirelli et al. (55) in 1984 treated 41 elderly patients with NHL with teniposide 100 mg/m² weekly infusion for at least 3 weeks. CR was obtained in 32% with a median overall survival lasting 10 months. At 3 years 40% of patients in CR were alive. No treatment-related deaths occurred. In a subsequent study Zagonel et al. (56) reported the results of treatment of 37 patients with etoposide and prednimustine 100 mg/m² p.o. for 5 days both every 21 days. CR was 46% with a 12-month median duration. The objective response rate in the 22 previously untreated patients reached nearly 70%. Median survival was 14 months. The overall toxicity was acceptable. Two patients died, however, after the first cycle of treatment. In a successive study the Aviano Group (57) treated 52 patients over 70 years with a new combination of drugs specifically planned for elderly NHL patients. In this treatment etoposide and prednimustine p.o. were combined with mitoxantrone i.v. (VMP) Mitoxantrone, an anthracenedione derivative, was chosen because it appeared to have comparable antineoplastic activity to that of doxorubicin, with lower risk of cardiotoxicity. Forty-eight patients were evaluable for response; CR was obtained in 46% and the overall response rate was 81%. Median overall survival was 12 months. Severe hematological toxicity (grade 3–4 WHO) was reported on 31% of administered cycles and one patient died due to sepsis. Extra-hematological toxicity was mild. In particular, no cardiac toxicity was observed. The authors tried to relate toxicity, clinical characteristics (PS, stage) and relative dose intensity (RDI) of medications and found that the only grade 4 WHO hematological toxicity occurred in a patient who had received a lower than planned RDI of chemotherapy.

A number of other chemotherapy regimens specifically designed for elderly with NHL appeared in the early nineties.

O'Reilly et al. of the Vancouver Group (58) used two brief weekly chemotherapy regimens: LD-ACOP-B (low-dose adriamycin, cyclophosphamide, vincristine, prednisone and bleomycin) and VABE (etoposide, adriamycin, vincristine, bleomycin and prednisone). In the former study from March '83 to September '85, 40 patients (age limit 65–85 years) were accrued. CR was achieved in 65%, two toxic deaths were reported. Actuarial failure-free survival and overall survival with a maximum follow-up of 6 years were 19% and 28% respectively. With the VABE regimen (etoposide, adriamycin, vincristine, bleomycin and prednisone) 32 patients were accrued: 63% achieved CR; two toxic deaths were observed, actuarial failure-free survival was 34% and overall survival with a maximum follow-up of 4 years was 36%. Hematological toxicity was greater in the VABE regimen than in the LD-ACOP-B. The two regimens share advantage of brevity, outpatient administration and acceptable long-term survival.

More recently, the same group presented the results of a new regimen named POCE (59) involving five drugs given over 8 weeks (epirubicine, vincristine, cyclophosphamide, etoposide and prednisone). Of the 61 patients, 56% achieved a CR. Median follow-up was 2 years. After 3 years the overall survival was 44%; 64% of CRs was disease free. A significant difference in WHO grade 3 and 4 leukopenia occurred in patients

Table 43.6 Prospective single arm studies in elderly patients with aggressive NHL.

Author, Year (reference)	# Patients	Median Age (Range)	Therapy	CR (%)	Overall Survival	Treatment-Related Deaths (%)
Tirelli et al. 1984 (55)	41	75 (70–84)	VM26	32	10 mo.	0
Zagonel et al. 1990 (56)	37	80 (71–84)	VP16-PRM	46	14 mo.	5
Tirelli et al. 1992 (57)	52	75 (71–92)	VMP	46	12 mo.	2
O'Reilly et al. 1991 (58)	40	72 (65–85)	LD-ACOP-B	65	20 mo.	5
O'Reilly et al. 1991 (58)	32	73 (65–84)	VABE	63	25 mo.	7
O'Reilly et al. 1992 (59)	61	75 (65–85)	POCE	56	44% at 3 yrs.	10
Kitamura et al. 1990 (60)	43	73 (65–84)	THP-COP	30	54% at 18 mo.	0
McMaster et al. 1990 (61)	26	75 (55–84)	BECALM	42	8 mo.	15
Tigaud et al. 1991 (69)	21	75 (70–81)	IFO-VP16	42	47% at 1 yr.	0
Sonneveld et al. 1990 (62)	30	70 (57–83)	CNOP	60	50% at 1 yr.	0
Salvagno et al. 1992 (63)	55	75 (64–93)	MVP	48	33% at 2 yrs.	4
Landys et al. 1992 (64)	61	77 (70–92)	NOSTE	72	22% at 2 yrs.	0
Torello et al. 1992 (65)	10	71 (66–77)	MINE	50	nr	0
Ansell et al. 1992 (66)	36	72*	CEMP ± GM-CSF	58	23 mo.	0
Hainsworth et al. 1993 (67)	19	73 (68–84)	EMCMV	69	nr	0
Goss et al. 1993 (88)	32	74 (66–92)	PEN	33	nr	0
Liang et al. 1993 (70)	141	66 (61–69)	COPP	50	40% at 2 yrs.	7
Zinzani et al. 1993 (71)	29	66 (60–78)	VNCOP-B	76	75% at 16 mo.	0
Martelli et al. 1993 (72)	60	67 (60–80)	P-VABEC	75	64% at 2 yrs.	0
Bertini et al. 1993 (73)	50	70 (65–80)	P-VEBEC MEMID	58 65	77% at 1 yr.	0

* range not reported

treated with LD-ACOP-B (24%), VABE (91%) and POCE (62%). The authors also compared the results of POCE with those obtained in elderly patients with MACOP-B and found that the two regimens produced comparable survival (Figure 43.2). This observation is extremely important, as it suggests that elderly individuals may be treated with less aggressive regimens of chemotherapy, without compromising overall survival.

A novel derivate of doxorubicin, THP-adriamycin, in combination with cyclophosphamide, vincristine and prednisone was used by Kitamura (60) to treat 43 patients. Thirteen of them (30%) achieved CR. Even though a better response rate was achieved in previously untreated patients, 4 patients previously treated with an adriamycin-containing regimen had a new response to the treatment. The median overall survival was 54% at 18 months. No patients had cardiac toxicity.

McMaster et al. (61) treated 26 patients with a novel 8-week chemotherapy regimen containing bleomycin, etoposide, cyclophosphamide, adriamycin, metho-

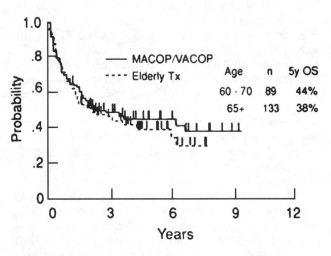

Figure 43.2 Survival of patients aged 60 and over treated with high dose chemotherapy (MACOP-B) and with regimens specifically designed for older individuals. From ref 59 with permission.

trexate with leucovorin and prednisone (BECALM). Eleven patients (42%) achieved a CR and 7 remain in continuous CR at a median follow-up of 37.5 months. There were 4 treatment-related deaths although only one of these resulted from neutropenia and subsequent sepsis.

Mitoxantrone, has been used in several combination therapies instead of doxorubicin. This drug, more attractive than anthracyclines for the treatment of elderly patients, has been mainly combined with etoposide in seven studies. Sonneveld *et al.* (62) used mitoxantrone in combination with cyclophosphamide, vincristine and prednisone (CNOP) and treated 30 consecutive patients, median age 70 years, with six courses of therapy. Of 30 patients 18 (60%) obtained a CR, while the total number of responders was 27 (90%). The overall survival was 50% at 1 year. Transient hematological toxicity was commonly observed but no dose-reductions were applied. No toxic deaths were reported.

A modified VMP regimen (prednisone instead of prednimustine) was used by Salvagno *et al.* (63) in 55 elderly patients. Median age was 75 years. Fourteen patients were pretreated (4 with adriamycin or etoposide-based chemotherapy, 12 with other types of combination chemotherapy, 2 with radiotherapy): 12 patients had a bulky disease and bone marrow involvement. In the previously untreated 40 patients CR rate was 55% and median duration of CR 12 months. In pretreated patients CR rate was 29% and duration of CR ranged from 4+ to 16+ months. Overall survival and relapse-free survival at 2 years of 40 previously untreated patients were 54% and 31% respectively. In pretreated patients overall survival was 15%. Two toxic deaths were reported (pneumonia, possible myocardial infarction) but no difference in myelodepression between untreated and pretreated patients was seen.

Landys *et al.* (64) treated 61 patients with NOTE (Mitoxantrone and Sterecyt). Thirty-one had aggressive NHL and 30 low-grade NHL; 11/27 pretreated patients had received doxorubicin. CR was obtained in 72% of patients (71% in aggressive NHL and 67% in low-grade NHL). Five-year disease-free survival was 25% in aggressive NHL, 20% in low-grade NHL and median time to relapse was 13 months and 23 months, respectively. Overall survival at 5 years was 37% (35% in aggressive NHL and 40% in low-grade NHL).

Torello *et al.* (65) used MINE (mesna, ifosfamide, novantrone and etoposide) in 10 refractory or relapsing patients older than 65 years. All cases had been pretreated with at least one anthracycline-containing regimen and 3 also received radiotherapy (RT). An overall 80% response rate was achieved with a 50% CR rate. Myelosuppression of grade 3–4 was reported in 40% of patients, most frequently in those with prior RT (67% vs 25%). This regimen turned out to be effective as a salvage treatment, with acceptable toxicity, but the number of patients is too small to draw any conclusion.

Ansell *et al.* (66) treated 36 patients with CEMP (cyclophosphamide, etoposide, mitoxantrone and prednisone). To five of these patients was given G-CSF, to prevent myelotoxicity. CR was reached in 58% of cases, 47% continuous disease-free, but life-threatening hematological toxicity was observed in 52% of cases with 6 treatment-related deaths. Median overall survival was not reached with a median follow-up of 23 months. This treatment showed to be effective but toxic; addition of G-CSF in 5 patients shortened the duration of hematological toxicity but did not affect the nadir neutrophil count.

In another report by Hainsworth *et al.* (67) 19 previously untreated NHL patients, median age 73, received a chronic schedule of oral etoposide with other active agents (metotrexate, leucovorin, cyclophosphamide, mitoxantrone and vincristine). Of 13 patients who completed therapy there were 9 CRs (69%) and 7 of these remained disease-free 8–22 months after diagnosis. No treatment-related deaths occurred, but six hospitalizations for neutropenic fever were required.

Goss *et al.* (68) treated with a combination of prednisone, etoposide (both at 50 mg p.o. for 14 days) and novantrone (PEN) 32 elderly patients with NHL (7 non-responders to prior therapy and 4 at relapse). Of the 21 evaluable patients, 7 (33%) achieved a CR with an overall response of 75%. Of the 11 previously treated patients, one had a CR. Five episodes of febrile neutropenia requiring hospitalization occurred.

When one compares mitoxantrone-including combinations of chemotherapy with those including doxorubicin, the incidence of cardiotoxicity, but not of myelotoxicity, appeared to have decreased with mitoxantrone. No comparisons can be made among the various mitoxantrone-based regimens because of the different criteria of selection and patient characteristics in the various case series.

In order to avoid or minimize cardiotoxicity from anthracyclines other approaches have been chosen. A prospective phase II study was performed by Tigaud *et al.* (69) to evaluate efficacy and toxicity of continuous infusion of ifosfamide plus etoposide. The 21 patients included, whose median age was 75 years, were unable to receive the usual front-line chemotherapy because of cardiac illness, relapse or no response to conventional chemotherapy. Nine CRs were observed, mostly in previously untreated patients. The overall survival rate was 47% at 1 year. No severe toxicities were reported.

The COPP regimen, consisting of cyclophosphamide, vincristine, procarbazine and prednisone, commonly used for treating Hodgkin's disease, was chosen by Liang *et al.* (70) to treat 141 elderly patients of all clinical stages. The authors reported the clinical outcome by stage of disease, showing an evident decrease in CR rate from stage I (76%) to stage II and III (53% and 50%) and to more advanced disease (22%). In agreement, the survival rate at 5 years ranged from 76% for stage I to 20% for stage IV. Although this regimen was, on the whole, well tolerated by this group of patients, there was still a 7% treatment-related mortality so that dosage reduction and treatment delay were often required. Compared to the adriamycin-containing regimen used by the same authors in younger patients the clinical outcome following COPP was inferior. However, the overall CR rate of 37.5% was similar to that of other investigators, who had treated elderly patients with anthracycline based combination chemotherapy.

Zinzani et al. (71) designed an 8-week outpatient chemotherapy regimen called VNCOP-B (a MACOP-B-like schedule, where the treatment was completed in 8 weeks and included mitoxantrone and etoposide instead of adriamycin and methotrexate. Twenty-nine untreated patients older than 60 years (12 stage II; 17 stage III-IV), completed therapy. Twenty-two (76%) patients obtained a CR with an overall response rate of 93%. Seventeen of 22 complete responders remained in continuous CR at a median follow-up of 13 months and the overall survival was 75% at 16 months. All 29 patients completed the entire course of treatment and received most or all of the planned dose of each drug. Although in 12 patients neutropenia led to temporary interruption of the sequential weekly treatment, there were no deaths related to drug side effects; non-hematological toxicity was minimal. The high CR rate and good tolerance of the VNCOP-B regimen in comparison with those seen in other prospective studies may be partially explained by the relatively low median age (66 years) of these patients. On the contrary, the previously mentioned regimens, with the only exception of that of Liang (70), were all administered to patients with a median age of 70 years or more.

A similar schedule of six-drug weekly combination chemotherapy regimen was used by Martelli et al. (72) in untreated elderly patients with aggressive NHL. Sixty patients entered the study. The first cohort of 26 patients was treated for a total of 8 weekly courses of P-VABEC regimen (prednisone, vincristine, adriamycin, bleomycin, etoposide, cyclophosphamide) and a second cohort of 34 patients received 12 weekly courses of treatment. Of 60 patients, 45 (75%) achieved a CR with an overall response rate of 92%. The projected overall survival (OS) rate at 2 years was 64%, while the projected disease free survival (DFS) and event free survival (EFS) rate were 57% and 55% respectively. The differences of OS, DFS and EFS between patients treated with 8 or 12 courses were not statistically significant. By univariate analysis, none of the standard prognostic factors was able to statistically influence CR rates, OS, DFS and EFS durations. Hematologic toxicity was acceptable: no patients experienced nadir counts lower than 500/μl for neutrophils or lower than 50000/μl for platelets. Debility, fatigue, peripheral neurotoxicity and cardiovascular symptoms were more common in patients treated with 12 courses compared with those treated with 8 courses of chemotherapy. One treatment-related toxic death of a 75-year-old woman who died while in CR of lung fibrosis, presumably related to bleomycin, was reported. The average relative dose-intensity was 88.6%: delivery of P-VEBEC treatment in 8 or 12 courses did not significantly affect the dose intensity of treatment. Even for patients enrolled in this study the median age was low (67 years). As in the

study by Martelli (72), the results may not be applicable to people over 75.

A slightly different treatment schedule was used by Bertini et al. (Italian Multiregional non-Hodgkin Lymphoma Study Group) (73) who treated 50 patients (median age 70.6, B-symptoms in 24% of patients, bulky disease in 66% of patients, LDH >500 in 30% and stage IV in 45%) with P-VEBEC (prednisone, vinblastine, epirubicin, bleomycin, etoposide and cyclophosphamide). Of 50 patients, 18 also received recombinant G-CSF s.c. at 5 μg/kg doses starting on day 2 of every week for 4 consecutive days to assess whether the growth factors may allow the administration of more dose intense chemotherapy. Twenty-nine cases (58%) achieved CR with an overall response of 94%. With a median follow-up of 12 months from initiation of treatment, overall survival and DFS were 77% and 66% respectively. No toxic death was observed. The use of G-CSF reduced the episodes of neutropenia with a nadir below 500/μl (5 patients compared to 19 cases not receiving growth factors, p < 0.02). The dose intensities were significantly higher in 18 patients receiving G-CSF (0.94 vs 0.79) but the CR rate was not different between the two groups. The authors believe that the short follow-up precludes a meaningful comparison of the two groups of patients, in terms of survival and DFS.

Hemopoietic growth factors were also used in elderly patients by Gaspard et al. (74) with the twofold aim to mitigate myelotoxicity and to increase the dose/intensity of chemotherapy. These authors treated 26 patients older than 65 years (median age 73) with a combination of mitoxantrone, etoposide, methylglyoxal, ifosfamide and dexametasone (MEMID) plus GM-CSF (5 μg/Kg/day for 8 days). GM-CSF was given during the first, but not during the second course of chemotherapy, so that each patient acted as his/her own control. The median time interval between two courses was 20 days with GM-CSF versus 25 days without GM-CSF. Grade III and IV leukopenia were observed in 70% of the courses and clinically relevant infections (4 of which were septicemias) occurred in 21 cases. No comparison of the infection rate with and without GM-CSF has been performed yet. A response rate of 75% (CR 65%) was seen among 20 valuable patients.

In order to determine whether the administration of full dose VMP at the scheduled intervals can be improved by G-CSF, Monfardini et al. (75) have studied 20 elderly patients (median age 75, range 70–88) treated with VMP with and without G-CSF administration. Also in this study G-CSF was administered every other cycle to all patients. The preliminary analysis of 78 cycles of therapy showed a statistically significant difference in terms of delayed treatment (78% VMP alone vs 9% VMP + G-CSF) and mean neutrophil counts at the 21st day. Three infectious episodes requiring hospitalization were reported during treatment without G-CSF vs none when G-CSF was added to chemotherapy. No toxic death was observed and an objective response was seen in 68% of patients (75).

Table 43.7 Randomized studies in elderly patients with aggressive NHL.

Author, Year (reference)	# Patients	Median Age (Range)	Therapy	CR (%)	Overall Survival	Treatment-Related Deaths (%)
Dumontee *et al.* 1992 (76)	242		CVP vs	17	40% at 2 yrs	9
	253	≥*	CVP + THP-ADM	26	50% at 2 yrs	9
Sonneveld *et al.* 1994 (62)	100	70 (60–86)	CHOP vs CNOP	43	10 mo.	10
Myer *et al.* 1994 (78)	19	>65*	CHOP vs	68	66% at 18 mo.	0
	19		"Chop"	74	51% at 18 mo.	

* Median not reported

Randomized Clinical Trials

Randomized studies in elderly patients with NHL have been rare (Table 43.7).

The GELA Group (Group d'Etudes de Lymphomes de l'Adult) (76) performed a large randomized study in patients older than 69 years with aggressive NHL. Four-hundred and ninety-five patients were entered in a prospective trial comparing CVP (cyclophosphamide, teniposide, prednisolone) with CVP + THP-adriamycin (pirarubicine) (CTVP). Two-hundred and forty-two patients received the CVP regimen and 253 received the CTVP treatment. The two groups were well balanced according to histological grade, clinical stage, performance status, B-symptoms, serum LDH and bone marrow involvement. The overall response rate was significantly higher in patients receiving the adriamycin-containing regimen (58%, CR 26%) than in the CVP group (48%, CR 17%), although the CR rates were quite low in both arms. There was a trend to longer overall survival in patients receiving THP-adriamycin (50% vs 40% at 2 yrs) with a longer disease-free survival (p < 0.02). Despite the better response, the CTVP group experienced more frequent and more severe hematological toxicity and a relatively greater rate of toxic deaths (9% compared to 4.5% of CVP groups).

In another study headed by the Dutch Hematology-Oncology Study Group (77) 148 NHL elderly patients (≥60; median age 71; age range: 60–84) were randomized to receive either CHOP or CNOP (where doxorubicin was replaced by mitoxantrone) using an every-4-week schedule. At least three courses were planned prior to evaluation of response. Responding patients received 3 or 5 more cycles. The overall complete response rate was 41% for CHOP and 31% for CNOP respectively (p = 0.03). At three year follow-up 42% of patients treated with CHOP and 26% of those treated with CNOP were alive (p = 0.034) (Figure 43.3). Thirty-one percent of the CNOP patients and 45% of the CHOP patients completed six courses of treatment. The relative dose intensity was the same for the two groups of treatment (92 ± 13 for CHOP and 90 ± 12 for CNOP). Likewise, the incidence and the severity of myelotoxicity was the same with the two regimens. The incidence of cardiotoxicity, as measured by a decline ≥15% in ejection fraction was observed in 9 of 23 CNOP patients and 10

of 22 CHOP patients. Symptomatic congestive heart failure developed in 2 CNOP and 4 CHOP patients. The number of treatment-related deaths was 11 in both groups. Two observations are noteworthy in this study. First, the complete response rate to CNOP and CHOP was the same during the first three courses of treatment; the superiority of CHOP emerged in the number of partial responders who became complete responders after three courses of treatment. Second, the survival of patients <70, 70–75 and >75 was the same, which suggest that in the case of lymphoma age 60 may indeed be an adequate cutting point in term of prognosis, i.e. the prognosis for patients aged 60 and over is the same, irrespective of age, as long as other prognostic factors are comparable. In a recent study, standard CHOP has been compared by Meyer (78) versus one third of the dose of CHOP given weekly ("chop") in a randomized phase II study. Patients aged >65 with advanced stage intermediate grade lymphoma were randomized to receive CHOP (19 patients) or "chop" (19 patients). No statistical differences were seen on CR rate between the two groups of treatment (CHOP 68% vs '"chop" 74%) (P = 1.0). At 18 months progression-free survival was 66% with CHOP and

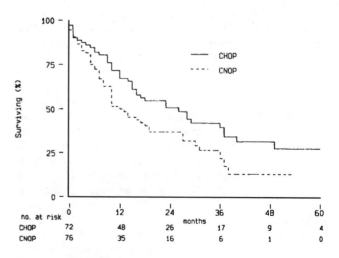

Figure 43.3 Survival of elderly patients with diffuse large cell lymphoma treated with CHOP and CNOP. From ref 77 with permission.

Table 43.8 Age and response in low grade NHL.

Author, Year (Reference)	N° Patients	Age Groups	Therapy	CR (%)	Difference in Survival
Aviles, *et al.* 1991 (81)	42	<50	CT or CT + IF or TNI	90	p 0.87
	76	>50		91	
Soubeyran, *et al.* 1991 (82)	133	<60	IF (stage I-II-III),	87	
	148	>60	CVP or CHOP (stage IV)	78	p < 0.0001
Bastion, *et al.* 1991 (83)	62	<50	RT ± CT (stage I-II)	79	p 0.58
	36	50–65	CT (stage III-IV)	81	p 0.46
	23	>65		79	p 0.33
Epelbaum, *et al.* 1991 (84)	48	<65 >65	RT ± CT (stage I-II)	/	p 0.16

CT = chemotherapy; IF = involved field irradiation; TNI = total nodal irradiation; RT = radiotherapy

50% with "chop" (P = 0.2). Mean dose intensities did not differ between the two schedules. CHOP produced more episodes of grade 4 ECG leukopenia, but no toxic death was reported. The authors came to the conclusion that, although "chop" is less toxic, progression-free and overall survival may be worse than after CHOP, which remains the standard therapy also for elderly patients.

Management of Low-grade Lymphomas

Unlike aggressive NHL, low-grade lymphomas are not potentially curable with current forms of treatment. The progression is slow and seemingly not influenced by age; median survival of advanced disease is 5–8 years (45). Therapeutic options consist in treating low grade NHL at the time of diagnosis or in waiting until the disease becomes symptomatic or causes serious problems (disfiguration, edema, pancytopenia, hemolytic anemia, autoimmune thrombocytopenia etc). There is no proof that early treatment may improve the survival of these patients, nor is there proof that aggressive combination chemotherapy (eg. CHOP), is preferable to less aggressive multi-agent regimens or even single agent therapy. In fact, according to the well-known Stanford study comparing chlorambucil with CVP, no difference in disease status and survival at 4 years was observed, even though the CR rate was higher in the group of patients treated with CVP (79). In another study of the Stanford Group comparing treatment at diagnosis and treatment at the time of disease progression, treatment at diagnosis did not appear to improve the patient OS or DFS and EFS. On the other hand a more aggressive treatment may be indicated for patients presented with a more virulent disease. For patients with stage I and II, extended field radiotherapy may provide prolonged control of the disease and is considered the treatment of choice by some investigators (80).

It is a matter of controversy whether old age adversely affects results of treatment in low-grade NHL (Table 43.8). In a randomized study comparing CVP versus CVP plus involved field irradiation or CVP plus total nodal irradiation in 118 untreated patients with stage III and IV nodular lymphoma, Aviles *et al.* (81) could not detect any difference in CR rate and survival between patients younger and older than 50 years. No information was, however, made available on how many patients were older than 65 or 70 years. In another study, 281 patients with stage I, II and III received involved field irradiation, while CVP or CHOP were used in patients with stage IV (82). The CR rate between patients older and younger than 60 years was not significantly different, while overall survival was significantly higher in patients younger than 60 years. However, in another French study (83) in which patients were treated with RT alone for stage I and II and with various chemotherapy regimens in advanced stages (CVP, procarbazine-COP, procarbazine-adriamycin-COP, CHOP, others), results were influenced only by the classical clinical and biological parameters of high tumor mass and response to treatment but not by age. In a further retrospective study addressed only to stage I and II patients, no differences could be found in survival between patients either older or younger than 65 years (84).

A recent addition to the therapeutic armamentarium may provide some new options in the treatment of low-grade NHL. The new purine derivatives fludarabine and 2-chlorodeoxyadenosine (2-CDA), have demonstrated high efficacy in the management of indolent lymphoid malignancies such as CLL and low-grade NHL (85).

Seemingly, these drugs, alone or in combination with other agents may improve the prognosis of these diseases. These drugs are being actively investigated in ongoing clinical trials. Among the experimental forms of treatment for low-grade NHL the use of tagged monoclonal antibodies (86) and recombinant alpha interferon and interleukins (86) are of particular interest, as they have demonstrated activity in small clinical trials.

Finally, it should be mentioned that the majority of Maltomas (Low-grade lymphoma) of the stomach have been associated to H. Pylori infection and may regress after eradication of the microorganism with antibiotic therapy (87). The antibiotic therapy is unsuccessful, however, when the disease has spread beyond the stomach.

Lessons Learned from Clinical Trials

The clinical trials reviewed in our analysis showed that advanced age is an adverse prognostic factor, at least in aggressive NHL. Through the cumulative analysis of several case series of aggressive NHL carried out in "The International Non-Hodgkin Lymphoma Prognostic Factors Project" it has been demonstrated that patients older than 60 years have a worse prognostic outcome compared with younger patients (88). The authors of this analysis established five independent prognostic factors for large cell NHL. These included, in addition to age ≥60, stage (I and II vs III and IV); PS (ECG 0-1 vs >1), serum LDH, and number of extranodal sites involved by the lymphoma (1vs >1). Of interest, age was not only associated with decreased response rate, but also with decreased DFS of the responders. Possibly, the inclusion of patients treated with MACOP-B, which caused a high incidence of severe myelotoxicity requiring dose reduction among the elderly, might have been responsible for the shorter DFS.

This analysis does not provide any clue as to the best management of older individuals with aggressive NHL and the questions related to the treatment are still unsolved, in spite of 10 years of clinical trials devoted to the elderly.

The conclusions concerning the relative value of the various chemotherapy regimens tried in elderly patients with intermediate and high grade NHL are controversial, due to some bias in both the conduction and the interpretation of each trial (89). As a whole, elderly patients seem to have a lower rate of durable CR than adults. The direct comparison of response of elderly with younger patients entered in trials where no age limit had been fixed is, however, complicated by the fact that older patients were often excluded from these studies. Another obstacle to the analysis of the results obtained in elderly with NHL consists of the fact that the upper age limits of various trials are not uniform. Some authors included in their trials patients older than 60, other authors cases older than 65 or 70 years. In some studies, median age was not even reported. As a consequence, a comparison of the results among these different groups of patients is difficult and there is still a doubt that a higher response rate obtained with some regimens (71, 72) may be attributable to the selection of a "younger" population of elderly patients. In the attempt to make a rough comparison of the CR rate of the trials previously reported, the data have been subdivided by lower limits of age in Table 43.9.

The last two studies on patients treated with hematopoietic growth factors have been excluded from this comparison (74, 75). The trials grouping patients older than 60 years showed a mean complete response rate of 53%, whereas in the studies grouping patients older than 65 the mean CR rate was 41% and in the trials with patients older than 70 yrs the mean CR rate was 30%. These differences were statistically significant. Age appears associated both with decreased CR

Table 43.9 Complete remission rate of elderly patients with aggressive NHL: Comparison of three groups with different lower age limits based on 29 trials (47–78).

Age Group	N° Patients	N° CR	CR%	P	
> 60 years	617	330	53	<0.001	0.001
> 65 years	705	286	41	<0.001	
>70 years	706	211	30		

rate and decreased survival of complete responders. Seemingly, the poorer outcome of older patients with aggressive NHL may be related not only to a poorer initial response for all regimens, but probably to an increased treatment-related toxicity. Another possibility should be examined too, and that is a higher prevalence of tumor cells expressing the multidrug resistance (MDR) gene in older individuals. As MDR may be modulated by Ca++ channel blockers, cyclosporine, and cyclosporine analogue, this information may be important in planning future clinical trials.

Certainly, clinical trials of lymphoma treatment in older individuals allow us to conclude that a higher incidence of severe or lethal toxicity occurs in elderly patients. Myelosuppression with subsequent neutropenic infection and sepsis was the most common drug-related complication. The risk of infection seems directly related both to severity and duration of leukopenia. The use of hematopoietic growth factors (G-CSF) may shorten the myelosuppression induced by chemotherapy. Even though not completely tested in elderly patients, hemopoietic growth factors may allow the appropriately dose intense treatment of the aged patients.

In the last few years combination chemotherapy regimens specifically designed for elderly patients with aggressive lymphomas have been tested. Some of them include adriamycin and cyclophosphamide, administered at different doses and schedules. More recently, mitoxantrone, considered less cardiotoxic than the anthracyclines, and etoposide, a drug with an oral formulation that allows treatment on an outpatient basis, were introduced. All these novel regimens have been reported to be active and relatively well tolerated. The CR rate has been widely variable even if usually no more than 50 patients were treated in each trial. The different characteristics of the patients in terms of performance status, prognostic factors related to the NHL and comorbidity do not allow a meaningful comparison among the results of these trials. In the only randomized trial in which doxorubicin and mitoxantrone were compared, doxorubicin appeared more effective than mitoxantrone (77).

To now, it is not yet clear whether regimens specifically designed for older individuals present any real advantage over standard treatment with CHOP in terms of therapeutic response and toxicity. The observation by O'Reilly et al. that PDOCE caused a response rate comparable to that of MACOP-B with significantly less toxicity is the only suggestion that these regimens may be better tolerated in older individuals. (59)

In NHL of favorable histology it is not clear whether prognosis is worse for elderly patients. The lack of a clear-cut difference in the results of therapy between younger and older patients compared with that of unfavorable NHL is not surprising, since a similar outcome could be due, in the elderly, to the lack of need of an intensive approach (either no therapy or single agents instead of combination chemotherapy regimens, involved field RT instead of extended RT plus combination chemotherapy) in a disease for which the induction of a CR is not essential to improve survival as it is in aggressive NHL.

Conclusions

In conclusion, overall pathological data indicate that the elderly (>70 years) form a relevant proportion (about 30%) of patients developing NHL. The patterns of presentation of NHLs in the elderly does not differ significantly from their younger counterparts in terms of histologic features and extranodal disease. Since an increase in "diffuse" vs "follicular" histologic patterns is observed with advancing age, a careful but active therapeutic approach is needed. For patients with aggressive forms of lymphomas, under treatment should be avoided as it may reduce the chances of cure.

Interestingly, some differences in the occurrence of distinct clinicopathologic entities included in the R.E.A.L. classification are observed between patients younger or older than 70 years: the immunohistologically defined CD30 positive ALCL and mediastinal B large cell lymphomas occur predominantly or exclusively in the group of patients younger than 70 years, whereas MCL cases seem to be restricted to the older patients. For what concerns the immunophenotype of NHL, most NHL cases in the elderly express B-cell markers. The relationship between immunesenscense and NHL is poorly understood (90).

The same staging procedures used in younger adults should be considered in the elderly. This goal is achieved through persuasion (and a certain degree of patience), by the health care providers.

In the frail elderly it may be reasonable to perform staging procedures while they are inpatient, to avoid the discomfort of repeated travel. The first course of chemotherapy should be administered at full doses, whenever possible. The tolerance of the first cycle of treatment will be a guide for the prosecution of therapy. The optimal management of aged patients with NHL should require a proper evaluation of the existing age-related limitations to intensive treatment such as comorbidity, possible deterioration of mental status and decreased physical fitness (91–92). The same intensive combination chemotherapy used for adults can probably be administered to patients with aggressive

NHL between 60 and 70 years in the absence of signs of organ function impairment, better if with the possibility of resorting to the hematopoietic growth factors in case of neutropenic sepsis.

After 70 years of age, various specifically designed or standard regimens are available. The choice of the combination should be made according to the individual experience of every medical oncologist with that specific combination in elderly patients with NHL, rather than adopting each time the newest regimen with the highest percentage of CR reported in a freshly published abstract. In the absence of comorbidity, therapy should be started at full dosage, especially when, in case of neutropenic sepsis, hematopoietic growth factors are available. Oral antibiotic prophylaxis may be a reasonable alternative to hematopoietic growth factors in some circumstances. Starting at reduced doses with subsequent increase in absence of severe toxicity seems, otherwise, an important option in case hematopoietic growth factors are not available and antibiotic prophylaxis is excluded.

In patients older than 80 years, chemotherapy should probably be administered at dosages reduced of 20–30%, even in the absence of associated diseases (93).

Limitations to trial entries for elderly patients with cardiac, renal, liver impairments are well known, and guidelines for dose reduction are available only for renal and liver insufficiency. In presence of cardiovascular diseases anthracycline-containing regimens should be avoided. Suggested regimens are those without anthracyclines (es. CVP and COPP) or those including the least cardiotoxic drug, i.e. mitoxantrone. In this instance the main mitoxantrone-including regimens are VMP, CNOP, MINE, CEMP, PEN (57, 62, 65, 66, 68).

Patients with stage I-II disease of unfavorable histology may be treated with only 2–3 cycles of chemotherapy before RT.

The management of low-grade NHL in elderly patients, compared to that of intermediate and high grade NHL, is easier since an aggressive approach is generally not needed. In clinically indolent cases no treatment may be a reasonable choice, while in patients with B-symptoms or more aggressive disease combination chemotherapy is indicated. To control local symptoms RT can be an alternative option.

No indications are at present at hand for the management of NHL in presence of the multiple associated pathologic conditions so frequently encountered in elderly patients. While awaiting the results of specific "pattern of care studies" (94), the way remains open to an enlightened empiricism.

References

1. Siegel JS. Recent and prospective demographic trends for the elderly population and some implications for health care. In Proceedings of the 2nd Conference on Epidemiology of Ageing; NIH Publication No. 80–696, edited by Heynes & Feinleib. Washington DC, 1980.
2. National Cancer Institute Update. Annual Cancer Statistics Update December 8, 1986. Bethesda, MD, National Cancer Institute, 1986.

3. National Cancer Institute. Cancer statistics review 1973–1987. *J Natl Cancer Inst* 1990; **82**: 1238–1240.

4. Horm JW, Asire AJ, Young JL Jr. SEER program: cancer incidence and mortality in the United States 1973–1981, US Department of Health, Education and Welfare Publication (NIH) 85–1837. Bethesda, National Cancer Institute, 1984.

5. Devesa SS, Silverman DT, Young JL, Jr, Pollack ES, Brown CC, Horm JW, Percy CL, Myers MH, McKay FW, Fraumeni JF Jr. Cancer incidence and mortality trends among whites in the United States. *J Natl Cancer Inst* 1987; **79**: 701–770.

6. Barnes N, Cartwright RA, O'Brien CO, Richards IDG, Roberts B, Bird CC. Rising incidence of lymphoid malignancies — True or false? *Br J Cancer* 1986; **53**: 393–398.

7. Rabkin CS, Devesa SS, Zahm S, *et al.* Increasing incidence of non-Hodgkin's lymphoma. *Semin Hematol* 1993; **30**: 286–296.

8. Jones SE, Fuks Z, Bull M, *et al.* Non-Hodgkin's lymphomas: IV. Clinicopathologic correlation in 405 cases. *Cancer* 1973; **31**: 806–823.

9. Patchefsky AS, Brodovsky HS, Menduke H, *et al.* Non-Hodgkin's lymphomas: A clinicopathologic study of 293 cases. *Cancer* 1974; **34**: 1173–1186.

10. Nathwani BN, Kim H, Rappaport H, Solomon J, Fox M. Non-Hodgkin's lymphomas: A clinicopathologic study comparing two classifications. *Cancer* 1978; **41**: 303–325.

11. Anderson T, Chabner BA, Young RC, *et al.* Malignant lymphoma: I. The histology and staging of 473 patients at the National Cancer Institute. *Cancer* 1982; **50**: 2699–2707.

12. Carbone A, Tirelli U, Volpe R, Zagonel V, Manconi R, Menin A, Trovó MG, Grigoletto E. Non-Hodgkin's lymphoma in the elderly: A retrospective clinicopathologic study of 50 patients. *Cancer* 1986; **57**: 2185–2189.

13. Elias L. Differences in age and sex distribution among patients with non-Hodgkin's lymphoma. *Cancer* 1979; **43**: 2540–2546.

14. Coiffier B. What treatment for elderly patients with aggressive lymphoma? *Ann Oncol* 1994; **5**: 873–875.

15. D'Amore F, Brincker H, Christensen BE, Thorling K, Pedersen M, Lanng Nielsen J, Sandberg E, Pedersen NT, Sorensen E, for the Danish LYFO-study group. Non-Hodgkin's lymphoma in the elderly. A study of 602 patients aged 70 or older from a Danish population-based registry. *Ann Oncol* 1992; **3**: 379–386.

16. Moller Jensen O, Estève J, Moller H, *et al.* Cancer in the European Community and its member states. *Eur J Cancer* 1990; **12**: 1167–1256.

17. Muir C, Waterhouse J, Mack T, Powell J, Whelan S. Cancer Incidence in Five Continents. Volume V. IARC Scientific Publication no. 88. International Agency for Research on Cancer, Lyon 1987.

18. Ballester OF, Moscinski L, Spiers A, Balducci L. Non-Hodgkin's lymphoma in the older person: a review. *J Am Geriatr Soc* 1993; **41**: 1245–1254.

19. Goss PE. Non-Hodgkin's lymphomas in elderly patients. *Leuk Lymphoma* 1993; **10**: 147–156.

20. Salminen EK. The outcome of > or = 70-year-old non-Hodgkin's lymphoma patients. *Int J Radiat Oncol Biol Phys* 1995; **32**: 349–353.

21. Neilly IJ, Ogston M, Bennett B, Dawson AA. High grade non-Hodgkin's lymphoma in the elderly – 12 year experience in the Grampian region of Scotland. *Hematol Oncol* 1995; **13**: 99–106.

22. Franceschi S. Epidemiology of non-Hodgkin's lymphomas in Europe. In *The Management of Non-Hodgkin's Lymphomas in Europe*, edited by S Monfardini. Eso Monograph. Berlin: Springer-Verlag, pp. 3–12, 1990.

23. Lipschitz DA, Goldstein S, Reis R, Weksler ME, Bressler R, Neilan BA. Cancer in the elderly: Basic science and clinical aspects. *Ann Int Med* 1985; **102**: 218–228.

24. Björkstén B, Svanborg C. Age and immunity. In *Cancer and Aging*, edited by A Macieira-Coelho, B Nordenskjöld. Boca Raton, Florida: CRC Press, Inc., pp. 86–96, 1990.

25. Lukes RJ, Collins RD. Immunological characterization of human malignant lymphomas. *Cancer* 1974; **34**: 1488–1503.

26. Stansfeld AG, Diebold J, Kapanci Y, Kelényi G, Lennert K, Mioduszewska O, Noel H, Rilke F, Sundstrom C, van Unnik JAM, Wright DH. Updated Kiel classification for lymphomas. *Lancet* 1988; **1**: 292–293.

27. The non-Hodgkin's lymphoma pathologic classification project. National Cancer Institute sponsored study of classification of non-Hodgkin's lymphomas. Summary and description of a working formulation for clinical usage. *Cancer* 1982; **49**: 2112–2135.

28. Harris NL, Jaffe ES, Stein H, Banks PM, Chan JKC, Cleary ML, Delsol G, De Wolf-Peeters C, Falini B, Gatter KC, Grogan TM, Isaacson PG, Knowles DM, Mason DY, Muller-Hermelink H-K, Pileri SA, Piris MA, Ralfkiaer E, Warnke RA. A revised European-American classification of lymphoid neoplasms: a proposal from the International Lymphoma Study Group. *Blood* 1994; **84**: 1361–1392.

29. Carbone A, Volpe R, Gloghini A, Trovó M, Zagonel V, Tirelli U, Monfardini S. Non-Hodgkin's lymphoma in the elderly. I. Pathologic features at presentation. *Cancer* 1990; **66**: 1991–1994.

30. Stein H, Mason DY, Gerdes J, O'Connor N, Wainscoat J, Pallesen G, Gatter K, Falini B, Delsol G, Lemke H, Schwarting R, Lennert K. The expression of the Hodgkin's disease associated antigen Ki-l in reactive and neoplastic lymphoid tissue: evidence that Reed-Sternberg cells and histiocytic malignancies are derived from activated lymphoid cells. *Blood* 1985; **66**: 848–858.

31. Banks PM, Chan J, Cleary ML, *et al.* Mantle cell lymphoma: a proposal for unification of morphologic, immunologic and molecular data. *Am J Surg Pathol* 1992; **16**: 637–640.

32. Isaacson PG. Lymphomas of mucosa-associated lymphoid tissue (MALT). *Histopathology* 1990; **16**: 617–619.

33. Tirelli U, Zagonel V, Serraino D, *et al.* Non-Hodgkin's lymphomas in 137 patients aged 70 years or older: A retrospective European organization for research and treatment of cancer lymphoma group study. *J Clin Oncol* 1988; **6**: 1708–1713.

34. Tirelli U, Carbone A, Zagonel V, Veronesi A, Canetta R. Non-Hodgkin's lymphomas in the elderly: prospective study with specifically devised chemotherapy regimens in 66 patients. *Eur J Cancer Clin Oncol* 1987; **23**: 535–540.

35. Barnes N, Cartwright RA, O'Brien C, Roberts B, Richards IDG, Hopkinson JM, Chorlton I, Bird CC. Variation in lymphoma incidence within Yorkshire Health Region. *Br J Cancer* 1987; **55**: 81–84.

36. Otter R, Gerrits WB, Kluin-Nelemans JC, Kluin PM, Stjinen T. NHL in a population based registry; elderly patients included. Third Int Conference on Malignant Lymphomas, Lugano, June 10–13, 1987 (Abs T61); 128.

37. Hancock BW, Aitken M, Ross CMD, Dunsmore IR. Non-Hodgkin's lymphoma in Sheffield 1971–1980. *Clin Oncol* 1983; **9**: 109–119.

38. Hoerni B, Sotto JJ, Eghbali H, Sotto MF, Hoerni-Simon G, Pegourié B. Non-Hodgkin's malignant lymphomas in patients older than 80: 70 cases. *Cancer* 1988; **61**: 2057–2059.

39. Otter R, Gerrits WBJ, Sandt MMVD, Hermans J, Willemze R. Primary extranodal and nodal non-Hodgkin's lymphoma: A survey of a population-based registry. *Eur J Cancer Clin Oncol* 1989; **25**: 1203–1210.

40. Monfardini S, Yancik R. Cancer in the elderly: meeting the challenge of an aging population. Commentary. *J Natl Cancer Inst* 1993; **85**(7): 532–538.

41. Raghavan D, Findlay MPN, McNeil EB. Cancer in the elderly. In *Oxford Textbook of Oncology*, Vol. 2, edited by M Peckham, H Pinedo, U Veronesi. Oxford: Oxford University Press, pp. 2169–2189, 1995.

42. Begg CB, Carbone PP, *et al.* Clinical trials and drug toxicity in the elderly: the experience of the Eastern Cooperative Oncology Group. *Cancer* 1983; **52**(11): 1986–1992.

43. Connors MJ. Infusions, age and drug dosages: Learning about large-cell lymphoma. *J Clin Oncol* 1988; **6**(3): 407–408.

44. Balducci L, Mowry K. Pharmacology and Organ Toxicity of Chemotherapy in Older Patients. *Oncology-Williston-Park* 1992; **6**(2 suppl): 62–68.

45. Lo Re G, Zagonel V, Monfardini S. Non-Hodgkin's lymphomas in the elderly. *Research and Clinical Forums* 1993; **15**(6) 9–18.

46. Sacco C, Zagonel V, Monfardini S. Clinical trials in older patients with intermediate and high-grade lymphomas. *Cancer Control* March/April 22–29, 1995.

47. Armitage JO, Potter JF. Aggressive chemotherapy for diffuse histiocytic lymphoma in the elderly: Increased complications with advancing age. *J Am Geriatr Soc* 1984; **32**(4): 269–273.

48. Dixon DO, Neilan B, Jones SE, *et al.* Effect of age on therapeutic outcome in advanced diffuse histiocytic lymphoma: The Southwest Oncology Group experience. *J Clin Oncol* 1986; **4**(3): 295–305.

49. O'Connel JD, Harrington DP, Johnson GJ, *et al.* Initial chemotherapy doses for elderly patients with malignant lymphoma. *J Clin Oncol* 1986; **4**: 1418 (letter).

50. Solal-Celigny P, Chastang C, Herrera A, *et al.* Age as the main prognostic factor in adult aggressive non-Hodgkin's lymphoma. *Am J Med* 1987; **83**(6): 1075–1079.

51. Vose JM, Armitage JO, Weisenburger DD, *et al.* The importance of age in survival of patients treated with chemotherapy for aggressive non-Hodgkin's lymphoma. *J Clin Oncol* 1988; **6**(12): 1838–1844.

52. Orlandi E, Lazzarino M, Brusamolino E, *et al.* Non-Hodgkin's lymphoma in the elderly: the impact of advanced age on therapeutic opinions and clinical results. *Hematologica* 1991; **76**(3): 204–208.

53. Bruno S, Santarelli MT, Corrado C, *et al.* Age-related results in intermediate and high-grade non-Hodgkin's lymphoma (NHL) patients (pts). First International Conference on Geriatric Oncology, Buenos Aires, October 28–30, 1992. 4.5. Abstract.

54. Grogan L, Corbally N, Dervan PA. Comparable prognostic factors and survival in elderly patients with aggressive non-Hodgkin's lymphoma treated with standard-dose adriamycin-based regimen. *Ann Oncol* 1994; **5**(S2): 47–51.

55. Tirelli U, Carbone A, Crivellari D, *et al.* A phase II trial of Teniposide (VM26) in advanced non-Hodgkin's lymphoma with emphasis on the treatment of elderly patients. *Cancer* 1984; **54**: 393–396.

56. Zagonel V, Tirelli U, Carbone A, *et al.* Combination chemotherapy specifically devised for elderly patients with unfavorable non-Hodgkin's lymphoma. *Cancer Invest* 1990; **8**(6): 577–582.

57. Tirelli U, Zagonel V, Errante D, *et al.* A prospective study on a new combination chemotherapy regimen in patients older than 70 years with unfavorable non-Hodgkin's lymphoma. *J Clin Oncol* 1992; **10**(2): 228–236.

58. O'Reilly S, Klimo P, Connors JM. Low dose-ACOP-B and VABE: weekly chemotherapy for elderly patients with advanced stage diffuse large cell lymphoma. *J Clin Oncol* 1991; **9**(5): 741–747.

59. O'Reilly SE, Hoskins P, Howdle S. POCE chemotherapy phase II trial in elderly patients with advanced stage diffuse large cell lymphoma. Proceedings of ASCO 1992. 116. Abstract.

60. Kitamura K, Takaku F. Pirarubicin, a novel derivative of doxorubicin. THP-COP therapy for non-Hodgkin's lymphoma in the elderly. *Am J Clin Oncol* 1990; **13**(suppl.l): S15–S19.

61. McMaster ML, Johnson DH, Greer JP, *et al.* A brief-duration combination chemotherapy for elderly patients with poor-prognosis non-Hodgkin's lymphoma. *Cancer* 1991; **67**(6): 1487–1492.

62. Sonneveld P, Michiels JJ. Full-dose chemotherapy in elderly patients with non-Hodgkin's lymphoma: a feasibility study using a mitoxantrone containing regimen. *Br J Cancer* 1990; **62**: 105–108.

63. Salvagno L, Contu A, Fiorentino MV, *et al.* A combination of mitoxantrone, etoposide and prednisone in elderly patients with non-Hodgkin's lymphoma. *Ann Oncol* 1992; **3**: 833–837.

64. Landys K, Hultén U, Toss L. Mitoxantrone in combination with prednimustine (NOSTE) in treatment of elderly patients with non-Hodgkin's lymphoma. First International Conference on Geriatric Oncology, Buenos Aires, October 28–30, 1992. 4.1. Abstract.

65. Torello E, Savignano R, Sutter M, *et al.* MINE: mesna (M), ifosfamide (I), novantrone (N), etoposide (E) in elderly patients (pts) with relapsed or refractory intermediate and high grade non-Hodgkin's lymphoma study. First International Conference on Geriatric Oncology, Buenos Aires, October 28–30, 1992. 4.7. Abstract.

66. Ansell SM, Falkson G, Uys A. A phase II study of a new chemotherapeutic combination in elderly patients with aggressive lymphoma. First International Conference on Geriatric Oncology, Buenos Aires, October 28–30, 1992. 4.2. Abstract.

67. Hainsworth JD. Effective, well-tolerated combination chemotherapy for elderly patients with aggressive non-Hodgkin's lymphoma. Proceedings of ASCO 1992. 1151. Abstract.

68. Goss P and the Metro Toronto Lymphoma Group. PEN (prednisone, etoposide and novantrone) for treatment of non-Hodgkin's lymphoma in elderly patients. Proceedings of ASCO 1993. 1259. Abstract.

69. Tigaud JD, Demolombe S, Coiffier B. Ifosfamide continuous infusion plus etoposide in the treatment of elderly patients with aggressive lymphoma: A phase II study. *Hematol Oncol* 1991; **9**: 225–233.

70. Liang R, Todd D, Chann TK. COPP therapy for elderly patients with intermediate and high grade non-Hodgkin's lymphoma. *Hematol Oncol* 1993; **II**: 43–50.

71. Zinzani PL, Bendani M, Gherlinzoni F. VNCOP-B regimen in the treatment of high-grade non-Hodgkin's lymphoma in the elderly. *Hematologica* 1993; **78**: 378–382.

72. Martelli M, Guglielmi C, Colussi S. P-VABEC: A prospective study of a new weekly chemotherapy regimen for elderly aggressive non-Hodgkin's lymphoma. *J Clin Oncol* 1993; **12**: 2362–2369.

73. Bertini M for the Italian Multiregional non-Hodgkin's lymphoma Study Group. Therapeutic strategies in intermediate grade lymphomas in elderly patients. In: Hematological Malignancies in the Elderly. *Hematol Oncol* 1993; **II**(Sl): 52–58.

74. Gaspard MH, Rossi GF, Thyss A, *et al.* Polychemotherapy with GM-CSF for aggressive non-Hodgkin's lymphoma (NHL) in elderly patients. *Ann Oncol* 1992; **3**(S5). 476. Abstract.

75. Monfardini S, Sacco C, Babare R, *et al.* VP-16, mitoxantrone and prednimustine (VMP) with or without G-CSF in patients with non-Hodgkin's lymphomas (NHL) older than 70 years. Proceedings of ASCO, 1994. 1277. Abstract.

76. Dumantee C, Bourdesoulle D, Coiffier B, *et al.* TPA-adriamycin in the treatment of elderly patients with aggressive non-Hodgkin's lymphoma. Results of the NHL-87 protocol. *Ann Oncol* 1992, **3**(S5). 474. Abstract.

77. Sommerveld P, deRidder M, van der Lelie H, *et al.* Comparison of doxorubicin and mitoxantrone in the treatment of elderly patients with advanced diffuse Non-Hodgkin's Lymphoma using CHOP versus CNOP chemotherapy. *J Clin Oncol* 1995; **13**: 2530–2539.

78. Meyer RM, Bauger A, Browman G. A randomized phase II comparison of standard CHOP with weekly "chop" for elderly patients with intermediate grade lymphoma. Proceedings of ASCO, 1994. 1245. Abstract.

79. Portlock CS, Rosenberg SA, Glatstein E, *et al.* Treatment of advanced non-Hodgkin's lymphomas with favorable histologies. Preliminary results of a prospective trial. *Blood* 1976; **47**: 747.

80. Rosenberg SA. The low-grade non-Hodgkin lymphomas: challenges and opportunities. *J Clin Oncol* 1985; **3**: 299.

81. Avilos A, Diaz-Maqueo JC, Sanchez E, Cortes HD, Ayala JR. Long-term results in patients with low-grade nodular non-Hodgkin's lymphoma. A randomized trial comparing chemotherapy plus radiotherapy with chemotherapy alone. *Acta Oncologica* 1991; **30**(3): 329–333.

82. Souberyan P, Eghbali H, Bonichon F, Trojani M, Richaud P, Hoerni B. Low-grade follicular lymphomas: analysis of prognosis in a series of 281 patients. *Eur J Cancer* 1991; **27**(12): 1606–1613.

83. Bastion Y, Berger F, Bryon PA, Felman P, French M, Coiffier B. Follicular lymphomas: assessment of prognostic factors in 127 patients followed for 10 years. *Ann Oncol* 1991; **2**(S2): 123–129.

84. Epelbaum R, Kuten A, Coahman NM, Faraggi D, Ben-Aire Y, Ben-Sharar M, Haim N, Leviov M, Cohen Y. Stage I-II low grade non-Hodgkin's lymphoma: prognostic factors and treatment results. *Strahlenther Onkol* 1992; **168**(2): 66–72.

85. Tallman MS, Hakimian D. Purine nucleoside analog: emerging roles in indolent lymphoproliferative disorders. *Blood* 1995; **86**: 2463–2474.

86. Fisher RI, Oken MM. Clinical Practice Guidelines: non-Hodgkin's Lymphomas. *Cleveland Clinic J Med.* **62** (Suppl l); SI6–SI41.

87. Roggero E, Zucca E, Pinotti G, *et al.* Eradication of Helicobacter Pylori Infection in Primary Low-Grade Gastric Lymphoma of Mucosa-associated Lymphoid Tissue. *Ann Int Med* 1995; **22**: 767–769.

88. The International Non-Hodgkin's Lymphoma Prognostic Factors Project. A predictive model for aggressive non-Hodgkin's lymphoma. *N Engl J Med* 1993; **329**(14): 87–994.

89. Tirelli U and Monfardini S. Non-Hodgkin's lymphoma. In *Cancer In The Elderly. Treatment And Research*, edited by IS Fentiman, S Monfardini. Oxford: Oxford Medical Publications, 144–151, 1994.

90. Tirelli U, Franceschi S, Carbone A. Malignant tumors in patients with HIV infection. *Br Med J* 1994; **308**: 1148–1153.

91. Monfardini S, Ferrucci L, Saran D, *et al*. Multidimensional Geriatric Evaluation in elderly with cancer. *Proc ASCO* 1995; 891 Abstract.

92. Monfardini S, Ferrucci L, Fratino L, Del Lungo I, Saran D, Zagonel V. Validation of a multidimensional evaluation scale for use in elderly cancer patients. *Cancer* 1996; **77**(2): 395–401.

93. Schneider M, Thyss A, Ayela P, *et al*. Chemotherapy for patients aged over 80. In *Cancer In The Elderly. Treatment And Research*, edited by IS Fentiman, S Monfardini. Oxford: Oxford Medical Publications, 53–60, 1994.

94. Monfardini S. What do we know on variables influencing clinical decision-making in elderly cancer patients? *Eur J Cancer* 1996; **32A**(1): 12–14.

44. Multiple Myeloma

Oscar F. Ballester, Claudia Corrado and David Vesole

Introduction

Multiple myeloma represents 1% of all cancers occurring in the US every year (1). A most striking feature of the disease is its age-dependant incidence (Figure 44.1A), from less than 1 case per 100,000 in individuals younger than 45, to more than 60 cases per 100,000 in those older than 80 (2, 3).

This chapter will focus on three specific areas pertinent to multiple myeloma in the older patient. First, we will review recent advances in the biology of the disease as they relate to the process of aging. Interpretation of the value of prognostic factors and outcomes of standard therapies for myeloma are currently based on data from clinical trials where older patients are under represented (Figure 44.1C) (4). In the second section of this chapter we will present an evaluation of prognostic factors and results of standard therapies in older patients with multiple myeloma. Patients younger than 65 (representing approximately 50% of the myeloma population, Figure 44.1B), may benefit from the use of high-dose therapy with autologous hematopoietic stem cell transplantation. With significant improvements in the safety of these procedures, the age-limit can be extended to individuals older than age 65. In the final section, we will present an analysis of outcomes of high-dose therapy in the older myeloma patient.

The reader is referred to several excellent recent reviews for a more detailed discussion on other aspects of the disease (5, 6, 7).

Role of Aging in the Biology of Multiple Myeloma

The development of multiple myeloma appears to be dependent on the interplay of three major factors: a genetically susceptible host, certain environmental exposure(s), and the process of aging. In the first section of this chapter, we will review recent information in these three areas, to base our hypothesis on the role of aging in this disorder.

Epidemiological studies have linked a higher risk for myeloma to certain environmental (primarily occupational) exposures. This would suggest that the initial oncogenic event may occur as early as in the third or fourth decade of life. However, the incidence of myeloma does not increase significantly before the sixth decade. A long latency period from exposure to clinical overt disease would be compatible with a slow and

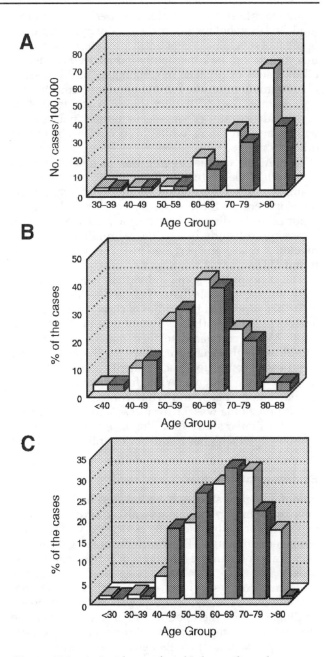

Figure 44.1 A: Incidence of multiple myeloma by age group (males: clear bars, females: dark bars).
B: Distribution of myeloma cases by age in the general population (males: clear bars, females: dark bars).
C: Distribution of myeloma cases by age in the general population (clear bars) and in clinical trials (dark bars) (4).

multistep oncogenic process, including the need for a permissive environment for the tumor to develop. Such a permissive environment could be created by the loss of immune mediated anti-tumor mechanisms associated with aging. While little is known regarding the first issues, data has accumulated over the past several years on the changes occurring with aging in the host's immune system that will promote tumor progression.

Genetic Factors

A genetic predisposition for the development of myeloma is best demonstrated in experimental animal models. The spontaneous or chemically induced development of myeloma is genetically predetermined. Plasmacytomas can be consistently induced with mineral oil injections or pristane in certain genetically susceptible strains of mice, like the BALB/c, while other strains are resistant. The C57BL mice shows an age-dependent high incidence rate of spontaneous monoclonal gammopathies and myeloma, while this occurrence is rare in other strains (8).

In humans, familial aggregation of myeloma cases is rare (9). While relatives of patients with hematological malignancies have a significant increased risk for the development of these disorders, this risk has been reported to be disease non-specific (10). However, in a case-control study of first degree relatives from 239 myeloma cases, an increased risk for myeloma was found (11).

The concept that some individuals may be genetically more susceptible than others to develop myeloma is further supported by studies of class I and II human leukocyte antigens (HLA) distribution in affected patients. When compared to their matched controls, a significant higher gene frequency for Bw65, Cw2 and Drw14 was found for black patients and for A3 and Cw2 for white patients. While frequency of Cw2 was similar among black and white controls, the relative risk for myeloma was 5.7 for blacks and 2.6 for whites (12). In a similar study from Russia, myeloma patients demonstrated a higher frequency of antigens A11 and B7 (13).

Environmental Factors

Epidemiological studies have linked a higher risk for developing multiple myeloma with certain occupational exposures or with conditions associated with chronic antigenic stimulation. These include ionizing radiation, chemicals and chronic infectious or inflammatory disorders.

Atomic bomb survivors, individuals with occupational exposure to radiation, as well as those exposed to diagnostic or therapeutic x-rays have an increase risk for developing myeloma. Workers in agriculture, rubber, petroleum and fuels, benzene and other chemical industries are, similarly, at higher risk for myeloma (1).

In a study of 1,098 myeloma cases from Denmark, the risk for myeloma was significantly elevated with certain occupations and specially with the duration of employment in these occupations. A near 5 fold increase in risk for myeloma was found among workers exposed to vinyl chloride for 5 or more years (14).

An increased risk for myeloma was also found for painters, particularly for those employed for 10 years or more. Similarly an excess risk was found among agricultural workers exposed to pesticides for 10 years or longer (15). High concentrations of polychlorinated dibenzo-p-dioxins and dibenzofurans in blood from consumption of fatty fish, was associated with a higher mortality from myeloma in Swedish fishermen (16). In a case-control study, an association was found between rheumatic diseases in general, and rheumatoid arthritis in particular with the occurrence of myeloma (17).

When multiple risk factors were considered including allergies, autoimmune disorders, chronic bacterial infections and inflammatory conditions, the rate of myeloma occurrence increased with the number of risk factors. Interestingly, there was also a significant increase with time (18).

Some epidemiological associations are controversial. For example, there are studies that have denied the role of chronic infections, autoimmune, allergic, musculoskeletal disorders (19) and rheumatoid arthritis (20). Similarly, some recent studies have failed to demonstrate an increase risk for myeloma in agricultural workers in Ireland (21), Iowa (22) and Denmark (14) and among atomic bomb survivors (23).

Aging, Immune Dysfunction and B Cell Proliferation

The process of aging in healthy individuals is associated with profound changes in the immune system (24, 25). A T lymphocyte deficit develops, probably as a consequence of thymic involution. Changes also extend to other elements of the immune system including natural killer (NK) cells, B lymphocytes and macrophages as well as to the regulation of cytokine expression.

T Lymphocytes

In mice, accumulation of memory T cells at the expense of naive T cells may account for the decline in the proportion of cells that secrete and respond to interleukin-2 (IL-2) (26). Memory CD8+ were increased in the splenic T cell pool of older mice at the expense of naive CD8+ cells, which may significantly contribute to their increased interferon-γ production capacity (27). In older mice, splenic T cells bearing the IL-2 receptor have an impaired proliferative and clonogenic ability in response to IL-2 stimulation. This is observed for both CD4+ and CD8+ subsets (28).

The physiologic involution of the thymus appears to be the central event in the changes occurring in humans with aging. Peripheral blood T cells from the aged had decreased proliferative responses, decreased number of high affinity IL-2 receptors and produced 10 fold less IL-2, but 3 fold higher amounts of interleukin-6 (IL-6) (29).

In a different study, the number of cells expressing the IL-2 receptor was comparable in peripheral blood mononuclear cells of older and younger healthy individuals, but older subjects showed a reduced *in-vitro* proliferative response to IL-2 (30).

Certain pathways of T cell activation may be more compromised in the elderly than others: T cells from elderly individuals have decreased proliferative response and secrete less IL-2 when stimulated with anti-CD3 antibodies, while responses to anti-CD2 antibodies are comparable to those of younger subjects (31). T cell receptor beta chain mRNA levels were comparable in younger and older individuals stimulated with either anti-CD3 or anti-CD2 antibodies. The proliferative response of peripheral blood mononuclear cells after allogeneic stimulation (mixed lymphocyte culture) was impaired in elderly subjects (32).

Particularly relevant to anti-tumor responses is the ability to generate cytotoxic T lymphocytes (33), which has been shown to experience an age-related decline.

T cell subsets in individuals older than 65, frequently contain expanded populations of CD8+ TCR (T cell receptor) V beta populations, which are mono or oligoclonal (34). This phenomenon may represent the T cell equivalent to the monoclonal gammopathies seen in older individuals (see below).

NK Cells

Aged mice were found to have a 50% reduction in the number of splenic NK (natural killer) cells. *In-vivo* IL-2 administration could not restore normal function or numbers of NK cells (35).

In humans, older subjects have normal or increased numbers of NK cells (36). This results from a significant increase in the CD16+/CD57+ cell subset, with a moderated decrease of the CD56+/CD57-cells (37). Higher innate NK lytic activity was found in elderly healthy individuals as compared with young controls. Interferon-α induced lytic activity, however, was found to be decreased in older individuals (38). In a different study, the lytic activity of NK cells was found to be decreased. *In-vitro*, Interferon-β or IL-2 were shown to restore normal function (36).

Interestingly, a negative correlation was found between NK cell numbers and blood levels of organochlorine compounds in Swedish fishermen, which was associated with a high mortality rate from myeloma (16).

B Lymphocytes

Some studies in experimental animal models have suggested that aging is associated with a decreased frequency of B cell precursors in the bone marrow (39). However, most abnormalities described in humoral immunity appear to be secondary to changes in T cell function (40).

Aged individuals demonstrate a restriction in immunoglobulin heterogeneity, with a decrease in some immunoglobulin subtypes and increases in others. The antibody responses to certain antigens are preserved, while those dependant on T cell regulation may be impaired. Regulatory auto-anti-idiotypic antibodies, also T cell dependent phenomenon, are increased with

age. This mechanism may be responsible for down regulating the production of antibody responses seen in older individuals (41).

Overall, a state of dysregulated B cell proliferation ensues in healthy older individuals, reflected in increased concentrations of serum polyclonal immunoglobulins and other measures of B lymphocyte mass, such as serum b-2-microglobulin levels (42). The incidence of spontaneously developing EBV-infected lymphoblastoid cell lines was significantly increased among healthy sero-positive donors aged 80 or older, when compared to younger controls (43). Whether this occurs as a consequence of defective T cell function had not been further clarified. On this background autoantibodies and monoclonal proteins are detected with increasing frequency. The later are particularly relevant to the development of multiple myeloma.

MGUS

The incidence of serum monoclonal gammopathies increases with age (44, 45), reaching 1% or more of the population older than 65. In the absence of other evidence of disease, these monoclonal gammopathies may remain stable and asymptomatic for years (monoclonal gammopathies of undetermined significance, MGUS).

Extended follow up studies in patients with MGUS have demonstrated that 8.5% by 5 years, 17% to 19.2% by 10 years and 33% by 20 years, have evolved into a malignant process, primarily multiple myeloma (46–7). Myeloma developed at a median of 10 years after the detection of a monoclonal protein (48). Retrospective analysis documented a MGUS stage in 58% of patients with newly diagnosed multiple myeloma (49). At least in humans, MGUS are considered the premyelomatous pathological state.

Macrophages and Cytokines

Macrophages are an important part of the immune system, because of their role as antigen presenting cells (APC) and in the production of a variety of cytokines that regulate both T and B cell proliferation and differentiation. While no significant and consistent abnormalities have been reported in APC with aging, *in-vitro* as well as *in-vivo* data suggests that their patterns of cytokine expression may be altered.

In mice experiments, older animals produced higher levels of IL-2 and interleukin-4 (IL-4) *"in vivo"* after exposure to staphylococcal enterotoxin B, which induced lethal toxic shock in these animals but was not observed in younger mice (50). Interleukin-1 (IL-1), IL-6 and tumor necrosis factor (TNF) production by unstimulated and Freund's adjuvant elicited peritoneal macrophages was decreased in older mice. However, some pathways of activation appear to be preserved since there were no differences in the production of these cytokines in thioglycollate-elicited macrophages (51).

In humans, monocytes from aged individuals had decreased responses to activation with LPS, had reduced cytotoxicity against tumor cells, and secreted less IL-1 than monocytes from young donors (52).

The production of interferon-γ by peripheral blood mononuclear cells stimulated with phytohemagglutinin was reduced in older heathy individuals, while the production of IL-4 and IL-6 was comparable to that of young controls (53). In a separate report, mononuclear cells from individuals older than 55 years produced higher levels of IL-1, both unstimulated as well as when stimulated with LPS. No differences were found in IL-1 production stimulated with 1, 25 hydroxivitamin D, or with TNF under any culture condition (54). In the culture supernatants of mixed lymphocyte cultures, elderly subjects had higher levels of IL-2, IL-1 and TNF-α, cytokines predominantly secreted by macrophages (32).

IL-6 and Aging

IL-6 is a multifunctional cytokine with important functions in hematopoiesis, inflammation and immunity (55, 56).

IL-6 levels increase with age in the sera of certain strains of mice such as the MRU/lpr which are susceptible to polyclonal B cell activation and autoimmune glomerulonephritis, but not in other strains including the BALB/c (57). The increased IL-6 synthesis observed with age in C57BU6 mice can be prevented by dietary restrictions that prolong the life-span of the animals (58).

In humans and in rhesus monkeys serum IL-6 levels increase with age. In the absence of infection or inflammation, interleukin-6 levels in serum are low or undetectable in young individuals, however, with advancing age serum IL-6 levels became detectable (59).

Administration of IL-6 to aged non-human primates resulted in a less significant, but more protracted decrease in certain immune functions as compared to middle-aged animals (60).

It must be pointed out that IL-6 is but only one of a host of cytokines dysregulated with normal aging (61, 62). Because of its reported role in multiple myeloma, it will be discussed in some detail.

IL-6 and Multiple Myeloma

Experiments with transgenic mice able to suppress or overexpress IL-6 production are illustrative of the potential role of this cytokine in the pathogenesis of myeloma.

Homozygous mice for the IL-6-null gene mutation (IL-6 deficient), failed to develop plasma cell tumors after induction with pristane and *myc-raf*-containing J3V1 retrovirus. This protocol induced plasmacytomas in 34 to 38% of heterozygous and wild type animals (63). Transgenic mice overexpressing human IL-6 develop massive but polyclonal plasmacytosis. Animals that were then backcrossed to BALB/c (one of the few strains known to be highly susceptible to plasmacytoma induction), developed transplantable monoclonal plasmacytomas (64).

Some myeloma cell lines have been shown to be dependent on exogenous IL-6 for "in-vitro" survival and/or proliferation, while others are IL-6 independent (65).

IL-6 has been proposed as a major growth factor for human myeloma cells (66, 67). The evidence for this is derived from: a) the prognostic significance of elevated serum IL-6 levels in patients with myeloma, and b) the ability of exogenous IL-6 to induce myeloma cell proliferation *in-vitro*.

Serum IL-6 levels have been shown to predict poor outcome of myeloma patients in some (68, 69), but not in all studies (70, 71). Elevated serum IL-6 levels are also found in a number of other hematological malignancies and solid tumors. In non-Hodgkin's lymphomas and prostate cancer increased serum IL-6 are associated with poor prognosis (72, 73). The origin of circulating serum IL-6 is unclear. Peripheral blood T lymphocytes from myeloma patients, particularly those untreated, produced significantly higher levels of IL-6 when stimulated with PHA than normal controls. No correlations were found, however, with disease stage or other prognostic factors (74).

Myeloma cells grow and proliferate in the bone marrow micro-environment. Therefore, bone marrow levels of IL-6 expression and secretion may be more relevant than serum levels. Myeloma cells from some, but not all patients, express the gp80 protein identified as the IL-6 receptor (IL-6R) in their surface. IL-6R is expressed in myeloma cells with a more immature phenotype. While 40% of myeloma cells expressed IL-6 mRNA, secretion of IL-6 in rather minute amounts was demonstrated in only 4 of 22 cases (75).

Signal transduction via IL-6/IL-6R is dependent on a second membrane protein, gp130, upon interaction of IL-6 and IL-6R. gp130 is shared as the signal transducer for several other molecules, including oncostatin M, interleukin-11, NCGT.

Stromal cells in the marrow microenvironment, such as macrophages, fibroblast, endothelial cells and T lymphocytes are rich sources of IL-6. The paracrine secretion of IL-6 appears quantitatively more important than the autocrine (Figure 44.2).

Studies have shown that stromal cells can produce very large amounts of I-6 after cell-to-cell contact with myeloma cells (76, 77).

Neither bone marrow plasma IL-6 levels (78), nor the levels of IL-6R saturation in freshly isolate myeloma cells (79), were correlated with an aggressive biological behavior of the disease.

Myeloma cells from experimental animal models undergo spontaneous cycles of cell proliferation and differentiation when transplanted into a normal host. After an initial phase characterized by the loss of the most differentiated cells, there is an expansion of the proliferative pool and subsequent repopulation of the tumor burden (79). When freshly obtained human myeloma cells are studied "in-vitro," an increase spontaneous cell proliferation is observed after several days in culture. Previous reports have suggested that this proliferation is dependent on endogenous IL-6 secretion and that is enhanced by exogenous IL-6 administration (66, 67). We have reported from our laboratory, that this type of cultures produce, indeed, very large amounts of IL-6. In our experience, exogenous IL-6 did

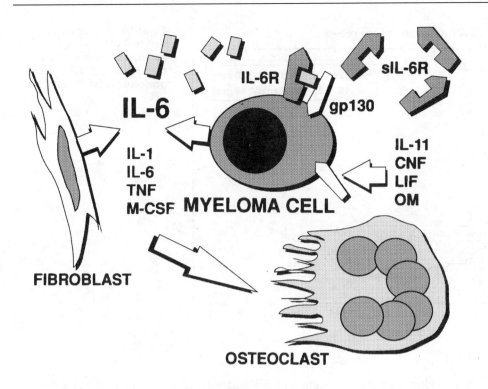

Figure 44.2 Biology of IL-6 in multiple myeloma.

not produce detectable changes in the growth fraction of the tumor (81).

In our study, high IL-6 levels spontaneously secreted in bone marrow cultures were correlated with low tumor mass (low % myeloma cells in bone marrow, low serum b-2 microglobulin), low growth fraction (percentage of Ki 67+ cells), and higher rates of immunoglobulin production (82). We interpreted our data to indicate, that tumors growing in a IL-6 abundant media were biologically less aggressive and more differentiated. These preliminary findings were recently confirmed by a study of 107 patients with plasma cell disorders. The highest median values for IL-6 were observed in patients with MGUS and indolent myelomas, and during the remission. The lowest IL-6 values were found in patients with plasma cell leukemia. Among newly diagnosed patients, high IL-6 levels resulted in significantly improved survival (83). In serial studies, IL-6 production in bone marrow cultures significantly increased after significant cytoreductions induced by chemotherapy (84).

Our interpretation of these results indicates that IL-6 secretion in the marrow environment depends largely upon the paracrine mechanism. A low tumor to stromal cell density ratio will favor the optimal secretion of IL-6. With tumor progression, a high tumor cell density will impair the interaction of tumor and stromal cells, with decreased IL-6 production.

Recently, it has been reported that IL-6 prevents programmed cell death (apoptosis) of myeloma cells (85). Preventing apoptosis of the most differentiated cells could inhibit the tumor's proliferative pool *in vivo*, maintaining the tumor relatively well differentiated and at a low tumor burden.

Immune Dysfunction and Myeloma Progression

The immune changes associated with aging significantly affect the anti-tumor responses of the host. In the experimental animal, manipulation of the immune response can clearly modulate myeloma growth.

In experimental animal models, T cell mediated tumor regression is significantly impaired in older mice (86). Aged mice with spontaneous high levels of memory CD4 and/or CD8 cells, low levels of naive CD4 cells and low T cell proliferative responses to IL-2 were more likely to experience early death than their littermates. Cases of lymphoid malignancies were predominant within this group (87). The ability of aged mice to induce T cell mediated regression of experimental tumors (L5178Y lymphoma and SA1 sarcoma cells) was profoundly impaired, as compared to young animals. This response is induced by preferential destruction of tumor-induced CD4+ suppressor T cells after the administration of anti-CD4 antibodies and vinblastine (88, 89).

In the experimental myeloma model, the generation of specific T helper or suppressor activity can profoundly affect the establishment and progression of inoculated myeloma cells (90). Similarly, passive anti-idiotype treatment prevented the growth of myeloma cells when the tumor mass was small: either early after inoculation or after tumor cytoreduction with cyclophosphamide (91). The development of an active idiotype-specific antibody response by subcutaneous immunization, either prevented the myeloma growth or significantly prolonged the survival of animals after inoculation with myeloma cells (92).

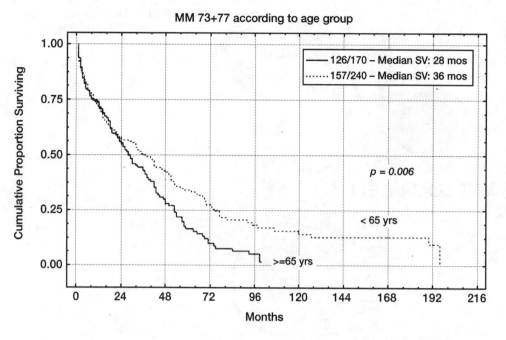

Figure 44.3 Actuarial survival of myeloma patients older and younger than 65 in GATLA's early protocols (MM-73, and MM-77).

Humans with MGUS or early stage myeloma appear to have clear evidence of cellular as well as humoral anti-myeloma immune activity, which is lost in patients with advanced disease. Whether tumor progression is the cause or the consequence of the loss of immune functions is not clear. Multiple myeloma and multiple plasmacytomas have been reported in recipients of solid organ transplants. Malignant cells in one case, contained EBV RNA transcripts, as frequently found in cases of non-Hodgkin's lymphoma seen more frequently in this setting (93, 94). Among 5 patients with a pre-existing MGUS, who were recipients of solid organ transplants (4 kidney, 1 heart), 2 cases evolved into myeloma with a follow up of 3 to 9 years (95).

Peripheral blood lymphocytes from normal controls, in particular a CD3+, CD16+ subset, can inhibit the *in vitro* growth of the RPMI 8226 human myeloma cell line. This process, which requires cell-to-cell contact, was found to be significantly impaired in patients with myeloma (96). T cell clones, mainly CD8+ cells, were found to bind the Fab fragments of the monoclonal protein and proliferated in response to the idiotype in patients with MGUS or stage I myeloma, but decreased or disappeared with advanced disease (97). Idiotype-specific CD4+ T cells were also described in 7 out of 8 patients with stage I myeloma (98). CD4+ are also important for the generation of cytotoxic T cells stimulated with anti-C monoclonal antibodies (99). Untreated myeloma patients have significantly decreased numbers of CD4+ in peripheral blood. Low numbers of CD4+ were associated with advanced stage and short survival, and were found of independent prognostic value (100).

NK cells (CD16+, CD56+) were increased in patients with MGUS, as was a subset of T cells with NK phenotype (CD16+, CD3+) (101). High NK activity and numbers was found in patients with low tumor bur-

den, but NK activity was low in patients with advanced disease. Spontaneous or IL-2 induced NK activity was normal in patients with myeloma, but interferon-stimulated was significantly depressed compared to controls (102).

Anti-idiotype antibody production has high with low tumor burden, but significantly decreases with advanced disease (103). Similarly, B cell lines producing anti-idiotypic antibodies to the monoclonal immunoglobulin were detected in peripheral blood of patients with MGUS and stage I myeloma, but not in patients with untreated advanced disease (97).

Recently, a novel anti-myeloma immune mechanism was described. CD16+ cells, either CD8+ or CD56+, present in untreated myeloma patients secrete a soluble form of the Fc receptor (sCD16). This molecule can bind surface immunoglobulin on the surface of myeloma cells, resulting in suppression of tumor growth, monoclonal protein secretion and eventually tumor cell cytolysis (104).

Aging and Multiple Myeloma: A Hypothesis

The primary role of aging in myeloma may be related to reduced anti-tumor immunity (Figure 44.3). Repeated exposure of a susceptible individual to oncogenic stimuli is necessary, but not sufficient for the development of progressive myeloma. The aging process creates the immunologic permissive conditions for the tumor to develop. In experimental models, the ability of T cell mediated immunity and anti-idiotype antibodies to modulate myeloma growth was clearly demonstrated. The preliminary observations in humans are compatible with this notion. This is perhaps best illustrated in the case of MGUS. MGUS, a monoclonal proliferation easily detectable by routine clinical techniques, will not progress to myeloma in the majority of cases, even after several decades of follow up. MGUS clones have a low tumor mass, very low proliferative compartment and are well differentiated as evidenced by high rates of monoclonal lg synthesis. These patients have preserved or increased NK activity as well as specific T and B cell immune responses to the tumor. Dysregulation of IL-6 expression (and that of other cytokines) may provide further support to halt tumor progression by maintaining myeloma cell differentiation. Indeed we have demonstrated high bone marrow IL-6 production in these individuals.

While in some experimental tumor systems, tumor growth can be inhibited by the age-related decline in immune function (105), progression to active myeloma is associated with the suppression or loss of anti-tumor immune mechanisms, and with the suppression of IL-6 secretion (and possibly other cytokines) in the marrow microenvironment. The role of IL-6 in the development and survival of myeloma tumors could be best exploited in patients with smoldering myeloma at high risk for progression. Similarly, modulation of immune function to enhance or stimulate anti-tumor responses could be most useful at the time of profound tumor cytoreduction, such as after high-dose therapy programs with stem cell transplantation.

Prognostic Factors and Standard Therapy of Older Patients with Multiple Myeloma

Prognostic Factors

Given the heterogeneity of clinical and biological behavior of this disorder, treatment recommendations for patients with multiple myeloma should be based on careful evaluation of disease-related characteristics as well as of patient-related variables. Among the former, the most useful prognostic indicators have been traditionally, measures of tumor burden such as Salmon-Durie clinical stage and serum β-2-microglobulin levels, as well as estimates of the tumor's proliferative compartment (106, 107, 108). Table 44.1 lists some of the clinical and laboratory characteristics associated with

Table 44.1 Clinical and laboratory characteristics associated with poor prognosis in multiple myeloma.

Clinical	Laboratory
Stage III	hypodiploidy
Renal failure elevated serum β-2 microglobulin	increased growth fraction
	Immunophenotype
elevated serum LDH	cytogenetics
elevated serum C-reactive protein	low RNA content
elevated serum IL-6 levels	
elevated serum IL-6R levels	
plasmablastic morphology	

a poor outcome. Numerous "staging" systems have been developed on the basis of these measurements that can discriminate patients with different prognoses (109). A rather simple system, based on the measurements of serum β-2-microglobulin and C-reactive protein alone, can discriminate patients with low risk (median survival 54 months), intermediate risk (median survival 27 months) and high risk (median survival 6 months) (110).

There is no agreement among different investigators as if age *per se* constitutes an independent prognostic factor. The poor prognosis in elderly patients, as reported in some studies, could be due to differences in the intrinsic biological behavior of the disease (such as a higher incidence of primary drug resistance), or to host-related factors such as poorer tolerance to chemotherapy and a higher incidence of deaths due to comorbid conditions.

The median age of myeloma patients in clinical trials reporting treatment results is often <65, suggesting that elderly patients might have been underrepresented in these studies. Age is an important cause for active and passive exclusion of patients from clinical trials, which may significantly impact on outcomes (111).

Since 1973, GATLA (Argentine Group for the Treatment of Acute Leukemia), has conducted four subsequent randomized protocols for patients with newly diagnosed multiple myeloma. A total of 527 patients have been entered in these protocols. The three initial protocols are currently closed to accrual, while protocol MM-89 is still open. The following analysis was carried out in order to compare retrospectively the initial characteristics, response and survival of patients according to their age. For this purpose, a follow-up analysis of a previously published report (112) has been updated as of December 1995.

Three hundred and two patients were below 65 years (range 20–64, median 56 yrs), and 225 above 65 yrs (range 65–90, median 71 yrs). Table 44.2 shows the distribution of these patients according to initial clinical characteristics and age group. Sex, ECOG performance status, renal function, type of "M" protein, Durie-Salmon stage, hemoglobin and albumin level were evenly distributed among the younger and elderly populations.

When rate of objective responses were analyzed (defined as a 50% decrease in initial "M" component), it could be observed that 189 of 302 young patients (63%) achieved a response, compared to 133 of 225 (59%) of patients above 65 yrs (p not significant), suggesting that myeloma in the elderly population is not intrinsically more resistant to standard dose chemotherapy.

Through the analysis of four subsequent randomized protocols, the comparison of patients below and above the age of 65, showed that elderly patients had similar clinical characteristics and response rates as the younger population. Actuarial median survival in the older group was significantly shorter only in our initial two protocols (28 months versus 36 months), primarily related to a higher number of myeloma unrelated deaths

Table 44.2 Distribution of clinical characteristics at diagnosis by age group (GATLA protocols).

		Age < 65 (n = 302) N	%	Age ≥ 65 (n = 225) N	%	p value
Sex	F	144	48	122	54	ns
	M	158	52	103	46	
Performance Status	0–2	267	80	192	85	ns
	> 2	59	20	33	15	
Renal Function	A	267	80	192	86	ns
	B	35	12	32	14	
"M" Protein	G	188	62	134	60	ns
	A	66	22	60	27	
	BJ	40	13	25	11	
	NS	4	1	4	1	
	D	2	1	1		
	M	2	1			
Stage	I	34	11	29	13	ns
	II	76	25	68	30	
	III	192	64	128	57	
Hg (gr/dL)	median	10.0		9.9		ns
Albumin (gr/dL)	median	3.5	3.4			ns

in the older population. Similar results have been reported by the Southeastern Cancer Cooperative Study Group (4).

Standard-Dose Therapy

When considering treatment for myeloma, three groups of patients need to be identified at the time of diagnosis: I) high risk individuals whose survival is limited with standard therapies and therefore could be candidates for innovative treatment protocols, II) patients who are likely to achieve good results with standard therapies, and III) patients who require no initial therapy.

Asymptomatic patients with no demonstrable bone abnormalities on conventional radiographs and small monoclonal protein peaks will remain stable for long periods of time. While they will eventually show evidence of disease progression, the median time to progression and need for therapeutic intervention was 61 months (113). While age was not a factor in predicting disease progression, this issue is particularly relevant to older patients since their life expectancy is already limited and quality of life issues may be more important. These individuals, as well as those with indolent and smoldering myeloma, will benefit from a close follow up withholding therapy until evidence of disease progression.

Since the development of melphalan and prednisone (MP) as an effective regimen for the treatment of multiple myeloma more than 25 years ago, the outcome of patients who require therapy has not changed significantly. The incorporation of multiple alkylating agents, vinca alkaloids and anthracyclines have, in some

studies, improved response rates, but generally without affecting the survival rates. A meta-analysis review of 3814 patients from 18 published randomized trials comparing MP to multidrug combinations revealed no overall differences in survival rates (114). Individual trials showing a benefit for multidrug combinations had low survival rates for the MP arm compared to those reported in other studies. This could be explained on the basis of differences in the proportion of high and low risk patients incorporated in each trial. High risk patients defined as those with Salmon-Durie clinical stage III, severe anemia, hypercalcemia or renal failure fared worse when treated with MP. Therefore, trials including a larger proportion of high risk patients will tend to show a difference in favor of multidrug combinations. It is still unclear, however, if multidrug combinations should be recommended for all patients with high risk myeloma outside their participation in clinical trials.

A single institution review of consecutive trials comparing MP, combination chemotherapy including bolous doxorubicin and VAD (continuous infusion doxorubicin, vincristine and high dose oral dexamethasone) revealed no differences in survival by treatment arm when patients were stratified by tumor mass (115).

In the GATLA studies previously discussed, protocol MM-73 compared the standard combination of MP versus the combination of MP plus methylCCNU and cyclophosphamide; protocol MM-77, MP versus MP plus methylCCNU, cyclophosphamide and vincristine; protocol MM-85, MP versus MP plus alpha-interferon, and protocol MM-89, high-dose methylprednisolone and melphalan, versus the addition of adriamycin to

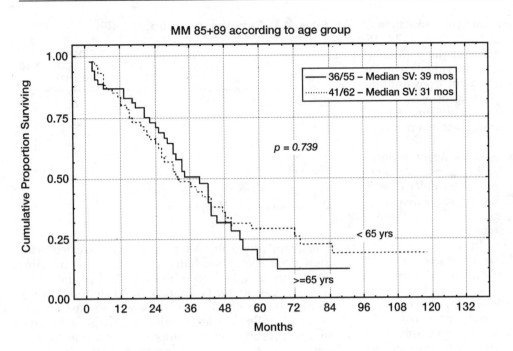

Figure 44.4 Actuarial survival of myeloma patients older and younger than 65 in GATLA's recent protocols (MM-85 and MM-89).

the same regimen. None of the protocols demonstrated any advantage favoring the different combinations versus the standard regimen. Actuarial survival curves show that patients <65 years treated with the initial protocols (MM-73 and 77) had a projected median survival of 36 months, versus 28 months for the elderly group (p = 0.006) (Figure 44.3). When only myeloma-related mortality was compared, no significant differences were observed suggesting that the survival

difference could be attributed to a higher number of non myeloma deaths in the older population. Though, when the two recent protocols are considered (MM-85 and MM-89), no survival difference was observed: median survival of 39 months versus 31 months between younger and older patients respectively (Figure 44.4).

The optimal therapy for the older myeloma patient remains undefined. As mentioned earlier, most clinical

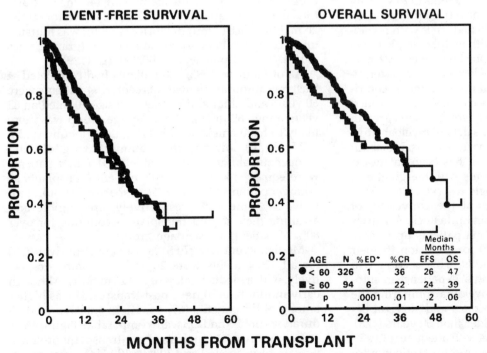

Figure 44.5 Autotransplants for multiple myeloma (N = 420). Event-free and overall survival from transplant according to age. Higher early mortality in the patients >60 years without significant differences in EFS and OS.

trials are biased in favor of the younger population. If we examine population-based trials (116, 117, 118) which may be more representative of the population at large (median age 67–70 years), individuals over the age of 65–70 do not appear to benefit from multiple drug combinations over MP. In fact, at least two of these studies suggested an inferior outcome for patients treated with multiple drug combinations (117, 118).

High dose dexamethasone as single agent in previously untreated patients produced response rates similar to MP and only 15% lower than those of VAD, with identical survival rates (119). It is unclear however, if older patients can tolerate high-dose dexamethasone as well as younger patients, since this regimen is not devoid of significant toxicities. In a study of 32 relapsed or refractory patients, 26 of whom were >60 years, moderate to severe side effects were documented in 55% of the cases (120).

α-interferon added to MP did not improve response rates, duration of response or overall survival of newly diagnosed patients (121). However, some subsets of patients may benefit from α-interferon maintenance after induction with standard chemotherapy regimens (122, 123). While some studies have failed to confirm this data, maintenance therapy with α-interferon significantly prolonged remission duration, and in one of the trials also survival, of patients who have responded to standard chemotherapy.

High Dose Therapy with Autologous Hematopoietic Transplantation in Older Patients with Multiple Myeloma

The late Tim McElwain was the first to demonstrate a dose-response effect for alkylating agents in MM using melphalan 140 mg/m2 without transplant (124). Barlogie *et al.* subsequently initiated trials with myeloablative chemoradiotherapy with melphalan plus total body irradiation with autologous bone marrow transplant, reasoning that most myeloma cells were terminally differentiated and would not be a major contributor to relapse (125). The use of chemotherapy-primed peripheral blood stem cells and hematopoietic growth factors has greatly increased the safety of myeloablative therapy due to shortening of marrow aplasia to about one week, so that this approach has been safely extended to include elderly patients with marginal performance status and physiologic reserve (126–127).

The group of investigators at the University of Arkansas for Medical Sciences in Little Rock, Arkansas have included multiple myeloma patients up to and, on occasion, exceeding age 70 for inclusion in their tandem autotransplant protocols. This section will review the University of Arkansas' experience in autotransplantation for multiple myeloma comparing the prognostic features, remission rates and survival between patients younger and older than 60 years (128).

Since 1990, myeloma patients with adequate physiologic organ reserve were considered for tandem auto-

Table 44.3 Patient characteristics (N = 420).

Parameter	< 60 (N = 326)	≥ 60 (N = 94)	p
	Age		
B2M > 2.5 mg/dL pre Tx-1	40*	63	.0001
Albumin ≤ 3.5 mg/dL pre Tx-1	59	85	.0003
Abnormal Karotype	46	71	.02

*Percent

NO DIFFERENCE: Months of Prior Therapy, Stage, CRP, Drug Resistance, LDH, Ig Isotype.

transplant protocols. All patients were treated with high dose cyclophosphamide 6g/m2 with hematopoietic growth factors, initially GM-CSF, and more recently, G-CSF, for peripheral blood stem cell mobilization (126, 130). Bone marrow was also harvested, predominantly in patients with extensive prior therapy, to procure sufficient hematopoietic stem cells to support future tandem transplantation. Initial treatment consisted of melphalan 200 mg/m2 with autologous transplant with the intention to proceed to a second high dose therapy within 3 to 6 months. Tumor cytoreductive response was evaluated prior to second transplant: those patients who had a sustained partial response (PR), as defined by tumor mass reduction by at least 75% including less than 100 mg/day of Bence Jones proteinuria and a bone marrow plasmacytosis of less than 5%, received a second cycle of melphalan 200 mg/m2. The remaining patients who either did not achieve a PR or relapsed from PR or complete response (CR) by the time of a second transplant, were offered chemoradiotherapy with melphalan 140 mg/m2 and total body irradiation (850–1125 cGy). Interferon-alpha 2b maintenance (3 mu/m2 thrice weekly) was initiated upon complete hematopoietic recovery (granulocytes > 1000/(L and platelets > 100,000/(L) (129).

As of January, 1995, 420 patients had completed at least one autotransplant at this center: 94 patients were 60 years and older and 4 were over age 70 (median 63 years; range 60 to 76). The older age group was more likely to have an elevated beta-2-microglobulin (B2M; > 2.5 mg/L), lower serum albumin (<3.5 g/dL) and cytogenetic abnormalities (Table 44.3). Older patients were equally likely to complete 2 autotransplants as younger patients (55% vs. 62%, respectively) and, similarly, 34% and 21%, respectively, are eligible and awaiting their second transplant accounting for over 80% of patients in each age group.

Median event-free (EFS) and overall survival (OS) for all 420 patients were 26 and 40 months, respectively, with a median follow-up of 16 months. Although early mortality (<30 days post-transplant) was higher among older patients (6% vs. 1%, p = .0001), median durations of EFS and OS were comparable (Figure 44.5).

In a multivariate analysis of pre-transplant prognostic variables, age (60 and LDH >190 U/L were recog-

Table 44.4 Multivariate analysis (n = 420).

Early Death	p value	Complete response	p value
Age ≥ 60	.0009	Sensitive	.0001
LDH > 190	.02	Age < 60	.02

Event free	p value	Survival	p value
Mos ≤ 12	.0003	B2M ≤ 2.5	.0001
B2M ≤ 2.5	.0004	Mos ≤ 12	.03
LDH ≤ 190	.009	LDH ≤ 190	.02
Non IgA	.05	Sensitive	.07

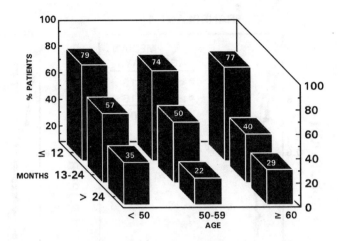

Figure 44.6 Stem cell mobilization following high dose cyclophosphamide. Shown are the percentage of patients with >5 × 10⁶ CD34+ cells/kg according to age and duration of prior therapy. Stem cell reserve is similar among age groups but decreases with more extensive prior therapy.

nized as predictors of early death (Table 44.4). Complete response was associated with chemotherapy-sensitive disease and younger age. Neither EFS nor OS, however, were adversely influenced by advanced age (>60 years). When the multivariate analysis was restricted to the older age groups, elevated LDH was identified as the sole significant feature for EFS and OS.

Stem cell reserve was well preserved in older patients. PBSC mobilization potential (defined as >5 × 10⁶ CD34+ cells per kilogram body weight in the apheresis product following high dose cyclophosphamide plus GM-CSF) was independent of age (Figure 44.6). The predominant feature associated with compromised stem cell reserve was the duration of prior therapy, particularly with alkylating agents (130). The median days to hematologic engraftment post-transplant was comparable in younger and older age groups for granulocyte recovery and minimally delayed for platelet recovery (Table 44.5). In both age groups, patients with more extensive prior therapy (>12 months) exhibited delayed granulocyte and platelet recovery. In addition, whereas granulocyte recovery was independent of the number of CD34+ cells infused, platelet recovery to >50,000/l was dependent upon the quantity of CD34+ cells infused, which is directly related to the duration of prior therapy.

The myeloablative therapy was generally well tolerated by both age groups. Older patients demonstrated

a higher incidence of any Grade III/IV non-hematologic toxicity 85% vs. 50%, p = .001 for transplant-1 and 74% vs. 59%, p = .9 for transplant-2, respectively, for the older vs. younger age groups. Although the extramedullary toxicities were more severe in the older patients, the median days of hospitalization for both groups were virtually identical for the first and second transplant, indicating the rapid reversal of these toxicities (Figure 44.7). Finally, due to the rapid hematologic recovery utilizing primed peripheral blood stem cells with hematopoietic growth factors and the well-tolerated and transient extramedullary toxicities post-transplant, the Arkansas group has piloted a study in 118 myeloma patients to evaluate the feasibility and safety of performing autotransplants completely in the outpatient setting (131). The initial analysis indicated that older patients tolerated outpatient autotransplant equally well as the younger patients: the incidence of hospital admission was 23% and 22%, respectively.

From these data, we conclude: 1) tandem autotrans-

Table 44.5 Median days to hematologic recovery according to age and duration of prior therapy.

Parameter	Median days to			
	Gran > 500 μL		PLt > 50,000/μL	
≤ 12 Mos from diagnosis				
Age ≤ 60	11	⎫ p = .9	12	⎫ p = .01
Age > 60	10	⎭	13	⎭
		p = .0001		p = .0001
> 12 Mos from diagnosis				
Age ≤ 60	12	⎫ p = .4	19	⎫ p = .02
Age > 60	12	⎭	22	⎭

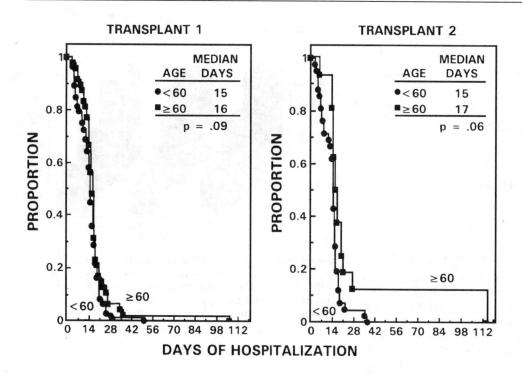

Figure 44.7 Duration of hospitalization following autotransplantation. Kaplan-Meier curves of total days of hospitalization for first and second transplant in patients <60 and >60 years showing similar median days of hospitalization.

plants are feasible and safe in patients over 60 years of age; 2) compared to younger patients, no significant difference in event-free and overall survival was observed, although older patients did exhibit higher transplant-related mortality and lower complete remission rate; 3) stem cell mobilization and post-transplant hematopoietic engraftment are independent of age; 4) high dose therapy was associated with a higher morbidity, yet the duration of hospitalization of older patients and the tolerance of outpatient transplants was similar in both age groups. Since 50% of myeloma patients are over age 65, the promising strategy of myeloablative therapy with autotransplantation should not be withheld from those patients with adequate stem cell reserve and physiologic organ function.

References

1. Riedel DA, Pottern LM. The epidemiology of multiple myeloma. *Hematol/Oncol Clin North Am* 6: 225–247, 1992.
2. Bergsagel D. The incidence and epidemiology of plasma cell neoplasms. *Stem Cells* 13(suppl 2): 1–9, 1995.
3. Kyle RA, Beard CM, O'Fallon WM, Kurland LT. Incidence of multiple myeloma in Olmsted County, Minnesota: 1978 through 1990, with a review of the trend since 1945. *J Clin Oncol* 12: 1577–1583, 1994.
4. Cohen HE, Bartolucci A. Age and the treatment of multiple myeloma. *Am J Med* 79: 316–324, 1985.
5. Barlogie B, Epstein J, Selvanayagam, Alexanian R. Plasma cell myeloma – New biological insights and advances in therapy. *Blood* 73: 865–879, 1989.
6. Greipp PR. Advances in the diagnosis and management of myeloma. *Semin Hematol* 29(suppl 2): 24–45, 1992.
7. Alexanian R, Dimopoulos M. The treatment of multiple myeloma. *N Engl J Med* 330: 484–489, 1994.
8. Potter M. Perspectives on the origins of multiple myeloma and plasmacytomas in mice. *Hematol/Oncol Clin of North Am* 6: 211–223, 1992.
9. Loth TS, Perrotta AL, Lima J, Whiteaker RS, Robinson A. Genetic aspects of familial multiple myeloma. *Military Medicine* 156: 430–433, 1991.
10. Shpilberg O, Modan M, Modan B, Chetrit A, Fuchs Z, Ramot B. Familial aggregation of haematological neoplasms: a controlled study. *Brit J Hematol* 87: 75–80, 1994.
11. Eriksson M, Hallberg B. Familial occurrence of hematologial malignancies and other diseases in multiple myeloma: a case control study. *Cancer Causes & Control* 3: 63–67, 1992.
12. Pottern LM, Gart JJ, Nam JM, Dunston G, Wilson J, Greenberg R, Schoenberg J, Swanson GM, Liff J, Schwartz AG. HLA and multiple myeloma among black and white men: evidence of a genetic association. *Cancer Epidemiology, Biomarkers & Prevention* 1: 177–182, 1992.
13. Golenkov AK, Nazarova IN, Petrochenkov AN, Serova LD, Sibiriakova LG, Starkov AE. The distribution of class-I HLA antigens in patients with multiple myeloma. *Gematologiia i Transfuziologiia* 38: 10–12, 1993.
14. Heineman EF, Olsen JH, Pottern LM, Gomez M, Raffn E, Blair A. Occupatioinal risk factors for multiple myeloma among Danish men. *Cancer Causes & Control* 3: 555–568, 1992.
15. Demers PA, Vaughan TL, Koepsell TD, Lyon JL, Swanson GM, Greenberg RS, Weiss NS. A case-control study of multiple myeloma and occupation. *Am J Industrial Medicine* 23: 629–639, 1993.
16. Svensson B. Human exposure and certain health implications of some toxic and essential compounds in fish. *Diss Abstr Int* 55: 551, 1994.
17. Eriksson M. Rheumatoid arthritis as a risk factor for multiple myeloma: a case control study. *European J Cancer* 29: 259–263, 1993.
18. Bourguet CC, Logue EE. Antigenic stimulation and multiple myeloma. A prospective study. *Cancer* 72: 2148–2154, 1993.
19. Doody MM, Linet MS, Glass AG, Friedman GD, Pottern LM, Boice JD, Fraumeni JF. Leukemia, lymphoma, and multiple myeloma following selected medical conditions. *Cancer Causes & Control* 3: 449–456, 1992.
20. Flipo RM, Deprez X, Fardellone P, Duquesnoy B, Delcambre B. Rheumaotid arthritis and multiple myeloma. Apropos of 22 cases. Results of a multicenter survey. *Revue du Rhumatisme* 60: 269–273, 1993.
21. Dean G. Death from primary brain cancer, lymphatic and haematopoietic cancers in agricultural workers in the Republic of Ireland. *J Epidemiology & Community Health* 48: 364–368, 1994.
22. Brown LM, Burmeister LF, Everett GD, Blair A. Pesticide exposures and multiple myeloma in Iowa men. *Cancer Causes & Control* 4: 253–156, 1993.

23. Preston DL, Kusumi S, Tomonaga M, Izumi S, Ron E, Kuramoto A, Kamada N, Dohy H, Matsuo T, Nonaka H. Cancer Incidence in atomic bomb survivors. Part III. Leukemia, lymphoma and multiple myeloma, 1950–1987. *Radiation Research* **137**: S68–97, 1994.

24. Cinader B, Doria G, Facchini A, Kurashima C, Thorbecke GJ, Weksler ME. Aging and the immune system: workshop #4 of the 8th Iternational Congress of Immunology, Budapest, Hungary. *Aging, Immunology and Infectious Disease* **4**: 47–65, 1993.

25. Fillit H, Meyer L, Bona C. Immunology of aging. In *Texbook of Geriatric Medicine and Gerontology*, edited by JC Brocklehurst, RC Tallis and HM Fillit. New York, New York: Churchill Livingstone, pp. 61–90, 1992.

26. Miller R. Aging and immune function: cellular and biochemical analyses. *Experimental Gerontology* **29**: 21–35, 1994.

27. Ernst DN, Weigle WO, Noonan DJ, McQuitty DN, Hobbs MV. The age associated increase in IFN-gamma synthesis by mouse CD8+ T cells correlates with shifts in the frequencies of cells defined by membrane CD44, CD45RB, 3G11, and MEL-14 expression. *J Immunol* **151**: 575–587, 1993.

28. Thoman ML. Impaired responsiveness of IL-2 receptor expressing T lymphocytes from aged mice. *Cellular Immunology* **135**: 410–417, 1991.

29. Negoro S. The characteristic changes of immune function with aging – analysis of the mechanisms. *Japanese Journal of Thoracic Diseases* **30**: 187–194, 1992.

30. Ferrero E, Manfredi A, Bianchi E, Schinheit A, Sabbadini MG, Rugarli C. Age related changes in interleukin 2 responsiveness of resting and activated human mononuclear cells. *Haematologica* **76**: 14–19, 1991.

31. Song LJ, Nagel LE, Chrest FJ, Collins GD, Adler WH. Comparison of C and CD2 activation pathways in T cells from young and elderly adults. *Aging* **4**: 307–315, 1992.

32. Molteni M, Della Bella S, Mascagni B, Coppola C, De Micheli V, Zulian C, Birindelli S, Vanoli M, Scorza R. Secretion of cytokines upon allogeneic stimulation: effect of aging. *J Biological Regulators & Homeostatic Agents* **8**: 4147, 1994.

33. Schreiber H. Tumor immunology. In *Fundamental Immunology*, edited by WE Paul. New York, New York: Raven Press, pp. 1143–1178, 1993.

34. Posnet DN, Sinha R, Kabak S, Russo C. Clonal populations of T cells in normal elderly humans: the T cell equivalent to "benign monoclonal gammopathy." *J Experimental Medicine* **179**: 609–618, 1994.

35. Dussault I, Miller SC. Decline in natural killer cell-mediated immuosurveillance in aging mice. *Mechanisms of Ageing & Development* **75**: 115–129, 1994.

36. Mariani E, Monaco MC, Sinoppi M, Facchini A. Distribution and Iytic activity of NK cell subsets in the elderly. *Mechanisms of Ageing & Development* **76**: 177–87, 1994.

37. Krishnaraj R, Svanborg A. Preferential accumulation of mature NK cells during human immunosenescence. *J of Cellular Biochemistry* **50**: 386 391, 1992.

38. Kutza J, Murasko DM. Effects of aging on natural killer activity and activation by interleukin-2 and IFN-alpha. *Cellular Immunology* **155**: 195–204, 1994.

39. Riley RL, Kruger MG, Elia J. B cell precursors are decreased in senescent BALB/c mice, but retain normal mitotic activity *in vivo* and *in vitro*. *Clinical Immunology & Immunopathology* **59**: 301–313, 1991.

40. Ben-Yehuda A, Weksler ME. Immune senescence: mechanisms and clinical implications. *Cancer Investigation* **10**: 525–531, 1992.

41. Valderrama R, Eggers AE, Revan S, Moomjy M, Frost M, Pipia P, Di Paola M. Idiotyic controls of the immune response. *J Neuroimmunol* **20**: 269–276, 1988.

42. Garewal H, Durie BGM, Kyle RA, Finley P, Bower B, Serokman R. Serum beta-2 microglobulin in the initial staging and subsequent monitoring of monoclonal plasma cell disorders. *J Clin Oncol* **2**: 51–57, 1984.

43. Rangan SR, Armantis P. Enhanced frequency of spontaneous B cell lines from Epstein-Barr virus (EBV) seropositive donors 80 years and older. *Experimental Gerontology* **26**: 541–547, 1991.

44. Crawford J, Eye MK, Cohen HJ. Evaluation of monoclonal gammopathies in the "well" elderly. *Am J Med* **82**: 39–45, 1987.

45. Blade J, Kyle RA. Monoclonal gammopathies of undetermined significance. In *Myeloma, biology and management*, edited by JS Malpas, DE Bergsagel and RA Kyle. Oxford, England: Oxford Medical Publications, 1995.

46. Kyle RA. Monoclonal gammopathy of undetermined significance. *Blood Reviews* **8**: 135–141, 1994.

47. Blade J, Lopez A, Rozman C, Cervantes F, Salgado C, Aguilar JL, Vives JL, Monserrat E. Malignant transformation and life expectancy in monoclonal gammopathy of undetermined significance. *Brit J Haematol* **81**: 391–394, 1992.

48. Kyle RA. "Benign" monoclonal gammopathy: after 20 to 35 years of follow-up. *Mayo Clinic Proceedings* **68**: 26–36, 1993.

49. Kyle RA, Beard CM, O'Fallon WM, Kurland LT. Incidence of multiple myeloma in Olmsted County, Minnesota: 1978 through 1990, with a review of the treand since 1945. *J Clin Oncol* **12**: 1577–1583, 1994.

50. Aroeira LS, Williams O, Lozano EG, Martinez AC. Age-dependent changes in the response to staphylococcal endotoxin B. *International Immunology* **6**: 1555–1560, 1994.

51. Chen Y, Bradley SF. Aging and eliciting agents: effect on murine peritoneal macrophage monokine bioactivity. *Experimental Gerontology* **28**: 145–159, 1993.

52. McLachlan JA, Serkin CD, Morrey KM, Bakouche O. Anti-tumoral properties of aged human monocytes. *J Immunol* **154**: 832–843, 1995.

53. Candore G, DiLorenzo G, Melluso M, Cigna D, Colucci AT, Modica MA, Caruso C. Gamma-interferon, interleukin-4 and interleukin-6 in vitro production in old subjects. *Autoimmunity* **16**: 275–280, 1993.

54. Riancho JA, Zarrabeitia MT, Amado JA, Olmos JM, Gonazales-Macias J. Age related differences in cytokine production. *Gerontology* **40**: 8–12, 1994.

55. Kishimoto T. The biology of interleukin-6. *Blood* **74**: 1–9, 1989.

56. Weber J. Interleukin-6: multifunctional cytokine. In *Biologic Therapy of Cancer Updates, volume 3*, edited by VT DeVita, S Hellman, SA Rosenberg. JB Lippincott publishers, 1993.

57. Tang B, Matsuda T, Akira S, Nagata N, Ikehara S, Hirano T, Kishimoto T. Age-associated increase in interleukin 6 in MRL/LPR mice. *International Immunology* **3**: 273–278, 1991.

58. Ershler WB, Sun WH, Binkley N, Gravenstein S, Volk MJ, Kamoske G, Klopp RG, Roecker EB, Daynes RA, Weindruch R. Interleukin-6 and aging: blood levels and mononuclear cell production increase with advancing age and *in vitro* production is modifiable by dietary restriction. *Lymphokine & Cytokine Resarch* **12**: 225–230, 1993.

59. Ershler WB. Interleukin-6: a cytokine for gerontologists. *J Am Geriat Soc.* **41**: 176–181, 1993.

60. Sun WH, Binkley N, Bidwell DW, Ershler WB. The influence of recombinant interleukin-6 on blood an immune parameters in middle-aged and old rhesus monkeys. *Lymphokine & Cytokine Research* **12**: 449–455, 1993.

61. Heine JW, Adler WH. The quantitative production of interferon by mitogen stimulated mouse lymphocytes as function of age and its effect on the lymphocytes proliferative response. *J of Immunol* **118**: 1366–1369, 1977.

62. Zhou D, Chrest FJ, Adler WH, Munster AM, Winchurch RA. Increased production of TGF-β and IL-6 by aged spleen cells. *Immunology Letters* **36**: 7–12, 1993.

63. Hilbert DM, Kopf M, Mock BA, Kohler G, Rudikoff S. Interleukin-6 is essential for in-vivo development of B lineage neoplasms. *J Experimental Medicine* **182**: 243–248, 1995.

64. Suematsu S, Matsusaka T, Matsuda T, Ohno S, Miyazaki J, Yamamura K, Hirano T, Kishimoto T. Generation of plasma-cytomas with the chromosomal translocation t(12;15) in interleukin-6 transgenic mice. *Proc Natl Acad Sci USA* **89**: 232–235, 1992.

65. Hitzler JK, Martinez-Valdez H, Bergsagel DB, Minden MD, Messner HA. Role of interleukin-6 in the proliferation of human multiple myeloma cell lines OCI-My 1 to 7 established from patietns with advanced stage of the disease. *Blood* **78**: 1996–2004, 1991.

66. Klein B, Zhang XG, Jourdan M, Content J, Houssiau F, Aarden L, Piechaczyk M, Bataille R. Paracrine rather than autocrine regulation of myeloma-cell growth and differentiation by interleukin-6. *Blood* **73**: 517–526, 1989.

67. Zhang XG, Klein B, Bataille R. Interleukin-6 is a potent myeloma-cell growth factor in patients with aggressive multiple myeloma. *Blood* **74**: 11–13, 1989.

68. Reibnegger G, Krainer M, Herold M, Ludwing H, Wachter H, Huber H. Predictive value of interleukin-6 and neopterin in patients with multiple myeloma. *Cancer Research* **51**: 6250–6253, 1991.

69. Pelliniemi TT, Irjala K, Mattila K, Pulkki K, Rajamaki A, Tienhaara A, Laasko M, Lahtinen R. Immunoreactive inter-leukin-6 and acute phase proteins as prognostic factors in multiple myeloma. *Blood* **85**: 765–771, 1995.

70. Kiss TL, Lipton JH, Bergsagel DE, Meharchand JM, Jamal N, Minden MD, Messner HA. Determination of IL-6, IL-1 and IL-4 in the plasma of patients with multiple myeloma. *Leukemia and Lymphoma* **14**: 335–340, 1994.

71. Ballester O, Corrado C, Moscinski LC, Bruna S, Burgess J. Cli-nical significance of serum interleukin-6 (IL-6) levels in patients with multiple myeloma (MM). *Proceedings ASCO* **11**: 98, 1992.

72. Seymour JF, Talpaz M, Cabanillas F, Wetzler M, Kurzrock R. Serum interleukin 6 levels correlate with prognosis in diffuse large-cell lymphoma. *J Cain Ankle* **13**: 575–582, 1995.

73. Twillie D, Eisenberger MA, Carducci MA, Hseih W, Kim WY, Simons JW. Interleukin-6: a candidate mediator of human prostate cancer morbidity. *Urology* **45**: 542–549, 1995.

74. Lapena P, Prieto A, Garcia-Suarez J, Reyes E, San Miguel J, Jorda J, Alvarez Mon M. Increased production of interleukin-6 by T lymphocytes from patients with multiple myeloma. *Experimental Hematology* **24**: 26–30, 1996.

75. Hata H, Xiao H, Petrucci MT, Woodliff J, Chang R, Epstein J. Interleukin-6 gene expression in multiple myeloma: a charac-teristic of immature tumor cells. *Blood* **81**: 3357–3364, 1993.

76. Caligaris-Cappio F, Bergui L, Gregoretti MG, Gaidano G, Gaboli M, Schena M, Zallone AZ, Marchisio PC. Role of bone marrow stromal cells in the growth of human multiple myeloma. *Blood* **77**: 2688–2693, 1991.

77. Uchiyama H, Barut BA, Mohrbacher AF, Chauhan D, Anderson KC. Adhesion of human myeloma-derived cell lines to bone marrow stromal cells stimulates interleukin-6 secretion. *Blood* **82**: 3712–3720, 1993.

78. Bell JB, Montes A, Gooding R, Riches P, Cunningham D, Millar BC. Comparison of interleukin-6 levels in the bone marrow of multiple myeloma patients with disease severity and clono-genicity in vitro. *Leukemia* **5**: 958–962, 1991.

79. Brown RD, Gorenc B, Gibson J, Joshua D. Interleukin-6 receptor expression and saturation on the bone marrow cells of patients with multiple myeloma. *Leukemia* **7**: 221–225, 1993.

80. Rohrer JW, Vasa K, Lynch RG. Myeloma cell immunoglobulin expression during *in vivo* growth in diffusion chambers: evidence for repetitive cycles of differentiation. *J Immunol* **11**: 861–866, 1977.

81. Moscinski LC, Ballester OF, Hill B, Farmelo MJ. Exogenous IL-6 induces IL-6 secretion in bone marrow supernatants from patients with multiple myeloma. *Proceedings of the 5th International workshop on multiple myeloma*. Le Baule, France, September 10–13, 1995.

82. Ballester OF, Moscinski LC, Lyman GH, Chaney JV, Saba HI, Spiers ASD. Klein C. High levels of interleukin-6 are associated with low tumor burden and low growth fraction in multiple myeloma. *Blood* **83**: 1903–1908, 1994.

83. Ballester OF, Moscinski LC, Farmelo MJ, Mullen MG, Hill B. Clinical significance of interleukin-6 and soluble interleukin-6 receptor expression in the bone marrow of patients with plasma cell disorders *Blood* **86(suppl 1)**: 63a, 1995.

84. Ballester OF, Janssen W, Moscinski L, Saba H, Farmelo M, Hil B. Interleukin-6 levels in the marrow of multiple myeloma patients after intensive chemotherapy with DC-IE. *Blood* **82(suppl 1)**: 559a, 1993.

85. Lichtenstein A, Tu Y, Fady C, Vescio R, Berenson J. Interleukin-6 inhibits apoptosis of malignant plasma cells. *Cellular Immunology* **162**: 248–255, 1995.

86. Dunn PL, North RJ. Effect of advanced age on the ability of mice to cause tumour regression in response to immunotherapy. *Immunology* **74**: 355–359, 1991.

87. Miller R, Turke P, Chrisp C, Ruger J, Luciano A, Peterson J, Chalmers K, Gorgas G, VanCise S. Age-sensitive T cell pheno-types covary in genetically heterogeneous mice and predict early death from lymphoma. *J Gerontol* **49**: 255–262, 1994.

88. Dunn PL, North RJ. Effect of advanced aging on the ability of mice to cause regression of an immunogenic lymphoma in response to immunotherapy based on depletion of suppressor T cells. *Cancer Immunology, Immunotherapy* **33**: 421–423, 1991.

89. Dunn PL, North RJ. Effect of advanced ageing on the ability of mice to cause tumour regression in response to immuno-therapy. *Immunology* **74**: 355–359, 1991.

90. Hoover RG, Kornbluth J. Immunoregulation of murine and human myeloma. *Hematol/Oncol Clin North Am* **6**: 407–424, 1992.

91. Croese JW, Van den Enden MH, Radl J. Immune regulation of 5T2 mouse myeloma. II Immunological treatment of 5T2 MM residual disease. *Neoplasma* **38**: 467–474, 1991.

92. Croese JW, Vissinga CS, Boersma WJ, Radl J. Immune regulation of mouse 5T2 multiple myeloma. I. Immune response to 5T2 MM idiotype. *Neoplasma* **38**: 457–466, 1991.

93. Joseph G, Barker RL, Yuan B, Martin A, Medeiros J, Peiper SC. Post-transplantation plasma cell dyscrasias. *Cancer* **74**: 1959–1964, 1994.

94. Chucrallah AE, Crow MK, Rice LE, Rajagopalan S, Hudnall SD. Multiple myeloma after cardiac transplantation: an unusual form of post-transplant lymphoproliferative disorder. *Human pathology* **25**: 541–545, 1994.

95. Rostaing L, Modesto A, Abbal M, Durand D. Long term follow-up of monoclonal gammopathy of undetermined significance in transplant patients. *Am J Nephrology* **14**: 187–191, 1994.

96. Amano T, Katagiri S, Tominaga N, Oritani K, Tamaki T, Kanayama Y, Yonezawa T, Tanuri S. Growth inhibition of RPMI 8226 human myeloma cells by peripheral blood lympho-cytes. *Acta Haematologica* **87**: 37–44, 1992.

97. Holm G, Bergenbrant S, Lefvert AK, Yi Q, Osterborg A, Mellstedt H. Anti-idiotype immunity as a potential regulator in myeloma and related diseases. *Annals of the New York Academy of Sciences* **636**: 178–183, 1991.

98. Osterborg A, Yi Q, Bergenbrant S, Holm G, Lefvert A, Mellstedt H. Idiotype specific T cells in multiple myeloma stage l: an evaluation by four different functional test. *Brit J Haematol* **89**: 110–116, 1995.

99. Bianchi A, Montacchini L, Barral P, Attisano C, Orsini E, Boccadoro M, Pileri A, Massaia M. C-induced T-cell activation in the bone marrow of myeloma patients: major role of CD4+ cells. *Brit J Haemato* **90**: 625–632, 1995.

100. San Miguel JF, Gonzalez M, Gason A, Moro MJ, Hernandez JM, Ortega F, Jimenez R, Guerras L, Romero M, Casanova F. Lymphoid subsets and prognostic factors in multiple myeloma. Cooperative group for the study of monoclonal gammopathies. *Brit J Haematol* **80**: 305–309, 1992.

101. Famularo G, D'Ambrossio A, Quintieri F, DiGiovanni S, Parzanese 1, Pizuto F, Giacomelli R, Pugliese O, Tonietti G. Natural killer frequency and function in patients with monoclonal gammopathies. *Journal of Clinical & Laboratory Immunology* **37**: 99–109, 1992.

102. Nielsen H, Nielsen HE, Tvede N, Klarlund K, Mansa B, Moesgaard F, Drivsholm A. Immune function in multiple myeloma. Reduced natural killer cell activity and increased levels of soluble interleukin-2 receptors. *APMIS* **99**: 340–346, 1991.

103. Osterborg CA. Clonal B cells and immunoregulatory functions in monoclonal gammopathies: an *in vitro* immunological study. *Diss Abstr Int* **52**: 569, 1991.

104. Hoover RG, Lary C, Page R, Travis P, Owens R, Flick J, Kornbluth J, Barlogie B. Autoregulatory circuits in myeloma. Tumor cell cytotoxicity mediated by soluble C16. *J Clinical Investigation* **95**: 241–247, 1995.

105. Ershler WB. Tumors and aging: the influence of age-associated immune changes upon tumor growth and spread. In *The underlying molecular, cellular and immunological factors in cancer and aging*, edited by SS Yang and HR Warner. New York, NY: Plenum Press, 1993.

106. Greipp PR. Advances in the diagnosis and management of myeloma. *Semin Hematol* **29(suppl 2)**: 24–45, 1992.

107. Kyle RA. Why better prognostic factors for multiple myeloma are needed. *Blood* **83**: 1713–1716, 1994.

108. Greipp PR, Lust JA, O'Fallon WM, Katzmann JA, Witzing TE, Kyle RA. Plasma cell labeling index and beta-2 microglobulin predict survival independent of thymidine kinase and C-reactive protein in multiple myeloma. *Blood* **81**: 3382–3387, 1993.

109. Ong F, Hermans J, Noordijk EM, Kluin-Nelemans JC. ls the Durie and Salmon diagnostic system for plasma cell dyscracias still the best choice. *Ann Hematol* **70**: 19–24, 1995.

110. Bataille R, Boccadoro M, Klein B, Durie B, Pileri A. C-reactive protein and β-2 microglobulin produce a simple and powerful myeloma staging system. *Blood* **80**: 733–737, 1992.

111. Hjorth M, Holmberg E, Rodjer S, Westin J. Impact of active and passive exclusions on the results of a clinical trial in multiple myeloma. The myeloma group of Western Sweden. *Brit J Haematol* **80**: 55–61, 1992.

112. C.Corrado, Santarelli M, Bezares R, Salslasky J, Bruno S, Pavlosky S and Grupo Argentino de Tratamiento de la Leucemia Aguda (GATLA). Effect of age on survival in multiple myeloma. *Proceedings of the IV International Workshop on Multiple Myeloma*. Rochester, Minnesota: 1993.

113. Dimopoulos MA, Moulopoulos A, Smith T, Dekasakke KB, Alexanian R. Risk of disease progression in asymptomatic multiplemyeloma. *Am J Med* **94**: 57–61, 1993.

114. Gregory WM, Richards MA, Malpas JS. Combination chemotherapy versus melphlan and prednisone in the treatment of multiple myeloma: an overview of published trials. *J Clin Oncol* **10**: 334–342, 1992.

115. Alexanian R, Barlogie B, Tucker S. VAD-based regimens as primary treatment for multiple myeloma. *Am J Hematol* **33**: 86–89, 1990.

116. Hjorth M, Hellquist L, Holmberg E, Magnusson B, Rodjer S, Westin J. Initial treatment in multiple myeloma: no advantage of multidrug chemotherapy over melphalan-prednisone. *Brit J Haematol* **74**: 185–190, 1990.

117. Ostenborg A, Ahre A, Bjorkholm M, Bjoreman M, Brenning G, Gahrton G, Gyllenhammer H, Johansson B, Juliusson G, Jarnmark M, Killander A, Kimby E, Lerner R, Nilsson B, Paul C, Simonsson B, Stalfelt AM, Strander H, Smedmyr B, Smednyr E, Uden AM, Wadman B, Wedelin C, Mellstedt H. Alternating combination chemotherapy (VMCPNBAP) is it superior to melphalan/prednisone in the treatment of multiple myeloma patients stage III – a randomized study from MGSC. *Eur J Haematol* **43**: 54–62, 1989.

118. Hannisdal E, Kildahl-Andersen O, Grottum KA, Lamvik J. Prognostic factors in multiple myeloma in a population-based trial. *Eur J Haematol* **45**: 198–202, 1990.

119. Alexanian R, Dimopoulos MA, Delasalle K, Barlogie B. Primary dexamethasone treatment of multiple myeloma. *Blood* **80**: 887–890, 1992.

120. Friedenberg WR, Kyle RA, Knospe WH, Bennett JM, Tsiatis A, Oken MM. High dose dexamethasone for refractory or relapsing multiple myeloma. *Am J Hematol* **36**: 171–175, 1991.

121. Cooper MR, Dear K, McIntyre OR, Ozer H, Ellerton J, Canellos G, Berhardt B, Duggan D, Faragher D, Schiffer C. A randomized clinical trial comparing melphalan/prednisone with or without interferon alpha-2b in newly diagnosed patients with multiple myeloma: a Cancer and Leukemia Group B study. *J Clin Oncol* **11**: 155–160, 1993.

122. Mandelli F, Awisati G, Amadori S, Boccadoro M, Gernone A, Lauto VM, Marmont F, Petruci MT, Tribalto M, Vegna ML, Dammacco F, Pileri A. Maintenanace treatment with recombinant interferon alpha-2b in patients with multiple myeloma responding to conventional induction chemotherapy. *N Engl J Med* **322**: 1430–1434, 1990.

123. Browman GP, Bergsagel D, Sicheri D, O'Reilly S, Wilson KS, Rubin S, Belch A, Shustik C, Barr R, Walker L. Randomized trial of interferon maintenance in multiple myeloma: a study of the National Cancer Institute of Canada Clinical Trials Group. *J Clin Oncol* **13**: 2354–2360, 1995.

124. McElwain TJ, Powles RJ. High-dose intravenous melphalan for plasma-cell leukemia and myeloma. *Lancet* **2**: 822–824, 1983.

125. Jagannath S, Barlogie B, Dicke K, Alexanian R, Zagars G, Cheson B, Lemaistre FC, Smallwood L, Pruitt K, Dixon DO. Autologous bone marrow transplantation in multiple myeloma: Identification of prognostic factors. *Blood* **76**: 1860–1866, 1990.

126. Jagannath S, Vesole D, Glenn L, Crowley J, Barlogie B. Low-risk intensive therapy for multiple myeloma with combined autologous bone marrow and blood stem cell support. *Blood* **80**: 1666–1672, 1992.

127. Vesole D, Barlogie B, Jagannath S, Cheson B, Tricot G, Alexanian R, Crowley J. High-dose therapy for refractory multiple myeloma: Improved prognosis with better supportive care and double transplants. *Blood* **84**: 950–956, 1994.

128. Vesole D, Jagannath S, Tricot G, Miller L, Cheson B, Bracy D, Barlogie B: 400 autotransplants (AT) for multiple myeloma (MM). *Blood* **84:** 535a, 1994 (abstr).

129. Jagannath S, Vesole D, Tricot G, Crowley J, Salmon S, Barlogie B: Hemopoietic stem cell transplants for multiple myeloma. *Oncology* **8**: 89–100, 1994.

130. Tricot G, Jagannath S, Vesole D, Nelson J, Tindle S, Miller L, Cheson B, Crowley J, Barlogie B: Peripheral blood stem cell transplants for multiple myeloma: Identification of favorable variables for rapid engraftment in 225 patients. *Blood* **85**: 588–596, 1995.

131. Jagannath S, Vesole D, Tricot G, Barlogie B: 118 outpatient (OPT) autotransplants in multiple myeloma (MM). *Blood* **84**: 212a, 1994 (abstr).

45.   Lung Cancer

Scott J. Antonia, Lary A. Robinson, John C. Ruckdeschel and Henry Wagner

Introduction

Lung cancer is a disease that frequently occurs in the elderly (1). It is a disease that often presents at an advanced stage and therapy often has only limited benefit with an overall survival of less than 15% (2). Also, therapy that has been shown to have some efficacy in lung cancer is potentially associated with significant toxicity. In some elderly patients with more advanced stages of disease, who have significant co-morbid conditions, careful consideration of the limited benefits and the potential for toxicity must be made. However, elderly patients who are physiologically sound and have early stage disease, benefit greatly from therapy. Even those patients with more advanced stages of disease, as long as they are medically fit, can be treated with the same degree of aggressiveness as younger patients with similar levels of toxicity and can obtain a similar outcome.

Surgical Treatment of Lung Cancer in the Older Patient

The most effective method for controlling lung cancer is widely felt to be complete surgical resection of the primary tumor, which generally provides the best chance of long-term cure (69). In determining which patients are candidates for surgery, the two independent factors that must be considered are the suitability of the host for surgery (operability) and the stage and resectability of the tumor.

Age alone as an isolated factor is not an absolute indicator of operability. Rather, the physiologic condition of the patient is of paramount importance rather than the chronological age. In general, older patients have a significant life expectancy: at age 65 it is 17.5 years, at age 75 it is 11.2 years and at 85 years it is still 6.2 years (4). Clearly, when lung cancer develops in the older patient, the disease, not their age, is the primary threat to their longevity.

Physiologic Changes with Aging

In relation to lung cancer, the most important change that occurs with aging is the gradual decline in pulmonary function (5). Maximal flow rates such as forced expiratory volume at one second (FEV_1), vital capacity (VC) and maximal voluntary ventilation (MVV) all slowly decrease leaving the older patient with less ventilatory reserve and a reduced ability to generate a strong cough to clear secretions. The lungs become less compliant with decreased elastic recoil resulting in an increased residual volume and a decreasing $P(A-a)O_2$, averaging 0.4 mmHg less per year (6). Postoperatively, this decrease in pulmonary reserve and declining PaO_2 results in more potential problems with hypoxemia with advancing age (7). If obesity accompanies advanced age, the propensity for postoperative hypoxemia further increases, particularly when the patient is in the supine position (8). This adverse effect of obesity is probably caused by elevated diaphragms associated with clinically significant atelectasis and a reduced expiratory reserve volume. Since almost all lung cancer patients are current or former smokers, the adverse effects of long-term tobacco use in the older patient can only aggravate the gradual decline in pulmonary function that accompanies aging.

Cardiac complications account for the other major source of morbidity and mortality following lung resection. Significant coronary artery disease and its associated cardiac dysfunction tend to occur more frequently in the lung cancer population. In addition, heart disease increases in frequency with advancing age and is the most frequent cause of death in all people over the age of 65 (9). Therefore, assessment of cardiac risk is extremely important in the preoperative evaluation of the older patient.

Older patients tend to have other complex medical problems such as cerebrovascular or peripheral vascular disease, diabetes mellitus, decreased renal function, and arthritis. Advancing age slows the hepatic metabolism of drugs and therefore the effect of various anesthetic agents including narcotics are frequently prolonged. Often older patients are also taking multiple medications preoperatively which may interfere with the pharmacokinetics of various anesthetic drugs. The immune system and wound healing rates tend to decline with age, as does muscle strength and limb mobility, often resulting in a relatively sedentary lifestyle. Postoperatively, the risk of venous thromboembolism increases with age, especially after the age of 70 years (10) and, in part, is caused by the common, postoperative delay in mobilizing the older patients.

Despite these recognized risk factors for the older patient, the extremely poor prognosis of medically-treated lung cancer in this age group mandates that each patient be evaluated individually for surgery, in a manner similar to younger age groups. Performance status and physiologic operability are far more important determinants of surgical risk than just chronological age.

Determining Operability

Pulmonary Evaluation

Cardiopulmonary complications account for the majority of the mortality and morbidity from lung resections (11). The most immediate postoperative threat is that of respiratory compromise, and for this reason it is critical the patients of all ages undergo a thorough evaluation of their pulmonary function prior to any lung resection.

Bronchospirometry

The first structured study of pulmonary function testing of lung resection candidates was reported in 1955, in which pulmonary tuberculosis patients with a maximal voluntary ventilation (MVV)< 50% of predicted and a forced vital capacity (FVC) < 70% of predicted were found to be at high risk for mortality with surgery (12). Over the intervening years, multiple other investigators have tried to correlate preoperative lung function testing with operative risk. Using split lung function studies, Block and Olsen (13, 14) in 1973 reported their criteria for an elective pneumonectomy that has held up well over the years: FVC > 50% of predicted, MVV > 50% of predicted, FEV_1 > 2 liters, ratio of FEV_1/FVC > 50% of predicted, and a predicted post-resectional FEV_1 > 800 ml.

One of the most recent and comprehensive studies of the predictive value of bronchospirometry in evaluating the lung resection candidate was by J. I. Miller who reviewed a series of 2340 patients undergoing thoracotomy, correlating their preoperative spirometry with postoperative morbidity and mortality (15). The criteria developed, which were considered independent of patient age, are similar to those proposed by prior authors and are shown in Table 45.1. Borderline candidates for any of these resections were then referred for additional testing using split differential radionuclide perfusion lung scanning to calculate residual FEV_1. A calculated postoperative FEV_1 > 800 ml or 40% of predicted was considered borderline although minimally acceptable for the planned resection.

Wernley and associates (16) and later Kearney and coworkers (17) verified the importance of differential

Table 45.1 Bronchospirometric criteria for various lung resections by open thoracotomy.

	Pneumonectomy	Lobectomy	Wedge/Segmental
FEV_1 (liters)	>2.0	>1.0	>0.6
FEV_{25-75} (liters)	>1.6	>0.6	>0.6
MVV (% of predicted)	>55%	>40%	>35%

FEV_1 = Forced expiratory volume in one second.

FEV_{25-75} = Forced expiratory volume between 25% to 75% of vital capacity.

MVV = Maximal voluntary ventilation.

Adapted from: Miller JI. Physiologic evaluation of pulmonary function in the candidate for lung resection.
J Thorac Cardiovasc Surg 1993; **105**: 347–352 (15).

perfusion lung scanning to aid in predicting post pneumonectomy lung function, but also described an easy yet accurate method of predicting residual FEV_1 after lobectomy. They gave all functional lung segments equal weight and counted the number removed (for example, 3 segments are removed during a right upper lobectomy) and divided by the total number of segments in both lungs (10 on the right and 9 on the left = 19 total segments). This equation accurately gave the expected fractional loss of lung function after lobectomy and could be used to calculate residual FEV_1. Adding split differential lung perfusion scanning to this calculation improved the accuracy of predicting residual FEV_1. The surgeon could then reliably determine whether the surgical candidate would retain at least a FEV_1 of 800 ml or 40% of predicted postoperatively following a lobectomy.

Diffusing Capacity of Carbon Monoxide

The diffusing capacity of the lung for carbon monoxide (DL_{co}) is another lung function test that appears to be an accurate predictor of postoperative survival and pulmonary complications that is independent of respiratory mechanics. This test assesses the basic gas exchange function of the lungs as opposed to measuring only the flow rates and lung volumes in the airways with spirometry. Ferguson and colleagues (18) retrospectively reviewed their results of lung resection in 237 patients with attention to various preoperative variables and found that a patient with a preoperative DL_{co} corrected for lung volume and hematocrit ($DL_{co}corr$) of less than 60% of predicted had a postoperative morbidity of 45% and a mortality of 25%. The risks were much lower when the $DL_{co}corr$ was greater than 60% of predicted.

Arterial Blood Gases

Arterial blood gases are commonly measured preoperatively and traditionally have be used as a discriminator of operability. Generally, a P_aO_2 < 60 mmHg (or O_2 saturation < 90%, especially with exercise) and a P_aCO_2 > 45 mmHg have been felt to indicate an unsuitable candidate for pulmonary resection (15,19). However, recent clinical studies have questioned whether these traditional arterial blood gas limits are too stringent. In their prospective study of 331 lung resection patients, Kearney and associates (17) found that a P_aCO_2 > 45 mmHg or an arterial oxygen saturation < 90% with exercise were not predictive of postoperative complications, and in their study only a low predicted postoperative FEV_1, was an indicator of patients at high risk for complications.

Exercise Pulmonary Function Testing

When there is any concern that the lung cancer patient has borderline pulmonary function for surgery based on spirometry or other baseline testing, then exercise pulmonary function testing appears to offer predictive capability that may help answer the question of operability. Using exercise to evaluate physiologic capacity in this setting is based on the theory that it stresses the oxygen delivery system and evaluates whether there is impaired cardiac function or significant pulmonary hypertension. In turn, exercise testing would therefore assess the cardiopulmonary reserve that will be necessary intraoperatively and postoperatively. Many studies have attempted to substantiate this theory and to a large part they have been successful. The first widely reported effort at exercise testing was that of J. Reichel in 1972 when he retrospectively correlated preoperative exercise testing in 75 patients with their tolerance for pneumonectomy and its complications (20). None of the 31 patients who successfully completed the six stages of the exercise test had postoperative complications, but 57% of the remaining patients experienced significant morbidity.

In the more recent studies, the preoperative measurement of the maximal uptake of oxygen at exercise (VO_2 max) has consistently been found in various studies to correlate well with morbidity and mortality with major lung resection (21,22,23,24). Morice and associates (22) reported on a series of 37 high risk candidates for lobectomy who normally would have been denied surgery and found that patients with a VO_2 max > 15 ml/kg/min experienced no mortality and a 25% complication rate. This substantiated earlier studies by Coleman and colleagues (21) who found that the best discriminatory test for postoperative complications was VO_2 max: < 15 ml/kg/min gave a 100% complication rate and 17% mortality; 15–20 ml/kg/min gave a 66% complication rate and 17% mortality; when > 20 ml/kg/min the complication rate was only 10% with no deaths. Generally, it is felt that exercise pulmonary function testing is a useful and predictive adjunct to other cardiopulmonary evaluation in selecting acceptable candidates for pulmonary resection. It is not necessary, however, when routine testing demonstrates more than adequate pulmonary reserve.

In view of studies demonstrating an elevated risk of complications with advanced age (23), Gerson and associates (25) prospectively analyzed a cohort of 177 patients greater than 65 years old who were scheduled to undergo elective noncardiac thoracic surgery or major abdominal surgery. They found that patients unable to exercise using routine supine bicycle ergometry with a goal of pedaling two minutes raising the heart rate above 99 beats/minute was highly predictive of major postoperative cardiopulmonary complications, seen in 42% of these patients with a 7.2% mortality. In the patient group where the exercise test was successfully completed, the complication rate was only 9.3% and the mortality was 0.9%. However despite its proponents (25,26), routine exercise testing has not been accepted as common practice in the preoperative evaluation of lung resection candidates but remains a highly useful tool to evaluate selected high risk patients.

Cardiac Testing

Once a lung cancer patient has been found to be a candidate for pulmonary resection, the other major source of morbidity and mortality, the heart, needs to be assessed. Any intrathoracic procedure, in addition to major upper abdominal or great vessel surgery is felt to be high risk and has a higher incidence of myocardial infarction and congestive heart failure than other general surgical procedures (27). Goldman and associates (27) developed a set of criteria applied to a set of patients with a relatively low prevalence of coronary artery disease, which was later enhanced by a list of clinical factors developed by Eagle and colleagues (28) (angina, diabetes requiring drug therapy, age > 70, Q wave on ECG and history of ectopic activity requiring treatment) who focused on higher risk vascular surgery patients. The criteria developed were predictive of major postoperative cardiac morbidity. Exercise stress testing was subsequently applied to selected patients meeting any of these criteria in an effort to find those patients at high risk for a perioperative event.

Based on these criteria, various cardiac stress tests have been applied including exercise treadmill testing with or without thallium-201 imaging which gives a specificity of approximately 90% and 95% respectively and SPECT (single photon emission computed tomography) imaging (29). When patients are unable to exercise, intravenous dipyridamole-thallium or adenosine-thallium imaging have been advocated and have been found to have good specificity for significant coronary artery disease (29).

The newest cardiac test for preoperative risk evaluation is dobutamine stress echocardiography. Despite the semiquantitative nature of the exam and the potential dependence on operator experience, dobutamine stress echocardiography has been demonstrated in multiple studies to be an extremely reliable test with a 93–100% sensitivity for detecting significant cardiac ischemia and a 100% negative predictive value (patients with a negative dobutamine echocardiogram were 100% free of perioperative cardiac events) (30,31,32, 33,34). Besides its high sensitivity, it has the advantages of being a relatively brief test (approximately 30 minutes) with results available almost immediately upon completion, the patient does not have to walk (an important consideration in the older population), and much lower costs than any of the myocardial radionuclide imaging tests. In addition, the earliest indicator of ischemia is wall motion change which occurs prior to ECG changes. Therefore, the test can be stopped immediately by the cardiologist in attendance, unlike the other stress tests which must progress longer or be completed before ischemia is recognizable. Dobutamine stress echocardiography is an exceedingly safe procedure (35) that is rapidly becoming the screening test of choice for preoperative cardiac risk stratification (30,34), and in our opinion is the procedure of choice for evaluating pulmonary resection candidates.

Based on the criteria previously developed, we currently advocate preoperative cardiological evaluation with dobutamine stress echocardiography for any of the indications listed on Table 45.2. Advanced age by itself is not included in those criteria. If a reversible wall motion abnormality or other cardiac problem is found during this test, the patient should undergo further evaluation which often includes cardiac cath-

Table 45.2 Indications for preoperative cardiac stress testing in the pulmonary resection candidate.

1. Prior cardiac surgery or invasive coronary procedure (coronary angioplasty, altherectomy, stenting or thrombolysis).

2. Prior hospitalization for cardiac problems or myocardial infarction.

3. Cardiac symptoms, including congestive heart failure.

4. Physical finding suggesting cardiac disease, such as a S3 gallop or jugular venous distension.

5. Abnormal resting ECG including significant Q waves and arrythmias.

6. Chest radiograph abnormalities suggesting cardiac disease, such as biventricular enlargement or pulmonary edema.

7. Presence of peripheral vascular disease.

8. Coronary artery calcification seen on chest computed tomography performed during the lung cancer evaluation.

9. Evidence of cardiac ischemia on exercise pulmonary function testing.

Table 45.3 Perioperative measures to decrease surgical risk.

1. Smoking cessation prior to surgery.

2. Use of preoperative inhaled bronchodilators, oral antibiotics, and/or corticosteriods in selected patients.

3. Prophylactic subcutaneous heparin and intermittent pneumatic compression stockings.

4. Antibiotic prophylaxis.

5. Selective administration of digoxin, especially for pneumonectomy patients.

6. Judicious intravenous fluid administration.

7. Continuous epidural analgesia postoperatively.

8. Muscle sparing thoracotomy incisions whenever possible.

eterization to assess the advisability of a cardiac intervention such as coronary artery bypass grafting or angioplasty prior to treating the lung cancer. If the patient is otherwise a pulmonary resection candidate yet the cardiac lesion is deemed mild to moderate and a cardiac intervention is not recommended, this higher risk patient will generally undergo lung surgery but various risk-reduction strategies will be employed (36). Invasive perioperative monitoring and drug therapy using a pulmonary artery catheter, preoperative hydration, preoperative aspirin, use of perioperative coronary vasodilators and/or short-acting beta-adrenergic blocking agents, and employing anesthetic techniques commonly used for open heart surgery may be used, but the benefits of these interventions in this setting have not been well proven.

However whenever the issue of operability in lung cancer arises, the question asked by Berggen and associates (37) must be considered: "What surgical mortality is acceptable in a disease that has a [nearly] 100% mortality rate?" The significant advancements in perioperative care, surgical technique (video-assisted thoracoscopic surgery, postoperative analgesia, lung volume reduction surgery), and understanding and treating cardiopulmonary physiology has led G. I. Olsen to suggest almost all patients with a resectable cancer are operable (38).

Decreasing Perioperative Risk

Once the decision has been made to proceed with a pulmonary resection, a variety of measures have been described to decrease the perioperative risks and they

are listed on Table 45.3. Smoking, a significant risk factor for postoperative pulmonary complications in several studies (25) should be discontinued if at all possible. Current or recent smokers or those with significant improvements in spirometry with bronchodilators are usually placed on a course of inhaled bronchodilators and occasionally a short course of steroids is added with a significant expectation of a short-term improvement in pulmonary function without increasing the operative risk (39). In addition, a course of preoperative oral antibiotics is frequently added to this regimen, especially if the patient has regular sputum production, although there is no definite evidence that this alters the postoperative course.

Ziomek and associates demonstrated a 19% incidence of deep venous thrombosis or pulmonary embolism in prospectively-studied patients undergoing lung resections who did not have any specific prophylactic measures employed (40). We and others recommend routine use of subcutaneous heparin 5000 units subcutaneously every 12 hours starting preoperatively and also the routine use of intermittent pneumatic compression stockings intra- and postoperatively in these high risk thoracotomy patients (10).

Antibiotic prophylaxis in pulmonary surgery has proven to be of benefit in reducing wound infections and possibly empyemas and pneumonia. Cefuroxime given just prior to surgery and continued for 48 hours postoperatively in a prospective trial by Bernard and associates demonstrated that this regimen offered significant protection against deep infections, particularly empyemas, in a large series of lung resection patients (41). Most thoracic surgeons generally employ some type of antibiotic prophylaxis with a cephalosporin in their lung cancer patients.

Cardiac dysrhythmias after major lung resections, especially pneumonectomy, are common. Although generally benign, they may present significant risks in some patients. Krowka and colleagues found a 22% incidence of supraventricular tachydysrhythmias following pneumonectomy in a series of 236 patients which, however, resulted in a 25% mortality (42). The origin of these arrhythmias may be high perioperative catecholamine levels, traumatizing and possible cutting of the autonomic nerves to the heart, or increased right heart pressure. However, the arrhythmias did not appear to be associated with an age over 70 alone (43). Earlier studies in the literature suggest that prophylactic digitalization of all pneumonectomy patients, which we tend to employ, decreases the incidence and complications of postoperative atrial tachyarrhythmias (44).

Perioperative intravenous fluid administration is an important consideration in managing the lung resection patient, especially when a pneumonectomy is performed. Patel and associates reported in a series of 141 pneumonectomy patients that infusion of greater than 3 liters of intravenous fluid over the first 24 hours after surgery was significantly related to increased morbidity and mortality (45). Although an unusual complication, post pneumonectomy pulmonary edema is best prevented by judicious fluid administration (11). In general, we try to limit intravenous fluid administration intraoperatively to less than 1.5 liters on all lung resections, especially pneumonectomies, and we keep all patients cautiously "dry" for the first 48 hours. This strategy tends to prevent hypoxemia and respiratory insufficiency.

In recent years, the muscle-sparing thoracotomy incision has been advocated for major lung resections as a method of reducing postoperative pain that traditionally has been the hallmark of the standard posterolateral thoracotomy incision. In addition, the pain from cutting the major chest muscles often leads to splinting, reduced pulmonary function and an increased incidence of pneumonitis. Hazelrigg and colleagues objectively evaluated the putative positive effects of a muscle-sparing thoracotomy versus the standard posterolateral thoracotomy incision in a prospective randomized blinded study of 50 lung resection patients (46). They found that this alternative muscle-sparing approach resulted in significantly less postoperative pain, decreased narcotic requirements, and maintenance of shoulder girdle strength, when compared to the standard thoracotomy incision. The muscle-sparing thoracotomy incision provides satisfactory exposure for most pulmonary resections but offers the advantages that may result in decreased morbidity, especially in the borderline surgical patient. For these reasons, we advocate the routine use of this less painful incision for almost all thoracotomies, including those in the older patient.

Post-thoracotomy pain management has seen distinct improvements in recent years, particularly with the more frequent use of continuous epidural analgesia. Lubenow and associates in 1994 reported a prospective series of 1324 thoracotomy patients treated postoperatively with continuous epidural anesthesia for 1–3 days (47). They encountered only a small number of minor side effects and 96.4% of patients reported adequate pain control with this method. Good post-thoracotomy pain control results in measurable improvements in FEV_1 (48). If in the immediate postoperative period lung function is improved in most patients, then it may be possible to offer surgery to even more high risk candidates with the expectation that they could now better tolerate lung resection with good pain control. Finally, less perioperative pain resulting from epidural anesthesia results in lower catecholamine levels, and this may lead to a lower incidence of arrhythmias and other myocardial events. Therefore, we advocate the routine use of continuous epidural analgesia in all of our thoracotomy patients because of its proven effectiveness, safety, and the avoidance of intravenous narcotic administration with its propensity for sedation and respiratory depression in the older patient.

Surgery for Early Stage Lung Cancer

Surgical Series in the Older Patient

Resectable Stage I, II and IIIA non-small cell lung cancer that is untreated has a poor outlook in all age groups, with a median survival of 17, 11, and 7–10 months, respectively (49). However, in the elderly lung cancer patient treated without resection, there is only a 7% one year survival (50) since this cancer appears to be progressively more lethal with advancing age (51). Therefore, when considering surgery for resectable lung cancer in the older patient, their mildly elevated operative risk over younger patients must be viewed in the context of the dismal outlook they face without surgery. When the older patient successfully undergoes resection, his prognosis for long-term survival is just as good as the younger patient (52). This fact should encourage an attitude toward curative therapy (surgery) whenever possible in the older patient.

Over the last two decades, the perioperative management of the lung resection patient has greatly improved resulting in decreased morbidity and mortality. These improvements are particularly noticeable in the results of three decades of surgical series of pulmonary resection in older patients (45, 50, 53, 54, 55, 56, 57, 58, 59, 60, 61, 62), as summarized in Table 45.4. It is apparent from these studies that pulmonary surgery including major resections such as lobectomy and pneumonectomy in the older patient population have become decidedly safer over the last two decades, such that now operative mortalities are well within acceptable limits. In almost all studies of long term survival after lung resection for lung cancer, age is not a risk factor and only the stage of the cancer predicts survival (60,61).

Resectability

If age by itself need not be considered a significant consideration in determining operability, then what lung cancers are resectable in the older patient? Staging of the tumor is the critical factor that needs the closest attention and evaluation (26). In the asymptomatic

Table 45.4 Mortality and morbidity of pulmonary resection in the older patient.

Series, Year	No. Patients	Stages	Procedure	Mortality	Morbidity
Hepper, *et al.*, 1960; (53)	21 (>70yrs.)	NA	Lobectomy	8.6%	NA
			Pneumonectomy	29.6%	NA
Bates, 1970; (54)	89 (>70yrs.)	NA	Lobectomy	13.8%	NA
			Pneumonectomy	23.0%	NA
Thompson Evans, *et al.*, 1973; (50)	69 (65–69 yrs.)	NA	All	16.0%	NA
	30 (70–74 yrs.)	NA	All	26.6%	NA
	15 (75–84 yrs.)	NA	All	26.6%	NA
Weiss, 1974; (55)	403 (60–69 yrs.)	NA	All	12.9%	NA
	105 (70–80 yrs.)	NA	All	19.4%	NA
Kirsch, *et al.*, 1976; (56)	75 (70–80 yrs.)	I-III	Lobectomy	14.3%	NA
			Pneumonectomy	16.7%	NA
Harviel, *et al.*, 1978; (57)	22 (>70 yrs.)	NA	All	18.2%	NA
Breyer, *et al.*, 1981; (58)	150 (70–93 yrs.)	NA	Lobectomy	5%	41.2%
			Pneumonectomy	5%	41.2%
Ginsberg, *et al.*, 1983; (59)	920 (60–69 yrs.)	NA	All	4.1%	NA
	416 (70–79 yrs.)	NA	All	7.0%	NA
	37 (>80 yrs.)	NA	All	8.1%	NA
	368 (>70yrs.)	NA	Lobectomy	7.3%	NA
	85 (>70 yrs.)	NA	Pneumonectomy	5.9%	NA
Patel, *et al.*, 1992; (45)	109 (60–69 yrs.)	I-III	Pneumonectomy	10%	NA
	32 (70–79 yrs.)	I-III	Pneumonectomy	13%	NA
Thomas, *et al.*, 1993; (60)	47 (70–79 yrs.)	I-III	All	12.8%	40.4%
Geibitekin, *et al.*, 1993; (61)	145 (70–81 yrs.)	I-II	All	8.9%	19.3%
Osaka, *et al.*, 1994; (62)	33 (80–92 yrs.)	I-IV	All	3.1%	67%

NA = Not Available

patient with a lung mass, the workup should include chest computed tomography (CT) to include the liver and the adrenal glands, routine blood chemistries, and a complete blood count. A bone scan or brain magnetic resonance imaging are not of significant benefit in early stage, asymptomatic patients (63).

However, the concern about potential mediastinal node metastases is real. Once the fundamental genetic changes occur that allow a tumor to permit its malignant daughter cells to migrate and successfully grow in lymph nodes even at a minimal distance away from the primary tumor, the possibility of obtaining a cure with surgery or other treatment modalities decreases significantly. Mediastinoscopy is perhaps the most sensitive method of documenting superior mediastinal node metastases, even better than high resolution chest CT scanning (64). Some authors advocate routine mediastinoscopy (65), but most prefer a selective ap-

proach recommending that this procedure be performed with mediastinal nodes greater than 1.0–1.5 cm diameter, larger central tumors, and adenocarcinoma or large cell carcinoma histology (66,67). If nodes are negative for metastatic tumor on frozen section at mediastinoscopy and the primary tumor appears operable, then the thoracotomy and lung resection should proceed during the same anesthetic.

Stage I

Early lung cancers without lymph node involvement are classified as Stage I. They commonly present as small asymptomatic peripheral masses discovered on a routine chest radiograph performed for another unrelated medical condition. The excellent five year postresection survival of $T_1N_0M_0$ patients is 80% and for $T_2N_0M_0$ patients it is 62% (68). No adjuvant therapy has yet been shown to improve upon these postoperative survival rates in Stage I lung cancer. The expected 5 year survival rate from death from all causes in a cohort of patients without lung cancer matched for age and sex is only 84%. Older patients with Stage I lung cancer should undergo the same physiologic evaluation as younger patients and be offered surgery with equal enthusiasm.

Lobectomy along with a mediastinal lymph node dissection has generally been considered the treatment of choice in Stage I lung cancer (69). Over the years, lesser resections such as segmentectomy or wedge resection have been advocated for small peripheral T_1 tumors, with the rationale that the survival rates are similar to lobectomy. Hoffmann and Ransdell retrospectively reviewed 199 pulmonary resections for lung cancer and found no significant difference in long term survival between wedge resection and lobectomy patients (70). However, this and subsequent studies of limited resection were flawed in that there was a significant selection bias, no consistent intraoperative nodal staging, especially in the mediastinum, and the analyses were retrospective. This issue was finally addressed by the Lung Cancer Study Group in a prospective, randomized series of 247 patients allocated to lobectomy or lesser resections for T_1 tumors (127). The data clearly shows that there is a significantly higher local recurrence rate with limited resections compared to lobectomy for Stage I lung cancer. Therefore, we recommend limited resections only for small peripheral tumors in patients with very limited pulmonary reserve, significant comorbid conditions, or synchronous primary lung cancers.

The advent of video assisted thoracic surgery (VATS) with its reduced morbidity over the open thoracotomy has been shown to allow the safe performance of wedge resections of peripheral lung cancers in high risk patients who might not otherwise qualify for the standard surgical approach (71,72,73).

Nevertheless, the treatment of choice for the best chance of long-term cure in Stage I disease is a lobectomy, and this is our recommendation regardless of patient age. Although a VATS lobectomy is technically possible in highly selected patients, randomized trials fail to show any advantages for this approach in terms of morbidity or mortality over an open muscle-sparing thoracotomy and the VATS lobectomy has potential major drawbacks (74). Therefore, a VATS lobectomy is still considered investigational and is not currently recommended.

Stage II

Stage II lung cancer is a tumor confined to the lung with involvement of the intrapulmonary or hilar lymph nodes (N_1 nodes). This group constitutes only about 10% of all resectable cancers. Usually it is not possible to make a diagnosis of Stage II lung cancer clinically prior to surgery and confirmation awaits the final pathology report or occasionally an intraoperative frozen section. Complete resection is the treatment of choice since all tumor and involved nodes should be removed. This usually requires a lobectomy or pneumonectomy depending upon the location of the primary tumor and the involved nodes.

Survival after complete resection of Stage II lung cancer is lower, as expected, compared to Stage I. In a large recent series of 214 Stage II tumors, Martini and associates found a 39% overall five-year survival (75). This long term survival rate depended upon the number of nodes involved, and was as high as 48% if only one lymph node was positive. Investigational trials are currently in progress addressing the role of adjuvant therapy with Stage II lung cancer (76). For the older age group, patients with Stage II tumors should undergo the same physiological testing and evaluation as for Stage I cancers, bearing in mind that resections less than a lobectomy are inadvisable with Stage II cancers.

Synchronous Primary Lung Cancer

Synchronous primary lung cancers are relatively uncommon, with an incidence 1–7% of all lung cancer patients (77). Frequently, it may be difficult to determine with certainty that two or more lesions are all primary malignancies versus metastases from a single primary, especially if the histologies are similar. Complete pulmonary function testing is important for planning to determine if all lesions may be removed yet leaving adequate pulmonary reserve. Pulmonary tissue should be conserved as much as possible often with wedge or segmental resections when removing multiple lesions, especially when they are bilateral. The mediastinum should be evaluated by mediastinoscopy just prior to thoracotomy, generally during the same anesthetic.

Bilateral primary cancers may be removed by staged bilateral thoracotomies with sequential resection starting with the most advanced or largest lesion. If the lesions are small and peripheral, then a median stemotomy or bilateral submammary ("clamshell") thoracotomy may be possible for complete resection. In patients with synchronous Stage I lung cancers (no nodal spread), one series found a median survival of 27 months after complete surgical resection of all known disease (77). Survival was less when one of the lesions was a higher stage. Whenever feasible, the patient should be given the benefit of the doubt and the second lesion should be considered a second primary rather than a metastasis.

Curative Radiation Therapy for Patients with Early Stage NSCLC

Table 45.5 summarizes the results of the published series describing results of radical radiation therapy for patients with early stage NSCLC. There is considerable variation in the stages of the patients treated (as well as the techniques used for ascertaining stage), and the clinical characteristics of the patients (Table 45.6). It is clear that for selected patients, particularly those with Tl lesions, long term survival can be achieved in a reasonable percentage with non surgical therapy, that inoperablilty and incurability are not synonymous. It is also clear that the survival reported with definitive

Table 45.5 Radiation therapy for patients with clinically resectable NSCLC.

Author	Pts	Stage (clinical)	Dose (Gy)	Median	2-yr. Survival	5-yr. Survival	Local Failure (%)
Morrison, 1963 (128)	28	operable	45/4 wks	n/a	14%	6% 4 yr.	n/a
Smart, 1966 (129)*	40	operable	50–55 (250kv)	~30 mo	~50%	22%	n/a
Coy, 1980 (130)*[1]	141	T1–3Nx	50–57.5 Gy	n/a	31%	11%	45[2]
Cooper, 1985 (131)	72	T1–3N0–1	variable	9 mo	n/a	6%	n/a
Haffty, 1988 (132)	43	T1–2N0–1	54–59	28 mo	60%	21%	39
Noordijk, 1988 (84)	50	T1–2N0	60	25 mo	56%	16%	70
Zhang, 1989 (81)	44	T1–2N0–2 (80% T1–2N0)	55–70	>36 mo	~55%	32%	27% for those w/data
Talton, 1990 (133)	77	T1–3N0	60	17 mo	36%	17%	n/a
Sandler, 1991 (134)	77	T1–2	60	20 mo	30%	~10%	56+
Ono, 1991 (85)	38	T1N0	60–70	~40 mo	68%	42%	-n/a
Dosoretz, 1992,1993	152	T1–3N0–1	50–70	17 mo	40%	10%	70%
(80,135)	44	T1	50–70	not reached	~60%	~60%	30%
	63	T2	50–70	~12 mo	~30%	~10%	80%
	41	T3	50–70	~12 mo	~30%	~10%	86%
Hayakawa, 1992 (82)	17	Stage I	60–80[3]		75%	31%	n/a
	47	Stage II	60–80[3]		44%	22%	n/a
Rosenthal, 1992 (136)	62	T1–2N1	18–65 (median 60)	17.9 mo	33%	12%	60%
Kaskowitz, 1993 (137)	53	T1–2N0	50–70 (median 63)	20.9 mo	43%	6%	55%
Graham, 1995 (119)	103	T1–2N0–1	18–60 (median 60)	16.1 mo	35%	14%	
	35[4]	T1N0–1	18–60 (median 60)	n/a	n/a	29%	

* Includes some patients with small cell carcinoma.

[1] Includes some patients with unresectable proximal T3 lesions.

[2] Data from autopsies of 31 patients (22% of entire series), of whom 14 had loco-regional disease, 17 disseminated disease, and 6 with no evidence of disease.

[3] Dose received by "majority of patients." Some received lower doses and 13 patients showing good response at 70 Gy were boosted to 80 Gy or higher.

[4] Subset of entire series of 103.

Modified with permission from Wagner H. Radiotherapeutic Management of Stage I and Stage II Lung Cancer in Lung *Cancer: Principles and Practice*, edited by Pass HI, Mitchell JB, Johnson DH, and Turrisi AT. Lippincott-Raven Publishers, Philadelphia (1966).

radiotherapy are not as good as those reported for surgery. This reflects both the imbalance of the two groups in stage of disease, in the general selection of patients with less co-morbidity for surgery rather than radiotherapy (the survival figures reported are for overall, not disease-specific survival), but also clearly the poorer local control achieved with radiation therapy than with surgery. For T1 lesions the best local control reported with radiotherapy is 70%, while for these patients local control with lobectomy is 95% and even with wedge resection 85%. Improvements in local control with radiotherapy may be possible in selected patients with dose escalation using conformal therapy (78,79).

Table 45.6 Radiation therapy for patients with clinically resectable NSCLC: clinical characteristics.

Author	Pts.	Stage (clinical)	Median Age	% with KPS <70 or ECOG (2–3)	% with Weight Loss > 5%	Squam Cell (%)	Exclusions
Morrison, 1963 (128)	28	operable	n/a	n/a	n/a	60.7	Included 25% with anaplastic Ca. Excluded patients unable to undergo pneumonectomy.
Smart, 1966 (129)	40	operable	57.7 (average)	n/a	n/a	63.1	Included 25% with SCLC
Coy, M1980 (130)	141	T1–T3 "localized"	60–69	0	n/a	68.1	KPS< 70
Cooper, 1985 (131)	72	T1–T3	66	n/a	n/a	72	N2 nodes on mediastinoscopy
Haffty, 1988 (132)	43	T1,T2	64 (mean)	n/a	n/a	53	any attempt at surgery before or after RT
Noordijk, 1988 (84)	50	T1,T2	74 (mean)	0	n/a	n/a	KPS < 80
Zhang, 1989 (81)	44	T1–2N0–2 (only 2 N2 pts.)	57.1	n/a	n/a	63.6	n/a
Talton, 1990 (133)	77	T1–3N0	n/a	n/a	n/a	84.0	< 60 Gy
Sandler, 1991 (134)	77	T1,T2	70+	18.2	n/a	57.1	prior malignancy
Ono, 1991 (85)	38	T1N0	n/a	n/a	n/a	50	n/a
Dosoretz, 1992 (80)	152	T1–T3	74	<17	n/a	n/a	non-curative intent
Hayakawa, 1992 (82)	17	Stage I-III	70+	39.5	n/a	100	n/a
Rosenthal, 1992 (136)	62	T1–2N1	68	33.8	40.2	64.5	pts. receiving chemo. or altered fractionation
Kaskowitz, 1993 (137)	53	T1–2N0	73	9.4	32.1	60.4	failure to complete RT
Graham, 1995 (119)	103	T1–2N0–1	67	33	13	48	n/a

Modified with permission from Wagner H. Radiotherapeutic Management of Stage I and II Lung Cancer in *Lung Cancer: Principles and Practice*, edited by Pass HI, Mitchell JB, Johnson DH, and Turrisi AT. Lippincott-Raven Publishers, Philadelphia (1966).

Dose, Fractionation, and Volume Considerations

With the exception of patients with T1 lesions, local control has been uniformly poor in these series. This is not terribly surprising, considering that tumor masses greater than 3 cm are difficult to control with doses of 60 Gy or so in any site. There has been a suggestion in several series (80,81,82) that local control is improved with higher radiation doses. This is certainly biologically logical but may in these series be due in part to selection of more favorable (smaller, peripheral) lesions to receive the higher doses. A clear benefit for continuous vs. split-course radiation has not been observed in these series. The heterogeneity of the patient population would make such analyses difficult. It should be remembered, however, that in other curative settings such as head and neck radiotherapy split course treatment has been consistently inferior to continuous and it should probably be avoided in treating lung cancer except for palliation.

The question of appropriate target volume has not been addressed in any prospective trials. Review of the various institutional series, some of which used fields encompassing only the primary tumor and others larger fields which also electively irradiated hilar and mediastinal nodes, suggests that, particularly for patients with peripheral Tl tumors, treatment to small fields is appropriate and elective nodal irradiation can be omitted. A recent series by Krol (83) which updated the earlier series of Noordijk (84) noted that only 4% of patients treated to fields encompassing only the primary tumor volume recurred in regional nodes, compared with 34% failing at the primary site. Treatment to small fields will clearly improve both acute tolerance to treatment, by avoiding irradiation of midline structures such as the esophagus, and also reduce late morbidity of cardiac and lung irradiation.

Complications of Radical Radiation Therapy

Most series have reported good tolerance to radiation therapy in this population, with significant complications in fewer than 10% of patients. The report by Ono (85) is an exception, with 7/38 patients (18%) developing fatal radiation pneumonitis. This complication was seen in 5/12 (42%) of patients whose fields included the primary tumor, hilum, and mediastinum, but only 2 of 26 (8%) of patients whose treatment volume encompassed only the primary tumor. Other series have reported occasional problems with late pulmonary fibrosis, pericarditis, or esophageal stricture, but these have occurred in only about 5% of cases. As with surgery, improvements in radiation therapy technique over the years have led to a reduction in such complications. One review of the toxicity of postoperative radiation therapy following pneumonectomy has noted a reduction in complication rates from 18% to 4% and of lethal complications from 12% to 4% with a shift from treatment planning with orthogonal radiographs and treatment with ^{60}Co beams to CT based treatment planning and treatment on linear accelerators (86). An additional improvement may come with treatment planning which explicitly minimizes not only the volume of lung irradiated but the volume of functioning lung based on regional ventilation-perfusion studies (87).

Summary

The data from these series indicate that radical radiation therapy is an appropriate form of treatment for patients with clinically resectable NSCLC who, by virtue of other medical conditions or personal insistence are not surgical candidates. They do not suggest that radiation therapy should replace surgery in patients who are good operative candidates. In the patient whose physiologic age, concurrent medical problems, or preference make him or her a poorer surgical candidate, the present data lead to the following conclusions and recommendations. Radical radiation therapy, as a single modality, is curative in a worthwhile proportion of patients, with 5-year survivals as high as 40% for patients with clinical Stage I disease, and should be offered as the present standard of care for patients with medically inoperable Stage I-II NSCLC.

While there are no prospective trials which address issues of optimal radiation dose, fractionation, and volume, data would suggest the following guidelines. The primary tumor should receive a dose of at least 65 Gy (as calculated without correction for lung density, with appropriate adjustments made if lung corrections are used) if conventional fractionation of one daily fraction of 1.8–2.0 Gy is used. Good results have been reported with both split-course and continuous fractionation schemes. In either case, undue protraction of treatment time, either by a long planned split or by frequent or long treatment interruptions for bothersome but not life threatening acute toxicities such as esophagitis is likely to decrease local control. The appropriate treatment volume remains undefined. It is reasonable at least for patients with T1N0 lesions to treat the primary tumor volume only without elective nodal irradiation. With current treatment techniques, both local and systemic failure are major causes of treatment failure, and both need to be addressed in order to improve treatment outcomes.

Surgery for Locally Advanced Lung Cancer

Of the locally advanced tumors, direct extension into the chest wall (T_3) in the absence of nodal spread ($T_3N_0M_0$) offers the greatest chance for complete resection and long-term cure. Any tumor cell type may demonstrate this locally aggressive behavior. Following complete resection with microscopically negative margins, patients with T_3N_0 (Stage IIIA) tumors may achieve as much as a 50% 5-year survival (88). With N_1 nodal metastases in the lung or hilum, the survival declines but surgical resection is still indicated. T3 patients with positive mediastinal N_2 nodes treated surgically only rarely survive long-term.

Commonly, the patient will present with complaints of local chest wall pain, although occasionally they will be asymptomatic. Unless there is obvious rib destruction, the plain chest radiograph will not be helpful to assess invasion. Chest computed tomography (CT) frequently suggests invasion only if a soft tissue mass is seen extending into the chest wall. Rib destruction, unless it is extensive, is difficult to judge on chest CT since the ribs pass through each image at an angle and a long length of any one rib is not seen on a single image. The appearance of the tumor in the lung directly abutting the pleural surface does not necessarily mean that there is chest wall invasion, even if some pleuritic pain is present. The preferred surgical approach to handle chest wall invasion is an en bloc resection of ribs and musculature along with the pulmonary resection, striving for macroscopically and microscopically negative margins. A mediastinal lymph node dissection should routinely be included with the surgery. If N_1 nodes appear to be present, surgical resection is still advisable. However, the presence of N_2 nodes suspected clinically or proven by mediastinoscopy, with its dismal outlook when accompanying a

T_3 tumor, may indicate that the patient is best treated in a multimodality neoadjuvant protocol or by non-operative means (88).

Almost all T_4 lesions are unresectable and removing the tumor for palliation is of questionable value and has never demonstrated any survival benefit. Rarely, limited involvement of the atrial wall, phrenic nerve, superior vena cava or esophagus might be amenable to an extended resection, although the mortality is greatly elevated and rarely indicated in the older patient (11).

Superior Sulcus Tumors (Stage IIIA, T_3 N_0 M_0)

Superior sulcus T_3 tumors (Pancoast tumors) are completely resectable for cure in selected patients with an overall 30% 5-year survival (89). Detailed staging is important in these patients and should always include mediastinoscopy. The 30% overall survival is composed of a mix of patients with no nodal involvement (45% 5-year survival) and patients with N_2 involvement with virtually no chance for long-term survival. MRI of the upper chest to determine vascular or vertebral invasion as well as the extent of brachial plexus involvement is often critical. If the tumor is actually T_4 or there is C-8 (or more) nerve root or stellate ganglion involvement, then only an incomplete resection is possible and the prognosis is poor. Commonly, preoperative radiation therapy up to 4500 cGy is given, and more recently it is often combined with a platin-based chemotherapy regimen. These regimens offer the possibility of improved resectability and long term cure, but the results of multimodality trials testing these approaches are still pending (76). For the older patient, these aggressive combination protocols may be too rigorous and perhaps inadvisable. Still, each patient needs to be considered for treatment based on his own physiologic age, personal desires, and expectations.

Stage IIIA with Mediastinal Node Metastases

If normal-sized, ipsilateral (N_2) nodes are found to be positive with microscopic foci of tumor at the time of thoracotomy but the nodes are completely resectable, then a lung resection with mediastinal node sampling or dissection should be performed. This finding places patients in the most favorable category of N_2 node positive lung cancers, with as much as a 30% 5-year survival (65). Unfortunately, probably only 10–20% of the entire Stage IIIA group presents with unsuspected nodal metastases.

The majority of Stage IIIA patients have enlarged (> 1.5 cm diameter) or even bulky N_2 nodes on chest CT scan. Mediastinoscopy should always be performed in this setting to document that these nodes actually contain metastatic tumor, since nodes may be enlarged for many other benign causes, especially if there is an associated recent pneumonitis. Adverse prognostic factors associated with positive mediastinal nodes include extracapsular spread of tumor, multiple levels of involved lymph nodes, and bulky enlarged nodes (90). Of special note is the location of the N_2 nodes, in that involvement of the higher superior mediastinal nodes (nodes found positive at mediastinoscopy) portends a worse prognosis than patients with a negative mediastinoscopy yet who are found to have positive nodes at thoracotomy (91).

Metastases to contralateral mediastinal nodes or any supraclavicular nodes (N_3 nodes) constitutes Stage IIIB lung cancer. Generally, this presentation has precluded long-term survival following surgical resection and positive N_3 nodes usually are a contraindication to surgery.

The Neoadjuvant Approach to Locally Advanced Lung Cancer

Recent attempts at improving the outcome of patients with Stage IIIA lung cancer have been performed which include various combinations of neoadjuvant therapy (chemotherapy and radiation therapy) followed by resection. There have been many phase II trials reporting 3 year survival rates from 20%-40% using this approach (69,92,93,94,95). For example, Martini and collegues (65) gave induction chemotherapy with mitomycin, vindesine or vinblastine, and cisplatin to Stage IIIA patients with bulky mediastinal nodal metastases or multilevel node disease and found a 65% complete resection rate, a 15% treatment-related mortality, and a 28% 3-year survival, which was far better than historic controls (8% 3-year survival).

Two randomized trials have been performed to evaluate the role of neoadjuvant chemotherapy in patients with potentially resectable Stage IIIA disease. Rosell et al. randomized patients to receive 3 cycles of pre-operative chemotherapy followed by resection or resection alone (96). There was a statistically significant improvement in disease-free survival at three years, with no patients who were treated with resection alone surviving at 3 years, but 23% of the resected patients who received pre-operative chemotherapy surviving at 3 years. The reported median age of patients enrolled was 60 with patients as old as 78 included. The authors report that the difference in survival did not depend on age. Roth et al. similarly randomized Stage IIIA patients to receive 3 cycles of pre-operative chemotherapy or immediate resection (97). This group reported an improvement in disease-free survival for the patients who received neoadjuvant chemotherapy. A third of the patients studied were over the age of 60. The specific outcome based on age was not reported.

The question that remains to be answered is whether there is a benefit of neoadjuvant therapy followed by resection beyond the results that can be achieved with a combination of radiation and chemotherapy without resection. Additionally this approach can be associated with considerable toxicity. Therefore the routine application of this approach to elderly patients is not acceptable. The most reasonable approach is to enroll eligible patients in ongoing clinical trials such as the current Intergroup Trial (76) designed to address these issues.

Adjuvant Therapy for Resected NSCCa of the Lung

The use of adjuvant radiation therapy in patients with completely resected disease has not been shown to prolong survival, regardless of stage, but does significantly improve local control in lymph node positive patients (98). The use of adjuvant chemotherapy in patients with completely resected Stage I disease also does not prolong survival (99). The benefit of adjuvant chemotherapy, or combined radiation and chemotherapy in patients with completely resected Stage II and III disease is unknown, and is an area of active investigation. In 1986 the LCSG reported the results of a study where patients with resected Stage II and III adenocarcinoma and large cell carcinoma were randomized to receive adjuvant CAP chemotherapy (cyclophosphamide, doxorubicin and cisplatin) or BCG-levamisole immunotherapy (100). The latter group received therapy which has subsequently been shown to have no effect on survival. An update of this study was reported in 1994 (101). It was found that the group of patients who received CAP chemotherapy had a statistically significant prolonged disease free survival and a trend toward improved overall survival (not statistically significant). In this study approximately one half of the patients were older than 60 years of age. The significance of the outcome did not change when adjustments for age were performed.

Combinations of Radiation and Chemotherapy for Stage III NSCLC

The addition of chemotherapy to radiation therapy for patients with NSCLC might improve survival either through improvement in local control or reduction in distant metastases. Several studies which reported improved survival for patients with Stage III disease by treating with induction chemotherapy followed by radiation found no improvement in local control (102,103). The use of concurrent daily cisplatin during radiation therapy was reported to improve local control and survival in one study, although another study of similar chemotherapeutic regimen but different radiation dose intensity showed no benefit for either endpoint (104,105). The effectiveness of present chemotherapy against NSCLC is modest, and its benefits appear restricted to prognostically favorable patients with excellent performance status and minimal weight loss (106), so its role in the treatment of elderly patients, or patients with significant non-neoplastic medical problems, with medically inoperable Stage I-II NSCLC may be limited. The development of drug analogues with lowered toxicity, such as carboplatin in place of cisplatin, or navelbine in place of vinblastine, as well as more effective anti-emetic agents and the use of hematopoietic growth factors to ameliorate myelosuppression may broaden the applicability of chemotherapy in these marginal patients.

Several recent trials have confirmed survival benefit for combined chemoradiotherapy compared to radiation alone for patients with Stage IIIA and IIIB NSCLC compared to radiation alone (107,108). These have largely been limited to individuals of excellent performance status, ECOG 0-1, and weight loss of <5%. While combined chemoradiation should be the current standard of care for such favorable patients, it should be used with greater caution in patients with poorer prognostic factors.

Chemotherapy for Patients with Metastatic Non-Small Cell Lung Cancer

In recent years it has been demonstrated that chemotherapy has a palliative role as well as providing a survival benefit for patients with metastatic non-small cell lung cancer. In 1988, the results of a National Cancer Institute of Canada Clinical Trials Group study was reported that included patients with Stage IIIB or IV non-small cell lung cancer with the majority of patients having metastatic disease (109). All patients enrolled had an ECOG performance status of 0 or 1. Approximately one half of the patients were between the ages of 60 and 70. Depending on the institution, patients were randomized to receive best supportive care (BSC), CAP, or VP (vindesine, cisplatin). There was a statistically significant prolongation of median survival by 3.9 months for the group of patients who received VP chemotherapy compared to the group of patients who received BSC. This result did not vary with age.

In 1993 Cartei *et al.* reported a study where patients with metastatic non-small cell lung cancer were randomized to receive BSC or chemotherapy with cisplatin, cyclophosphamide, and mitomycin (110). There was a statistically significant prolongation in survival by 5.2 months for the group receiving chemotherapy. Only 8% of the patients enrolled in this study were between 65 and 75 years of age; and their specific outcome was not reported.

In 1994 Le Chevalier *et al.* reported a study where patients were randomized to receive single agent vinorelbine, vinorelbine combined with cisplatin, or cisplatin combined with vindesine (111). The median age of patients was 59 with patients up to 75 years old being eligible. The most active regimen was found to be vinorelbine combined with cisplatin, with a two-month prolongation of median survival compared to the cisplatin/vindesine combination, and a 2.3 month prolongation of survival compared to single agent vinorelbine. The latter was statistically significant, and the significance persisted when adjustments for age were made.

The recently studied combination chemotherapy regimen of paclitaxel and carboplatin is intriguing, with a suggestion of increased efficacy with reduced toxicity in patients with metastatic non-small cell lung cancer. Langer *et al.* reported a phase II study where patients with Stage IIIB with malignant pleural effusion or Stage IV non-small cell lung cancer were treated with paclitaxel and carboplatin (112). The median age of patients enrolled was 62, with patients as old as 84 included. The overall response rate was 62% with a median survival of 13.3 months. By way of historical comparison, the patients in the best supportive care of the Canadian study had a median survival of 4.3 months. The response rate was found not to vary with age. Phase III trials studying this drug combination are ongoing.

Analyses have been reported that suggest that elderly patients with lung cancer who receive systemic

Table 45.7 Palliation of symptoms of NSCLC with external beam irradiation (percent of patients with symptom palliated).

Symptom	Standard RT (24–30 Gy in 6–10 fractions)[1]	17 Gy in 2 Fractions (first trial/second trial)[1]	1 Fraction of 11 Gy [1]
Cough	56	65/48	56
Hemoptysis	86	81/75	72
Chest Pain	80	75/59	72
Anorexia	64	68/45	55
Depression	57	72/na	n/a
Anxiety	66	71/na	n/a
Breathlessness	57	66/41	43

n/a = data not available

[1.] Bleehen NM, Girling DJ, Fayers PM, Aber VR, and Stephens RJ. (1991) Inoperable non-small cell lung cancer (NSCLC): a Medical Research Council randomized trial of palliative radiotherapy with two fractions or ten fractions. Report to the Medical Research Council by its Lung Cancer Working Party. *Br J Cancer*, **63**: 265–270.

Bleehen NM, Bolger JJ, Hasleton PS, Hopwood P, *et al.* (1992). A Medical Research Council (MRC) randomized trial of palliative radiotherapy with two fractions or a single fraction in patients with inoperable non-small -cell-lung cancer and poor performance status. *Br J Cancer* **65**: 934–941.

chemotherapy have at least as good, or a better outcome than younger patients. There is no evidence that elderly patients treated with chemotherapy have a worse outcome. Multivariate analysis of the SWOG data base of metastatic non-small cell lung cancer patients treated with chemotherapy has been reported (113). Also, Hickish *et al.* analyzed the influence of age on outcome in 290 patients who were treated with chemotherapy (114). Elderly patients had no different outcome than younger patients when survival or symptom relief was the outcome measure. Additionally there was a greater likelihood of achieving an objective response to chemotherapy in elderly patients. Many other analyses have been reported which have shown that age is not an independent prognostic factor (115).

Palliative Radiation Therapy for Symptoms of Local and Distant Disease

Most patients with lung cancer have distressing local symptoms either at presentation or at some point in their illness. These may arise from airway obstruction from the primary tumor, compression of mediastinal structures by nodal metastases, or metastatic involvement of distant organs. Radiation therapy is effective in palliating most local symptoms as well as symptoms of common metastatic sites such as bone and brain. For selected patients with a solitary brain metastasis and controlled disease in other sites, resection followed by radiation appears superior to radiation therapy alone. In the US, most radiation oncologists have used doses in the range of 30 Gy/10 fractions for palliative treatment. For many older patients and their families, travel to and from the radiation therapy center represents a substantial difficulty, and hospitalization in order to receive radiation therapy keeps the patient away from home (and is increasingly disapproved of by third-party payers). Randomized trials conducted in the UK indi-

cate that similar efficacy in palliating the common symptoms of lung cancer without greater toxicity is achieved with abbreviated schedules such as 17 Gy/ 2 fractions 1 week apart, or with single fractions of 10 Gy (Table 45.7). Similar trials have shown the effectiveness of single fraction treatment (4–8 Gy) for the palliation of painful bone metastases. On the other hand, treatment of brain metastases with a single fraction has been associated with acute toxicity, probably from cerebral edema, and is not recommended. These patients should be treated with fractionated regimens of 20 Gy in 5 fractions to 30 Gy in 10 fractions.

Endobronchial irradiation with ^{60}Co or ^{192}Ir has been used to palliate symptoms arising from partial airway obstruction including cough, dyspnea, and hemoptysis. The dosimetric advantage of being able to deliver a high radiation dose to the obstructing endobronchial tumor while sparing adjacent normal structures such as lung, spinal cord, and esophagus, has clear appeal, particularly in the patient who has recurred following prior external beam irradiation. While good rates of palliation have been reported, significant complications including fatal hemoptysis are seen in 5–10% of patients. Endobronchial irradiation should be considered one approach along with laser excision, cryotherapy, and stent placement in the management of patients with symptomatic airway obstruction and management individualized. All of these approaches are more suited for patients with partial rather than complete airway obstruction.

Surgery for Patients with Metastatic Non-Small Cell Lung Cancer

Occasionally, patients will present with a resectable lung cancer and no evidence of mediastinal node metastases, but will be found to have a solitary brain metastasis (M_1) that may or may not be producing symptoms. If after a thorough but unsuccessful search for other sites of metastases (including the use of mediastinoscopy) is negative, then it is reasonable to proceed with surgical resection of the brain lesion and soon after resect the lung mass. Using this strategy, cure rates up to 20% at 5 years have been reported, with survival dependent upon the intrathoracic stage of the primary cancer (116). With recent advances in focused radiation therapy, stereotactic radiosurgery with its excellent local control of solitary brain metastases may permit substitution of this modality when the brain lesion is not in an accessible location for surgical excision (117).

Resection of an isolated metastasis to the adrenal gland with curative intent followed by resection of the lung primary has been reported and occasionally results in a long term survival (118). True solitary adrenal or other solid organ metastases from lung cancer are quite rare so that most series have few patients. Any patient who is being considered for this type of sequential resection for M_1 disease should be extensively evaluated for other metastatic foci. However, surgery may be reasonable in an occasional patient, regardless of their age.

Small Cell Lung Cancer

Surgery for Small Cell Lung Cancer

Small cell lung cancer is staged and managed differently than non-small cell lung cancer. Small cell lung cancer is more frequently systemically distributed at diagnosis. Occasionally, a small cell carcinoma will present as a limited small peripheral tumor that clinically may be staged as T_1N_0 or T_2N_0. Various surgical series of resection with adjuvant chemotherapy have yielded five year survivals as high as 85% in Stage I disease, although substantially lower survival rates are seen with nodal spread (119). Surgery alone is generally not considered curative even in Stage I disease and adjuvant chemotherapy is recommended. Radiotherapy should also be added if nodal spread is found at thoracotomy but a complete resection is performed. Older patients should be considered for this approach provided they are physiologic candidates for surgery.

Combined Radiation and Chemotherapy for Small Cell Lung Cancer

More commonly, limited stage disease is not surgically resectable, but there is potential for long term survival by treating patients with concurrent combined modality chemotherapy with radiation therapy. Randomized trials comparing chemotherapy alone to chemotherapy plus thoracic irradiation (T1) have been compiled in two meta-analyses and show a clear benefit for the addition of T1 in improving both local control and survival (120,121). While important questions remain as to the optimum radiation doses, volumes, and timing with regard to chemotherapy, a reasonable present standard is to deliver a dose of 45 Gy in 25 fractions

over five weeks concurrent with chemotherapy consisting of cisplatin and etoposide. The use of BID irradiation may be modestly more effective but was associated in an ECOG/RTOG/SWOG Intergroup trial with a significant (16% to 31%) increase in grade 3 and 4 esophagitis (122). Excellent results have been achieved with radiation given either at the outset of therapy for concurrent with the third and fourth cycles of chemotherapy, but should not be delayed further (123). There is not at this time any clear evidence that late intensification, maintenance chemotherapy, or the use of alternating non-cross-resistant drug regimens is of benefit, and some of the best results have been achieved with short but intensive regimens (122).

Few investigators have looked specifically at the applicability of such regimens to the older patient. In the US/Canadian Intergroup trial mentioned above, the median age of patients was 62 and there were not striking differences in severe toxicity based on age. More detailed analyses of the influence of age on outcome are currently underway. It should be remembered, of course, that patients on this trial were selected by themselves and their physicians as being suitable for aggressive treatment and may not be representative of all patients (in any age group). It would seem at this time reasonable to consider older patients for such aggressive and potentially curative regimens but to pay particular attention to their nutritional status and be willing to provide aggressive supportive care. We routinely place venous access devices in these patients and are aggressive in parenteral fluid and caloric support in patients with substantial treatment associated esophagitis.

Chemotherapy for Extensive Stage Disease

Extensive stage small cell lung cancer is treated with chemotherapy. The combination of cisplatin and etoposide appears to have the most efficacy. There is a relatively high response rate with a prolongation of survival, though very little chance for long term survival. Given these very limited benefits, oral single agent etoposide is a reasonable alternative, particularly for frail, elderly patients. This drug has significant activity and may have less toxicity than combination chemotherapy.

Prophylactic Cranial Irradiation (PCI)

The role of PCI for patients with SCLC remains controversial. Most trials have shown a substantial reduction in CNS relapse rates but at best a modest effect on survival (124). There has been concern about the contribution of PCI to the neurologic deterioration seen in some patients with SCLC, although it is becoming increasingly clear that this is in part a paraneoplastic phenomenon which can be measured prior to PCI (125). When PCI is to be used, current data suggest that only patients with complete or near-complete response of disease outside the CNS be offered PCI, that chemotherapy with agents having known toxicity to the CNS (e.g. Methotrexate, procarbazine, nitrosoureas) be avoided, and that chemotherapy not be administered during or after the administration of PCI. Radiation doses for PCI should probably be in the range of 25 to 30 Gy with a daily fraction size of 2 to 3 Gy. Animal models using old rats are being developed which should be of help in evaluating the toxicity of PCI in the older human, which is probably not well predicted from data on pediatric or adolescent brain irradiation (126).

References

1. Zagonel V, Tirelli U, Serraino D, LoRe G, Merola M, Mascorin M, Trovo M, Carbone A, Monfardini S. The aged patient with lung cancer. *Drugs and Aging* 1994; **4**: 34–46.

2. Beckett WS. Epidemiology and etiology of lung cancer. *Clin Chest Med* 1993, **14**: 1–15.

3. Martini N, Kris MG, Flehinger BJ, *et al*. Preoperative chemotherapy for stage IIIa (N$_2$) lung cancer: The Sloan-Kettering experience with 136 patients. *Ann Thorac Surg* 1993; **55**: 1365–1374.

4. U.S. Department of Commerce. Statistical Abstract of the United States, 115th ed. September, 86, 1995.

5. Reilly JJ, Mentzer SJ, Sugarbaker DJ. Preoperative assessment of patients undergoing pulmonary resection. *Chest* 1993; **103**: 342S–345S.

6. Sorbini CA, Grassi V, Solinas E, Muiesan G. Arterial oxygen tension in relation to age in healthy subjects. *Respiration* 1968; **25**: 3–13.

7. Kitamura H, Sawa T, Ikezono E. Postoperative hypoxemia: The contribution of age to the maldistribution of ventilation. *Anesthesiology* 1972; **36**: 244–252.

8. Vaughn RW, Engelhardt RC, Wise L. Postoperative hypoxemia in obese patients. *Ann Surg* 1974; **180**: 877–882.

9. U.S. Department of Commerce. Statistical Abstract of the United States, 115th ed. September, 94, 1995.

10. Clagett GP. Prevention of postoperative venous thromboembolism: An update. *Amer J Surg* 1994; **168**: 515–522.

11. Shields TW. General features and complications of pulmonary resections. In *General Thoracic Surgery*, 4th ed., edited by TW Shields. Baltimore: Williams & Wilkins, 391–414, 1994.

12. Gaensler EA, Cugell DW, Lindgren I, *et al*. The role of pulmonary insufficiency in mortality and invalidism following surgery for pulmonary tuberculosis. *J Thorac Cardiovasc Surg* 1955; **29**: 163–187.

13. Olsen NO, Block AJ. Pulmonary function testing in evaluation for pneumonectomy. *Hosp Pract* 1973; **9**: 137–144.

14. Olsen GN, Block AJ, Tobias JA. Prediction of postpneumonectomy pulmonary function using quantitative macroaggregate lung scanning. *Chest* 1994; **66**: 13–16.

15. Miller JI. Physiologic evaluation of pulmonary function in the candidate for lung resection. *J Thorac Cardiovasc Surg* 1993; **105**: 347–352.

16. Wernly JA, DeMeester TR, Kirchner PT, *et al*. Clinical value of quantitative ventilation-perfusion scans in the surgical management of bronchogenic carcinoma. *J Thorac Cardiovasc Surg* 1980; **80**: 535–543.

17. Kearney DJ, Lee TH, Reilly JJ, *et al*. Assessment of operative risk in patients undergoing lung resection: Importance of predicted pulmonary function. *Chest* 1994; **105**: 753–759.

18. Ferguson MK, Little L, Rizzo L, *et al*. Diffusing capacity predicts morbidity and mortality after pulmonary resection. *J Thorac Cardiovasc Surg* 1988; **96**: 894–900.

19. American College of Physicians. Preoperative pulmonary function testing. *Ann Intern Med* 1990; **112**: 793–794.

20. Reichel J. Assessment of operative risk of pneumonectomy. *Chest* 1972; **62**: 570–576.

21. Coleman NC, Schraufrasel DE, Rivington RN, *et al*. Exercise testing in evaluation of patients for lung resection. *Am Rev Resp Dis* 1982; **125**: 604–606.

22. Morice RC, Peters EJ, Ryan MB, *et al*. Exercise testing in the evaluation of patients at high risk for complications from lung resection. *Chest* 1992; **101**: 356–361.

23. Dales RE, Dionne G, Leech JA, Lunau M, Schweitzer I. Preoperative prediction of pulmonary complications following thoracic surgery. *Chest* 1991; **104**: 155–159.

24. Walsh GL, Morice RC, Putman JB, *et al*. Resection of lung cancer is justified in high-risk patients selected by exercise oxygen consumption. *Ann Thorac Surg* 1994; **58**: 704–711.

25. Gerson MC, Hurst JM, Hertzberg VS, *et al*. Prediction of cardiac and pulmonary complications related to elective abdominal and noncardiac thoracic surgery in geriatric patients. *Amer J Med* 1990; **88**: 101–107.

26. Miller JD, Gorenstein LA, Patterson GA. Staging: The key to rational management of lung cancer. *Ann Thoracic Surg* 1992; **53**: 170–8.

27. Goldman L, Caldera DL, Nussbaum SR, *et al*. Multifactorial index of cardiac risk in non-cardiac surgical procedures. *N Engl J Med* 1977; **297**: 845–50.

28. Eagle KA, Boucher CA. Cardiac risk of noncardiac surgery. *N Engl J Med* 1989; **321**: 1330–1335.

29. Alazraki N, Vansant J, Taylor A, *et al*. Myocardial perfusion imaging. *Emory J Med* 1991; **3**: 181–188.

30. Takase B, Younis LT, Byers SL, *et al*. Comparative prognostic value of clinical risk indices, resting two dimensional echocardiography, and dipyridamole stress thallium-201 myocardial imaging for perioperative cardiac events in major nonvascular surgery patients. *Am Heart J* 1993; **126**: 1099–1106.

31. Mazeika PK, Nadazadin A, Oakley CM. Dobutamine stress echocardiography for detection and assessment of coronary artery disease. *J Am Coll Cardiol* 1992; **19**: 1203–1209.

32. Poldermans D, Fioretti PM, Forster T, *et al*. Dobutamine stress echocardiography for assessment of perioperative cardiac risk in patients undergoing major vascular surgery. *Circ* 1993; **87**: 1506–1512.

33. Eichelberger JP, Schwarz KQ, Black ER, Green RM, Ouriel K. Predictive value of dobutamine echocardiography just before noncardiac vascular surgery. *Am J Cardiol* 1993; **72**: 602–607.

34. Poldermans D, Mariaosaria A, Fioretti PM, *et al*. Improved cardiac risk stratification in major vascular surgery with dobutamine-atropine stress echocardiography. *J Amer Coll Cardiol* 1995; **26**: 648–653.

35. Tanimoto M, Pai RG, Jintapakorn W, Shah PM. Dobutamine stress echocardiography for the diagnosis and management of coronary artery disease. *Clin Cardiol* 1995; **18**: 252–260.

36. Mangano DT. Perioperative cardiac morbidity. *Anesthesiology* 1990; **72**: 153–184.

37. Berggen H, Ekroth R, Malmberg R, Naucler J, William-Olsson G. Hospital mortality and long term survival in relation to preoperative function in elderly patients with bronchogenic . carcinoma. *Ann Thorac Surg* 1984; **38**: 633–636.

38. Olsen GN. Lung cancer resection: Who's inoperable. *Chest* 1995; **108**: 298–299.

39. Oh SH. Surgery in cortico-steroid dependent asthmatics. *J Allergy Clin Immunol* 1974; **53**: 345–349.

40. Ziomek S, Read RC, Tobler HG, *et al*. Thromboembolism in patients undergoing thoracotomy. *Ann Thorac Surg* 1993; **56**: 223–227.

41. Bernard A, Pillet M, Goudet P, Viard H. Antibiotic prophylaxis in pulmonary surgery. *J Thorac Cardiovasc Surg* 1994; **107**: 896–900.

42. Krowka MJ, Pairolero PC, Trastek VF, Payne WS, Bernatz PE. Cardiac dysrhythmia following pneumonectomy. *Chest* 1987; **91**: 490–495.

43. Amar D. Increased right heart pressure linked to arrhythmias after thoracic surgery. *Adv Cardiovasc Surg Anesthesiol* 1995; **2**: 13–15.

44. Shields TW, Ujiki GT. Digitalization for prevention of arrhythmias following pulmonary surgery. *Surg Gynecol Obstet* 1968; **126**: 743–746.

45. Patel RL, Townsend ER, Fountain SW. Elective pneumonectomy: Factors associated with morbidity and operative mortality. *Ann Thorac Surg* 1992; **54**: 84–88.

46. Hazelrigg SR, Landreneau RJ, Boley TM, *et al*. The effect of muscle-sparing versus standard posterolateral thoracotomy on pulmonary function, muscle strength, and postoperative pain. *J Thorac Cardiovasc Surg* 1991; **101**: 394–401.

47. Lubenow TR, Faber LP, McCarthy RJ, *et al.* Postthoracotomy pain management using continuous epidural analgesia in 1324 patients. *Ann Thorac Surg* 1994; **58**: 924–930.

48. Berrisford RG, Sabenathan SS, Mearns AJ, *et al.* Pulmonary complications of lung resection: The effect of continuous extrapleural intercostal nerve block. *Eur J Cardiothorac Surg* 1990; **4**: 407–411.

49. Vrdoljak E, Mise K, Sapunar D, Rozga A, Marusic M. Survival analysis of untreated patients with non-small cell lung cancer. *Chest* 1994; **106**: 1797–1800.

50. Thompson-Evans, EW. Resection of bronchial carcinoma in the elderly. *Thorax* 1973; **28**: 86–88.

51. Yellin A, Benfield JR. Surgery for bronchogenic carcinoma in the elderly. *Am Rev Respir Dis* 1985; **131**: 197.

52. Foucher P, Coudert B, Arveux P, *et al.* Age and prognosis of non-small cell lung cancer: Usefullness of a relative survival model. *Eur J Cancer* 1993; **29A**: 1809–1813.

53. Hepper NGG, Bernatz PE. Thoracic surgery in the aged. *Chest* 1960; **37**: 298–303.

54. Bates M. Results of surgery for bronchial carcinoma — Patients aged 70 and older. *Thorax* 1970; **25**: 77–78.

55. Weiss W. Operative mortality and five year survival rates in patients with bronchogenic carcinoma. *Amer J Surg* 1974; **128**: 799–804.

56. Kirsh MM, Rotman H, Bove E, *et al.* Major pulmonary resection for bronchogenic carcinoma in the elderly. *Ann Thorac Surg* 1976; **22**: 369–373.

57. Harviel JD, McNamara JJ, Straehley CJ. Surgical treatment of lung cancer in patients over the age of 70. *J Thorac Cardiovasc Surg* 1978; **75**: 802–805.

58. Breyer RH, Zippe C, Pharr WF, *et al.* Thoracotomy in patients over seventy years. *J Thorac Cardiovasc Surg* 1981; **81**: 187–93.

59. Ginsberg RJ, Hill LD, Eagan RT, *et al.* Modern thirty day operative mortality for surgical resection in lung cancer. *J Thorac Cardiovasc Surg* 1983; **86**: 654–658.

60. Thomas P, Sielezneff I, Ragni J, Giudicelli R, Fuenties P. Is lung cancer resection justified in patients over 70 years? *Eur J Cardio-Thorac Surg* 1993; **7**: 246–251.

61. Gebitekin C, Gupta NK, Martin PG, Saunders NR, Walker DR. Long-term results in the elderly following pulmonary resection for non-small cell lung carcinoma. *Eur J Cardio-Thorac Surg* 1993; **7**: 653–656.

62. Osaki T, Shirakusa T, Kodate M, *et al.* Surgical treatment of lung cancer in the octogenarian. *Ann Thorac Surg* 1994; **57**: 188–193.

63. Hatter J, Kohman LJ, Mosca RS, *et al.* Preoperative evaluation of stage I and stage II non-small cell lung cancer. *Ann Thorac Surg* 1994; **58**: 1758–1741.

64. Patterson GA, Ginsberg RJ, Poon PY, *et al.* A prospective evaluation of magnetic resonance imaging, computed tomography, and mediastinoscopy in the preoperative assessment of mediastinal node status in bronchogenic carcinoma. *J Thorac Cardiovasc Surg* 1987; **94**: 679–684.

65. Martini N, Kris MG, Flehingen BJ, *et al.* Pre-operative chemotherapy for stage IIIa (N₂) lung cancer: The Sloan-Kettering experience with 136 patients. *Ann Thorac Surg* 1993; **55**: 1365–74.

66. Thermann M, Bluemm R, Schroeder U, Wassmuth E, Dohmann R. Efficacy and benefit of mediastinal computed tomography as a selection method for mediastinoscopy. *Ann Thorac Surg* 1989; **48**: 565–567.

67. Sugarbaker DJ, Strauss GM. Advances in surgical staging and therapy of non-small cell lung cancer. *Sem Oncol* 1993; **20**: 163–172.

68. Williams DE, Pairolero PC, Davis CS, *et al.* Survival of patients surgically treated for Stage 1 lung cancer. *J Thorac Cardiovasc Surg* 1981; **82**: 70–76.

69. Martini N. Operable lung cancer. *CA* 1993; **43**: 201–215.

70. Hoffman TH, Ransdell HT. Comparison of lobectomy and wedge resection for carcinoma of the lung. *J Thorac Cardiovasc Surg* 1980; **79**: 211–217.

71. Hazelrigg SR, Nunchuck SK, LoCicero J. Video assisted thoracic surgery study group data. *Ann Thorac Surg* 1993; **56**: 1039–1044.

72. Landreneau RJ, Hazelrigg SR, Mack MJ, *et al.* Postoperative pain-related morbidity: Video-assisted thoracic surgery versus thoracotomy. *Ann Thorac Surg* 1993; **56**: 1285–1289.

73. Shennib HAF, Landreneau R, Mulder DS, Mack M. Video-assisted thoracoscopic wedge resection of Tl lung cancer in high-risk patients. *Ann Surg* 1993; **218**: 555–560.

74. Kirby TJ, Mack MJ, Landreneau RJ, Rice TW. Lobectomy–Video-assisted thoracic surgery versus muscle-sparing thoracotomy. *J Thorac Cardiovasc Surg* 1995; **109**: 997–1002.

75. Martini N, Burt ME, Bains MS, *et al.* Survival after resection of Stage II non-small cell lung cancer. *Ann Thorac Surg* 1992; **54**: 460–465.

76. Rusch VW, Feins RH, Thoracic Intergroup. Summary of current cooperative group clinical trials in thoracic malignancies. *Ann Thorac Surg* 1994; **57**: 102–106.

77. Ferguson MK, DeMeester TR, DesLauriers J, *et al.* Diagnosis and management of synchronous lung cancers. *J Thorac Cardiovasc Surg* 1985; **89**: 378–385.

78. Hazuka MB, Turrisi AT, Lutz ST, *et al.* Results of high-dose thoracic irradiation incorporating beam's eye view display in non-small cell lung cancer: a retrospective multivariate analysis. *Int J Radiation Oncology Biol Phys* 1993; **27**: 273–284.

79. Hazuka MB, Turrisi AT, Martel MK, *et al.* Dose escalation in non-small cell lung cancer (NSCLC) using conformal three-dimensional radiation treatment planning (3DRTP): Preliminary results of a phase I study. *Prac Am Soc Clin Oncol* 1994; **13**: 337.

80. Dosoretz D, Galmarini D, Rubenstein J, *et al.* Local control in medically inoperable lung cancer: an analysis of its importance in outcome and factors determining the probability of tumor eradication. *International Journal of Radiation Oncology Biol Phys* 1993; **27**: 507–516.

81. Zhang H, Yin W, Yang Z. Curative Radiotherapy of Early Operable Non-Small-Cell Lung Cancer. *Cancer* 1989; **14**: 89–94.

82. Hayakawa K, Mituhashi N, Nakajima N, *et al.* Radiation therapy for Stage I-III epidermoid carcinoma of the lung. *Lung Cancer* 1992; **8**: 213–224.

83. Krol ADG, Aussems P, Noordijk EM, *et al.* Local irradiation alone for peripheral Stage I lung cancer: could we omit the elective nodal irradiation? *Int J Radiation Oncology Biol Phys* 1996; **34**: 297–302.

84. Noordijk E, Poest C, Hermans J, *et al.* Radiotherapy as an alternative to surgery in elderly patients with resectable lung cancer. *Radiother Oncol* 1988; **13**: 83–89.

85. Ono R, Egawa S, Suemasu K, *et al.* Radiotherapy in inoperable Stage I lung cancer. Japanese *Journal of Clinical Oncology* 1991; **21**: 125–128.

86. Philips P, Rocmans P, Vanderhoeft P, *et al.* Postoperative radiotherapy after pneumonectomy: Impact of modern treatment facilities. *International Journal of Radiation Oncology Biol Phys* 1993; **27**: 525–529.

87. Marks LB, Spencer DP, Sherouse GW, *et al.* The role of three dimensional functional lung imaging in radiation treatment planning: the functional dose-volume histogram. *Int J Radiation Oncology Biol Phys* 1995; 33: 65–75.

88. Piehler JM, Painder OPC, Weiland LH, *et al.* Bronchogenic carcinoma with chest wall invasion: Factors affecting survival following "en bloc" resection. *Ann Thor Surg* 1982; **34**: 684–691.

89. Hilaris DS, Martini N, Wong GW, *et al.* Treatment of superior sulcus tumors (Pancoast tumors). *Surg Clin N Am* 1987; **67**: 965–977.

90. Rusch VW. Surgery for stage III non-small cell lung cancer. *Cancer Control* 1994; **1**: 455–466.

91. Pearson FG, DeLarue NC, Ilves R, Todd TRJ, Cooper JD. Significance of positive superior mediastinal nodes identified at mediastinoscopy in patients with resectable cancer of the lung. *J Thorac Cardiovasc Surg* 1982; **83**: 1–11.

92. Burkes RL, Ginsberg RJ, Shepherd FA, Blackstein ME, Goldberg ME, Waters PF, Patterson GA, Todd T, Pearson F, Cooper JD, Jones D, Lockwood G. Induction chemotherapy with mitomycin, vindesine, and cisplatin for Stage III unresectable non-small-cell lung cancer: Results of the Toronto Phase II trial. *J Clin Onco* 1992; **10**: 580–586.

93. Strauss GM, Herndon JE, Sherman DD, Mathisen DJ, Carey RW, Choi NC, Rege VB, Modeas C, Green MR. Neoadjuvant chemotherapy and radiotherapy followed by surgery in Stage IIIA non-small-cell carcinoma of the lung: report of a cancer and leukemia group B Phase II study. *J Clin Oncology* 1992; **10**: 1237–1244.

94. Skarin A, Jochelson M, Sheldon I, Malcolm A, Oliynyk P, Overholt R, Hunt M, Frei E. Neoadjuvant chemotherapy in marginally resectable stage III Mo Non-small cell lung cancer: Long-term follow-up in 41 patients. *J of Surgical Oncology* 1989; **40**: 266–274.

95. Bonomi P, Faber LP. Neoadjuvant chmeoradiation therapy in non-small cell lung cancer: the Rush University experience. *Lung Cancer* 1993; **9**: 383–390.

96. Rosell R, Gomez-Codina J, Camps C, Maestre J, Padille J, Canto A, Mate J, Li S, Roig J, Olazabal A, Canela M, Ariza A, Skacel Z, Morera-Prat J, Abad A. A randomized trial comparing preoperative chemotherapy plus surgery with surgery alone in patients with non-small-cell lung cancer. *N England J Med* 1994; **330**: 153–158.

97. Roth JA, Fossella F, Komaki R, Ryan M, Putnam JB, Lee JS, Dhingra H, DeCaro L, Chasen M, McGavran M, Atkinson EN, Hong WK. A randomized trial comparing perioperative chemotherapy and surgery with surgery alone in resectable Stage IIIA non-small-cell lung cancer. *J Natl Cancer Inst* 1994; **86**: 673–680.

98. The Lung Cancer Study Group. Effects of post operative mediastinal radiation on completely resected Stage II and Stage III epidermoid cancer. *New England J of Medicine* 1986, **315**: 1377–1381.

99. Feld R, Rubinstein L, Thomas PA and The Lung Cancer Study Group. Adjuvant chemotherapy with cyclophosphamide, doxorubicin, and cisplatin in patients with completely resected Stage I non small-cell lung cancer. *J Natl Cancer Inst* 1993; **85**: 299–306.

100. Holmes EC, Gail M and The Lung Cancer Group. Surgical adjuvant therapy for Stage II and III adenocarcinoma and large cell undifferentiated carcinoma. *J Clin Oncol* 1986; **4**: 710–715.

101. Holmes E. Surgical adjuvant therapy for Stage II and Stage III adenocarcinoma and large cell undifferentiated carcinoma. *Chest* 1994; **106**: 293S–296S.

102. LeChevalier T, Arriagada R, Tarayre M, *et al.* Significant effect of adjuvant chemotherapy on survival in locally advanced non-small-cell lung cancer. *J Natl Cancer Inst* 1992; **84**: 58.

103. Dillman R, Seagren S, Propert K, *et al.* A randomized trial of induction chemotherapy plus high-dose radiation versus radiation alone in stage III non-small cell lung cancer. *N Engl J Med* 1990; 940–945.

104. Schaake-Koning C, Van Den Bogert W, Dalesio O, *et al.* Effects of concomitant cisplatin and radiotherapy in inoperable non-small-cell lung cancer. *N Engl J Med* 1992; **326**: 524–530.

105. Trovo M, Zanelli G, Minatel E, *et al.* Radiotherapy Versus Radiotherapy enhanced by Cisplatin in Stage III Non-Small Cell Lung Cancer. *Int J Radiation Oncology Biol Phys* 1992; **24**: 573–574.

106. Ruckdeschel J, Findelstein D, Ettinger D, *et al.* A randomized trial of the four most active regimens for metastatic non-small cell lung cancer. *J Clin Oncol* 1986; **4**: 14–22.

107. Dillman RO, Seagren SL, Herndon J, *et al.* Randomized trial of induction chemotherapy + radiation therapy versus RT alone in stage III non-small-cell lung cancer (NSCLC): 5-year follow-up of CALGB 84-33. Proceedings of *ASCO* 1993; **12**(A1092).

108. Sause WT, Scott C, Taylor S, *et al.* Radiation therapy oncology group (RTOG) 88–08 and eastern cooperative oncology group (ECOG) 4588: Preliminary results of a Phase III trial in regionally advanced unresectable non-small-cell lung cancer. *J Nat Cancer Inst* 1995; **87**: 198–205.

109. Rapp E, Pater JL, Willan A, Cormier Y, Murray N, Evans WK, Hodson DI, Clark DA, Feld R, Arnold AM, Ayoub JI, Wilson KS, Latreille J, Wierzbicki RF, Hill DP. Chemotherapy can prolong survival in patients with advanced non-small-cell lung cancer - Report of a Canadian multicenter randomized trial. *J Clinical Oncology* 1988; **6**: 633–641.

110. Cartei G, Cartei F, Cantone A, Cansarano D, Genco G, Tobaldin A, Interlandi G, Giraldi T. Cisplatin-Cyclophosphamide mitomycin combination chemotherapy with supportive care versus supportive care alone for treatment of metastatic non-small-cell lung cancer. *J Natl Cancer Inst* 1993; **85**: 794–800.

111. Le Chevalier T, Brisgand D, Douillard J, Pujol J, Alberola V, Monnier A, Riviere A, Lianes P, Chomy P, Cigolari S, Gottfried M, Ruffie P, Panizo A, Gaspard M, Ravaioli A, Besenval M, Besson F, Mertinez A, Bethand P, Tursz T. Randomized study of vinorelbine and cisplatin versus vindesine and cisplatin versus vinorelbine alone in advanced non-small-cell lung cancer: Results of a european multicenter trial including 612 patients. *J Clinical Oncology* 1994; **12**: 360–367.

112. Sabanathan S, Richardson J, Mearns AJ, Goulden C. Results of surgical treatment of Stage III lung cancer. *Eur J Cardio-thorac Surg* 1994; **8**: 183–187.

113. Albain KS, Crowley JJ, LeBlanc M, Livingston RB. Survival determinants in extensive-stage non small-cell lung cancer: The Southwest Oncology Group Experience. *J Clinical Oncology* 1991; **9**: 1618–1626.

114. Hickish TF, Smith IE, Middleton G. Chemotherapy for elderly patients with lung cancer. *Lancet* 1995; **346**: 580.

115. Paesmans M, Sculier JP, Libert P, Bureau G, Dabouis G, Thiriaux J, Michel J, Van Cutsem O, Sergysels R, Mommen P, Klastersky J. Prognostic factors for survival in advanced non-small cell lung cancer. Univariate and multivariate analyses including recursive partitioning amalgamation algorithms in 1,052 patients. *J Clinical Oncology* 1995; **13**: 1221–1230.

116. McGilligan DJ. Treatment of lung cancer metastatic to the brain: Results of combined excision. *Surg Clin N Am* 1987; **67**: 1073–1080.

117. Black PMcL. Solitary brain metastases: radiation, resection, or radiosurgery. *Chest* 1993; **103(Suppl 4)**: 367S–369S .

118. Raviv G, Klein E, Yellin A, *et al.* Surgical treatment of solitary adrenal metastases from lung carcinoma. *J Surg Oncol* 1990; **43**: 123–124.

119. Graham BL, Balducci L, Khansur T, Dalton ML, Lambuth B. Surgery for small cell lung cancer. *Ann Thorac Surg* 1988; **45**: 687–692.

120. Warde P, Payne D. Does thoracic irrradiation improve survival or local control in limited stage small cell carcinoma of the lung? A Meta-analysis. *J Clin Oncol* 1992; **10**: 890–895.

121. Pignon JP, Arriagada R, Ihde DC, *et al.* A meta-analysis of thoracic radiotherapy for small-cell lung cancer. *New Eng J Med* 1992; **327(23)**: 1618–1624.

122. Johnson DH, Kim K, Turrisi AT, *et al.* Sisplatin (P) and Etoposide (E) + concurrent thoracic radiotherapy (TRT) administered once versus twice daily for limited-stage (LS) small cell lung cancer (SCLC): Preliminary results of an intergroup trial (Meeting Abstract). Proceedings of *ASCO* 1994; **13**(A1105).

123. Murray N, Coy P, Pater JL, *et al.* Importance of timing for thoracic irradiation in the combined modality treatment of limited-stage small-cell lung cancer. The National Cancer Institute of Canada clinical trials. *J Clin Oncol* 1993; **11**: 336–344.

124. Arriagada R, LeChevalier T, Borie F, *et al.* Prophylactic cranial irradiation for patients with small-cell lung cancer in complete remission. *J Nat Cancer Inst* 1995; **87**: 183–190.

125. Komaki R, Meyers CA, Shin DM, *et al.* Evaluation of cognitive function in patients with limited small cell lung cancer prior to and shortly following prophylactic cranial irradiation. *Int J Radiation Oncology Biol Phys* 1995; **33**: 179–182.

126. Lamproglou I, Chen QM, Boisserie G, *et al.* Radiation-induced cognitive dysfunction: An experimental model in the old rat. *Int J Radiation Oncology Biol Phys* 1995; **31**: 65–70.

127. Ginsberg RJ, Rubinstein L. The comparison of limited resection to lobectomy for T_1N_0 non-small cell lung cancer. *Chest* 1994; **106**: 318S–319S.

128. Morrison R, Deeley TJ, Cleland W. The treatment of carcinoma of the bronchus: A clinical trial to compare surgery and supervoltage radiotherapy. *Lancet* 1963; **1**: 683–684.

129. Smart J. Can lung cancer be cured by irradiation alone? *JAMA* 1966; **195**: 158–159.

130. Coy P, Hodson I, Payne D, *et al.* The effect of dose of thoracic irradiation on recurrence in patients with limited stage small

cell lung cancer: Initial results of a Canadian multicenter randomized trial. *Int J Radiat Oncol Biol Phys* 1988; **14**: 219–226.

131. Cooper JD, Pearson FG, Todd TRJ, *et al.* Radiotherapy alone for patients with operable carcinoma of the lung. *Chest*, 1865; **87**: 289–292.

132. Haft, B, Goldberg N, Gerstley J, *et al.* Results of radical radiation therapy in clinical stage I, technically operable non-small cell lung cancer. *Int J Radiat Oncol Biol Phys* 1988; **15**: 69–73.

133. Talton B, Constable W, Kersh C. Curative radiotherapy in non-small cell carcinoma of the lung. *Int J Radiation Oncology Biology Phys* 1990; **19**: 15–21.

134. Sandler H, Curran W, Turrisi A. The influence of tumor size and pre-treatment staging on outcome following radiation therapy alone for Stage I non-small cell lung cancer. *Int J Radiation Oncology Biology Phys*, 1991; **19**: 9–13.

135. Dosoretz D, Katin M, Blitzer P, *et al.* Radiation therapy in the management of medically inoperable carcinoma of the lung: Results and implications for future treatment strategies. *Int J Radiation Oncology Biology Phys* 1992; **24**: 3–9.

136. Rosenthal S, Curran WJ, Herbert S, *et al.* Clinical Stage II non-small cell lung cancer treated with radiation therapy alone: The significance of clinically staged ipsilateral hilar adenopathy. *Cancer* 1992; **70**: 2410–2417.

137. Kaskowitz B, Graham M, Emami B, *et al.* Radiation therapy alone for stage I non-small cell lung cancer. *International Journal of Radiation Oncology Biol Phys* 1993; **27**: 517–523.

46. Breast Cancer: An Oncological Perspective – Part 1

Lodovico Balducci, Rebecca A. Silliman and Paul Baekey

Introduction

Breast cancer is the most common malignancy and the most common cause of cancer death in women over 65 (1–4). The control of breast cancer in older individuals may be improved by the study and the understanding of some critical questions which are still unanswered (5–6). These include: age-related changes in the biology of breast cancer; age-related barriers to cancer prevention and treatment; value of screening asymptomatic older women for breast cancer; optimal management of primary breast cancer; optimal duration of adjuvant treatment with tamoxifen; place of adjuvant chemotherapy; optimal management of metastatic disease. We will explore these questions after an overview of the epidemiology of breast cancer in the older woman.

Extent of the Problem

General Epidemiology

The incidence of breast cancer increases with age (6–7). According to the SEER data (Figure 46.1), the incidence of breast cancer increases up to age 80, plateaus between ages 80–85, and may decline thereafter (6). Lack of reliable information in persons over 85 may explain the late decline. Some autopsy data from Trieste, Italy, described in more details elsewhere in this book, support a real decrement in the incidence of breast cancer in the oldest old (8). The pathologists from Trieste regularly searched for occult breast cancer all women coming to autopsy. In an autopsy population of approximately 30000 women they found that the prevalence of occult breast cancer was highest between ages

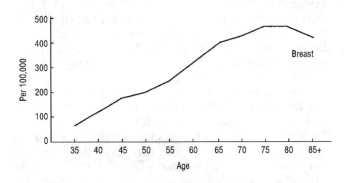

Table 46.1 Risk factors for breast cancer.

Age
Familiarity
Endocrine History
Age at menarch and menopause
Age of first pregnancy
Number of pregnancies
Therapeutic use of estrogens
Body shape
Nutritional factors
Ionizing radiations

50–60 and declined progressively thereafter; virtually no cases of occult breast cancer were detected in women aged 80 and older. More data is needed to confirm these preliminary findings: at present the information related to the incidence of breast cancer after age 85 is inadequate.

Two thirds of breast cancers occur after age fifty; 50% after age 65; 56% of breast cancer-related deaths affect women aged 65 and older (1–8). At the present rate of growth of the older population, one can expect 65% of all breast cancers and 70% of all breast cancer deaths in women aged 65 and over by the year 2010.

Risk Factors

Breast cancer has been associated with a number of conditions (Table 46.1), some of which may be relevant to the elderly (1). Madigan *et al.* studied the proportion of breast cancer cases in the USA that may be explained by well established risk factors and found that family history, reproductive history and higher income may account for as many as 47% of cases (9). Of interest, the relative risk for breast cancer for women aged ≥ 70 was 2.4 in the presence of positive family history, 1.9 for nulliparity, 3.0 for first pregnancy after age 30, and 2.3 for income. This project stemmed from the National Health and Nutrition Examination Survey I (NHANES I), and consequently had a limited scope. In particular it could not include other risk factors such as hormone replacement therapy (for lack of information) or body size (that was dealt with in a separate study). Still,

Figure 46.1 Age-related incidence of breast cancer. From reference 6, with permission.

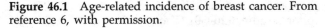

these results are very important as they demonstrate that many risk factors remain significant throughout old age.

Family history

Frequently, breast cancer appears a familial disease. Goldstein and Amos calculated that approximately 60% of postmenopausal ductal breast cancers detected in the "Cancer and Steroid Hormone Study" (CASH) were familial (10). Thus, family history is an important risk factor even for older women. The relation of familial and inheritable cancer is complex. Familiarity does not necessarily imply inheritance (11). Environmental conditions prevalent in the same household may cause a cluster of cancers in the same family. For a long time it was hold that inheritable cancers tend to occur in a population younger than that in which sporadic cancers occur (11). A new insight of the different categories of persons at risk for cancer (oncodemes) may explain how inheritable cancer develop in older persons (12). Recently four type of oncodemes have been defined (12). These include:

1. Background oncodeme. In these persons cancer is independent of both genetic and environmental factors.
2. Genetic oncodeme. In these persons cancer is inheritable.
3. Environmental oncodeme. In these persons cancer is due exclusively to environmental factors.
4. Interactive oncodeme. In these persons cancer requires both inherited predisposition and environmental influences.

It is not unreasonable to construe an interactive oncodeme for women with family history of breast cancer, who develop cancer late in life. It should be underlined that even genetic oncodemes may occasionally include older persons. Two recently defined breast cancer oncodemes appear to be genetic, in that the majority of the population carrying the gene develop breast cancer (13). Though independent from each other, both are associated with increased incidence of breast and ovarian cancer in the same family. One oncodeme involves mutations in the BRCA1 gene, on chromosome 17q, which has been recently cloned (14). The penetrance of BRCA1 (or cumulative risk of developing breast cancer for members of a breast cancer family carrying the mutation) was calculated 59% by age 50 and 87% by age 70 (15). The other oncodeme involves a mutation of the BRCA2 gene on chromosome 13q (16). This gene, that has not been cloned at the time of this writing, implies increased risk of prostate and male breast cancer, in addition to female breast and ovary (16). In one BRCA2 family, 17% of breast cancers occurred after age 60. Breast cancers associated with BRCA1 and BRCA2 mutations occur mostly in women under 50, but a sizable portion of older women with the mutations are also at risk.

Both BRCA1 and BRCA2 are antioncogenes. Other mutations, such as alterations of oncogenes and of DNA repairing genes are also likely to cause inheritable breast cancer (13) Seemingly, other inheritable genetic mutations leading to breast cancer have not been yet recognized, as neither BRCA1 and BRCA2 mutations were found in some families at high risk of breast cancer.

The practical implications of the discovery of the BRCA1 and BRCA2 mutations are not clear yet. Ideally, these mutations may be used to screen individuals at high risk of breast cancer and to institute prophylactic measures, which may involve bilateral mastectomy, intensive mammographic screening, and chemoprevention (17). Several parameters need to be defined prior to recommending molecular screening of the general population. These include positive and negative predictive value of BRCA1 and BRCA2 mutations for risk of breast cancer in the general population, and efficacy of prophylactic interventions. At present, the prevalence of BRCA1 and BRCA2 mutations in the general population, and their implications in terms of breast cancer risk are unknown.

Endocrine factors

Of the endocrine factors, hormone replacement therapy is of particular concern to older women. This issue involves two major questions: does estrogen replacement increase the risk of breast cancer? Does the addition of progestins to estrogen modulate the risk of breast cancer? Two meta-analyses of case-control studies related to estrogen replacement have recently been performed (18–19).

Dupont *et al.* (18) failed to demonstrate a definitive association between postmenopausal estrogens and breast cancer but found that the relative risk of breast cancer increased with prolonged use of estrogens, at doses equivalent to ≥ 1.25 mg conjugated estrogens. The risk of breast cancer declined almost immediately after discontinuance of the hormones. Most important, these authors also established that doses equal to or lower than 625 mg of conjugated estrogens did not increase the risk of breast cancer, irrespective of treatment duration. The low doses of estrogen were effective in preventing osteoporosis and coronary artery disease, but did not ameliorate disabling symptoms of menopause, such as hot flashes and vaginal atrophy. Colditz *et al.* found a small but definitive increase in the risk of breast cancer for women receiving estrogen replacement therapy (relative risk 1.40; 95% CI 1.20–1.63) (19). The risk abated upon treatment cessation. Previous estrogen users who had discontinued the therapy had a relative risk of 1.02 (CI 0.93–1.12). Of interest, progestins did not protect from breast cancer, according to these authors.

The combination of estrogen and progestins has been proposed as hormone replacement therapy to reduce the risk of endometrial cancer. Recent studies showed that progestins did not lessen the benefits of estrogen on osteoporosis, lipid profile, coronary artery disease and postmenopausal symptoms (20). The effects of this promising combination of hormones on breast cancer risk has been explored both in case-control (21–25) and cohort studies (26–30) (Table 46.2). These studies in-

Table 46.2 Hormone replacement therapy with estrogen and progestins, and risk of breast cancer.

A. Case Control

Study	#Subjects*	Age Range	Odd Ratio (CI)
Ewertz et al. (21)	2822	all ages	1.36 (0.98–1.87)
Kaufman et al. (22)	3763	40–69	1.7 (0.9–3.3)
Palmer et al. (23)	1821	<70	0.9 (0.6–1.2)
Yang et al. (24)	1384	<75	1.2 (0.6–2.2)
Stanford et al. (25)	1029	50–64	0.9 (0.7–1.3)

B. Cohorts

Study	#Subjects*	Age Range	Relative Risk (CI)
Bergkvist et al. (26)	23,244	35–UP	4.1 (0.9–22.1)
Hunt et al. (27)	4,544	45–54	1.59 (1.18–2.10)
Risch & Howe (28)	33,003	43–49	NR (p=0.48)
Schairer et al. (29)	49,017	55–UP	1.2 (1.0–1.6)
Colditz et al. (30)	121,700	54–UP	1.41 (1.15–1.74)

NR=non reported: there were no cases of breast cancer.

* Includes all study subjects;untreated controls, those treated with estrogen only, and those recevieing combinations of estrogens and progestins.

volved different populations, of different ages and at different times; not surprisingly the results were highly variable. With the exception of the study by Stanford et al. (25), involving 537 patients aged 55–64 and 492 matched and randomly selected controls, all other studies included women taking both estrogen and estrogen-progestins in combination. The study of Stanford is a model case-control study in terms of methodology. However, the small number of subjects might have limited the statistical power to detect small differences. Also, the selection of women in a relatively narrow age-range, close to the menopause, might have prevented adequate assessment of long term hormone-replacement. In most studies, patients treated with combination therapy were a minority and the results of these studies are not conclusive (21–24; 26–27). For example, Risch and Howe (28) did not find a single case of breast cancer among women receiving combination hormonal therapy, but only 171 of 33,003 women were treated exclusively with combination therapy. An additional 646 women received both estrogen alone and estrogens in combination with progestins at sometimes in their postmenopausal years; of these, 3 developed breast cancer. The Swedish study reported a staggering relative risk of 4.1 for women using combination hormonal replacement therapy (26). Several reasons make this study an outlier. The large confidence interval indicates that the relative risk is far from precise. Also, the Swedish used a combination of estradiol compounds and levonorgestrel, for hormone

replacement. This treatment is quite different from the combinations of hormones used in the USA and may have a more pronounced carcinogenic effect (26). Two studies deserve special attention (29–30). Schairer et al. followed a cohort of 49,017 postmenopausal women involved in the Breast Cancer Detection Demonstration Project (29) for a total of 10 years; 85% of the patients completed the study, and of those who failed to complete the study 5% did so because of death. Approximately 40% of these women received estrogen alone, and 7% estrogen and progestins in combination. These authors reported two interesting results: relative risk of breast cancer was definitely increased by the combination treatment but not by estrogen alone and most cancers related to hormone replacement were "carcinomas in situ." The lack of estrogen effect cannot be ascribed to inadequate sample and poor follow-up; it may reflect however a higher prevalence of low-dose estrogen users among health conscious women. The higher prevalence of "carcinomas in situ" may reflect the increased utilization of screening mammography by this population.

The study of Colditz et al. is particularly important for several reasons (30). Is this a cohort study with a large number of patients and with a particularly prolonged follow-up (16 years), involving professional individuals (nurses) with a high comprehension of the nature and the goals of the study, so that the compliance was unusually high and the data collection very reliable. The authors had the opportunity to study the effects of both estrogen alone (until 1986) and estrogens in combination with progestins (after 1986). It was found that the relative risk of breast cancer increased with estrogen alone (1.32; CI:1.14–1.54) and with the combination (1.41; CI 1.15–1.74). Also, the relative risk increased with the duration of treatment and with the age of the patients; for women aged 60–65 the relative risk was 1.71. Seemingly, there was a relation between age and treatment duration. The addition of progestins to estrogen appeared to enhance the risk of breast cancer. The risk of breast cancer declined almost immediately upon discontinuance of the hormones, both in the case of estrogen and of combination treatment. Of special concern is the high breast cancer-related mortality in this population, suggesting that hormone-replacement may cause invasive and aggressive cancers in the majority of cases. This report may have a major impact on the quality of life of millions of women, should the use of hormone replacement therapy be discouraged by the fear of breast cancer. It is necessary to highlight important issues which were not addressed and deserve special comments. First, the authors did not address the issue of estrogen doses. As found in previous meta-analyses, doses lower than or equivalent to 625 mg of conjugated estrogen don't appear to increase the risk of breast cancer and may be reasonably safe. The timing of treatment was also not addressed. Most women start receiving estrogen replacement at the time of menopause. It is not unusual, however, to institute estrogen replacement later in life, to delay the development of rapid osteoporosis or to reverse menopausal symptoms which might have become unbearable. It is not clear whether late hormone replacement poses a risk of breast cancer.

A common question related to hormone replacement therapy concerns the effects of therapy in women with personal or familial history of breast cancer. None of the studies here reviewed has been able to clarify this issue. At present, there is no proof that the risks of these women to develop a new breast cancer is enhanced by exogenous estrogens. Likewise, there is no proof that estrogen- or combination therapy-replacement increases the risk of recurrence of breast cancer after surgery.

In conclusion, existing evidence indicates that hormone replacement therapy may be associated with an increased risk of breast cancer. This increment may vary between 16 and 71%. The risk of breast cancer is modulated by the duration of treatment and by the doses of estrogen.

With the aging of the population the issue of hormone replacement is becoming more and more critical in terms of quality of life, function, survival and cost of chronic care. The majority of menopausal women are sexually, professionally, and socially active and the symptoms of menopause represent a serious threat in each area of activity. Also, the more prolonged life expectancy involves more prolonged risk for coronary artery disease and for osteoporotic fractures, which in turn are a cause of cost and disability. By preventing these conditions, hormone-replacement therapy plays a major role in the function, the survival, the quality of life and the cost of care of these patients (31).

The current recommendations are to use hormone-replacement therapy in women with a history of or at high risk for coronary artery disease, and in women at risk for osteoporosis, determined from measurement of the bony mass (31). In addition, hormone replacement improves the quality of life in a number of women, by relieving menopausal-related symptoms. For those women who may benefit from hormone replacement but are seriously concerned about the risk of breast cancer, a reasonable treatment strategy may involve hormone replacement for 8–10 years following menopause. This treatment may be adequate to prevent osteoporosis and to relieve the menopausal symptoms at the most critical time, and may minimize the risk of breast cancer, which increases with more prolonged use. It is not clear however whether this strategy may prevent coronary artery disease later in life. For women with minimal menopausal symptoms, low-dose estrogen replacement (625 mg conjugated estrogen daily) may be beneficial. It is not clear at this point whether there are definite indications for the combination of estrogen and progestins as hormone-replacement therapy.

Body shape

The association of breast cancer and central (android) obesity was reported in several studies and was related to decreased concentrations of circulating sexual hormone-binding globulin in the presence of android obesity (32–35). Android obesity was defined as a ratio ≥ 0.71 between the body circumferences measured at the waists and at the hips (34). As the prevalence of android obesity increases with age, this association is of special concern for older women. Sellers *et al.* described an association between the prevalence of breast cancer and of android fat distribution in the same family (36). Android obesity is due to accumulation of fat in preexisting adipose cells and is easily reversed by a negative caloric balance through diet and exercise (37).

Diet

Of the dietary factors alcohol has a definite etiologic role (38–40), while controversy persists concerning the role — if any — of dietary fat (41). Several studies have documented an association between animal fat intake and incidence of breast cancer in different populations (42–44). Likewise, immigrant studies showed that the incidence of breast cancer among Asian women increased after they moved to the United States and adopted an American diet, which was richer in fat than in their country of origin (45–46). However, large cohort studies of fat intake, including the Iowa Study (47), the NHANES I (48), the Nurse Health Study (49), and the Amsterdam Study (50) failed to show a relationship between individual fat intake and individual risk of breast cancer. Only a cohort study from Canada suggested a marginal increase in breast cancer risk related to fat intake (51). Possibly, a high baseline fat content of most Western diets, even in those that are "low fat" may account for the lack of a dose/effect of fat on breast cancer. In other words, there may be a "threshold" for fat intake, beyond which the risk of breast cancer is uniformly increased. Another hypothesis is gaining some credit, however, and that is that in most diets fat and fiber intakes are inversely related (52). Thus, the scarcity of fiber rather than the excess of fat may be responsible for enhanced breast cancer risk. This hypothesis is supported by the recent discovery of a group of natural dietary components, called phytoestrogen, with antiestrogenic activity, that are abundant in soya and tofu (53). Interestingly, the phytoestrogens do not seem to interfere with a woman's reproductive life, and their antiestrogenic activity may be limited to breast and endometrium. Whereas it is prudent to limit the percentage of fat-related calories in one's diet, it may also be advisable to enhance the intake of phytoestrogen-rich fiber. This issue is very pertinent to older individuals. Phytoestrogens may represent a physiological, non toxic form of chemoprevention of breast cancer. Possibly, phytoestrogens may also prevent systemic recurrence of primary breast cancer, without the toxicity of adjuvant chemotherapy.

Influence of Age on Diagnosis and Treatment of Breast Cancer

Controversy exists as to whether breast cancer is more advanced at presentation in older women (54–56). In 1986, a report from the New Mexico Tumor Registry (55) suggested that such was the case in women over

65, while a review of the Rhode Island Cancer Registry over ten years failed to demonstrate any correlation between patient age and stage of the disease at presentation (56). More recently, a review of the SEER data also failed to demonstrate a correlation between age and stage of breast cancer at presentation (6). There are two possible, non mutually exclusive explanations for this discrepancy. The first is regional variation in the pursuance of medical care and cancer screening in general and in particular among the aged (57–58). The second is an improved utilization of screening mammography by older women in recent years (59–60). More widespread awareness of breast cancer in older women among public and professionals alike played a major role in increased detection. Clearly, ethnic and socioeconomic factors influence the presentation of breast cancer. In most reviews of this issue, breast cancer was more advanced at presentation among low income, Afro-American, and Hispanic women (61–62).

The SEER data showed that the percentage of breast cancers inadequately staged increased with the age of the patient (6). This finding indicates that some older individuals do not receive standard cancer care and reiterates previous observations that the pattern of cancer care tends to become less aggressive with the age of the patient (63–65). The central question raised by these reports is whether and when less aggressive care is appropriate. The appropriateness of the treatment received by individual patients is determined by considerations of life-expectancy and quality of life, for the elderly. Aging is highly individualized: different persons develop disability and diseases at different ages (66). Clearly, the number of breast cancer patients who die of unrelated conditions increases with age (67–68), and is strictly related to the prevalence and seriousness of comorbid conditions. Likewise, deteriorating functional status is associated with higher mortality and poorer tolerance of antineoplastic treatment (66). Thus, in many cases, departure from standard care is justified and commendable. It is important to underline, however, that in the absence of serious comorbidity or functional impairment, age itself does not represent an indication for substandard care. The average life expectancy of an 85 year old woman is more than 6 year (69). Breast cancer may rob such a woman of several years of quality life.

Biology of Breast Cancer in the Aged

A common view holds that breast cancer becomes more indolent in the aged. We will address this issue with three questions: do older women develop a form of breast cancer that is intrinsically less aggressive? Does the older organism represent an unfavorable soil for the growth of breast cancer? Is the clinical course of breast cancer more indolent in older individuals?

Theoretical considerations suggest that older individuals may have a higher prevalence of more indolent tumors than younger individuals. In general the growth rate of a tumor is related to its aggressiveness: if more

Table 46.3 Markers of tumor aggressiveness.

High Nuclear Grade

High histologic grade

Low concentration of estrogen and progesteron receptors

High tumor cell proliferation rate

High expression of the HER/2 oncogene

High vascularization and concentration of angiogenic factor

indolent tumors take more time to grow, they are also more likely to become manifest later in life and to be more prevalent among older individuals (70). Clinical observations support this hypothesis. A number of tumor markers (Table 46.3) may be used to assess the aggressiveness of breast cancer (71–73). Nixon *et al.* (74) and Lyman (75) *et al.*, among others, have shown that the prevalence of poorly differentiated (grade 3) tumors decreases, while the prevalence of hormone-receptor-rich tumors increases with the age of the patient population. Valentinis *et al.* (76) have shown in more than 1400 women, that the proliferation rate of breast cancer cells, measured by the incorporation of tritiated thymidine, decreased with the patient's age. The relation of other tumor markers to age is currently under study.

Circumstantial evidence suggests that the growth and the metastatic spread of breast cancer are slower in older than in younger organisms. In a series of 819 Finnish women, Holmberg *et al.* found that for tumors of similar size, the prevalence of axillary lymph node involvement decreased with the age of the patient, after age 55 (77). Kurtz *et al.* studied the relationship between the growth of primary breast cancer and the degree of mononuclear cell infiltration of the tumor in a group of French women (78). They found a direct correlation between tumor growth rate and degree of mononuclear cell infiltration and they hypothesized that mononuclear cells produced a tumor growth-stimulating cytokine. They also found that the degree of mononuclear cell response was inversely related to the age of the patient. This study is particularly important as it contradicts the common tenet that immunesenescence favors cancer development (79). At least in the case of breast cancer the opposite appears to be true. Nixon *et al.* confirmed the observation of Kurtz in a group of American women (74). They also found that the likelihood of lymphatic invasion decreased with the age of the patient. An area of research that appears particularly promising is the study of tumor growth factors in persons of different ages (80). Of special interest are age-related variations in the concentration of Insulin-Like Growth Factor I (IGF-I) and IGF-I binding proteins (IGFBP) (81). Lonning *et al.* reported that the concentration of IGFBP increased during treatment with tamoxifen and speculated that one of the mechanisms of action of tamoxifen was a blockage of IGF-I activity (82). Age-related variations in the serum concentration of these substances appear likely. Another growth factor of interest is the Transforming Growth Factor — beta (TGF-beta). In this designation a family of proteins opposing the growth of breast cancer are comprehended (83). Age-related variations in the production and in the serum concentration of TGF-beta are unknown. Tamoxifen stimulates the release of TGF-beta from stromal tissues, and this response may be enhanced in older individuals (84). A special mention deserves the factor responsible for tumor angiogenesis. The concentration of new vessels appears one of the most powerful prognosticators of recurrence in breast cancer (73). This factor has not been identified yet for breast cancer. In other tumors, the Vascular Permeability Factor appears to have an important role in tumor neovascularization (85). Other factors of interest include interleukin 6 (IL-6) and interleukin-4 (IL-4) (86).

For what concerns the natural course of breast cancer, several investigators have found that soft tissue, bony, and nodular pulmonary metastases are associated with a more prolonged survival than hepatic and lymphangitic lung metastases. The former become more prevalent and the latter rarer with the age of the patient (87). Also, in a review of older series of patients, studied prior to the modern chemotherapy era, Holmes found that the risk of dying of breast cancer among patients with metastatic disease decreased with the age of the patient (Table 46.4). This finding may indicate that breast cancer is more indolent in older women or, alternatively, that serious and lethal comorbid conditions are more prevalent. Satariano and Ragland explored the role of comorbidity in causing the death of older women with breast cancer (67). These authors found that the relative risk of breast cancer death declined with the number of comorbid conditions.

In conclusion, there is clear evidence that the prevalence of more indolent tumors increases with the age of the population and there is a reasonable suggestion that older individuals present somewhat unfavorable conditions to tumor growth. It is uncertain whether this translates into a more benign natural course of breast cancer in older individuals.

It is important at this point to underline that breast cancer is frequently lethal in older women. The detection of more benign biological characteristics may open important insight into the interactions of the tumor and the tumor-host and may provide new important prognostic clues. They should not deceive the clinician however into complacency. Breast cancer is a lethal disease at any age and should be treated timely and aggressively. A simple mathematic calculations may highlight this point. Let's assume that the prevalence of hormone-receptor rich tumors is 80% for women aged 70 and older and 20% for women under 35. If the prevalence of breast cancer is 400/100000 in the older group of women and 30/100000 in the younger, the prevalence of aggressive tumors will be 80/100000 and 24/100000 respectively.

Prevention and Early Detection

Primary prevention of breast cancer involves elimination of breast carcinogens or administration of substances which block carcinogenesis in the late stages (chemoprevention) (88).

Known carcinogens include alcohol (38) and estrogen or estrogen/progesterone in combination (30). Seemingly, these factors account only for a minority of breast cancer cases. Reduction of alcohol intake to less than three ounces of whisky daily or equivalent amounts of other alcoholic drinks is advisable. Complete abstinence from alcohol may have adverse impact on a person lifestyle without appreciable health benefits. For what concerns hormone replacement therapy, one has to balance a modest increase in the risk of breast cancer with the benefits of hormone replacement on osteoporosis and coronary artery diseases, as well as on the general well being and the sexual function of the older woman. Grady et al. (31) estimated gains and losses of hormone replacement therapy for a postmenopausal woman aged 50, taking into accounts personal risk of coronary artery disease, hip fractures, and breast cancer. Hormone replacement therapy may provide an additional year of life-expectancy for women with no known risk factors; 2.1 years for those with history of coronary artery disease and 0.7 years for those at risk for breast cancer. These estimates are conservative as they don't take into account the effects of hormone replacement on quality of life.

Thus, elimination of known carcinogens does not appear at present as a realistic form of cancer control.

Chemoprevention of breast cancer with estrogen antagonists appears promising. The Oxford meta-analysis showed a 36% reduction in new contralateral breast cancers in women treated with adjuvant tamoxifen (89), over a follow-up period of 15 years. Three ongoing clinical trials in the USA, the UK and Italy explore prospectively chemoprevention of breast cancer in postmenopausal women with tamoxifen (90). These studies have been surrounded by the controversy related to the risks of prolonged tamoxifen treatment, as outlined later in this chapter. Other substances which may have a chemopreventative effect include retinoids, DMFO, and oltripaz (90–91). Older individuals may represent ideal candidates for chemoprevention, because aging is associated with a number of carcinogenic changes which may be arrested or reversed with chemoprevention (92–93). However, chemoprevention of breast cancer should be considered experimental, at present.

The best established form of breast cancer prevention is secondary prevention, which involves screening asymptomatic persons. The aim of screening is detection of breast cancer at early stages (94). With aging, a number of factors influence the value of screening tests for breast cancer:

Aging is associated with increasing prevalence of breast cancer: consequently, the positive predictive value of screening tests improves with the age of the population screened.

Table 46.4 Prospective clinical trials of screening mammography.

Trial	Age Range	Interval	N. of Examinations	RR Cancer Death
HIP (102)	40–64	12	4	.65 (.46–.92)
MALMO (103)	45–69	18–24	6	.81 (.62–1.07)
EDINBURGH (104)	45–64	24	4	.84 (.63–1.12)
KOPPARBERG (103)	40–74	24–33	5–6	.64 (.45–.90)
OSTERGOTLAND (103)	40–74	24–33	5–6	.74 (.55–.99)
CANADIAN 2 (105)	50–59	12	5	.97 (.62–1.52)
STOCKOLM (103)	40–64	28	2	.8 (0.53–1.22)
GOTHENBURG (103)	40–59	18	2	.86 (.54–1.37)

By the time they are 65 and older, most women have already undergone some screening for breast cancer. This initial screening generally detect the "prevalence cases", whereas follow-up screening detects new, "incidence cases." Thus, serial screening tests in older women may become less and less productive.

The clinical course of breast cancer may become more indolent with age. Thus, breast cancer detected through screening may never become clinically relevant in older women.

The life expectancy of a person progressively decreases with age and the risk of comorbid conditions increases (67, 95–96). In women with limited life expectancy from advanced age and severe comorbidity, early detection of breast cancer may have only marginal impact on cancer specific mortality.

Currently, screening tests include breast self-examination (BSE), clinical examination of the breast (CBE), and mammography.

The value of BSE is controversial (97–98). None of 2 cohort and 11 case-control trials assessing BSE could demonstrate a reduction in breast-cancer related mortality (98–99). In developing countries, where radiological facilities may not be readily available, BSE may represent an effective form of cancer screening, but in the USA and other Western countries, the value of this practice is marginal at best. The main potential benefit of BSE is enhanced awareness of the risk of breast cancer and of the need of health maintenance. The main risk of BSE is a false sense of security from a negative examination which may dissuade more effective screening strategies.

CBE by a trained health professional is a valuable form of cancer screening, both alone and in combination with mammography. Approximately 5–10% of early breast cancers diagnosed at CBE escape mammographic detection (90–91). CBE may be particularly productive in older women for the following reasons:

- With age, the breast atrophies, and the physical exam of the breast becomes more sensitive of cancer — related abnormalities.

- With age, health care consumption increases dramatically. Most older women attend a physician office several times a year. These office visits represent an unique opportunity for breast cancer screening, and may spare the inconvenience of an additional trip to a screening center, which may become particularly burdensome for older individuals.

In a very poignant editorial Mitra made the case for breast cancer screening with CBE only and without mammography (100). His main argument was that the majority of cancers diagnosed at mammography only both in the Breast Cancer Detection Demonstration Project (BCDDP) (101) and in the Canadian study (105) were "Carcinoma In situ" with negligible malignant potential. In addition, the Canadian study randomized women aged 50–59 to mammography and CBE and CBE only, and could not demonstrate any decrement in mortality from the addition of mammography to the screening program. The issue whether CBE may substitute for mammography in the general population is highly charged and certainly beyond the scope of this chapter. For our purposes it is important to underline that in the older population CBE may have a major role as screening tool.

The best established strategy for breast cancer screening is serial mammography. Eight prospective control trials conducted worldwide (Table 46.4) showed a reduction in breast cancer — related mortality between 20–30% for women aged 50–70 and in three cases the difference was statistically significant (102–103). Several historically controlled studies supported these findings (Table 46.5) (101; 106–109). In the BCDDP study the reduction in breast cancer death rate was approximately 26% for women aged 59–74. A recent meta-analysis of these trials showed a relative risk (RR) of breast cancer death of .77 (C.I.: .69–.87) for the prospective trials and .45 (.29–.70) for case-control trials (110). The benefits of screening mammography over age 70 are less well established. Only two prospective trials involved women aged 70–74 and these showed a trend

Table 46.5 Historically controlled clinical trials of screening mammography.

Trial	Age Range	Interval	N of Exminations	RR Cancer Death
BCDDP (101)	59–74	yearly	5	–
DOM (106)	50–64	25	5	.52 (.32–.83)
FLORENCE (107)	40–70	30	3–7	.53 (.33–.85)
NIJIMEGEN (108)	35–65	24	4	.51 (.26–.99)
UK (109)	45–64	24	4	.76 (.54–1.08)

BCDDP= Breast Cancer Detection Program

toward reduced mortality (RR:.94;CI:.60–1.64) (103). The meta-analysis of these trials failed to demonstrate a statistically significant reduction in mortality for older women (RR 0.89; CI 0.67–1.42) (110).

Especially provocative are the results of the Nijmegen study, recently published (108). This trial had started more than a decade ago as a historically controlled trial, and involved only subjects up to age 70. In the last seven years the invitation to participate into the screening program was extended to women of all ages. The most recent analysis of the trial revealed a significant reduction in cancer specific mortality for women aged 65–75 (RR 0.89; CI: 0.71–0.98). Interestingly, after age 75 the breast cancer mortality increased with the utilization of screening mammography (108). Seemingly, the majority of women who underwent mammography after age 75 had a personal history of breast cancer, which explains the increased mortality.

Some considerations of the design of the clinical trials of mammography are necessary to outline the limits of our information and to formulate a reasonable program for screening asymptomatic older women. First, the majority of the trials involved serial CBEs in addition to mammography. The respective contribution of the two procedures to early detection of breast cancer has not been always well established, especially in older women. Second, most studies involved a limited number of mammographic examinations (between 4 and 7): the advantages of additional examinations has not been demonstrated. Third, the intervals between screening tests varied between 1 and 3 years in different studies. Mammogaphy appeared equally effective at two years and at shorter intervals. In terms of convenience and cost an interval of two years appears most appropriate for older women, whose cancer may have a more indolent natural course. Fourth, the benefits of screening in terms of mortality reduction became apparent 3–7 years since the beginning of the screening program (99,110). Seemingly, only women with a life expectancy of three years or longer may benefit from screening.

Clearly, the decision whether to screen asymptomatic older women for breast cancer is not based on conclusive evidence but rather on common sense consideration. We favor some type of screening program for the following reasons:

- Mammography and CBE are harmless and relatively inexpensive.
- Early diagnosis and timely treatment of breast cancer in older women may lead to significant reduction in morbidity and management cost, even if it has minimal effects on mortality.
- Older women were under represented or completely excluded from previous trials of screening mammography. It is reasonable to postulate that the failure to demonstrate the effectiveness of screening in older individuals might have been due to inadequate numbers.
- The life-expectancy of the older population is in continuous expansion. This expansion is associated with improved functional preservation. Thus, early detection of breast cancer may play an increasingly important role in reducing the mortality and in preserving the quality of life of older women.
- A decision analysis estimated that screening mammography may prolong life expectancy of women as old as 85 (96).

In our opinion, any screening program should be limited to subjects with a life expectancy of three years and longer, should involve CBE at any physician visit and mammography at biennial intervals.

In the mean time more information about the value of screening older women should be gathered. New randomized clinical trials of CBE or mammography in older individuals are unlikely and even undesirable, because the results of these trials may not be available for a decade, and when they have matured, new, more effective screening strategies, such as molecular screening, may be available. Important information may be generated by analyzing the results of current practices. These practices may be validated by answers to crucial questions such as: how many cancers are diagnosed with CBE of older women? How many are diagnosed with mammography? How many of these cancers are carcinomas "in situ" and how many invasive cancers? How many of the women who have undergone screening develop metastatic cancer during their lifetimes and die from cancer?

An unique problem related to older individuals involves cultural and social barriers to cancer screening (111). Several studies have examined this problem.

Lack of information and motivation, economic restrictions, inadequate transportation and poor social support have been responsible for a sharp decline in women undergoing breast cancer screening after age 65. In a very well documented study in Southern California, Fox *et al.* showed that lack of physician support was the weightiest factor in preventing the screening of older women (111). Fortunately, these barriers have been largely overcome in recent years. Coleman *et al.* reported in 1994 that for the first time the majority of women aged 65–74 have undergone at least one screening mammography throughout the Institutions belonging to the Breast Cancer Screening Consortium (60). Professional and public education, as well as decreased cost of mammography and implementation of mobile mammographic units might have played a central role in this change (94). It is also important to recognize the effort that many professional centers and voluntary organizations, like the American Cancer Society, have focused on older women in recent years. Programs involving individualized interventions, such as personal yearly letters reminding older women of screening deadlines have been particularly successful.

The massive participation of older women to screening programs in recent years represent a new opportunity to study issues of effectiveness and cost/effectiveness.

In the future, the screening of asymptomatic persons for cancer will certainly involve molecular screening (112). In the case of breast cancer one may predict two different approaches to molecular screening: identification of carriers of genotypes associated with breast cancer, and discovery of early carcinogenic changes in breast tissue. Seemingly, the latter approach may be of interest to older women. As the techniques for molecular diagnosis of cancer are developed, validated, and evaluated in clinical trials, serial mammographies and CBE will remain the mainstay of diagnosis of breast cancer at early stages.

Pathological and Clinical Aspects of Breast Cancer

A detailed discussion of the pathology of breast cancer is beyond the scope of this book. It is important however to mention pathological findings with prognostic and therapeutic implications and to recognize special histologic forms of breast cancer, with unique clinical course.

The most common histologic form of invasive breast cancer is infiltrating ductal carcinoma, which represent approximately 70–80% of cases. Important pathologic characteristics include size, histologic and nuclear grade, proliferation rate, degree of neovascularization, and the concentration of estrogen and progesterone receptors (ER and PR) (71–73). Other findings of clinical relevance are ploidy, S fraction, HER/neu2 oncogene amplification, and concentration of cathepsin D (71–73).

The second most common form of invasive breast cancer is invasive lobular carcinoma. This histologic subtype represent approximately 5 to 15% of cases.

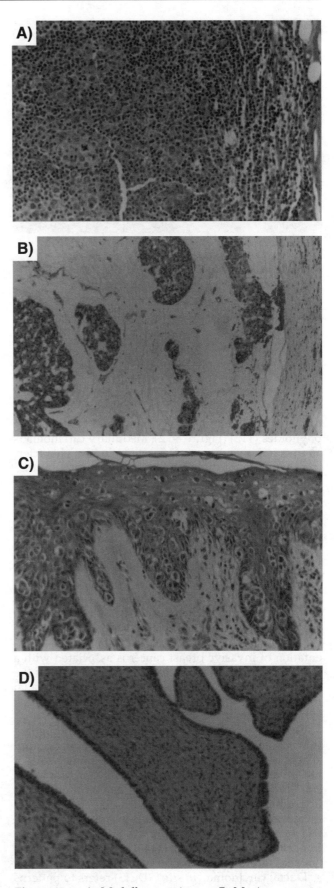

Figure 46.2 A: Medullary carcinoma; B. Mucinous carcinoma; C. Paget's disease; D. Cystosarcoma Phylloides.

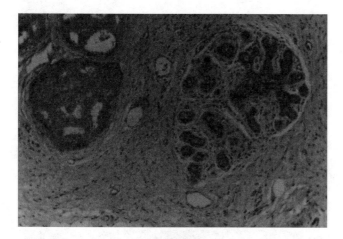

Figure 46.3 Ductal Carcinoma *"in situ"* (DCIS) contrasted with normal breast tissue.

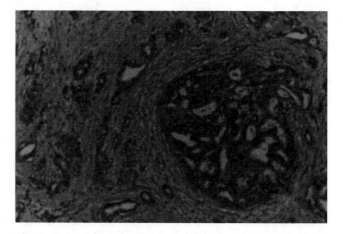

Figure 46.4 Coexistence of DCIS and infiltrating ductal carcinoma.

Infiltrating lobular carcinoma is often more poorly circumscribed in presentation and is usually positive for steroid hormone receptors. Stage for stage the prognosis is approximately equivalent to moderately differentiated infiltrating ductal carcinoma.

Less frequently occurring subtypes of invasive breast neoplasms include medullary carcinoma, mucinous carcinoma, inflammatory carcinoma, and cystosarcoma phylloides (113) (Figure 46.2). Medullary carcinoma is an uncommon subtype of breast carcinoma, characterized by sheets of high grade cells with a pronounced lymphocytic infiltrate forming a well circumscribed mass. Despite the high nuclear grade, medullary carcinoma has a relatively good prognosis if the axillary lymph nodes are uninvolved. Mucinous carcinoma of the breast is also a relatively infrequent subtype. It is generally well circumscribed and histologically is composed of epithelial cells suspended in a mucoid matrix. The risk of systemic spread is low. Inflammatory carcinoma refers to a clinical-pathologic presentation of breast carcinoma which has permeated lymphatic spaces, including dermal lymphatics, giving the clinical impression of induration and erythema. This presentation of invasive breast cancer is associated with a very poor prognosis. Cystosarcoma phylloides of the breast is a tumor of connective tissue and epithelial elements which may reach large dimensions but has a low risk of systemic spread.

Carcinoma *"in situ"* of the breast refers to malignant cells contained within basement membrane-bound spaces of the ductal and lobular epithelial network of the breast parenchyma (Figure 46.3). Carcinoma *"in situ"* is becoming an increasingly more common and important clinical problem (114–115). The apparent increasing frequency may be due to more widespread use of screening mammography and represents an important clinical problem (114–115). Most carcinomas *"in situ"* are ductal, lobular, or Paget's disease.

Ductal carcinoma *"in situ"* (DCIS) refers to patterns of non-invasive breast carcinoma which are believed to be precursors of infiltrating ductal carcinoma and ac-

counts for approximately 85% of all carcinomas *"in situ"*. DCIS is frequently multifocal and has a tendency to recur after wide margin resection; also, DCIS may undergo invasive transformation at the rate of 1% per year (114). Certain characteristics of DCIS predict higher likelihood of local recurrence and invasive transformation. These include size (diameter ≥ 2.5 cm), aneuploidy, high nuclear grade, and presence of necrosis. According to a recent report, tumors of high grade accounted for 25% of all cases and 60% of all recurrences; low grade DCIS accounted for 70% of all cases and 40% of all recurrences (115). Once recurrence occurred, however, the risk of invasive transformation was the same in all tumors, irrespective of histology (114).

Lobular Carcinoma *"in situ"* (LCIS) accounts for 15% of all tumors *"in situ."* It represent a therapeutic challenge in that the risk for developing subsequent invasive carcinoma following biopsy is relatively low and not restricted to the site of the biopsy. LCIS is uniformly identified as an incidental finding in biopsies done for other clinical or mammographic findings. For these reasons treatment recommendations for LCIS have varied from observation to bilateral simple mastectomy. Currently, close observation is gaining favor in the management of uncomplicated LCIS.

Paget's disease of the breast is also a form of *"in situ"* carcinoma in which tumor cells are present at the dermal/epidermal junction of the nipple, resulting in nipple erosion. The histologic pattern probably represents spread of *"in situ"* (usually ductal) carcinoma from underlying lactiferous sinuses. The prognosis of Paget's disease is determined by the characteristics of the accompanying neoplasm, either DCIS or associated invasive carcinoma.

Frequently, *"in situ"* and invasive carcinoma coexist in the same tumor (Figure 46.4). This coexistence presents a clinical challenge, because tumor size is an important prognostic factor in invasive carcinoma. It is customary to measure only the size of the invasive component to establish the risk of systemic metastasis and to assess the need for adjuvant treatment.

Neoplastic involvement of regional lymph nodes is harbinger of systemic tumor recurrence. The diagnosis of lymph node involvement is trusted to light microscopy, at present. The polymerase chain reaction (PCR), may be used to identify minuscule amounts of neoplastic genome in the lymph nodes and promises to provide a much more sensitive diagnostic technique (116).

Tumor markers of breast cancer include CEA and CA15-3. CA-27.29 is both more specific and more sensitive for breast cancer than CEA and is increased in approximately 90% of cases (117). It is not clear whether the measurement of CEA levels add any information to that obtained from CA-27.29. Most practitioners don't use CEA anymore.

The proper clinical use of tumor markers is controversial. A rise in the serum concentration of CA-27.29 is often the first sign of recurrence of breast cancer after surgery and adjuvant therapy. In the follow-up of patients with metastatic disease receiving systemic treatment, variations on serum CA-27.29 levels may reflect therapeutic response and obviate the need of more expensive imaging tests (117).

The diagnosis of breast cancer is established by biopsy; fine needle aspiration biopsy is performed for palpable lesions, wire-guided core biopsy for mammographic lesions (118). The staging of the patient involves a complete physical exam, CBC, automatized chemical panel, tumor markers and chest radiograph. More extensive staging, such as bone scan, brain and liver imaging, is indicated when physical or chemical abnormalities suggest involvement of these organs or for locally advanced (Stage III) disease.

The optimal follow-up of patients after treatment of localized or locally advanced breast cancer is controversial. In most practices, patients are followed every three-four months for two years, every six months for three years, and yearly thereafter. Follow-up includes physical exam, chemical panel and tumor markers at each visit, chest radiograph and mammography yearly (1). Some authors feel that even this limited approach is excessive and that chemical panel, tumor markers and chest radiograph could be eliminated. They support a minimalistic approach for two considerations. First, the majority of recurrences are diagnosed because the patient presents new complains, not as a result of follow-up visits. Second, the early diagnosis of systemic recurrences does not seem to improve the prognosis of breast cancer (119).

Treatment

General Considerations

The treatment of breast cancer is according to the stage of the disease (Table 46.6). For each stage we will describe standard treatment and we will illustrate specific issues related to older individuals.

Carcinoma "in situ"

DCIS entails a high risk of local recurrence, because it is often multicentric (120). The treatment of DCIS

Table 46.6 Clinical staging of breast cancer.

Stage 0	:	TIS	N0	M0
Stage I	:	T1	N0	M0
Stage II	:	T0	N1	M0
		T2	N0	M0
		T2	N1	M0
		T3	N0	M0
Stage IIIA	:	T0	N2	M0
		T1	N2	M0
		T2	N2	M0
		T3	N1	M0
		T3	N2	M0
Stage IIIB	:	T4	any N	M0
		any T	N3	M0
Stage IV	:	T4	any N	any M
		any T	N3	any M
		any T	any N	M1

Tx = Primary tumor cannot be assessed

T0 = No evidence of primary tumor

TIS = Paget's disease without a tumor; Carcinoma "in situ"

T1 = Largest diameter primary tumor ≤2cm

T2 = Largest diameter primary tumor 2–5 cm

T3 = Largest diameter primary tumor > 5 cm

T4 = Tumor of any size with extension to the chest wall or to the skin.

Nx = Regional lymph nodes cannot be assessed

N1 = Metastases to ipsilateral movable lymph nodes

N2 = Metastases to ipsilateral axillary lymph nodes fixed to each other or to other structures.

N3 = Metastases to ipsilateral internal mammary lymph nodes.

Mx = Presence of distant metastases cannot be assessed.

M0 = No evidence of distal metastases.

M1 = Distant metastases including ipsilateral supraclavicular lymph nodes.

involves mastectomy, or partial mastectomy followed by postoperative irradiation. The advent of mammography has been associated with a dramatic increase in the incidence of DCIS (from 3% to 30%) and with important changes in the clinical presentation of this neoplasm (101,114;121). Prior to mammography most DCIS were large tumors necessitating mastectomy. The majority of DCIS detected at mammography are small

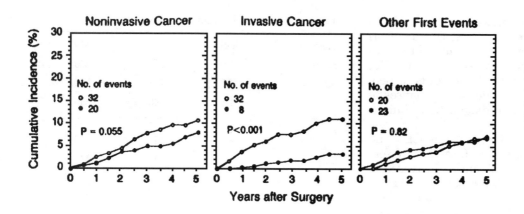

Figure 46.5 Incidence of recurrence of non-invasive and invasive cancer after treatment of DCIS with lumpectomy with (closed circles) and without (open circles) postoperative irradiation. From ref. 120, with permission.

tumors which might be completely excised with partial mastectomy. From the new presentation of DCIS stemmed the question whether DCIS could be managed with partial mastectomy only. The NSABP addressed this question in 1985, by comparing lumpectomy with and without postoperative irradiation in 818 women with DCIS (120). Radiation consisted of 50 Gy administered at the rate of 2 Gy a day five days a week. Patients were stratified according to age, type of tumor (DCIS or LCIS), axillary lymph node dissection and method of diagnosis. The risk of local recurrences of both DCIS and invasive cancer during the first five postoperative years was reduced by postoperative irradiation (Figure 46.5). Postoperative irradiation did not affect the risk of lymph node and distant metastases, contralateral breast cancer, second primary cancers and non-cancer deaths. Of special interest to the readers of this book, 36% of women were over 60.

The NSABP study left some important questions unanswered. The trial did not assess how different risk factors affected recurrence. In particular it did not explore the possibility that poor histologic differentiation and aneuploidy were associated with higher recurrence rate after partial mastectomy, as suggested by a recent review of the subject (115). These questions are important because radiation therapy adds substantial cost and inconvenience to the treatment. A new intergroup study has been planned to examine the need of irradiation in women with tumors which are ≤2.5 cm in diameter and without comedocarcinoma. As postoperative irradiation appears to have minimal, if any, impact on survival, another important issue is whether postoperative irradiation is preferable to local reexcision upon recurrence. This question is critical for older women for whom the daily trips to the radiation therapy treatment unit may be very burdensome.

Another unresolved issue in the management of DCIS is the role of axillary dissection. Since the cumulative incidence of microscopic lymph node involvement in several studies is <1% many practitioners feel that lymph node dissection and its related morbidity are not warranted in this disease.

The management of LCIS involves either local excision or bilateral mastectomy. Postoperative irradiation of the breast is not indicated in this condition, given the likelihood of recurrence in both breasts. As the

benefits of bilateral mastectomy in terms of survival have never been demonstrated, local excision with mammographic follow-up appears the most sensible treatment.

Treatment of localized breast cancer (Stages I and II)

The treatment of localized breast cancer is a multidisciplinary task that often requires a combination of surgery, radiation therapy and systemic treatment (chemotherapy or hormonal therapy).

Several controlled studies from the USA (122;123) and Europe (124;125) have clearly demonstrated the equivalence of total mastectomy and partial mastectomy in combination with postoperative irradiation in the management of primary breast tumors. It should be underlined that different forms of partial mastectomy were used in these trials: in some cases a quadrantectomy and in other cases a lesser procedure was employed. Also, some studies involved only women with a tumor diameter ≤2.5 cm (124) and others women with tumor diameters ≤5cm (122,123). Thus, the results of these studies may not be comparable with each others. Based on these studies a recent consensus conference recommended that breast conserving surgery be performed when adequate esthetic result may be assured and wound healing is not impaired by underlying diseases (126). The conference properly did not address issues related to the size of the tumor. It should be emphasized that both partial and total mastectomy are nowadays simple surgical procedures that can be performed under local anesthesia, with minimal risk even for the oldest old (127, 128). Last, but not least, the preference of individual patients should be accommodated whenever possible. It should not be assumed that breast preservation is preferred by the vast majority of women. A recent meta-analysis of several quality of life-studies comparing simple and partial mastectomy, failed to demonstrate a clear gain in quality of life with partial mastectomy (129).

Axillary dissection is part of the management of localized invasive breast cancer. The aim of axillary dissection is twofold: staging, and elimination of residual disease (126). Axillary dissection may be associated with increased morbidity, such as lymphedema of the arm and brachial neuropathy. Furthermore, axillary dissection may prolong the duration of surgery and mandate the use of general anesthesia in patients who might have otherwise been managed with local anesthesia. According to the NIH consensus conference the extent of the dissection may be limited to axillary levels I and II when the lymph nodes at these levels are free of tumor (126). A new diagnostic technique, which was pioneered at the University of South Florida may obviate the need of axillary dissection in women with uninvolved lymph nodes, in the near future. Lymphnode mapping uses a radioactive tracer to identify the so called "sentinel lymphnode", that is the first axillary node to receive lymphatic drainage from the breast tumor area (130). Several surgical groups around the country are studying the correlation between neoplastic involvement of the sentinel node and other axillary nodes. If a sentinel lymph node free of tumor predicts a tumor-negative axilla, many women may be spared the morbidity and the cost of axillary dissection. In some trials, sentinel lymph nodes are studied with both light microscopy and PCR for cytokeratin (116).

The practice to irradiate the chest wall after simple mastectomy has been largely abandoned with the advent of adjuvant chemotherapy. In specific conditions involving high risk of chest wall recurrence adjuvant radiotherapy may still have an important role. These conditions include tumor size ≥5 cm in diameter, involvement of more than 4 axillary lymph nodes (131) and extranodal spreading of the tumor.

In a randomized controlled study of adjuvant radiation therapy to the chest in patients receiving adjuvant chemotherapy, by Griem *et al.* (132) radiation therapy reduced the local recurrence rate in patients with more than 4 positive lymph nodes, without affecting the overall survival of that population. The authors concluded that adjuvant chemotherapy alone is not very effective in preventing local recurrences. It should be noticed that the chemotherapy used in that study might have been inadequate for present standards. The Early Breast Cancer Trialists' Collaborative Group performed a meta-analysis of clinical trials comparing breast cancer surgery with and without postoperative irradiation (133). A total of 64 clinical trials were reviewed (36 comparing radiation and surgery with the same type of surgery alone, 10 comparing more extensive surgery and less extensive surgery, and 18 comparing more extensive surgery and less extensive surgery plus radiation), including 29,175 women. The general conclusion was that radiation therapy prevented local recurrences and deaths from breast cancer, but had no impact on overall survival as it was associated with more deaths unrelated to cancer. A very important age-related trend emerged from this study (Table 46.7): the number of deaths associated with breast irradiation and unrelated to breast cancer increased with the patient age and was highest for women ≥60. In this group of patients the number of non cancer deaths almost doubled in the presence of breast irradiation. Presumably, the non-cancer deaths were mainly due to heart failure in patients who received radiation therapy of the left

Table 46.7 Age related incidence of non breast cancer+breast cancer-related deaths/total number of patients, in women trated with and without breast irradiation according to the Oxford Meta-analysis (133).

Age	Radiation	No Radiation
< 50	62+798/2524	49+851/2486
50–59	126+747/2062	93+796/2089
≥ 60	339+778/2221	249+865/2241

chest. New techniques to shield the heart from irradiation may prevent a number of these deaths in the future.

We recommend that postoperative irradiation after mastectomy be limited to those women who have a definite indication, for the following reasons:

- lack of a definitive survival benefit
- lack of a demonstrable effect on local recurrences in the majority of cases
- substantial increase in the risk of non-cancer deaths in patients over 60 receiving radiotherapy.

In specific clinical situations, adjuvant systemic therapy prolongs the disease-free survival (DFS) and the overall survival (OS) of patients with localized breast cancer (126; 89). Adjuvant chemotherapy prolongs (DFS) and (OS) of premenopausal women with involved axillary lymph nodes (89), while adjuvant hormonal therapy with tamoxifen prolongs DFS and OS of postmenopausal women with localized breast cancer (89). In other clinical situations, the use of adjuvant chemotherapy is controversial. The St Gallien Conference has recently met and has proposed some guidelines for the use of adjuvant chemotherapy (Table 46.8) (134).

Table 46.8 St Gallien Conference Recommendations for adjuvant chemotherapy of breast cancer (134).

A. Node-Negative Patients
   Postmenopausal Patients.

	Low risk	High Risk
ER + :	**Tamoxifen**	**Chemotherapy** ±Tamoxifen
ER − :	Not Applicable	**Chemotherapy** ±Tamoxifen

   Elderly (>70)

ER + :	**Tamoxifen**	**Tamoxifen**
ER − :	Not Applicable	**Chemotherapy** ±Tamoxifen

B. Node-Positive Patients
   Postmenopausal Patients.

ER +:	**Tamoxifen** ± Chemotherapy
ER − :	**Chemotherapy** ±Tamoxifen

   Elderly (>70)

ER +:	**Tamoxifen**
ER − :	**Chemotherapy** ±Tamoxifen

Age may affect all the areas of management of localized breast cancer. We will examine the following questions: role of postoperative radiation after partial mastectomy; role of axillary dissection; primary treatment of localized breast cancer with tamoxifen, role of chemotherapy and hormonal therapy in the adjuvant treatment of breast cancer.

Postoperative irradiation reduces the local recurrence rate of breast cancer and allows preservation of the breast, but does not appear to affect the overall patient survival (122–126). This practice adds significant cost and inconvenience to the management of breast cancer especially for older individuals with limited resources and limited access to transportation. Toxicity of radiotherapy does not appear as an issue in older women. Wyckoff et al. reported that women aged 65 and older tolerated breast irradiation as well as younger women (135).

Morrow et al. (136) reviewed the randomized studies comparing lumpectomy with and without radiation therapy. They found that the local recurrence rate in the absence of radiation varied widely from one study to the other, but they were unable to identify a subset of patients in whom radiation was not necessary to prevent local recurrences. The issue is of serious consequence to older women. We would like to review existing data and draw our conclusions, that somehow differ from those of Morrow et al., for what concerns elderly individuals. Several authors studied the influence of patient's age on the local recurrence rate of breast cancer after partial mastectomy (Table 46.9) (137–143). In three of the studies (137–138; 143), there was a definite decline in local recurrence rate with the patient age. In two studies (139–140), the local recurrence rate was similar in patients of different ages, but significantly lower than the 38% originally reported by the NSABP (123). One may argue that a local recurrence rate <20% in the absence of radiation therapy may be an acceptable price for some patients to avoid cost and inconvenience of radiation. The study by Kantorovitz et al. is an outlier (141). These authors reported a staggering local recurrence rate of 27% in women over 60, in the absence of radiation therapy. These results must be seen with caution given the nature of the study. This is a retrospective study reviewing local recurrence rate of breast cancer in patients treated at different hospitals of New York State and involved women treated by different surgeons with different techniques at the beginning of the era of breast preservation, when the standards of partial mastectomy had not yet been established. Furthermore, many patients were lost to follow-up. Those who had experienced recurrence were more likely to return for further treatment, and might have biased the overall assessment of the local recurrence rate. Of some concern is the recent report from the Joint Center for Radiation Therapy (142). These authors addressed specifically the issue of age. They studied the incidence of local recurrences in absence of radiation therapy in a population of 90 women, median age 67, with T1 (<1 cm diameter) tumor and negative lymphnodes. All pa-

Table 46.9 Local recurrence rate of breast cancer and patient age.

A.	With radiotherapy	Age	Recurrrence Rate
	JCRT (137)	<35	21%
		35–50	10%
		51–65	9%
		>65	2%

B.	Without Radiotherapy Authors	Age	Recurrence rate
	Nemoto et al. (138)	30–39	40%
		40–49	24%
		50–59	28%
		60–69	11%
		70+	2%
	Clark et al. (139)	>50	13%
	Liljegren et al. (140)	35–72	18%
	Kantorowitz et al. (141)	>60	27%
	Hayman J et al. (142)	>60	16%
	Veronesi et al. (143)	≤ 45	17.5%
		46–55	8.7%
		> 55	3.8%

JCRT = Joint Center for Radiation Therapy

tients were managed with partial mastectomy and had no tumor cells within one cm of the specimen margin. The local recurrence rate was 16% with a median follow-up of 57 months. One may question whether the surgery, which was less than a quadrantectomy, was adequate. Veronesi et al. compared prospectively the local recurrence rate of breast cancer after partial mastectomy with and without radiotherapy (142). They found that the local recurrence rate decreased dramatically after age 55 from 19% to 3%, in the absence of postoperative irradiation (Figure 46.6). It should be noticed that only patients with tumor diameters ≤2.5 cm were enrolled in this trial and that the surgical procedure was in all cases a quadrantectomy. Thus, the conclusions of the trial are not necessarily valid for women with larger tumors or women undergoing a lesser procedure.

One may conclude from this review that the local recurrence rate of breast cancer declines with age and that postoperative irradiation may not be necessary in older women. In women over 55 with small tumors (≤2.5 cm) undergoing segmentectomy, and without extensive DCIS component, postoperative irradiation appears avoidable.

Three ongoing prospective studies explore the need of postoperative irradiation after partial mastectomy (126). The NSABP B-21 compares the local recurrence rate in women of any age with a tumor ≤1 cm largest

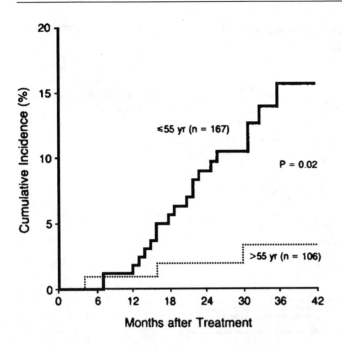

Figure 46.6 Local recurrence of breast cancer after quadrantectomy without postoperative irradiation in women aged >55 and in younger women. From ref.143, with permission.

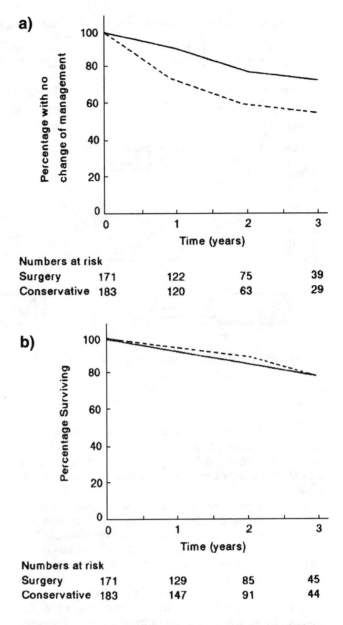

Figure 46.7 a) progressive disease in women aged 70 and over treated with mastectomy and tamoxifen (–) or tamoxifen only (...); b) survival of women aged 70 and older treated with surgery and tamoxifen (–) or tamoxifen only (...). From reference 145, with permission.

diameter treated postoperatively with breast irradiation and placebo, breast irradiation and tamoxifen and tamoxifen only. The CALGB 9343 concerns women ≥70 with a tumor size ≤4 cm and clinically negative nodes and compares postoperative irradiation and tamoxifen with tamoxifen alone. The EORTC 10932 involves women aged ≥50 with an invasive tumor ≤2 cm, histologic grade I, minimal or absent DCIS component and negative axillary lymph nodes, and compares postoperative treatment with irradiation alone or observation.

The need of lymph node dissection in older women was called into question when tamoxifen first appeared as the only effective form of adjuvant treatment for postmenopausal women. As all patients were destined to receive tamoxifen, while chemotherapy was not indicated, the staging of the axilla appeared unnecessary. Two series of women aged 70 and older, prospectively treated with lumpectomy and no lympnode dissection were reported, one from the Tufts Medical Center (144), the other from the Istituto Nazionale dei Tumori in Milano, Italy (128). The main difference in treatment plan was inclusion of postoperative irradiation in the Boston series. In both cases more than 80% of the women were free of disease at five years. The main problem with this approach is that lack of information related to axillary involvement. This information is vital to study the value of adjuvant chemotherapy in older women. The extent of axillary involvement may also determine the necessity of radiotherapy to prevent locoregional recurrences (126,133). Hopefully, the development of lymph node mapping may allow

to distinguish women whose lymph nodes are free of tumor with minimal morbidity, and will put to rest the controversy related to axillary dissection.

Several studies explored primary treatment of localized breast cancer with tamoxifen in women aged 70 and older. Of these, the Breast Cancer Campaign Trial (BCCT) produced the most definitive results (145). In 347 women, the BCCT compared tamoxifen and partial mastectomy followed by adjuvant tamoxifen. After three years of follow-up approximately 40% of patients treated without surgery experienced local progression which required excision (Figure 46.7).

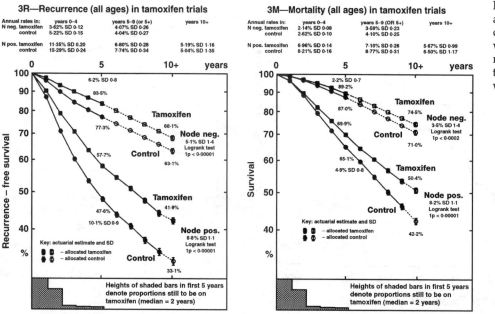

Figure 46.8 Recurrence rate and mortality of breast cancer in postmenopausal women receiving and not receiving adjuvant tamoxifen. From ref. 89, with permission.

It is difficult to see the advantage of pure medical management of localized breast cancer, given the safety of both partial and total mastectomy. Medical treatment may be an alternative for women who refuse surgery.

Adjuvant systemic treatment of the older woman with localized breast cancer is an area of major controversy. This include indications and durations of tamoxifen treatment and indications of adjuvant chemotherapy.

Several studies have demonstrated that adjuvant tamoxifen prolongs both DFS and OS of postmenopausal women with localized breast cancer (146–148;95). The Early Breast Cancer Trialists' Collaborative Group performed a meta-analysis of all randomized tamoxifen trials and demonstrated an overall reduction of 25% in recurrence rate and of 16% in mortality for postmenopausal women treated for two years or longer (89). Of interest, there was a reduction in recurrence rate and mortality also for women with uninvolved axillary lymphnodes (Figure 46.8). A pertinent problem with these trials is that they generally had an upper age limit for enrollment (80 for the Scottish trial, 70 for the others). Thus, it is not clear whether the results may be applied to the oldest old.

Two questions are left unanswered by this meta-analysis: the value of tamoxifen in women with hormone-receptor negative tumors (ER concentration<5 fm/mg), and the optimal treatment duration.

Conceptually, tamoxifen may be beneficial even in the case of hormone-unresponsive neoplasms. The antineoplastic activity of tamoxifen includes enhanced production of Transforming Growth Factor Beta (TGF-beta), a substance which opposes tumor growth, from the tumor stroma; inhibition of the secretion of Insulin-like growth factor 1 (IGF-1), and increased production of IGF-1 binding proteins, that lessen the concentration of free, active, IGF-1 (149–150). These mechanisms of action are independent from the antiestrogenic activity of tamoxifen. Both the NATO and the Scottish Trial demonstrated an advantage of adjuvant tamoxifen in tumors poor in hormone receptors, albeit not as pronounced as in receptor-rich tumors (146–147). These results are of difficult interpretation, however, because the concentration of progesterone receptors had not been measured and even the concentration of estrogen receptors was unknown in approximately half of the patients. Also, the assays used in those old studies might have not been as accurate as newer assays. Thus, some of the tumors reported as hormone-receptor poor might have contained a modest but significant concentration of receptors. A recent randomized and controlled study failed to demonstrate any survival advantage from adjuvant tamoxifen in postmenopausal women with hormone receptor poor tumors, but the power of the study for small survival differences was low (150). In view of the additional benefits of tamoxifen, we recommend adjuvant hormonal therapy in all postmenopausal women irrespective of the receptor status, with the caveat that the survival benefits may be negligible for receptor negative neoplasms.

The Early Breast Cancer Trialist Collaborative Group Meta-analysis found that at least two years of treatment were necessary for improving the patient survival (89). Several groups explored more prolonged treatment. The current information is derived from four trials, none of which produced conclusive results (152). In the NSABP-B09 trial women were randomized to receive melphalan and fluorouracil with or without tamoxifen for two years; those who had received tamoxifen were allowed to receive tamoxifen for one more year. The decision to continue tamoxifen treatment was based on patient preference, not on a randomized process (153). This trial reported further decrement in tumor recurrences for an additional year of tamoxifen treatment. The results of this study cannot be considered conclusive, as patients were not randomized to more or less prolonged tamoxifen treatment, and two years of chemotherapy might have influenced the outcome independently from tamoxifen. In ECOG E-4181, postmenopausal women were randomized to receive combination chemotherapy with or without tamoxifen for 12 months; at the end of 12 months, women originally treated with tamoxifen were randomized to continue tamoxifen or to undergo observation. After a 5 year follow-up the disease-free interval was superior for women receiving tamoxifen for a more prolonged period of time (154). These results are also fraught with two problems: chemotherapy as a confounding factor and comparison of five years of tamoxifen treatment, with one year, which is clearly a suboptimal duration. Two subsequent Swedish studies compared two and five years of tamoxifen in postmenopausal women with tumors ≤ 3 cm in diameter, positive hormone receptors and negative lymph nodes (155). There was only a marginal reduction in recurrence rate for patients treated longer. It should be underlined that this study was limited to patients with excellent prognosis, for whom it would appear very problematic to demonstrate any difference in survival or disease-free survival, especially during the initial years of adjuvant treatment. None of these studies could demonstrate a survival advantage for more prolonged tamoxifen treatment. The power to detect survival differences is clearly low in patients at relative low risk for recurrence of breast cancer and at risk for competitive causes of death, as are many older individuals (67;95).

The final results of the NSABP-B14 (156) trials were recently reported (B.Fisher, Personal Communication, American Society of Clinical Oncology, Philadelphia, PA, May, 1996). This study compared five and ten years of tamoxifen in women with hormone-receptor rich tumors and uninvolved lymph nodes and failed to show any advantage for the more prolonged treatment period. However, the power of the study might have been inadequate to detect small differences. Ongoing clinical trials that explore the value of prolonging the administration of tamoxifen beyond five years include the Scottish Cancer Trials Group (157) that compares 5 and 10 years of tamoxifen, and the ECOG E4181 (154) compares 5 years with a lifetime of tamoxifen treatment. Of these, only the E4181 include women with neoplastic involvement of regional lymph nodes.

While the results of these studies are maturing, the practitioner must decide the optimal duration of tamoxifen treatment in postmenopausal patients on the basis of incomplete data. In our opinion, several factors support prolongation of tamoxifen treatment for at least 5 years, and longer for women with involved lymph nodes. First, virtually all studies showed a reduction in tumor recurrence rate fairly constant in time, among patients treated with tamoxifen (89;156–157), which suggests consistent activity of tamoxifen over time. Second, tamoxifen has additional important health benefits for older women. These include

reduction in the risk of contralateral breast cancer (89), reduction in the rate of osteoporosis development (158–160), improved lipid profile (161–162) and possibly reduction in coronary deaths (163–164).

The Early Breast Cancer Trialists' Cooperative Group meta-analysis reported a 37% reduction in the incidence of contralateral breast cancer among women randomized to adjuvant tamoxifen treatment (89). Similar reductions were also reported in individual trials of long term adjuvant tamoxifen treatment, such as the Stockholm trial (165) and the NSABP-B14 (156).

In the Wisconsin pilot tamoxifen trial, Love et al. reported preservation of the bone density of the radium and improvement of the bone density of the spine for postmenopausal women with breast cancer receiving tamoxifen (158). These observations were reproduced by other authors (159–160) and relieved the concern of many practitioners that tamoxifen might have aggravated postmenopausal osteoporosis because of its antiestrogenic activity.

Love et al. also reported that tamoxifen decreased the concentration of serum cholesterol, VLDL and fibrinogen in postmenopausal women after 6–12 months of treatment (161). Though the concentration of HDL was also decreased by tamoxifen, the VLDL/HDL ratio was maintained in a favorable range. These changes predict a decline in cardiovascular morbidity. Other authors reported similar modifications of the lipid profile (162, 164). A decreased number of fatal myocardial infarctions was observed in the Scottish trial among tamoxifen-treated patients (163).

A decision analysis study (166) explored the cost/effectiveness of prolonged tamoxifen treatment. In most circumstances tamoxifen may prolong the survival of older patients of one year or longer at the cost of approximately $15000.00 per year, which is a very favorable figure when compared to other life-prolonging intervention, such as biennial screening mammography (96).

The possible complications of long-term tamoxifen treatment have been recently reviewed (167). Approximately 5–10% of women do not complete treatment because of discomfort from hot flashes, vaginal discharge, mild nausea, dizziness and lightheadedness. Of these symptoms the most bothersome is hot flashes, in our experience, and these may be relieved by clonidine or lorazepam. Cobleigh proposed simultaneous treatment with tamoxifen and estrogen, to mitigate the disabling symptoms of tamoxifen (168). This idea is interesting for several reasons. Not only would estrogen reduce the postmenopausal symptoms of tamoxifen. They would also increase the level of circulating HDL, which are decreased by tamoxifen, and further reduce the coronary risk of these women. An ongoing ECOG trial explores the feasibility and the safety of this approach. Until completion of the trial the combination treatment does not appear justified. Retinal damage has been reported almost exclusively for doses of tamoxifen of 180 mg/daily, and is very rare for doses ≤ 30 mg/day. At our institution we don't recommend routine eye examination to patients on tamoxifen. The risk of deep vein thrombosis is also low (<1%), though it may increase after age 70 (Bernard Fisher, personal; communication, American Society of Clinical Oncology, Philadelphia, PA, May 1996), and appears related to a decline in circulating antithrombin III.

The major concerns related to long term tamoxifen treatment is carcinogenicity, especially carcinoma of the endometrium (156, 165, 168). Rutqvist et al. reported a six-fold increase in the incidence of endometrial cancer and a twofold increase in the incidence of gastrointestinal cancer (colorectal and gastric) among women treated with 30 or 40 daily mg of tamoxifen for two years respect to untreated controls in Sweden and Denmark (165). It should be underlined that the doses of tamoxifen in this study were noticeably higher than those commonly used. Fisher et al. also found a similarly increased risk of endometrial cancer among women treated with 20 daily mg of tamoxifen for five years or longer (156). This report deserves two comments. First, of several NSABP studies using tamoxifen in the adjuvant setting, only this one found increased incidence of endometrial cancer; the prolonged duration of treatment might have effected this result. Second, the incidence of endometrial cancer in the placebo treated patients was unusually low, approximately half the risk reported by SEER and by previous NSABP studies. This occurrence might have generated an unusually high relative risk for tamoxifen-related endometrial cancer. Of interest, these authors failed to find any increment in other types of cancer. The Early Breast Cancer Trialist Collaborative Group did not find any increase in the risk of any type of cancer for women treated with tamoxifen, in their meta-analysis (89). Endometrial cancer might have been under reported in the trials reviewed, especially in the earliest trials. Of special concern Magriples et al. reported that tamoxifen related-endometrial cancer was particularly aggressive and lethal (169). Most likely, the increased incidence of multiple neoplasms in the Scandinavian study was a random occurrence and did not reflect a real therapeutic risk. Tamoxifen-related endometrial cancer appears as a real risk, to be reckoned with prior to recommending long-term antiestrogenic treatment. The following questions need an answer: does tamoxifen increase the incidence of endometrial cancer? the risk of advanced aggressive endometrial cancer? is this carcinogenic effect a function of treatment duration? These questions were addressed by Jordan in a series of comprehensive reviews (personal communication, ECOG biannual meeting, Denver, Colorado, February 1995, 169, 170). He could find 168 cases of endometrial cancer in tamoxifen-treated women worldwide. The overall relative risk with respect to the SEER data is 1.4. It should be noted however that the SEER population may not represent an appropriate control. Women with breast cancer are already at increased risk of endometrial cancer and the contribution of tamoxifen to this risk may be marginal. In 156 cases the stage of the tumor and in 165 the histologic grade of the tumor was provided. In 80% of tamoxifen-related endometrial cancer and in 79% of

the SEER cases the tumor presented at an early stage (I and II). The incidence of well differentiated and poorly differentiated endometrial cancer was also similar for patients treated with tamoxifen and SEER cases. Thus, the concern that tamoxifen may induce a more aggressive form of cancer may be dismissed. For what concerns treatment duration, the Stockolm experience showed that 13 of the 15 cases of endometrial cancer occurred during the first two years of treatment and only two additional cancers were detected in women randomized to an additional year of tamoxifen. A cluster of endometrial cancers developed during the first two years of treatment. It is even possible to speculate that in some cases tamoxifen precipitates the diagnosis of a preexisting cancer by causing endometrial sloughing and abnormal vaginal bleeding. More data are clearly necessary to establish the risk of tamoxifen-induced endometrial cancer. Given the widespread use of the drug, and the limited number of cancer so far reported, it is unlikely that the risk of endometrial cancer may have a major impact on current practices. We advise women receiving tamoxifen therapy to undergo yearly gynecological examination with transvaginal ultrasound.

Another concern related to prolonged tamoxifen treatment is development of resistance (172). In murine models of mammary carcinoma, Osborne et al. reported that after prolonged treatment with tamoxifen (4–6 months), tamoxifen resistance developed. This was mainly due to an alteration in tamoxifen metabolism which led to a predominance of the weak metabolite cis-hydroxytamoxifen over the powerful antiestrogen trans-hydroxytamoxifen. These experiments also suggested the possibility that tamoxifen itself may start stimulating tumor growth. Circumstantial evidence suggests that tamoxifen resistance may also develop in human tumors. Osborne et al. found a high ratio of tumoral concentrations of cis- and trans-hydroxytamoxfen in tumors resistant to tamoxifen (172). Also, the response of approximately 20% of tamoxifen-resistant breast cancer to tamoxifen withdrawal (173) suggests that tamoxifen may stimulate tumor growth in certain circumstances. Other causes of tamoxifen resistance may include decreased absorption and increased catabolism of tamoxifen after prolonged use (174). The relevance of these observations to long term adjuvant therapy are unknown. Tumor resistance does not appear a significant problem for at least five years, according to the NSABP-B14 (156), the Scottish (163) or the Stockolm trials (165). As data are accruing on more prolonged adjuvant treatment, the questions of tamoxifen resistance should be put into perspective: what is the incidence of this problem? How does it affect the future treatment of metastatic tumor? Does the risk of tamoxifen resistance deny other benefits of prolonged tamoxifen treatment, such as delay in breast cancer recurrence, prevention of osteoporosis, contralateral breast cancer and possibly of coronary deaths? The balance of risk and benefits seems to favor the benefits of long-term treatment. It appears unlikely that tamoxifen resistance may result in higher morbidity than earlier recurrence of breast cancer. Rather, awareness that resistance may develop should stimulate research on how to prevent resistance. This may include the use of different estrogen-antagonists (176) and intermittent treatment.

Recently, the NCI has released a recommendation that adjuvant treatment of breast cancer with tamoxifen be not prolonged beyond five years. This recommendation, which is based on an interim analysis of NSABP-B14 is premature in our opinion. As Peto has observed (Personal communication, Breast Cancer Conference, San Antonio, Texas, December, 1995) NSABP-B14 involved women with receptor-rich tumors and uninvolved lymph node, that is a group of patients with particularly favorable prognosis, in whom it may be difficult to assess differences in mortality, and for whom the benefits of adjuvant therapy may be less evident than in women with more advanced disease.

There is general agreement that the optimal dose of tamoxifen is 20 daily mg, which may be administered as a single dose. A recent report of the EORTC (Piero Mustacchi, Societa' Medica Triestina, Trieste, Italy, December, 13, 1995) suggests that a high induction dose at the beginning of treatment, may be beneficial. These authors randomized women with early breast cancer to receive 20 mg of tamoxifen daily or 160 mg daily for a week followed by 20 mg daily. An interim analysis of this study showed a substantial reduction in distant metastases for the women treated with the induction dose. This issue clearly needs further investigation.

There is very limited information on adjuvant hormonal therapy other than tamoxifen. Jones *et al.* randomized 354 postmenopausal women with node-positive breast cancer to observation or two-year treatment with aminogluthetimide (176). After 8 years of follow-up no benefits in terms of survival or disease-free survival were seen for patients receiving aminoglutethimide.

The issues related to adjuvant chemotherapy involve three questions: is chemotherapy of value to older women? which drugs are effective in older women? which conditions warrant adjuvant chemotherapy? The question whether adjuvant chemotherapy was beneficial to older women was originally proposed by the work of Bonadonna *et al.* (177). Studies initiated more than 20 years ago showed that eight years after diagnosis CMF improved by 11% the disease free survival (DFS) and by 23% the overall survival of premenopausal women with 1–3 lymph nodes involved by cancer, but had no effects in postmenopausal women. Since then, the adjuvant treatment of postmenopausal women with chemotherapy has been controversial.

The Early Breast Cancer Trialists Cooperative Group explored the activity of adjuvant chemotherapy in the meta-analysis (89) (Table 46.10). Clearly, the benefits of adjuvant chemotherapy both in terms of freedom from progression and of survival declined with the patient age, and no benefits were seen in patients aged 70 and

Table 46.10 Reduction in recurrence rate (Re R) and mortality by adjuvant chemotherapy in postmenopausal women with breast cancer.

Age Group	#of Patient	Re R	Mortality
50–59	3128	29% ± 5	13% ± 7
60–69	3874	20% ± 5	10% ± 6
70 +	274	–	–

older. The oldest group of patients represented less than 4% of the total postmenopausal population and this number is too small to draw firm conclusions. The age-related decline in mortality reduction for women aged 50–70 may best be explained by competitive causes of death (67,95); another possible explanation deserves some attention, however, and that is excessive treatment related toxicity. Although clinical trials exclude acute therapeutic toxicity as a major cause of death in older women, information on long term toxicity is scarce and is being collected in ongoing studies. Also of interest, Olivotto *et al.* (178) compared disease free survival and overall survival of breast cancer patients aged 50–89 treated in British Columbia prior to and after the introduction of adjuvant chemotherapy. They found a statistically significant 7% improvement in DFS and 6% improvement of OS at 7 years from the diagnosis. A number of factors, including more widespread use of screening mammography and earlier pursuance of medical attention may have contributed to such improvement. Adjuvant chemotherapy may well have been one of these factors.

The exam of individual clinical trials of adjuvant chemotherapy in postmenopausal women shed some light concerning the most effective agents and the conditions that warrant adjuvant treatment (Tables 46. 11 and 46.12).

Table 46.11 summarizes major clinical trials in postmenopausal women with involvement of axillary lymph nodes. Clearly, only treatment regimens employing doxorubicin (adriamycin) have produced improvement in both disease free and overall survival with some consistency (182–183;188–189). It is important to outline some questions elicited by these trials. The NSABP first explored the value of adriamycin in postmenopausal women in the trials B-11 and B-12. From the result of previous studies, the NSABP has defined as tamoxifen-unresponsive, postmenopausal women aged 50–59 with progesterone-receptor poor tumors, and tamoxifen-responsive all postmenopausal women aged 60 and over and those under 60 with progesterone-receptor rich tumors. In B11, tamoxifen-unresponsive women were randomized to receive melphalan and fluorouracil (PF) or melphalan, adriamycin and fluorouracil (PAF). PAF proved superior to PF both in terms of DFS and overall survival. In B-12, tamoxifen-responsive women were randomized to receive PF and tamoxifen (PFT) or PAF and tamoxifen

Table 46.11 Main clinical trials of adjuvant chemotherapy in postmenopausal women with positive lymph nodes (+LN).

Trial	#	Upper Age	P Characteristics	Regimen(s)	DFS	SUR
NSABP-B07 (179)	1863	70	+LN	P vs PF	32%	27% (8y)
NCCTG (180)	234	75	+LN	CFPvsCFPT vs O	18% (5Y)	–
ECOG (181)	265	65	+LN	CFMP vs CFMPT vs O	ER+: ER–: 18%	– –
ECOG (181)	962	80	+LN	CMFPT × 12 vs CMFPTX4	–	–
NSABP-B11 (182)	281	59	+LN–PR	PF vs PAF	7%	6%
NSABP-B12 (182)	758	70	+LN+PR	PFT vs PAFT	–	–
NSABP-B16 (183)	1245	70	+LN+PR	T vs ACT	17%	10%
GROCTA (184)	267	65	+LN+ER	T vs CMFE vs CMFET	–25%	–12%
GBSG (185)	546	70	+LN	CMF × 3 vs CMF × 6 ± T	–	–
SWOG (186)	214	NS	+LN	P vs CMFVP	14%	12%
SWOG (187)	966	87	+LN	CMFVP vs +ER CMFVPT vs T	–	–
CALGB (188)	723	65	+LN	Cah vs CAi vs CAl	18%	8%
Milan (189)	188	65	≥4+LN	A → CMF vs A/CMF	12%	30%
GABGG (190)	456	65	Low risk High risk	T vs CMFT AC vs ACT	–23% 21%	– 10%
Canada (191)	705	NS	+LN +ER or PR	T vs CMFT	ND	ND
Ludwig III (197)	463	NS	+LN (+) – (–)HR	O vs pT vs CMFpT	20%	8%*

NS = not stated
ND = no difference

Cooperative Groups
GABGG = Gynecological adjuvant Study Group Germany
GROCTA = Gruppo Ricerca Oncologico Chemoterapia Adiuvante
GBSG = German Breast Cancer Study Group
CALGB = Cancer Acute Leukemia Group B
ECOG = Eastern Cooperative Oncology Group
NCCTG = North Central Cancer Treatment Group
NSABP = National Surgical Adjuvant Breast and Bowel Project.
SWOG = South West Oncology Group

Treatment regimens
A → CMF = Adriamycin followed by Cyclophosphamide, Methotrexate, Fluorouracil
A/CMF = Adriamycin alternated with Cyclophosphamide, Methotrexate, Fluorouracil
ACT = Adriamycin, Cyclophosphamide, Tamoxifen
CAh = Cyclophosphamide, Adriamycin, high dose intensity
CAi = Cyclophosphamide, Adriamycin, intermediate dose intensity
CAl = Cyclophosphamide, Adriamycin, low dose intensity
CFMP = Cyclophosphamide, Fluorouracil, Methotrexate, Prednisone
CFMPT = Cyclophosphamide, Fluorouracil, Methotrexate, Prednisone, Tamoxifen
CFP = Cyclophosphamide, Fluorouracil, Prednisone
CFPT = Cyclophosphamide, Fluorouracil, Prednisone, Tamoxifen
CMF = Cyclophosphamide, Methotrexate, Fluorouracil
CMFE = Cyclophosphamide, Methotrexate, Fluorouracil, Epirubicin
CMFET = Cyclophosphamide, Methotrexate, Fluorouracil, Epirubicin, Tamoxifen.
CMFpT = Cyclophosphamide, Methotrexate, Fluorouracil prednisone, Tamoxifen.
CMFVP = Cyclophosphamide, Methotrexate, Fluorouracil, Vincristine, Prednisone
CMFVPT = Cyclophosphamide, Methotrexate, Fluorouracil, Vincristine, Prednisone, Tamoxifen.
O = Observation.
P = Melphalan
PAF = Melphalan, Adriamycin, Fluorouracil
PAFT = Malphalan, Adriamycin, Fluorouracil, Tamoxifen
PF = Melphalan/Fluorouracil
PFT = Melphalan, Fluorouracil, Tamoxifen
pT = Prednisone, tamoxifen
T = Tamoxifen

*survival advantage limited to HR poor tumors

Table 46.12 Randomized clinical trials of adjuvant chemotherapy in postmenopausal women: node (–) patients.

Study	Patient #	Upper Age	Characteristics	Regimen	Outcome DFS	S
Milan Node (–) (192)	90	65	–LN; –ER	CMF vs O	40%	28%
NSABP-B13 (193)	280	60	–LN; –ER	O vs M → F	17%	14%
Intergroup (194)	153	70	–LN	O vs CMFP	12%	–

NSABP = National Surgical Adjuvant Breast and Bowel Project

CMF = Cyclophosphamide, Methotrexate, Fluorouracil

CMFP = Cyclophosphamide, Methotrexate, Fluorouracil, Prednisone.

M → F = Sequential Methotrexate Fluorouracil

O = Observation

(PAFT). The addition of adriamycin did not appear beneficial to these patients. In a subsequent trial, however (B-16) (183), tamoxifen-responsive women were randomized to receive adriamycin, cyclophosphamide and tamoxifen (ACT), and tamoxifen alone (T). In B16, ACT was superior to T both in terms of disease free and overall survival. There is an apparent discrepancy between the results of B-12 and B-16. One may ask why the ACT combination was not compared to PFT rather than to tamoxifen alone. There were two main reasons for the design of B-16. First, it was important to establish whether the combination of chemotherapy and tamoxifen was superior to tamoxifen alone in this group of women. Second, it was important to try a combination of chemotherapy of shorter duration and lesser toxicity than PF. PF was administered for 17 treatment cycles and AC only for four. The question whether PF is comparable to AC is a moot question, as AC proved to be much more manageable. The CALGB compared high (60/m2 and 600/m2), intermediate (40/m2 and 400/m2) and low (30/m2 and 300/m2) doses of adriamycin and cyclophosphamide in breast cancer patients with positive axillary lymph-nodes (188). The highest doses were administered for a total of 4 courses of treatment; the intermediate and low doses for six courses. Both high and intermediate doses were superior to low doses in both pre and postmenopausal women. High doses of chemotherapy were superior to intermediate doses for patients with high tumoral expression of the c-erb-2 oncogene (196). From our standpoint this study is important as it demonstrates the benefit of adjuvant adriamycin-containing combination chemotherapy in postmenopausal women.

Bonadonna et al. compared adriamycin at 75mg/m2 for three courses followed by six courses of CMF with adriamycin at the same doses, alternated with CMF (189). They demonstrated the superiority of the sequential over the alternate treatment both in pre and postmenopausal women with 4–8 lymph nodes positive for breast cancer. The main aims of the study were to prove the validity of the theoretical principle "best drug first" in clinical practice and to demonstrate the benefits of adjuvant chemotherapy in women with more than three axillary lymph-nodes involved by the tumor. From our standpoint the study proves once more the value of doxorubicin-based adjuvant chemotherapy in postmenopausal women.

Of interest is also the GABSG study (190); these investigators divided patients into "low risk" (1–3 involved lymph nodes, ER and/or PR positive) and "high risk" (≥4 positive lymph nodes or 1–3 positive lymph nodes and negative ER and/or PR). In low risk patients, tamoxifen proved superior to CMF chemotherapy; in high risk patients the combination of doxorubicin, cyclophosphamide and tamoxifen was superior to doxorubicin/cyclophosphamide without tamoxifen.

Only one study, which was carried out in Italy (183), failed to demonstrate the advantages of an anthracycline in the adjuvant treatment of postmenopausal women. In fact, Boccardo et al. found that a combination of cyclophosphamide, fluorouracil, methotrexate and epirubicin (CFME), resulted in poorer disease free and overall survival than tamoxifen alone or CFME plus tamoxifen (CFMET). The findings of this well controlled study are disturbing; the lack of benefits of chemotherapy may be explained to some extent by the design of the treatment program, with epirubicin being given after 6 courses of CMF; in other words the design contradicted the principle of the "best drug first." It is also possible that the significant toxicity of chemotherapy prevented the administration of effective dose/intensity of the drugs.

The SWOG investigators run two subsequent studies in postmenopausal women. In the first study (186) women were randomized to melphalan for two years or CMFVP for one year. The combination appeared superior to single agent melphalan both in terms of disease free and overall survival. In the second study, which included only women with tumors rich in hormone receptors, these investigators compared tamoxifen and CMFVP plus tamoxifen and found that the chemotherapy did not enhance the benefits of tamoxifen.

With the exception of the PF regimen in NSABP-B07 (178) of the fist SWOG study, and of the Ludwig III study (197) no other drug combination excluding doxorubicin proved conclusively active in the adjuvant treatment of postmenopausal women with positive lymphnodes. The results of B-07 should be scrutinized very carefully. This is an old study, published first in 1977, in which patients were divided by age (under 50 and 50 and over) rather than by menopausal status. Probably only a handful of those women were older than 60. It is possible that the benefits seen in B-07 concern mainly old premenopausal women. Likewise, the first SWOG study was also an old study, with a relatively small population of patients, in many of whom the value of hormone receptor was unknown. The subsequent study of this group denied the benefit of adjuvant chemotherapy, at least in the case of hormone receptor-rich tumors. The Ludwig III study is a relatively small study (456 patients), comparing observation, prednisone and tamoxifen, and cyclophosphamide, fluorouracil, methotrexate, prednisone and tamoxifen: after 13 year of follow-up a small survival advantage emerged, but limited to women with hormone-receptor poor tumors. One may question the validity of a subset analysis in a three arm study with a limited patient sample.

The situation of women with negative lymph nodes is even less clear (Table 46.2). The Milan node (–) study (192) reported an improvement of survival for postmenopausal women with negative lymph nodes, but this study had two major flaws: the small number of patients and the inadequate patient selection. The only adverse prognostic factor recognized in that old study was absence of estrogen receptors: no consideration was given to nuclear grade, tumor size, and more recently identified prognostic factors, such as tumor cell proliferation, c-erb-2 concentration, and neovascularization. It is very possible that the marked survival differences resulted from the accidental comparison of different patient populations and not from the effects of treatment. A recent update of NSABP B-13 study (193–194) indicates a small advantage in overall survival for postmenopausal women with node (–) tumor who received adjuvant chemotherapy with methotrexate and fluorouracil. The Intergroup study reported improved disease free survival but not overall survival with CMF. It is very possible that no difference in survival has emerged yet due to the low number of cancer-related deaths expected in the controls, in this patient population with a relatively good prognosis. Thus, adriamycin may not be required in node-negative postmenopausal women.

An important consideration related to these trials of postmenopausal women concerns the under representation of women over 70, who were included only in the SWOG trial (186), a trial which failed to demonstrate the benefits of adjuvant chemotherapy.

From the preceding discussion one can draw the following conclusions:

• Adjuvant chemotherapy containing adriamycin may prolong both disease free and overall survival of postmenopausal women with positive lymph nodes. The most effective of these regimens has not been established; at our institution we prefer to use the

AC combination of the NSABP (183), which involves doxorubicin 60/m2 IV and cyclophosphamide 600/m2 IV every three weeks for a total of four courses. Even for patients in their 70s we found this regimen very tolerable.
• Non-doxorubicin based combination chemotherapy may improve the prognosis of node (–) patients, as it may delay disease recurrence and possibly improve the overall survival.
• Non doxorubicin-based combination chemotherapy represents a valid alternative for node (+) patients with tumors poor in hormone receptors who cannot tolerate doxorubicin. These regimens may prolong the disease free survival of the patients.

More information is needed in women over 70; until the time this information is accrued, it is reasonable to treat the oldest women like other postmenopausal women as long as coexisting conditions don't enhance the risk of treatment toxicity or limit the patients' life-expectancy to one year or less.

Seemingly, the main benefit of adjuvant chemotherapy in older women may be prolongation of the disease-free survival; it is important to ask whether this prolongation results into a quality of life improvement. Gelber et al. (197) devised a quality of life-assessing instrument to address this problem. The TWiST (Time without symptoms and treatment) is currently used by the International Breast Cancer Study Group, and assesses quality of life as the time during which the patient is not bothered by symptoms of cancer or by the inconvenience and the complications of treatment. These authors found that most patients achieve a substantial gain in quality of life from adjuvant chemotherapy even when there is no appreciable survival gain. In other words, the delay in breast cancer recurrence is worthy the transient symptoms of adjuvant treatment. The main advantage of TWiST is to be an objective measurement. The main disadvantage is also to be an objective measurement, unable to accommodate individual reactions to treatment. Altogether we believe that the TWiST reflects faithfully the reactions of most patients with early breast cancer and validates the benefits of adjuvant chemotherapy when a prolongation of survival is not clearly evident.

As doxorubicin has a central role in the adjuvant treatment of postmenopausal patients, concern about cardiotoxic complications in women aged 70 and older may arise. These women appear more susceptible to anthracycline-related cardiotoxicity (198). The use of the cardioprotector desrazoxane (199) or the substitution of doxorubicin with mitoxantrone (200) may be considered. Clinical trials employing these compounds in postmenopausal women, especially in the population over 70, appear advisable.

The more widespread use of adjuvant chemotherapy in older women may involve a substantial increase in treatment cost. Desch et al. have studied the cost and cost/effectiveness of adjuvant chemotherapy in elderly women with node (–) breast cancer (201). As expected, they found that the cost increases and the effectiveness decreases with the patient age: for example, the cost for 1 year of quality/adjusted life would be $28200 for a 60 year old; $44400 for a 75 year old, and $57100 for a 80 year old. These figures should not discourage the use of adjuvant therapy, but should rather stimulate definition of criteria for a better patient selection, so that only patients at high risk for recurrence and low risk of treatment complications, enter the chemotherapy program.

Stage III Disease

Stage III A

The standard treatment of Stage IIIA breast cancer involves surgery, which generally requires mastectomy, followed by adjuvant chemotherapy and, in the majority of cases, adjuvant irradiation. A number of investigators have explored the feasibility to treat these patients with neoadjuvant chemotherapy (202–204). The theoretical advantages of this approach include "in vivo" documentation of tumor chemosensitivity, earlier treatment of micro metastatic disease, prior to development of multidrug resistance, treatment of patients in better general conditions and more able to tolerate dose/intensive chemotherapy, possibility of breast-conserving surgery from reduction of the size of the primary tumor. The main potential disadvantage is inadequate surgical staging (205).

Stage III B

The management of stage III B breast cancer involves the combination of chemotherapy, generally administered as initial treatment, followed by mastectomy and chest wall irradiation. With this approach a 5 year survival of 30–40% is obtainable (206–207). Chemotherapy is critical in the management of stage IIIB breast cancer. Prior to chemotherapy the 5 year survival with local treatment only was less than 5% (208). In the majority of cases combination chemotherapy involves an anthracycline (doxorubicin or epirubicin); the role of new drugs such as mitoxantrone, paclitaxel, docetaxel, and navelbine is not established yet. An ongoing clinical trial at the University of South Florida/H Lee Moffitt Cancer Center, explores induction therapy with high dose mitoxantrone and maintenance treatment with paclitaxel and navelbine, in women aged 65 and older. The rationale of this trial is to obtain adequate cancer control with less myelotoxicity and cardiotoxicity. Generally, inflammatory breast cancer is poor in hormone receptor, and tamoxifen or other hormonal manipulations are not indicated. In the presence of hormone receptor rich tumors, hormonal therapy should be added to combination chemotherapy.

Stage IV breast cancer

The management of metastatic breast cancer is tailored to the location of the metastases and the hormone-responsiveness of the tumor.

The location of the metastases is important for several reasons, such as tumor sanctuaries, risk of local complications, management of single recurrence to the chest walls, and specific life expectancy. Tumor sanctuaries include the central nervous system and possi-

bly the eye. Metastases to the brain are treated with surgical excision and radiotherapy when single; with radiotherapy when multiple; spinal metastases are treated with radiotherapy; the treatment of meningeal metastases which may cause neoplastic meningitis, includes intrathecal administration of cytotoxic agents such as methotrexate, cytarabine or tiothepa; radiation therapy is reserved for chemotherapy-resistant tumors. The management of retinal and choroidal metastases is controversial. Although many authors advocate radiotherapy, as the penetration of systemic treatment in these areas is unpredictable, there are reports of good responses to systemic treatment (209). When the patient is asymptomatic, the risk of retinal detachment is not imminent and the patients general conditions allow it, we prefer to use systemic treatment first, to provide systemic coverage of metastatic cancer and to prevent radiation toxicity to the eye. Close ophthalmological follow-up is imperative in these circumstances.

Local complications may be seen with metastases to the long bones, to the spine and to the skin. Metastases to the long bones involve the risk of pathological fractures, whereas metastases to the spine may involve the risk of spinal cord compression. Whenever 50% or more of the cortex of the long bones is involved by tumor, emergent orthopedic fixation of the bone is indicated (210). While waiting for surgery, the patient should be instructed not to bear weight with the bone at risk; the use of crutches or of a wheelchair is highly recommended. Painful metastases to the spine should be evaluated with myelogram or MRI; in the presence of epidural extension, emergency radiation therapy and steroid treatment are indicated.

Metastases to the skin may grow into fungating and ulcerative tumors: timely and aggressive local management of skin metastases resistant to systemic treatment with surgery and radiation therapy may prevent this dreadful complication.

Single chest wall metastases require both local and systemic treatment (211–213; 89). Local treatment involves surgery, when feasible, or radiation therapy. The duration of systemic treatment is not definitely established. We choose to administer hormonal therapy for at least five years for hormone-receptor-rich tumors, and six courses of chemotherapy, for hormone-receptor-poor tumors. With this approach, more than 50% of patients are alive and free of disease five years from the time of chest wall recurrence (211–213).

Metastases to different organs imply different life-expectancies (87). For example, hepatic metastases, or lymphangitic metastases to the lung are associated with a short median survival (3–6 months), when untreated. In these circumstances the use of hormonal therapy may be inappropriate, even for hormone-sensitive tumors, because responses to endocrine therapy are seen after 6 weeks of treatment or longer. Bone, skin, and nodular lung metastases, on the other side, are associated with a survival longer than 2 years.

The hormone-responsiveness of a tumor is determined by the concentration of hormone-receptors (214). Responses to frontline hormonal treatment as high as 80% may be seen in tumors rich both in estrogen and

Table 46.13 Hormonal agents for the treatment of metastatic breast cancer.

Class	Doses	Complications
Estrogen Antagonists		
Tamoxifen	20 mg qd	Hot flashes
		Vaginal secretions
		DVT
		Retinopathy
		Hypercalcemia*
Progestins		
Megestrol Acetate	40 mg qid	Weight gain
		Nausea
		Fluid retention
Aromatase Inhibitors		
Aminoglutethimide	250 mg bid+	Somnolence
		Skin rash
		Hypoadrenalism
Estrogens		
Diethylstilbestrol	5 mg tid	DVT
		Fluid retention
		Hypercalcemia*
Androgens		
Halotestin	10 mg tid	Virilization
		Fluid retention

DVT = Deep vein thrombosis

* In patients with bony metastases

+ Always combine with hydrcortisone 20mg bid.

progesterone receptors; the response rate of tumors which are rich in only one of the two types of receptors is around 30–50%. Tumors poor in both estrogen and progesterone receptors may be responsive to tamoxifen, in 15–20% of cases, as some of the antineoplastic effects of tamoxifen are independent from estrogen antagonism.

The hormonal treatment of breast cancer in the older woman includes the agents listed in Table 46.13 (1, 214). Estrogens in high doses, which act as estrogen antagonists, and androgens are now seldom used, due to toxicity. They may have a role in patients who require symptom palliation, have failed other forms of hormonal treatment and are not good chemotherapy candidate. The administration of tamoxifen as a daily dose is more convenient especially for older individuals and equally effective as in divided doses (215). Higher doses of progestins have been tried with substantial increase in toxicity, but no improvement in antineoplastic activity (216). Two new aromatase inhibitor, 4-hydroxy androstendione and letrozol, are undergoing clinical trials with very promising results:

they appear much more active and less toxic than aminoglutethimide (217). In particular, they do not cause hypoadrenalism and consequently do not require replacement therapy with corticosteroids. As frontline hormonal agents, both megestrol acetate and aminoglutethimide have an activity comparable to that of tamoxifen (218–219). Aminoglutethimide may be preferable in patients with bone metastases (218). The combination of two hormonal agents does not appear more effective than single drugs, and is not recommended (220).

Cytotoxic chemotherapy of breast cancer involves a number of drugs or drug combinations (221–222). Some of the most popular regimens are listed in Table 46.14. Generally, CMF, CAF or CNF are chosen as initial treatment. In patients who did not receive doxorubicin in the adjuvant setting we prefer to use CNF to CAF. The antineoplastic activity of both regimens is similar and is somewhat superior to CMF (223–224), but CNF is better tolerated in terms of nausea, alopecia, cardiotoxicity and possibly myelotoxicity. Anthracycline induced myelotoxicity and cardiotoxicity are of special concern in the aged, as the incidence of these complications increases with the age of the population. We like to treat women aged 65 and older with a hemopoietic growth factor, either G-CSF or GM-CSF. In this patient population both the incidence of neutropenic infection and the risk of dying from infection is higher than in younger women (225).

The combination of doxorubicin and a taxane appears very promising. Gianni *et al.* reported an astounding 41% CR rate in women treated with paclitaxel and doxorubicin (226), and this combination was active also in women who had previously received an anthracycline. Unfortunately, the incidence of cardiotoxicity was prohibitively high (75% of patients experienced a decline in the left ventricular ejection fraction measured by radionuclide angiography). This interesting combination cannot be recommended to older women, until the issue of cardiotoxicity is addressed. Interestingly, docetaxel and doxorubicin produced also a very high response rate, but with substantially less cardiotoxicity (227).

Several drugs and drug combinations have proved effective as second line chemotherapy, with a response rate of 30–35% (Table 46.14). We have found weekly navelbine well tolerated by older women, even without the addition of growth factors. The combination of methotrexate/fluorouracil (Larry Norton, personal communication), and infusional fluorouracil (Charles Vogel, personal communication) are also of interest because they appear to cause minimal myelotoxicity. Mucosal toxicity, however, which is generally more severe in older individuals, may be dose-limiting (198).

How well do older breast cancer patients tolerate combination chemotherapy? Three studies have addressed this question (228–230). Gelman and Taylor compared the effectiveness and toxicity of CMF in women younger than 65 and in older patients. In older patients they modified the doses of methotrexate and cyclophosphamide according to the patient's creatinine clearance. They found that the response rate was simi-

Table 46.14 Common combinations of cytotoxic chemotherapy in metastatic breast cancer.

Drugs	Doses (m2 BSA)	Interval
Cyclophosphamide	100 day 1–14 p.o.	
Methotrexate	40 day1&8 I.V.	28 days
Fluorouracil	600 day 1&8 I.V.	
Cyclophosphamide	500 day 1 I.V.	
Adriamycin	50 day 1 I.V.	21 days
Fluorouracil	500 day 1 I.V.	
Cyclophosphamide	500 day 1 I.V.	
Novantrone	10 day 1 I.V.	21 days
Fluorouracil	500 day 1 I.V.	
Methotrexate	160 day 1 I.V.	
Fluorouracil	600 day 2 I.V.	14 days
Leucovorin	25 q6h p.o. x6 start 24 hrs after methotrexate	
Fluorouracil	200 day1–24 CIVI	42 days
Paclitaxel	125 day 1 3 h infusion	21 days
Doxorubicin	60 day 1	
Docetaxel		
Doxorubicin		
Paclitaxel	220 day 1 I.V.	21 days
Docetaxel	75 day 1 I.V.	21 days
Navelbine	30 day 1 I.V.	weekly
Mitomycin C	10 day 1 I.V.	28–42 days

CIVI= continuous IV infusion

I.V.= intravenously

p.o.= orally

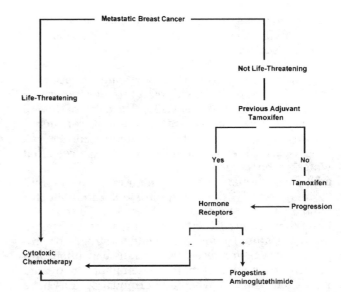

Figure 46.9 Our current approach to the treatment of metastatic breast cancer in older women.

lar in the two groups of patients, but the incidence and severity of myelotoxicity were lower for the older patients (228).

Christman *et al.* compared the response to chemotherapy and the incidence of complications among three groups of women, subdivided by age, treated according various protocols of the Piedmont Oncology Group and found no difference between the women younger than 45 and those older than 65 (229). Ibrahim *et al.* compared response rate and toxicity of chemotherapy in younger and older women treated at the M D Anderson Cancer Center in Houston and again they could not demonstrate age-related differences (230). These results should be looked at with caution for two reasons. First, the subjects of these studies were enrolled in clinical trials, in virtue of their excellent general conditions. They may not represent the majority of older individuals. Second, very few of the patients were aged 80 and older. For practical purposes there is no information concerning chemotherapy in the oldest old.

In addition to the use of growth factors to prevent myelotoxicity, two other recent advances may ameliorate the toxicity of chemotherapy in older women. These involve the cardiotoxicity of the anthracyclines, whose incidence increases with age (198). Cardiotoxicity may be lessened with the administration of desrazoxane (231), or with the use of liposomal doxorubicin (232). Desrazoxane is a free radical scavenger that was studied in a randomized placebo-controlled trial in patients with metastatic breast cancer. Those patients who received desrazoxane were able to receive a substantially higher total dose of doxorubicin with a substantially lower incidence of cardiotoxicity (231). The exact timing of desrazoxane therapy is controversial (198). The current recommendation to institute desrazoxane treatment after a total dose of doxorubicin of 300 mg/square meter of body surface area, stems from two considerations: cardiotoxicity is minimal at lower doses of doxorubicin and there is some concern, probably unfunded, that desrazoxane may prevent the antineoplastic activity of the drug during the early phases of treatment (198). Liposomal doxorubicin is associated with lower risk of cardiotoxicity, due to the slow release of the drug. Currently, the experience with liposomal doxorubicin in breast cancer is extremely limited.

Our most common treatment strategy for women aged 65 and older is illustrated in Figure 46.9. If the patient has life-threatening metastases, defined as lymphangitic metastases to the lung, or hepatic metastases involving more than 50% of the liver parenchyma, we use chemotherapy as frontline treatment. We treat all other patients with tamoxifen, irrespective of receptor-status, unless metastatic disease developed during adjuvant treatment with tamoxifen or within one year from cessation of such treatment. Our approach is supported by two studies. Taylor *et al.* showed that women over 65 may be treated initially with tamoxifen, irrespective of receptor status, as approximately 20% of patients with receptor-poor tumor will respond to such a treatment (233). The delay of chemotherapy in unresponsive patients was approximately 3 months and did not affect the patient overall survival. Muss *et al.* (234) and Fourander *et al.* (235) showed that women who experience recurrence after cessation of adjuvant treatment with tamoxifen may still respond to this agent. Patients who are not candidate for tamoxifen and patients who progress while receiving tamoxifen receive further treatment according to receptor status. Tumors rich in either estrogen or progesterone receptor receive progestins and upon progression aminogluthetimide. These tumors are treated with chemotherapy when all hormonal options have been exhausted. Tumors poor in both type of hormone receptors are treated with chemotherapy.

The only situations in which we may use a combination of chemotherapy and hormones is life-threatening metastases from receptor-rich tumors. In all other circumstances we avoid the simultaneous use of chemotherapy and hormones. This combination was not proven superior to either modality alone and may augment the cost and the complications of treatment (236).

Symptom palliation is an important part of the management of metastatic disease. Bone metastases may be excruciatingly painful. Several options exist when systemic treatment fails. These include external beam irradiation, radioactive strontium and diphosphonates. External beam irradiation is the simpler form of treatment of isolated painful bone metastases. Radioactive strontium is effective in controlling for 4–6 months the pain from multiple bone metastases is approximately 50% of cases (237). Diphosphonates are used mainly as adjuvant pain treatment in combination with other treatment modalities. Of the diphosphonates available in the USA, pamidronate is the most effective. At doses of 60–90 mg daily every three-four week pamidronate may help approximately 30% of patients with painful bony metastases (238).

Summary

In this section we will summarize the most important items of breast cancer in the older women and we will propose a research agenda.

Epidemiology

The incidence of breast cancer increases with age up to age 80 and plateaus thereafter. There may be a decline after age 85. Preliminary autopsy data suggest that the incidence of occult breast cancer declines after age 60.

The most important questions of future research concern:

- Real incidence of breast cancer in the oldest old.

- Mortality and morbidity of breast cancer in the oldest old.
- Incidence and prevalence of occult breast cancer after age 60. The answer to this question may have heavy impact on future screening practices.

Biology

The prevalence of cancers with less aggressive characteristics (high hormone receptor concentration, low histologic grade, low proliferation) increases with age. There is also evidence that the growth of breast cancer may be delayed in the older organism. In view of these findings screening mammography may be performed at longer interval in older than in younger women.

Important research questions include:

- Mechanisms that control the tumor growth in older individuals, with particular attention to IGF-1, IGF-1 Binding Proteins, IL-6, and TGF-beta.
- Mechanisms by which immunesenescense may delay tumor growth in older individuals.
- Predictive value of immunesenescense and host-derived growth factors on the outcome of breast cancer at different stages.

Prevention

A. Primary prevention

Primary prevention of breast cancer may involve abstinence from alcohol or only moderate consumption (< 3 daily ounces), and weight loss for persons who have an android type of obesity.

Of particular concern is hormone replacement therapy (HRT). Though HRT is definitely associated with breast cancer, we don't recommend avoidance of HRT, whose benefits seem to grossly outweigh the risks. We recommend the following however:

- Estrogen replacement seems preferable to the combination of estrogen and progestins, for what concerns the risk of breast cancer.
- For women who are not bothered by hot flushes, vaginal dryness, or depression, low doses of estrogen (equivalent to $\leq .625$ mg conjugated estrogen daily) may be adequate.
- HRT for a limited period of time (5–10 years post-menopausal)may be considered.

Important research issues include:

- Value of a diet low in fat in the prevention of breast cancer.
- Risks of HRT in women with family history of breast cancer.
- Durability of the benefits of HRT of limited duration on bones and coronary arteries.
- Chemoprevention of breast cancer with tamoxifen, retinoids, oltripaz and other substances.

B. Secondary prevention (screening)

The practice of screening women for breast cancer with serial mammograms and physical examinations of the breast has resulted in a 20–30% decline in breast cancer-related mortality for women aged 50–70. One start seeing the benefits of screening 3–7 years after the initial examination. According to the BCCDP study, the physical examination of the breast missed approximately 11% of the breast cancers detected at mammography, according to the Canadian study, the two examinations were approximately equivalent. Mammography at two year and at one year intervals yielded comparative results. The ideal number of mammographic examinations has not been established.

We recommend that all women be screened for breast cancer, irrespective of age, when the life expectancy is three years or longer.

As screening methods for women over 65 we recommend:

- Physical examination of the breast at each clinic visit.
- Mammography every two years.

Important research issues involve:

- Comparison of the predictive values of physical breast exam and mammography in older women.
- Incidence of new breast cancers detected at mammography after age 65, to determine the ideal number of mammograms that should be performed.
- Value of molecular screening in older women.

Treatment

A. Local disease (stages I & II)

The treatment of local disease is a multidisciplinary endeavor involving surgery, radiation therapy and systemic treatment.

In terms of local control, total mastectomy and partial mastectomy with postoperative irradiation have yielded similar results. Axillary dissection is part of current practice, to eliminate local disease, to establish the prognosis of the patients, to establish which patients are candidate for systemic adjuvant treatment and for irradiation of the chest wall. The identification of the "sentinel node" may help identify in the future patients who necessitate a full nodal dissection and may spare the morbidity of this treatment to the majority of patients. Systemic adjuvant treatment with tamoxifen and with chemotherapy may be indicated according to the circumstances. Adjuvant tamoxifen is beneficial for women with hormone receptor rich tumors; adjuvant chemotherapy is beneficial in terms of disease-free and overall survival for postmenopausal women up to age 70 who have positive lymph node, or negative lymph nodes and a tumor with the largest diameter ≥1 cm which is receptor poor. The benefits of adjuvant chemotherapy after age 70 have not been established.

As the rate of local recurrence may decline with the age of the patients, postoperative irradiation may not be necessary after partial mastectomy in older women, but it is difficult to establish a subgroup of patients in whom this practice may be forgone. Clearly, postoperative irradiation may be avoided for women over 55 when:

- The tumor has a largest diameter ≤2.5 cm
- There is minimal or no DCIS component.
- The surgical procedure was a quadrantectomy.
- In all other cases the treatment needs to be individualized according to patient preferences.

For what concerns adjuvant systemic treatment we adhere to the recommendations of the St Gallien conference (Table 46.8). The duration of tamoxifen treatment should be 5 years and possibly longer especially in women with involved lymph nodes. Adjuvant chemotherapy should involve doxorubicin or another anthracycline in women with positive lymph nodes.

Important research issues involve:

- Definition of subgroups of patients for whom breast irradiation may be avoided after partial mastectomy.
- Optimal duration of adjuvant tamoxifen treatment, including potential benefits on morbidity and mortality unrelated to breast cancer (osteoporosis, coronary artery diseases, contralateral breast cancer).
- Adjuvant chemotherapy of women aged ≥70.
- Role of mitoxantrone, taxanes and navelbine in the adjuvant treatment of postmenopausal women.

B. Advanced disease (stage IV)

The management of advanced disease involves systemic treatment and palliative treatment.

We recommend a trial of tamoxifen in all women who don't have life-threatening disease (lymphangitic lung metastases, hepatic metastases) irrespective of receptor status. Upon tamoxifen failure we recommend progestin and aromatase inhibitor in the presence of hormone-receptor rich tumor, and chemotherapy for receptor-poor tumors or receptor-rich tumors which have failed all hormonal options.

In our experience, a combination of cyclophosphamide, mitoxantrone and fluorouracil, navelbine as single agent and intermediate doses of methotrexate, with fluorouracil and leucovorin have been well tolerated by older individuals. The introduction of the cardioprotector desrazoxane and of liposomal doxorubicin may improve the tolerance of doxorubicin by older individuals with breast cancer.

References

1. Balducci L, Schapira DV, Cox CE, et al. Breast Cancer in the Older Woman: an Annotated Review. *J Am Ger Soc* 1991; **39**: 1113–1123.
2. Silliman RA, Balducci L, Goodwin J, et al. Breast cancer and old age: what we know, don't know, and do. *J Natl Cancer Inst* 1993; **85**: 190–199.
3. Balducci L, Lyman GH, Schapira DV. Trends in prevention and treatment of breast cancer in the older woman. In *Facts and Research in Gerontology*, edited by BJ Vellas, JL Albarede, PJ Garry. New York: Serdi Publishing Company, 179–192, 1994.
4. de Graaf H, Willemse PHB, Sleijfer DT. Review: breast cancer in elderly patients. *Age and Aging* 1994; **23**: 427–434.
5. Balducci L, Greenberg H. Breast cancer in the older woman: Therapeutic controversies. *Cancer Control* 1994; **1**, 350–356.
6. Yancik R, Ries LA. Cancer in older persons: magnitude of the problem. *Cancer* 1994; **74**: 1995–2003.

7. La Vecchia C, Franceschi S. International Variations and Trends in the incidence of cancer in older women. *Cancer Control* 1994; **1**: 327–333.

8. Stanta G. Morbid Anatomy of Age. In *Comprehensive Geriatric Oncology*, edited by L Balducci, GH Lyman, WB Ershler. London, England: Harwood Academic Press, 229–235, 1997.

9. Madigan MP, Ziegler RG, Benichou J, *et al*. Proportion of breast cancer cases in the United States explained by well established risk factors. *J Natl Cancer Inst* 1995; **87**: 1681–1685.

10. Goldstein AM, Amos CI. Segregation analysis of breast cancer from the cancer and steroid hormone study: histologic subtypes. *J Natl Cancer Inst* 1990; **82** 1911–1917.

11. Lynch HT, Watson P, Conway TA, *et al*. Clinical/genetic features in hereditary breast cancer. *Breast Cancer Res Treat* 1990; **15**: 63–71.

12. Knudson AG Jr. Hereditary cancers: from discovery to intervention. Monographs, *J Natl Cancer Inst* 1995; **17**: 5–7.

13. Peters J. Breast Cancer Genetics. Relevance to Oncology Practice. *Cancer Control* 1995; **2**: 195–208.

14. Shattuck-Eidens D, McClure M, Simard J, *et al*. A collaborative survey of 80 mutations in the BRCA1 breast and ovarian cancer susceptibility gene. *JAMA* 1995; **273**: 535–541.

15. Easton DF, Bishop DT, Ford D, *et al*. Genetic linkage analysis in familial breast and ovarian cancer: results from 214 families: the Breast cancer Linkage Consortium. *Am J Hum Gen* 1993; **52**: 678–701.

16. Goldgar DE, Neuhausen SL, Steele L, *et al*. A 45 year follow-up of kindred 107 and the search for BRCA2. Monographs, *J Natl Cancer Inst* 1995; **17**: 15–19.

17. Holtzman NA. Scale-up technology: moving predictive tests for inherited breast, ovarian, and colon cancers. From the bench to the bedside and beyond. Monographs. *J Natl Cancer Inst* 1995; **17**: 91–94.

18. Dupont WD, Page DL. Menopausal estrogen replacement therapy and breast cancer. *Arch Int Med* 1991; **151**: 67–72.

19. Colditz GA, Egan KM, Stampfer MJ. Hormone replacement therapy and risk of breast cancer: results from epidemiologic studies. *Am J Obstet Gynecol* 1993; **168**: 1473–1480.

20. Nabulsi AA, Folsom AR, White A, *et al*. Association of hormone-replacement therapy with various cardiovascular risk factors in postmenopausal women. *N Engl J Med* 1993; **328**: 1069–1075.

21. Ewertz M. Influence of non-contraceptive exogenous and endogenous sex hormones on breast cancer risk in Denmark. *Int J Cancer* 1988; **42**: 832–838.

22. Kaufman DW, Palmer JR, deMonzon J, *et al*. Estrogen replacement therapy and the risk of breast cancer: results from the case-control surveillance study. *Am J Epidemiol* 1991; **134**: 1375–1385.

23. Palmer JR, Roenberg L, Clarke EA, *et al*. Breast cancer study after estrogen replacement therapy: results from the Toronto Breast Cancer Study. *Am J Epidemiol* 1991; **34**: 1386–1395.

24. Yang CP, Daling JR, Band PR *et al*. Noncontraceptive hormone use and risk of breast cancer. *Cancer Causes Control* 1992; **3**: 475–479.

25. Stanford JL, Weiss NS, Voigt LF, *et al*. Combined estrogen and progestin hormone replacement therapy in relation to risk of breast cancer in middle-aged women. *JAMA* 1995: **274**: 137–142.

26. Bergkvist L, Adami H-O, Persson I, *et al*. The risk of breast cancer after estrogen and estrogen-progestin replacement. *N Engl J Med* 1989; **321**: 293–297.

27. Hunt K, Vessey M, McPherson K, *et al*. Long-term surveillance of mortality and cancer incidence in women receiving hormone replacement therapy. *Br J Obstetr Gynecol* 1987; **94**: 620–635.

28. Risch HA, Howe GR. Menopausal hormone usage and breast cancer in Saskatchewan: a record-linkage study. *Am J Epidemiol* 1994; **139**: 670–683.

29. Schairer C, Byrne C, Keyl PM, *et al*. Menopausal estrogen and estrogen-progestin replacement therapy and risk of breast cancer. *Cancer Causes Control* 1994; **5**: 491–500.

30. Colditz GA, Hankinson SE, Hunter DJ, *et al*. The use of estrogens and progestins and the risk of breast cancer in postmenopausal women. *N Engl J Med* 1995; **332**: 1589–1593.

31. Grady D, Rubin SM, Petitti DB, *et al*. Hormone therapy to prevent disease and prolong life in postmenopausal women. *Ann Int Med* 1992; **117**: 1013–1017.

32. Ballard-Barbash R, Shatzkin A, Carter CL, *et al*. Body fat distribution and breast cancer in the Framingham Study. *J Natl Cancer Inst* 1990; **82**: 286–290.

33. Folsom AR, Kaye SA, Prineas RJ, *et al*. Increased incidence of carcinoma of the breast associated with abdominal adiposity in postmenopausal women. *Am J Epidemiol* 1990; **131**: 794–803.

34. Schapira DV, Kumar NB, Lyman GH, *et al*. Abdominal obesity and breast cancer risk. *Ann Int Med* 1990; **112**: 182–186.

35. Kirschner MA, Samojic E, Drejka M. Androgen-estrogen metabolism in women with upper body vs lower body adiposity. *J Clin Endocrinol Metab* 1990; **70**: 473–479.

36. Sellers TA, Kushi LM, Potter JD, *et al*. Effect of family history, body fat distribution, and reproductive factors on the risk of postmenopausal breast cancer. *N Engl J Med* 1992; **326**: 1323–1325.

37. Schapira DV, Kumar NB, Lyman GH. Estimate of breast cancer risk reduction with weight loss. *Cancer* 1991; **67**: 2622–2625.

38. LaVecchia C, Decaru A, Franceschi S, *et al*. Alcohol consumption and the risk of breast cancer in women. *J Natl Cancer Inst* 1985; **75**: 61–65.

39. Le MG, Hill C, Kramar A, *et al*. Alcohol beverage consumption and breast cancer in a French case-control study. *Am J Epidemiol* 1984; **120**: 350–357.

40. Schatzkin A, Jones Y, Hoover RN, *et al*. Alcohol consumption and breast cancer in the epidemiologic follow-up study of the First Health and Nutrition Examination Survey. *N Engl J Med* 1987; **376**: 1169–1173.

41. Kushi LH, Sellers TA, Potter JD, *et al*. Dietary fat and postmenopausal breast cancer. *J Natl Cancer Inst* 1992; **84**: 1092–1099.

42. Kitchevski D. Nutrition and breast cancer. *Cancer*: 1990; **66**: 1321–1326.

43. Toniolo P, Riboli E, Protta F, *et al*. Calorie-providing nutrients and risk of breast cancer. *J Natl Cancer Inst* 1989; **81**: 278–286.

44. Howe GR, Hirohata T, Hislop TG, *et al*. Dietary factors and risk of breast cancer: combined analysis of 12 case-control studies. *J Natl Cancer Inst* 1990; **82**: 561–569.

45. Boyle P, Leake R. Progress in understanding breast cancer. epidemiological and biological interactions. *Breast Cancer Res Treat* 1988; **111**: 91–112.

46. Ziegler RG, Hoover RN, Pike ML, *et al*. Migration pattern and breast cancer risk in Asian-American women. *J Natl Cancer Inst* 1993; **85**: 1819–1827.

47. Mills PK, Beeson WL, Phillips RL, *et al*. Dietary habits and breast cancer incidence among seventh day adventist. *Cancer* 1989; **64**: 582–590.

48. Jones DY, Schatzkin A, Green SB, *et al*. Dietary fat and breast cancer in the National Health and Nutrition Examination Survey I. Epidemiologic follow-up study. *J Natl Cancer Inst* 1987; **79**: 465–471.

49. Willett WC, Stampferer MJ, Colditz GA, *et al*. Dietary fat and the risk of breast cancer. *N Engl J Med* 1987; **316**: 22–28.

50. van den Brandt PA, van't Veer P, Goldbohm A, *et al*. A prospective cohort study on dietary fat and the risk of post-menopausal breast cancer. *Cancer Res* 1993; **53**: 75–82.

51. Howe GR, Friedenreich CM, Jain M, *et al*. A cohort study of fat intake and risk of breast cancer. *J Natl Cancer Inst* 1991; **83**: 336–340.

52. Herman C, Adlercreutz H, Goldin BR, *et al*. Soybean phytoestrogen intake and cancer risk. *J Nutr* 1995; **125**: 757S–770S.

53. Adlercreutz H, Mousavi Y, Hockerstedt K. Diet and breast cancer. *Acta Oncol* 1992; **31**: 175–181.

54. Yancik R, Ries LG, Yates GW. Breast cancer in aging women. a population-based study of contrasts in stage, surgery, and survival. *Cancer* 1989; **63**: 973–981.

55. Goodwin JS, Samet JM, Key CR, *et al*. Stage at diagnosis of cancer varies with the age of the patient. *J Am Geriatr Soc* 1986; **34**: 20–26.

56. Mor V, Guadagnoli E, Masterson-Allen S, *et al*. Lung, breast and colorectal cancer: the relationship between extent of disease and age at diagnosis. *J Am Ger Soc* 1988; **36**: 873–876.

57. Nattinger AB, Gottlieb MS, Veum J, *et al.* Geographic variations in the use of breast-conserving treatment for breast cancer. *N Engl J Med* 1992; **327**: 1102–1107.

58. Farrow DC, Hunt WC, Samet JM. Geographic variations in the treatment of localized breast cancer. *N Engl J Med* 1992; **326**: 1097–1101.

59. Fletcher SW, Harris RP, Gonzalez JG, *et al.* Increasing mammography utilization: a controlled study. *J Natl Cancer Inst* 1993; **85**: 112–120.

60. Coleman EA, Feuer EJ. Breast Cancer screening among women from 65 to 74 years of age in 1987–88 and 1991. *Ann Int Med* 1992; **117**: 961–966.

61. Fox SA, Roetzheim RG. Screening mammography and older Hispanic women: current status and issues. *Cancer* 1994; **74**: 2028–2033.

62. Roberson NL. Breast cancer screening in older black women. *Cancer* 1994; **74**: 2034–2041.

63. Greenfield S, Blanco DH, Elashoff RM, Ganz PA. Patterns of care related to age of breast cancer patients. *JAMA* 1987; **257**: 2766–2770.

64. McKenna RJ. Clinical aspects of cancer in the elderly. *Cancer* 1994; **74**: 2107–2117.

65. Goodwin JS, Samet JM. Care received by older women diagnosed with breast cancer. *Cancer Control* 1994; **1**: 313–319.

66. Balducci L. Perspectives on quality of life of older patients with cancer. *Drugs and Aging* 1994; **4**: 313–324.

67. Satariano WA, Ragland DR. The effect of comorbidity on 3-year survival of women with primary breast cancer. *Ann Intern Med* 1994; **120**: 104–110.

68. Havlik RJ, Yancik R, Long S, *et al.* The national Institute on Aging and National Cancer Institute SEER collaborative study on comorbidity and early diagnosis of cancer in the elderly. *Cancer* 1994; **74**: 2101–2106.

69. Life Tables. USA government printing office, 1995.

70. Ershler WB. Tumor Host Interactions, Aging and Tumor Growth. In *Comprehensive Geriatric Oncology*, edited by L Balducci, GH Lyman, WB Ershler. London, England: Harwood Academic Press, 201–211, 1997.

71. Figueroa JA, Yee D, McGuire WL. Prognostic indicators in early breast cancer. *Am J Med Sci* 1993; **305**: 176–182.

72. Costantino J, Fisher B, Gunduz N, *et al.* Tumor size, ploidy, S-phase, and ERB B-2 markers in patients with node-negative Er-positive tumors. Findings from NSABP B-14. *Proc Am Soc Clin Oncol* 1994; **13**: 64.

73. Gasparini G, Barbareschi M, Boracchi P, *et al.* Tumor angiogenesis predicts clinical outcome of node-positive breast cancer patients treated with adjuvant hormone therapy or chemotherapy. *The Cancer J Sci Am* 1995; **1**: 131–141.

74. Nixon AJ, Neuberg D, Hayes DF, *et al.* Relationship of patients age to pathologic features of the tumor and prognosis for patients with stage I or II breast cancer. *J Clin Oncol* 1994; **12**: 888–894.

75. Lyman, *et al.* Breast cancer in the older woman: a comparative study of younger and older women with breast cancer. *J Gerontol*, in press.

76. Valentinis B, Silvestrini R, Daidone MG, *et al.* 3H-Thymidine labeling index, hormone receptors and ploidy in breast cancer from elderly patients. *Breast Cancer Res Treat* 1991; **20** 19–24.

77. Holmberg L, Lindgren A, Norden T, *et al.* Age as a determinant of axillary node involvement in invasive breast cancer. *Acta Oncol* 1992; **31**, 533–538.

78. Kurtz JM, Jacquemier J, Amalric R, *et al.* Why are local recurrences after breast-conserving therapy more frequent in younger patients. *J Clin Oncol* 1990; **10**: 141–152.

79. Burns E, Goodwin J. Immunological Changes of Aging. In *Comprehensive Geriatric Oncology*, edited by L Balducci, GH Lyman, WB Ershler. London, England: Harwood Academic Press, 213–222, 1997.

80. Ethier SP. Growth Factor Synthesis and Human Breast Cancer Progression. *J Natl Cancer Inst* 1995; **87**: 964–973.

81. Yee D, Sharma J, Hilsenbeck SG. Prognostic significance of Insulin-like growth factor binding protein expression in axillary lymph node-negative breast cancer. *J Natl Cancer Inst* 1994; **86**: 1785–1789.

82. Lonning PE, Hall K, Aakvaag A, *et al.* Influence of tamoxifen on plasma levels of insulin-like growth factor I and insulin-like growth factor I binding proteins in breast cancer patients. *Cancer res* 1992; **52**: 4719–4723.

83. Roberts A.B, Sporn M.B. Physiological actions and clinical applications of transforming growth factors beta. *Growth Factors* 1993; **8**: 1–9.

84. Butta A, Maclennan K, Flanders KC, *et al.* Induction of transforming growth factor beta in human breast cancer *"in vivo"* following tamoxifen. *Cancer Res* 1992; **52**: 4261–4264.

85. Guidi AJ, Abu-Jawdeh G, Berse B, *et al.* Vascular Permeability Factor (Vascular Endothelial Growth Factor) expression and angiogenesis in cervical neoplasia. *J Natl Cancer Inst* 1995; **87**: 1237–1245.

86. Ershler WB. Interleukin 6: a cytokine for gerontologists. *J Am Ger Soc* 1993; **41**: 176–181.

87. Holmes FF. Clinical Course of cancer in the elderly. *Cancer Control* 1994; **1**: 108–114.

88. Hong WK, Lippman SM. Cancer Chemoprevention. Monographs. *J Natl Cancer Inst* 1995; **17**: 49–54.

89. Early Breast Cancer Trialists' Collaborative Group. Systemic treatment of early breast cancer by hormonal, cytotoxic or immune therapy. *Lancet* 1992; **339**: 1–15, 71–85.

90. LaFollette S, Cobleigh M. Dietary and chemoprevention strategies for breast cancer prevention. *Cancer Control* 1995; **2**: 218–223.

91. Atiba JO, Meyskens FL. Chemoprevention of breast cancer. *Sem Oncol* 1992; **19**: 220–229.

92. Anisimov VN. Age as a Risk Factor in Multistage Carcinogenesis. In *Comprehensive Geriatric Oncology*, edited by L Balducci, GH Lyman, WB Ershler. London, England: Harwood Academic Press, 157–178, 1997.

93. Fernandes-Pol JA. Growth Factors, Oncogenes and Aging. In *Comprehensive Geriatric Oncology*, edited by L Balducci, GH Lyman, WB Ershler. London, England: Harwood Academic Press, 170–196, 1997.

94. Beghe' C, Balducci L, Cohen HJ. Secondary prevention of breast cancer in the older woman: issues related to screening. *Cancer Control* 1994; **1**: 320–326.

95. Castiglione M, Gelber RD, Goldhirsch A. Adjuvant systemic therapy for breast cancer in the elderly. Competing causes of mortality. *J Clin Oncol* 1990; **8**: 519–526.

96. Mandelblatt JS, Wheat ME, Monane M, *et al.* Breast cancer screening for elderly women with and without comorbid conditions. *Ann Int Med* 1992; **116**: 722–730.

97. Champion V. Breast self-examination in women 65 and older. *J Gerontol* 1992; **47**: 75–79.

98. O'Malley MS, Fletcher SW. US Preventive Services Task Force: screening for breast cancer with breast self-examination. a critical review. *JAMA* 1987; **257**: 2196–2203.

99. Fletcher SW, Black W, Harris R, *et al.* Report of International Workshop on screening for breast cancer. *J Natl Cancer Inst* 1993; **85**: 1644–1656.

100. Mitra I. Breast screening: the case for physical examination without mammography. *Lancet* 1994; **343**: 342–344.

101. Morrison AS, Brisson J, Khalid N. Breast cancer incidence and mortality in the Breast Cancer Detection Demonstration Project. *J Natl Cancer Inst* 1988; **80**: 1540–1547.

102. Shapiro S. Periodic screening for breast cancer: the health insurance pilot project and its sequelae, 1963–1986. Baltimore Md: Johns Hopkins University Press, 1988.

103. Nystrom L, Rutquvist LE, Wall S, *et al.* Breast cancer screening with mammography: overview of Swedish randomized trials. *Lancet* 1993; **341**: 973–978.

104. Wald N, Chamberlain J, Hackshaw A and EUSOMA evaluation committee. Report of the European society for mastology breast cancer screening evaluation committee. *J Eur Soc Mastology* 1993; **13**: 1–25.

105. Miller AB, Baines CJ, To T, *et al.* Canadian National Breast Screening Study 2: breast cancer detection and death rates among women aged 50 to 59 years. *Can Med Ass J* 1992; **147**: 1477–1488.

106. Collette HJA, deWaard F, Collette C, et al. Further evidence of benefits of a (non randomized) breast cancer screening programme: the DOM project. *J Epidemiol Community Health* 1992; **46**: 382–386.

107. Palli D, Del Turco MR, Buiatti E, et al. Time interval since last test in a breast cancer screening programme: a case-control study in Italy. *J Epidemiol Community Health* 1989; **43**: 241–248.

108. van Dijck JAAM, Holland R, Verbeek, ALM, et al. Efficacy of mammographic screening in the elderly: a case-referent study in the Nijmegen program in the Netherlands. *J Natl Cancer Inst* 1994; **86**: 934–938.

109. Moss SM, Summerley ME, Thomas BT, et al. A case-control evaluation of the effect of breast-cancer screening in the United Kingdom Trial of Early Detection of Breast Cancer. *J Epidemiol Community Health* 1992; **46**: 362–364.

110. Kerlikowske K, Grady D, Rubin SM, et al. Efficacy of screening mammography: A meta-analysis. *JAMA* 1995; **273**: 149–154.

111. Fox SA, Roetzheim RS, Kingston RS. Barriers to Cancer Prevention in the Older Person. In *Comprehensive Geriatric Oncology*, edited by L Balducci, GH Lyman, WB Ershler. London, England: Harwood Academic Press, 353–363, 1997.

112. Sidransky D. Molecular markers in cancer diagnosis. *Monographs J Natl Cancer Inst* 1995; **17**: 27–30.

113. Rosen PP. The pathology of invasive breast carcinoma. In *Breast Diseases*, edited by JR Harris, S Hellman, IC Henderson, DW Kinne. JB Lippincott, 245–296, 1991.

114. Berg JW, Hutter RVP. Breast cancer. *Cancer* 1995; **75**: 257–269.

115. Silverstein MJ, Poller DN, Waisman JR, et al. Prognostic classification of breast ductal carcinoma "*in situ*." *Lancet* 1995; **345**: 1154–1157.

116. Field K, Moscinski L, Trudeau W, Elfenbein G. The use of polymerase chain reaction (PCR) for amplification of cytokeratin 19 (K19) to detect bone marrow metastases in breast cancer. *Am Soc Clin Oncol Proc* 1994; **13**: 115.

117. Hayes DF. Tumor Markers for breast cancer. *Hematol/Oncol Clin N America* 1994; **8**: 485–506.

118. Phillips DL, Balducci L. Breast cancer: a practical review. *Am Fam Phys* 1995, in press.

119. Shapira DV, Urban N. A minimalistic policy for breast cancer surveillance. *JAMA* 1991; **256**: 380–383.

120. Fisher B, Costantino J, Redmond C, et al. Lumpectomy compared with lumpectomy and radiation therapy for the treatment of intraductal breast cancer. *N Engl J Med* 1993; **328**: 1581–1586.

121. Ries LAG, Hankey BF, Miller BA, et al. Cancer Statistics Review 1973–1988, Bethesda MD, National Cancer Institute, 1991.

122. Jacobson JA, Danforth DN, Cowan KH, et al. Ten-year results of a comparison of conservation with mastectomy in the treatment of stage I and II breast cancer. *N Engl J Med* 1995; **332**: 907–911.

123. Fisher B, Anderson S, Redmond CK, et al. Reanalysis and results after 12 years of follow-up in a randomized clinical trial comparing total mastectomy with lumpectomy with or without irradiation in the treatment of breast cancer. *N Engl J Med* 1995; **333**: 1456–1461.

124. Veronesi U, Banfi A, Salvadori B, et al. Breast conservation is the treatment of choice in small breast cancer: long term-results of a randomized trial. *Eur J Cancer* 1990; **26**: 668–670.

125. van Dongen JA, Bartelink H, Fentiman IS, et al. Randomized clinical trial to assess the value of breast conserving therapy in stage I and II breast cancer. EORTC 10801 trial. *Monogr Natl Cancer Inst* 1992; **11**: 15–18.

126. Abrams JS, Phillips PH, Friedman MH. Meeting highlights: a reappraisal of research results for the local treatment of early stage breast cancer. *J Natl Cancer Inst* 1995; **87**: 1837–1845.

127. Foster RS. Management of primary breast cancer in older patients: treatment options. *Cancer Control* 1994; **1**: 339–343.

128. Galante E, Cerrotta AM, Crippa A. Outpatient treatment of clinically node-negative breast cancer in elderly women. *Cancer Control* 1994; **1**: 344–349.

129. Kiebert GM, de Haes JCJM, van der Velde CJH, et al. the impact of breast conserving treatment and mastectomy on the quality of life of early stage breast cancer patients: a review. *J Clin Oncol* 1991; **9**: 1059–1070.

130. Giuliano AE, Kirgan DM, Gunther JM, et al. Lymphatic mapping and sentinel lymphadenectomy for breast cancer. *Ann Surg* 1994; **220**: 391–398.

131. Harris JR. Postmastectomy radiotherapy. In *Breast Diseases*, edited by JR Harris, S Hellman, IC Henderson, DW Kinne. JB Lippincott, 383–387, 1992.

132. Griem KL, Henderson IC, Gelman R, et al. The 5 year results of a randomized trial of adjuvant radiation therapy after chemotherapy in breast cancer patients treated with mastectomy. *J Clin Oncol* 1987; **5**: 1546–1555.

133. Early Breast Cancer Trialists' Collaborative Group. Effects of radiotherapy and surgery in early breast cancer. *N Engl J Med* 1995; **333**: 1444–1455.

134. Goldhirsch A, Wood WC, Senn H-J, et al. Meeting highlight: International Consensus Panel on the treatment of primary breast cancer. *J Natl Cancer Inst* 1995; **87**: 1441–1445.

135. Wyckoff J, Greenberg H, Sanderson R, et al. Breast irradiation in the older woman: a toxicity study. *J Am Ger Soc* 1994; **42**: 153–156.

136. Morrow M, Harris JR, Schnitt SJ. Local control following breast cancer conserving surgery: results of clinical trials. *J Natl Cancer Inst* 1995; **87**: 1669–1673.

137. Harris JR, Recht A. Conservative surgery and radiotherapy. In *Breast Diseases*, edited by JR Harris, S Hellman, IC Henderson, DW Kinne. JB Lippincott, 388–419, 1992.

138. Nemoto T, Patel JK, Rosner D, et al. Factors affecting recurrence in lumpectomy without irradiation for breast cancer. *Cancer* 1991; **67**: 2079–2082.

139. Clark RM, McCulloch PB, Levine MN. Randomized clinical trial to assess the effectiveness of breast irradiation following lumpectomy and axillary dissection for node-negative breast cancer. *J Natl Cancer Inst* 1992; **84**: 683–689.

140. Liljegren G, Holmberg L, Adami H-O, et al. Sector resection with or without postoperative radiotherapy for stage I breast cancer. Five-Year results of a randomized trial. *J Natl Cancer Inst* 1994; **86**: 717–722.

141. Kantorowitz D.A, Poulter C.A, Sischy B, et al. Treatment of breast cancer among elderly women with segmental mastectomy or segmental mastectomy plus postoperative radiotherapy. *Int J Radiat Oncol Biol Phys* 1988; **15**: 263–270.

142. Hayman J, Schnitt S, Gelman R, et al. A prospective trial of conservative surgery (CS) alone without radiation therapy (RT) in selected patients with early stage breast cancer. *Int J Radiat Oncol Biol Phys* 1995; **32 (suppl 1)**: 209.

143. Veronesi U, Luini A, Del Vecchio M, et al. Radiotherapy after breast preserving surgery in women with localized cancer of the breast. *N Engl J Med* 1993; **328**: 1587–1591.

144. Wazer DE, Erban JK, Robert NJ, et al. Breast conservation in elderly women for clinically negative axillary lymph nodes without axillary dissection. *Cancer* 1994; **74**: 878–883.

145. Bates T, Riley DL, Houghton J, et al. Breast cancer in elderly women: a cancer research campaign trial comparing treatment with tamoxifen and optimal surgery and optimal surgery with tamoxifen alone. The elderly breast cancer working party. *Br J Surg* 1991; **78**: 591–594.

146. Nolvadex Adjuvant Trial Organization. Controlled trial of tamoxifen as single adjuvant agent in the management of early breast cancer. *Lancet* 1985; **1**: 836–840.

147. Report from the breast cancer trial committee, Scottish Cancer Trials Office (MRC) Edinburgh. Adjuvant tamoxifen in the management of operable breast cancer: the Scottish trial.

148. Ribeiro G, Swindell R. The Christie Hospital Adjuvant Tamoxifen Trial. Monograph, *J Natl Cancer Inst* 1992; **11**: 121–126.

149. Looming PE, Hall K, Aakvaag A, et al. Influence of tamoxifen on plasma levels of insulin-like growth factor I and insulin-like growth factor-binding proteins in breast cancer patients. *Cancer Res* 1992; **52**: 4719–4723.

150. Butta A, MacLennan K, Flanders KC, et al. Induction of transforming growth factor beta in human breast cancer "*in vivo*" following tamoxifen. *Cancer Res* 1992; **52**: 4261–4264.

151. Vermorken JB, Burgers JMV, Taat CW, et al. Adjuvant tamoxifen in breast cancer: interim results of a comprehensive cancer center Amsterdam trial. *Proc Amer Soc Clin Oncol* 1994; **13**: 76.

152. Tripathy D. How long should adjuvant tamoxifen be continued? *Oncology* 1994; **8 (10)**: 25–38.

153. Fisher B, Brown A, Wolmark N, et al. Prolonging tamoxifen therapy for primary breast cancer. *Ann Intern Med* 1987; **106**: 649–654.

154. Falkson HC, Gray R, Wolberg WH, *et al*. Adjuvant trial of 12 cycles of CMFPT followed by observation or continuous tamoxifen vs four cycles of CMFPT in postmenopausal women with breast cancer: an Eastern Cooperative Oncology Group phase III study. *J Clin Oncol* 1990; **8**: 599–607.

155. Rutqvist LE, Cedermark B, Glas U, *et al*. Randomized trial of adjuvant tamoxifen in node negative postmenopausal breast cancer. Stockholm Breast Cancer Study Group. *Acta Oncol* 1992; **31**: 265–270.

156. Fisher B, Costantino JP, Rewdmond CK, *et al*. Endometrial Cancer in tamoxifen-treated breast cancer patients: findings from the National Surgical Adjuvant Breast and Bowel Project (NSABP) B-14. *J Natl Cancer Inst* 1994; **86**: 527–537.

157. Stewart HJ. The Scottish Trial of adjuvant tamoxifen in node-negative breast cancer. *Monogr Natl Cancer Inst* 1992; **11**: 105–116.

158. Turken S, Siris E, Seldin D, *et al*. Effects of Tamoxifen on spinal bone density in women with breast cancer. *J Natl Cancer Inst* 1989; **81**: 1086–1088.

159. Wright CDP, Mansell RE, Gazet J-C, *et al*. Effect of long term tamoxifen treatment on bone turn-over in women with breast cancer. *Br Med J* 1993; **306**: 429–430.

160. Love RR, Mazess RB, Barden HS, *et al*. Effects of tamoxifen on bone mineral density in postmenopausal women with breast cancer. *N Engl J Med* 1992; **326**: 852–856.

161. Love RR, Wiebe DA, Feyzi JM, *et al*. Effects of tamoxifen on cardiovascular risk factors in postmenopausal women after 5 years of treatment. *J Natl Cancer Inst* 1994; **86**: 1534–1539.

162. Schapira DV, Kumar NB, Lyman GH. Serum cholesterol reduction with tamoxifen. *Breast Cancer Res Treat* 1990; **17**: 3–7.

163. McDonald CC, Stewart HJ. Fatal myocardial infarction in the Scottish Adjuvant Tamoxifen Trial. The Scottish Breast Cancer Committee. *J Natl Cancer Inst* 1994; **86**: 1534–1539.

164. Rutqvist LE, Mattsson A. Cardiac and thromboembolic morbidity among postmenopausal women with early-stage breast cancer in a randomized trial of tamoxifen. The Stockholm Breast Cancer Study Group. *J Natl Cancer Inst* 1994; **86**: 1534–1539.

165. Rutqvist LE, Johansson H, Signomklao T, *et al*. Adjuvant tamoxifen therapy for early stage breast cancer and second primary malignancies. *J Natl Cancer Inst* 1995; **87**: 645–651.

166. Extermann M, Balducci L, Lyman GH. Optimal duration of adjuvant Tamoxifen treatment in elderly breast cancer patients: influence of age, comorbidities, and various effectiveness hypotheses on life-expectancy and cost. *Breast Disease* 1996; **9**: 327–339.

167. Jayesimi IA, Buzdar AU, Decker DA, *et al*. Use of Tamoxifen for breast cancer: twenty-eight years later. *J Clin Oncol* 1995; **13**: 513–529.

168. Cobleigh MA, Berris RF, Bush T, *et al*. Estrogen replacement therapy in breast cancer survivors. A time for change. Breast Cancer Committees of the Eastern Cooperative Oncology Group. *JAMA* 1994; **272**: 540–545.

169. Magriples U, Naftalin F, Schwartz PE, *et al*. High-grade endometrial carcinoma in tamoxifen-treated breast cancer patients. *J Clin Oncol* 1993; **11**: 485–490.

170. Jordan VC, Morrow M. Should clinicians be concerned about the carcinogenic potential of tamoxifen? *Eur J Cancer* 1994; **11**: 1714–1721.

171. Jordan VC. Tamoxifen and tumorigenicity: a predictable concern. *J Natl Cancer Inst* 1995; **87**: 623–625.

172. Osborne CK, Wiebe VJ, Mcguire WL, *et al*. Tamoxifen and the isomers of 4-hydroxytamoxifen in Tamoxifen-resistant tumors from breast cancer patients. *J Clin Oncol* 1992; **10**: 304–310.

173. Taylor SG, Gelman RS, Falkson G, *et al*. Combination chemotherapy compared with tamoxifen as initial therapy for stage IV breast cancer in elderly women. *Ann Int Med* 1986; **104**: 455–461.

174. Langan-Fahey SM, Tormey DC, Jordan VC. Tamoxifen metabolites in patients on long term adjuvant therapy for breast cancer. *Eur J Cancer* 1990; **26**: 883–888.

175. DeGregorio MW, Ford JM, Benz CC, *et al*. Toremifene: pharmacologic and pharmacokinetic basis of reversing multidrug resistance. *J Clin Oncol* 1989; **7**: 1359–1364.

176. Jones AL, Powles TJ, Law M, *et al*. Adjuvant aminoglethimide for postmenopausal patients with primary breast cancer: analysis at 8 years. *J Clin Oncol* 1992; **10**: 1547–1552.

177. Bonadonna G, Valagussa P, Moliterni A, *et al*. Adjuvant cyclophosphamide, methotrexate and fluorouracil in node-positive breast cancer. *N Engl J Med* 1995; **332**: 901–906.

178. Olivotto IA, Bajdic CD, Penderpleith IH, *et al*. Adjuvant systemic therapy and survival after breast cancer. *N Engl J Med* 1994; **330**: 805–810.

179. Fisher B, Redmond C, Fisher ER, *et al*. Systemic adjuvant treatment of primary breast cancer. National Surgical Adjuvant Breast and Bowel Project Experience. *NCI Monograph* 1986; **1**: 35–43.

180. Ingle JN, Everson LK, Wieand HS, *et al*. Randomized trial of observation vs adjuvant therapy with Cyclophosphamide, Fluorouracil, Prednisone with or without tamoxifen, following mastectomy in postmenopausal women with node-positive breast cancer. *J Clin Oncol* 1988; **6**: 1388–1396.

181. Taylor SG, Knuiman MW, Sleeper LA, *et al*. Six-Year results of the Eastern Cooperative Oncology Group Trial of observation versus CMFP versus CMFPT in postmenopausal patients with node-positive breast cancer. *J Clin Oncol* 1989; **7**: 879–889.

182. Fisher B, Redmond C, Wickerham DL, *et al*. Doxorubicin containing regimens for the treatment of stage II breast cancer: the National Surgical Adjuvant Breast and Bowel Project experience. *J Clin Oncol* 1989; **7**: 572–582.

183. Fisher B, Redmond C, Legault-Poisson S, *et al*. Postoperative chemotherapy and tamoxifen compared with tamoxifen alone in the treatment of positive-node breast cancer patients aged 50 years and older with tumors responsive to tamoxifen: results from the National Breast and Bowel Project B-16. *J Clin Oncol* 1990; **8**: 1005–1018.

184. Boccardo F, Rubagotti A, Bruzzi P, *et al*. Chemotherapy versus tamoxifen versus chemotherapy plus tamoxifen in Node-positive, Estrogen-receptor positive breast cancer patients: results of a multicenter Italian study. *J Clin Oncol* 1990; **8**: 1310–1320.

185. Schumacher M, Bastert G, Bojar H, *et al*. A randomized 2 × 2 trial evaluating hormonal treatment and the duration of chemotherapy in node-positive breast cancer patients. *J Clin Oncol* 1994; **12**: 2086–2093.

186. Rivkin SE, Glucksberg H, Foulkes M. Adjuvant therapy of breast cancer: a Southwest Oncology Group Experience. *Rec Res Cancer Res* 1984; **96**: 166–174.

187. Rivkin SE, Green S, Metch B, *et al*. Adjuvant CMFVP vs Tamoxifen vs concurrent CMFVP and Tamoxifen for post-menopausal Node-positive and Estrogen-Receptor-Positive breast cancer patients: a Southwest Oncology Group Study. *J Clin Oncol* 1994; **12**: 2078–2085.

188. Wood WC, Budman DR, Korzun AH, *et al*. Dose and dose intensity of adjuvant chemotherapy for stage II node-positive breast carcinoma. *N Engl J Med* 1994; **330**: 1253–1259.

189. Bonadonna G, Zambetti M, Valagussa P, *et al*. Sequential or Alternating Doxorubicin and CMF regimens in Breast Cancer with more than three positive nodes. *JAMA* 1995; **273**: 542–547.

190. Kaufmann M, Abel JU, Hilfrich J, *et al*. Adjuvant randomized trials of doxorubicin/Cyclophosphamide vs doxorubicin, Cyclophosphamide, tamoxifen and CMF chemotherapy versus tamoxifen in women with node-positive breast cancer. *J Clin Oncol* 1993; **11**: 454–460.

191. Pritchard KI, Zee B, Paul N, *et al*. CMF added to tamoxifen as adjuvant therapy in post-menopausal women with node positive estrogen and/or progesterone receptor-positive breast cancer: negative results of a randomized clinical trial. *Proc Am Soc Clin Oncol* 1994; **13**: 65.

192. Bonadonna G. Evolving Concepts in the Systemic Adjuvant Treatment of Breast Cancer. *Cancer Res* 1992; **52**: 2127–2137.

193. Fisher B, Redmond C, Dimitrov N.V, *et al*. A randomized clinical trial evaluating sequential methotrexate and fluorouracil in the treatment of patients with node-negative breast cancer who have estrogen-receptor-negative tumors. *N Engl J Med* 1989; **320**: 473–478.

194. Fisher B, Costantino J, Wickerman L, *et al*. Adjuvant therapy for node-negative breast cancer. An update of NSABP findings. *Proc Am Soc Cli Oncol* 1993; **12**: 69.

195. Mansour EG, Gray R, Shatila AH, *et al*. Efficacy of adjuvant chemotherapy in high-risk node-negative breast cancer patients. *N Engl J Med* 1989; **320**: 485–490.

196. Muss HB, Thor AD, Berry DA, *et al*. C-erbB-2 expression and response to adjuvant therapy in women with node-positive early breast cancer. *N Engl J Med* 1994; **330**: 1260–1266.

197. Gelbes RD, Goldhirsch A, Cavalli F. Quality-of-Life adjusted evaluation of adjuvant therapies for operable breast cancer. *Ann Int Med*: 1991; **114**: 621–628.

198. Cova D, Beretta G, Balducci L. Cancer Chemotherapy in the Older Patient. In *Comprehensive Geriatric Oncology*, edited by L Balducci, GH Lyman, WB Ershler. London, England: Harwood Academic Press, 431–444, 1997.

199. Speyer JL, Green MD, Kramer E, *et al*. Protective effect of the bispiperazinedione ICRF-187 against doxorubicin induced cardiac toxicity in women with advanced breast cancer. *N Engl J Med* 1988; **319**: 756–752.

200. Henderson IC, Allegra JC, Woodcock T, *et al*. Randomized clinical trial comparing mitoxantrone with doxorubicin in previously treated patients with metastatic breast cancer. *J Clin Oncol* 1989; **7**: 560–571.

201. Desch CE, Hillner BE, Smith TJ, *et al*. Should elderly receive chemotherapy for node-negative breast cancer? A cost-effectiveness analysis examining total and active life-expectancy outcome. *J Clin Oncol* 1993; **11**: 777–782.

202. Powles TJ, Hickish TF, Makris A, *et al*. Randomized trial of chemoendocrine surgery started before or after surgery for treatment of primary breast cancer. *J Clin Oncol* 1995; **13**: 547–552.

203. Fisher B, Rockette H, Robidoux A. Effect of preoperative therapy for breast cancer on local-regional disease: first report of NSABP B-18. *Proc Am Soc Clin Onol* 1994; **13**: 64.

204. Scholl SM, Fourquet A, Asselain B, *et al*. Neoadjuvant vs adjuvant chemotherapy in premenopausal patients with tumors considered too large for breast-conserving surgery. Preliminary results of a randomised trial. S6 *Eur J Cancer* 1994; **30A**: 645–652.

205. Fisher B, Mamounas EP. Preoperative chemotherapy: a model for studying the biology and therapy of primary breast cancer. *J Clin Oncol* 1995; **13**: 537–540.

206. Hortobagy GN. Comprehensive management of locally advanced breast cancer. *Cancer* 1990; **66**: 1387–1391.

207. Mourali N, Tabbane F, Muenz LR, *et al*. Ten-year results utilizing chemotherapy as primary treatment in non-metastatic, rapidly progressive breast cancer. *Cancer Invest* 1993; **11**: 363–370.

208. Booser DJ, Hortobagyi GN. Treatment of locally advanced breast cancer. *Sem Oncol* 1992; **19**: 278–285.

209. Brady LV, Shields JA, Augsburger JJ, *et al*. Malignant intraocular tumors. *Cancer* 1982; 578–585.

210. Jardines L, Callans LS, Torosian MH. recurrent breast cancer: presentation, diagnosis and treatment. *Sem Oncol* 1993; **20**: 538–550.

211. Crow JP, Gordon NH, Antunez AR, *et al*. Locoregional breast cancer recurrence following mastectomy. *Arch Surg* 1991; **126**: 429–432.

212. Janjan NA, McNeese MD, Buzdar AU, *et al*. Loco-regional recurrent breast cancer treated with radiation or a combination of radiation and chemotherapy. *Int J Rad Biol Phys* 1985; **11 (suppl 1)**: 152–153.

213. Borner M, Bacchi M, Goldhirsch A, *et al*. First isolated loco-regional recurrence following mastectomy for Breast Cancer. results of a Phase III multicenter study comparing systemic treatment with observation after excision and radiation. *J Clin Oncol* 1994; **12**: 2071–2077.

214. Ziegler LD, Buzdar AU. Recent advances in the treatment of breast cancer. *Am J Med Sci* 1991; **301**: 337–349.

215. Buzdar AU, Hortobagyi GN, Frye D, *et al*. Bioequivalence of 20-mg once-daily tamoxifen relative to 10 mg twice daily tamoxifen regimens for breast cancer. *J Clin Oncol* 1994; **12**: 50–54.

216. Muss HB, Case LD, Capizzi RL, *et al*. High versus standard dose megestrol acetate in women with advanced breast cancer. A phase III trial of the Piedmont Oncology Association. *J Clin Oncol* 1990; **8**: 1797–1805.

217. Hoffken K, Passinger JR, Kolbel M, *et al*. Aromatase inhibition with 4-hydroxy-androstendione in the treatment of postmenopausal patients with advanced breast cancer. A phase II study. *J Clin Oncol* 1990; **8**: 875–880.

218. Miller WR. Aromatase inhibitors in the treatment of advanced breast cancer. *Cancer Treat Rev* 1989; **16**: 83–93.

219. Peterson AHG, Hanson J, Pritchard KI, *et al*. Comparison of antiestrogen and progestogen therapy for initial treatment and consequences of their combination for second line treatment of recurrent breast cancer. *Sem Oncol* 1990; **17**: 52–62 (suppl 9).

220. Glauber JG, Kiang DT. The changing role of hormonal therapy in advanced breast cancer. *Sem Oncol* 1992; **19**: 308–316.

221. Sledge GW, Antman KH. Progress in chemotherapy for metastatic breast cancer. *Sem Oncol* 1992; **19**: 317–332.

222. Hayes DF, Henderson IC, Shapiro CL. Treatment of metastatic breast cancer: present and future prospects. *Sem Oncol* 1995; **22(suppl.5)**: 5–21.

223. A' Hern RP, Smith IE, Ebbs SR. Chemotherapy and survival in advanced breast cancer. The inclusion of doxorubicin in Cooper's like regimens. *Br J Cancer* 1993; **67**: 801–808.

224. Bennett JM, Muss HB, Doroshow JH, *et al*. A randomized multicenter trial comparing mitoxantrone, cyclophosphamide and fluorouracil with doxorubicin, cyclophosphamide, and fluorouracil in the therapy of metastatic breast carcinoma. *J Clin Oncol* 1988; **6**: 1611–1620.

225. Balducci L, Lyman GH. Effectiveness and cost-effectiveness of hemopoietic growth factors in cancer treatment. *Adv Oncol*, In press.

226. Gianni L, Munzone E, Capri G, *et al*. Paclitaxel by eight-hour infusion in combination with bolus doxorubicin in women with untreated metastatic breast cancer: high antitumor efficacy and cardiac effects in a dose-finding and sequence-finding study. *J Clin Oncol* 1995; **13**: 2688–2699.

227. Gruia G, Misset JL, Giacchetti S, *et al*. A phase I-II study of taxotere in combination with adriamycin as first line chemotherapy in patients with metastatic breast cancer. *Proc Am Soc Clin Oncol* 1995; **14**: 140.

228. Gelman RS, Taylor SG. Cyclophosphamide, methotrexate and fluorouracil chemotherapy in women more than 65 year old with advanced breast cancer: the elimination of age trends in toxicity by using doses based on creatinine clearance. *J Clin Oncol* 1984; **2**: 1406–1414.

229. Christman K, Muss HB, Case D, *et al*. Chemotherapy of metastatic breast cancer in the elderly. *JAMA* 1992; **268**: 57–62.

230. Ibrahim N, Buzdar A, Frye D, *et al*. Should age be a determinant factor in treating breast cancer patients with combination chemotherapy? *Proc Am Soc Clin Oncol* 1993; **12**: 68.

231. Speyer JL, Green MD, Zeleniuch-Jacquotte A, *et al*. ICRF-187 permits longer treatment with doxorubicin in women with breast cancer. *J Clin Oncol* 1992; **10**: 117–127.

232. Fonseca GA, Valero V, Buzdar A, *et al*. Decreased cardiac toxicity by TLC D-99 (liposomal doxorubicin) in the treatment of metastatic breast carcinoma. *Am Soc Clin Oncol Proceeding* 1995; **14**: 99.

233. Taylor SG, Gelman RS, Falkson G, *et al*. Combination chemotherapy compared to tamoxifen as initial therapy for stage IV breast cancer in elderly women. *Ann Intern Med* 1986; **4**: 455–461.

234. Muss HB, Smith LR, Cooper MR. Tamoxifen rechallenge: response to tamoxifen following relapse after adjuvant chemohormonal therapy for breast cancer. *J Clin Oncol* 1987; **5**: 1556–1558.

235. Fournander T. Rutqvist LE, Glas U. Response to tamoxifen and fluoxymesterone in a group of breast cancer patients with disease recurrence after cessation of adjuvant tamoxifen. *Cancer Treat Rep* 1987; **71**: 685–688.

236. Kiang DT, Gay J, Goldman A, *et al*. A randomized trial of chemotherapy and hormonal therapy in advanced breast cancer. *N Engl J Med* 1985; **313**: 1241–1246.

237. Reddy EK, Robinson RG, Mansfield CM. Strontium-89 therapy for palliation of bone metastases. *J Natl Med Assoc* 1986; **78**: 27.

238. Peterson AHG, Powles TJ, Kanis JA, *et al*. Double blind controlled trial of Oral clodronate in patients with bone metastases from breast cancer. *J Clin Oncol* 1993; **11**: 59–65.

46. Breast Cancer: A Geriatric Perspective – Part 2

Rebecca A. Silliman and Lodovico Balducci

Introduction

Breast cancer is a disease primarily of older women, with its incidence reaching a maximum well into the ninth decade of life (1). It is also a serious disease in older women. For example, five-year breast cancer-specific survival rates are similar for women <35 years and ≥85 years of age with local and regional disease, and are worse than for women between these ages (1). Furthermore, although the approximate 10-year risk of recurrence for women ≥70 years of age who are node negative with 1–5 cm tumors is 20–30%, the risk for women with 1–3 positive nodes and tumors of any size is 50%, and the risk for women with ≥4 positive nodes and tumors of any size is 80% (2). These risks have become increasingly important because recent gains in life expectancy have occurred at the end of life: the average life expectancy of a 75 year old woman is nearly 12 years, and the average life expectancy of an 8 5 year old woman is nearly 6.5 years (3). Recurrences have important negative consequences for this group of patients who are often frail; recurrences complicate medical and personal care and are difficult for patients, their families, and their physicians to manage. Furthermore, because of gender disparities in life expectancy, older women are frequently single and have diminished family support (4).

Early Stage Disease: Management of the Primary Tumor

The 1990 NIH Consensus Development Conference on the treatment of early stage breast cancer concluded that, "Breast conservation treatment is an appropriate method of primary therapy for the majority of women with stage I and II breast cancer and is preferable because it provides survival rates equivalent to those of total mastectomy and axillary dissection while preserving the breast." Total mastectomy should therefore be reserved for those whose cancer is multicentric or in whom cosmetic results are likely to be unacceptable (5).

Although breast conserving surgery and axillary dissection, followed by post-operative radiation therapy, is recommended for the majority of women regardless of age and should be offered as a treatment option, several considerations are likely to influence older women's decisions. First, for many, a mastectomy will seem to be a more definitive procedure, particularly when the risk of disease recurrence within the breast is considered to be an important outcome. Second, by choosing mastectomy, the need for post-operative radiation therapy is generally eliminated. Third, body image considerations are less important to certain subsets of older women. Fourth, and perhaps most importantly, physicians' recommendations have a powerful influence on older women's decisions. Our own data indicate their physicians' recommendations and minimizing the risk of recurrence are the two most important factors influencing older women's treatment decisions (6).

The problem for physicians trying to use an evidence-based approach to caring for older women with breast cancer is that there are few scientific data on which to base therapeutic recommendations, since they have generally been excluded from clinical trials addressing treatment efficacy. As a result, there are two important unresolved controversies involving primary tumor management in older women. These are: 1) the need for post-operative radiation therapy following breast conserving surgery in older women; and 2) the need for axillary dissection in older women, regardless of the surgical management of the breast.

With respect to post-operative radiation, there is no evidence that such therapy prevents the development of systemic disease or that it prolongs survival (5). In addition, because older women appear to have lower recurrence rates than younger women (7–11), it is not clear whether radiation is effective in preventing disease recurrence in older women. Furthermore, although the side effects of radiation are probably no different on older women than in younger women, their impact may be greater for several reasons. First, a several week schedule of daily radiation treatments may be difficult because of the need to rely on others for transportation, because of the physical fatigue associated with the treatments themselves, and because of travel and waiting times. Second, positioning may be uncomfortable for women with arthritis or who have had vertebral fractures. Third, underlying cardiopulmonary comorbidities may be exacerbated by radiation treatments and these effects which may be manifested several years following treatment.

Although the lack of definitive data do not lead us to recommend that breast conserving surgery *not* be followed by post-operative radiation therapy for all, or even most older women, this approach is a reasonable option for those older women in whom a lesser surgical procedure would be preferable because of increased perioperative risk. Although data are lacking, adjuvant if tamoxifen may be a prudent addition to therapy in this circumstance.

Axillary dissection has been advocated as a therapeutic intervention that both eliminates residual disease and stages patients. Whether either is necessary in older women remains open to question. First, the goal of eliminating residual disease has not been studied in women ≥70 years of age. Furthermore, data from NSABP protocol B-04 that address this issue do not provide a *definitive answer* because about 40% of women assigned to the total mastectomy without lymph node dissection or radiation to the axilla group actually received some form of axillary dissection (12). Second, axillary dissection is only necessary if the decision to prescribe adjuvant therapy is based on pathologically proven involvement of the regional lymph nodes. If adjuvant tamoxifen is indicated more broadly (see discussion below), then axillary dissection may not be necessary (5, 13).

Decision-making with respect to choosing mastectomy versus breast conserving surgery, with or without radiation, and with or without axillary dissection, must take into account body image and upper body function, the logistical difficulties associated with radiation therapy, the emotional impact of disease recurrence, and the ability to tolerate mastectomy at some point in the future should there be an in-breast recurrence (14). Regardless of the type of surgical procedure chosen, careful attention should be paid to preserving upper body, shoulder, and arm function. Ideally, women should receive exercise instructions prior to surgery, as has become the standard approach to patients undergoing elective hip and knee replacement. An exercise program and the judicious use of analgesics in the early postoperative period will help women regain upper body function as quickly as possible. This is particularly important if an axillary lymph node dissection has been performed.

Primary medical, rather than surgical treatment, is an additional consideration in the initial management of early stage breast cancer. Although studies comparing outcomes of women initially treated with tamoxifen with those surgically treated have found that mortality rates are comparable, patients treated with tamoxifen alone have experienced more local progression than those treated surgically (15–17). These findings suggest that tamoxifen should only be considered as a primary treatment option when women are too frail or refuse to undergo surgery.

Early Stage Disease: Adjuvant Treatment

Tamoxifen

Adjuvant tamoxifen therapy has been shown to decrease both rates of recurrence and mortality in older women with early stage breast cancer. A meta-analysis of clinical trials worldwide that included 2656 women ≥70 years of age, documented decreases in both recurrence (28%) and overall mortality (21%) rates among patients with node-positive disease treated with adjuvant tamoxifen. Similar proportional risk reductions were found for node negative patients, although the absolute risk reduction was greater for women who were node positive. In addition, the magnitude of risk reduction, both with respect to recurrence and mortality, was similar across three postmenopausal age groups: 50–59, 60–69, and 70+. Adjuvant tamoxifen therapy also was beneficial for women with hormone receptor-poor tumors, albeit to a lesser extent than in those with hormone receptor-rich tumors. Furthermore, treatment with tamoxifen also prevented the development of contralateral breast cancer (18).

There may be non-breast cancer benefits of therapy for postmenopausal women as well. Tamoxifen may prevent osteoporosis (19) and lower cholesterol levels (20). Indeed, recent reports from Europe suggest that tamoxifen reduces the risk of hospitalization for cardiovascular disease and for fatal myocardial infarction (21, 22).

Although the benefits of tamoxifen are clear, treatment with tamoxifen also increases the risk of rare, but serious illnesses. Deep vein thrombosis can complicate the use of tamoxifen and this risk appears to be greater in women ≥65 years (23). In addition, recent studies from Europe and the United States are relatively consistent in demonstrating an increased risk of endometrial cancer among tamoxifen users (24, 25). About 75% of endometrial cancers occur in women ≥60 years of age, and this already elevated base rate appears to be increased by the addition of tamoxifen treatment. Whether this increase is because tamoxifen actually causes endometrial cancer, or because it unmasks silent disease by causing bleeding is not known (26). Furthermore, although annual gynecological examinations, ranging from a history and physical examination to pelvic and/or endovaginal ultrasound and/or endometrial sampling are recommended for patients if receiving tamoxifen (25), there is uncertainty as to the best approach to surveillance (27–29), particularly since most uterine cancers associated with tamoxifen therapy have been diagnosed at an early stage (25).

In summary, the benefits of adjuvant treatment with tamoxifen have been proven in older women and outweigh its risks (30). Until more sensitive indicators of recurrence risk are identified, treatment of most older women with early stage disease with adjuvant tamoxifen should be recommended, excepting perhaps those with tumors ≤1 centimeter in size. Treatment for longer than two years is probably also indicated, not only because more prolonged therapy delays recurrence (18), but because it may reduce a woman's risk of developing osteoporosis and coronary heart disease.

Menopausal symptoms, either caused by or exacerbated by tamoxifen may limit its use, particularly in the young old. Hot flashes are the most common and bothersome of side effects, occurring in up to one fourth of patients (31). Although transdermal clonidine or oral progesterone derivatives are side effect treatment options, their own side effects may be equally problematic for older women. This therapeutic dilemma raises the question of whether estrogen replacement therapy might be a reasonable alternative for the management of menopausal symptoms in these patients, some of whom may have been receiving such treatment prior to the diagnosis of their cancer. A recent thoughtful review by Cobleigh and colleagues (32) argues for clinical trials to study the effects of hormone replacement therapy in breast cancer survivors. The accumulated evidence does not support the continued prohibition of estrogen replacement therapy in breast cancer survivors. Pending the conduct of definitive clinical trials, estrogen replacement therapy can be recommended at least for breast cancer survivors receiving adjuvant tamoxifen therapy because it does not appear to increase the risk of recurrence or the development of contralateral disease, it will decrease the duration and severity of menopausal symptoms, and it may accentuate the cardiovascular and bone benefits of tamoxifen.

Chemotherapy

Adjuvant chemotherapy alone or in conjunction with tamoxifen has not been well-studied in women over 70 years of age. The meta-analysis of studies worldwide included only 274 women in this age group who were entered into trials testing the efficacy of adjuvant chemotherapy, In these women, adjuvant chemotherapy did not appear to be of benefit, either with respect to recurrence or mortality (33). Whether chemotherapy is efficacious, particularly in high-risk subsets of older patients, is not known. What is known is that older women who are otherwise generally healthy are able to tolerate combination chemotherapy (34, 35). Clinical trials of combination chemotherapy that are specifically designed for women in this age group are very much needed.

Metastatic Disease

Survival rates in older women diagnosed with metastatic disease decrease with age. Although the one year survival rate for women 65–74 years of age is similar to that in the first postmenopausal age decade (about 60%), this rate declines to 54% in those 75–84 years and to 44% in those ≥85 years of age (1). Five year survival rates across all age groups are very low, ranging from 16 to 20%. These rates provide a compelling argument for continued efforts to improve access and use of screening mammography in older women.

Although endocrine treatment in older women has only a modest effect on survival, symptom palliation is usually possible (36, 37). Because it is well-tolerated in general, tamoxifen is the preferred first line of treatment. The average response rate to tamoxifen is about 30%. The highest response rates are observed in those women who have tumors with positive hormone receptors, those who have had a long disease-free interval, and those who have soft tissue or bony metastases. If bony metastases are present, calcium

levels should be monitored initially since transient hypercalcemia can occur. Other endocrine agents, such as megestrol acetate, aromatase inhibitors (aminoglutethimide), or stilbestrol may be useful when patients relapse, although the side effects of these agents, especially nausea, weight gain, fluid retention, and fatigue may be troublesome.

The use of chemotherapy in older women with metastatic disease has not been widely studied. Nonetheless, recent reports indicate that there are probably no important age-related differences in response rates, time to progression, survival, and toxic side-effects (34, 35). Until more definitive studies have been performed, older women whose disease has become refractory to endocrine treatments should be considered for treatment with combination chemotherapy. Although complete response is rare, partial responses that last 6–12 months can be expected in about 40% of such patients (2).

As with all patients with life-threatening disease, treatment decision-making in women with metastatic disease must take into account risk and benefits and patient preferences. End of life care, including advance directives, hospice care, and preferences for site of death should be discussed with patients and their families, ideally earlier rather than later. However, patient and families need to understand that the therapeutic plan can be flexible as patient's needs change.

Care of Breast Cancer Survivors

As more women with treated breast cancer survive into old age, new questions arise for clinicians caring for them. One question that has received considerable attention in recent years is, "What kind and duration of follow-up care should breast cancer survivors receive?" Although the question has not been answered for older women *per se*, studies of the value of routine follow-up testing demonstrate that such testing neither improves survival nor influences health-related quality of life (38–40). It is doubtful that studies specifically of older women would reach different conclusions.

However, other question are especially germane to older women and should be addressed by carefully conducted follow-up studies of older long-term survivors. These include, but are not limited to: 1) How long should surveillance mammography be continued? 2) What are the long-term musculoskeletal complications of mastectomy and axillary dissection? 3) What are the long-term pulmonary complications of post-operative radiation therapy? 4) What are the long-term psychosocial issues that influence older women's quality of life?

Summary and Conclusions

Breast cancer is becoming an increasingly important disease in older women. Although the knowledge base on which to base therapeutic recommendations is incomplete, most older women with early stage disease should be given the same options as younger postmenopausal women. Nonetheless, patient preferences, comorbidity, functional status, life expectancy, risks and benefits of treatment, and family support are all important considerations when developing a treatment plan. Older women should be encouraged to participate in clinical trials and outcomes studies specifically designed to expand the scientific knowledge on which to base recommendations for their care.

References

1. Yancik R, Ries LB, Yates JW. Breast cancer in aging women: a population-based study of contrasts in stage, surgery, and survival. *Cancer* 1989; **63**: 164–69.
2. Muss HB. The role of chemotherapy and adjuvant therapy in the management of breast cancer in older women. *Cancer* 1994; **74**: 2165–2171.
3. Manton K. Cross-sectional estimates of active life expectancy for the US elderly and oldest-old populations. *J Gerontol* 1991; **46**: S170-S182.
4. *The aging population in the twenty-first century*, edited by DM Gilford. Washington, DC: National Academy Press, 1988.
5. NIH consensus conference. Treatment of early stage breast cancer. *JAMA* 1991; **265**: 391–95.
6. Silliman RA, Dukes KA, Kaplan SH. Family and social support. Cancer in the Elderly: Second International Conference on Geriatric Oncology, 1994.
7. Fisher B, Redmond C, Poisson R, et al. Eight year results of a randomized clinical trial comparing total mastectomy and lympectomy with or without irradiation in the treatment of breast cancer. *N Engl J Med* 1989; **320**: 822–28.
8. Nemoto T, Patel JK, Rosner D, et al. Factors affecting recurrence in lumpectomy without irradiation for breast cancer. *Cancer* 1991; **67**: 2079–2082.
9. Clark RM, McCulloch PB, Levine MN. Randomized clinical trial to assess the effectiveness of breast irradiation following lumpectomy and axillary dissection for node negative breast cancer. *J Natl Cancer* 1992; **84**: 683–689.
10. Kantorowitz DA, Poulter CA, Sischy B, et al. Treatment of breast cancer among elderly women with segmental mastectomy of segmental mastectomy plus postoperative radiotherapy. *Int J Radial Oncol Biol Phys* 1988; **15**: 263–270.
11. Veronesi U, Luini A, Del Vecchio M, et al. Radiotherapy after breast-preserving surgery in women with localized cancer of the breast. *N Engl J Med* 1993; **328**:1587–91.
12. Harris JR, Osteen RT. Patients benefit from effective axillary treatment. *Breast Cancer Res Treat* 1985; **5**: 17–21.
13. Balducci L, Schapira DV, Cox CE, Greenberg HM, Lyman GH. Breast cancer of the older woman: an annotated review. *J Am Geriatr Soc* 1991; **39**: 1113–1123.
14. Lichter AS. Conservative treatment of primary breast cancer: How much is required? *J Natl Cancer Inst* 1992; **84**: 659–660.
15. Robertson JF, Ellis IO, Elston CW, Blarney RW. Mastectomy or tamoxifen as initial therapy for operable breast cancer in elderly patients: 5-year follow-up. *Eur J Cancer* 1992; **28A**: 908–10.
16. Gazet JC, Markopoulos C, Ford HT, et al. Prospective randomized trial of tamoxifen versus surgery in elderly patients with breast cancer. *Lancet* 1988; **1**: 679–681.
17. Bates T, Riley DL, Houghton J, et al. Breast cancer in elderly women: a Cancer Research Campaign trial comparing treatment with tamoxifen and optimal surgery with tamoxifen alone. The Elderly Breast Cancer Working Party. *Br J Surg* 1991; **78**: 591–594.
18. Early breast cancer trialists' collaborative group. Systemic treatment of early breast cancer by hormonal, cytotoxic, or immune therapy: 133 randomized trials involving 31,000 recurrences and 24,000 deaths among 75,000 women. Part 1. *Lancet* 1992; **339**: 1–15.
19. Love RR, Mazess RB, Barden HS, et al. Effects of tamoxifen on bone mineral density in postmenopausal women with breast cancer. *N Engl J Med* 1992; **326**: 852–56.
20. Love RR, Wiebe DA, Newcomb PA, Cameron L, Leventhal H, Jordan VC. Effects of tamoxifen on cardiovascular risk factors in postmenopausal women. *Ann Intern Med* 1991; **115**: 860–64.
21. McDonald CC, Stewart HJ. Fatal myocardial infarction in the Scottish adjuvant tamoxifen trial. *BMJ* 1991; **303**: 435–437.
22. Rutqvist LE, Mattsson A. Cardiac and thromboembolic morbidity among postmenopausal women with early-stage breast cancer in a randomized trial of adjuvant tamoxifen. *J Natl Cancer Inst* 1993; **85**: 1398–1406.
23. Fisher B, Brown A, Wolmark N, Redmond C, Wickerham DL, Wittliff J. Prolonging tamoxifen therapy for primary breast cancer. *Ann Intern Med* 1987; **106**: 649–54.
24. Fornander T, Cedermark B, Mattson A, et al. Adjuvant tamoxifen in early breast cancer. Occurrence of new primary cancers. *Lancet* 1989; **1**: 117–120.
25. Fisher B, Costantino JP, Redmond CK, et al. Endometrial cancer in tamoxifen-treated breast cancer patients. Findings from the National Surgical Adjuvant Breast and Bowel Project (NSABP) B-14. *J Natl Cancer Inst* 1994; **86**: 527–537.
26. Fritsch M, Wolf DM. Symptomatic side effects of tamoxifen therapy. In: Jordan VC, ed. *Long-term tamoxifen treatment for breast cancer*, Madison: The University of Wisconsin Press, 1994; 235–255.
27. Hulka CA, Hall DA. Endometrial abnormalities associated with tamoxifen therapy for breast cancer: Sonographic and pathologic correlation. *AJR* 1993; **160**: 809–812.
28. Cohen I, Rosen DJD, Tepper R, et al. Ultrasonographic evaluation of the endometrium and correlation with endometrial sampling in postmenopausal patients treated with tamoxifen. *J Ultrasound Med* 1993; **5**: 275–280.
29. Cohen I, Rosen DJD, Shapira J, et al. Endometrial changes in postmenopausal women treated with tamoxifen for breast cancer. *Brit J Obs Gynecol* 1993; **100**: 657–570.
30. Ragaz J, Goldman A. Age-matched survival impact (SI) of adjuvant tamoxifen in long term breast cancer survivors (LTBCS) taking into analysis contralateral breast cancer (CBC), cardiovascular events (CVS), uterine cancer (UC) and pulmonary emboli (PE). *Proc ASCO* 1995; **14**: 112 (abstract).
31. Love RR, Cameron L, Connell BL, et al. Symptoms associated with tamoxifen treatment in postmenopausal women. *Arch Intern Med* 1991; **151**: 1842–1847.
32. Cobleigh MA, Berris RF, Bush T, et al. Estrogen replacement therapy in breast cancer survivors: A time for change. *JAMA* 1994; **272**: 540–545.
33. Early breast cancer trialists' collaborative group. Systemic treatment of early breast cancer by hormonal, cytotoxic, or immune therapy: 133 randomized trials involving 31,000 recurrences and 24,000 deaths among 75,000 women. Part 2. *Lancet* 1992; **339**: 71–85.
34. Gelman RS, Taylor SG. Cyclophosphamide, methotrexate and 5-fluorouracil chemotherapy in women more than 65 years old with advanced breast cancer: the elimination of age trends in toxicity by using doses based on creatinine clearance. *J Clin Oncol* 1984; **2**: 1404–1413.
35. Christman K, Muss HB, Case LD, et al. Chemotherapy of metastatic breast cancer in the elderly. The Piedmont Oncology Association experience. *JAMA* 1992; **268**: 57–62.
36. Pritchard RI, Sutherland DJA. The use of endocrine therapy. *Hematol Oncol Clin* 1989; **3**: 765–806.
37. Ziegler LD, Buzdar AU. Recent advances in the treatment of breast cancer. *Am J Med Sci* 1991; **301**: 337–349.
38. Marrazza A, Solina G, Puccia V, Fiorentino E, Bazan P. Evaluation of routine follow-up after surgery for breast carcinoma. *J Surg Oncol* 1986; **32**: 179–181.
39. Zwaveling A, Albers GHR, Fulthuis W, Hermans J. An evaluation of routine follow-up for detection of breast cancer recurrences. *J Surg Oncol* 1987; **34**: 194–197.
40. The GIVIO Investigators. Impact of follow-up testing on survival and health-related quality of life in breast cancer patients: A multicenter randomized controlled trial. *JAMA* 1994; **271**: 1587–1592.

47. Cancer of the Large Bowel

Barbara A. Neilan

Epidemiology and Etiology

Incidence

Cancer of the large bowel is presently the second most common malignancy in the United States. The estimated number of new cases of colon and rectal cancer in 1997 is 131,200, and the number of cancer deaths is estimated at 54,900 (1).

Colorectal cancer is of special interest to geriatricians since it occurs primarily in older persons. More than 90% of cancers of the large bowel occur in people over 50 years of age, and about 75% in people older than 65 years. Moreover, in women and men over age 75 years, this carcinoma represents the first and the third site for cancer mortality, respectively (2).

With respect to sex, cancer of the large bowel occurs slightly more often in women than in men (1). There is little difference in the incidence of cancer of the colon compared to cancer of the rectum. The incidence in blacks is slightly lower than in whites. Unfortunately however, mortality is increasing in black men.

Risk Factors

Several definite and possible risk factors have been identified for colorectal cancer (Table 47.1).

Age is a leading risk factor for cancer of the large bowel. Risk begins at 40 years of age, but it increases sharply at 50 years of age, doubling each decade until age 80 years (3).

There is considerable evidence that most colorectal cancers develop from adenomas. The chance of an adenoma becoming malignant depends on size and histology. About 5% of adenomas that reach 5 mm will become malignant (4). On average, a 1 cm adenoma will become an invasive cancer within 7 years (range,

0 to 14 years) (4). Patients who have had polyps of 1 cm or greater in size removed are at increased risk for cancer in other areas of the bowel (5). Villous adenomas have a higher frequency of developing invasive carcinoma than tubular adenomas. In addition to histology and size, it appears that the greater the number of polyps, the higher the risk of cancer (5).

Another major risk factor is a history of cancer of the large bowel. Persons with colon cancer are at increased risk for having a second colon cancer either at initial presentation (synchronous) or at a later date (metachronous). Synchronous lesions occur with a frequency of 1.5 to 2.5% (6). The frequency of metachronous lesions is even higher, 5–10% (3).

Inflammatory bowel disease is associated with an increased risk of colorectal carcinoma. In ulcerative colitis, the risk increases with duration of the disease and extent of bowel involvement. Patients with granulomatous colitis are also at increased risk, although this risk is less than with ulcerative colitis.

There are also hereditary conditions associated with colorectal cancer. The role of inheritance is most evident in two syndromes: familial adenomatous polyposis and hereditary nonpolyposis colorectal cancer. Familial adenomatous polyposis is characterized by hundreds of adenomas. Prophylactic colectomy is recommended for these patients since a small number of these adenomas progress to carcinoma in the fourth decade. Hereditary nonpolyposis colorectal cancer consists of the Lynch I syndrome (only includes inherited colorectal cancer) and the Lynch II syndrome (includes other tumors, such as pancreatic, gastric, endometrial and ovarian).

Etiology

The cause of cancer of the large bowel is not known, however, it has been suggested that genetic, environmental, and diet-related factors may all play a role. The hereditary nature of colorectal cancer has suggested a genetic basis for this disease. The identification of specific genetic mutations in hereditary colorectal cancer syndromes gives further support to this.

Epidemiologic studies suggest that environmental factors, especially diet, are causative. The incidence of colon cancer is lower in African countries compared to Western nations. When Africans migrate to developed countries, the incidence of colorectal cancer rises which may be related to dietary change. The diets of African populations contain more fiber and less refined carbo-

Table 47.1 Risk factors.

Age	>40 years old
Adenomas	villous > tubula
Previous colon cancer	metachronous > synchronous
Inflammatory bowel disease	ulcerative > granulomatous
Hereditary	familial polyposis coli, Gardner syndrome, and familial colon cancer without polypos

Table 47.2 WHO guidelines for the prevention of colorectal cancer.

1. Fat consumption shoud be low, not exceeding 20% of total calories. Both animal and vegetable fat should be reduced to achieve this goal.

2. A balanced diet should be consumed. It should include at least 5 to 8 servings daily of fruits and vegetables, legumes, and whole grain cereals and breads in order to provide adequate fiber, vitamins and other components with potential anticarcinogenic effects.

3. Dietary fiber from all sources should be at least 25 g/day.

4. Consumption of excess calories and being overweight should be avoided.

5. Tobacco use should be avoided.

6. Physical activities should be incorporated into daily routine (walk rather than drive short distances. Climb the stairs rather than take the lift or elevator).

hydrates and fats. High fiber diets may be protective by causing a faster intestinal transit time resulting in less exposure to potential carcinogens. In addition, it has been suggested that the high fat content of Western diets may change the activity of intestinal micro flora and the concentration of bile acids, leading to production of tumor promoting substances in the colon.

A variety of lifestyles may be associated with development of large bowel cancer. Beer consumption has been labeled a risk factor (3,7). Substantial consumption of alcohol (>2 drinks daily), when combined with inadequate intakes of folate and methionine, may increase colon cancer risk (8). Physical inactivity may predispose to colon cancer (9,10). In addition, height and obesity, particularly abdominal adiposity are associated with an increased risk of cancer of the large bowel (10).

Prevention

Studies suggest that the risk of cancer of the large bowel can be reduced by various dietary measures. Risk can be reduced by a low intake of animal derived fat and high intake of vegetables and fiber. The WHO Collaborating Center for the Prevention of Colorectal Cancer at Memorial Sloan-Kettering Cancer Center in conjunction with an International Advisory Committee has published guidelines for primary prevention of colorectal cancer (Table 47.2) (11).

Dietary factors may account for the different mortality rates from colon cancer in Florida and in the northeastern United States (12). The mortality rate of people who lived in the northeastern U. S. but retired to Florida is lower than the mortality rate of the population still living in the Northeast. This decrease in mortality may be due to a change in lifestyle in Florida, possibly diet. Since the decrease happens in a relatively short time, dietary change may be able to lower the

incidence of colorectal cancer, even in elderly individuals such as reside in Florida.

Calcium may be beneficial because of binding to fatty and bile acids in the gut, forming insoluble soaps which may then prevent potential carcinogens from contacting the bowel (13). Although two studies have shown an inverse relationship between calcium intake and colorectal mortality (14,15), four of five case-control studies have not shown a beneficial effect (7).

Regular use of aspirin appears to decrease the risk of cancer of the large bowel. One study involving 47,900 male health professionals who responded to a mailed questionnaire showed that regular intake of aspirin (>2 times per week) decreased the risk of colorectal cancer (16). In the Nurses' Health Study the rates of colorectal cancer were determined according to the number of consecutive years of regular aspirin use (17).This study showed that regular aspirin use substantially reduced the risk of colorectal cancer in women also, but the benefit may not be evident until after a decade of aspirin consumption.

Postmenopausal use of estrogens may result in a decreased risk of cancer of the large bowel. A large prospective study of women taking estrogen replacement therapy found that estrogen therapy, particularly recent and long-term use, was associated with a decreased risk of fatal colon cancer (18).

Detection and Diagnosis

Screening

Cancer of the large bowel is curable if detected in the early stages. Screening of asymptomatic persons is one of the primary ways to detect early colorectal cancer and reduce mortality. It is estimated that early detection can save the lives of 75% of patients with cancer of the colon and rectum. As the population to the United States grows older and more people are at risk for colorectal cancer, the number of lives saved can be increased.

Screening for colorectal cancer is feasible since it is a common disorder, screening tests are readily available, and early detection decreases mortality. Three basic tools are used for screening: the digital rectal examination, fecal occult blood testing, and sigmoidoscopy. The American Cancer Society has developed guidelines for screening asymptomatic persons using these tests (Table 47.3).

The digital rectal examination can detect low rectal lesions as well as prostatic cancer. It can be done as part of the annual physical examination without advance

Table 47.3 Screening for cancer of the large bowel (American Cancer Society guidelines).

Digital rectal examination yearly after age 40 years

Fecal occult blood test yearly after age 50 years

Sigmoidoscopy every 3–5 years after age 50 years

preparation and does not involve additional expense. However, since proximal colon lesions are now more common than distal lesions, the rectal examination will uncover only a small percentage of colorectal cancers.

The fecal occult blood test is the most commonly used screening test. Five controlled trials have been done in asymptomatic persons (19–23). One of these studies showed a reduction in colorectal cancer mortality as a result of fecal occult blood testing (22). In addition, a shift to earlier stage cancers was reported in this trial. In the screened group there were 20% more Dukes' A cancers and only half as many Dukes' D tumors compared with controls. Similar staging shifts were seen in some of the other studies.

Two interesting observations have been made with respect to age and fecal occult blood testing (24). One observation was that the number of positive test results increased with age. Secondly, the percentage of adenomas and cancer found in persons with positive fecal occult blood tests increased with advancing age. Thus, this test may be more sensitive in asymptomatic geriatric patients.

The third screening test for cancer of the large bowel is sigmoidoscopy. Although periodic sigmoidoscopy is currently recommended by several national groups starting at age 50 years, the effectiveness of this test is still being evaluated. Currently, there are no prospective, randomized studies demonstrating that sigmoidoscopy reduces colorectal cancer mortality. One randomized trial of rigid sigmoidoscopy screening showed a decrease in colon cancer mortality (25), however, a number of problems have been cited with this study. Two case-control studies using rigid sigmoidoscopy showed a reduction in mortality resulting from tumors within reach of the sigmoidoscope (26,27). Another study evaluated the risk of colorectal cancer after removal of rectosigmoid adenomas (28).This study showed that sigmoidoscopy may not only reduce mortality through polypectomy, but may be predictive of colorectal cancer risk by characterization of the polyps. To further confirm the value of sigmoidoscopy, the National Cancer Institute is conducting a large, prospective trial of flexible sigmoidoscopy screening. However, these results will not be available for several years (29).

All three screening tests are important to detect early cancer. If any one of these tests is abnormal, further evaluation for colorectal cancer should be carried out.

When the importance of early diagnosis is emphasized by physicians, patient compliance with screening studies is generally good. In this regard elderly individuals appear also to be cooperative. When evaluating fecal occult blood tests, one study found no difference in compliance in younger and older individuals (24).

Clinical Presentation

It is important to recognize the presenting symptoms of cancer of the large bowel. One-half of patients present with bleeding, abdominal pain, change in bowel habits, anorexia, or weight loss. Symptoms may differ depending on location of the cancer. Cancer of the right side of the colon may present with abdominal pain or fatigue secondary to iron deficiency anemia. Left-sided colon cancers are associated with crampy abdominal pain, signs of obstruction, or bleeding. Rectal cancers most often present with bleeding, a sense of incomplete evacuation and urgency, or constipation.

In the elderly, the presenting symptoms may be more vague. Weight loss, change in bowel habits, increased bearing down during evacuation, or fatigue may be the only symptoms. These symptoms must be fully evaluated and not attributed simply to age.

It is unclear whether the distribution of colon cancers is affected by age. In one study the location of cancers in the right or left colon was not affected by age . However, a retrospective review of 922 patients with colorectal cancer showed that female patients with right-sided colon cancer are significantly older (31). Therefore, the increasing incidence of proximal colorectal cancer may be related in part to an aging population, especially in women.

Diagnostic Studies

When cancer of the large bowel is suspected from the above symptoms, or a positive result from one of the three screening tests, further diagnostic studies are indicated.

Sigmoidoscopic examination can be performed using either the rigid or flexible sigmoidoscope. The rigid sigmoidoscope can be passed through 25 cm of the colon, although the average length visualized is about 17 cm. The flexible scope has improved visualization (up to 60 cm.) and patient comfort.

Barium enemas can be done with or without air contrast. Polyps can be detected better with air contrast studies. The lower sigmoid is not well visualized by barium enema, and sigmoidoscopy may be done in addition to evaluate this segment of colon.

Colonoscopy allows for direct visualization of the entire colon, and may be done in place of sigmoidoscopy and barium enema. Colonoscopy is also indicated preoperatively to rule out synchronous lesions.

Carcinoembryonic antigen (CEA) has been studied to evaluate its role in screening for cancer of the large bowel. However, CEA testing is not sensitive or specific enough to be useful in screening. CEA levels are useful in predicting the presence of liver metastases in the preoperative setting, or can be used to monitor for recurrent cancer postoperatively.

When colorectal cancer is suspected in geriatric patients, the possible risks of these diagnostic procedures must be considered. One study indicated that these tests can be done without major complications in patients over 60 years of age as well as in patients under 60 years (30).

Another consideration is whether geriatric patients will be less cooperative with diagnostic work-ups. No difference was found in the compliance with testing, including both radiographic studies and colonoscopy, between patients over 60 years and those under 60 years (30). In fact, the percentage of patients who re-

Table 47.4 Modified Astler-Coller classification of the Dukes staging system for cancer of the large bowel.

Stage	Description
A	Lesion not penetrating submucosa
B1	Lesion up to, but not through, serosa
B2	Lesion through serosa, with involvement of adjacent organs
C1	Lesion up to, but not through, serosa; regional lymph node metastasis
C2	Lesion through serosa, with involvement of adjacent organs; regional lymph node metastasis
D	Distant metastatic disease

fused studies decreased with age, even though these patients had more medical problems.

Classification

Pathology

Adenocarcinomas account for greater than 90% of colorectal cancers. Other histologic variants include mucinous (colloid) carcinoma, signet-ring carcinoma, adenosquamous carcinoma, and undifferentiated carcinoma. Adenocarcinomas are graded by the degree of differentiation, nuclear pleomorphism, and the number of mitoses. Grade 1 tumors have the most developed glandular structures and the least number of mitoses.

Staging

Staging of cancers of the large bowel is important to determine prognosis and potential treatment options. These cancers are staged according to whether the cancer has remained within the intestine or has spread to other sites. One commonly used staging system is the Dukes staging system (Table 47.4).

Older patients with colorectal cancer present with similar stage of disease as younger patients according to one study (30). However, when the cancers were detected by fecal occult blood testing, older patients had earlier stage disease than patients under age 60 years.

Prognosis

The prognosis for cancer of the large bowel is based primarily on the stage of disease. The two most important predictors of prognosis are depth of invasion and the presence or absence of regional lymph node involvement. Early stage lesions are readily cured by surgery. Dukes stage A cancer is curable in 80–90% of patients. However, in later stage disease, the prognosis decreases markedly. The 5-year survival in Dukes stage C cancer is 35–50%.

The degree of histologic differentiation has also been shown to have prognostic significance. Other factors influencing prognosis include the presence of obstruction, perforation, and rectal bleeding (32).

Geriatric patients do not appear to have an adverse prognosis on the basis of age. In one report older patients fared as well as younger patients when matched by stage, with the exception of a small fraction of patients less than 45 or over 75 years with localized disease (33).

Management

Although few studies have specifically evaluated treatment of older patients, no biologic difference has been found between younger and older patients with colorectal cancer (34). Therefore, treatment decisions should not be based on age, but rather on stage of disease and the medical condition of the patient.

Surgery

The goal of surgery is to remove the cancer in the bowel, draining lymph nodes, and contiguous organs. In colon cancer, procedures entailing wide surgical resection and anastomosis are done. In rectal cancer, the standard surgery has been an abdominal-perineal resection which requires a permanent sigmoid colostomy. Recent advances have led to the use of sphincter-preserving surgery for mid and some distal rectal cancers.

Age in itself does not appear to increase surgical risk. Several retrospective studies indicate that operative risk is not increased in older patients (35,37). When intercurrent illness is present, preoperative attention to correctable problems can reduce the adverse effects of these coexisting diseases. However, in some patients, disability from other medical conditions may be such that aggressive surgical resection is not advisable.

In older patients, surgical resection has a higher risk for rectal cancer than for colon cancer. Postoperative mortality in patients over age 70 years was two-thirds higher for rectal cancers than for colon lesions. However, in elderly patients with rectal cancer, surgery may give better results than alternative treatments. Local extirpation or diathermy destruction resulted in half the survival rate for surgical resection (33).

Adjuvant Therapy

Adjuvant therapy has been studied in patients at high risk for relapse after surgery, Dukes stage B2 or C disease. These recurrences may result from the presence of micrometastases or from tumor cell dissemination at surgery. For these reasons, adjuvant therapy has been tried before, during, and immediately after surgery. Radiotherapy, chemotherapy and immunotherapy, either alone or in combination, have been evaluated.

Colon Cancer

Most relapses after surgery for colon cancer occur in distant sites. To decrease the risk of distant failures, adjuvant chemotherapy has been studied in patients at high risk for recurrence, Dukes B2 and C stage disease. Adjuvant chemotherapy refers to the administration of systemic therapy after curative resection. Adjuvant clinical trials with fluorouracil (5-FU) and the immunomodulatory drug levamisole have shown significant decrease in recurrence and mortality in patients with positive lymph nodes (Dukes C) (39,40).

Age was not an exclusion criterion in this study, and patients as old as 84 years were entered. Age did not affect treatment outcome. Similar disease-free survivals and overall survivals were found in patients over 60 years and in those under 60 years.

Likewise, age does not appear to affect tolerance of adjuvant chemotherapy. Preliminary results of a study done on 1014 patients with Dukes stage B2, B3 or C colon cancer who were randomized to receive 5-fluorouracil plus levamisole or 5-fluorouracil plus leucovorin and levamisole suggest that patients over 70 years do not have greater toxicity than younger patients (41). However, the percentages of patients that had their treatment discontinued was higher in the elderly. This lower adherence to treatment plans in the older patients may have been due to a bias that geriatric patients are more likely to experience toxicity.

Rectal Cancer

Unlike colon cancer, when rectal cancer recurs, the failures are more often local. The principal reasons for local recurrence appear to be anatomic constraints in obtaining wide radial margins at surgery, and the lack of an adequate serosa in the rectum. Radiotherapy has been shown to reduce the risk of locoregional failure, but does not improve overall survival (42). The tolerance and response of older patients to radiation therapy has not been sufficiently studied. Therefore, treatment decisions regarding adjuvant radiotherapy in older patients should be made on the basis of available data and not age alone. However, older patients may be at higher risk of radiation-induced small bowel complications, requiring special attention to limiting small bowel exposure (43).

Radiotherapy plus 5-FU based chemotherapy has been shown to significantly reduce recurrence and improve survival in rectal cancer (44). The best method of administering fluorouracil for radiosensitization is still being investigated. An Intergroup trial comparing 5-FU by protracted venous infusion to bolus 5-FU found that infusional 5-FU was associated with improved relapse free and overall survival (45).

Surveillance

One of the first principles of follow-up is to ensure that the entire large bowel is clear of adenomas or synchronous cancers. Therefore, if colonoscopy or double contrast barium enema was not done prior to surgery, these studies are done within a few months after surgery.

After surgery patients should be followed closely for the possibility of recurrent disease. Eighty-five percent of recurrent disease is manifested during the first 2.5 years after surgery, while the remaining 15% recur during the subsequent 2.5 years. Therefore, patients require close monitoring for possible recurrence. Patients should be seen every three months for the first 3 years and have fecal occult blood tests and blood tests (liver function tests, CBC, and CEA) done. Chest X-rays should be obtained every 6 months for two years,

and then yearly. Colonoscopy should be performed yearly. A baseline CT scan of the abdomen and pelvis should be obtained about 3 months after surgery, but the value of routine CT scans has not been demonstrated.

CEA levels may be followed to detect recurrent disease prior to clinical manifestations. After complete surgical resection, the CEA level returns to normal in 4 to 6 weeks. If the CEA level does not normalize, all of the cancer may not have been removed. If a normal postoperative CEA level subsequently rises, the possibility of recurrent disease should be further investigated. If diagnostic studies do not reveal the site of recurrent disease, second-look surgery may be indicated.

Recurrent and Metastatic Disease

Metastatic cancer of the large bowel is not considered a curable disease. Instead, the goals of treatment are to relieve symptoms. Palliative therapy may include surgery, radiotherapy, chemotherapy, or a combination of these modalities.

Chemotherapy

Fluorouracil.   Fluorouracil (5-FU) is the primary chemotherapeutic agent for treatment of advanced colorectal cancer. The response rate to single agent 5-FU is about 20%. When 5-FU is combined with leucovorin, the response rate increases to about 40% (46).

Hepatic Artery Infusion.   Hepatic artery infusion of chemotherapy has been tried for hepatic metastases. Infusion of floxuridine has a high response rate, but is associated with significant toxicity. Cholangiocyte and hepatocyte toxicity, gastritis and peptic ulcerations have been seen.

Age.   Until recently, older patients were excluded from treatment protocols or given dose reductions of chemotherapy based on age alone. This age-related treatment bias was based primarily on anecdotal experience, and has not been substantiated. A retrospective analysis of patients with colorectal cancer enrolled on Eastern Cooperative Oncology Group trials showed that patients age 70 years or older tolerated chemotherapy as well as younger patients (47). Therefore, it appears that the same principles for prescribing chemotherapy should be used for younger and older patients.

Hepatic Resection

Since metastatic disease from colorectal cancer occurs primarily in the liver, resection of liver metastases has been evaluated. Resection of a solitary metastatic lesion has given 5-year survival rates of 37% (48). Although there are no randomized studies evaluating the role of hepatic resection, two studies with matched controls showed no survivors at three years in the unresected group (49,50).

Is complicated surgery such as hepatic resection contraindicated in the elderly? Although this may have been true in the past, age alone should not deter a potentially life-prolonging operation. In a retrospective analysis of liver resection for colorectal metastases performed between 1985 and 1994, there was no significant difference in morbidity and mortality in patients over 70 years compared to younger patients (51).This study suggests that properly selected geriatric patients can tolerate major surgical procedures for cancer.

Summary

Cancer of the large bowel is one of the leading causes of death in older individuals. Therefore, this age-related cancer is of particular importance to geriatricians.

Although etiology is unknown, it has been suggested that cancer of the large bowel results from genetic, environmental, and diet-related factors. Modifications of diet and life-style, and intake of aspirin may be helpful in preventing the development and progression of large bowel cancer.

Screening of older asymptomatic persons is currently one of the most important available techniques for decreasing mortality from colorectal cancer. Because age is the leading risk factor for cancer of the large bowel, the American Cancer Society has developed screening guidelines for older patients.

When cancer of the large bowel is detected, patients require staging studies to determine prognosis and potential treatment options. For localized disease, surgical resection with or without adjuvant therapy is the primary therapy. In advanced disease, palliative treatment may include the use of surgery, radiotherapy, chemotherapy, or a combination of these modalities. More studies addressing treatment outcomes in older patients are needed. However, the few available studies suggest that age alone should not be a factor in treatment decisions. Principles of management can be applied similarly in geriatric and younger patients.

References

1. Parker SL, Tong T, Bolden S, et al. Cancer Statistics: CA — A Cancer Journal for Clinicians 1996; **46**(1): 5–27.
2. Ziegler RG, Devesa SS, Fraumeni JF, et al. Epidemiologic patterns of colorectal cancer. In Important Advances in Oncology, edited by VT DeVita, S Hellman, SA Rosenberg. Philadelphia, Pa: JB Lippincott, 209–232, 1986.
3. Winawer SJ, Miller DG, Sherlock P. Risk and screening for colorectal cancer. Adv Intern Med 1984; **30**: 471–496.
4. Morson BC. Genesis of colorectal cancer. Clin Gastroenterol 1976; **5**: 505–25.
5. Lotfi AM, Spencer RJ, Ilstrup DM, et al. Colorectal polyps and the risk of subsequent carcinoma. Mayo Clin Proc 1986; **61**: 337–343.
6. Cutler SJ, Young JL Jr. Third national cancer survey incidence data (monograph). Natl Cancer Inst 1975; **41**: 1–454.
7. Faivre J, Wilpart M, Boutron MC. Primary prevention of large bowel cancer. Recent Results Cancer Res 1991; **122**: 85–99.
8. Giovannucci D, Rimm EB, Ascherio A, et al. Alcohol, low-methionine-low-folate diets, and risk of colon cancer in men. J Natl Cancer Inst 1995; **87**: 265–273.
9. Garabrant DH, et al. Job activity and colon cancer risks. Am J Epidemiol 1984; **199**: 1005–1014.
10. Giovannucci E, Ascherio A, Rimm EB et al. Physical activity, obesity, and risk for colon cancer and adenoma in men. Ann Intern Med 1995; **122**: 327–334.
11. Winawer SJ, St. John DJ, Bond JH, et al. Prevention of colorectal cancer: guidelines based on new data. Bulletin of the World Health Organization. 1995; **73**(1): 7–10.
12. DeVita VT. Opening remarks. In Perspectives on Prevention and Treatment of Cancer in the Elderly, edited by R Yancik, PP Carbone. New York: Raven Press, 1–3, 1983.
13. Slattery ML, Sorenson AW, Fora MH. Dietary calcium intake as a mitigating factor in colon cancer. Am J Epidemiol 1988; **128**: 504–514.
14. Garland C, Shekelle RB, Barrett-Connore E, et al. Dietary vitamin D and calcium and risk of colorectal cancer a 19-year prospective study in men. Lancet 1985; **1**: 307–309.
15. Garland C, Garland F. Do sunlight and vitamin D reduce the risk of colon cancer? Int J Epidemiol 1980; **9**: 227–231.
16. Giovannucci E, Rimm EB, Stampfer MJ, et al. Aspirin use and the risk for colorectal cancer and adenoma in male health professionals. Ann Intern Med 1994; **121**: 241–246.
17. Giovannucci E, Egan KM, Hunter DJ, et al. Aspirin and the risk of colorectal cancer in women. N Engl J Med 1995; **333**: 609–14.
18. Calle EE, Miracle-McMahill HL, Thun MJ, et al. Estrogen replacement therapy and risk of fatal colon cancer in a prospective cohort of postmenopausal women. J Natl Cancer Inst 1995; **87**: 517–523.
19. Winawer SJ, Schottenfeld D, Flehinger BJ. Colorectal cancer screening. J Natl Cancer Inst 1991; **83**: 243–253.
20. Hardcastle JD, Chamberlin J, Sheffield J, et al. Randomized trial of fecal occult blood screening for colorectal cancer. Results for the first 107,349 subjects. Lancet 1989; **1**: 1160–1164.
21. Kewenter J, Bjork S, Haglind E, et al. Screening and rescreening for colorectal cancer. A controlled trial of fecal occult blood testing in 27,700 subjects. Cancer 1988; **62**: 645–650.
22. Mandel JS, Bond JH, Church TR, et al. Reducing mortality from colorectal cancer by screening for fecal occult blood. N Engl J Med 1993; **328**: 1365–1371.
23. Kronborg L, Fenger C, Sondergaard O, et al. Initial mass screening for colorectal cancer with fecal occult blood test. Scand J Gastroenterol 1987; **677**: 22–28.
24. Winawer SJ, Andrews M, Flehinger B, et al. Progress report on controlled trial of fecal occult blood testing for the detection of colorectal neoplasia. Cancer 1980; **45**: 2959–2964.
25. Dales LG, Friedman GD, Collen MF. Evaluating periodic multiphasic health check up: A controlled trial. J Chron Dis 1979; **32**: 385–404.
26. Selby JV, Friedman GD, Quesenberry CP, et al. A case-control study of screening sigmoidoscopy and mortality from colorectal cancer. N Engl J Med 1992; **326**: 653–657.
27. Newcomb PA, Norfleet RG, Storer BE, et al. Screening sigmoidoscopy and colorectal cancer mortality. J Natl Cancer Inst 1992; **84**: 1572–1575.
28. Atkin WS, Morson BC, Cuzick J. Long term risk of colorectal cancer after excision of rectosigmoid adenomas. N Engl J Med 1992; **326**: 658–662.
29. Kramer BS, Gohagan J, Prorok PC, et al. A National Cancer Institute sponsored screening trial for prostatic, lung, colorectal and ovarian cancers. Cancer 1993; **71**: 589–593.
30. Winawer SJ, Baldwin M, Herbert E, et al. Screening experience with fecal occult blood testing as a function of age. In Perspectives on Prevention and Treatment of Cancer in the Elderly, edited by R Yancik, PP Carbone. New York: Raven Press, 265–274, 1983.
31. Fleshner P, Later G, Aufes A Jr. Age and sex distribution of patients with colorectal cancer. Dis Colon Rectum 1989; **32**: 107–111.
32. Steinberg SM, Barkin JS, Kaplan RS, et al. Prognostic indicators of colon tumors: The Gastrointestinal Tumor Study Group experience. Cancer 1986; **57**: 1866–1870.
33. Five-year relative survival rates: White patients, both sexes 1967–73. From Cancer Patient Survival, Report No. 5, DHEW Pub. No. (NIH) 77–992.
34. Patterson W. Oncology perspective on colorectal cancer in the geriatric patient. In Perspectives on Prevention and Treatment of Cancer in the Elderly, edited by R Yancik, PP Carbone. New York: Raven Press, 105–112, 1983.
35. Calabrese CT, Adam YG, Volk H. Geriatric colon cancer. Am J Surg 1973; **125**: 181–184.

36. Irvin GL, Robinson DS, Hubbard S. Operative risks in patients with colorectal cancer. *Am J Surg* 1985; **51**: 418–422.

37. Jensen HE, Nielsen J, Balslev I. Carcinoma of the colon in old age. *Ann Surg* 1970; **171**: 107–115.

38. Jensen HE, Balslev 1, Fenger HJ, *et al.* Carcinoma of the rectum in old age. *Acta Chir Scand* 1973; **139**: 563–567.

39. Laurie JA, Moertel CG, Fleming TR, *et al.* Surgical adjuvant therapy of large bowel carcinoma: An evaluation of levamisole and the combination of levamisole and fluorouracil. *J Clin Oncol* 1989; **7**: 1447–1456.

40. Moertel CG, Fleming TR, Macdonald, JS, *et al.* Fluorouracil plus levamisole as effective adjuvant therapy after resection of stage III colon carcinoma: A final report. *Ann Intern Med* 1995; **122**: 321–326.

41. Aschele C, Guglielmi A, Tixi LM, *et al.* Adjuvant treatment of colorectal cancer in the elderly. *Cancer Control* 1995; 36–38.

42. Rosenthal SA, Trock BJ, Coia LR. Randomized trials of adjuvant radiation therapy for rectal carcinoma: A review. *Dis Colon Rectum* 1990; **33**: 335–343.

43. Farniak KE, Levitt SH. The role of radiation therapy in the treatment of colorectal cancer. Implications for the older patient. *Cancer* 1994; **74**: 2154–2159.

44. Krook JE, Moertel CG, Gunderson LL, *et al.* Effective surgical adjuvant therapy for high-risk rectal carcinoma. *N Engl J Med* 1991; **324**: 709–715.

45. O'Connell MJ, Martenson JA, Wieand HS, *et al.* Improving adjuvant therapy for rectal cancer by combining protracted-infusion fluorouracil with radiation therapy after curative surgery. *N Engl J Med* 1994; **331**: 502–507.

46. Petrelli N, Herrera L, Rustum Y *et al.* A prospective randomized trial of 5-fluorouracil versus 5-fluorouracil and high-dose leucovorin versus 5-fluorouracil and methotrexate in previously untreated patients with advanced colorectal carcinoma. *J Clin Oncol* 1987; **5**: 1559–1565.

47. Begg CB, Carbone PP. Clinical trials and drug toxicity in the elderly: The experience of the Eastern Cooperative Oncology Group. *Cancer* 1983; **52**: 1986–1992.

48. Hughes K, Simon R, Songhorabodi S, *et al.* Resection of the liver for colorectal carcinoma metastases: A multi-institutional study of indications for resection. Registry of hepatic metastases. *Surgery* 1988; **103**: 278–288.

49. Wilson SM, Adson MA. Surgical treatment of hepatic metastases from colorectal cancers. *Arch Surg* 1976; **111**: 330 334.

50. Scheele J, Stangl R, Altendorf-Hofmann A. Hepatic metastases from colorectal carcinoma: Impact of surgical resection on the natural history. *Br J Surg* 1990; **77**: 1241–1246.

51. Fong Y, Blumgart LH, Fortner JG, *et al.* Pancreatic or liver resection for malignancy is safe and effective for the elderly. *Ann Surg* 1995; **222**: 426–437.

48.   Head and Neck Oncology

James N. Endicott

Introduction

There are approximately 95,140 cases of cancer of the head and neck each year in the United States with the average age at 59 (1). A five year review of analytic cases of head and neck cancer over age 65 ending in December 1994. At the H. Lee Moffitt Cancer and Research Institute found that 114 (30%) patients were in their 70's and that 32 (10%) were over 80 years old. Eighty percent of these cancers are of the squamous cell type and occur primarily in the upper aerodigestive system. The remaining 20% of cancers are adenocarcinomas and sarcomas and occur primarily in the glandular tissue or mesodermal elements of the head and neck. The majority of the patients surviving treatment have residual morbidity as a result of their therapy. Although head and neck cancer comprises 7% of all cancers, its cosmetic deformity and functional, economic, and psychosocial consequences that affect quality of life warrant special attention (2).

The overall survival rate with standard therapy using surgery or radiation for localized disease is approximately 67% (Stage I) and 30% for those with regional metastasis (Stage III and IV). The cure rate for Stage IV patients with distant metastasis is negligible (3).

Pathogenesis

The induction and progression of head and neck cancer are probably part of a multistep process that occurs after long term exposure to carcinogens and promoters. The process is associated with a concomitant failure of natural immunologic homeostasis that is directly related to the aging process. Cytogenetic disruption is another factor in the initial event of carcinogenesis.

The mechanisms of exposure to carcinogens include natural and man-made irradiation, direct contact by respiration and alimentation, and iatrogenic causes (4). Exposure to irradiation in the form of ultraviolet rays from the sun may result in basal cell carcinomas, squamous cell carcinomas, malignant melanomas, and Merkel cell carcinomas in decreasing order of frequency. Melanoma accounts for 75% of deaths from all varieties of skin cancer. The risk of an individual developing malignant melanoma during their lifetime is expected to be 1 in 75 by the year 2001 (5). Skin cancers are increasing in frequency (6) and may be attributed to genetic factors and to the decrease in the ultraviolet filtering ozone layer of the atmosphere caused by air pollution. Protective clothing and sunscreen lotions can diminish the incidence of skin cancers. X-ray treatment for adenoids, as was done in the first part of this century in the Baltimore area or for acne or other head and neck lesions before the hazards of radiation were known, has left an older generation of aging patients at risk for head and neck cancer development. These sites include skin, thyroid, and upper aerodigestive mucosal and glandular sites.

Some assert that perhaps all cancers are caused by environmental factors (7). A single exposure to some carcinogens is enough to induce a cancer under laboratory conditions. However, there is usually a long time between exposure and the appearance of cancer, and even if a single exposure causes cancer in humans, carcinogen identification may not be possible. It is generally felt that few cancers occur in humans after a single exposure of a carcinogen.

A primary reason why cancer is an affliction of older people is their repeated exposures to carcinogens over time. As we eradicate infections, disease, and trauma that kill younger members of society, allowing the population to live longer, we see a relative increase in degenerative diseases that accompany aging, such as: heart disease, stroke, and cancer (7).

The largest single irrefutable causative factor in head and neck carcinogenesis today is tobacco use. Cigarette smoking accounts for 360,000 premature deaths annually, which could be avoided by eliminating this unnecessary social habit. One-half of these patients die of cancer; 25% of cancer victims succumb to lung cancer (8).

Genetic factors may play a role in cancer. Nasopharyngeal cancer (NPC) has a high prevalence in Chinese living in Southern China, as well as in Eskimos, North Africans in the Mediterranean area, and East Africans (9). Epstein-Barr virus is present in many cases of NPC and is also implicated in Burkitt's lymphoma and mononucleosis and is an example of an infectious agent that may play a role in the induction of some cancers. Human retroviruses, such as human immunodeficiency virus (HIV), which is responsible for AIDS, may also play a role in carcinogenesis. Kaposi's sarcoma, which is found in many patients afflicted with AIDS, may be viral induced.

Human papillomavirus (HPV) can induce wart-like surface lesions, including laryngeal papillomatosis. In 1986 human papillomavirus capsid antigens were identified in tissue taken by biopsy from 14 of 20 patients with carcinoma *in situ* of the larynx (10). Problems in identifying infectious agents as a cause of cancer lie in individual resistance or susceptibility to infection by virus, as well as synergism with other carcinogens. The increased incidence of cancer with age indicates that factors other than viruses are the major etiologic agents.

Heavy alcohol consumption when combined with cigarette smoking seems to be synergistic in causing an increased incidence of cancer of the upper aerodigestive tract, usually involving the oral cavity, esophagus, and pharynx (11,12). Theories explaining the carcinogenic effects of alcohol emphasize (1) the role of carcinogens other than ethanol as risk factors; (2) nutritional deficiency caused by the impaired absorption of nutrients and vitamins such as Vitamin A, which is important in the regulation of epithelial cell differentiation (11,12); (3) alcohol as a solvent for tobacco related carcinogens thereby permitting their easier passage through the gastrointestinal cellular membrane; and (4) decreased liver metabolism in a severely cirrhotic patient resulting in a decreased ability to detoxify carcinogens. Another possible cause involving ethanol is the diminution of the hepatic contribution to the immune system. A prospective study of 462 head and neck cancer patients had only 34 nondrinkers and eight nonsmokers (13).

A major component of the aging process is a gradual senescence of the immune system, which has been associated with an increased incidence of neoplasia, autoimmune disorders, and infectious diseases (14,15). New knowledge about immune mechanisms has been achieved through advances in biochemistry, molecular biology, and hybridoma technology. The function of T lymphocytes as mediators of tumor rejection and the role of regulatory lymphokines (eg, interleukins) as important co-factors in the maintenance and amplification of the immune response have been recognized (16).

Many changes in the cellular immune system that are associated with aging are attributed to the gradual loss of a cell's ability to proliferate; for example, a decrease in antigen-specific T-cell cytotoxic function (eg, CD8-cytotoxic suppressor cell) and the decline of Interleukin-2 production with increasing age (17,18). These deficits are similar to immune deficits in patients with head and neck cancer and may be related to the senescence of the thymus gland (19). Strategies of immunorestorative treatment that are used as an adjuvant to conventional treatment and might benefit the older patient with cancer include adaptive replacement of affected cell populations and lymphokines or stimulation of appropriate lymphokine production and lymphocyte proliferation in vitro. These techniques have been used in preliminary studies with advanced renal cell carcinoma and melanoma, but were associated with severe toxicities (20). Immunorestorative measures that employ better tolerated natural products, such as thymic hormones (thymosin alpha$_1$), retinoids, or essential trace elements, may be used for older tumor-free or cancer patients.

Chromosomal mutations of specific genes which affect cell growth (oncogenes) or genes of immunologic regulation are now thought to play a role in the development of cancer (21). Aging may play an important role in chromosomal fragility or mutagenic capa-

bility. Gene splicing using retrovirus technology may be a useful potential therapeutic strategy.

Management

In the past, advanced age was considered a relative contraindication to major surgery and these patients were treated with alternative, less effective modes of therapy (22). The prospect of locally and regionally uncontrolled head and neck cancer with its slow progression resulting in a gradual increase in pain, disfigurement and loss of function should be weighed against the surgical and anesthetic risks in the elderly patient. Studies of surgery in aging patients have demonstrated acceptable morbidity and mortality in the geriatric population. Physiologic age and concurrent illness are more closely associated with mortality and complication rates than is chronologic age alone. Surgery of the head and neck, in general, is better tolerated than surgery of the body cavities. Mortality occurs more often when there is more than one peri-operative complication, i.e., the domino effect. Cardiac and pulmonary problems are the leading causes of postoperative death in older patients. Therefore, close attention to all details of preoperative, intraoperative, and postoperative management is critical. Head and neck surgery is equally tolerated in patients both above and under the age of 65 (23).

The older head and neck cancer patient requires more specific preoperative considerations than the younger patient. The etiologic risk factors for head and neck cancer — smoking and alcohol use — are also causes of major systemic and organ system diseases. Aging may result in variable degrees of renal impairment, decreased cardiac and pulmonary reserve, atherosclerosis, and diminished wound healing (24). Therefore, medical and specialty preoperative consultations often are necessary when intercurrent disease is present or a lengthy surgical case is anticipated. A metastatic work-up is necessary, including chest x-ray, liver enzyme analysis, and CT scans with selected CT-guided needle biopsy for remote disease. Frequently, the head and neck cancer patient is malnourished. Caloric, protein, vitamin, and mineral depletion result from alcoholism and pain, dysphagia, and metabolic derangements secondary to cancer. Malnutrition results in poor wound healing and secondary surgical complications (25,26). Nutritional evaluation and aggressive enteral feeding by PEG tube or G tube are essential in the dysphagic patient, particularly when an ablative surgical procedure is necessary that would result in a severe postoperative swallowing impairment with an unpredictable functional recovery or when radiation therapy may be interrupted due to dysphagia. Patients with extreme visceral protein loss may have inefficient gastrointestinal absorption and require parenteral nutrition.

Advances in technology, pharmacology, and anesthesia methods now allow major surgery to be performed routinely in the older patient. The elderly patient has, with careful attention and timely physiologic support, as good a chance of surviving as a similarly ill younger patient, although his or her course may be more prolonged (27). Intraoperatively, volume status and cardiac and pulmonary function can be monitored precisely using pulmonary artery and radial artery catheters and SaO_2, SvO_2, and $PaCO_2$ measurements. Optimal management of the cardiac and pulmonary systems is possible. Studies of the risk of reinfarction after myocardial infarction show that the time from the infarction to anesthesia is the most critical factor determining the reinfarction rate (28).

Similarly, advances in postoperative management of major head and neck surgery patients enable the successful management of the older patient. Intensive care facilities can monitor cardiac rhythm and hemodynamics, oxygen saturation, bronchial hygiene, airway and fluid status, and the suction drainage apparatus in the immediate postoperative recovery phase. Postoperative broad spectrum antibiotics and the rapid resumption of nutritional therapy are now routine. Ambulation can begin within 48 hours in most head and neck surgery patients, thus diminishing the risk of pulmonary embolism and postoperative pneumonia. Medical support for intercurrent disease management is useful.

Rehabilitative surgical reconstructive techniques for communication and improved function have been developed to further improve the quality of life of older patients. The most simple yet effective means of reconstruction are favored for rehabilitation. Complications are largely related to intercurrent disease and previous radiation (29). For limited defects of the oral cavity and oropharynx, split-thickness skin grafts, local mucosal flaps, and primary closure are the best reconstructive methods. More extensive reconstructive methods may be necessary when there is limited tongue, palate, or upper pharynx function. Skin or skin muscle flap reconstruction uses local or regional soft tissue flaps nourished by a specific arterial supply to replace the surgically ablated anatomic site. Local flaps, such as tongue and nasolabial flaps, are useful for limited defects. However, for larger defects, or in some heavily radiated patients, regional flaps are indicated. The popular pectoralis musculocutaneous flap, based on the thoracoacromial artery, was developed in the 1970s and has revolutionized head and neck reconstruction. Microvascular free flaps add a versatility to head and neck reconstruction, allowing the selection of different thicknesses of skin and muscle and enabling vascularized bone to be used for reconstruction. Limitations of this technique include flap reliability, the need for suitable recipient vessels, technical demands and length of the procedure, and the variable donor site morbidity.

In the elderly, conservation surgery of the larynx is available for early lesions at specific glottic and supraglottic sites, thereby allowing preservation of the physiologically functional voice. Supraglottic laryngectomy requires adequate pulmonary reserve with a good cough so that postoperative aspiration pneumonia can be avoided. Total laryngectomy is traditionally necessary to effect a cure in cases of radiation failure of most patients with small supraglottic lesions (T_1 and T_2) and for more advanced cancers of the larynx. Total loss of one's voice has a profound impact on the quality of life. Speech rehabilitation can be accomplished in one or more of three ways. Only 20% of patients can successfully acquire the traditional esophageal speech, a technique of releasing air from the esophagus in a controlled manner (30). The hand-held, battery-operated mechanical "electro larynx" produces an electronic voice and may be used by most patients successfully. Sound is directed into the vocal tract either by placement of the device against the side of the neck or through a small plastic tube directly into the mouth. Speech is produced when the sound is articulated by the lips and tongue. In 1980, Singer and Blom (23) described the tracheoesophageal puncture procedure for patients who do not develop acceptable esophageal speech or do not wish to use the electro-larynx. Voice is produced when exhaled air is directed through the stoma Silastic prosthesis during momentary tracheostoma occlusion, with expulsion through the mouth giving the patient lung-powered speech. Successful prosthesis use requires good manual dexterity and sufficient visual acuity to enable the patient to learn how to remove, clean, and reinsert a small device in the stomal airway. Some geriatric patients may not meet these criteria. A speech therapist plays an important rehabilitative role in the alaryngeal patient's future functional recovery.

Ninety-five percent of all cases of oral cancer occur in individuals over 40. Although early cancers of the oral cavity may be managed solely by surgery or radiation therapy with similar outcomes, surgery is the treatment of choice because radiation will leave permanent significant dryness as a sequela. This side effect in an older patient contributes to dysphagia and poor appetite (31). Good nutritional status has prognostic and therapeutic importance in oncology (32).

Fedele *et al.* states that, "screening for oral cancer is a simple, non-invasive procedure which can be easily incorporated into the comprehensive assessment of older patients. Oral cancer screening can detect early, localized lesions which are associated with an improved prognosis. Five-year survival rates are more than four times greater in individuals with localized lesions than those with distant metastases. Since older Americans visit their physician more often than their dentist, the physician's medical examination provides an excellent opportunity to screen for oral cancers (33)".

Older patients with loco-regional oropharyngeal cancer, or at least a subset of them, appear to be able to tolerate radical courses of radiotherapy, and have similar outcomes as do younger patients (22). When partial or total pharyngectomy is necessary for primary hypopharyngeal, oropharyngeal, and some laryngeal tumors and for most peristomal recurrences, rehabilitation by the pectoralis myocutaneous flap or jejunal microvascular free flap (34) is favored when primary closure cannot be effected. Gastric transposition has an 11% mortality rate (35) as a reconstructive procedure and may not be suitable for the older patient.

Thyroid nodules in the elderly are more frequent and more frequently malignant. Fine needle aspiration is the first step to diagnose these type of nodules, and thyroid scans and ultrasounds may be obtained in special cases. Thyroid suppression is frequently not effective in decreasing the size of the nodule and may cause subclinical or clinical thyrotoxicosis. Between 2 and 10% of thyroid nodules are noted to be carcinomatous (36).

Patients with a maxillectomy, rhinectomy, and/or orbital exenteration may be rehabilitated successfully by an intraoral or extraoral prosthesis made by a skilled maxillofacial prosthodontist. The unusually good cosmetic result and subsequent patient self-acceptance are important in the older patient thereby allowing aggressive surgical management of cancer of the nose, paranasal sinuses, and large facial carcinomas. However, these patients should be observed for several years for early recurrence before facial reconstruction is performed (37).

Radiation therapy plays an important role in management of malignancy in the head and neck cancer patient. Radiation used as an optional single modality of treatment in the range of 7,000 rads for attempted cure in Stage I or II carcinomas, has a higher rate of success depending upon the site of the lesion. Early glottic larynx lesions can have a cure rate as high as 97% (Stage I) and 85% (Stage II) using surgery for salvage (38). However, a T_1 lesion (Stage I) of the hypopharynx (pyriform sinus) has a cure rate of 80%, and this rate is lower for a Stage II lesion treated solely by radiation. More advanced carcinomas — Stage III and Stage IV — often require planned surgery, as well as postoperative radiation in the range of 5,000 rads, for the best cure rates. Preoperative radiation is generally avoided because of the high incidence of postoperative complications and loss of visible original tumor margins at most sites. Newer developments in radiation include hyperfractionation techniques, the use of radiation sensitizers, and oxygen radical enhancement for unresectable advanced or recurrent disease. Investigations are ongoing of concomitant chemotherapy and radiation and various fractionation radiation schedules for advanced disease. With the aid of new imaging techniques and preradiation dosimetry planning by radiation physicists, cure rates can be improved.

Aging patients with head and neck cancer usually have complex problems that affect their function and self-image after treatment. Equally important in determining outcome are the functional and social situations of the patient. The needs and abilities of a self-sufficient patient who lives alone are different from those of an institutionalized patient suffering from senile dementia. Other factors of importance are the patient's psychologic state, communicative abilities and disabilities, available social resources, and the perception of quality-of-life issues. It should be apparent that each case must be thoughtfully individualized to ensure the

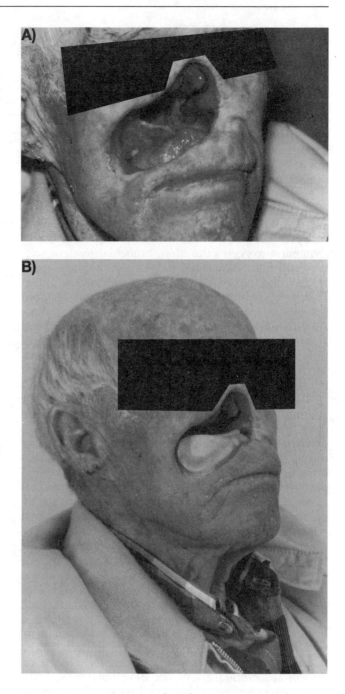

Figure 48.1 A. Patient with right midface and palatal resection; B. Intraoral prosthesis.

best possible outcome (23). Doing so requires several health professionals, working as a team in a comprehensive systematic fashion, to effect the treatment and rehabilitation of the patient.

Case Reports

Case 1 (Figure 48.1)

84 year old white male with arthritic knees and hypertension developed intranasal squamous cell carcinoma. He received radiation therapy for the primary

disease which recurred and required midline maxillectomy. Over 6 years, he recurred locally in 3 midface sites requiring three more operative procedures. He then developed right neck metastasis (N_2B Level II and III) and received 7000 cGy to his neck, but disease persisted requiring a right selective neck dissection. At age 92, he had been disease-free for two years. He is very alert, vigorous, and enjoys his life with his family especially his 8 year old grandson. He wears a prosthesis allowing him to talk and eat a normal diet. He chooses not to wear his external prosthesis.

Case 2:

A vigorous 88 year old white male developed a T_1 squamous cell carcinoma of one left true vocal cord. Two years later, (after a recent marriage), he developed a subglottic recurrence. A total laryngectomy was performed and required a return to surgery later the same day because of a large hematoma thought to be secondary to a hypertensive episode in the recovery room. The hematoma was evacuated under local anesthesia and the patient recovered uneventfully. He is speaking with an electro-larynx and will soon receive a Blom-Singer prosthesis for improved speech.

Case 3:

An 84 year old white male received radiation therapy to a T_1 spindle cell carcinoma of the left true vocal cord. He was in good health and he played 18 holes of golf 3 days/week and carried his own clubs using no golf cart, did pushups every morning and evening. He developed a recurrence of his cancer and had a hemilaryngectomy with a resulting hoarseness no worse that his preoperative symptom. He is again playing golf over 1 year from his surgery.

All patients were cleared for major surgery by the medicine service and all were physiologically much younger than their stated age. They felt that their psychosocial quality of life was impaired in a minor way because of the strong support from close family members and their resulting functional impairments have been corrected by prosthetic rehabilitation or conservation surgery.

Current therapeutic research protocol strategies using neoadjuvant chemotherapy are now prevalent throughout the country. Carboplatinum, an active analogue of cisplatinum can be given safely in elderly patients or patients with renal impairment (39). Organ preservation is now a major goal in many of these multidisciplinary protocols, which are designed to improve the quality of life in the older patient by avoiding the standard treatment of ablative surgery plus radiation for advanced head and neck cancer. The VA 268 Cooperative Study for cancer of the larynx demonstrated the efficacy of this approach in 266 prospectively randomized patients using triple-cycle chemotherapy (CP/5-FU) and postoperative radiation therapy, with surgery used for salvage on the study arm (13).

Multidisciplinary research into new treatment strategies for advanced and relapsed disease, such as adjuvant immunotherapy and other newer modalities of treatment, is not as prevalent. Rehabilitative interdisciplinary research in speech pathology, swallowing, prosthetics, physical therapy, and psychosocial and dietary disciplines is extremely important for the advancement of our knowledge and ability to improve the quality of life of the posttreatment head and neck cancer patient. Both basic science and clinical research should be supported. A series of scientifically rigorous, carefully executed clinical trials, performed in a multi-institutional framework, could provide reasonably rapid answers to important scientific questions (2). From such research we would learn how the aging immune system affects the development of head and neck cancer and where interventions could be applied to correct age-related defects. We would better understand the pathophysiology of these disorders; develop new cytologic, diagnostic, and prognostic tests; establish better-defined hypotheses for future studies; and thus enhance our ability to prevent and treat head and neck cancer (23).

References

1. American Cancer Society. Estimated new cancer cases and deaths by sex for all sites, United States, 1996. *Cancer Facts & Figures* — 1996, p. 7.
2. Endicott JN, Cantrell R, Kelly J, Neel H, Gordon A, Zajtchuk J. Head and neck surgery and cancer in aging patients. *Otolarnygol Head Neck Surg* 1989; **100**: 290–291.
3. Conley J. Oncology and aging. Introduction. In *Geriatric Otorhinolaryngology*, edited by JC Goldstein, HK Kashima, CF Koopman. Philadelphia: BC Decker, 146–147, 1989.
4. Cantrell RW. Etiologic factors in the development of cancer. In *Geriatric Otorhinolaryngology*, edited by JC Goldstein, HK Kashima, CF Koopman. Philadelphia: BC Decker, 148–157, 1989.
5. Brozena SJ, Fenske NA, Perez IR. Epidemiology of malignant melanoma, world wide incidence, and etiologic factors. *Semin Surg Oncol* 1993; **9**: 165–167
6. Cantrell RW. Malignant neoplasms of the skin of the head. In *Otolaryngology*, edited by GM English. Philadelphia: Harper & Row, 1982, vol 5, Chapter 59: 1.
7. Cairns J. The cancer problem. *Scientific Am* 1975.
8. Warner KE. Health and economic implications of a tobacco-free society. *JAMA* 1987; **258**: 2080–2086.
9. de The G. Role of Epstein-Barr virus in human diseases. Infectious mono nucleosis, Burkitt's lymphoma, and nasopharyngeal carcinoma. In *Viral Oncology*, edited by G Klein. New York: Raven Press, 769, 1980.
10. Kashima H, Mounts P, Kuhajda F, *et al.* Demonstration of human papillomavirus capsid antigen in carcinoma *in situ* of the larynx. *Ann Otol Rhinol Laryngol* 1986; **95**: 603–607.
11. Kabat GC, Chang CJ, Wynder EL. The role of tobacco, alcohol use, and body mass index in oral and pharyngeal cancer. *International Journal of Epidemiology* 1994; **23(6)**: 1137–1144.
12. Baron AE, Franceschi S, Barra S, Talamini R, La Vecchia C. A comparison of the joint effects of alcolol and smoking on the risk of cancer across sites in the upper aerodigestive tract. *Cancer Epidemiology, Biomarkers & Prevention* 1993; **2(6)**: 519–523.
13. Endicott JN, Jensen R, Lyman G, *et al.* Adjuvant chemotherapy for advanced head and neck squamous carcinoma. Final report of the head and neck contracts program. *Cancer* 1987; **60**: 301–311.
14. Weksler ME. Senescence of the immune system. *Med Clin North Am* 1983; **67**: 263–272.
15. Ford PM. The immunology of ageing. *Clin Rheum Dis* 1986; **12**: 1–10.
16. Gillis J. Interleukin-2. Biology and biochemistry. *J Clin Immunol* 1983; **3**: 1–15.

17. Wolf GT, Schmaltz S, Hudson J, *et al*. Alterations in T-lymphocyte subpopulations in patients with head and neck cancer. Correlations with prognosis. *Arch Otolaryngol Head Neck Surg* 1987; **113**: 1200–1206.

18. Wu W, Pahlavani M, Cheung HT, Richardson A. The effect of aging on the expression of interleukin-2 messenger ribonucleic acid. *Cell Immunol* 1986; **100**: 224–231.

19. Wolf GT. Aging, the immune system, and head and neck cancer. In *Geriatric Otorhinolaryngology*, edited by JC Goldstein, AK Kashima, CT Koopman. Philadelphia: BC Decker, 161, 1989.

20. Rosenberg SA, Lotze MT, Muul LM, *et al*. A progress report on the treatment of 157 patients with advanced cancer using lymphokine-activated killer cells and interleukin-2 or high dose interleukin-2 alone. *N Engl J Med* 1987; **316**: 889–897.

21. Lester EP, Tharapel SA. Chromosome abnormalities in squamous carcinoma cell lines of head and neck origin, abstract. Third International Head and Neck Oncology Research Conference, September 1990.

22. Chin R, Fisher RJ, Smee Rl, Barton MB. Oropharyngeal cancer in the elderly. *Int J Radiat Oncol Biol Phys* 1995; **32(4)**: 1007–1016.

23. Sanders A, Blom E, Singer M, Hamaker R. Reconstructive and rehabilitative aspects of head and neck cancer in the elderly. *Otolaryngol Clin North Am* 1990; **23**: 1159–1168.

24. Robinson DS. Head and neck considerations in the elderly patient. *Surg Clin North Am* 1994; **74(2)**: 431–439.

25. Daly JM, Dudrick SJ, Copeland EM. Parenteral nutrition in patients with head and neck cancer. Techniques and results. *Otolaryngol Head Neck Surg* 1980; **88**: 707.

26. Hooley RD, Levine H, Toribio CF, *et al*. Predicting postoperative head and neck complications using nutritional assessment. *Arch Otolaryngol* 1983; **109**: 83.

27. Watters JM, Bessey PQ. Critical care for the elderly patient. *Surg Clin North Am* Feb 1994; **74(1)**: 187–197.

28. Steen PA, Tinker JH, Tarhan S. Myocardial reinfarction after anesthesia and surgery. *JAMA* 1978; **239**: 2566.

29. Johnson JT, Rabuzzi DD, Tucker HM. Composite resection in the elderly. A well tolerated procedure. *Laryngoscope* 1977; **87**: 1509.

30. Gates GA, Ryan W, Cooper JC, *et al*. Current status of laryngectomee rehabilitation. Results of therapy. *Am J Otolaryngol* 1982; **3**: 1.

31. Silverman S Jr. Precancerous lesions and oral cancer in the elderly. *Clin Geriatr Med* 1992; **8(3)**: 529–541.

32. Tchekmedyian NS, Zahyna D, Halpert C, Canchola A, Heber D. Clinical staging or nutrional status of cancer patients (meeting abstract). *Proc Annu Meet Am Soc Clin Oncol* 1992; **11**: A1388.

33. Fedele DJ, Jones JA, Niessen LC. Oral cancer screening in the elderly. *J Am Geriatr Soc* 1991; **39(9)**: 920–925.

34. Robinson DW, MacLeon AM. Microvascular free jejunal transfer. *Br J Plast Surg* 1982; **35**: 258.

35. Harrison DFN. Surgical management of hypopharyngeal cancer. Particular reference to the gastric "pull-up" operation. *Arch Otolaryngol* 1979; **105**: 149.

36. Rolla AR. Thyroid nodules in the elderly. *Clin Geriatr Med* 1995; **11(2)**: 259–269.

37. Teichgraber JF, Goepfert H. Rhinectomy. Timing and reconstruction. *Otolaryngol Head Neck Surg* 1990; **102**: 362–369.

38. Wang CC. Radiation therapy of laryngeal tumors. In *Comprehensive Management of Head and Neck Cancers*, edited by Thawley, Panje, Batsakis, Liudberg. Philadelphia: WB Sanders Co, 911, 1987.

49. Prostate Cancer in the Elderly

Timothy D. Moon

Introduction

Adenocarcinoma of the prostate has, for several years now, had the dubious distinction of being the most commonly diagnosed nonskin cancer in men (1). In 1995, the American Cancer Society estimated that 244,000 men would be diagnosed with prostate cancer and 40,400 would die from their disease (1). Indeed these numbers reflect part of the problem in that the diagnosis rate has risen from 56,000 per year in 1975 (2) to 244,000 now while the mortality rate during the same period has increased from 18,700 to 40,400. Thus in the past 20 years, the diagnosis of prostate cancer has risen fourfold while the mortality rate has doubled. Several hypotheses might be developed from these data. The first is that prostate cancer is being successfully treated as evidenced by the more slowly rising mortality rate. Another contrarian hypothesis is that most cancers are indolent with the patients dying of other causes rather than from prostate cancer. Implied in this latter hypothesis is a lack of relevance of treatment to these statistics.

The major factor in this increasing diagnosis rate has been the introduction of serum prostate specific antigen measurement for screening or at least case finding (3). In addition, we have a population with a rapidly expanding aged population who form the primary cohort for the diagnosis of prostate cancer. Thus, while it is clear that for most patients the disease runs an indolent course, prostate cancer is the second-most common cause of cancer death in men. At a time when resources are diminishing, while the aged population expands, it is important to define the efficacy of therapy especially in the context of quality of life. Surprisingly, surgical treatments for prostate cancer were first performed over 90 years ago (4), yet without any scientific demonstration of their efficacy. This position is no longer tenable and the National Cancer Institute recognized the importance of economics in patient treatment when they held their first economic conference. The integration of economic outcome measures into National Cancer Institute sponsored therapeutic trials (5). Finally, in a discussion of treatment for the gerontologic patient, we must also recognize that neither the approach of the physician nor the wishes of the patient are necessarily the same as they might be for a younger person.

Etiology

An increasing number of influences upon the development of prostate cancer are being described and ad-

Table 49.1 Factors influencing the development of prostate cancer.

Heredity

Chromosomal Alterations

Oncogenes

Tumor Suppressor Genes

Programmed Cell Death

Growth Factors

Androgens / Androgen Receptors

Chemical Carcinogens

Infection

vances in molecular biology have greatly expanded our knowledge (Table 49.1).

Hereditary Prostate Cancer

The concept of genetic influences upon the development of prostate cancer has been around for many years. A computerized database of the Mormon population has defined clustering within families (6). Additional studies using case-control methods have shown significant increases in the cancer risk for first degree relatives (7,8). This risk increases from twofold with one relative involved or affected to elevenfold with three affected probands (9). Segregation analysis suggested an autosomal dominant model affecting 0.36% of the population but accounting for 43% of cancers occurring in men less than 55 years of age (10). At present a specific gene or genes associated with hereditary cancer have not been identified.

Cytogenetic Data

Multiple chromosomal aberrations have been defined in prostate cancer. Loss of chromosomes 1, 2, 5, and Y, together with gains in chromosomes 7, 14, 20, and 22 have been described (11). Multiple rearrangements have also been described including chromosomes 2p7q and 10q (11).

Molecular analysis of alleles using restricted fragment length polymorphism and tumor associated loss of heterozygosity has been used to demonstrate loss of heterozygosity at 11 sites, namely 3p, 7q, 9q, 10p, 10q, 11p, 13q, 16p, 16q, 17p, and 18q. The highest frequency losses are found at 10q and 16q. Of interest is the finding of the decreased expression of the cell adhesion molecule E-cadherin in high grade prostate tumors (12,13). E-cadherin is located on chromosome 16q.

Oncogenes

A proto-oncogene is a normal gene sequence coding for a normal cellular protein required for normal cell growth and proliferation (14). The altered form of gene sequence is the oncogene. The alterations may be point mutations, replications (extra copies of the gene resulting in amplification), or translocations on the gene such that gene promoters or regulators do not act correctly. Several oncogenes have been studied. Studies of myc and fos have not been fruitful (15–17). *Ras* family mutations have been studied by many investigators. American studies have rarely shown aberrations (18–21) while Japanese studies have shown alterations in about 25% of cases (22,23). C-cerbB-2 protein expression has been studied with many investigators finding significant expression (24–26). However, C-cerbB-2 DNA amplification or mRNA expression has not been demonstrated (24–26).

Tumor Suppressor Genes

The p53 gene is currently the gene of preeminence for study in prostate cancer. Located at 17p13 it encodes for a nuclear phosphoprotein which arrests the cell from entering the S-phase of cell cycle (14,27). It may also be involved with regulation of apoptosis (28). Mutations in the p53 may therefore permit DNA damaged cells in G1 to enter the S phase resulting in genetically unstable cells more likely to be associated with the development of malignancy (29). Additionally, mutated p53 exhibits an increased half-life giving the appearance of increased expression (14). Most studies have shown alterations in p53 expression with the greatest expression in higher grade tumors (30). A recent study using tissue from hormonally untreated patients demonstrated no abnormal p53 staining in patients with cancers confined to the gland while 10% of locally advanced tumors showed abnormal p53 accumulation and 20% of patients with metastatic disease demonstrated abnormal p53 concentration (31). Interestingly, in the majority of these patients the p53 abnormality was only detected at the metastatic site and not in the primary tissue (31).

Programmed Cell Death (Apoptosis)

Cell death occurs as a result of many signals including DNA fragmentation secondary to activation of Ca^{2+}/Mg^{2+} dependent nuclear endonuclease (32). Castration causes androgen levels to fall with a simultaneous reduction in androgen receptors (33). These changes in hormonal milieu allow for expression of normally repressed genes such as TPRM-2 and TGF-β (34,35). TGF-β1 has been associated with increased intracellular calcium levels and an increase in expression of the calcium binding protein calmodulin. Calmodulin levels have also been found to be increased in other tumors (36).

The oncoprotein Bcl-2 has been shown to provide protection from apoptotic stimuli (37). Bcl-2 is located in the basal epithelial cells and is highly expressed in the prostate (38, 39). Bcl-2 upregulation occurs maximally 10 days after castration in the rat (37). Conversely, Bcl-2 expression is greater in androgen resistant human prostate specimens. Interestingly, it is hypothesized that as Bcl-2 is produced by the hormonally insensitive basal-layer cells that these may represent the subpopulation of androgen independent cells (32). Thus there are significant implications for the management of hormonal resistant prostate cancer through Bcl-2 mediated mechanisms (32).

Growth Factors

One of the earlier growth factors to be studied was epidermal growth factor (EGF). EGF receptors are located on the basement membrane side of the glandular epithelial cells (39). Unfortunately while the receptor is present in 90% of the benign prostatic hyperplasia tissue, it is absent from prostatic adenocarcinoma tissue (40,41). However, transforming growth factor α(TGF-α) which is structurally and functionally related to EGF and which reacts with EGF receptors has been demonstrated in prostate cancer tissue (42). TGF-β is expressed in most prostate cells but primarily in the mesenchyme (43). TGF-β alone appears to have inhibitory growth effects yet when co-cultured with EGF is stimulatory in action (32). TGF-β has also been found to regulate fibroblast growth factor (44). Acidic FGF may be required to support growth of malignant epithelium through a paracrine mechanism (45).

Androgens and Androgen Receptors

Androgens are essential for the normal growth and function of prostatic tissue (46). Both testosterone and dihydrotestosterone mediate their effects through the same androgen receptor protein and function as a nuclear transcriptional activator. Dihydrotestosterone is 10 times more powerful than testosterone as a receptor transcriptional activator. This difference results from the much higher binding affinity of dihydrotestosterone to the androgen receptor. This receptor is encoded by the X chromosome between the centromere and 13q (47). Mutation of the androgen receptor has been shown to inactivate antiandrogens (48,49). While the androgen receptor cannot be viewed as a proto-oncogene the importance of its presence and its transcriptional regulation of a host of gene products proven to be more important in cellular transformation cannot be overlooked.

However, although androgens and androgen receptors are obviously required from normal prostatic growth, the place of androgens as carcinogens is less clear. Noble in an attempt to define a carcinogenic role for hormones in the induction of prostate cancer-treated rats with testosterone and markedly increase the incidence of tumors from 0.45% to 18% (50). Further, he found that if the testosterone was administered concurrently with estrone, the tumors developed after a shorter lag time, suggesting a more complex hormonal interrelationship than androgen stimulation alone. Additionally, further the work demonstrated that with one exception transplants from these tumors were hormone independent (51).

Synergism between androgens and estrogens has been noted in benign prostatic hypertrophy (52) and leads to the question of whether benign prostatic hyperplasia increases the risk of developing prostate cancer. The evidence is unclear and opposing viewpoints are available in the literature (53,54).

Chemical Carcinogens

Because of the high level of pollutants in our industrial society the question of chemical carcinogenesis is always present. The only tool available for the study of humans is epidemiological research; this has uncovered several facts suggesting a significant environmental impact. First generation Japanese migrants to the United States have been noted to have an increased incidence of prostate cancer compared with native Japanese (55,56). Similarly the mortality ratio for foreign-born versus native-born U.S. caucasian males was found to be 89:100 (57). It has been suggested that automobile exhaust fumes, cadmium, fertilizer, and chemicals in the printing, painting, and ship fitting industries may act as carcinogens or promoters (58–60). On the other hand, no association has been found for smoking tobacco (61).

Many attempts have been made to induce prostatic adenocarcinoma in animals using chemical carcinogens. As early as 1937, Moore and Melchionna (62) injected benzpyrene into the prostates of rats but only squamous carcinoma of the prostate developed. Other investigators injected methylcholanthrene and they too only achieved the development of squamous carcinoma (63–65). Finally, Horning (66), enlarging on work by others, developed a method for producing adenocarcinoma. Sheets of prostatic epithelium were wrapped around methylcholanthrene pellets and grafted subcutaneously into the abdomens of syngeneic mice. This technique was refined by the addition of estrogens that enhanced the carcinogenic potentials (67). The most successful technique, using a combination of hormonal manipulation followed by subsequent treatment with a carcinogen, consisted of castrating rats and then treating them with 9,10 dimethyl-1,2 benzanthracene (68). All of these animals developed adenocarcinoma of the prostate. The pathogenic hypothesis for this model presumes that "old" atrophic prostate glands are more susceptible to developing adenocarcinomas than "younger" normal glandular tissue.

Infection

Various investigators have looked at a variety of infections for causal relationships for adenocarcinoma. Venereal disease has been suggested (69), but other studies have failed to show any relationship (70). Likewise a higher frequency has been reported for prostate cancer in patients with prostatitis. It is unclear whether this relationship is causal or merely a consequence of common factors. Bacteria and viruses have also been found in prostate cancer specimens but their significance is unclear. Paulsen et al. (71) induced a neoplastic transformation of hamster prostatic cells in vitro with the SV40 virus. Herpes simplex II virus and cytomegalovirus virus have also been demonstrated in prostatic carcinoma tissue (72–74). Reverse transcriptase NC-type viral particles have been found as suggested evidence for RNA virus involvement (75–77). However, at the present time there is no good direct evidence of a viral cause for prostate cancer.

Screening for Prostate Cancer

The basic requirement for a screening program is that it results in a reduction of mortality and/or morbidity from the disease. As will be discussed later in the treatment section, it has yet to be conclusively demonstrated that active (with curative intent) intervention alters patient outcome. It is a rather sad commentary that the intergroup PIVOT study (78) started in 1994, 90 years after the first radical prostatectomy was performed (4). The PIVOT study randomizes men with clinically localized disease to radical prostatectomy vs. watchful waiting (no active treatment). In addition to the medical requirements of a screening program, economics have clearly begun to impact how we treat disease. With health care costs in the United States reaching 12.1% of GNP in 1990 (79), it is clear that there are finite fiscal limits. Discussions about how limited resources will be allocated, will eventually be made, and will be termed rationing by politicians. For comparison, European countries spent 6.2% to 8.8% of GNP on health care during the same period (79). The National Cancer Institute first formally addressed this issue in 1994, when they held their first conference on the integration of economic outcome measures into NCI-sponsored therapeutic trials (5).

Current Recommendations

In 1992, the American Cancer Society recommended as part of health screening that "every man aged 50 years and older should undergo an annual PSA determination and digital rectal examination (Table 49.2) Men at high risk, such as African-Americans, or those with a strong family history, may start at a younger age. Men with a life expectancy of at least 10 years may benefit from examination (3)." These recommendations have also been endorsed by the American Urologic Association.

Table 49.2 Screening for prostate cancer.

Recommendations of American Cancer Society/American Urological Association

Annual	• Digital Rectal Examination
	• Prostate Specific Antigen
	Men over 50 years unless high risk (e.g. African American then annually after aged 40 years)
	Life expectancy of at least 10 years

Table 49.3 Controversy over prostate cancer screening

Pro	Con
• Prostate cancer most common cancer in men	• Most men die *with* cancer rather than *of* cancer
• Prostate cancer second most common cause of cancer death in men	• Patients with well differentiated cancers do just as well without treatment
• Allows detection of cancer while still localized (and asymptomatic)	• Patients with poorly differentiated cancers do poorly with or without treatment
• Allows curative treatment while still localized	• Competing causes of death overwhelm deaths from prostate cancer
	• Curative treatments not proven over expectant therapy in controlled trials

This position is not held universally, however, as the U.S. preventative services task force does not recommend for or against screening for prostate cancer (80). Additionally, the Canadian task force on the periodic health examination has recommended against use of PSA in prostate cancer screening as has the Canadian Urological Association (81). The controversy over screening is summarized in Table 49.3.

Screening Tests

At the present time, screening for prostate cancer consists of digital rectal examination (DRE) and prostate-specific antigen determination (PSA) (82). Prostatic ultrasound has been tested and rejected as a screening tool.

The DRE is time-honored examination not only for prostate cancer but also for detection of rectal cancer. DRE is limited in its effectiveness. One can only palpate the posterior surface, and while the majority of cancers are located in this region, they will only be palpable when quite large. About half of the cancers detected in this manner have already spread beyond the capsule when diagnosed. In a recent study of men over 50 years of age, 15% had an abnormal rectal examination (83,84). Of these men, 21% were diagnosed with cancer for a detection rate of 3.2%. The real detection rate, however, was only 1.3%, as the remainder were diagnosed from biopsies taken elsewhere in the gland. A review of the studies evaluating DRE as diagnostic tool has recently been published with detection rates varying from 0.1% to 2.5% (82).

PSA is a 34 kD serine kinase produced by normal as well as malignant prostatic epithelium (85). Its function is for the liquefaction of semen. PSA levels in semen are in milligram amounts, while in serum, are in nanogram amounts. There is thus, a million-fold difference between these concentrations. Any cellular changes which allow PSA to "leak" into the blood, will cause increased levels. Inflammatory changes (86,87), together with those associated with malignancy (such as the abnormal blood vessels associated with malignant neovascularity) are associated with such leaks. Prostatic biopsy may also cause an increase in PSA

levels, such that repeat serum measurements within several weeks of biopsy may reveal artifactually elevated levels.

Several assays are clinically available. Abbotts IMx assay and hybritech tandem assays utilize monoclonal antibodies and have normal levels at 0 to 4 ng/ml, while the Yang Pros-check assay utilizes a polyclonal antibody and has values about 1.6-fold higher than the other two assays (82). It is thus important, to know which assay one's lab uses and any changes that are made.

Of recent interest have been the studies demonstrating PSA in free and complex forms. PSA may complex with α-chymotrypsin and also α2-macroglobulins, the latter of which completely envelops the PSA molecule, making it undetectable (88). Suggestions have recently been made that measuring the free PSA is a more sensitive method for detecting prostate cancer (89).

PSA — Density

As an aid to cancer detection, PSA has been calculated in various ways. PSA density (PSAD) is PSA per unit volume of prostate and values of greater than 0.15 have been suggested to indicate cancer (90). This, of course, requires prostatic ultrasound determination, raising the financial cost of patient evaluation. The value of PSAD has, however, more recently been brought into question (91).

PSA — Velocity

Another method of evaluating PSA is PSA velocity (i.e., changes in PSA with time). It is suggested that increases of greater than 0.5 ng/ml/year are important (92). Other studies have shown that in periods of less than one year, changes of greater than 30% are common, making PSA velocity of very limited clinical value (93). However, as men collect PSA data about themselves over 5- to 10-year periods, then PSA changes may become of more importance.

PSA — Age-Specific Ranges

Finally, PSA age-specific reference ranges have been proposed and even utilized by some clinical labs. These suggest normal ranges up to 5.4 ng/ml for men in their 60's and 6.5 ng/ml for men in their 70's (94,95) Others have questioned the utility of these ranges suggesting that it would result in detection of fewer organ confined cancers (96).

Studies utilizing PSA for cancer detection have yielded higher results, than DRE studies. The PSA cutoff value for the studies has been 4 ng/ml. All U.S. studies have been invitational in nature, immediately rendering them non-population based (82). However, two large U.S. studies both detected prostate cancer in 2.6% and 3.1% (97,98) of their population groups. This compares favorably with a population-based Swedish study, where the detection rate was 2.9% (99). A review of PSA-based screening studies has recently been published with detection rates varying from 1.5% to 4.1% (82).

The final issue which should be addressed concerns the effects of repeated screening of the same population. Relatively little data exist, and suggest a decreasing yield, but with a higher likelihood of diagnosing organ-confined disease (82).

Combination Testing

Patients are routinely evaluated with both PSA and DRE. Studies clearly demonstrate that PSA testing will identify more cancers than will DRE (83,84). However, of patients diagnosed with prostate cancer, up to 20% will have a normal PSA value, indicating unique patients may be identifiable by each method.

The Need for Treatment

Arguably, the greatest debate in urology at the present time concerns the need, or lack thereof, for treatment. While it has long been the case that European urologists have taken a more passive line toward therapy, their U.S. counterparts have taken a much more active approach. The debate over treatment heated up following the publication by Johansen in 1992 (100). In this study, men with prostate cancer were merely followed, with the resultant mortality rate from prostate cancer of 10% at 10 years. More recently, Chodak performed a meta analysis of watchful waiting series with the conclusion that low grade cancers may be watched, while high grade cancers will have a poor outcome with such management (101).

The prostate Patient Outcome Research Team (PORT) utilized published treatment result data in a Markov computer decision analysis model to measure the effects of radiation therapy or radical prostatectomy vs. outcomes with watchful waiting (102). The results for 65-year-old men revealed a quality of life adjusted benefit of –0.34 year for well-differentiated cancer with 0.33 year and 1.0 years, respectively for moderately- and poorly-differentiated cancers. The Baylor group have recently revised these outcomes, inputting more recent clinical data into the model. Their results now show quality of life adjusted benefits of radical prostatectomy of 1.01, 2.41 and 2.18 years for well-, moderately- and poorly-differentiated cancers, respec-

tively (103). Again, these figures represent benefits for 65-year-old men. As men get older, these benefits will shrink accordingly. The reasons are threefold: (1) that carcinoma of the prostate is generally slow growing, (2) that life expectancy is shrinking, and (3) that competing causes of death are becoming more prominent.

However, the contrarian view states that 61% of prostate cancer deaths are in men older than 74 years of age (104). Older men are also at higher risk of harboring large or more poorly-differentiated cancers that are locally extensive at diagnosis. Unfortunately, these cancers do poorly with or without treatment.

Diagnosis and Staging

Prostate Biopsy

The diagnosis of prostate cancer is usually made by biopsying the prostate. This is normally performed by transrectal ultrasound-guided biopsies. Several years ago, the Stanford group calculated that by taking sextant biopsies, one had less than a 5% chance of missing a significant cancer (105). Thus, it is usual practice for most urologists to biopsy the whole gland, even if the prostate biopsy was driven by a palpable nodule with a normal PSA level. Previous work suggests that at least 16% of cancers would have been missed if only the nodule had been biopsied. Prostate biopsy is usually indicated because of a prostate nodule or elevated PSA level. Occasionally, the finding of metastatic adenocarcinoma requires prostate biopsy in the search for the primary tumor. Ten percent of patients undergoing transurethral prostatectomy for presumptively benign disease are found, after histologic analysis, to have adenocarcinoma in the prostate. The other main method of diagnosis is measurement of PSA levels. Routine measurement of PSA is performed by many internists and gerontologists. While the American Cancer Society recommends annual PSA and DRE for men over 50 years of age, it also suggests that a longevity of 10 years is necessary for treatment benefit (3). At age 75 years, men have a less than 10-year life expectancy (104), yet it is not uncommon to be referred asymptomatic patients in their 80's with elevated PSA levels. This is often true for patients with multiple medical problems and not just for those in good health and with a genetic pedigree suggestive of long survival. The general sense among U.S. urologists is that radical prostatectomy is questionable for septuagenarians (at least in academic circles). This being the case, then routine measurement of PSA in these men (over 75 years of age) must be brought into question.

At a statistical level, PSAs in normal range of 0 to 4 ng/ml in the absence of rectal abnormality will have a very low yield. PSA levels between 4 and 10 ng/ml will overall have a 25% likelihood of being associated with carcinoma of the prostate. If the DRE is negative, then positive predictive value is about 10% while if positive, it is about 40%. Above 10 ng/ml the positive predictive value is about 67%(106). BPH is probably

Table 49.4 Prostate cancer staging.

Tumor

$T_{1a\&b}$	Incidentally found at surgery for benign disease
T_{1c}	Elevated PSA
T_2	Clinically localized to the prostate
T_3	Local extension beyond the prostate
T_4	Involves other organs or pelvic side wall

Nodes

N_1	Single positive node < 2 cm
N_2	One or more nodes 2–5 cm
N_3	One or more nodes > 5 cm

Metastases

| M_0 | No distant metastases |
| M_1 | Distant metastases present |

the most common cause of benign elevations in this range, though values up to 80 ng/ml have been seen in patients with acute prostatitis (86).

Staging

After several years of trying, use of the tumor, nodes, and metastases method of staging prostate cancer is now commonplace and will soon completely replace the old ABCD system (107). The staging system is summarized in Table 49.4. Essentially T1 tumors are incidently found subsequent to surgery for benign disease or because of an elevated PSA. T2 tumors are localized to the prostate. T3 tumors have clinically spread beyond the prostatic capsule, and T4 tumors involve other organs or the pelvic side wall.

T1   Tumors

T1a Clinically benign prostate found incidentally at surgery (usually transurethral prostatectomy). Well differentiated tumor involving less than 5% of resected tissue.

T1b Incidentally found tumor. Poorly differentiated tumor or involving more than 5% of resected tissue.

T1c Clinically benign prostate with tumor diagnosed because of elevated PSA level.

T2   Palpable tumor clinically localized to the prostate

T2a Involves less than half of one prostatic lobe.

T2b Involves more than half of one prostatic lobe.

T2C Involves both lobes of the prostate.

T3   Tumor extends beyond the capsule of prostate

T3a Unilateral extension beyond prostate.

T3b Bilateral extension beyond prostate.

T3C Tumor invades one or both seminal vesicles

T4	**Tumor involves other organs or pelvic side walls**
T4a	Tumor involves bladder neck + external sphincter + rectum.
T4b	Tumor involves additional adjacent organs.

N	**Nodal Metastases**
N0	No nodal metastases.
N1	Metastases in single node <2 cm in diameter.
N2	Metastases in one or more nodes 2–5 cm in diameter.
N3	Metastases in one or more nodes >5 cm in diameter.

M	**Metastases**
M0	No distant metastases present.
M1	Distant metastases present.

Grading

Numerous grading systems have been proposed for prostate cancer. The most common of these is the Gleason grading system (108). The basis for this system is a low power microscopic evaluation of the prostatic glands. The glands are graded from one, where there is an increase in the number of glands which are slightly smaller than normal, to five where only sheets of anaplastic cells exist.

Gleason also noted that prostatic tumors are generally heterogeneous in nature with areas of different degrees of differentiation. For that reason, the Gleason system has two numbers attached to it. The first number represents the primary tumor grade while the second number represents the secondary pattern (which must represent more than 5% of the total area). Generally, tumors with a combined score of 2–4 are considered well differentiated, 5–6/7 moderately differentiated, and 7/8–10 poorly differentiated. The other less commonly utilized grading systems use the more common cytologic abnormalities such as mitotic figures, nuclear to cytoplasmic ratios, and nucleoli, etc. Approximately 10% to 20% of tumors will be well differentiated, 70% to 80% moderately differentiated, and 10% poorly differentiated.

Treatment

The treatment of prostate cancer has generated more heated debate in the urologic community and from a position of less certainty than the average debate in Washington. The treatment spectrum runs the gamut from no treatment (watchful waiting) to radical prostatectomy with radiation therapy and (possibly cryotherapy) in between (Table 49.5).

Watchful Waiting

To rationalize this disparity one must realize that most cancers run a protracted course such that competing causes of death overwhelm the likelihood of the cancer actually being the cause of death (109,110). The hazard

Table 49.5 Treatment options.

No Treatment	(Watchful waiting)
Radical Prostatectomy	Retropubic
	Perineal
Radiation Therapy	External beam
	Conformational external beam
	Interstitial radiation
Hormonal Therapy	
	(other — cryotherapy, proton therapy)

ratio for progression (and presumably clinical problems) continues to increase such that U.S. standards have defined a 10-year life expectancy as the threshold for treatment. Thus treatments with intent to cure will have limited benefit for men over age 70 years. The meta analysis performed by Dr. Chodak *et al.* from six watchful waiting studies has 10-year disease specific survivals of 87%, 87%, and 34% for grades 1, 2, and 3 tumors respectively (101). The nonmetastatic rate at 10 years is 81%, 58%, and 26% respectively for grades 1, 2, and 3 tumors. These data do not separate by stage at diagnosis and higher stage disease not surprisingly is associated with higher progression rates. The above data demonstrate that even with grade 1 disease about 20% of patients will have metastases by 10 years. A reasonable implication of this is patient morbidity and a decrease in quality of life. For Grade 2 tumors the progression rate is 52% over 10 years making active intervention a much more attractive proposition.

From a patient decision making process this should be balanced by the upfront morbidity associated with active intervention. A complex subjective evaluative process is necessary for the patient to make the right choice of treatment for him as opposed to the right choice for the physician (Table 49.6).

It is also clear that many patients are poorly informed of these choices but many are also unable to grasp complex issues for themselves making it important for the physician to try and interpret the patients wishes and help him toward those goals. In many

Table 49.7 Radical prostatectomy.

Pro	Con
• Cancer Removed	• Major Surgery
	• 90% Impotence rate (50% of population over 70 years impotent)
	• 30% will have some alteration in continence

respects, watchful waiting trades lack of morbidity now for possible morbidity later (if they live that long). When a patient makes that choice, there appears little benefit (in terms of reduction of quality of life) for focusing in on tumor progression (whether by DRE or PSA) in the absence of symptomatic change. Despite the above, current practice advises routine follow-up which may vary from quarterly to annually where changes in DRE and PSA will be measured. As part of the natural history, one might anticipate that nodules will enlarge and PSA will rise over time inevitably having a negative impact upon the patients quality of life yet not benefitting the patient in any way.

An extreme example seen recently was an octogenarian unable to walk because of severe cardiac disease but who, along with his relatives, obsessed about his PSA and/or changes in rectal examination despite an absence of change in urinary symptoms. Interestingly, such patients become conditioned by practice of care such that they are offended by the notion that specific urologic follow-up is not helpful in the absence of a change in symptoms.

Radical Prostatectomy (Table 49.7).

Radical prostatectomy was first performed in 1904, yet it is only in the last 15 years that it has seen an explosive growth in popularity. During the 1980's, the primary approach was radical retropubic prostatectomy. This technique was championed by Walsh *et al.* demonstrating that with anatomic dissection of the prostate, the penile nerves could be preserved and with it potency (111). As a medical text, complete surgical descriptions are not given but may be found in many surgical textbooks (111). Briefly the retroperitoneum is exposed

Table 49.6 Watchful waiting.

Pro	Con
• No side effects of treatment	• Patients quality of life negatively impacted by worrying over untreated cancer
• Disease may not impact patients quality of life	• Disease has high likelihood of spreading given long enough time
• Treatment unlikely to affect survival in less than 10 years	• PSA will rise • Tumor will enlarge • Local symptoms may develop

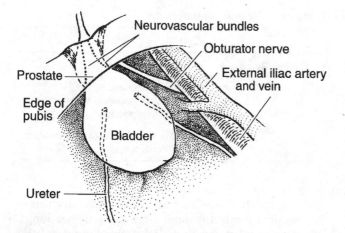

Figure 49.1 Operative view of pelvis during exposure for radical retropubic prostatectomy. Note neurovascular bundles posterolateral to prostate which is deep in pelvis below pubic symphysis.

Table 49.8 Complications of radical prostatectomy and radiation therapy.

	Radical Prostatectomy	Radiation Therapy
Death	1%	0.2%
Any Incontinence	27	6
Total Incontinence	6	1
Any Bowel Injury	3	11
Bowel Injury requiring long-term treatment		
Stricture	12	5
Impotence	85	42
Diarrhea	–	4
Rectal Bleeding		1

From: Wassan *et al. Arch Fam Med.* **2**:487–493, 1993 and Reference 120.

through a lower midline incision. The peritoneum is swept cephalad such that the lymph nodes surrounding the external iliac vessels are exposed and may be dissected along with the obturator nodes (Figure 49.1).

If the nodes are negative, then the prostate is removed. The neurovascular bundles lie posterolateral to the prostate. Blood loss during the procedure seems to have generally declined such that autologous blood donation, commonplace during the 80's, has recently come under fire as not being effective (112). Autologous blood donation at this institution costs $250 per unit but is variably covered by insurance companies. Hospitalizations have also shrunk from a week or more a decade ago to about 3 or 4 days today with the patient being admitted to hospital postoperatively. The patient is discharged with a foley catheter indwelling with removal 2 to 3 weeks after surgery depending upon surgeon preference. Recovery time is about 2 months though continence (if a problem) may continue to improve for up to 6 months following surgery. The main complications of this procedure are shown in Table 49.8.

Urinary incontinence (16) has recently been reviewed and found to be much more prevalent than heretofore published (113,114). However, a recent study at our institution demonstrated significant incontinence prior to treatment (115). It is important that the patient understand that their continence mechanism will be different and that while one-third of patients will lose some urine during stress, for most this will have a trivial impact upon their quality of life. A major problem with urinary control should occur in less than 5% of patients. Indeed of the one-third of patients affected, many place a pad in their underwear merely for self-confidence rather than because they have any significant leakage.

The other major issue with radical retropubic prostatectomy concerns potency. The early work from Walsh and his group suggested that about three quarters of

patients with localized disease would maintain potency. A recent review of medicare patients found that about 90% were functionally impotent (114). Thus while potency preservation is age and stage dependent and while penile engorgement is different from rigidity, and with it the ability for vaginal penetration, when one looks at the overall patient population the majority will be impotent following surgery. Indeed, in a patient group over 70 years of age, it would only be the rare patient potent before surgery who would maintain this following surgery. For perspective, we recently found that in general for men in their 60's about 25% were impotent and by their 70's 50% were impotent (116).

Radical Perineal Prostatectomy

Over the last several years there has been a major resurgence in the performance of radical perineal prostatectomy (Figure 49.2).

There have been two major driving forces for this change. The first developed out of better prognostic information about nodal status based upon biopsy histology and PSA (117). If the biopsy demonstrated well or moderately differentiated cancer while the PSA is less than 10 ng/ml, then the likelihood of node positive disease is less than 5% making surgical evaluation of the nodes unnecessary. The second reason is because radical perineal prostatectomy is a less morbid procedure with very little postoperative pain (118). Patients are routinely discharged on the second postoperative day and many could probably be discharged on postoperative day one. The catheter is likewise removed at 2 to 3 weeks but full recovery is quicker without an abdominal wound.

Additionally, the neurovascular bundles may be preserved equally as well (or as poorly) with a perineal approach as with a retropubic approach. Blood loss for the procedure is generally less than with radical retro-

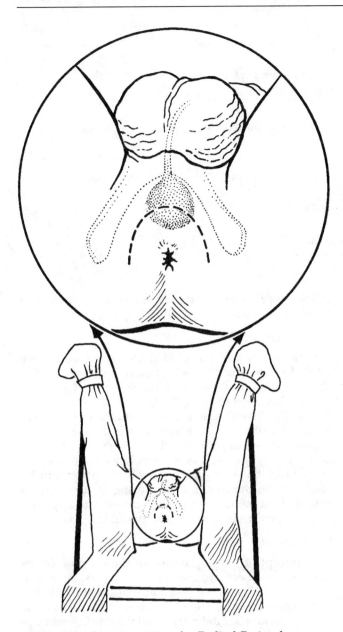

Figure 49.2 Patient position for Radical Perineal Prostatectomy. Insert shows incision line with position of prostate relatively superficial to skin.

pubic prostatectomy as one stays away from the dorsal vein complex which is a potential source of significant bleeding with the radical retropubic prostatectomy (118). Finally, because of the approach to the gland the prostatic apex is superficial in the wound and therefore the vesicourethral anastomoses is more easily performed and with a greater degree of control and precision. Two practical issues limit the perineal approach. If a patient has hip problems, than he probably will not be able to be placed in the exaggerated lithotomy position. Secondly, if the prostate is large or the inferior pubic ramus angle is narrow, then this too may preclude such an approach (Figure 49.2).

A practical approach to technique selection for patients who desire radical prostatectomy is as follows.

Table 49.9 Radiation therapy.

Pro	Con
• Not Surgery	• Efficacy debated
	• Impotence
	• Incontinence

If the PSA is less than 10 ng/ml and their glands small or moderately differentiated, then radical perineal prostatectomy is suggested as this is a very small likelihood of finding positive nodes. If these do not apply, then I suggest radical retropubic prostatectomy as the probability of finding positive nodes increases at which point the prostatectomy would not be performed. As recently as one year ago, I would have added that if the PSA was greater than 25 to 30 ng/ml, then I would suggest laparoscopic pelvic lymph node dissection with subsequent radical prostatectomy if the nodes were negative. Recently, the appropriateness of radical prostatectomy for patients with PSA's above 30 ng/ml has been increasingly questioned. However, for the exceptions to every rule I might still recommend laparoscopic pelvic lymph node dissection in this situation where the node postive rate will be at least 25% (119). The benefits of laparoscopic lymphs node dissection are very little postoperative discomfort with full return to normal activity in a few days.

Radiation Therapy (Table 49.9).

Radiation therapy is the other main type of therapy for prostate cancer. The radiation may be delivered in several forms (Table 49.10), conventional external beam, conformational external beam, interstitial radiation therapy, and particle therapy.

The most commonly utilized method of delivery is conventional external beam. Modern therapy units utilize linear accelerators. With increasing energy, side effects from radiation therapy have decreased. The primary acute side effects (Table 49.8) are radiation proctitis and cystitis (120). Chronic radiation cystitis and proctitis are much less common but may be debilitating. Incontinence and impotence, while less than radical prostatectomy, are still significant.

Good studies comparing efficacy between radical prostatectomy and radiation therapy do not exist but a recent evaluation of RTOG studies suggests that external beam radiation therapy is 50% effective for T2 disease when viewed from 15-year follow-up data.[121] Patients with T1 disease show 15-year survivals in keeping with life table expectant survivals although this is also true for the watchful waiting group (121).

In an attempt to improve on survival data (especially stage T2 patients), the idea of conformational radiation therapy was developed (121). In order to increase the delivered radiation dose, in excess of 7000 cGy, the scientific disciplines of medical physics, radiation dosimetry, computer science, statistics and probability, radiology, and radiation oncology have been

Table 49.10 Methods of radiation therapy.

Conventional External Beams

Four field or rotational fields delivered using pelvic x-rays (pubic symphysis) to define treatment fields

Conformational External Beam

Computer-guided using CT reconstructed images for more precise localization to the prostate

Interstitial Radiation

Radioactive pellets placed permanently or temporarily in the prostate for radiation delivery. Seeds placed using ultrasound or CT guidance.

Particle Therapy

Experimental and limited due to lack of equipment availability

combined to deliver increased doses of radiation precisely (conforming) to the prostate (122). Three-dimensional images of the prostate are developed with computed tomography from which pseudo three-dimensional images of the prostate are developed. With these models it is now possible to deliver radiation precisely to the prostate and therefore at greater doses. Standard techniques use 7-cm by 7-cm to 8-cm by 8-cm boxes centered 1-cm superior to the symphysis in the AP dimension and over the femoral neck for the lateral projection. Using such techniques, there is a 25% geographic miss of part of the prostate (123). Preliminary reports suggest that dose escalations to 7400–8040 cGy are possible using conformational radiation without an increase in normal tissue side effects. However, long-term studies will be required to define improvements in efficacy.

Prostate Brachytherapy

The insertion of radioactive seeds into the prostate now has a long history. A variety of isotopes have been inserted with I^{125} being the most common. One of the largest series utilizing manually placed seeds came from Memorial Sloan Kettering in New York (124). In this series, a formal retropubic dissection was performed and the seeds placed manually with a trocar. Dosimetry reconstructions have suggested significant problems with underdosing such that long-term results have been poor (70% progression at 10 years). In an attempt to improve on these results, seeds have been placed using ultrasound or CT guidance. Preliminary data have suggested encouraging results but until long-term data are available, one cannot conclude that the results are different and improved from the older Memorial data (125).

Most recently, new higher dose rate seeds such as Palladium-103 have become available (122,125). Others have utilized removable implants such as Iridium-192 (122,125). Palladium provides different radiation characteristics from I^{125}. Its tissue penetration is similar but its half-life is only 17 days. Thus, it delivers its dose more quickly than I^{125} providing very different radiobiological effects. Iridium, on the other hand, provides

much more penetrating gamma energy mandating temporary implantation only.

Particle Therapy

Particle therapy in the United States has been very limited because of the lack of equipment availability (Boston, Massachusetts and Loma Linda, California only) (122). Protons have the benefit of a similar biological effectiveness as photons but a more selective energy distribution. Little radiation is delivered to the superficial tissues with deposition in the deeper tissues of a high energy peak and thereafter a complete dissipation of the energy. This peak of energy can be "focused" to the tumor with sparing of surrounding tissues. Comparative studies of proton therapy with conventional radiation are not available.

Cryotherapy

The concept of freezing tissue for the purpose of destruction has been around for many years. As a consequence of this fact, cryotherapy of the prostate has not required FDA controlled trials. Interestingly, the medical insurance industry has taken a different approach and generally has not accepted cryotherapy as a covered benefit. Thus, patients have been treated in multiple centers around the country without even appropriate animal studies being conducted. Animal studies were recently conducted in our institution and demonstrated a failure to destroy all prostatic tissue (126).

Essentially the procedure consists of inserting multiple probes perineally into the prostate under transrectal ultrasound guidance. A transurethral warming catheter is placed in order to preserve the prostatic urethral mucosa and the prostate is frozen by circulating liquid nitrogen through the cryoprobes. The iceball thus created is monitored with transrectal ultrasound. Recent clinical data from salvage radical prostatectomy after cryotherapy have confirmed the lack of destruction of prostatic tissue despite the obvious "iceball" appearance involving the complete prostate (127). This same group found that 59% of treated patients suffered from complications. The most frequent of these were

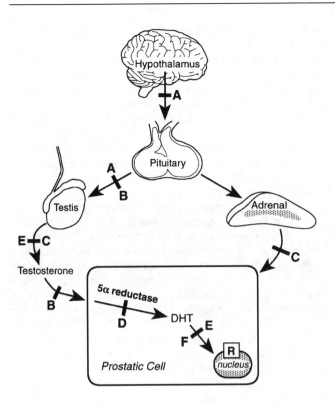

Figure 49.3 The sites of action for drugs controlling androgen production or activity on the prostate cell.
A. GnRH
B. Estrogens
C. Ketoconazole
D. Megestrol Acetate
E. Cyproterone Acetate
F. Non steroidal anti Androgens
R. Androgen receptor

urinary retention (29%), urinary incontinence (27%), tissue slough (19%), and perineal pain (11%) (128). Cryotherapy has also been utilized for radiation failures but the conclusion of the study was that it was not effective (129).

At the present time, therefore, cryotherapy appears to have a questionable future. No comparative or long-term studies are available. Current data suggest ineffectiveness in tissue destruction along with a high immediate complication rate.

Metastatic Disease

Once prostate cancer spreads beyond the prostate, cure is not possible. Indeed even for localized disease, palliative therapy may be used as the primary treatment for older patients (70–75 years and older). In 1941, Huggins and Hodges noted the hormone sensitivity of prostate cancer (130). Over the past 40 years newer methods of hormonal manipulation have been developed, but the fundamental outlook of patients with metastatic prostate cancer has not significantly changed.

All clinical methods for hormonal therapy for metastatic prostate cancer work by blocking the various steps of androgen production, secretion, or action (Figure 49.3).

Orchiectomy is the most basic form of androgen ablation and is the standard against which all other therapies should be compared. Because the testes produce 95% of serum testosterone, bilateral orchiectomy results in an immediate decrease in androgen blood levels. This fall will sometimes give overnight "relief" from painful metastases. No chemical methods can provide such an immediate effect.

For those patients who refuse orchiectomy, the standard treatment, until recently, was diethyl stilbestrol (DES). In the 1960's, studies were conducted by the veterans administration cooperative urologic research group (VACURG). These studies looked at all stages of prostate cancer (131–136). For patients with focal localized disease, they found that the addition of estrogen treatment to radical prostatectomy decreased survival, presumably owing to the estrogen side effects (131). Patients who refused participation in this study were offered participation in the second study, randomizing placebo, DES, and orchiectomy with and without estrogen (133). No significant differences were seen between the groups or with the radical prostate group in the other study. This study also demonstrated that only 6.8% of patients progressed during the study (mean age 73 years). More recent studies have shown progression rates for stage A1 disease for stage T1 disease of 9% in 16%. Patients with metastatic disease were treated with placebo, orchiectomy with and without stilbestrol or stilbestrol alone, 5 mg per day (134). No significant differences were seen in patients survival over 5 years. It should be noted that patients who progressed were taken off study and treated individually. Thus, most placebo patients were treated hormonally at progression. This suggests that delayed hormonal treatment is not detrimental to patient survival. One other observation from the first VACURG study was the excess number of deaths occurring in the estrogen-treated patients from cardiovascular causes. This led the investigators to evaluate different doses of DES, namely 0.2 mg, 1 mg, and 5 mg per day (134). This study revealed that 0.2 mg per day was not sufficient in controlling the prostate cancer while 5 mg per day caused an excess of cardiovascular deaths (137,138). Subsequent studies demonstrated that 1 mg per day did not reliably suppress testosterone production while 1 mg three times daily did not cause an increase in cardiovascular deaths. Combined, the data for DES or orchiectomy show that 10% of patients die within 6 months, 50% within 2-1/2 years, and 10% are alive 10 years later (139).

More recently, the morbidity associated with estrogen therapy has been studied further. One nonrandomized study evaluated 48 patients treated with stilbestrol 1 mg three times daily. Over a four-year period, 14 cardiovascular complications were seen (140). The control arm of 37 patients who underwent a bilateral orchiectomy suffered only three cardiovascular complications. In an attempt to understand the mechanism for this increased risk, investigators measured serum levels of antithrombin-3. Antithrombin-3 is an alpha globulin synthesized in the liver and is the single most important physiologic inhibitor of blood coagulation. In one study, antithrombin-3 levels were reduced by 25% in patients on 5 mg DES per day while no changes were seen with 1 mg per day (141). In another small study, no differences were seen between 1 and 3 mg per day in the effected antithrombin-3 levels, though the numbers were very small (142). Interestingly, when the GnRH agonist Goserelin was studied, no change was seen, while the antiandrogen cyproterone acetate increased anti-thrombin-3 levels (143,144).

GnRH analogues produce castrate levels of testosterone through their action on the pituitary gland (145). Although 50 to 100 times more potent than the natural hormone, chronic administration depletes pituitary LH and down regulates GnRH receptors making the pituitary refractory to further stimulation. Extra pituitary effects of GnRH analogues include the desensitization of the gonad to LH and direct gonadal steroid enzyme inhibition, further decreasing testosterone production (145).

In a multicenter study, leuprolide was compared with DES 3 mg per day. Ninety-eight patients and 101 patients, respectively, were assigned to each arm (146). In the DES group, testosterone levels fell to anorchic levels within 2 weeks while in the leuprolide group testosterone levels rose during the first week and only by 4 weeks did they reach anorchic levels. No difference in progression rates or survival was seen between the two arms. Nausea, vomiting, and edema were significantly increased in the DES group (16% vs. 5%), and, while not significant, thrombosis or phlebitis and pulmonary embolus were also increased in the DES group (7% vs 1%). This study demonstrated that daily leuprolide injections were equally as effective as DES in treating prostate cancer but with fewer side effects.

Current formulations of the available GnRH agonists (leuprolide, lupron, Goserelin acetate, and zoladex) require monthly injections.

One problem with the GnRH analogues concerns their agonistic properties. Prior to blocking testosterone production they stimulate the testes to increase the output of testosterone. This may be associated with increased pain from metastasis and anecdotally has resulted in paralysis and even death. This is the so-called flare phenomenon. In an attempt to control this problem and to block the effects of adrenal androgens Labrie pioneered the combination treatment of GnRH analogues together with the antiandrogen flutamide (147). Flutamide is a nonsteroidal antiandrogen that acts by blocking the effects of dihydro testosterone on the cell nucleus. This phenomenon will negate the effects of initial rise in testosterone levels and permanently block the effects of adrenal steroids. This type of combination has been termed complete androgen blockade. A national cooperative study group compared the response to the GnRH analogue leuprolide with or without the addition of flutamide (148). The study with more than 600 patients demonstrated an improved overall survivorship for patients treated with leuprolide plus flutamide. When the data were analyzed relative to extent of metastases, those patients with minimal metastatic disease did markedly better with the addition of flutamide. This difference was not seen for patients with large volume metastatic disease. Flutamide has two major problems. Diarrhea has been a problem for 12% of patients. Much less common, but more serious, is hepatic dysfunction. A recent report from the FDA demonstrated the mortality rate from flutamide of 3 per 10,000 patients treated (149). It is thus extremely important that patients have liver function tests checked for the first few months after starting treatment and also that patients be instructed to report any problems with nausea, vomiting, fatigue, and jaundice.

Another nonsteroidal antiandrogen bicalutamide (Casodex) has recently been approved by the FDA. The drug is a once-a-day dosing (as compared with three times a day for flutamide). In a recently published 800 patient study, bicalutamide was compared with flutamide with both being used in combination with a GnRH agonist (150). Bicalutamide was shown to be as least as effective as flutamide. The severe diarrhea rate for bicalutamide was much less than that for flutamide (0.5% vs. 6%). Of note, however, the abnormal liver function test rate was similar for both drugs. Thus, it is extremely important to evaluate liver function when any nonsteroidal antiandrogen is being used for therapy.

In summary, hormonal manipulation will benefit approximately 75% of patients with newly diagnosed metastatic prostate cancer. The median duration of response is approximately 15 months. Following failure of hormonal therapy to control the disease, median survival is less than one year. The spectrum of survival from diagnosis of metastatic disease is wide. In the veterans study conducted during the 1960's, 10% of patients survived less than 6 months, 10% longer than 10 years while median survival was about 2.5 years. Furthermore, when "off study" patient data were analyzed those initially treated with placebo fared no worse than those actively treated at the beginning of the study (151). The intergroup study from the 1980's comparing leuprolide with or without flutamide for treatment of metastatic disease found median survival times were 28 months for leuprolide alone and 35 months for leuprolide plus flutamide. While the two studies are not truly comparable, one might question the level of advancement with this treatment.

Recently, anecdotes have arisen that patients failing complete androgen blockade have had a symptomatic, and PSA, response to the withdrawal of flutamide (152). The precise mechanism is not clear but this is now the subject of clinical cancer group investigation.

One complication common to the various hormonal manipulations is the phenomenon of hot flashes. After orchiectomy this problem is rarely reported, yet when patients are specifically questioned, its prevalence appears much higher. Studies of GNRH agonists and DES have shown incidences of 51% and 11% respectively. The etiologic mechanism remains obscure. The only common events to the described treatments is a rapid reduction in androgen levels. Orchiectomy causes an increase in GNRH and LH as a consequence of loss of feedback inhibition. GnRH agonists exogenously increases GnRH while decreasing LH and testosterone levels. Estrogen suppressed GnRH, LH, and testosterone production. The treatment for men (and women) is estrogen therapy. After orchiectomy it was suggested that this worked by suppression of GnRH and LH production. For some patients, estrogens are contraindicated for cardiovascular reasons. For these patients, the antiandrogen cyproterone acetate has been used successfully (143,153). As a progestational agent, cyproterone acetate inhibits GnRH production, and it is probably this mechanism that is active rather than its antiandrogen activities at the cellular level. More recently clonidine and megestrol acetate have been reported to be successful in the treatment of hot flashes (154,155). Clinically, they are rarely a problem though their prevalence is much greater when patients are questioned about them than if they are not. Again, the severity of the hot flashes tends to diminish with time.

Chemotherapy

Active chemotherapeutic agents are urgently needed for prostate cancer. To date, no drug has achieved a standard "therapy" status. At the present time, Suramin has achieved the status of most promising drug (156). Suramin is a polysulfonated naphthylurea. Originally evaluated as an AIDS drug because of its ability to inhibit reverse transcriptase of RNA viruses, it was subsequently found not to be useful in that disease. Through interaction with glycosaminoglycan function it inhibits binding of various growth factors including $TGF\beta$, FGF, and EGF. It also appears to affect TNF, IL2, and Topoisomerase-2. Finally, it reduces bone reabsorption which may account for the pain relief seen in some patients.

The drug is excreted unchanged through the kidneys and with a long half-life. Dose limiting neurotoxicity has been found and occasionally irreversible adrenal insufficiency. Dose limiting toxicity in the 20% to 60% range has been seen between the various studies. The best results have been seen in continuous infusion studies with 30% to 50% of patients having measurable responses. Studies with hormone naive patients are now ongoing to continue the evaluation of this drug.

Current Research Studies — Areas for Investigation

Localized Prostate Cancer

PIVOT study

This study randomizes patients with clinically localized prostate cancer to radical prostatectomy versus expectant management.

Regionalized Cancer

Radical prostatectomy ± radiation therapy for pathologic T3 cancers

Over the past decade numerous articles pro and con the addition of radiation therapy for patients with pathologic T_3 cancers after radical prostatectomy have been published. The study is attempting to answer the question as to whether or not adjuvant radiation therapy is helpful.

Total androgen blockade ± pelvic irradiation

This study will evaluate the benefit of adding pelvic irradiation to complete androgen blockade for patients with locally advanced (N_0M_0) patients.

Metastatic Prostate Cancer

Intermittent androgen deprivation

This study will randomize patients initially responding to complete androgen blockade (3 months) to continuous versus intermittent androgen blockade. Animal studies together with pilot human study suggests that patients do at least as well with intermittent hormonal therapy with some suggestion that they may even do better than with continuous therapy. Therapy is reinstituted for rising PSA's or other evidence of progression.

Suramin

Suramin studies evaluating different doses of suramin alone over the complete androgen blockade are being evaluated.

Flutamide withdrawal

Anecdotally, patients failing complete androgen blockade hormonal therapy have been found to subjectively respond to withdrawal of flutamide therapy. This study will evaluate this phenomenon.

Areas for Research

The fundamental problem with carcinoma of the prostate is that most people with histologic prostate cancer die with and not from their disease. Conversely, adenocarcinoma of the prostate is the second leading cause of cancer death in men. The challenge, therefore, is to diagnose those cancers destined to have a malignant course early in the disease process such that interventions with curative intent will be successful. Compounding the problem is molecular heterogeneity between multiple cancers within the same prostate. Genetic studies of multiple foci of cancer within the prostate have demonstrated multiple different abnormalities. The problem has thus been seen that a metastasis has a genetic abnormality which may not be seen on a biopsy of only one area of tumor. Thus, even with the development of relevant molecular probes there will still remain many hurdles in being able to prognosticate from the diagnosis of prostate cancer to its outcome.

References

1. Wingo PA, Tong T, Bolden S. Cancer statistics, 1995. *C A Cancer J Clin* 1995; **45**: 8–30.
2. Cancer statistics, 1975. *CA Cancer J Clin* 1975; **25**: 8–26.
3. Mettlin C, Jones G, Averette H, Gusberg SB, Murphy GP. Defining and updating the American Cancer Society guidelines for the cancer-related checkup: Prostate and endometrial cancers. *CA Cancer J Clin* 1993; **43**: 42–46.

4. Young H. A Surgeon's autobiography. New York: Harcourt, Brace and Co., 1940.

5. National Cancer Institute economic conference: The integration of economic outcome measures into NCI-sponsored therapeutic trials. *Monograph J Natl Cancer Inst.* 1995:19.

6. Cannon L, Bishop DT, Skolnick M, Hunt S, Lyon JL, Smart CR. Genetic epidemiology of prostate cancer in the Utah Mormon genealogy. *Cancer Surv* 1982; **1**: 47.

7. Steinberg GD, Carter BS, Beaty TH, Childs B, Walsh PC. Family history and the risk of prostate cancer. *Prostate* 1990; **17**: 337–347.

8. Spitz MR, Currier RD, Fueger JJ, Babaian RJ, Newell GR. Familiar patterns of prostate cancer: a case-control analysis. *J Urol* 1991; **146**: 1305–1307.

9. Carter BS, Beaty TH, Steinberg GD, Childs B, Walsh PC. Mendelian inheritance of familial prostate cancer. *Proc Am Soc Clin Oncol* 1992; **89**: 3367–3371.

10. Carter BS, Bova GS, Beaty TH, et al. Hereditary prostate cancer: epidemiologic and clinical features. *J Urol* 1993; **150**: 797–802.

11. Brothman AR, Peehl DM, Patel AM, McNeal JE. Frequency and pattern of karyotypic abnormalities in human prostate cancer. *Cancer Res* 1990; **50**: 3795–3803.

12. Carter BS, Ewing CM, Ward WS, Treiger BF. Allelic loss of chromosomes 16q and 10q in human prostate cancer. *Proc Natl Acad Sci USA* 1990; **87**: 8751–8755.

13. Bergerheim USR, Kunimi K, Collins VP, Ekman P. Deletion mapping of chromosomes 8, 10 and 16 in human prostate carcinoma. *Genes Chromosom Cancer* 1991; **3**: 215–220.

14. Moul JM, Gaddipati J, Srivastava S. Molecular biology of prostate cancer: Oncogenes and tumor suppressor genes. In *Prostate cancer*, edited by NA Dawson, NJ Vogelzang. New York: Wiley-Liss, Inc., 19–46, 1994.

15. Peehl DM, Wehner N, Stamey TA. Activated Ki-*ras* oncogene in human prostatic adenocarcinoma. *Prostate* 1987; **10**: 281–289.

16. Buttyan R, Sawczuk IS, Benson MC, Siegal JD, Olsson CA. Enhanced expression of the *c-myc* proto-oncogene in high-grade human prostate cancer. *Prostate* 1987; **11**: 327–337.

17. Habib FK, Chisholm GD. The role of growth factors in the human prostate. *Scand J Urol Nephrol Suppl* 1991; **126**: 53–58.

18. Pergolizzi RG, Kreis W, Rottach C, Susin M, Broome JD. Mutational status of codons 12 and 13 of the N and K *ras* genes in tissue and cell lines derived from primary and metastatic prostate carcinomas. *Cancer Invest* 1993; **11**: 25–32.

19. Carter BS, Epstein JI, Isaacs WB. *ras* gene mutations in human prostate cancer. *Cancer Res* 1990; **50**: 6830–6832.

20. Gumerlock PH, Poonmallee UR, Meyers FJ, de Vere White RW. Activated *ras* alleles in human carcinoma of the prostate are rare. *Cancer Res* 1991; **51**: 1632–1637.

21. Moul JW, Lance RS, Friedrichs PA, Theune SM, Chang EH. Infrequent *ras* oncogene mutations in human prostate cancer. *Prostate* 1992; **20**: 327–338.

22. Konishi N, Enomoto T, Buzard G, Ohshima M, Ward JM, Rice JM. K-*ras* activation and *ras* p21 expression in latent prostatic carcinomas in Japanese men. *Cancer* 1992; **69**: 2293–2299.

23. Anwar K, Nakakuki K, Shiraishi T, Naiki H, Yatani R, Inwua M. Presence of *ras* oncogene mutations and human papillomavirus DNA in human prostate carcinomas. *Cancer Res* 1992; **52**: 5991–5996.

24. Zhau HE, Wan DS, Zhou J, Miller GJ, Von Eschenbach AC. Expression of *c-erbB–2/neu* proto-oncogene in human prostatic cancer tissues and cell lines. *Mol Carcinog* 1992; **5**: 320–327.

25. Ware JL, Maygarden SJ, Koontz WW, Strom SC. Immunohistochemical detection of *c-erb*B-2 protein in human benign and neoplastic prostate. *Hum Pathol* 1991; **22**: 254–258.

26. Kuhn EJ, Kurnot RA, Sesterhenn IA, Chang EH, Moul JW. Expression of the *c-erb*B-2 (HER-2/neu) oncoprotein in human prostatic carcinoma. *J Urol* 1993; **150**: 1427–1433.

27. Volgelstein B, Kinzler KW. p53 function and dysfunction. *Cell* 1992; **70**: 523–526.

28. Lowe SW, Schmitt EM, Smith SW, Osborne BA, Jacks T. p53 is required for radiation induced apoptosis in mouse thymocytes. *Nature* 1993; **362**: 847–849.

29. Levine AJ, Momand J, Finlay CA. The p53 tumor suppressor gene. *Nature* 1991; **351**: 453–456.

30. Hamdy FC, Thurrell W, Lawry J, Anderson JB. p53 mutant expression correlates with hormone sensitivity and prognosis in human prostatic adenocarcinoma. *J Urol* 1993; **149**: 377A.

31. Eastham JA, Stapleton AM, Gousse AE, et al. Association of p53 mutations with metastatic prostate cancer. *Clin Res* 1995; **1**: 1111–1118.

32. Habib FK. The biology of benign prostatic hyperplasia and prostate cancer. In *Trends in experimental and clinical medicine*, edited by M Pavone-Macaluso, PH Smith. Genova: 1995.

33. Kyprianou N, Isaacs JT. Identification of a cellular receptor of transforming growth factor beta in rat ventral prostate and its negative regulation by androgens. *Endocrinology* 1988; **123**: 2124–2131.

34. Montpetit ML, et al. Androgen repressed messages in the rat from ventral prostate. *Prostate* 1986; **8**: 25–36.

35. Kyprianou N, Isaacs JT. Expression of transforming growth factor beta in the rat ventral prostate during castration induced programmed cell death. *Mol Endocrinol* 1989; **3**: 1515–1522.

36. Moon TD, Morley JE, Levine A, Vessella RL, Peterson G, Lange PH. The role of calmodulin in human renal cell carcinoma. *Biochem Biophys Res Commun* 1983; **114**: 843–849.

37. McDonnell TJ, et al. Expression of the protooncogene *bcl-2* in the prostate and its association with emergence of androgen independent prostate cancer. *Cancer Res* 1992; **52**: 6940–6944.

38. Colombel M, et al. Detection of the apoptosis-suppressing oncoprotein Bcl-2 in hormone-refractory human prostate cancers. *Am J Pathol* 1993; **143**: 390–340.

39. Maddy SQ, et al. Localization of epidermal growth factor receptors in the human prostate by biochemical and immunocytochemical methods. *J Endocrinol* 1987; **112**: 147–153.

40. Mellon K, et al. p53, C-erbB-2 and the epidermal growth factor receptor in the benign and malignant prostate. *J Urol* 1992; **147**: 496–499.

41. Maddy SQ, et al. Epidermal growth factor receptors in human prostate cancer: Correlation with histological differentiation of the tumor. *Br J Cancer* 1989; **60**: 41–44.

42. Yang Y, et al. Epidermal growth factor and transforming growth factor alpha concentrations in BPH and cancer of the prostate: Their relationships with tissue androgen levels. *Br J Cancer* 1993; **67**: 152–155.

43. Timme TL, et al. Mesenchymal/epithelial interaction and transforming growth factor beta expression during prostate morphogenesis. *Endocrinology* 1994; **134**: 1039–1045.

44. Story MT, et al. Influence of androgen in transforming growth factor beta on basic fibroblast growth factor levels in human prostate derived fibroblast cell cultures. *J Urol* 1990; **143**: A211.

45. Thomson TC. Growth factors and oncogenes in prostate cancer. *Cancer cells* 1990; **2**: 345–354.

46. Moon TD, Sloane BB. Prostatic adenocarcinoma: Carcinogenesis and growth. *J Am Geriatr Soc* 1989; **37**: 55–64.

47. Lubamn DB, Joseph DR, Sullivan PM, Willard HF, French FS, Wilson EM. Cloning of human androgen receptor complimentary DNA and localization to the X chromosome. *Science* 1988; **240**: 327–330.

48. Wilding G, Chen M, Gelmann EP. Aberrant response *in vitro* of hormone-responsive prostate cancer cells to antiandrogens. *Prostate* 1989; **14**: 103–115.

49. Harris S, Harris MA, Rong Z, et al. Androgen regulation of HβGF-I (αFGF) mRNA and characterization of the androgen-receptor mRNA in the human prostate carcinoma cell line-LNCaP/A-DEP. In *Molecular and cellular biology of prostate cancer*, edited by JP Karr, DS Coffey, RG Smith, DJ Tindall. New York: Plenum Press, 315–330, 1991.

50. Noble RL. The development of prostatic adenocarcinoma in Nb rats following prolonged sex hormone administration. *Cancer Res* 1977; **37**: 1929–1933.

51. Noble RL, Hoover L. A classification of transplantable tumors in Nb rats controlled by estrogen from dormancy to autonomy. *Cancer Res* 1975; **35**: 2935–2941.

52. Coffey DS. The biochemistry and physiology of the prostate. In *Campbell's urology*, edited by PC Walsh, RF Gittes, AD Perlmutter. Philadelphia: WB Saunders, 1986.

53. Greenwald P, Vincenne K, Polan AK, et al. Cancer of the prostate among men with benign prostatic hyperplasia. *J Natl Cancer Inst* 1974; **53**: 335–340.

54. Armenian HK, Lilienfeld AM, *et al.* Relationship between benign prostatic hyperplasia and cancer of the prostate: A prospective and retrospective study. *Lancet* 1974; **2**: 115–117.

55. Haenszel W, Kurichara W. Studies of Japanese migrants: 1. Mortality from cancer and other diseases among Japanese in the United States. *J Natl Cancer Inst* 1968; **40**: 43–68.

56. Akazaki K, Stemmerman GN. Comparative study of latent carcinoma of the prostate among Japanese in Japan and Hawaii. *J Natl Cancer Inst* 1973; **50**: 1137–1144.

57. Haenszel W. Cancer mortality among the foreign born in the United States. *J Natl Cancer Inst* 1961; **26**: 37.

58. Winkelstein W, Ernster VL. Epidemiology and etiology. In *Prostatic cancer*, edited by GP Murphy. Littleton: PSG Publishing, 1974.

59. Kipling MD, Waterhouse JA. Cadmium and prostate carcinoma. *Lancet* 1967; **1**: 730.

60. Winkelstein W, Kantor S. Prostatic cancer, relationship to suspended particulate air pollution. *Am J Public Health* 1969; **59**: 1134–1138.

61. Wynder EL, Mabuchi K, Whitmore WF. Epidemiology of cancer of the prostate. *Cancer* 1971; **28**: 344–360.

62. Moore RA, Melchionna RH. Production of tumors of the prostate in the white rat with 1,2-benzpyrene. *Am J Cancer* 1937; **30**: 731.

63. Dunning WF, Curtis MR, Segaloff A. Methyl cholanthrene squamous cell carcinoma of the rat prostate with skeletal metastases and failure of the rat liver to respond to the same carcinogen. *Cancer Res* 1946; **6**: 256.

64. Horning ES, Dmochowski C. Induction of prostate tumor in mice. *Br J Cancer* 1947; **1**: 54.

65. Gupta SK, Mathur IS, Karr AB. Chemical induction of prostatic tumors in random bred rats. *Indian J Exp Biol* 1971; **9**: 296–299.

66. Horning ES. Induction of glandular carcinomas of the prostate in the mouse: Preliminary communication. *Lancet* 1946; **2**: 829.

67. Horning ES. The local action of 20-methylcholanthrene and sex hormones on prostatic grafts. *Br J Cancer* 1952; **6**: 80.

68. Fingerhut B, Veenema R. An animal model for the study of prostatic adenocarcinoma. *Invest Urol* 1977; **15**: 42–48.

69. Ravich A, Ravich RA. Prophylaxis of cancer of the prostate, penis, and cervix by circumcision. *NY Med J* 1951; **51**: 1514.

70. Kaplan GW, O'Connor VJ. The incidence of carcinoma of the prostate in jews and gentiles. *JAMA* 1966; **196**: 123.

71. Paulson DF, Rabson AS, Fraley EE. Viral neoplastic transformation of hamster prostate tissue in vitro. *Science* 1968; **159**: 200–201.

72. Centifano YM, Kaufman HE, Zam ZS, *et al.* Herpes virus particles in prostatic carcinoma cells. *J Virol* 1973; **12**: 1608–1611.

73. Lang DJ, Kummer JF, Hurley JH. Cytomegalovirus in semen: Persistence and determination in extracellular fluids. *N Engl J Med* 1974; **291**: 121–123.

74. Sanford EJ, Gedar L, Laychock A. Evidence for the association of cytomegalovirus with carcinoma of the prostate. *J Urol* 1977; **118**: 789–792.

75. Farnsworth WE. Human prostatic reverse transcriptase and RNA virus. *Urol Res* 1973; **1**: 106–112.

76. Dmochowski L, Maruyama K, Ohtsuki Y. Virologic and immunologic studies of human prostatic carcinoma. *Cancer Chemother Rep* 1975; **59**: 17–31.

77. McCombs RM. Role of oncornoviruses in carcinoma of the prostate. *Cancer Treat Rep* 1977; **61**: 131–132.

78. Moon TD, Brawer MK, Wilt TJ. Prostate intervention versus observation trial (PIVOT): a randomized trial comparing radical prostatectomy with palliative expectant management for treatment of clinically localized prostate cancer. *J Natl Cancer Inst* 1995; **19**: 69–71.

79. Holtgrewe HL. The economics of urological care in the 21st century. *Urology* 1995; **46**: 1–3.

80. The US Preventive Taskforce. Screening for prostate cancer: commentary on the recommendations on the Canadian Task Force on the periodic health examination. *Am J Prev Med* 1994; **10**: 187–193.

81. Feightner JW. The early detection and treatment of prostate cancer: the perspective of the Canadian Task Force on the periodic health examination. *J Urol* 1994; **152**: 1682–1684.

82. Coley CM, Barry MJ, Fleming C, Wasson JH, Fahs MC, Oesterling JE. Should medicare provide reimbursement for prostate-specific antigen testing for early detection of prostate cancer? Part II: Early detection strategies. *Urology* 1995; **46**: 125–141.

83. Catalona WJ, Richie JP, Ahmann FR, *et al.* Comparison of digital rectal examination and serum prostate specific antigen in the early detection of prostate cancer: results of a multicenter clinical trial of 6,630 men. *J Urol* 1994; **151**: 1283–1290.

84. Richie JP, Ratliff TL, Catalona WJ, *et al.* Effect of patient age on early detection of prostate cancer with serum prostate-specific antigen and digital rectal examination. *Urology* 1993; **42**: 365–374.

85. McCormack RT, Rittenhouse HG, Finlay JA, *et al.* Molecular forms of prostate-specific antigen and the human kallikrein gene family: A new era. *Urology* 1996; **45**: 729–742.

86. Neal DE, Clejan S, Sarma D, Moon TD. Prostate specific antigen and prostatits I. Effect of prostatitis on serum PSA in the human and nonhuman primate. *Prostate* 1996; **20**: 105–112.

87. Moon TD, Clejan S, Neal DE. Prostate specific antigen and prostatitis II. PSA production and release kinetic in vitro. *Prostate* 1996; **20**: 113–116.

88. Brawer M. How to use prostate-specific antigen in the early detection or screening for prostatic carcinoma. *CA Cancer J Clin* 1995; **45**: 148–164.

89. Stenman UH, Hakama M, Knekt P, Aromaa A, Teppo L, Leinonen J. Serum concentrations of prostate specific antigen and its complex with alpha 1-antichymotrypsin before diagnosis of prostate cancer. *Lancet* 1994; **344**: 1594–1598.

90. Benson MC, Whang IS, Pantuck A, *et al.* Prostate specific antigen density: A means of distinguishing benign prostatic hypertrophy and prostate cancer. *J Urol* 1992; **147**: 815–816.

91. Brawer MK, Aramburu EA, Chen GL, Preston SD, Ellis WJ. The inability of prostate specific antigen index to enhance the predictive value of prostate specific antigen in the diagnosis of prostatic carcinoma. *J Urol* 1993; **150**: 369–373.

92. Carter HB, Pearson JD, Metter EJ, *et al.* Longitudinal evaluation of prostate-specific antigen levels in men with and without prostate disease. *JAMA* 1992; **267**: 2215–2220.

93. Riehmann M, Rhodes PR, Cook TD, Grose GS, Bruskewitz RC. Analysis of variation in prostate-specific antigen values. *Urology* 1993; **42**: 390–397.

94. Oesterling JE, Cooner WH, Jacobsen SJ, Guess HA, Lieber MM. Influence of patient age on the serum PSA concentration. An important clinical observation. *Urol Clin North Am* 1993; **20**: 671–680.

95. Dalkin BL, Ahmann FR, Kopp JB. Prostate specific antigen levels in men older than 50 years without clinical evidence of prostatic carcinoma. *J Urol* 1993; **150**: 1837–1839.

96. Catalona WJ, Hudson A, Scardino PT, *et al.* Selection of optimal prostate specific antigen cutoffs for early detection of prostate cancer: Receiver operating characteristic curves. *J Urol* 1994; **152**: 2037–2042.

97. Brawer MK, Chetner MP, Beatie J, Buchner DM, Vessella RL, Lange PH. Screening for prostatic carcinoma with prostate specific antigen. *Urology* 1992; **147**: 841–845.

98. Catalona WJ, Smith DS, Ratliff TL, Basler JW. Detection of organ-confined prostate cancer is increased through prostate-specific antigen-based screening. *JAMA* 1993; **270**: 948–954.

99. Gustafsson O, Norming U, Almgard LE, *et al.* Diagnostic methods in the detection of prostate cancer: A study of a randomly selected population of 2,400 men. *J Urol* 1992; **148**: 1827–1831.

100. Johansson JE, Adami HO, Andersson SO, Bergstron R, Holmbert L, Krusemo UB. High 10-year survival rate in patients with early, untreated prostatic cancer. *JAMA* 1992; **267**: 2191–2196.

101. Chodak GW, Thisted RA, Gerber GS, *et al.* Results of conservative management of clinically localized prostate cancer. *N Engl J Med* 1994; **330**: 242–248.

102. Fleming C, Wasson JH, Albertsen PC, Barry MJ, Wennberg JE. A decision analysis of alternative treatment strategies for clinically localized prostate cancer. *JAMA* 1993; **269**: 2650–2658.

103. Beck JR, Kattan MW, Miles BJ. A critique of the decision analysis for clinically localized prostate cancer. *J Urol* 1994; **152**: 1894–1899.

104. Barry MJ, Fleming C, Coley CM, Wasson JH, Fahs MC, Oesterling JE. Should medicare provide reimbursement for prostate specific antigen testing for early detection of prostate cancer? Part I: Framing the debate. *Urology* 1995; **46**: 2–46.

105. Hodge KK, McNeal JE, Terris MK, Stamey TA. Random systematic versus directed ultrasound guided transrectal core biopsies of the prostate. *J Urol* 1989; **142**: 71–74.

106. Stamey TA, McNeal JE. Adenocarcinoma of the prostate. In: AnonymousCampbell's Urology, Philadelphia: W.B. Saunders and Co. 1992: 1159–1221.

107. Montie JE. 1992 Staging system for prostate cancer. *Semin Oncol* 1992; **11**: 10–13.

108. Gleason DF. Classification of prostatic carcinomas. *Cancer Chemother Rep* 1966; **50**: 125–128.

109. Woolf SH. Public health perspective: The health policy implications of screening for prostate cancer. *J Urol* 1994; **152**: 1685–1688.

110. Wilt TJ, Brawer MK. The prostate cancer intervention versus observation trial: A randomized trial comparing radical prostatectomy versus expectant management for the treatment of clinically localized prostate cancer. *J Urol* 1994; **152**: 1910–1914.

111. Walsh PC. Radical retropubic prostatectomy. In *Campbell's Urology*, edited by PC Walsh, AB Retik, TA Stamey, ED Vaughan. Philadelphia: W.B. Saunders and Co., 2865–2886, 1992.

112. Goad JR, Eastham JA, Fitzgerald KB, *et al*. Radical retropubic prostatectomy: Limited benefit of autologous blood donation. *Urology* 1995; **154**: 2103–2109.

113. Jønler M, Messing EM, Rhodes PR, Bruskewitz RC. Sequelae of radical prostatectomy. *Br J Urol* 1994; **74**: 352–358.

114. Fowler FJ, Barry MJ, Lu-Yao G, Roman A, Wasson J, Wennberg JE. Patient-reported complications and follow-up treatment after radical prostatectomy. *Urology* 1993; **42**: 622–629.

115. Jønler M, Madsen FA, Rhodes PR, Bruskewitz RC. Urinary incontinence in patients undergoing radical prostatectomy. *Proc Am Urol Assoc* 1995; **153**: A506.

116. Jønler M, Moon TD, Brannan W, Stone NN, Heisey D, Bruskewitz RC. The effect of age, ethnicity and geographical location on impotence and quality of life. *Urology* 1995; **75**: 651–655.

117. Partin AW, Yoo J, Carter HB, *et al*. The use of prostate specific antigen, clinical stage and gleason score to predict pathological stage in men with localized prostate cancer. *Urology* 1993; **150**: 110–114.

118. Carlin BI, Resnick MI. The craft of urologic surgery. *Urology* 1995; **22**: 461–473.

119. Wolf JS, Shinohara K, Kerlikowske KM, Narayan P, Stoller ML, Carroll PR. Selection of patients for laparoscopic pelvic lymphadenectomy prior to radical prostatectomy: A decision analysis. *Urology* 1993; **42**: 680–688.

120. Shipley WU, Zietman AL, Hanks GE, *et al*. Treatment related sequelae following external beam radiation for prostate cancer: A review with an update in patients with stages T1 and T2 tumor. *J Urol* 1994; **152**: 1799–1805.

121. Hanks GE, Hanlon A, Schultheiss T, Corn B, Shipley WU, Lee WR. Early prostate cancer: The national results of radiation treatment from the patterns of care and radiation therapy oncology group studies with prospects for improvement with conformal radiation and adjuvant androgen deprivation. *J Urol* 1994; **152**: 1775–1780.

122. Russell KJ. Current research directions in the radiation therapy of localized prostate cancer. *Prostate* 1994; 133–149.

123. Roach M, Pickett B, Holland J, Zapotowski KA, Marsh DL, Tatera BS. The role of the urethrogram during simulation for localized prostate cancer. *Int J Radiat Oncol Biol Phys* 1993; **25**: 299–307.

124. Whitmore WF, Hilaris B. Treatment of localized prostate cancer by interstitial 125-I. In *Prostate Cancer: The second Tokyo symposium*, edited by JP Karr, H Yamanaka. New York: Elsevier Science Publishing Co, 1989.

125. Porter AT, Blasko JC, Grimm PD, Reddy SM, Ragde H. Brachytherapy for prostate cancer. *CA Cancer J Clin* 1995; **45**: 165–178.

126. Lee F, Kryger JV, Messing EM, Zarvan N, Chin D, Siders D. Cryosurgical ablation of the prostate in a canine model. *In Preparation* 1996; 127. Grampsas SA, Miller GJ, Crawford ED.

128. Cox RL, Crawford ED. Complications of cryosurgical ablation of the prostate to treat localized adenocarcinoma of the prostate. *Urology* 1995; **45**: 932–935.

129. Bales GT, Williams MJ, Sinner M, Thisted R, Chodak GW. Short-term outcomes after cryosurgical ablation of the prostate in men with recurrent prostate carcinoma following radiation therapy. *Urology* 1995; **46**: 65.

130. Huggins C, Hodges CV. Studies on prostatic cancer. The effect of castration, of estrogen and of androgen injection on serum phosphatases in metastate carcinoma of the prostate. *Cancer Res* 1941; **1**: 293–297.

131. Arduino LJ, Bailar JC, Becker LE, *et al*. Carcinoma of the prostate: Treatment comparisons. *J Urol* 1967; **98**: 516–522.

132. Arduino LJ, Bailar JC, Becker LE, *et al*. Factors in the prognosis of carcinoma of the prostate: A cooperative study. *J Urol* 1968; **100**: 59–65.

133. Byar DP. Survival of patients with incidentally found microscopic cancer of the prostate: Results of a clinical trial of conservative treatment. *J Urol* 1972; **108**: 908–913.

134. Byar DP. The veterans administration cooperative urological research group's studies of cancer of the prostate. *Cancer* 1973; **32**: 1126–1130.

135. Lowe BA, Listrom MB. Incidental carcinoma of the prostate: An analysis of the predictors of progression. *J Urol* 1988; **140**: 1340–1344.

136. Epstein JI, Paull G, Eggleston JC, Walsh PC. Prognosis of untreated stage A_1 prostatic carcinoma: A study of 94 cases with extended followup. *J Urol* 1986; **136**: 837–839.

137. Beck PH, McAninch JW, Goebel JL, Stutzman RE. Plasma testosterone in patients receiving diethylstilbestrol. *Urology* 1978; **XI**: 157–160.

138. Shearer RJ, Hendry WF, Sommerville JF, Fergusson JD. Plasma testosterone: An accurate monitor of hormone treatment in prostatic cancer. *Br J Urol* 1973; **45**: 668–677.

139. Jordan WP, Blackard CE, Byar DP. Reconsideration of orchiectomy in the treatment of advanced prostatic carcinoma. *South Med J* 1977; **70**: 1411–1413.

140. Glashan RW, Robinson RG. Cardiovascular complications in the treatment of prostatic carcinoma. *Br J Urol* 1981; **53**: 624–627.

141. Buller HR, Boon TA, Henny CP, Dabhoiwala NF, Ten Cate JW. Estrogen-induced deficiency and decrease in antithrombin III activity in patients with prostatic cancer. *J Urol* 1981; **128**: 72–74.

142. Dobbs RM, Barber JA, Weigel JW, Bergin JE. Clotting predisposition in carcinoma of the prostate. *J Urol* 1980; **123**: 706–709.

143. Varenhorst E, Wallentin L, Risberg B. The effects of orchiectomy, oestrogens and cyproterone-acetate on the antithrombin-III concentration in carcinoma of the prostate. *Urol Res* 1981; **9**: 25–28.

144. Blackledge G, Emtage LA, Trethowan C, *et al*. "Zoladex" depot vs DES 3 mg/day in advanced prostate cancer: A randomized trial comparing efficacy and tolerability. *J Urol* 1989; **141**: 347.

145. Trachtenberg J. The effect of the chronic administration of a potent luteinizing hormone releasing hormone analogue on the rat prostate. *J Urol* 1982; **128**: 1097–1100.

146. Leuprolide study group. Leuprolide versus diethylstilbestrol for metastatic prostate cancer. *N Engl J Med* 1984; **311**: 1281–1286.

147. Labrie F, Dupont A, Belanger A, *et al*. New approach in the treatment of prostate cancer: Complete instead of partial withdrawal of androgens. *Prostate* 1983; **4**: 579–594.

148. Eisenberger M, Crawford ED, Blumenstein B, *et al*. Significance of pre-treatment stratification by extent of disease (ED) in stage D_2 prostate cancer (PC) patients treated with leuprolide + flutamide (LF) or leuprolide + placebo (LP). *Proc Am Soc Clin Oncol* 1989; A515.

149. Wysowsik DK, Fourcroy JL. Flutamide hepatotoxicity. *Urology* 1996; **155**: 209–212.

150. Schellhammer P, Sharifi R, Block N, *et al*. A controlled trial of bicalutamide versus flutamide, each in combination with luteinizing hormone-releasing hormone analogue therapy, in patients with advanced prostate cancer. *Urology* 1995; **45**: 745–752.

151. Hurst KS, Byar DP. An analysis of the effects of changes from the assigned treatment in a clinical trial of treatment for prostatic cancer. *J Chronic Dis* 1973; **26**: 311–324.

152. Small EJ, Srinivas S. The antiandrogen withdrawal syndrome. *Cancer* 1995; **76**: 1428–1434.

153. Moon TD. Letter to the editor: Cyproterone acetate for treatment of hot flashes after orchiectomy. *J Urol* 1985; **134**: 155–156.

154. Loprinzi CL, Goldberg RM, O'Fallon J, *et al*. Transdermal clonidine for ameliorating post-orchiectomy hot flashes. *Urology* 1994; **151**: 634–636.

155. Loprinzi CL, Michalak JC, Quella SK, *et al*. Megestrol acetate for the prevention of hot flashes. *N Engl J Med* 1994; **331**: 347–352.

156. Eisenberger MA, Reyno L, Sinibaldi V, Sridhara R, Carducci M, Egorin M. The experience with suramin in advanced prostate cancer. *Cancer* 1995; **75**: 1927–1934.

50. Transitional Cell Carcinoma of the Bladder

Julio Pow-Sang, Jay Friedland and Albert B. Einstein

Introduction

Bladder cancer is the second most common urologic malignancy in the USA (1). Transitional cell carcinoma (TCC) accounts for 75 to 90% of the cases of bladder cancer (2). The other histologic subtypes (squamous cell and adenocarcinoma are relatively rare in this country). The incidence of TCC increases with age and over 50% of cases occur in persons over 65 (1). The most common cause of TCC of the bladder in the US is tobacco smoke. Over 75% of TCC present as superficial tumors (Ta, Tl, Tcis) (Table 50.1), 20% present as invasive cancer and 5% of cases are metastatic at diagnosis. Eventually 15–30% of superficial bladder cancer and up to 70% of invasive cancer will give origin to metastases (3). The treatment of bladder cancer is according to stage (Table 50.1). The stage at diagnosis of bladder cancer does not appear affected by the age of the patient.

Superficial Bladder Cancer

Evaluation

The initial presentation is usually gross, painless hematuria. This finding mandates a complete urological evaluation including history, physical exam, urinalysis, urine cytology, cystoscopy, and intravenous pyelogram (4). The presence of irritative voiding symptoms, such as dysuria, frequency and urgency in the presence of negative urine culture should alert the practitioner to the presence of "carcinoma *in situ*" (*cis*) (5). Flexible cystoscopes make the evaluation of these patients simple and pain-free. The procedure is well tolerated by

Table 50.1 Stages of TCC of the bladder.

T stages	
CIS	Carcinoma *"in situ."*
Ta	Polypoid lesions, not involving the *"lamina propria."*
Tl	Lesions involving the *"lamina propria."*
T2	Lesions infiltrating the superficial half of the *muscularis.*
T3a	Lesions involving the deeper half of the *muscularis.*
T3b	Lesions invading the peripheral fat.
T4a	Lesions involving adjacent organs.
T4b	Lesions involving the pelvic and the abdominal wall.

patients of advanced ages (even in their 90s, at our institution). The location, number, size and configuration of the lesion or lesions has prognostic and therapeutic implications and should be carefully documented.

Treatment

The first step in treatment is complete transurethral resection of the lesion or lesions under anesthesia. Selected biopsies of the right and left lateral bladder wall, trigone, and in the man of the prostate urethra should be performed to determine the presence of non-obvious lesions. The histopathology should include the grade of the tumor and the depth of invasion. These findings and the configuration, number and size of lesion(s), the presence or absence of *cis* and the number of previous recurrences allow the allocation of patients to groups at high or low risk for recurrence and progression. Patients at low risk undergo surveillance with periodic cystoscopic and cytologic examinations. Approximately 70% of patients experience recurrence within the first two years of initial diagnosis (7). Patients at high risk for recurrence, and patients whose tumor was incompletely excised are treated with intravesical therapy. The most common agents for intravesical therapy are *Bacillus* Calmette Guerin, Mitomycin C and Thiotepa.

Invasive Bladder Cancer

Evaluation

The initial evaluation of these patients is similar to that for superficial bladder cancer. A careful and thorough examination of the bladder under anesthesia is essential to staging as the presence of a palpable mass after transurethral resection is indicative of deep muscle invasion or perivesical extension. The biopsy indicates the presence of invasive cancer. Initial staging includes a CAT scan of the abdomen and of the pelvis to assess the presence of lymphadenopathy and of liver metastases.

Treatment

When the cancer invades the bladder muscles intravesical treatment is no longer effective (8). A selective group of patients may be managed with transurethral resection only (8). These patients are recognized as follows:

- presentation of a solitary papillary lesion;

- absence of an appreciable mass during bimanual examination under anesthesia after resection of the tumor;
- no visible residual tumor after resection.

A second resection is generally performed in these patients four to six weeks after the initial resection. If no tumor is documented at re-resection, these patients can be carefully followed up with surveillance cystoscopies and cytologies.

Another groups of patients are amenable to partial cystectomy. These patients have a solitary, invasive lesion in non-fixed areas of the bladder away from the trigone. In the majority of cases, management of invasive bladder cancer involves more radical interventions. Radical cystectomy is still the standard treatment for invasive bladder cancer, and radical radiation therapy is the alternative treatment for poor surgical candidates. In the last few years, several programs for combined modality treatment of bladder cancer were developed, with the aims to improve the cure rate and to obtain organ preservation. These combined modality treatment programs may be of special interest for older individuals and will be discussed in a separate section.

Radical cystectomy is the standard treatment for bladder cancer in the USA. With improvement in anesthesia and postoperative care, the mortality of this procedure has decreased from 15 to <2% (9); Similarly, the morbidity of this procedure has also decreased with improvement in surgical techniques (10). The quality of life of patients is also markedly improved with the use of bladder replacement in the majority of patients undergoing cystectomy. When bladder replacement is contraindicated a continent urinary diversion or ileal conduit may be offered to the patient.

Radiation therapy is typically administered as external beam irradiation, although brachytherapy has been utilized in the past (11). Radiotherapy may be administered either preoperatively, postoperatively, in conjunction with chemotherapy or alone. Ongoing clinical trials evaluate altered radiotherapy fractionation regimens (ECOG consortium) and altered chemoradiation fractionation regimens (RTOG 95-06). In both cases the goal of therapy is bladder preservation. Using modern techniques with high energy (>MV photons) linear accelerators, multiple fields, custom blocking to spare normal tissues and appropriate fractionation, the rate of severe complications is quite low (<5%). Complications of radiation therapy include radiation cystitis, radiation proctitis/colitis, impotence, and small intestinal obstruction. Recent pilot data from our institution (unpublished) indicate that pentoxifylline may ameliorate radiation cystitis and proctitis/colitis in the majority of patients. Approximately 50% of sexually active men will develop impotence.

Local-regional tumor control in many published radiation therapy alone series was not well documented, but was estimated in the range of 10–40% for T2–T4 tumors (12). Complete clinical response rate with conventional radiotherapy alone is in the order of about 45% (13), while with accelerated, hyperfractionated radiotherapy alone or chemoradiation the response rate is about 70% (14–17). Radiotherapy alone is preferred for patients who are unfit for major surgery or chemotherapy and is well tolerated. However, newer techniques incorporating accelerated and/or hyperfractionated radiotherapy may prove to be both tolerable and more efficacious than conventional radiotherapy and may become the treatment of choice for older individuals.

Response to radiotherapy is affected by several parameters including: clinical stage, presence of ureteral obstruction. tumor morphology (papillary vs solid), tumor grade, completeness of transurethral resection, response to treatment, and dose (11).

Combined Therapy for Invasive Disease and Chemotherapy for Metastatic Disease

Invasive transitional cell carcinoma (TCC) of the bladder is a potentially life threatening problem. The management of invasive disease (stages T2–T4) remains controversial and the subject of multiple clinical trials. Radical cystectomy continues to be the cornerstone for treatment of muscle-invading transitional cell carcinoma of the bladder in the U.S. whereas full-dose radiation therapy is more commonly employed in Great Britain and Canada. The best results obtainable with either therapy alone is 45–50% five-year survival with patients that have a lower T stage tumor having a better prognosis (18–23). Preoperative radiation therapy followed by radical cystectomy does not improve survival rates compared to surgery alone (24–27). Failure of primary therapy has been due to the development of metastases following cystectomy and local bladder failure and/or metastases following radiation therapy. Because of the availability of a number of active chemotherapeutic agents for transitional cell carcinoma, new therapeutic strategies have included combining systemic chemotherapy with surgery and/or radiotherapy with the primary goal of increasing survival by treating micro-metastases and in some cases with the secondary goal of preserving the bladder.

Systemic chemotherapy may be used as adjuvant therapy after primary tumor treatment or as neoadjuvant therapy, prior to treatment of the primary tumor. In either ease, the primary objective is to treat micrometastases that could lead to recurrence and death. In addition, neoadjuvant therapy potentially may downsize the primary tumor and render it more treatable by surgery or radiation therapy as well as providing an "in vivo" indication of the chemosensitivity of the disease. Adjuvant chemotherapy has been difficult for the elderly population that tends to get bladder cancer and compliance in clinical trials has been poor. On the other hand, neoadjuvant chemotherapy has been well tolerated, making this approach more appealing in current trials.

Clinical trials utilizing single agent or multiple agent adjuvant chemotherapy either have shown no survival benefit or suggest a delay in recurrence of tumor and prolonged survival. The National Bladder Cancer Group phase III trial evaluating cisplatin following preoperative radiation therapy and radical cystectomy had poor compliance with the chemotherapy and failed to demonstrate a survival advantage for patients receiving cisplatin (28). Logothetis and his colleagues at M.D. Anderson did a retrospective analysis of patients receiving CISCA (cisplatin, cyclophosphamide, and doxorubicin) following cystectomy and reported that the survival of high risk patients receiving adjuvant chemotherapy was similar to low risk patients and better than high risk patients not receiving chemotherapy (29). Skinner and colleagues reported on a randomized trial utilizing cyclophosphamide, doxorubicin, and cisplatin (CAP) and concluded that adjuvant chemotherapy prolonged survival in patients with one positive node, but not in patients with two or more positive nodes (30). Stockle et al. randomized patients post cystectomy to receive adjuvant methotrexate, vinblastine, doxorubicin, and cisplatin (MVAC) or methotrexate, vinblastine, epirubicin, carboplatin (MVEC) versus no chemotherapy even at time of relapse for stages pN1or2, pT3b, or pT4a, and reported a significant reduction in tumor recurrence and a significant improvement in survival for patients receiving chemotherapy (31–32). These trials are suggestive that adjuvant chemotherapy has value for patients at high risk of recurrence following cystectomy based on adverse pathologic indicators (extra vesical extension, positive nodes, and vascular invasion) but no trial to date can unfortunately be considered definitive.

Neoadjuvant chemotherapy prior to definitive surgery or radiation therapy is currently the most promising approach to positively impacting survival of patients with invasive bladder cancer. In the Memorial-Sloan Kettering Cancer Center phase II trial, neoadjuvant MVAC (4 cycles) followed by cystectomy downstaged the disease in the bladder to endoscopic complete remissions in 48% of patients and pathologically eradicated the disease (pT0) in 23% (33–35). A SWOG phase II study evaluating extensive TURB and neoadjuvant cisplatin, methotrexate, and vinblastine followed by definitive radiation therapy and concurrent cisplatin in patients who were not candidates for cystectomy achieved 56% clinical CR following all treatment with a median overall survival of 21 months and 18% 57 months survival (36). In this study aggressive clinically complete resection of a tumor by the initial TURB was associated with prolonged survival. An M.D. Anderson study comparing two courses of neoadjuvant MVAC followed by cystectomy plus five courses of adjuvant MVAC versus adjuvant MVAC alone found no difference in median survival (22 months) (37). Likewise, the RTOG 89-03 study randomized patients to receive radiation therapy with or without neoadjuvant chemotherapy. Only 40% of the patients randomized to neoadjuvant treatment received the planned dose of chemotherapy, and the survival of these patients did not appear improved (J. Friedland, personal communication). A Scandinavian trial randomizing patients to preoperative radiation therapy followed by cystectomy

or two courses of cisplatin and doxorubicin followed by the same preoperative radiation therapy and cystectomy demonstrated a 10–15% five-year survival advantage for the neoadjuvant group (38).

Most neoadjuvant trials have demonstrated 20–80% major clinical response of the primary tumor and 25–30% pathologic eradication of disease (39). This disparity between the clinical and pathologic results underscores the difficulty in adequately evaluating the tumor prior to surgery. The ability to achieve pT0 has been found to be greater in T2 and T3a tumors compared to T3b and T4. The optimal number of neoadjuvant courses to achieve maximum tumor response has not been ascertained but some suggest that more than two courses are necessary (40). A significant response of the primary tumor seems to predict a better survival. Multi-variate analyses suggest that pretreatment tumor stage and size and the response to chemotherapy are the most important prognostic factors for survival (41–43). Currently, two large randomized phase III neoadjuvant trials are being performed; one, the SWOG-Intergroup study evaluating preoperative MVAC and the other, the EORTC study comparing cystectomy and curative radiation therapy with and without neoadjuvant CMV chemotherapy. The results of these trials will help establish the value of neoadjuvant chemotherapy for bladder cancer.

There are also theoretical problems associated with the use of neoadjuvant chemotherapy. The first concern is toxicity. In the RTOG 89-03 trial there were some cases of lethal toxicity. Second, some investigators have speculated that neoadjuvant chemotherapy may induce accelerated tumor repopulation within a given individual tumor, thus rendering conventional radiation therapy less effective. Theoretically, this problem could be compensated for by the use of accelerated radiotherapy fractionation schemes.

While prolongation of survival remains the primary goal for neoadjuvant trials, a secondary goal for some clinical trials has been bladder preservation. Kaufman et al. reported on the Massachusetts General Hospital phase II trial employing TURB, two cycles of neoadjuvant CMV, and 4000 cGy radiation therapy plus concurrent cisplatin followed by reevaluation of the tumor. If no tumor was present, patients completed curative radiation therapy to the tumor site, total dose 6480 Cgy, but if a tumor was present, they had a radical cystectomy (15). Five-year overall actuarial survival was 48% with 38% surviving with bladder preservation. Multi-variate analyses indicated that the presence or absence of hydronephrosis and tumor stage independently predicted outcome. The RTOG utilizing the same protocol in a multi-institutional setting achieved similar results (44). Houssett et al. at the University of Paris developed a treatment program utilizing concomitant cisplatin, 5-fluorouracil, and twice-a-day irradiation of 300 cGy for three weeks has yielded 70% CR, confirmed at cystectomy (45). This program is now being evaluated as a bladder sparing treatment by the RTOG. All of these multi-modality bladder sparing protocols have been well tolerated by the elderly patients.

Table 50.2 Combination chemotherapy of common use in TCC of the bladder.

CMV:	Methotrexate 30 mg/m^2
	Cisplatin 70 mg/m^2 every three weeks
	Vinblastine 3 mg/m^2
MVAC:	Methotrexate 30 mg/m^2 days 1,15,21
	Vinblastine 3 mg/m^2 days 1,15,21 every 4 weeks
	Doxorubicin 30 mg/m^2 day 2
	Cisplatin 70 mg/m^2 day 2
VIG:	Etoposide
	Ifosfamide
	Galliun
	Mesna

While combination treatment appears promising for bladder preservation, it is important to mention that bladder preservation has also been accomplished by using altered radiotherapy fractionation schemes. Edsmyr *et al.* randomized patients with T2–T4 TCC to receive either 84 Gy in 8 weeks (1.OGy thrice daily, split course, two weeks rest), or 64 Gy in 6.5 weeks (2 Gy once daily, continuous course) (l4). Local control rates of 24–46% were noticed with conventional fractionation (total dose 64Gy). In contrast, the complete clinical response rate with hyperfractionated radiotherapy was 62–67%. The hyperfractionation was associated with improved survival of patients with T3 carcinoma. Another study demonstrating the effectiveness of altered fractionation was reported by Plataniotis *et al.* (17). In a phase II study patients with T2–T3b bladder cancer received 62–65 Gy in 32–38 days. Local control was achieved in 66.7% of patients, and all T2 patients responded to treatment. The 3 year disease free survival was approximately 60%.

The treatment of metastatic transitional cell carcinoma of the bladder remains combination chemotherapy (Table 50.2). Phase I and II trials have identified a number of single agents with significant activity including cisplatin, methotrexate, doxorubicin, vinblastine, gallium, ifosfamide, paclitaxel, docetaxel, trimetrexate, and gemcitabine (46–58). MVAC was the first combination regimen to yield significant results better than single agents with 39–72% response rates, 13–35% complete responses, and 12–13 month median survival (59–61). Though never directly compared with MVAC, CMV yielded similar results in a phase II trial and has the advantage of not inducing cardiac toxicity, a potentially significant problem for older patients (62). The combination of vinblastine, ifosphamide, and gallium (VIG) has yielded 67% response rate and a median survival of 43 weeks but with formidable hematologic and renal toxicities (63). Cisplatin plus paclitaxel and the same two drugs plus ifosphamide are currently being evaluated. Utilization of these newer combinations of drugs in the neoadjuvant setting provide

hope of better survival results for patients with invasive stage of the disease. It is important to underline that approximately 50% of these patients were aged 65 or older, and age did not appear associated with excessive therapeutic toxicity.

Conclusions

The two major challenges related to bladder cancer are:

- Control of systemic disease
- Preservation of a functional bladder.

Previous clinical trials indicate that chemotherapy may be beneficial to the treatment of localized invasive bladder cancer, but the best setting in which to use chemotherapy, whether preoperatively (neoadjuvant), postoperatively (adjuvant) or both, is not clear. Ongoing clinical trials explore this issues.

Organ preservation may be achieved by a combination of chemotherapy and radiation or by hyperfractionated radiation therapy. Which of these approaches produces better functional results is not clear at present. As chemotherapy may control systemic disease, a combined approach appears theoretically advantageous. Current clinical trials are addressing this problem. Another issue related to organ preservation is whether this approach is preferable to surgical bladder replacement.

TCC of the bladder is a highly chemosensitive tumors and a number of new agents appear to have activity in this disease and may improve current treatment options.

Age does not seem to alter the clinical presentation or the effectiveness of treatment.

References

1. Parker SL, Tong T, Bolden S, Wingo PA. *Cancer Statistics*, 1996. CA, a *Cancer Journal for Clinicians* 1996; **46**: 5–27.
2. Murphy WM, Beckwith JB, Farrow GM. Grading system for transitional cell neoplasms. *Atlas of Tumor pathology* 1994; **11** 199.
3. Catalona WJ. Bladder Cancer. In *Adult and Pediatric Urology*, edited by JY Gillenwatwer, JT Grayhack, SS Howards, JW Duckett. 1135–1183, 1991.
4. Cummings KB, Barone JG, Ward WS. Diagnosis and staging of bladder cancer. *Urol Cli N America* 1992; **19**: 455–465.
5. Utz BC, Hanash KA, Farrow DM. The plight of the patient with carcinoma *"in situ"* of the bladder. *J Urol* 1970; **103**: 160–164.
6. Heney NM, Ahmed S, Flanagan MJ, *et al.* Superficial bladder cancer: progression and recurrence. *J Urol* 1983; **130**: 1083–1086.
7. Ro JY, Staerkel GA, Ayala AG. Cytologic and histologic features of superficial bladder cancer. *Urol Clin N America* 1992; **19**: 435453.
8. Herr HW. Conservative management of muscle-infiltrating bladder cancer: prospective experience. *J Urol* 1987; **138**: 1162–1163.
9. Dreicer R, Cooper CS, Williams RD. Management of prostate cancer and bladder cancer in the elderly. *Urol Clin N America* 1996; **23**: 87–97.
10. Pow-Sang JM, Lockhart JL. Continent urinary diversion: the Florida pouch. *Problems in Urology* 1992; **6**: 581–586.
11. Porter AT. the role of radiotherapy in the treatment of muscle invasive bladder cancer. *Progr Clin Biol Res* 1990; **353**: 23–34.

12. Zietman AL, Shipley WM, Kaufman DS. The combination of cisplatin based chemotherapy and radiation in the treatment of muscle-invading transitional cell carcinoma of the bladder. *Int J rad Oncol Biol Phys* 1993; **17,**

13. Duncan W, Quilty PM. The results of a series of 963 patients with transitional cell carcinoma of the urinary bladder, primarily treated by radical megavoltage X-Ray therapy. *Rad Oncol* 1986; **7**: 299–310.

14. Edsmyr F, Anderson L, Esposti PL, *et al.* Irradiation therapy with multiple small fractions per day in urinary bladder cancer. *Rad Oncol* 1985; **4** 197–203.

15. Kaufman DS, Shipley WM, Griffin PP, *et al.* Selective bladder preservation by combination treatment of invasive bladder cancer. *N Engl J Med* 1993; **329**: 1377–1382.

16. Russell KJ, Boilean MA, Higano C, *et al.* Combined 5–FU and irradiation for transitional cell carcinoma of the bladder. *Int J Radiol Oncol Biol Phys* 1990; **19**: 693–699.

17. Plataniotis G, Michalopoulos E, Kouvaris J, *et al.* A feasibility study of partially accelerated radiotherapy for bladder cancer. *Rad Oncol* 1994; **33**: 84–87.

18. Lerner SP, Skinner E, Skinner DG. Radical cystectomy in regionally advanced bladder cancer. *Uro Clin North Am* 1992; **19**: 713–723.

19. Skinner DG, Lieskovsky G. Management of invasive and high-grade bladder cancer. In *Diagnosis and Management of Genitourinary Cancer*, edited by DG Skinner, G Lieskovsky G. Philadelphia, PA: WB Saunders, 295–312, 1988.

20. Blandy JP, England HR, Evans SJ, *et al.* T3 bladder cancer: The ease for salvage cystectomy. *Br J Urol* 1980; **52**: 506.

21. Quilty PM, Duncan W, Chishom GD, *et al.* Results of surgery following radical radiotherapy for invasive bladder cancer. *Br J Urol* 1986; **58**: 396.

22. Goffinet DR, Schneider NJ, Glastein EJ, *et al.* Bladder cancer: results of radiation therapy in 334 patients. *Radiology* 1975; **117**: 149.

23. Wallace DN, Bloom HJG. The management of deeply infiltrating bladder carcinoma: control trial of radical radiotherapy vs. preoperative radiotherapy and radical cystectomy. *Br J Urol* 1976; **48**: 587.

24. Crawford ED, Das S, Smith JA. Preoperative radiation therapy in the treatment of bladder cancer. *Urol Clin North Am* 1987; **14**: 781–787.

25. Smith JA Jr, Crawford ED, Blumenstein B, *et al.* A randomized prospective trial of preoperative irradiation plus radical cystectomy versus surgery alone for transitional cell carcinoma of the bladder. A Southwest Oncology Group study. *J Urol* 1988; **139**: 266A.

26. Blackard CE, Byar DP. Veterans Administration Cooperative Urological Research Group: results of a clinical trial of surgery and radiation in stages 11 and III carcinoma of the bladder. *J Urol* 1972; **108**: 875–878.

27. Gospodarowicz MK, Warde P. The role of radiation therapy in the management of transitional cell carcinoma of the bladder. *Hem Oncol Clin North AM* 1992; **6**: 147–168.

28. Einstein AB, Shipley WU, Coombs J, *et al.* Cisplatin as adjunctive treatment for invasive bladder carcinoma: tolerance and toxicities. *Urology* 1984; **23(suppl)**: 100–117.

29. Logothetis CJ, Johnsen DE, Chong C, *et al.* Adjuvant cyclophosphamide, doxorubicin, and cisplatin chemotherapy for bladder cancer: an update. *J Clin Oncol* 1988; **6**: 1590–1596.

30. Skinner G, Daniels JR, Russel CA, *et al.* The role of adjuvant chemotherapy following cystectomy for invasive bladder cancer: a prospective comparative trial. *J Urol* 1991; **145**: 459–464.

31. Stoekle M, Meyenburg W, Welleck S, *et al.* Advanced bladder cancer (stages pT3b, pT4a, pN1 and pN2): improved survival after radial cystectomy and 3 adjuvant cycles of chemotherapy. Results of a controlled prospective study. *J Urol* 1992; **148**: 302–307.

32. Stoekl M, Meyenburg W, Welleek S, *et al.* Role de la polychimiotherpie M-VAC dans le traitement du careinome urothelial avanee de la vesse. *Ann Urol* 1993; **27**: 51–57.

33. Scher HI, Norton L. Chemotherapy for urothelial tract malignancies: breaking the deadlock. *Semin Surg Oncol* 1992; **8**: 316–341.

34. Schultz PK, Herr HW, Zhang Z-F, *et al.* Neoadjuvant chemotherapy for invasive bladder cancer: prognostic factors for survival of patients treated with M-VAC with 5 year follow up. *J Clin Oncol* 1994; **12**: 1394–1401.

35. Scher Hl, Yagoda A, Herr HW, *et al.* Neoadjuvant M-VAC (methotrexate, vinblastine, doxorubiein, and cisplatin) effect on primary bladder lesion. *J Urol* 1988; **139**: 470–74.

36. Einstein AB Jr, Wolf M, Hallidya KR, *et al.* Combination transurethral resection, systemic chemotherapy, and pelvic radiotherapy for invasive (T24) bladder cancer unsuitable for cystectomy: a phase 1/11 Southwest Oncology Group study. *Urol* 1996; **47**: 652–657.

37. Logothetis CJ, Ogden S, Dexeus FH, *et al.* A prospective randomized trial comparing neoadjuvant (neo) to adjuvant (adj) MVAC in patients with high stage (vascular invasion, T3b, T4a) bladder carcinoma (Abstract). *Pro Am Soc Clin Oncol* 1991; **10**: 166.

38. Rintaka E, Hannisdahl E, Fossa SD, *et al.* Neoadjuvant chemotherapy in bladder cancer: a randomized study. *Scand J Urol Nephrol* 1993; **27**: 355–362.

39. Splinter TAW, Scher HI: Adjuvant and neoadjuvant chemotherapy for invasive (T3–T4) bladder cancer, in *Comprehensive Textbook of Genitourinary Oncology*, pp. 464–471.

40. Scher HI, Yagoda A, Herr HW, *et al.* Neoadjuvant M-VAC (methotrexate, vinblastine, doxorubiein and cisplatin) effect on the primary bladder lesion. *J Urol* 1988; **139**: 470–474.

41. Splinter TAW, Scher Hl, Denis L, *et al.* The prognostic value of the pathological response to combination chemotherapy before cystectomy in patients with invasive bladder cancer. *JUrol* 1992; **147**: 606–608.

42. Schultz PK, Herr HW, Zhang ZF, *et al.* Neoadjuvant chemotherapy for invasive bladder cancer: prognostic factors for survival of patients treated with M-VAC with 5-year follow-up. *J Clin Oncol* 1994; **12**: 1394–1401.

43. Fung CY, Shipley WU, Young RH, *et al.* Prognostic factors in invasive bladder carcinoma in a prospective trial of preoperative adjuvant chemotherapy and radiotherapy. *J Clin Oncol* 1991; **9**: 1533–1542.

44. Tester W, Caplan R, Heaney J, *et al.* Neoadjuvant combined modality program with selective organ preservation for invasive bladder cancer: results of Radiation Therapy Oncology Group phase 1I trial 8802. *J Clin Oncol* 1996; **14**: 119–126.

45. Housset M, Maulard C, Chretien YC, *et al.* Combined radiation and chemotherapy for invasive transitional cell carcinoma of the bladder. A prospective study. *J Clin Oncol* 1993; **1**: 2150–2157.

46. Yagoda A: Chemotherapy of urothelial tract tumors. *Cancer* 1987; **60**: 574–585.

47. Yagoda A, Watson RC, Kemeny H, *et al.* Diammine-dichloride platinum 11 and cyclophosphamide in the treatment of advanced urothelial cancer. *Cancer* 1978; **39**: 279–285.

48. Oliver RJD, England HR, Risdon RN, *et al.* Methotrexate in the treatment of metastatic and recurrent primary transitional cell carcinoma. *J Urol* 1984; **131**: 483.

49. Yagoda A, Watson RC, Whitmore WF, *et al.* Adriamycin in advanced urinary tract cancer. *Cancer* 1977; **39**: 279–285.

50. Blumenreich MA, Yagoda A, Natale RB, *et al.* Phase II trial of vinblastine sulfate for metastatic urothelial tract tumors. *Cancer* 1982; **50**: 435–438.

51. Crawford ED, Saiers JH, Bakaer LH, Costanzi JH, Bukowski RM. Gallium nitrate in advance bladder carcinoma: Southwest Oncology Group study. *Urology* 1991; **38**: 355 357.

52. Warrell RP, Coonley CJ, Straus DJ, Young CW. Treatment of patients with advanced malignant lymphoma using gallium nitrate administered as a seven-day continuous infusion. *Cancer* 1983: **51**: 1982–1987.

53. Seligman PA, Crawford ED. Treatment of advanced transitional cell carcinoma of the bladder with continuous-infusion gallium nitrate. *J Natl Cancer lnst* 1991; **83**: 1582–1584.

54. Witte R, Loehrer P, Dreicer R, Williams S, Elson P. Ifosfamide in advanced urothelial carcinoma: an ECOG trial. *Proc Am Soc Clin Oncol* 1993; **12**: 230.

55. Roth BJ, Dreicer R, Einhorn LH, *et al.* Significant activity of paclitaxel in advanced transitional cell carcinoma of the urothelium: a phase II trial of the Eastern Cooperative Oncology Group (E 1892). *J Clin Oncol* 1994; **12**: 2264–2270.

56. Sadan S, Bajorin D, Amsterdam A, Scher H. Docetaxel in patients with advanced transitional cell cancer who failed cisplatin-based chemotherapy: a phase II trial. *Proc. AM Soc Clin Oncol* 1994; **13**: 244.

57. Witte RS, Elson P, Khandaker J, Trump DL. An Eastern Cooperative Oncology Group phase 1I trial of trimetrexate in the treatment of advanced urothelial carcinoma. *Cancer* 1994; **73**: 688–691.

58. Pollera CF, Ceribelli A, Crecco M, Calabresi F. Weekly gemcitabine in advanced bladder cancer: a preliminary report from a phase I study. Ann *Oncol* 1994; **5**: 182–184.

59. Sternberg CN. Yagoda A, Scher Hl, *et al.* Preliminary results of methotrexate, vinblastine, Adriamycin and cisplatin (M-VAC) in advanced urothelial tumors. *J Urol* 1985; **133**: 403–407.

60. Sternberg CN, Yagoda A, Scher Hl, *et al.* M-VAC for advanced transitional cell carcinoma of the urothelium: efficacy and patterns of response an relapse. *Cancer* 1989; **64**: 2448–2458.

61. Conner JP, Olsson CA, Benson MC, *et al.* Long-term follow-up in patients treated with methotrexate, vinblastine, doxorubicin and cisplatin (M-VAC) for transitional cell carcinoma of the urinary bladder: cause for concern. *Urology* 1989; **34**: 353–356.

62. Harker WG, Meyers FJ, Fuad SF, *et al.* Cisplatin, methotrexate, and vinblastine (CMV), an effective chemotherapy regimen for metastatic transitional cell carcinoma of the urinary tract. A Northern California Oncology Group study. *J Clin Oncol* 1985; **3**: 1463–1470.

63. Einhorn LH, Roth BJ, Ansari R, Dreicer R, Gonin R, Loehrer PJ. Phase II trail of vinblastine, ifosfamide and gallium combination chemotherapy in metastatic urotherlail carcinoma. *J Clin Oncol* 1994; **12**: 2271–2276.

51. Brain Tumors

Alexandra Flowers

Introduction

Brain tumors are a group of neurologic diseases with high morbidity and mortality. In the spectrum of neurologic disorders, brain tumors are second only to strokes as the leading cause of death. The treatment of brain tumors requires the cooperative efforts of a multispecialty team, including neurologists, neurosurgeons, radiation therapists and medical oncologists. The incidence of brain tumors is increasing in the elderly, and the management needs to be adjusted to the specific needs of the older patients. The attitude of the medical community is changing, as more elderly patients desire and receive therapy for brain tumors. This change has been made possible by the recent advances in basic and clinical research regarding the management of brain tumors, and as treatment modalities are perfected. The overall prognosis remains poor, and there is an ongoing search for new, more effective therapies.

This chapter will discuss the epidemiology, clinical aspects and therapy of brain tumors, with emphasis on the specific problems in the elderly patient population.

Epidemiology

Over the last twenty years there has been an increase in the overall incidence of cancer of over 10% as reported in the NCI statistics, with an average annual percentage change of about 1%. The incidence of brain tumors has increased an average of 1.2%/year, lower than the other cancers, but significant in the context of its personal, social, and economic consequences. Brain tumors account for only 2.2% of all cancers, yet their effect on the patient's ability to function is dramatic, and their impact is devastating (1–3).

In the United States it is estimated (1993 NCI statistics) that 17,500 new cases of primary brain tumors are diagnosed every year (3). About 12, 000 patients are estimated to die every year due to brain tumors (3,4). While the overall incidence is increasing slowly, the incidence of brain tumors in patients over the age of 70 has more than doubled since 1973, and has increased over fivefold for patients older than 85 (5).

The epidemiologic factors that led to the increased incidence of brain tumors in all age groups are not well defined. The incidence of some genetically transmitted diseases associated with brain tumors, such as neurofibromatosis and the familial cancer syndromes such as Li-Fraumeni, has not increased. Also, there are no clearly established links between environmental factors such as pesticides, electromagnetic fields, radiation exposure, and the occurrence of brain tumors, except for higher risk for meningiomas in patients who had previously received radiation therapy to the head (6–9). Recently, the possible causative effect of prolonged use of cellular phones has received media attention, however there is no scientific proof to support this hypothesis. In some patients with a family history of malignancy there are abnormalities of tumor suppressor genes and over expression of oncogenes, which can be identified with molecular biology techniques (10,11).

The dramatic increase in incidence of brain tumors in the elderly reflects both the overall increase in the general population, the improved diagnostic techniques, and the changes in the attitude of society and of the medical community towards addressing the health care needs of the older population. The patients as health care consumers have become more educated, and there is an increased awareness of the symptoms and signs of brain tumors, which leads to earlier diagnosis (12–17). The number of reported cases will be higher in geographic areas with a higher concentration of senior citizens, like Florida or Arizona (18).

The survival rates for patients with malignant brain tumors are also age-dependent. The 5-year survival rate for patients with glioblastoma multiforme is about 20% in patients <35 years of age, 10% for patients ages 35–54, and only 1% in patients over 55 (19). Similar trends are noted for patients with anaplastic astrocytomas (70%, 22%, and 15% respectively) (Figure 51.1).

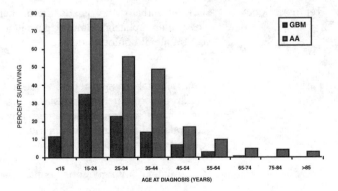

Figure 51.1 Survival of patients with malignant gliomas at 5 years by age (1980–1985 surveys).
(GBM-glioblastoma multiform; AA-anaplastic astrocytoma)

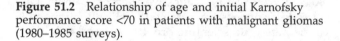

Figure 51.2 Relationship of age and initial Karnofsky performance score <70 in patients with malignant gliomas (1980–1985 surveys).

The age-based survival data parallel the survival rates based on performance status, as measured by Karnofsky score. About fifty percent of patients with malignant gliomas over the age of 55 are likely to have a Karnofsky performance score (KPS) <70 at diagnosis, as compared with only 20% in the younger patients group (Figure 51.2). The performance status is not the only determinant of survival in the elderly, but a low Karnofsky score will influence the type of treatment these patients will be offered (20).

Diagnosis

The diagnosis of brain tumors is based on the clinical presentation, imaging studies, and histology (21,22). In older patients, in the absence of focal signs, intellectual decline over a short period of time, gait disturbances, short term memory deficits, may be caused by a brain tumor, and must be differentiated from the "normal" phenomena of aging.

Symptoms and Signs

The symptoms and signs are dependent on the tumor location (Table 51.1). Headaches and seizures are the most common symptoms at presentation. Since in the older age groups brain tumors are most often located supratentorialy, the headaches are caused primarily by local increased pressure. Less commonly headaches are caused by invasion in the meninges, or hydrocephalus in the case of posterior fossa tumors. The seizures can be generalized, or focal, in which case they may have localizing value. The neurological examination can reveal cognitive and/or behavioral changes seen in patients with frontal, temporal or parietal lobe tumors, speech, reading or writing problems when the tumor involves the dominant hemisphere. The presence of focal neurologic deficits can help localize the lesion even before neuroimaging studies are performed. The degree of neurologic compromise is an important factor in deciding the therapeutic approach. Tumors in the anterior frontal lobes, anterior temporal lobes or base of skull can grow to significantly large size with very few or no symptoms, or nonspecific symptoms often ascribed to the aging process, such as memory loss or personality changes, or some gait difficulties.

Table 51.1 Symptoms and signs of brain tumors.

Tumor location	Symptoms and signs dominant hemisphere	Symptoms and signs nondominant hemisphere
Frontal lobe	Personality changes, apathy, impaired planning, disinhibition or apathy, expressive aphasia, contralateral motor weakness, motor seizures.	Personality changes, motor weakness, motor seizures, the personality changes are most marked with lesions in the right frontal lobe.
Temporal lobe	Loss of verbal memory, short term memory loss; fluent aphasia; complex partial seizures; contralateral homonymous superior quadrantanopia	Loss of visual spatial memory, complex partial seizures; contralateral homonymous superior quadrantanopia
Parietal lobe	Contralateral sensory deficit; aphasia syndromes conduction aphasia, Gerstman's syndrome, alexia, agraphia, contralateral homonymous inferior quadrantanopia; sensory seizures	Contralateral sensory deficit, contralateral homonymous inferior quadrantanopia; contralateral hemibody neglect, visual neglect, constructional apraxia, dressing apraxia; sensory seizures.
Occipital lobe	Contralateral homonymous hemianopia; alexia; prosopagnosia	Contralateral homonymous hemianopia
Posterior fossa	Headache due to obstructive hydrocephalus, focal findings depending on tumor location, vertigo, nystagmus, altered level of consciousness	

Over 60% of malignant gliomas arise in the frontal and temporal lobes.

Unilateral hearing loss, vertigo, mild face weakness are symptoms caused by acoustic neuromas, and imaging studies help differentiate from verebro-basilar insufficiency.

Radiologic Diagnosis

Neuroimaging studies are valuable tools in determining the location of the lesion (s), and may suggest the diagnosis and the malignant character of a tumor (23). Plain skull x-rays are only rarely performed in instances other than head trauma. Skull x-rays can reveal abnormalities of the sella turcica, suggesting a pituitary tumor, or erosion of the bone as seen in patients with meningiomas, also calcifications in low grade astrocytomas, oligodendrogliomas or meningiomas. Cerebral angiogram helps differentiate between tumors and vascular malformations or aneurysms, and also defines the blood supply of the tumor, and thus can assist with the surgical management. The cerebral angiography technique is used for the Wada test, to establish the dominant areas for speech and memory in left-handed patients with fronto-temporal lesions, in preparation for surgery. The most useful neuroimaging techniques are computed axial tomography (CAT) scan of the brain, and magnetic resonance imaging (MRI) of the brain. Nonenhanced CAT scan of the brain can reveal the presence of calcifications or hemorrhagic lesions, as well as hydrocephalus. Nonenhanced scans will show hypodense areas at the site of a tumor, but it is necessary to perform a contrast-enhanced scan to visualize the outline of the tumor and differentiate it from surrounding edema. Inferior frontal lobe or anterior temporal lobe lesions, as well as lesions in the posterior fossa may not be visualized on CAT scan due to bone artifact. MRI scan of the brain is becoming the imaging modality of choice for brain tumors. It allows visualization of the tumor in axial, coronal and sagittal planes, thus giving a three-dimensional view of the tumor and its relationship with the surrounding structures. MRI has greater tissue contrast resolution than CAT scan, and permits visualization of very small lesions, of lesions in the temporal tip, inferior frontal lobe, or posterior fossa, and at the base of the skull. The paramagnetic substance gadolinium diethylenetriamine pentaacetic acid (GdDPTA) is used as a contrast substance for MRI scan and it helps define the intracranial lesions, differentiate neoplasms from other lesions, and helps define even subtle changes in the appearance of a tumor during treatment. MRI scan with gadolinium is also useful in diagnosing leptomeningeal metastases, which are seen with increased frequency as brain tumor patients survive longer. Positron emission tomography (PET) scan and single positron emission computed tomography (SPECT) scan are less useful at diagnosis, but can help distinguish tumor necrosis from radiation induced necrosis in the follow-up of tumors after therapy (24,25). MR spectroscopy is still a research tool, however it has the potential to become a noninvasive diagnostic modality, in differentiating low grade from anaplastic gliomas.

Pathologic Diagnosis

While the imaging techniques can localize the tumor and at times suggest the pathologic diagnosis, in order to establish the final diagnosis and course of treatment it is necessary to obtain tumor tissue for histologic characterization. The pathologic examination of the tumor specimen, on frozen section and fixed material, defines the type of tumor, and the histologic grade. Brain tumors can be primary or metastatic. Primary brain tumors are classified histologically based on the World Health Organization classification. The most common primary brain tumors are gliomas, which are classified based on the cell type in astrocytic tumors, oligodendroglial tumors, and mixed gliomas. The grade of malignancy is defined based on the cellularity, the presence of mitoses, vascular endothelial proliferation, and necrosis. For an accurate grading, the pathologist needs to know whether or not the patient received radiation therapy or chemotherapy prior to the surgical procedure. Radiation therapy can cause tissue necrosis, just as some malignant tumors do, particularly glioblastoma multiforme. There are several classification schemes based on grading of gliomas (Table 51.2). The histologic features are important determinants of prognosis. In 1949 Kernohan noted the link between the histopathologic features of gliomas and patient survival, and introduced a four-tier grading system, which is still used today, with some modifications (26). Daumas-Duport determined that the length of postoperative survival is inversely proportional to the number of histologic features of malignancy, such as nuclear atypia, mitoses, vascular endothelial proliferation and necrosis found in the tumor (27,28). From a practical standpoint, in the older patients, a three-tier grading system is adequate, since even low-anaplastic tumors (grade II) tend to behave more aggressively and need to be treated as anaplastic tumors rather than low grade. Gliomas occurring before the age of 10 and after the age of 45 tend to be more undifferentiated and associated with more aggressive behavior and shorter postoperative survival (29). Oligodendrogliomas and mixed oligo-astrocytomas carry a better prognosis (30). Determination of tumor cell proliferation pattern, using mitotic index calculation by labelling with bromodeoxyuridine (BUdR) or Ki-67 nuclear antigen, or flow cytometry, is being investigated as a way to define prognosis (31–33).

In the recent years, research has focused on defining the genetic alterations, and the interactions between tumor-suppressor genes, oncogenes and their products, growth factors and enzyme systems. The goal of this research is to determine the mechanisms of oncogenesis, of cell resistance and repair mechanisms, and to develop new treatment modalities based on the molecular biology data. The p53 tumor suppressor gene, found on chromosome 17p, is frequently altered in gliomas, as it is in systemic cancers. Tumors with a high percentage of cells with mutated p53 gene are rapid-growing, and tend to recur faster and be more resistant to therapy. Alterations on chromosome 17p are the most common seen in gliomas, even in low-

Table 51.2 Grading of malignant gliomas.

Grading system and criteria	Grade 1	Grade 2	Grade 3	Grade 4
Kernohan				
• cell anaplasia	none	minimal	in half of cells	extensive
• cellularity	mild	mild	increased	marked
• mitoses	none	none	present	numerous
• vascular endothelial proliferation	none or minimal	none or minimal	more frequent	marked
• necrosis	none	none	regional	extensive
• transition zone to normal brain	broad	broad	narrowed	may be sharply delineated
WHO	**Pilocytic astrocytoma**	**Astrocytoma** (fibrillary, protoplasmic, gemystocytes, giant cell, combinations)	**Anaplastic astrocytoma** Astrocytoma with areas of anaplastic transformation	**Glioblastoma** anaplastic glial tumor with high cellularity and necrosis
• Based on cell type				
Daumas-Duport	None of the four criteria	One criterion	Two criteria	Three or four criteria
• nuclear abnormalities				
• mitoses				
• endothelial proliferation				
• necrosis				

Ringertz	**Astrocytoma** Tumor showing infiltrative growth pattern and mild to moderate hyper cellularity. Cytologic features resemble normal astrocytes with only mild nuclear abnormalities.	**Anaplastic astrocytoma** Cellular infiltrative astrocytic tumor containing astrocytes with moderate pleomorphism. Mitoses and moderate vascular proliferation may be seen. No necrosis.	**Glioblastoma multiform** Markedly pleomorphic astrocytic tumor with high Cellularity, frequent mitosis, increased vascularity and necrosis

grade tumors. With higher grade of malignancy, other chromosomal alterations are seen on chromosomes 9p, 19q, 4, 7, 13. Alterations on chromosome 10 are seen in 50% of glioblastomas. It is not known yet whether chromosome 10 is the site of a tumor suppressor gene. The loss of chromosome 10 has been directly correlated with amplification of the epidermal growth factor receptor (EGFR), which can be targeted for therapeutic interventions. Ploidy studies indicate that for astrocytomas, survival is better for patients with aneuploid tumors than with euploid tumors. No such correlation was found for oligodendrogliomas (34,35).

Meningiomas are more common in older patients (median age 59), with a female predominance. The 5-year survival is 92% for patients ages 45–74, and 70% for patients older than 75. From the statistics reviewed it is not clear whether the drop in survival rate is related to tumor progression or non-neurologic causes. The majority are benign tumors. Only 1% of meningiomas have malignant characteristics, either with brain parenchyma invasion, or with increased number of mitoses and necrosis, indicating a rapid growth pattern and high rate of local recurrence within a short time after complete resection (4).

Pituitary adenomas are also more common in the older age. In many cases asymptomatic microadenomas are found on scans of the brain done for other reasons, such as head trauma, headaches, dizziness. Some patients present with galactorrhea, and in such cases an elevated prolactin level will establish the diagnosis of prolactinoma. The treatment with bromocriptine can be curative in patients with small tumors, or may reduce the size of larger tumors to where a transsphenoidal resection can be safely performed. The majority of pituitary tumors are nonsecreting. Rarely, a growth hormone secreting adenoma can be suspected based on specific changes in the patient's appearance (acromegaly). In such cases, somatostatin or bromocriptin could control the growth hormone secretion. Surgery or stereotactic radiosurgery may be indicated in some patients.

Acoustic neuromas are benign tumors also seen in older patients, and should be suspected in patients with unilateral hearing loss and vertigo which does not resolve with medical treatment. In these patients, unlike the young age group, the acoustic neuromas are unilateral, and usually are isolated, not as part of neurofibromatosis. Depending on the patient's age, severity of symptoms, and the size of the tumor, the management can be conservative, with symptomatic treatment and follow-up with serial scans, or more definitive, with surgery or stereotactic radiosurgery.

Differential Diagnosis

In the older patients presenting with neurologic symptoms the differential diagnosis is primarily with cerebrovascular disease. Neuroimaging studies can differentiate between tumor and stroke when the lesion does not respect a vascular distribution. It can also help differentiate between hemorrhage due to hypertension and hemorrhage into a tumor. When the scan reveals enhancing lesions, the differential diagnosis is between primary and metastatic tumors. If the chest radiograph is normal, the most yielding procedure will be a biopsy of one of the lesions for tissue diagnosis. In this age group, infectious or vasculitic lesions are less common than in the younger patients.

Therapy

The treatment of brain tumors is determined by the histologic type, location in the cranial cavity, the patient's performance status and neurologic status, age, and life expectancy as defined not only by the neurologic status, but also by coexisting medical problems (36,38). Benign tumors, such as meningiomas, acoustic neuromas, or pituitary adenomas can be managed conservatively in the older patients, unless the symptoms warrant a more aggressive approach. Surgery and/or radiation therapy would be indicated for tumors extending into the cavernous sinus, compressing cranial nerves or vascular structures, or causing seizures which are not well controlled with anticonvulsants.

For gliomas, the conventional therapy involves surgery, radiation therapy, and chemotherapy (39–45). There are also new treatment modalities being developed (Table 51.3). The following sections will detail primarily the management of malignant gliomas, which are the most common, but also the most difficult to treat primary brain tumors. Age is an important factor influencing the results of brain tumor therapy protocols, and results are often analyzed separately for patients younger than 50 years of age and older. Age 50 is an arbitrary cut-off, and should not be construed as an absolute age limit to good response to therapy. Patients over the age of 50 with good performance status and resectable tumors may respond well to therapy, and have a survival rate better than the average for the age group. Such patients would benefit from aggressive therapeutic approaches.

Most primary brain tumors and metastatic tumors have surrounding vasogenic edema, which contributes to the neurologic symptoms. The edema is controlled with corticosteroids, diuretics, or, in some cases, mannitol. The dose of steroids is determined based on the amount of edema and mass effect. The duration of steroid treatment depends on the therapeutic intervention considered. Patients who undergo a wide resection of the tumor can be tapered off steroids relatively quickly. For patients on long-term steroids side-effects are gastric irritation, steroid myopathy, Cushingoid appearance, and in some patients osteoporosis, depression, or steroid psychosis. For patients with diabetes, if they need to be on steroids, the blood glucose must be monitored carefully, and they may need to start insulin therapy for control of the hyperglycemia. In cases where steroids are contraindicated, such as active peptic ulcer, heart failure or uncontrolled diabetes, diuretics such as acetazolamide or furosemide can decrease the edema.

Surgery

Surgery is usually the first therapeutic intervention for brain tumors. The decision regarding the extent of resection, considering the morbidity associated with an open resection, should be based on the extent and location of the tumor, the grade of malignancy, the presence of other medical problems, and the subsequent treatment plan (46,50). In patients with rapidly deteriorating neurologic status due to an expanding mass, surgical intervention can bring about significant improvement, while at the same time providing tissue for pathologic diagnosis, and recently for such experimental treatments as gene therapy or adoptive immunotherapy ("tumor vaccine").

For patients with multifocal lesions, infiltrating tumors, involvement of the corpus callosum, or subependymal or leptomeningeal spread, a stereotactic biopsy for tissue diagnosis will be sufficient. Biopsy would also be indicated in patients with deep seated lesions, or tumors involving the motor or speech areas, even when the tumor is well defined and appears to be localized. Patients with significant neurologic deficits, and serious medical problems such as heart disease or severe lung disease are at high risk for perioperative complications, and should be offered stereotactic biopsy for diagnosis (46).

When feasible, complete resection of the tumor has been shown to significantly increase the rate of survival, both by improving the patient's performance status, and by providing cytoreduction, with a better chance of response to subsequent therapy (49,52). This survival advantage is particularly significant for anaplastic astrocytomas. The 5-year survival rates are 50% in patients with astrocytomas who had total resection, but only 20% in patients who had biopsy only (52). The perfected neurosurgical techniques, such as computer-assisted minimal access surgery, have reduced the morbidity associated with the open craniotomies, and shortened the length of hospital stay. This has also made such interventions safer, and more accepted for older patients with resectable tumors (53).

Reoperation for recurrent or progressing tumors must be considered on a case-by-case basis, depending on the tumor type, expected survival, KPS, age, and plans for further therapy. Age is a factor that can influence the outcome. In one study, survival after reoperation for recurrent gliomas was 57 weeks for patients younger than 40 years, but only 36 weeks for older patients (54). Other authors found a correlation between age and overall survival from diagnosis, but no difference after reoperation (48).

For patients with hydrocephalus shunting procedures are sometimes necessary. Also for cystic tumors, an Ommaya-type reservoir can be inserted, which

Table 51.3 Treatment of brain tumors.

Therapy	Methods
Surgery	Biopsy • Open • Stereotactic, frame less stereotactic Resection • Craniotomy • Computer-assisted, minimally invasive
Radiation therapy	External beam • Conventional fractionation 180–200 cGy/day • Hyperfractionation 120–160 cGy twice a day, 100 cGy three times a day Radiosurgery • Linear accelerator, gamma knife, particle beam, conformal Brachytherapy Boron neutron capture therapy Radiosensitizers
Chemotherapy	Routes of administration • intravenous • oral • intraarterial, blood-brain barrier modification • interstitial • intracavitary • intraventricular/intrathecal Drugs • alkylating agents • antimetabolites • polyamine inhibitors • topoisomerase inhibitors, vinca alkaloids Drug combinations
Immunotherapy	Interferons Adoptive immunotherapy ("tumor vaccine") Monoclonal antibodies Immunoconjugates
Other agents	Retinoids Tamoxifen
Gene therapy	Herpes-virus thymidine kinase/gancyclovir Insulin-like growth factor antisense oligonucleotide
Combined modalities	Chemo-radiotherapy Chemotherapy and tamoxifen Retinoids and interferon Radioimmunotherapy

would allow easy access and drainage should the cyst reaccumulate.

The rate of complications and operative mortality are reduced when surgery is performed at centers with experience in the management of brain tumors. Reported morbidity rates average 10%, and mortality rates 6%. Postoperative complications are increased neurologic deficit due to increased edema, hemorrhage, CSF leak, infections. In patients with malignant gliomas there is an increased risk for thromboembolic complications, particularly in the postoperative period, and it is important to screen such patients for deep venous thrombosis, and provide prophylactic measures (early mobilization, elastic stockings). The treating physician needs to maintain a high index of suspicion, and obtain lung ventilation-perfusion scans if the patients complain of fatigue out of proportion with the degree of neurologic deficit, exertional dyspnea, or chest pain. The presence of a brain tumor is not a contraindication to anticoagulation therapy, except in the immediate postoperative period (first 7–10 days), or if there is recent hemorrhage present within the tumor. In such cases, low-dose subcutaneous heparin, placement of an inferior vena cava filter, and close observation in the hospital may be considered.

Radiation Therapy

Postoperative radiation therapy (RT) is a well established treatment modality for malignant brain tumors. For malignant gliomas RT with doses of 50–60 Gy increases survival compared with surgery alone (55).The role of RT is less well established for treatment of low-grade gliomas. It is clearly indicated for patients with seizures not controlled with anticonvulsants. When total resection is feasible, RT does not add to survival. For unresectable tumors, RT has a definite influence on survival rate (56,57). In older patients low-grade gliomas have a biologic behavior different from that in younger patients, and the progression to anaplastic tumors is more rapid. For this reason, older patients with low-grade gliomas should be offered RT. Oligodendrogliomas also benefit from RT.

For malignant gliomas the RT is delivered to the area of tumor as visualized on CAT or MRI scan, and an additional 3-cm margin. Whole brain RT, which was used in the past is associated with a high incidence of leukoencephalopathy and long term cognitive deficits. The total dose of radiation is delivered over 30–33 days, in daily fractions of 160–200 cGy. Age is an important prognostic factor. In one study the survival at 18 months was 64% in patients younger than 40, but only 8% in patients older than 60. The performance status is an independent variable. Patients with an initial Karnofsky score of 70 or greater have a survival rate at 18 months of 34%, as compared to 13% for patients with a score of 60 or below. The most important prognostic factor remains the extent of resection. The postoperative residual tumor volume (determined on enhanced CAT or MRI scans) correlates inversely with survival (49,58).

The results of conventional fractionation RT have been disappointing in terms of providing a cure, or at least long-term survival in patients with malignant gliomas. Reasons for failure are related to tumor cell resistance, particularly in hypoxic areas of the tumor, the presence of repair mechanisms, and also the pattern of spread of these tumors along white matter tracts, outside the radiation field. There are several different methods under investigation to enhance radiosensitivity, provide protection to the normal brain tissue, and to deliver higher doses of radiation to the tumor.

Radiosensitizers

Hypoxic cell sensitizers such as misonidazole or lonidamine in combination with RT were promising in experimental studies, however in randomized clinical trials showed no benefit in survival. Halogenated pyrimidine analogues such as bromo-dioxyuridine (BUdR) or idoxyuridine (IUdR) are incorporated into rapidly dividing cells and act as radiosensitizers. Phase II studies noted an increase in survival over conventional RT. There are now randomized studies to evaluate the efficacy of these agents with conventional RT and hyperfractionation schedules. Other studies have investigated the radiosensitizing effect of some chemotherapeutic agents, like hydroxyurea, vincristine, BCNU. The dif-

ference in survival compared with conventional RT is not significant. The patients under the age of 60 years seem to benefit most.

Hyperfractionation, hypofractionation, and accelerated fractionation schedules

In hyperfractionation schedules the RT is delivered in two or three daily treatments. This allows for smaller doses to be delivered at shorter time intervals, with the advantage that larger total doses could be used with less toxicity to the normal brain, since the radiation would preferentially affect the rapidly proliferating tumor cells. Using this approach, in two daily doses, the total dose could be escalated to 72–82 Gy. The survival in a randomized RTOG study was longer in the 72 Gy group than the 82 Gy group, probably due to excessive neurotoxicity of the higher dose. Ongoing hyperfractionation studies with chemotherapeutic agents as radiosensitizers are also in phase III trials.

Hypofractionation schedules, where RT is delivered in weekly doses of 500–650 cGy over 6 weeks, to a total dose of 36–39 Gy, together with administration of cisplatin or carboplatin as radiosensitizers, have been used for patients with a poor performance status (KPS of 60 or below). Such an approach was shown to be well tolerated, and improved both the performance status and survival in some of the patients (59).

In accelerated fractionation schedules, the conventional dose of radiation is delivered in two or three daily fractions. The rationale is that shortened treatment time (two to four weeks instead of six weeks) would improve the therapeutic ratio, with greater tumor control. In an RTOG study with twice daily doses given over four weeks with BCNU, there was no survival advantage over conventional fractionation. There are presently phase III trials conducted with acceleration hyperfractionation schedules of RT with carboplatin or BUdR as radiosensitizers. The toxicities in these studies are related to the myelosuppressive effect of the cytotoxic agents, skin rash with BUdR. These schedules are quite well tolerated, even by older patients. Accelerated fractionation has been used for hospitalized patients with poor performance status, to shorten the duration of treatment (60). It is not yet known whether such RT schedules will significantly improve survival.

Radiosurgery

Stereotactic radiosurgery (RS) is a noninvasive technique which allows delivery of high-dose single fractions of radiation to small, well circumscribed tumors. Stereotactic frames establish a coordinate system for precise definition of tumor location and tumor volume on computerized imaging studies. The radiation is delivered either by stationary multiple coplanar beams centered on the tumor, or similar noncoplanar arc rotations that converge the radiation on the tumor. The most commonly used radiation sources for RS are linear accelerators (Linac) and cobalt-60 gamma ray units (Gamma Knife). The treatment is safe, effective, and because it is done in one single dose, in an outpatient setting, is very convenient for the patient, and cost-effective. The morbidity associated with RS is primarily related to increased peritumoral edema, and is easily controlled with steroids. To date, no cognitive deficits have been described in patients who have received RS without conventional RT.

For treatment of malignant gliomas RS is used as adjuvant to external beam RT, to deliver high-dose radiation boost to areas of tumor with nodular, well circumscribed enhancement, usually indicative of more aggressive tumor. These areas have to be smaller than 5 cm. Because of the infiltrative pattern of growth of these tumors RS can not be used as the sole radiation modality (61). Radiosurgery can also be administered in fractionated doses (62). On the other hand, brain metastases, which displace rather than invade brain tissue, and are usually well circumscribed, are optimal candidates for RS.

Radiosurgery is also used for treatment of small but symptomatic meningiomas when resection is deemed too risky either because of the tumor location or the patient's medical condition. Acoustic neuromas are also treated with RS, especially in elderly patients. Pituitary adenomas, particularly the secreting ones, are successfully treated with RS.

Brachytherapy

Interstitial radiation therapy (brachytherapy) is a more invasive way of delivering high dose radiation to a tumor, while limiting the dose to the surrounding brain. A dose of 60 Gy or more can be delivered even after 60 Gy external beam RT. Brachytherapy refers to treatment with radiation sources placed directly into the tumor mass, or adjacent to tumors (e.g. in the surgical cavity). The most commonly used isotopes for brachytherapy are ^{192}Ir and ^{125}I. The implants can be placed permanently, or the sources can be removed after a few days, once the desired dose has been delivered (temporary implants). The dose distribution surrounding a radiation source decreases rapidly with distance away from the source and to attenuation of radiation as it passes through the tissue. The distance between sources and the depth of the implant can be thus calculated to deliver maximal radiation to the tumor tissue, with least damage to the normal brain.

Although more invasive than RS, and with significantly greater morbidity, brachytherapy in malignant gliomas has the advantage that it can be used for infiltrating or cavitary tumors, and tumors larger than 3 cm. The implants are placed surgically, under local or general anesthesia, using stereotactic coordinates. The radiation sources are shielded, and during the hospitalization the medical personnel and the visitors need to be protected by wearing a lead apron or by a lead screen. The implant removal can be performed at bedside. Brachytherapy can be done as a boost to external beam RT, or as salvage therapy at recurrence. Brachytherapy was shown to improve survival in patients with malignant gliomas (63,64).

Serious complications after brachytherapy include wound infections, cerebral edema, abscess into the tumor, hemorrhage, and radiation necrosis, which requires surgical intervention. These complications make brachytherapy a less attractive treatment modality for elderly patients, and for patients with poor performance status.

Side-effects of radiation therapy

Regardless of the radiation modality used, RT does have side effects of which the patients need to be informed, and monitored for. The reactions to RT are more significant when RT is administered to a large portion of the brain. The effects can be acute, early delayed, and late delayed (65). The acute effects occur during treatment or shortly after completion of radiation therapy. Some patients experience headaches, probably related to edema, or a worsening of the neurologic deficits. Fatigue is another complaint, and depending on the tumor location, the patients may experience nausea, sore throat, hearing loss, blurring of vision. These symptoms are transient, and can be controlled with steroids and reassurance. The early delayed effects appear in the first 3 months after completion of RT, and are marked by somnolence, loss of appetite, apathy. These effects are self-limiting, seem to be more severe in the older patients. The late-delayed radiation injury occurs months, or even years after completion of radiation. The patients notice loss of short term memory and cognitive decline. These effects were more significant with whole brain RT, but are also seen with limited field RT, particularly with large fields. The CAT or MRI scans reveal white matter changes bilaterally, or may show focal radiation necrosis. Areas of necrosis do enhance and can have surrounding edema, thus making them difficult to distinguish from recurrent tumor. PET and SPECT scans can be helpful, showing metabolically hypoactive areas of radiation necrosis, as compared with the increased metabolic activity in tumor tissue (24,25). The definitive differential diagnosis is done by biopsy (66). Focal radiation necrosis can cause focal neurologic deficits, and may require resection of the necrotic area for control. Corticosteroids may control the necrosis, but long-term use has its own complications. Results of treatment with low-dose anticoagulants have been mixed. The risk for radiation necrosis is high with brachytherapy. The degree of cognitive impairment varies, but can be more severe in patients with tumors involving the temporal lobes, and elderly patients with baseline mild dementia. In the later patient population, the decision regarding RT must be based on the type of tumor and the life expectancy. For patients with malignant gliomas, who have a very poor long-term prognosis, conventional fractionation or hypofractionation RT provides palliation and can improve the quality of life over the short term. The degree of cognitive impairment can be quantitated using neuropsychometric evaluation prior to RT, and at 6, 12, 18 months intervals (67–69).

Chemotherapy

Chemotherapy (CT) is now established as standard treatment for primary brain tumors (70–72). The addition of chemotherapy to RT has been shown to prolong survival by another 6–18 months, depending on the grade of the tumor. Longer term survivals have also been reported. Still, CT is not curative, and the side-effects in some patients can be dose-limiting.

There are several factors determining CT failure. Brain tumors are heterogeneous, and glioma cells have been shown to express the multidrug resistance gene (MDR-1). Repair enzymes such as glutathion-S-transferase and O^6-alkylguanine alkyl transferase counteract the cytotoxic effect of platinum compounds and nitrosoureas; and some of the tumor cells are in G_0 phase and are less susceptible to chemotherapy. The blood-brain barrier limits the brain tissue penetrance of drugs which are not liposoluble or nonionized. The drugs should attain and maintain in the tumor a cytocidal concentration (73–75). This is dependent on the physical and chemical properties of the drug, and its pharmacokinetics. The half-life of the drug, intracellular binding and capillary-to-cell diffusion are important factors. The dose, route of administration and schedule of administration can influence the drug concentrations.

Most of the drugs used for CT of primary brain tumors are the same drugs used for systemic cancer. There are only very few agents designed for treatment of gliomas, such as diazoquinone and temozolamide. There are several classes of drugs used for the CT of brain tumors: alkylating agents, antimetabolites, natural compounds, urea analogs, methylhydrazine derivatives, polyamine inhibitors. Nitrosoureas are the most effective drugs for treatment of malignant gliomas (72). These drugs are highly lipophilic, bifunctional alkylating agents, which cause DNA cross-linking and inhibit DNA repair and RNA synthesis. The most widely used nitrosoureas are 1,3-bis 2-chloroethyl-1 nitrosourea (BCNU), which is administered intravenously or intra-arterially, and 1-(2-chloroethyl)-3-cyclohexyl-1-nitrosourea (CCNU), given orally. The clinical activity is similar for the two drugs, with 40% response rates. Resistance to BCNU is determined by the activity of the enzyme O^6-alkylguanyl alkyl transferase, which is not age-dependent (76). Platinum compounds (cisplatin and carboplatin) are also very effective, but the duration of response is shorter than for nitrosoureas (77). Cisplatin can be also administered intraarterially, but the risk for neurotoxicity and optic nerve toxicity is higher (78). Dacarbazine (DTIC) is an agent used in combination CT for treatment of malignant meningiomas. Its derivative, temozolamide, which has been extensively studied in England, is a promising drug for treatment of malignant gliomas, and is now used in the United States in clinical trials. It is administered orally, and is well tolerated. Procarbazine, a cell-cycle nonspecific agent, is used in combination CT, or as single agent for malignant gliomas. It is an oral agent, related to disulfiram and monoamine oxidase inhibitors, which explains some of its specific dietary restrictions regarding alcohol and foods containing tyramine (79). The purine and pyrimidine analogs are used in drug combinations, as are the plant alkaloids vincristine and etoposide.

Chemotherapy is given traditionally after completion of radiation therapy, as adjuvant treatment, or at the time of tumor recurrence or progression (80–85). Some chemotherapeutic agents, such as BCNU, hydroxyurea, vincristine, also have a radiosensitizing effect, and there are clinical trials using CT in conjunction with RT. Recent reports suggest a benefit in using CT prior to RT, particularly in oligodendrogliomas. Newer agents, such as 9-aminocamptothecin, a topoisomerase I inhibitor, are also under investigation as pre-radiation CT for glioblastomas. Chemotherapy with the combination procarbazine, CCNU and vincristine (PCV) is at the present time the most effective for oligodendrogliomas, low-grade or anaplastic, and also for anaplastic astrocytomas (83,84). In low grade oligodendrogliomas, CT with PCV was shown to inhibit tumor growth and induce regression of the tumor on imaging studies (86). Pre-radiation CT can be used for palliation in patients with low performance status (87).

Age is an important factor in determining the response of brain tumors to chemotherapy. Patients over the age of 60 have a lower response rate and shorter duration of response than patients under 60 years of age (88,89). Rosenblum et al. demonstrated in vitro that the sensitivity to BCNU of tumor cells obtained from biopsy specimens correlates strongly with the age of the patient. Tumor cells from patients under 50 years old were sensitive in seven of eight cases, but cells from only one of eight patients over 50 years of age responded to BCNU. The reasons for this observed difference are not known (90). The outcomes for patients receiving CT are usually analyzed for the whole group. There are only a few studies evaluating age as parameter of response (Table 51.4). The differences in duration of response and survival are quite significant when comparing patients under the age of 50 and over the age of 50 (89).

Table 51.4 Response to chemotherapy for malignant gliomas based on patient's age.

Study	Chemo	No. Pts.	Response rate %		Median DOR wks		Med. survival wks.	
			<50	>50	<50	>50	<50	>50
Grant, 1995*(79)	BCNU/PCV	146	76	39	23	6	50	24
Sandberg, 1991 (87)	PCV+RT	171	NA	NA	81	23	124	51
Yung, 1992 (80)	BCNU+CDDP	45	NA	NA	35	31	128	55

[*Cut off ages <40, >40 (40–59 and >60)]

The most common side-effect of CT is myelosuppression, in some cases requiring blood transfusions or use of colony stimulating factors. Myelosuppression from chemotherapy occurs earlier in the course of treatment in older patients. No significant nitrosourea-induced pulmonary toxicity was noted in patients over the age of 60, possibly because their survival rates are low, and pulmonary fibrosis occurs after several courses of treatment. Other common side-effects of chemotherapy are nausea, fatigue, loss of appetite. These respond well to symptomatic treatment, are mild, and usually self-limiting. Procarbazine can cause allergic reactions, or if dietary restrictions are not observed, can cause paroxysmal hypertension. Peripheral neuropathy is a common side effect of vincristine, cisplatin and procarbazine. The symptoms are numbness in the hands and feet, constipation, and occasionally jaw pain or numbness. When the neuropathy affects the fine motor skills, the offending agent must be discontinued. Preexisting conditions such as diabetes, hypothyroidism, vitamin B12 deficiency, cause peripheral neuropathy, and the patients need to be evaluated neurologically before starting CT with these drugs, to avoid debilitating neuropathy. Cisplatin, cytarabine, fluorouracil and methotrexate have as potential side-effect central neurotoxicity, manifested by encephalopathy, seizures, or cerebellar dysfunction. Monitoring and correcting for hyponatremia, hypomagnesemia, and hypokalemia, can help prevent some of these serious problems. Patients treated with etoposide are at higher risk for second malignancies, mainly leukemia. In patients with malignant gliomas the long term survival is very low, and does not allow enough time for a second malignancy to develop.

Hormonal Therapy

Laboratory studies have shown that protein kinase C (PKC) is an important factor in promoting proliferation of malignant gliomas. Cell replication is inhibited by PKC inhibitors. Tamoxifen, an estrogen receptor blocking agent commonly used for treatment of breast cancer, has been shown to inhibit proliferation of malignant astrocytomas via non-estrogen receptor mediated PKC blockade. In clinical studies, the dose of tamoxifen shown to inhibit brain tumor growth is much higher than the dose used for breast cancer (40–100 mg b.i.d. vs. 10 mg b.i.d.). The effect appears to be dose-dependent, and is cytostatic rather than cytotoxic. Still, in patients with good performance status, tamoxifen was shown to increase survival. The antimitotic effect is not reversed by estrogen, indicating a non-estrogen receptor mediated mechanism of action. Tamoxifen does cross the blood-brain barrier (91,92). The drug is very well tolerated, even at these high doses. Tamoxifen is now being studied in combination with BCNU as adjuvant therapy after RT. Because of its good safety profile and ease of administration, tamoxifen can be offered as an alternative treatment to elderly patients with malignant gliomas who had received RT and do not wish to take chemotherapy, but would consider other forms of treatment. The incidence of thromboembolic complica-

tion from tamoxifen is higher in the brain tumor patients than in breast cancer patients, but these patients have an overall higher incidence of thromboembolism, even without tamoxifen.

Meningiomas are another group of tumors which can benefit from hormonal therapy. Meningiomas are more common in women, and there is a strong association between meningiomas and breast cancer. Meningiomas express hormone receptors, particularly progesterone receptors, which are present in 70% of the meningioma specimens studied. *In vitro* and clinical studies suggest that progestins can be modulators of meningioma growth (93). Mifepristone (RU 486), an oral nonsteroidal anti-progestative agent, has been shown to bring about subjective and objective improvement in meningioma patients (94). The side-effects are mild, and include fatigue, gynecomastia, thinning of hair, and skin rash. In premenopausal patients it also causes amenorrhea. The drug is now undergoing phase III studies, in a double-blind randomized trial. It is not yet commercially available, primarily because of its other use, as abortive agent.

Biologic Therapy

Biologic therapies with differentiating and immunomodulatory agents are presently under investigation as alternatives to the conventional forms of treatment (95). They can be used alone, or in combination with RT or chemotherapy. These agents are cytostatic rather than cytotoxic. The mechanisms of action are not yet completely elucidated.

Retinoids

The retinoids (13-cis-retinoic acid (CRA) and all-trans-retinoic acid (TRA) are natural and synthetic derivatives of vitamin A, and have proven efficacy in some premalignant and malignant conditions (96). *In vitro* studies demonstrated the differentiating and growth inhibitory effect of retinoic acid on glioma cells. The growth inhibition is related to decrease in EGF receptor-mediated phosphorylation activity. In clinical studies CRA showed activity against malignant gliomas (97,98). The side-effects were relatively mild: dryness of the skin and mucosa, and headache. In some patients, the headaches appeared to be due to increased intracranial pressure (pseudotumor cerebri-type), and responded to treatment with diuretics and glycerol. Similar problems, somewhat more severe, were noted with TRA. Another, potentially fatal, complication of treatment with retinoids is pancreatitis, and the enzymes amylase and lipase must be monitored carefully during therapy. Both TRA and CRA are administered orally in doses of 60–120 mg/m^2/day for three weeks, followed by one week rest. Presently retinoids are undergoing clinical trials in combination with interferon.

Immunemodulators

Interferons (IFN) are naturally produced glycoproteins with antiviral, antiproliferative and immunomodulatory properties (99). There are three main classes of IFN, alpha, beta and gamma, identified based on their cell of origin, and antigenic and biological differences. Interferons stimulate immune effector cells *in vitro* and *in vivo*, induce expression of MHC antigens, and can induce expression of some tumor-related antigens on the surface of tumor cells. IFN gamma is not effective against brain tumor cells. Both IFN alpha and beta have demonstrated activity against malignant gliomas *in vitro* and in clinical trials (100–104). IFN α-2b modulates the activity of PKC, downregulating it (100). There are reports of enhanced activity of IFN and other agents in combination against various tumors. The combination CRA and IFN beta is now studied in a randomized phase III trial. IFN was also reported to enhance the activity of fluorouracil, and may be useful in combination with chemotherapeutic agents (105,106).

Known side-effects of IFN therapy are flu-like symptoms and hypotension. Some patients develop low back pain or arthralgias, at times severe enough to warrant discontinuing the treatment. This can make IFN less well tolerated by elderly patients with arthritis.

Other immunemodulators, such as interleukin-2 and LAK cells, alone or in combination, yielded no objective responses when administered intravenously, but have shown promising results with intratumoral administration (107,108). The side-effects with systemic administration are similar with those seen with IFN. Capillary leak syndrome and allergic reactions can also occur. Complications of intratumoral administration are mainly related to local edema and necrosis, as well as the inherent potential complications of the surgical procedure.

Future Directions

The management of brain tumors continues to bring new challenges for the treating physicians, and there is ongoing research aimed at defining the biologic mechanisms of malignancy and developing new treatment modalities.

While there has been significant progress in identifying the genes responsible for oncogenesis and drug resistance, the progress has been less impressive in finding effective treatments, particularly for malignant gliomas. Some studies combine conventional therapies with some novel approaches, others introduce new experimental treatments.

Modification of Conventional Therapies

Radiation Therapy

Radiation therapy is still the most effective cytotoxic agent for brain tumors. Efforts are being made to improve the therapeutic ratio, by increasing the tumoricidal effect, and/or reducing the damage done to normal tissues. This is achieved by improving the existing radiation therapy machines, better tumor localization, and treatment planning. Also, radiation beams other than the usual photons and electrons are now under investigation. Beams of protons, neutrons, π-mesons, afford better dose localization on the tumor and radiobiological efficiency, with sparing of the surrounding normal tissues.

Another way of insuring dose localization is through radioimmunotherapy, where a monoclonal antibody coupled to a radionuclide is introduced into the tumor (109). The monoclonal antibody is designed to bind only to receptors expressed by tumor and not by normal cells, thus sparing normal tissue. There are some adjuvant methods, used to enhance the radiosensitivity of tumor cells, particularly the hypoxic cells (nitroimidazoles, hyperbaric oxygen, metabolic or pharmacologic manipulation, adjuvant hyperthermia), and methods of normal tissue radioprotection with hyperfractionation schedules or use of chemical compounds (aminothiol compounds).

Chemotherapy

The unique cytoarchitecture of the brain, with a very effective blood-brain barrier, as well as the infiltrative pattern of growth of some primary brain tumors and the heterogeneity of tumor cells are all factors which influence the efficacy or lack of it of chemotherapeutic agents. Unfortunately, the rat animal models used to develop chemotherapeutic drags, do not reproduce reliably these elements of human brain tumors, and the results of clinical trials have been rather disappointing. Also, most drugs used for the treatment of brain tumors have been borrowed from the general oncology arsenal, rather than being specifically designed for use against brain tumor cells. New approaches to chemotherapy are directed at circumventing the blood brain barrier, overcoming drug resistance mechanisms, and minimizing the systemic and neurotoxicity.

The BBB can be circumvented by increasing the dose of the drug, with subsequent increased toxicity, intraarterial chemotherapy with BBB modification, or use of new delivery systems. Intratumoral administration has the advantage that it allows delivery of cytotoxic concentrations of drugs in the tumor bed, with no systemic toxicity. The disadvantages are related to diffusion problems, and local toxicity (necrosis). Chemotherapy can be administered intratumorally via an Ommaya reservoir, or through liposomes or biodegradable polymers. There are phase I and II clinical studies under way using drugs such as BCNU, methotrexate, bleomycin (110–116). Immunoconjugates can also be used for intratumoral chemotherapy. Thus far such an approach has not been applied in clinical trials for brain tumors.

Bone marrow transplant has been used for treatment of pediatric brain tumors, and brain tumors in young adults. Because it involves very intensive chemotherapy, with high toxicity and high risk for infectious complications, it is doubtful that elderly patients could tolerate this modality.

Novel Therapies

Photodynamic therapy

Photodynamic therapy takes advantage of the selective uptake of photosensitizers such as hematoporphyrin derivatives (HpD) by tumor cells compared to the normal brain tissue. When exposed to light of an appropriate wavelength (630 nm) to activate the sensitizer, there is release of free radicals in the tumor cells, with subsequent damage to blood vessels and cell membranes. Highest uptake of HpD was noted in glioblastomas, with good local control. Patients with infiltrating tumors are less likely to benefit from this treatment (117,118).

Boron Neutron Capture Therapy (BNCT)

Boron neutron capture therapy (BNCT) is a form of radiation therapy presently under investigation for treatment of malignant gliomas. BNCT is mediated by short range (less than 10 microns) high energy particles resulting from neutron-induced disintegration of boron-10. There is preferential accumulation of boron-10 in conjunction with high thermal neutron flux at the tumor site. The bombardment of the boron nucleus with a slow neutron induces disintegration of boron, which yields ionizing radiation. Best results with BNCT were reported by Japanese investigators. The studies do not specify differences, if any, in response based on tumor types, age, performance status. The initial clinical trials have been marred by significant brain necrosis. The improved technologies have rekindled the interest in this treatment modality (119,120).

Gene Therapy

Gene therapy refers to introduction of new genetic material into cells, with beneficial effect to the patient. The preferred method for gene transfer is through viral vectors, which have a high efficiency in infecting host cells by inserting their own genetic material into the host cell genome. The viruses infect preferentially dividing cells, and this makes them attractive vectors for gene therapy for malignant brain tumors. The DNA sequence of interest is inserted into the viral genome from which the genes encoding for replication and capsule formation have been deleted. The virus becomes a harmless gene carrier. Both retroviruses and adenoviruses are studied for use as vectors for gene therapy (121–123).

The most publicized gene therapy clinical trial for brain tumors involves transfer of the herpes simplex virus thymidine kinase (Hstk) gene into tumor cells, using retroviral vectors. Hstk is an enzyme which phosphorilates the antiviral prodrug gancyclovir, which becomes virocydal and cytotoxic (124).

Another clinical trial involves transfection of glioblastoma cells with antisense insulin growth factor I cDNA sequence. The transfected cells injected subcutaneously trigger a powerful and specific antitumor-immune response (125). Results of these trials are not yet available.

Other gene therapy studies are still in experimental phase (126–129). There are still very few animal and clinical data regarding the efficacy of gene therapy for brain tumors, the long term effects, and the safety of viral vectors.

Antisense oligonucleotides therapy

Antisense therapy involves introduction into cells of oligonucleotide sequences complementary to mRNA,

thus achieving a highly specific inhibition of gene expression. The antisense DNA sequence forms complementary base pairing with the target mRNA. The antisense oligonucleotide can be introduced into cells through gene therapy techniques. There are many potential targets in brain tumor cells, such as growth factor receptors, oncogene products, etc. Experimental work is directed at investigating the efficacy of antisense gene therapy on inhibition of tumor growth by blocking EGF receptors, and inhibition of angiogenesis (130).

Immunotherapy

Most clinical trials with interferons or interleukins attempt to enhance the host's immunity in a nonspecific manner (131). Recent studies have focused on adoptive immunotherapy, utilizing sensitized T lymphocytes, lymphokine activated killer (LAK) cells or tumor-infiltrating lymphocytes (TIL). The brain is considered an immunologically privileged site, with no lymphatic drainage. There are immunocompetent cells into the brain at the site of brain tumors (macrophages, perivascular lymphocytes), however the immune response is not powerful enough to induce regression of the tumor (131–137). Adoptive immunotherapy is the transfer of tumor-reactive lymphoid cells into the tumor-bearing host, resulting in tumor regression. "Tumor vaccines" are presently being developed. There are phase I clinical trials under way to asses the efficacy and safety of adoptive immunotherapy of glioblastoma multiforme with tumor-sensitized ex vivo activated T lymphocytes. Following surgical resection of the tumor, the patients are vaccinated with a mixture of irradiated autologous tumor cells and BCG at a site close to a draining lymph node. The regional draining lymph node is resected, the T lymphocytes are extracted, and are activated and expanded ex vivo with anti-CD3 or a superantigen. The activated lymphocytes are then injected intravenously into the patient, who is followed up with serial scans of the brain to monitor the response. The patients do receive adjuvant radiation therapy after tumor resection for control of the tumor growth pending lymphocytes activation. To ensure maximal immune competence, the patients must be tapered off steroids as quickly as possible after resection (134,137,138). The immune status of the patient is evaluated prior to starting therapy. Optimal candidates are patients who are fully immunocompetent, and have a complete or near-complete resection of the tumor.

Immunoconjugates

Immunoconjugates are cytotoxic compounds which combine a ligand and a cytotoxic agent, which can be either a radioisotope, a chemotherapeutic drug, or a toxin (139). Clinical trials have been conducted on small numbers of patients with leptomeningeal carcinomatosis using immunoradiotherapy. Current clinical trials are under way for treatment of malignant gliomas. Glioma cells express transferrin receptors, which are targeted with immunoconjugates using as ligands either monoclonal antibodies to transferrin receptors, or transferrin, conjugated with a toxin. The toxins are ribosomal inhibitors, either of plant (ricin), or bacterial (CRM-107) origin. The dose of toxin necessary for tumoricydal effect is smaller than predicted by the tumor volume, which indicates a bystander effect. The results of these trials are not yet available (140–142). Other experimental studies investigate the combined effect of immunoconjugates and chemotherapeutic drugs (143).

Immunomodulators

Experimental studies investigate the feasibility of intratumoral administration of interferon, using biocompatible polymers. There are no clinical data yet on this method (144).

Other biologic agents

Recent studies evaluate other biologic agents for treatment of malignant gliomas, targeting factors which intervene in cell replication or angiogenesis.

Malignant gliomas utilize mevalonate for synthesis of cholesterol and intermediates for cell replication. Lovastatin and phenylacetates inhibit the enzymes HMG-CoA reductase and MVA-PP decarboxylase, and thus affect the mevalonate synthesis and utilization, and induce cytostasis and apoptosis. Both lovastatin (Mevacor) and phenylacetates are presently in clinical trials (145,146).

Angiogenesis is an important feature in malignant gliomas. There are multiple angiogenesis factors, which can be targeted specifically. Fumagillin, an antibiotic derived from the fungus Aspergillus fumigatus fresenius, was noted to inhibit angiogenesis in vitro The fumagillin analog AGM-1470 (TNP-470) is less toxic, and has greater potency in vivo than fumagillin. This compound is presently under investigation in clinical trials, alone or in combination with chemotherapeutic agents, for different malignancies, including gliomas.

These novel therapies are still in experimental phase. Larger studies and longer follow-up periods will be necessary to evaluate their safety and efficacy against brain tumors in all age groups, and the differences, if any, in the older patients. An attractive feature of these treatment modalities is the fact that many of them are administered intratumorally, with minimal systemic toxicity. The long-term potential for neurotoxicity will need to be evaluated.

Treatment of Brain Metastases

A detailed discussion regarding the management of brain metastases is beyond the scope of this chapter. The treatment modalities are similar for primary and metastatic brain tumors. For brain metastases, the choice of treatment is based also on the status of the systemic disease. When feasible, surgical resection will significantly improve the performance status and prolong survival. Brain metastases are optimal lesions for radiosurgery. Chemotherapy can be considered for control of both brain and active systemic metastatic disease (149,150).

Quality of Life Issues

Brain tumors are debilitating diseases, affecting both the cognitive and physical abilities of the patients. Therapy must be aimed at improving the symptoms and the patient's performance status (149). Even if the long-term prognosis is poor for patients with malignant gliomas, physical and occupational therapy will improve the patient's ability to perform activities of daily living. It is important to provide the necessary home equipment, and to actively involve the family in the rehabilitation process (151,152). The majority of brain tumor patients develop reactive depression, which seems to be more severe in elderly patients and needs to be treated with medications. The choice of the antidepressant depends on the patient's medical history (drugs with anticholinergic side-effects must be avoided in patients with prostate hypertrophy or hypotension), and the chemotherapy regimen (tricyclics and monoamine oxidase inhibitors should not be prescribed in patients taking procarbazine).

The nature of the tumor and the prognosis must be discussed with the patient and the family at the time of the diagnosis, in a manner which would not discourage therapy, but would not raise false hope. Therapy can prolong survival with reasonably good quality of life and all the options should be discussed, and the patient allowed the choice (153). The treating physicians need to involve actively the patients and family in management decisions, thus creating a support system for the patient (154).

Practical Considerations

In elderly patients brain tumors behave more aggressively, and tend to be more resistant to treatment. It is important however to consider each case in deciding on therapy. The goal of therapy is to control the tumor growth, and improve the patient's neurologic status (155). Age alone should not be the major determinant for therapeutic decisions. More aggressive therapy can benefit patients with good performance status, and relatively small tumors which can be resected (Figure 51.3). For patients with poor performance status, significant neurologic deficit which is not likely to improve with treatment, multi focal tumors, and debilitating medical problems, it is reasonable to limit the management to steroids and supportive care, or if desired by the patient, to palliative radiation therapy (Figure 51.4).

Conclusions

Brain tumors continue to carry a poor prognosis in spite of aggressive multimodality therapy. Age does influence negatively the prognosis. The treatment at the present time is not curative, except for low grade tumors such as meningiomas. New treatment modalities are being developed based on molecular biology data. At this time the long-term efficacy of these new therapies is not known.

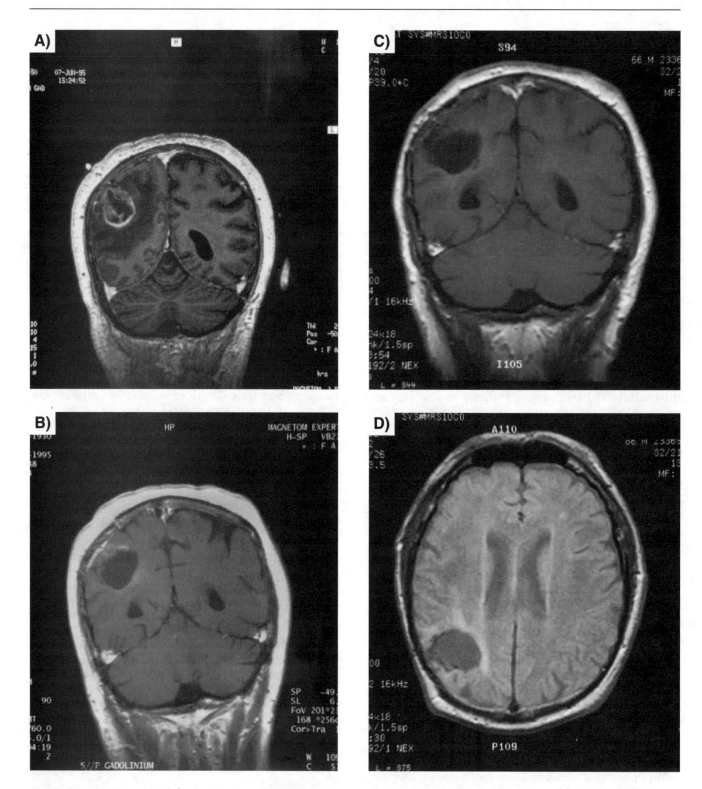

Figure 51.3 MRI scans of the brain of a 66 years old patient with glioblastoma multiform of the right parietal lobe, with good performance status and minimal neurologic deficit. He underwent surgery, RT and adoptive immunotherapy, and at 8 months since diagnosis has no recurrence of the tumor and has a normal neurologic examination and KPS 100.
a) Gadolinium-enhanced coronal T1 MRI at diagnosis, showing a necrotic mass in the right parietal lobe, with ring enhancement, with edema and mass effect.
b) Gadolinium enhanced coronal T1 MRI after surgery and RT, before adoptive immunotherapy. The edema and mass effect have resolved, and there is minimal enhancement at the edges of the surgical cavity, possibly related to surgery.
c) Gadolinium-enhanced coronal T1 MRI 6 months after adoptive immunotherapy. No evidence of tumor recurrence, no enhancement.
d) Axial T2 MRI showing gliosis around the surgical cavity.

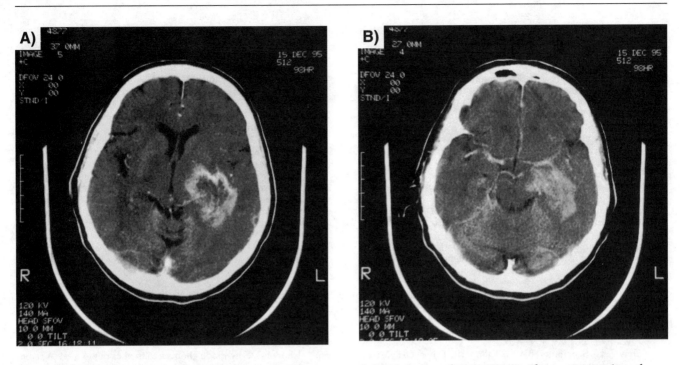

Figure 51.4   CAT scan of the brain of a 73 years old patient with hemiplegia, aphasia, KPS 60. The tumor involves the left temporal lobe, with extension into the midbrain. Because of her poor performance status, the family agreed with supportive care only.
a) Contrast-enhanced axial image, showing a large necrotic mass in the left temporal lobe, with ring enhancement, suggestive of a malignant glioma (GBM).
b) Contrast-enhanced axial image, showing extension of the tumor into the left cerebral peduncle and midbrain, which explains the patient's hemiplegia.

Elderly patients can benefit from therapy for brain tumors, and the treatment must be individualized. The recent advances in the treatment of brain tumors, with limited surgery, radiosurgery, controlled toxicities, have improved the access and acceptance of elderly patients to brain tumor therapy.

References

1.   Laws ER, Thapar K. Brain tumors. *CA Cancer J for Clinicians* 1993; **43**: 263–271.
2.   Boring CC, Squires TS, Tong T. Cancer Statistics. *CA Cancer J for Clinicians* 1991; **141**: 19–36.
3.   Boring CC, Squires TS, Tong T. Cancer Statistics. *CA Cancer J for Clinicians* 1993; **43**: 7–26.
4.   Giles GG, Gonzales MF. *Epidemiology of brain tumors and factors in prognosis*. In *Brain Tumors. An Encyclopedic Approach*, edited by AH Kaye, ER Laws. Edinborough: Churchill Livingstone, 47–68, 1995.
5.   Greig NH, Ries LG, Yancik R, Rappaport SI. Increasing annual incidence of primary brain tumors in the elderly. *J NCI* 1990; **82**: 1621–1624.
6.   Crawford J, Cohen HJ. Relationship of cancer and aging. *Clin Geriatric Med* 1987; **3**: 419–423.
7.   Bondy ML, Wrensch M. Update on brain cancer epidemiology. *Cancer Bull* 1993; **45**: 365–369.
8.   Mack W, Preston-Martin S, Peters JM. Astrocytoma risk related to job exposure to electric and magnetic fields. *Bioelectromagnetics* 1991; **12**: 57–66.
9.   Tsung RW, Laperierre NJ, Simpson WJ, *et al*. Glioma arising after radiation therapy for pituitary adenoma. A report of four patients and estimation of risk. *Cancer* 1993; **72**: 2227–2233.
10. Schoenberg BS, Christine BW, Whisnant JP. Nervous system neoplasms and primary malignancy of other sites. The unique association between meningiomas and breast cancer. *Neurology* 1975; **28**: 817–823.
11. Ahsan H, Neugut AJ, Bruce JN. Association of malignant brain tumors and cancers of other sites. *J Clin Oncol* 1995; **13**: 2931–2935.
12. Velma JP, Walker AM. The age curve of nervous system tumor incidence in adults: Common shape but changing levels by sex, race and geographic location. *Int J Epidemiol* 1987; **16**: 177–183.
13. Boyle P, Maisonneuve P, Saracci R, Muir CS. Is the increased incidence of primary malignant brain tumors in the elderly real? *J NCI* 1990; **82**: 1594–1596.
14. Larsen NS. Experts divided over rising incidence of brain tumors. *Primary care and Cancer* 1993; **13**: 26–29.
15. Desneules M, Mikkelsen T, Mao Y. Increasing incidence of primary malignant brain tumors. Influence of diagnostic methods. *J NCI* 1992; **84**: 442–445.
16. Bodan B, Wegener DK, Feldman JJ, *et al*. Increased mortality from brain tumors: A combined outcome of diagnostic technology and change of attitude towards the elderly. *Am J Epidemiol* 1992; **135**: 1349–1357.
17. Polednak AP. Time trends in incidence of brain and central nervous system cancers in Connecticut. *J NCI* 1991; **83**: 1679–1681.
18. Werner MH, Phupanich S, Lyman GH. Increasing incidence of primary brain tumors in the elderly in Florida. *Cancer Control* 1995; **2**: 309–314.
19. Mahaley MS, Mettlin C, Natarajan N, *et al*. National survey of patterns of care for brain tumor patients. *J Neurosurg* 1989; **71**: 826–835.
20. Hildebrand J, Thomas DGT. Report of a workshop sponsored by the European Organization for Research and Treatment of Cancer (EORTC) on the treatment of primary malignant brain tumors. *J Neurol Neurosurg Psych* 1991; **54**: 182–183.

21. McDermott MW. How to diagnose and manage adult astrocytomas. *Contemporary Oncology* 1993; **12**: 11–21.

22. Black PM. Brain tumors. (Part I) *New Engl J Med* 1991; **324**: 1471–1475.

23. Patronas NJ, Moore WD, Schellinger DR. Brain imaging in the diagnosis of intracranial neoplasms. In *Advances in Neuro-Oncology*, edited by PL Kornblith, MD Walker. Mount Kisco, NY: Futura Publ. Co., 197–247, 1988.

24. Mineura K, Sasajima T, Kowada M, *et al*. Perfusion and metabolism in predicting the survival of patients with central gliomas. *Cancer* 1994; **73**: 2386–2394.

25. Vertosick FT, Selker RG, Grossman SJ, Joyce JM. Correlation of Thallium–201 Single Photon Emission Computed Tomography and survival after treatment failure in patients with glioblastoma multiforme. *Neurosurg* 1994; **34**: 396–401.

26. Kernohan JN, Mabon RF, Suien HS, *et al*. A simplified classification of gliomas. *Proc Staff Mtg Mayo Clinic* 1949; **24**: 71–74.

27. Daumas-Duport C, Scheitauer B, O'Fallon J, *et al*. Grading of astrocytomas: A simple reproducible method. *Cancer* 1988; **62**: 2152–2165.

28. Kim TS, Halliday AL, Hedley-Whyte ET, *et al*. Correlates of survival and the Daumas-Duport grading system for astrocytomas. *J Neurosurg* 1991; **74**: 27–37.

29. Nelson DF, Nelson JS, Davis DR, *et al*. Survival and prognosis of patients with astrocytoma with typical anaplastic features. *J Neuro Oncol* 1985; **3**: 99–103.

30. Shaw EG, Scheitauer BW, O'Fallon JR, Davis DH. Mixed oligoastrocytomas: A survival and prognostic factor analysis. *Neurosurg* 1994; **34**: 577–582.

31. Saarinen UM, Pinko H, Makipernaa A. Prognostic factors for high-grade malignant glioma: Development of a prognostic index. A report of the Medical Research Council Brain Tumor Working Party. *J Neuro Oncol* 1990; **9**: 47–56.

32. Salmon I, Dewhite O, Pasteels JL, *et al*. Prognostic scoring in adult astrocytic tumors using patient age, histopathologic grade and DNA histogram type. *J Neurosurg* 1994; **80**: 877–883.

33. Bruner JM, Langford LA, Fuller GN. Neuropathology, cell biology, and newer diagnostic methods. *Current Opinion in Oncology* 1993; **5**: 441–449.

34. Steck PA, Bruner JM, Pershouse MA. Molecular, genetic and biologic aspects of primary brain tumors. *Cancer Bull* 1993; **45**: 365–369.

35. Kyritsis AP, Bondy ML, Hess KR, *et al*. Prognostic significance of p53 immunoreactivity in patients with glioma. *Clin Cancer Res* 1995; **1**: 1617–1622.

36. Salcman M, Scholtz H, Kaplan RS, Kulik S. Long-term survival in patients with malignant astrocytoma. *Neurosurg* 1994; **34**: 213–219.

37. Halperin EC. Malignant gliomas in older adults with poor prognostic signs. Going nowhere and taking a long time to do it. *Oncology* 1995; **9**: 229–234.

38. Jelsma R, Bucy PG. Glioblastoma multiforme, its treatment and some factors affecting survival. *Arch Neurol* 1969; **20**: 161–171.

39. Janus TJ, Kyritsis AP, Forman AD, Levin VA. Biology and treatment of gliomas. *Ann Oncol* 1992; **3**: 423–433.

40. Weingart J, Brem H. Current management of high grade gliomas. *Contemporary Oncology* 1993; **2**: 19–31.

41. Whittle IR, Gregor A. The treatment of primary malignant brain tumors. *Neurol Neurosurg Psych* 1991; **54**: 101–103.

42. Shapiro WR. Therapy of malignant brain tumors: What have the clinical trials taught us? *Seminars in Oncol* 1986; **1**: 38–45.

43. Mc Vic JC. The therapeutic challenge of gliomas. *Eur J Cancer* 1993; **29A**: 936–939.

44. Ushio Y. Treatment of gliomas in adults. *Current Opinions in Oncol* 1991; **3**: 467–475.

45. Duncan GG, Goodman GB, Ludgate CM, Rheaume DE. The treatment of adult supratentorial high grade astrocytoma. *J Neuro Oncol* 1992; **13**: 63–72.

46. Salcman M. Surgery for malignant glioma. In *Brain Tumors: A Comprehensive text*, edited by RA Morantz, JW Walsh. NY, Basel, Hong-Kong: Marcel Decker, Inc., 417–427, 1984.

47. Devaux BC, O'Fallon JR, Kelly PJ. Resection, biopsy and survival in malignant glial neoplasms: A retrospective study of clinical parameters, therapy and outcome. *J Neurosurgery* 1993; **78**: 762–775.

48. Ammirati M, Vick N, Liao Y, *et al*. Effect of the extent of surgical resection on survival and quality of life in patients with supratentorial glioblastomas and anaplastic astrocytomas. *Neurosurg* 1987; **21**: 201–206.

49. Berger MS, Deliganis AV, Dobbins J, Keles GE. The effect of extent of resection on recurrence in patients with low grade cerebral hemispheric gliomas. *Cancer* 1994; **74**: 1784–1791.

50. Andreou J, George AE, Wise A, *et al*. CT prognostic criteria of survival after malignant glioma surgery. *AJNR* 1983; **4**: 488–490.

51. Albert FK, Forsting M, Sartor K, *et al*. Early postoperative magnetic resonance imaging after resection of malignant glioma: Objective evaluation of residual tumor and its influence on regrowth and prognosis. *Neurosurg* 1994; **34**: 45–60.

52. Winger MJ, MacDonald DR, Cairncross JG. Supratentorial anaplastic gliomas in adults: The prognostic importance of extent of resection and low grade glioma. *J Neurosurg* 1989; **71**: 487–493.

53. Barnett GH, Kormos DW, Steiner CP, Weisenberger J. Use of a frameless, armless stereotactic wand for brain tumor localization with two-dimensional and three-dimensional neuroimaging. *Neurosurgery* 1993; **33**: 4.

54. Salcman M, Karvan RS, Ducker TB, *et al*. Effect of age and reoperation on survival in the combined modality treatment of malignant astrocytomas. *Neurosurg* 1982; **10**: 454–463.

55. Sheline GE. Radiation therapy of brain tumors. *Cancer* 1977; **39**: 873–881.

56. Ishow EG. Low-grade gliomas: to treat or not to treat. A radiation oncologist's viewpoint. *Arch Neurol* 1990; **47**: 1138–1139.

57. Leibel SA, Sheline GE, Wara NBM, *et al*. The role of radiation therapy in the treatment of astrocytomas. *Cancer* 1975; **35**: 1551–1557.

58. Kreth FW, Warnke PC, Scremet R, Ostertag CB. Surgical resection and radiation therapy versus biopsy and radiation therapy in the treatment of glioblastoma multiforme. *J Neurosurg* 1993; **78**: 762–766.

59. Hercberg AA, Tadmor A, Findler S, *et al*. Hypofractionated radiation therapy and concurrent cisplatin in malignant cerebral gliomas-rapid palliation in low performance status patients. *Cancer* 1989; **64**: 816–820.

60. Hernandez JC, Manuyama Y, Yates R, Chin HW. Accelerated fractionation radiotherapy for hospitalized glioblastoma multiforme patients with poor prognostic factors. *J Neuro Oncol* 1990; **9**: 41–46.

61. Brada M, Laing R. Radiotherapy/stereotactic external beam radiotherapy for malignant brain tumors. The Royal Marsden Hospital experience. *Recent Results in Cancer Research* 1994; **135**: 91–104.

62. Southam L, Olivier A, Podgorsak EB, *et al*. Fractionated streeotactic radiation therapy for intracranial tumors. *Cancer* 1991; **68**: 2101–2108.

63. Wen PY, Alexander E, Brack PM, *et al*. Long term results of stereotactic brachytherapy used in the initial treatment of patients with glioblastomas. *Cancer* 1994; **73**: 3029–3036.

64. Kitchen ND, Hughes SW, Taub NA, *et al*. Survival following brachytherapy for recurrent malignant glioma. *J Neuro Oncol* 1993; **18**: 33–39.

65. Sheline GE, Wara WM, Smith V. Therapeutic irradiation and brain injury. *Int J Radiat Oncol Biol Phys* 1980; **6**: 1215–1228.

66. Forsyth PA, Kelly PJ, Cascino TL, *et al*. Radiation necrosis or glioma recurrence: Is computer-assisted stereotactic biopsy useful? *J Neurosurg* 1995; **82**: 436–444.

67. Armstrong C, Ruffer J, Corn B, *et al*. Biphasic patterns of memory deficits following moderate-dose partial-brain irradiation: Neuropsychologic outcome and proposed mechanisms. *J Clin Oncol* 1995; **13**: 2263–2271.

68. Trouette R, Caudry M, Maire JP, Demeaux H. Adult mental deterioration, the main limiting factor in cerebral radiotherapy? *Bull Cancer/Radiother* 1993; **80**: 209–221. (Fr)

69. Crossen JR, Garwood D, Glatstein E, Neuwelt EA. Neurobehavioral sequelae of cranial irradiation in adults: A review of radiation-induced encephalopathy 1994; **12**: 627–642.

70. Yung WKA. Chemotherapy for malignant brain tumors. *Curr Opin Oncol* 1990; **2**: 673–678.

71. Kyritsis A. Chemotherapy for malignant gliomas. *Oncology* 1993; **7**: 93–100.

72. Flowers A, Levin VA. Chemotherapy of brain tumors. In *Brain Tumors: An Encyclopedic Approach*, edited by AH Kaye, ER Laws Jr. Edinburgh, Hong Kong, London, Madrid, New York, Tokyo: Churchill Livingstone, 349–360, 1995.

73. Donelli MG, Zuchetti M, Dincalci M. Do anticancer drugs reach the tumor target in the human brain? *Cancer Chemother Pharmacol* 1992; **30**: 251–260.

74. Boaziz C, Breau JL, Morere JF, Israel L. The blood-brain barrier: Implications for chemotherapy in brain tumors. *Path Biol* 1991; **39**: 789–794.

75. Vendrick CP, Berger JJ, DeJong WH, Steernberger PA. Resistance to cytostatic drugs at the cellular level. *Cancer Chemother Pharmacol* 1992; **29**: 413–429.

76. Yung WKA, Janus TJ, Maor M, Feung LG. Adjuvant chemotherapy with carmustine and cisplatin in patients with malignant glioma. *J Neuro Oncol* 1992; **12**: 131–135.

77. Belanich M, Pastor M, Randall T, et al. Retrospective study of the correlation between the DNA repair protein alkyltransferase and survival of brain tumor patients treated with carmustine. *Cancer Res* 1996; **56**: 783–787.

78. Rogers LR, Purvis JB, Lederman RJ, et al. Alternating sequential intracarotid BCNU and cisplatin in recurrent malignant glioma. *Cancer* 1991; **68**: 15–21.

79. Newton HB, Bromberg J, Junck L, et al. Comparison between BCNU and procarbazine chemotherapy for treatment of gliomas. *J Neuro Oncol* 1993; **15**: 257–263.

80. Chang CH, Horton J, Schoenfeld D, et al. Comparison of post-operative radiotherapy and combined postoperative radiotherapy and chemotherapy in the multidisciplinary management of malignant gliomas. *Cancer* 1983; **52**: 997–1007.

81. Fine HA, Dear KB, Loeffler JS, et al. Meta-analysis of radiation therapy with and without adjuvant chemotherapy for malignant gliomas in adults. *Cancer* 1993; **71**: 2585–2597.

82. Walker MD, Green SB, Byar DP, et al. Randomized comparison of radiotherapy and nitrosoureas for the treatment of malignant gliomas after surgery. *N Engl J Med* 1980; **303**: 1323–1329.

83. Levin VA, Silver P, Hannigan J, et al. Superiority of post-radiotherapy adjuvant chemotherapy with CCNU, procarbazine and vincristine (PCV) over BCNU for anaplastic glioma: NCOG 6C61 final report. *Int J Radiat Oncol Biol Phys* 1990; **18**: 321–324.

84. Sandberg WM, Malmstrom P, Stromblod LG, et al. A randomized study of chemotherapy with procarbazine, vincristine and lomustine with and without radiation therapy for astrocytoma grades 3 and/or 4. *Cancer* 1991; **68**: 22–29.

85. Krishnasamy S, Vokes EE, Dohrman G, et al. Concomitant chemoradiotherapy, neutron boost, and adjuvant chemotherapy for anaplastic astrocytoma and glioblastoma multiforme. *Cancer Investigation* 1995; **13**: 453–459.

86. Mason WP, Krol GS, DeAngelis LA. Low-grade oligodendroglioma responds to chemotherapy. *Neurology* 1996; **46**: 203–207.

87. Watne K, Nome O, Hager B, Hirschberg H. Pre irradiation chemotherapy in glioma patients with poor prognostic factors. *J Neurooncol* 1992; **13**: 261–264.

88. Eagon RT, Scott M. Evaluation of prognostic factors in chemotherapy of recurrent brain tumors. *J Clin Oncol* 1983; **1**: 38–44.

89. Grant R, Liang BC, Page MA, et al. Age influences chemotherapy response in astrocytomas. *Neurology* 1995; **5**: 929–933.

90. Rosenblum ML, Gerosa M, Dougherty DV, et al. Age, related chemosensitivity of stem cells from human malignant brain tumors. *Lancet* 1982; **1**: 885–887.

91. Vertosick FT, Selker RG, Pollack IF, Arena V. The treatment of intracranial malignant gliomas using orally administered tamoxifen therapy: preliminary results in a series of "failed" patients. *Neurosurgery* 1992; **30**: 897–903.

92. Couldwell WT, Weiss MH, DeGiorgio CM, et al. Clinical and radiographic response in a minority of patients with recurrent malignant gliomas treated with high-dose tamoxifen. *Neurosurg* 1993; **32**: 485–490.

93. Olson JJ, Beck DW, Schlechte J, et al. Hormonal manipulation of meningiomas *in vitro*. *J Neurosurg* 1986; **65**: 99–107.

94. Grunberg SM, Weiss MH, Spitz IM, et al. Treatment of unresectable meningiomas with the antiprogestational agent mifepristone. *J Neurosurg* 1991; **74**: 861–866.

95. Chatel M, Lebrun C, Frenay M. Chemotherapy and immunotherapy in adult malignant gliomas. *Curr Opin Oncol* 1993; **5**: 464–473.

96. Lippman SM, Kessler JF, Meyskens FL. Retinoids as preventive and therapeutic anticancer agents (Part II). *Cancer Treat Rep* 1987; **17**: 493–515.

97. Yung WKA, Lotan D, Lee P, et al. Modulation of growth and EGF receptor activity by retinoic acid in human glioma cells. *Cancer Res* 1989; **49**: 1014–1019.

98. Yung WKA, Simaga M, Levin VA. 13-Cis-retinoic acid. A new and potentially effective agent for recurrent malignant astrocytomas. (Abstr) *Proc ASCO* 1993; **12**: 175.

99. Schneider J, Hoffman FM, Appuzo MLJ, Hinton DR. Cytokines and immunoregulatory molecules in malignant glial neoplasms. *J Neurosurg* 1992; **77**: 265–273.

100. Acevedo-Duncan N, Zhang R, Byvoet P, et al. Interferon modulates human glioma protein kinase C II (Abstr), *Proc Am Assoc Cancer Res* 1993; **34**: 176.

101. Nagai M, Arai T: Clinical effect of interferon in malignant brain tumors. *Neurosurg Rev* 1984; **7**: 55–64.

102. Duff TA, Borden E, Bay J, et al. Phase II trial of interferon-β for treatment of recurrent glioblastoma multiforme. *J Neurosurg* 1986; **64**: 408–413.

103. Yung WKA, Castellanos AM, van Tassel P, et al. A pilot study of recombinant interferon beta (IFN β_{ser}) in patients with recurrent glioma *J Neurooncol* 1990; **9**: 29–34.

104. Yung WKA, Prados M, Levin VA, et al. Intravenous recombinant interferon beta in patients with recurrent malignant gliomas: A phase I/II study. *J Clin Oncol* 1991; **9**: 1945–1949.

105. Fine HA, Wen P, Alexander E, et al. Alpha interferon, BCNU and 5-fluorouracil in the treatment of recurrent high-grade astrocytomas. (Abstr), *Proc ASCO*; 1993; **12**: 175.

106. Buckner JC, Brown LD, Kugler JW, et al. Phase II evaluation of recombinant interferon alpha and BCNU in recurrent glioma. *J Neurosurg* 1995; **82**: 430–435.

107. Young HF. Treatment of recurrent malignant glioma by repeated intracerebral injections of human recombinant interleukin-2, alone or in combination with systemic interferon-α: Results of a phase — I clinical trial. *J Neurooncol* 1992; **12**: 75–83.

108. Moser RP, Bruner JM, Grimm EA. Biologic therapy for brain tumors. *Cancer Bull* 1991; **48**: 117–126.

109. Riva P, Arista A, Sturiale C, et al. Intralesional radio-immunotherapy of malignant gliomas. An effective treatment in recurrent tumors. *Cancer* 1994; **73**: 1076–1082.

110. Neuwelt EA, Frenkel EP, Diehl J, et al. Reversible osmotic blood-brain barrier disruption in humans: implications for the chemotherapy of malignant brain tumors. *Neurosurgery* 1980; **7**: 44–52.

111. Neuwelt EA, Specht HD, Barnett PA, et al. Increased delivery of tumor-specific monoclonal antibodies to brain after osmotic blood-brain barrier modification in patients with melanoma metastatic to the central nervous system. *Neurosurgery* 1987; **20**: 885–895.

112. Garfield J, Dayan AD. Postoperative intracavitary chemotherapy of malignant supratentorial astrocytomas using BCNU. *J Neurosurg* 1973; **39**: 315–322.

113. Avellanosa A, West C, Barua N, Patel A. Intracavitary combination chemotherapy of recurrent malignant glioma via Ommaya Shunt-a pilot study. *Proc Am Soc Clin Oncol* 1983; **2**: 234.

114. Bouvier G, Penn RD, Krohn JS, et al. Direct delivery of medication into a brain tumor through multiple chronically implanted catheters. *Neurosurgery* 1987; **20**: 286–291.

115. Firth G, Oliver AS, McKeran TO. Studies on the intracerebral injection of bleomycin free and entrapped with liposomes in the rat. *J Neurol Neurosurg Psychiatry* 1984; **47**: 585–589.

116. Brem H, Mahaley MS, Vick NA, et al. Interstitial chemotherapy with drug polymer implants for the treatment of recurrent gliomas. *J Neurosurg* 1991; **74**: 441–446.

117. Kaye AH, Morstyn G, Apuzzo MLJ. Photoradiation therapy and its potential in the management of neurological tumors. *J Neurosurg* 1988; **69**: 1–24.

118. Hill JS, Kaye AH, Sawyer WH, et al. Selective uptake of hematoporphyrin derivative into human cerebral glioma. *Neurosurgery* 1990; **26**: 248–254.

119. Barth RF, Soloway AH, Fairchild RG. Boron neutron capture therapy of cancer. *Cancer Res* 1990; **50**: 1061–1070.

120. Saris SC, Solares GR, Wazer DE, *et al.* Boron neutron capture therapy for murine malignant gliomas. *Cancer Res* 1992: **52**: 4672–4677.

121. Culver KW, Ram Z, Wallbridge S, *et al.* In vivo gene transfer with retroviral vector-producer cells for treatment of experimental brain tumors. *Science* 1993; **256**: 988–990.

122. Markert JM, Coen DM, Malick A, *et al.* Expanded spectrum of viral therapy in the treatment of nervous system tumors. *J Neurosurg* 1992; **77**: 590–594.

123. Takamya Y, Short MA, Moolten FL, *et al.* An experimental model of retroviral gene therapy for malignant brain tumors. *J Neurosurg* 1993; **79**: 104–110.

124. Zerbe LK, Hughes TL, Josephs SA, *et al.* Rapid cytotoxicity with gancyclovir following adenovirus transduction of glioma cells with herpes virus thymidine kinase. (Abstr) *Proc Am Assoc Cancer Res* 1995; **36**: 423.

125. Trojan J, Johnson TR, Rudin SD, *et al.* Treatment and prevention of rat glioblastoma by immunogenic C6 cells expressing antisense insulin-like growth factor I RNA. *Science* 1993; **259**: 94–96.

126. Yu JS, Wei MK, Chiocca A, *et al.* Treatment of glioma by genetically engineered interleukin-4-secreting cells. *Cancer Res* 1993; **53**: 3125–3128.

127. Sobol RE, Fakhrai H, Shawler D, *et al.* Immuno-gene therapy of glioblastoma. (Abstr) *Proc Am Assoc Cancer Res* 1995; **36**: 439.

128. Yung WKA, Shi YX, Zhang WW, *et al.* Growth suppression of human glioma cells by restoration of wild-type p53 gene utilizing an adenovirus vector. (Abstr) *Proc Am Assoc Cancer Res* 1995; **36**: 423.

129. Gomez-Manzano C, Fueyo J, Kyritsis AP, *et al.* Adenovirus-mediated transfer of the p53 gene produces rapid and generalized death of human glioma cells via apoptosis. *Cancer Res* 1996; **56**: 694–699.

130. Saleh M, Stacker SA, Wilks AF. Inhibition of growth of C6 glioma cells in vivo by expression of antisense vascular endothelial growth factor sequence. *Cancer Res* 1996; **56**: 393–401.

131. Hayes RL. The cellular immunotherapy of primary brain tumors. *Rev Neurol* 1992; **148**: 454–466.

132. Yanasaki T, Handa H, Yamashita J, *et al.* Specific adoptive immunotherapy with tumor-specific cytotoxic T lymphocytes clone for murine malignant gliomas. *Cancer Res* 1984; **44**: 1776–1783.

133. Holladay FP, Lopez GL, Morantz RA, Wood GW. Generation of cytotoxic immune response against a rat glioma by in vivo priming and secondary in vitro stimulation with tumor cells. *Neurosurgery* 1992; **30**: 499–505.

134. Merchant RE, Coquia EM, Novitzki MR, *et al.* Adoptive immunotherapy using glioma-sensitized cytotoxic T cells. *Proc Am Assoc Cancer Res* 1995; **36**: 474.

135. Merchant RE, Merchant LH, Cook SHS, *et al.* Intralesional infusion of lymphokine-activated killer (LAK) cells and recombinant interleukin-2 (rIL-2) for the treatment of patients with malignant brain tumor. *Neurosurgery* 1988; **23**: 725–732.

136. Merchant RE, Ellison MD, Young HF. Immunotherapy for malignant glioma using human recombinant interleukin-2 and activated autologous lymphocytes. *J Neurooncol* 1990; **8**: 173–188.

137. Granger G, Ioli G, Hiserodt J, *et al.* Basic and clinical studies of intralesional therapy of gliomas with allogeneic, lymphoid cells. (Abstr) *Proc Am Assoc Cancer Res* 1995; **36**: 472.

138. Lillehei KO, Mitchell DH, Johnson SD, *et al.* Long term follow-up of patients with recurrent malignant gliomas treated with adjuvant adoptive immunotherapy. *Neurosurgery* 1991; **28**: 16–23.

139. Hall WA, Fodstad O. Immunotoxins and central nervous system neoplasia. *J Neurosurg* 1992; **76**: 1–12.

140. Johnson VG, Wrobel C, Wilson D, *et al.* Improved tumor-specific immunotoxins in the treatment of CNS and leptomeningeal neoplasia. *J Neurosurg* 1989; **70**: 240–248.

141. Recht LD, Griffin TW, Raso V, Salimi AR: Potent cytotoxicity of an antihuman transferrin receptor-Ricin A-chain immunotoxin on human glioma cells in vitro. *Cancer Res* 1990; **50**: 6696–6700.

142. Hall WA, Godal A, Juell S, Fodstad O. In vitro efficacy of transferrin-toxin conjugates against glioblastoma multiforme. *J Neurosurg* 1992; **76**: 838–844.

143. Flowers A, Steck PA, Donato NJ, Yung WKA. Enhanced cytotoxicity of cisplatin and BCNU on glioma cell lines by pretreatment with an EGF receptor targeted immunoconjugate. (Abstr) *Proc Am Assoc Cancer Res* 1994; **35**: 504.

144. Wiranowska M, Ransohoff J, Naidu AK, *et al.* Interferon containing biocompatible polymers for localized cerebral immunotherapy of glioma. (Abstr) *Proc Am Assoc Cancer Res* 1994; **35**: 491.

145. Shack S, Prasanna P, Hudgins WR, *et al.* Experimental therapies for malignant gliomas: Targeting the mevalonate pathway of cholesterol synthesis. (Abstr) *Proc Am Assoc Cancer Res* 1994; **35**: 409.

146. Samid D, Shack S, Liu L, *et al.* Phenylacetate and related nontoxic differentiation inducers in treatment of prostate, brain and skin cancer. (Abstr), *Proc Am Assoc Cancer Res* 1993; **34**: 377.

147. Ingber D, Fujita T, Kishimoto S, *et al.* Synthetic analogues of fumagillin that inhibit angiogenesis and suppress tumor growth. *Nature* 1990; **348**: 555–557.

148. Teicher BA, Holden SA, Ara G, Brem H. Potentiation of cytotoxic cancer therapies by AGM-1470 (AGM) alone and with other angiogenic antiangiogenic agents. (Abstr) *Proc Am Assoc Cancer Res* 1994; **35**: 324.

149. Sawaya R, Ligon BL, Flowers A, Bindal R. Management of metastatic brain tumors: A review. *Neurosurg Quarterly* 1994; **4**: 140–157.

150. Noordjik EM, Vecht CJ, Haaxma-Reiche H, *et al.* The choice of treatment of single brain metastases should be based on extracranial tumor activity and age. *Int J Radiat Oncol Biol Phys* 1994; **29**: 711–718.

151. Trojanowski T, Peszynski J, Turowski K, *et al.* Quality of survival in patients with brain gliomas, treated; with postoperative CCNU and radiation therapy. *J Neurosurg* 1989; **70**: 18–23.

152. Weitzner MA, Meyers CA, Gelke CK, *et al.* The Functional Assessment of Cancer Therapy (FACT) Scale. Development of a Brain Subscale and revalidation of the general version (FACT-G) in patients with primary brain tumors. *Cancer* 1995; **75**: 1151–116.

153. Meyers CA, Boeke C. Neurobehavioral disorders in brain tumor patients: Rehabilitation strategies. *The Cancer Bull* 1993; **45**: 362–364.

154. Wegmann JA. CNS tumors. Supportive management of the patient and family. *Oncology* 1991; **5**: 109–113.

155. Balducci L, Ades T, Carbone P, *et al.* Issues in treatment. *Cancer* 1991; **68**; (Suppl): 2527–2529.

52. Gynecologic Cancers

Tate Thigpen

While cancers of the female genital tract can originate in virtually every portion of the tract, three lesions account for over 90% of all cases: celomic epithelial carcinomas of the ovary, carcinoma of the cervix, and endometrial carcinoma. These three lesions will form the focus of the following discussion.

Celomic Epithelial Carcinoma of the Ovary

Cancer of the ovary includes several different types of malignancy: celomic epithelial carcinomas, germ cell neoplasms, and stromal tumors. The celomic epithelial carcinomas (henceforth referred to as ovarian carcinoma) account for almost 90% of these and are the most common cause of death due to gynecologic cancers in the United States.

General Considerations

Proper management of ovarian carcinoma depends on an understanding of specific characteristics of the disease: etiology, the impact of age, and prognostic factors including especially stage.

Etiology

Although the etiology of ovarian carcinoma is not known, there is an association between uninterrupted ovulation and the disease (1). Familial factors are also evident from the identification of hereditary ovarian cancer syndrome, hereditary breast-ovarian syndrome, and Lynch II (colon carcinoma in association with ovarian cancer) (2). These syndromes characteristically produce ovarian carcinoma at a younger age (45–52 years old median versus 59 years old for other cases) and are associated with a positive family history.

Impact of age

Age is a significant factor in ovarian carcinoma. In terms of incidence, ovarian carcinoma becomes increasingly common from age 30 through age 80 (3). For women under age 50, the incidence of ovarian carcinoma is 20 per 100,000; whereas the incidence to 40 per 10,000 for women over age 50.

With reference to outcome, cancer registry data show that older patients exhibit a much higher incidence of advanced disease than do younger patients (41% of patients between 25 and 34 years of age with advanced disease as compared to 73% in patients older than age 85) (4). Extensive data from cooperative group trials also show that, independent of stage and comorbid conditions, older patients have poorer survival than younger patients; hence, older patients appear to have

more aggressive disease than their younger counterparts (5–6). Whether older patients respond more poorly to treatment than younger patients is obscured by the tendency of physicians to reduce chemotherapy dose intensity or to employ regimens regarded as less toxic but also less effective. The use of such "more conservative" regimens is contrary to scientific evidence which shows that older patients tolerate aggressive therapy as well as their younger counterparts (5,7–8).

Other prognostic factors

Other than age, the most significant prognostic factors for ovarian carcinoma are: histologic type and grade (9), extent of disease (stage), and volume of residual disease (10–13). Patients with serous or endometrioid tumors have a better prognosis than those with mucinous or clear cell lesions. More poorly differentiated tumors are associated with a poorer prognosis. The most important determinant of prognosis, however, is the extent of disease at the time of diagnosis as expressed in the FIGO staging system (Table 52.1) (4).

The FIGO staging system incorporates two important characteristics of ovarian carcinoma. First, the most common route of spread is peritoneal dissemination. Stage III, which includes those patients who have disseminated disease confined to the peritoneal cavity, is by far the most common stage at presentation. Secondly, among patients with stage III disease, volume of disease is an important determinant of response to chemotherapy and survival (those with nodules less than two centimeters have a higher response rate and a longer survival); hence, stage III is subdivided according to volume of disease at the time the abdomen is opened.

Clinical Presentation and Evaluation

Screening

Because ovarian carcinoma is an intraabdominal process with few specific early symptoms, a majority of patients present with advanced disease. Since regular pelvic examination has failed to yield a higher frequency of early diagnosis, more recent efforts have focused on serum CA-125 and transvaginal sonography (15).

CA-125 is a celomic epithelial marker elevated in more than 80% of patients with ovarian carcinoma, the frequency of elevation varying directly with the extent of disease from 50% in stage I to more than 90% in stages III and IV disease (16). The marker is also elevated in a number of benign gynecologic and other

Table 52.1 FIGO staging system for ovarian carcinoma (14).

Stage		Description
I		Growth limited to the ovaries
	A	One ovary; no ascites; capsule intact; no tumor on external surface
	B	Two ovaries; no ascites; capsule intact; no tumor on external surface
	C	One or both ovaries with either: surface tumor; ruptured capsule; or ascites or peritoneal washings with malignant cells
II		Pelvic extension
	A	Involvement of uterus and/or tubes
	B	Involvement of other pelvic tissues
	C	IIA or IIB with factors as in IC
III		Peritoneal implants outside pelvis and/or positive retroperitoneal or inguinal nodes
	A	Grossly limited to true pelvis; negative nodes; microscopic seeding of abdominal peritoneum
	B	Implants of abdominal peritoneum 2 cm or less; nodes negative
	C	Abdominal implants greater than 2 cm and/or positive retroperitoneal or inguinal nodes
IV		Distant metastases

conditions; hence, elevations are not specific for ovarian carcinoma. Two trials (15,17) assessing the value of CA-125 as a screening test demonstrate that the test can detect ovarian carcinoma with a specificity as high as 0.970; but sensitivity is lacking particularly in those patients with stage I disease where CA-125 is elevated in only 15–50% of clinically detectable tumors and even fewer with sonographically detectable tumors.

Transvaginal sonography is a second approach advocated for the early detection of ovarian carcinoma. In two trials of 1300 and 776 women respectively, a total of 5 stage I ovarian cancers were detected (18–19). In the larger of these two trials, 27 laparotomies were performed to detect two stage I cancers.

Because of the lack of sensitivity for early stage tumors and the relatively large number of laparotomies required to diagnose a single case of early stage ovarian carcinoma, CA-125 and transvaginal sonography cannot be recommended for routine screening at the present time. Randomized trials in a high-risk group are needed to determine whether these two approaches used together in a serial fashion constitute effective screen for ovarian carcinoma. Family history provides the means for selecting the high risk group to be investigated since patients with one or more relatives with ovarian carcinoma are at 2.9 to 4.5 fold increased risk for developing the disease.

Clinical presentation and evaluation

Patients usually present with non-specific symptoms such as a heavy sensation in the pelvis or increasing abdominal girth because of ascites. Although physical examination and various imaging techniques are employed in evaluation, all patients without demonstrated stage IV disease require an exploratory laparotomy to establish the diagnosis and extent of disease.

Management of Advanced Disease

Patients with advanced (stage III or IV) disease, unless stage IV is already established, undergo exploratory laparotomy which, in addition to establishing the extent of disease, affords the first step in therapy. The laparotomy is done through an incision sufficient to permit the exploration of the entire peritoneal cavity. In the absence of gross disease outside of the pelvis, multiple biopsies are taken to rule out microscopic disease. Finally, based on considerations noted above, an aggressive attempt at surgical cytoreduction is undertaken (20).

The mainstay of the treatment of advanced disease is systemic therapy. A number of drugs are active against ovarian carcinoma: platinum compounds, alkylating agents, taxol, doxorubicin, hexamethylmelamine, 5-fluorouracil, methotrexate, topotecan, oral etoposide, and tamoxifen (Table 52.2) (21–28). The standard of care for first-line therapy currently is a combination of paclitaxel 135 mg/m2 over 24 hours followed by cisplatin 75 mg/m2 with the combination repeated every three weeks for six cycles (Table 52.3) (29). This combination should yield regressions of 50% or greater in 75% of patients with large-volume disease, complete regression of disease in 40–50% of such patients, a pathologic complete response (disease-free at second-look laparotomy at the conclusion of chemotherapy) in

Table 52.2 Active systemic agents in celomic epithelial carcinoma of the ovary (21–28).

Patients	(Response Rate %)
Available Agents	
Alkylating Agents	1408 (33%)
Cisplatin	190 (32%)
Carboplatin	82 (24%)
Paclitaxel	189 (29%)
Doxorubicin	102 (33%)
5-Fluorouracil	126 (29%)
Methotrexate	34 (18%)
Mitomycin	49 (16%)
Hexamethylmelamine	215 (24%)
Oral Etoposide	70 (30%)
Topotecan	271 (19%)
Navelbine	38 (29%)
Gemcitabine	19 (16%)
Investigational Agents	
Prednimustine	36 (28%)
Dihydroxybusulfan	26 (27%)
Galactitol	39 (15%)
Hormones and Biologicals	
Progestins	176 (12%)
Antiestrogens	42 (19%)
Alpha Interferon	21 (19%)
Gamma Interferon	14 (29%)

Table 52.3 Gynecologic Oncology Group Protocol 111, a comparison of cisplatin plus either cyclophosphamide or paclitaxel (29).

Response	Cisplatin +* Cyclophosphamide	Cisplatin +** Paclitaxel
Complete Response	36 (31%)	51 (51%)
Partial Response	34 (29%)	22 (22%)
No Response	46 (40%)	27 (27%)
Response Rate	70 (60%)	73 (73%)
Total	116 (100%)	100 (100%)

*Cisplatin 75 mg/m2 plus Cyclophosphamide 750 mg/m2 intravenously every three weeks

**Taxol 135 mg/m2 intravenously over 24 hours followed by Cisplatin 75 mg/m2 intravenously every three weeks

***Clinical response and complete response (p=0.01) with cis/taxol are superior.

Table 52.4 Risk groups of patients with limited ovarian carcinoma (9).

Group	Characteristics
Low Risk	Grade 1 or 2 disease
	Intact capsule
	No tumor on external surface
	Negative peritoneal cytology
	No ascites
	Growth confined to ovaries
High Risk	Grade 3 disease
	Ruptured capsule
	Tumor on external surface
	Positive peritoneal cytology
	Ascites
	Growth outside ovaries

If any high-risk factors are present, the patient is considered high risk.

20–25%, a median progression-free survival of 18 months, and a median overall survival of 37 months. Modifications of this regimen under current investigation include: shortening (1–3 hour) or lengthening (96 hour) of the infusion length of paclitaxel, increasing the dose of paclitaxel (175 to 250 mg/m2), and substitution of carboplatin (AUC 5-7) for cisplatin. The value of these alterations remain investigational.

Other combinations which have been used, with somewhat less success, include: cisplatin plus cyclophosphamide, carboplatin plus cyclophosphamide, and cisplatin plus doxorubicin plus cyclophosphamide (30). In patients with small-volume disease, the frequency of pathologic complete response, the duration of response, and the overall survival will be significantly better than in patients with large-volume disease (10–13).

Management of Limited Disease

As is the case with advanced disease, exploratory laparotomy determines whether disease is truly confined to the ovaries (stage I) or pelvis (stage II) (9,31). Information from the laparotomy characterizes the patient as low risk for recurrence (grade 1 or 2, intracystic disease, no extraovarian disease, no ascites, and negative peritoneal cytology) or high risk (grade 3, extracystic disease, extraovarian disease, ascites, or positive peritoneal cytology) (Table 52.4) (9). Patients at low risk have a cure rate which exceeds 90% with total abdominal hysterectomy, bilateral salpingo-oophorectomy, and omentectomy alone and require no additional therapy. Those at high risk have a recurrence rate which may reach as high as 40% and should

Table 52.5 Recommendations for management of previously untreated patients.

Disease Status	Recommendation
Limited Disease	
Low Risk	Total abdominal hysterectomy, bilateral salpingo-oophorectomy, and observation
High Risk	Same surgery as low risk followed by adjuvant platinum-based chemotherapy
Advanced Disease	
Small Volume	Maximum surgical cytoreduction followed by Paclitaxel/Cisplatin
Large Volume	Paclitaxel/Cisplatin

receive additional therapy after surgical resection. Accepted therapy is intravenous platinum-based chemotherapy (32).

Table 52.5 summarizes the front-line management of both advanced and limited disease based on current evidence.

Salvage Therapy

For patients who recur after initial therapy, appropriate management is determined by response to initial treatment (Table 52.6) (33). Patients who initially respond to platinum-based chemotherapy and then recur more than six months after completion of initial treatment should be considered "platinum-sensitive." Such patients respond well to repeat treatment with platinum-based therapy. On the other hand, those who have progressive disease on platinum-based treatment, who exhibit persistent disease at the end of initial platinum-based therapy, or who recur within six months respond infrequently to repeat platinum-based treatment and should be considered "platinum-resistant." Such patients, if they have not received taxol as a part of initial therapy, should be treated with paclitaxel. Other agents which have been reported to yield at least some responses include: oral etoposide, topotecan, ifosfamide, hexamethylmelamine, navelbine, and tamoxifen.

Table 52.6 Gynecologic Oncology Group definitions of platinum-sensitive and platinum-resistant ovarian carcinoma (33).

Platinum Sensitive	Initial Response to Platinum
	Platinum-Free Interval >6 Months
Platinum Resistant	Progression on Platinum
	Stable Disease on Prior Platinum
	Relapse <6 Months after Prior Platinum

At the present time, data do not support the use outside of clinical trials of either intraperitoneal therapy or high-dose chemotherapy with autologous bone marrow support as a part of either first-line or salvage treatment. Intraperitoneal cisplatin can induce responses in patients who have had prior platinum-based chemotherapy and remain platinum sensitive; and one major randomized phase III trial suggests that intraperitoneal cisplatin yields a modest, statistically significant improvement in survival compared to intravenous cisplatin (34). Because of statistical problems with the phase III trial, routine clinical application of intraperitoneal therapy should await a confirmatory trial. The use of high-dose chemotherapy supported by stem cells has been tested only in phase II trials in patients who have had prior chemotherapy. This approach remains an interesting concept with insufficient evidence to support its use outside of clinical trials.

Management of the High-Risk Patient

Much attention has been recently directed to individuals at high risk for the development of ovarian carcinoma. The overall lifetime risk for the development of ovarian carcinoma for women in the United States is approximately 1.4% (one chance in 70). Reasonable evidence supports an enhanced risk for women with one first-order relative (mother or sibling) which approximates 5% (2). For women with two or more first-order relatives with ovarian carcinoma, the risk is considerably higher (estimates range from 10% to more than 50% with the actual level of risk not as yet clear) (35).

As has been noted earlier, no screening test of proven efficacy is available. In the absence of an effective screening test, some have suggested that women at high risk should undergo prophylactic oophorectomy (35–36). While such an approach certainly has appeal, recent reports of celomic epithelial carcinomas of the peritoneal surface in women who have undergone prophylactic oophorectomy raise questions about whether such an approach is truly effective. Six such cases have been reported among 324 high-risk women who have undergone prophylactic oophorectomy for an overall incidence of 1.8% (36). Although such a rate is lower than would be anticipated in a high risk group, further follow-up is needed before any conclusions are drawn.

For the present, no dogmatic recommendations can be made. Issues regarding the use of CA-125 and transvaginal sonography for screening and prophylactic oophorectomy in women at high risk for developing ovarian cancer should be discussed with patients, but such approaches cannot be recommended for widespread application based on currently available data.

Squamous Cell Carcinoma of the Uterine Cervix

Cancer of the uterine cervix includes a variety of histologies: squamous cell carcinoma, adenocarcinoma, adenosquamous carcinoma, small cell carcinoma, clear cell carcinoma, and mixed histologies. The most common of these is squamous cell carcinoma which accounts for more than 80% of all cases. The ensuing discussion does not address differences in management among the various histologies because the frequency of non-squamous histology is too low to permit separate studies.

General Considerations

Etiology

Although the etiology of squamous cell carcinoma of the uterine cervix is not fully understood, certain facts are clear. The process exhibits the epidemiology of a venereal disease (37) with associated factors including lower socioeconomic status, onset of coitus at an early age, frequent coitus, multiple sexual partners, and coitus with an uncircumcised partner or one who practices poor genital hygiene. There is also an intimate connection between the disease and human papilloma virus (HPV) which, as would be expected from epidemiologic evidence, is believed to be transmitted by sexual intercourse (38).

Preinvasive disease

Squamous cell carcinoma of the uterine cervix is associated with a well-described premalignant state which is variously described as cervical intraepithelial neoplasia (CIN 1–3) or a squamous intraepithelial lesion (SIL — low-grade or LGSIL and high-grade or HGSIL) (39). These lesions can be detected by cervical cytology, which constitutes the most effective screening test for cancer. The process by which cells go from mild through severe dysplasia and carcinoma-in-situ to frankly invasive cancer usually takes years; hence, there is a significant window of opportunity for early diagnosis and cure of the vast majority of women with the disease.

Staging

The most important prognostic feature of invasive disease is the extent of disease at the time of diagnosis as expressed in the FIGO staging system (Table 52.7) (40). This clinical staging system will form the basis for treatment selection. An appropriate staging evaluation should include: careful history and physical to include a thorough pelvic and rectal examination, complete blood count, tests to evaluate hepatic and renal status, urinalysis, flexible sigmoidoscopy, barium enema, intravenous pyelogram, computerized tomographic scan of the abdomen and pelvis, and histologic confirmation of malignancy and cell type. Histologic confirmation may require: cytologic smears, colposcopy, conization, punch biopsies of four quadrants of the cervix, or dilatation and curettage as well as cystoscopy. While the extent of the workup will be determined by findings of each procedure, it must yield sufficient information to stage the patient accurately.

Impact of age

Because of its relationship to sexual activity, carcinoma of the cervix tends to occur at a younger average age (50 years) than either ovarian or endometrial carcinoma. This has prompted physicians to perform fewer Pap smears in older women (11.8 per 1000 visits in

Table 52.7 FIGO staging system for cervix cancer (40).

Stage	Description
0	Carcinoma-in-situ
I	Cervix carcinoma confined to uterus (disregard extension to corpus)
IA	Invasive carcinoma diagnosed by microscopy only
IAI	Minimal microscopic stromal invasion
IA2	Invasive component less than 5mm depth from base of epithelium and 7mm or less horizontal spread
IB	Larger than IA2
II	Invasion beyond uterus but not to pelvic wall or lower third of vagina
IIA	No parametrial invasion
IIB	Parametrial invasion
III	Extension to pelvic wall and/or involvement of lower third of vagina or hydronephrosis or non-functioning kidney
IIIA	Lower third of vagina only
IIIB	Pelvic wall involvement or hydronephrosis or non-functioning kidney
IVA	Involvement of mucosa of bladder or rectum
IVB	Extension beyond true pelvis

women age 65 and older) than in younger women (121.3–143.4 per 1000 visits in women ages 25–44). As a result, the incidence of localized disease drops from 98% in younger women to 59% in older women with a corresponding rise in the death rate (41). Adding to this problem are technical difficulties in older women such as problems in identifying the squamocolumnar junction and the presence of a stenotic atrophic cervix.

The choice of therapy for older women also represents an age-related problem in carcinoma of the cervix. Current practice tends to avoid radical surgery in women over the age of 65 and to employ radiotherapy instead. Studies, however, do not support such practice. Two trials of radical hystrectomy and pelvic lymphadenectomy show similar survival rates in elderly and younger patients with no significant differences in morbidity and mortality from the surgery (42–43). In contrast, three studies showed an increase in complications in elderly patients with radiotherapy for carcinoma of the cervix (44–45). These data suggest that decisions regarding treatment in elderly patients should be based on factors other than age and, for those without major medical problems, should not differ from decisions in younger patients.

Management of Limited Disease

Patients who have disease confined to the cervix, detectable by microscopy only, and limited in invasion to 5 millimeters or less in depth taken from the base of

Table 52.8 Management of cervix cancer by stage of disease.

Disease Status	Recommendations
Preinvasive or IA	Total abdominal hysterectomy; lesser procedures in selected cases of preinvasive disease
Stage IB/IIA	Radiotherapy with or without surgery except in selected cases appropriate for radical hysterectomy; role of chemotherapy undetermined
Stage IIB/III/IVA	Radiotherapy; randomized trials support the use of concurrent chemoradiation with cisplatin/5-fluorouracil plus radiotherapy
Stage IVB or Recurrent	Systemic therapy with a combination to include a platinum compound plus ifosfamide

Table 52.9 Active drugs in cervix carcinoma (21,54).

Drug	Response (%)
Alkylating Agents	
Cyclophosphamide	38/251(15%)
Chlorambucil	11/44 (25%)
Melphalan	4/20 (20%)
Ifosfamide	25/157(15%)
Dibromodulcitol	23/102(29%)
Galactitol	7/36 (19%)
Heavy Metal Complexes	
Cisplatin	190/815(23%)
Carboplatin	27/175(15%)
Antibiotics	
Doxorubicin	45/266(20%)
Porfiromycin	17/78 (22%)
Antimetabolites	
5-Fluorouracil	29/142(20%)
Methotrexate	17/96 (18%)
Baker's Antifol	5/32 (16%)
Plant Alkaloids	
Vincristine	10/55 (18%)
Vindesine	5/21 (24%)
Other Agents	
ICRF-159	5/28 (18%)
Hexamethylmelamine	12/64 (19%)
Paclitaxel	9/52 (18%)

the epithelium and 7 millimeters or less in horizontal spread have either stage 0 (carcinoma-in-situ), stage IA1 (minimal microscopic stromal invasion), or stage IA2 (more invasive up to the limits described). The definitive treatment for these lesions is total abdominal hysterectomy, although non-surgical candidates can be treated with radiation therapy (46). Selected patients, in particular those with carcinoma-*in-situ* and those with minimally invasive lesions (less than one millimeter in depth), can be managed with more conservative measures such as conization provided all margins are clear (Table 52.8) (47).

Management of Locoregionally Advanced Disease

Patients with stages IB-IVA disease have more advanced disease still confined to the pelvis. In addition to the extent of pelvic disease, the status of the para-aortic lymph nodes is an important prognostic factor (48). Management of patients with uninvolved para-aortic nodes will be discussed stage-by-stage followed by consideration of the management of those with involved para-aortic nodes.

For patients with stage IB or IIA disease, either pelvic radiotherapy or radical hysterectomy constitutes reasonable treatment. Five-year survival should exceed 80% in carefully staged patients with either approach. Current research is directed to evaluation of combined modality regimens using either surgery plus radiation or platinum-based chemotherapy integrated with either surgery or radiation therapy (49–50).

For patients with more advanced locoregional disease (stages IIB-IVA), solid evidence from randomized trials supports the enhanced effectiveness of concurrent chemoradiation. GOG studies have demonstrated superiority for hydroxyurea 4 grams/m2 twice weekly during radiation over radiation alone and for radiation

concurrent with 5-fluorouracil plus cisplatin over concurrent hydroxyurea plus radiation. The standard of care is thus concurrent chemoradiation with cisplatin/5-fluorouracil plus radiation (48,51–52).

In patients with positive para-aortic nodes, survival is much worse (53). The standard approach to these patients is extension of the radiation port to include the para-aortic node area. Five-year survival is 10–15%. There are no well-designed randomized studies of systemic therapy in combination with radiation, although the rationale for such an approach is excellent.

Management of Advanced or Recurrent Disease

Patients who present with stage IVB disease or who recur after initial therapy for more limited disease are candidates for systemic therapy. There are a number of chemotherapeutic agents with moderate activity, (21,54) but two drugs in particular have consistently yielded single-agent response rates in excess of 20%: the platinum compounds and ifosfamide.

Table 52.10 Results of Gynecologic Oncology Group Protocol 110, a randomized trial of patients with advanced or recurrent squamous cell carcinoma of the cervix (58)

Regimen*	Response
Cisplatin 50 mg/m2 IV	9CR,16PR/140 (18%)
Cisplatin 50 mg/m2 IV + Ifosfamide 5 gm/m2 IV 24 hours	19CR,28PR/151 (31%)
Cisplatin 50 mg/m2 IV + Mitolactol 180 mg/m2 po days 2–6	14CR,17PR/147 (21%)

*Cisplatin is given as an infusion at a rate of 1 mg/min, ifosfamide as a 24 hour infusion with mesna. All regimens are repeated every three weeks.

**Progression-free survival (4–5 months) and overall survival (8 months) were not significantly different among the regimens.

A number of studies of combination chemotherapy have been reported; virtually all of these are uncontrolled trials in selected patients and are very difficult to interpret. Combinations which are of continuing interest include: ifosfamide plus a platinum compound with or without bleomycin (55–56) and a platinum compound plus 5-fluorouracil (57). The Gynecologic Oncology Group recently completed a randomized trial in which a combination of ifosfamide plus cisplatin produced a superior response rate as compared to cisplatin alone with no difference in progression-free or overall survival (Table 52.10) (58).

In summary, the treatment of choice for patients with advanced or recurrent disease at present is combination chemotherapy with ifosfamide plus cisplatin. This combination should yield a response rate of 31%, a clinical complete response rate of 13%, a progression-free survival of 4.6 months and an overall survival of 8.3 months.

Endometrial Carcinoma

The more than 30,000 new cases of endometrial carcinoma in the United States each year make this tumor the most common invasive malignancy of the female genital tract. Although the cure rate is high at 66%, a significant proportion of patients will recur and die of their disease; hence, efforts at treatment must focus on systemic therapy as well as the management of localized disease.

General Considerations

Endometrial carcinoma is a disease primarily of menopausal and postmenopausal women with a median patient age of 61 years. Personal risk factors include: obesity, nulliparity, late menopause, diabetes, hypertension, immunodeficiency, and exogenous estrogens (59). The most common presenting manifestation is dysfunctional uterine bleeding. Such bleeding in postmenopausal women results from malignancies approximately 20% of the time; a majority of these will be endometrial carcinoma. In contrast, over 90% of endometrial carcinomas present with dysfunctional bleeding.

Impact of age

Endometrial carcinoma is a disease of older women. There is no evidence, however, that age alone should be a consideration in management decisions. Differences in stage at presentation for older versus younger patients appear to relate entirely to a less aggressive approach to the evaluation of postmenopausal bleeding in older patients. Although adverse effects associated with treatment are more common in older patients, there is no evidence that survival is compromised. Factors other than age should drive management decisions.

Pathology

Endometrial carcinoma most commonly is adenocarcinoma which accounts for 70% of cases (60). Most of the remainder will have adenocarcinoma mixed with either squamous metaplasia (adenoacanthoma) or squamous carcinoma (adenosquamous carcinoma). After stage and grade are considered, the most common 3 cell types have little bearing on prognosis or approach to therapy.

Clinical course

Endometrial carcinoma arises from the glandular component of the endometrium. Development of malignant changes may be preceded by endometrial hyperplasia with dysplastic changes (adenomatous hyperplasia) (61). Early growth within the uterine cavity yields an exophytic, friable mass with spontaneous bleeding. Both vertical and horizontal spread occur with involvement of the myometrium and the cervix. Spreading beyond the uterus occurs as a result of: lymphatic spread to parametrial, pelvic, inguinal, and para-aortic nodes; hematogenous dissemination to distant sites such as the lungs, liver, and bones; and peritoneal implantation from either transtubal spread or vertical penetration of the entire thickness of the uterine wall.

Recurrence after initial treatment is most commonly extra pelvic in such locations as lungs, liver, bone, abdominal cavity, and lymph nodes. A majority of failures will occur within 2 years of initial treatment.

Prognostic Factors

The most important determinant of prognosis is the extent of the disease at presentation as reflected in the staging system of the International Federation of Gynecology and Obstetrics (FIGO) (Table 52.11) (62). Stage I disease is by far the most common stage at presentation (75%) with an excellent 5-year survival of 76%. Survival decreases dramatically as initial extent of disease increases, but the overall 5-year survival is 66% as a result of the frequency of stage I disease. Stage I and II disease is considered limited disease, whereas

Table 52.11 FIGO staging system for endometrial carcinoma (62).

Stage	Description
Stage 0	Carcinoma *in situ*. Histologic findings suspicious for malignancy
Stage I	Carcinoma confined to corpus
IAG123	Tumor limited to endometrium
IBG123	Invasion to <1/2 myometrium
ICG123	Invasion to >1/2 myometrium
Stage II	Carcinoma involving corpus and cervix but not extending outside uterus
IIAG123	Endocervical glandular involvement only
IIBG123	Cervical stromal invasion
Stage III	Carcinoma extending outside uterus but not outside true pelvis
IIIAG123	Tumor invades serosa or adnexae or positive peritoneal cytology
IIIBG123	Vaginal metastases
IIICG123	Metastases to pelvic or para-aortic lymph nodes
Stage IV	Carcinoma extending outside true pelvis or involving bladder or rectal mucosa
IVAG123	Tumor invasion of bladder and/or bowel mucosa
IVB	Distant metastases including intra-abdominal and/or inguinal lymph nodes

Table 52.12 Risk groups based on pathologic variables in patients with limited endometrial carcinoma (63).

Risk Category	Pathologic Features
High*	Grade 3 lesion
	Grade 1 or 2 lesion with deep myometrial invasion
	Positive pelvic and/or para-aortic lymph nodes
	Positive peritoneal cytology
	Stromal invasion of the cervix
	Extrauterine spread
Low**	Grade 1 or 2 lesion without deep myometrial invasion
	Negative peritoneal cytology
	No stromal invasion of the cervix
	No extrauterine spread

*One or more factors present

**All factors present

1 or 2 lesion with myometrial invasion, a grade 1 lesion with deep myometrial invasion, positive pelvic and/or para-aortic lymph nodes, positive peritoneal cytology, stromal invasion of the cervix, or extrauterine spread.

Factors in advanced disease

Patients who present with advanced (stage III or IV) or recurrent disease fall into two prognostic categories according to site of disease. Those with locoregional disease only (confined to the pelvis) account for 40% of these patients and have a distinctly better outlook than those with distant disease with or without locoregional involvement.

Diagnosis and Evaluation

Patients with dysfunctional uterine bleeding should have a thorough evaluation, the key to which is obtaining an adequate endometrial tissue sample. The Pap smear, the simplest technique, suffers from a low diagnostic accuracy of 40%. Aspiration techniques in the ambulatory setting yield better accuracy of 70%, but a negative result does not rule out endometrial carcinoma. A more accurate and complete evaluation is provided by dilatation and fractional curettage which allows for assessment for endocervical involvement.

Pretreatment evaluation should delineate those disease features essential to assignment of stage and prognostic category. This information will then be used to make appropriate management decisions.

Management of Limited Disease

Patients with limited (clinical stage I or II) endometrial

stage III and IV disease is regarded as advanced disease.

Factors in limited disease

Patients with limited disease are at low risk or high risk for recurrence based on features of the primary lesion and its regional spread (60,63). Six pathological features determine prognostic categories which form the basis for a rational approach to management: histologic grade, depth of myometrial invasion, involvement of pelvic and/or para-aortic lymph nodes, peritoneal cytology, adnexal spread, and involvement of the cervix (Table 52.12).

Using these pathologic features, patients at low risk for recurrence are those with all of the following features: either a grade 1 lesion without deep myometrial invasion or grade 2 lesion with no myometrial invasion, negative peritoneal cytology, no stromal invasion of the cervix, and no extrauterine spread. Those at high risk for recurrence include all other clinical stage I and all clinical stage II patients who will exhibit one or more of the following factors: a grade 3 lesion, a grade

Table 52.13 Management recommendations for endometrial carcinoma.

Disease Status	Recommendations
Limited Disease Low Risk	Total abdominal hysterectomy, bilateral salpingo-oophorectomy
High Risk	Same surgery as low risk followed by adjuvant therapy; no form of adjuvant therapy, however, shown to be of benefit
Advanced Disease Locoregional Disease	If confined to uterus, ovaries, and fallopian tubes, radical hysterectomy + pelvic node dissection followed by pelvic radiation; for others, radiotherapy
Disseminated Disease	Systemic therapy: progestins if well-differentiated or receptor positive, doxorubicin plus cisplatin for others

Table 52.14 Active single drugs in endometrial carcinoma (21,65–75).

Drug	Patients	Response Rate (%)
Medroxyprogesterone Acetate	609	20%
Tamoxifen	115	18%
Doxorubicin	161	26%
Cisplatin	124	24%
Carboplatin	52	31%
Ifosfamide	33	24%
Paclitaxel	28	36%

carcinoma constitute the vast majority of patients and have an excellent chance at cure. The management of an individual patient will depend upon the patient's risk status (Table 52.13). Virtually all patients with limited disease should have surgical resection of the primary disease unless the operative risk is unacceptably high. The surgical procedure should include a total abdominal hysterectomy and bilateral salpingo-oophorectomy as well as assessment of peritoneal cytology and pelvic and para-aortic lymph nodes.

Low-risk patients

Patients at low risk for recurrence have greater than 90% chance of remaining disease-free beyond 5 years when treated with surgery alone (63). Appropriate management is therefore total abdominal hysterectomy and bilateral salpingo-oophorectomy with assessment for high-risk features.

High-risk patients

Patients at high risk for recurrence have been treated with a variety of approaches combining surgery and radiotherapy including: surgery preceded by radium and/or external beam, surgery followed by radium and/or external beam, and surgery both preceded and followed by radiation therapy. Dose and schedule for radiation have varied widely. No concurrently controlled studies and no good uncontrolled data currently available show conclusive survival benefit from the use of radiation in combination with surgery, although preoperative radiotherapy does reduce the incidence of vaginal recurrence (from 12 to 2%) (64). Standard treatment for the high-risk patient, however, is a combination of surgery and radiation therapy. The use of systemic adjuvant therapy is not warranted.

Management of Advanced or Recurrent Disease

The management of patients with advanced (clinical stage III or IV) or recurrent endometrial carcinoma is determined by whether the disease is confined to the pelvis and/or abdomen or includes distant spread (Table 52.13).

Locoregional disease

Careful evaluation should rule out distant spread to such sites as the lungs, liver, abdominal cavity, and bone before assigning a patient to those with locoregional involvement only. Treatment is radiotherapy with or without surgery. Patients with the best outlook are those with disease confined clinically to uterus, ovaries, and/or fallopian tubes. Such patients should undergo a radical hysterectomy and bilateral pelvic lymphadenectomy followed by postoperative pelvic radiation with an expected five-year survival of 50%. For patients with parametrial extension, vaginal involvement, or other pelvic extension, radiotherapy is the initial treatment modality with expected five-year survivals between 25 and 50%.

Disseminated disease

Patients with disseminated disease are candidates for systemic therapy with either hormones or chemotherapy (Table 52.14). With regard to hormonal therapy, the most commonly employed agent is progestin. Recent series demonstrate response rates of 20–24% with oral preparations (65–66). Median duration of response is 3–4 months, median survival 9–10 months. A randomized trial looking at standard versus high-dose progestin therapy showed no advantage to the higher doses (66). Standard therapy is therefore either medroxyprogesterone 200 mg/day orally or megestrol acetate 160 mg/day orally.

A number of factors potentially predictive of response to hormonal therapy have been evaluated (67). The two factors which predict best are histologic grade (the better the differentiation the greater the frequency of response) and hormone receptor status (positive estrogen and progesterone receptor assays are associated with higher response rates) (21).

Table 52.15 Gynecologic Oncology Group Protocol 107: a randomized trial of doxorubicin with or without cisplatin (76).

Response Status	Doxorubicin	Doxorubicin/Cisplatin
Complete response	10 (8%)	23 (21%)
Partial response	25 (20%)	25 (23%)
Stable disease	60 (47%)	46 (42%)
Increasing disease	32 (25%)	16 (15%)
Total	127 (100%)	110 (100%)

*The overall response rate of 44% with the combination is significantly superior to the 27% with doxorubicin. The progression-free interval with the combination is also superior.

Among other hormonal therapies, only tamoxifen has been studied in endometrial carcinoma. Some studies suggest that tamoxifen is active; but a recent, larger trial shows insignifcant activity either in patients with no prior hormonal therapy or in patients with prior progestins (68–69).

Chemotherapy

Chemotherapy has been studied intensively only in the last two decades. Active drugs identified to date include doxorubicin, (65,70) the platinum compounds, (71–73) ifosfamide, (74) and paclitaxel, (75) each with response rates in excess of 20%, median durations of response ranging from four to seven months, and median survivals of nine to twelve months (Table 52.14).

Trials of combination chemotherapy in endometrial carcinoma have, for the most part, been single-arm studies of relatively small numbers of patients, trials that permit no definitive conclusions about the relative merits of the combination versus single agent therapy. A recently completed randomized trial comparing doxorubicin alone versus doxorubicin plus cisplatin showed superior response rate and progression-free survival for patients receiving the combination regimen (Table 52.15) (76). The treatment of choice for patients with advanced or recurrent disease no longer responsive to hormonal agents is therefore a combination of doxorubicin 60 mg/m2 plus cisplatin 50 mg/m2 intravenously every three weeks.

Summary

The proper clinical approach to endometrial carcinoma rests on attention to early diagnosis. Any patient with dysfunctional uterine bleeding must be evaluated with uterine tissue sampling and, in most instances, dilatation and fractional curettage. Once a diagnosis of endometrial carcinoma has been made, careful clinical staging is essential with attention to significant pathological factors in patients with clinical stage I disease: histological grade, depth of myometrial penetration, status of pelvic and para-aortic lymph nodes, peritoneal cytology, cervix involvement, and extrauterine spread.

Patients with limited (clinical stage I and II) disease will be managed with surgery and/or radiotherapy. Patients at low risk for recurrence require total abdominal hysterectomy and bilateral salpingo-oophorectomy only and should have a 5-year survival rate which exceeds 90%. High-risk patients are currently managed with a combination of surgery plus radiotherapy with the specifics of the regimen varying from institution to institution. Systemic therapy has no proven role in early disease.

Patients with advanced or recurrent disease should be evaluated to determine whether disease is confined to pelvis alone or involves extrapelvic sites. In the former case, radiotherapy with or without surgery has potential to yield long-term survivors. In the latter case, systemic therapy is required. Active systemic agents include progestins, doxorubicin, the platinum compounds, ifosfamide, and paclitaxel. Current recommendations are to use hormonal agents in patients with receptor positive or well-differentiated disease and to employ cytotoxic drugs in patients with receptor negative or poorly differentiated disease or those patients no longer responsive to hormonal therapy. The chemotherapy of choice is doxorubicin plus cisplatin.

References

1. Cassagrande JT, Pike MC, Russ RK, *et al.* Incessant ovulation and ovarian cancer. *Lancet* **2**: 170, 1979.
2. Lynch HT, Watson P, Lynch JF, *et al.* Hereditary ovarian cancer: heterogeneity in age at onset. *Cancer* **71**: 573–581, 1993.
3. Yancik R. Ovarian cancer: age contrasts in incidence, histology, disease stage at diagnosis, and mortality. *Cancer* **71**: 517–23, 1993.
4. Grover SA, Cook EF, Adam J, *et al.* Delayed diagnosis of gynecologic tumors in elderly women: relation to national medical practice patterns. *Am J Med* **86**: 151–7, 1989.
5. Thigpen T, Brady M, Omura G, *et al.* Age as a prognostic factor in ovarian carcinoma: the Gynecologic Oncology Group experience. *Cancer* **71**: 606–614, 1993.
6. Alberts DS, Dahlberg S, Green SJ, *et al.* Analysis of patient age as an independent prognostic factor for survival in a phase III study of cisplatin-cyclophosphamide versus carboplatin-cyclophosphamide in stages III (suboptimal) and IV ovarian cancer: a Southwest Oncology Group study. *Cancer* **71**: 618–27, 1993.
7. Edmondson J, Su J and Krook JE. Treatment of ovarian cancer in elderly women: Mayo Clinic — North Central Cancer Treatment Group studies. *Cancer* **71**: 615–7, 1993.
8. Bicher A, Sarosy G, Kohn E, *et al.* Age does not influence taxol dose intensity in recurrent carcinoma of the ovary. *Cancer* **71**: 594–600, 1993.
9. Young RC, Walton L, Ellenberg SS, Homesley HD, Wilbanks GD, Decker DG, Miller A, Park R and Major F Jr. Adjuvant therapy in stage I and stage II epithelial ovarian cancer. Results of two prospective randomized trials. *New Eng J Med* **322**: 1021–7, 1990.
10. Omura G, Blessing J, Ehrlich C, *et al.* A randomized trial of cyclophosphamide and doxorubicin with or without cisplatin in advanced ovarian carcinoma. *Cancer* **57**: 1725–1730, 1986.
11. Ehrlich C, Einhorn L, Williams S, *et al.* Chemotherapy for stage III-IV epithelial ovarian cancer with cis-dichlorodiammine-platinum (II), adriamycin, and cyclophosphamide: a preliminary report. *Cancer Treat Rep* **63**: 281–288, 1979.
12. Greco F, Julian C, Richardson R, *et al.* Advanced ovarian cancer: brief intensive combination chemotherapy and second-look operation. *Obstet Gynecol* **58**: 199–205, 1981.

13. Young R, Howser D, Myers C, et al. Combination chemotherapy (CHex-UP) with intraperitoneal maintenance in advanced ovarian adenocarcinoma. Proc ASCO 22: 465, 1981.

14. The new FIGO stage grouping for primary carcinoma of the ovary (1985). Gynecol Oncol 25: 383, 1986.

15. Van Nagell JR, DePriest PD, Gallion HH and Pavlik EJ. Ovarian cancer screening. Cancer 71: 1523–8, 1993.

16. Jacobs J and Bast R. The CA-125 tumor-associated antigen: a review of the literature. Hum Reprod 4: 1–12, 1989.

17. Jacobs I, Bridges J, Reynolds C, et al. Multimodal approach to screening for ovarian cancer. Lancet 2: 268–71, 1988.

18. Van Nagell JR, DePriest PD, Puls LE, et al. Ovarian cancer screening in asymptomatic postmenopausal women by transvaginal sonography. Cancer 68: 458–62, 1991.

19. Bourne TH, Whitehead M, Campbell S, et al. Ultrasound screening for familial ovarian cancer. Gynecol Oncol 43: 92–7, 1991.

20. Hoskins WJ. Surgical staging and cytoreductive surgery of epithelial ovarian cancer. Cancer 71: 1534–40, 1993.

21. Thigpen JT. Chemotherapy of cancers of the female genital tract. In: Perry M, ed, The Chemotherapy Source Book, Williams and Wilkins, Baltimore, pp. 1039–1065, 1992.

22. Rose P, Blessing J, Mayer A and Homesley H. Prolonged oral etoposide as second line therapy for platinum resistant and platinum sensitive ovarian carcinoma: a Gynecologic Oncology Group study. Proc ASCO 15: 282, 1996.

23. Gordon A, Bookman M, Malmstrom H, et al. Efficacy of topotecan in advanced epithelial ovarian cancer after failure of platinum and paclitaxel: International Topotecan Study Group trial. Proc ASCO 15: 282, 1996.

24. Carmichael J, Gordon A, Malfetano J, et al. Topotecan, a new active drug vs paclitaxel in advanced epithelial ovarian carcinoma: International Topotecan Study Group trial. Proc ASCO 15: 283, 1996.

25. Ten Bokkel Huinink W, Gore M, Bolis G, et al. A phase II trial of topotecan for the treatment of relapsed advanced ovarian carcinoma. Proc ASCO 15: 284, 1996.

26. Hochster H, Speyer J, Wadler S, et al. Phase II study of topotecan 21-day infusion in platinum-treated ovarian cancer: a highly active regimen. Proc ASCO 15: 285, 1996.

27. Burger R, Burman S, White R and DiSaia P. Phase II trial of navelbine in advanced epithelial ovarian cancer. Proc ASCO 15: 286, 1996.

28. Underhill C, Parnis F, Highley M, et al. A phase II study of gemcitabine in previously untreated patients with advanced epithelial ovarian cancer. Proc ASCO 15: 290, 1996.

29. McGuire WP, Hoskins WJ, Brady MF, et al. Cyclophosphamide and cisplatin compared with paclitaxel and cisplatin in patients with stage III and stage IV ovarian cancer. New Eng J Med 334: 1–6, 1996.

30. McGuire WP. Primary treatment of epithelial ovarian malignancies. Cancer 71: 1541–1550, 1993.

31. Day TG and Smith JP. Diagnosis and staging of ovarian carcinoma. Semin Oncol 2: 217, 1975.

32. Bolis G, Colombo N, Favalli G, et al. Randomized multicenter clinical trials in stage I epithelial ovarian cancer. Proc ASCO 11: 225, 1992.

33. Thigpen JT, Vance RB and Khansur T. Second-line chemotherapy for recurrent carcinoma of the ovary. Cancer 71: 1559–64, 1993.

34. Alberts D, Liu P, Hannigan E, et al. Phase III study of intraperitoneal cisplatin/intravenous cyclophosphamide vs IV cisplatin/IV cyclophosphamide in patients with optimal disease stage III ovarian cancer: a SWOG-GOG-ECOG intergroup study. Proc ASCO 14: 273, 1995.

35. Piver MS, Baker TR, Jishi MF, et al. Familial ovarian cancer: a report of 658 families from the Gilda Radner Familial Ovarian Cancer Registry (1981–1991). Cancer 71: 582–588, 1993.

36. Piver MS, Jishi MF, Tsukada Y, et al. Primary peritoneal carcinoma after oophorectomy in women with a family history of ovarian cancer. Cancer 71: 2751–2755, 1993.

37. Keighley E. Carcinoma of the cervix among prostitutes in a women's prison. Br J Vener Dis 44: 254–255, 1968.

38. Boon ME, Susanti I, Tasche MJA and Kok KP. Human papillomavirus-associated male and female genital carcinomas in a Hindu population: the male as a vector and victim. Cancer 64: 559- 565, 1989.

39. Richart RM and Wright TC. Controversies in the management of low-grade cervical intraepithelial neoplasia. Cancer 71: 1413–21, 1993.

40. Beahrs OH, Henson DE, Hutter RVP and Myers MH. Manual for Staging of Cancer, 3rd edition. Philadelphia: JB Lippincott, pp. 151–3, 1988.

41. Grover SA, Cook EF, Adams J, et al. Delayed diagnosis of gynecologic tumors in elderly women: relation to national medical practice patterns. Am J Med 86: 151–157, 1989.

42. Fuchtner C, Manetta A, Walker JL, et al. Radial hysterectomy in the elderly patient: analysis of morbidity. Am J Obstet Gynecol 166: 593–597, 1992.

43. Kinney WK, Egorshin EV and Podratz KC. Wertheim hysterectomy in the geriatric population. Gynecol Oncol 31: 227, 1984.

44. Grant PT, Jeffrey JF, Fraser RC, et al. Pelvic radiation therapy for gynecologic malignancy in geriatric patients. Gynecol Oncol 33: 185–188, 1989.

45. McGonigle KF, Lavey RS, Juillard GJF, et al. Complications of pelvic radiation therapy for gynecologic malignancies in elderly women. Int J Gynecol Cancer 6: 149–155, 1996.

46. Grigsby PW and Perez CA. Radiotherapy alone for medically inoperable carcinoma of the cervix: stage IA and carcinoma-in-situ. Int J Radiat Oncol Biol Phys 21: 375–378, 1991.

47. Kolstad P. Folow-up study of 232 patients with stage IA1 and 411 patients with stage IA2 squamous cell carcinoma of the cervix (microinvasive carcinoma). Gynecol Oncol 33: 265–272, 1989.

48. Stehman F, Bundy B, Keys H, et al. A randomized trial of hydroxyurea versus misonidazole adjunct to radiation therapy in carcinoma of the cervix. Amer J Obstet Gynecol 159: 87-94, 1988.

49. Averette HE, Nguyen HN, Donato DM, et al. Radical hysterectomy for invasive cervical cancer. Cancer 71: 1422–37, 1993.

50. Marcial VA and Marcial LV. Radiation therapy of cervical cancer. Cancer 71: 1438–45, 1993.

51. Hreshchyshyn M, Aron B, Boronow R, et al. Hydroxyurea or placebo combined with radiation to treat stages IIIB and IV cervical cancer confined to the pelvis. Int J Radiation Oncology Biol Phys 5: 317–322, 1979.

52. Bundy B. Personal communication based on GOG data.

53. DiSaia P, Bundy B, Curry S, et al. Phase III study on the treatment of women with cervical cancer, stage IIB, IIIB, and IVA (confined to the pelvis and/or periaortic nodes), with radiotherapy alone versus radio therapy plus immunotherapy with intravenous Corynebacterium parvum: a Gynecologic Oncology Group study. Gynecol Oncol 26: 386–397, 1987.

54. McGuire WP, Blessing JA, Moore D, et al. Paclitaxel has moderate activity in squamous cervix cancer: a Gynecologic Oncology Group study. J Clin Oncol 14: 792–795, 1996.

55. Lara P, Garcia-Puche J, Pedraza V. Cisplatin-ifosfamide as neoadjuvant chemotherapy in stage IIIB cervical uterine squamous-cell carcinoma. Cancer Chemother Pharmacol 26: S36-S38, 1990.

56. Buxton E, Meanwell C, Hilton C, et al. Combination bleomycin, ifosfamide, and cisplatin chemotherapy in cervical cancer. J Natl Cancer Inst 81: 359–61, 1989.

57. Bonomi P, Blessing J, Ball H, et al. A phase II evaluation of cisplatin and 5-fluorouracil in patients with advanced squamous cell carcinoma of the cervix: a Gynecologic Oncology Group study. Gynecol Oncol 34: 357-9, 1989.

58. Omura G, Blessing J, Vaccarello L, et al. A randomized trial of cisplatin versus cisplatin + mitolactol versus cisplatin + ifosfamide in advanced squamous carcinoma of the cervix by the Gynecologic Oncology Group. Gynec Oncol 60: 120, 1996.

59. MacMahon B. Risk factors for endometrial cancer. Gynecol Oncol 2: 122, 1974.

60. Creasman WT, Morrow CP, Bundy BN, et al. Surgical pathological spread patterns of endometrial cancer (a Gynecologic Oncology Group study). Cancer 60: 2035–2041, 1987.

61. Kurman RJ, Kaminski PF and Norris HJ. The behavior of endometrial hyperplasia: a long-term study of "untreated" hyperplasia in 170 patients. *CA* **56**: 403, 1985.

62. FIGO. Corpus cancer staging. *Int J Gynecol Obstet* **28**: 190, 1989.

63. Boronow RC, Morrow CP, Creasman WT, *et al.* Surgical staging in endometrial cancer: 1. Clinical-pathologic findings of a prospective study. *Obstet Gynecol* **63**: 825–832, 1984.

64. Moss WT, Brand WN and Battifora H. *Radiation Oncology — Rationale, Technique, Results*, 5th ed. St. Louis: CV Mosby, p. 492, 1979.

65. Thigpen T, Blessing J, DiSaia P, *et al.* A randomized comparison of adriamycin with or without cyclophosphamide in the treatment of advanced or recurrent endometrial carcinoma. *J Clin Oncol* **12**: 1408–1414, 1994.

66. Thigpen T, Blessing J, Hatch K, *et al.* Oral medroxyprogesterone acetate in the treatment of advanced or recurrent endometrial carcinoma: a dose-response study by the Gynecologic Oncology Group. Submitted to *J Clin Oncol* 1996.

67. Thigpen JT, Blessing J and DiSaia P. Oral medroxyprogesterone acetate in advanced or recurrent endometrial carcinoma: results of therapy and correlation with estrogen and progesterone receptor levels. The Gynecologic Oncology Group experience. In *Endocrinology of Malignancy*, edited by EE Baulieu, S Slacobelli and WL McGuire WL. Park Ridge, NJ: Parthenon, p. 446, 1986.

68. Thigpen T, Vance R, Lambuth B, *et al.* Chemotherapy for advanced or recurrent gynecologic cancer. *Cancer* **60**: 2104, 2116, 1987.

69. Thigpen T. Personal communication of Gynecologic Oncology Group data 1996.

70. Thigpen T, Buchsbaum H, Mangan C and Blessing J. Phase II trial of adriamycin in the treatment of advanced or recur rent endometrial carcinoma: a Gynecologic Oncology Group study. *Cancer Treat Rep* **63**: 21–27, 1979.

71. Thigpen T, Blessing J, Homesley H, Creasman W and Sutton G. Phase II trial of cisplatin as first-line chemotherapy in patients with advanced or recurrent endometrial carcinoma: a Gynecologic Oncology Group study. *Gynecol Oncol* **33**: 68–70, 1989.

72. Thigpen JT, Blessing JA, Lagasse LD, *et al.* Phase II trial of cisplatin as second-line chemotherapy in patients with advanced or recurrent endometrial carcinoma (a Gynecologic Oncology Group study). *Amer J Clin Oncol* **7**: 253–256, 1984.

73. Thigpen T. Systemic therapy with single agents for advanced or recurrent endometrial carcinoma. In *Endometrial Carcinoma*, edited by D Alberts and E Surwit. Boston: Martinus Nijhoff, 1989.

74. Sutton G, Blessing J, DeMars L, *et al.* A phase II Gynecologic Oncology Group trial of ifosfamide and mesna in advanced or recurrent adenocarcinoma of the endometrium. *Gynec Oncol* **63**: 25–27, 1996.

75. Ball H, Blessing J, Lentz S and Mutch D. A phase II trial of paclitaxel in patients with advanced or recurrent adenocarcinoma of the endometrium: a Gynecologic Oncology Group study. *Gynec Oncol* **62**: 278–281, 1996.

76. Thigpen T, Blessing J, Homesley H, *et al.* Phase III trial of doxorubicin +/– cisplatin in advanced or recurrent endometrial carcinoma: a Gynecologic Oncology Group study. *Proc ASCO* **12**: 261, 1993.

53. Management of Infectious Complications

John N. Greene

Introduction

Cancer and infection make up the leading causes of death among persons aged 65 and older. Serious infectious complications are the dose-limiting factor for the treatment of the aged cancer patient. Strategies to improve tolerance of intensive therapy is being explored especially with the use of cytokines and prophylactic antimicrobials. However, delay in diagnosis of infectious complications because of atypical clinical manifestations in the aged is a serious concern. Decremental biologic changes with age, often accelerated by coexisting diseases can influence the physiologic response to an acute illness and thus alter the clinical manifestations of a geriatric patient with a given disorder (1). Some elderly patients may exhibit minimal or no focal signs pointing to a specifically involved organ system as in acute appendicitis or cholecystitis (1). The high prevalence of multiple chronic and debilitating diseases may further complicate the therapy of infections in the elderly cancer patient. Peak temperatures, maximum white blood cell counts, and intensity of many clinical symptoms and signs are less marked in the elderly (2). The blunting of the febrile response in the elderly was cited by Hippocrates in his Aphorisms (1). The febrile response may be blunted or even absent in a small but significant number of older patients with common infections such as pneumonia (1). Afebrile bacteremia complicating pneumonia, urinary tract infections, and cellulitis occurred predominantly in aged patients (3). In another study, 90% of afebrile patients with culture proven bacteremia were elderly (3). In addition, medications frequently taken by older patients, such as antipyretics and corticosteroids may diminish the febrile response (1). Frequently, the elderly may have a low basal temperature. An oral temperature greater than 37.2°C (99°F) Should be regarded as elevated in patients older than 65 years of age (4). A temperature of 100°F may represent a significant increase if a low basal temperature was present (1). Ninety-five percent of elderly patients who have infection will show some febrile response (5). Elderly patients with fever are more likely to have serious bacterial infections in contrast to younger patients in whom fever usually signifies viral or benign bacterial infections (1). Occult bacterial infection should be suspected in the elderly patient with the new onset of fever and is a frequent cause of fever of unknown origin (FUO) in this population (2). Unlike FUO in the young, a cause for prolonged fever in older patients could be determined in most cases (1). In one series, 36% of cases

were treatable infections, 26% connective tissue diseases and 24% neoplasia (lymphoma and carcinoma) (2,5). Lymphoma is the most common neoplasm, and most lymphomas are intraabdominal (5).

Immunological and Structural Changes with Age

The process of aging leads to immune senescence and thus a moderate immunodeficient state. The susceptibility to and severity of certain viral and bacterial diseases is increased by the waning immunity of aging (6). B-cell dysregulation manifesting as clonal expansions and monoclonal gammopathies occur with higher frequency in older patients (7). Neoplastic transformation of the CD5+ B-cell lineage results in chronic lymphocytic leukemia, a disease almost exclusively seen in old age (7). No striking changes can be defined in antigen presenting cells such as macrophages and dendritic cells with age and in general, their function is preserved. (7). Information is inconclusive regarding changes in neutrophil function with increasing age (7). Other elements of the inflammatory response, leukocytosis, phagocytosis and intracellular killing have also been reported to be impaired with the elderly (8).

The strongest case for a causal relationship between immune senescence and infectious disease can be made for the reactivation of latent varicella zoster, mycobacterial disease, and some of the dimorphic fungal pathogens (6). Reactivation of these diseases is almost always associated with defects in cell-mediated immunity that occur with immunosuppressive drug therapy, the impaired immunity associated with neoplastic disease or with aging (6). The change in the distribution and function of T-cell subsets alters cell-mediated immunity with age (7). Helper T-cell activity and cytotoxic T lymphocytes declines with age, even though the percentage of CD4+ increases and the proportion of CD8+ decreases with age (7). The decline in cell-mediated immunity results in an increase in anergy to delayed hypersensitivity skin tests. An increase risk of all-cause mortality was noted in anergic individuals over 60 years of age (9).

Beginning at 45 years of age, the incidence of shingles increases markedly. Between 45 and 85 years of age, the incidence of shingles increases five fold despite well-maintained humoral immunity to the virus (6). Therefore, the increased incidence of shingles appears to be related to the loss of cell-mediated immunity to the varicella virus (6). Reactivation of varicella-zoster virus due to waning cellular immunity with age more commonly resulted in protracted and disabling pain in elderly patients (4).

The prevalence of bacteriuria in the elderly is approximately 10 percent in men and 20 percent in women (2). Structural changes in the urinary system e.g. prosthetic hypertrophy and relaxation of the pelvic floor, lead to the accumulation of residual urine (6). Urinary stasis from prostate hypertrophy and incomplete emptying in older adults enhances bacterial colonization and persistent bacteriuria (7).

The gastrointestinal tract maintains host resistance to a variety of pathogens, mainly by gastric acid secretion and by the gut-associated lymphoid tissue (7). Gastric acidity declines with age and Peyer's patches are reduced in number, but no data suggests that the function of the gut-associated lymphoid tissue decreases with age (7).

With age the epidermis becomes thinner and the dermis loses its density, vascularity and elasticity and the subcutaneous tissues decrease as well (7). The immunosenscence of the skin is attributed to the decline in the number and function of Langerhans' cells, especially in sun-exposed areas (7). Such skin changes place the older adult at greater risk for skin and soft tissue infections (7). Cellulitis in elderly individuals may resolve slower than cellulitis in younger patients (4).

There is a seven fold risk increase of adverse drug reactions in patients over seventy (10). However, the underlying physiologic condition of the individual patient should dictate selection of therapy and not age alone (10). Because of decreased renal and hepatic function in older individuals, doses of antimicrobials that are somewhat lower than the maximum dose used for younger patients can be used (4). Certain antimicrobials, such as aminoglycosides, are used cautiously in the elderly.

Pneumonia

Community acquired pneumonia occurred 50 times more frequently in individuals over the age of 75 as in 15–19 year olds (11) with a mortality rate as high as 30–40% (4). Community-acquired pneumonia in the aged is most commonly due to *Streptococcus pneumoniae* followed by gram-negative bacteria (*Haemophilus influenzae, Moraxella catarrhalis,* and *E. coli*) (4). Other serious causes of pneumonia in the elderly include *Staphylococcus aureus,* Legionella pneumophila, influenzae virus, and *Mycobacterium tuberculosis.* An altered mental status may be the first sign of pneumonia. The geriatric patient with pneumonia may not exhibit cough, pleuritic chest pain, fever, leukocytosis, or sputum production.

There is no evidence of a reduction in mucosal immunity or reduced function of alveolar macrophages with aging (7). The impaired cough reflex and more frequent aspiration increases the risk of pneumonia in the elderly (7). Changes in the lungs, e.g. loss of elastic recoil, decreased mucous production, impaired ciliary action, as well as depression of the cough reflex lead to less efficient pulmonary clearance (6). Hospitalized

patients above the age of 95 have a three fold higher incidence of nosocomial pneumonia compared with hospitalized younger individuals aged 18 to 24 (12). Gram-negative bacteria colonize the respiratory tract more frequently with advancing age, immobility, debility, chronic disease, and increasing level of care required for a patient (13). In general, both community- and hospital-acquired settings the risk of gram-negative or staphylococcal pulmonary infection appears increased in the elderly (11).

Prophylaxis of respiratory disease in the elderly by immunization with influenza vaccine and pneumococcal vaccine is recommended. Vaccinations recommended for those over 60 include diphtheria and tetanus toxoids every 10 years, influenza virus vaccine annually, and pneumococcal polysaccharide vaccine once or possibly every six years (14).

Tuberculosis

The reactivation of tuberculosis in the elderly appears to be related to the declining vigor of cell-mediated immunity, poor nutrition, diabetes or use of corticosteroid therapy (2,4,6) Viable bacteria in old granulomata escape to disseminate after breakdown of local barriers and cell-medicated immunity with age (6). Individuals over age 65 account for perhaps twice the number of cases of tuberculosis that one might predict given the numbers within the population (2). In Arkansas, 53% of the cases of tuberculosis occurred in the 14% of the population who were over age 65 (15). The occurrence of unexplained weight loss or fever, pulmonary symptoms, unexplained lymphadenopathy, or changes in renal function all should be clues to the possible presence of tuberculosis (2). Unique features of tuberculosis in the elderly includes more frequent disseminated disease at presentation and less frequent presentations with TB associated symptoms such as night sweats, cough, fever, and hemoptysis (40). Individuals with a recently converted tuberculin test, regardless of age, should be given isoniazid (INH) prophylaxis 300 mg in a once-a-day dose for 6–12 months (2). However, when patients of various ages with culture-proven tuberculosis have been skin tested, 10% of tubercular patients under the age of 55 were unresponsive while 30% of tubercular patients over 55 years of age were unresponsive (16).

Viral Pneumonia

Bacterial pneumonia and influenzae together comprise the fifth leading cause of death among persons older than 65 years (17). Influenza among persons aged 65 and older has a five fold excess death rate than among young adults (7). Factors related to this excess death rate is a decline in cell-mediated immunity, failure to provide the influenza vaccine, and failure to form protective antibodies (35% over 65 years of age) when vaccinated (7).

More than 80% of influenzae cases are symptomatic in older individuals and confusion may preclude an accurate history (17). After or during primary influenzae viral pneumonia, secondary bacterial pneumonias may supervene. These secondary bacterial pneumonias occur more often in elderly and chronically ill people. Recrudescence of fever and development of a productive cough and possibly pleuritic chest pain after initial improvement from the classic "flu" symptoms point to secondary bacterial pneumonia. *S. pneumoniae, S. aureus,* and *H. influenzae* are the most common pathogens.

Besides influenzae, RSV is the next most important cause of viral pneumonia in the elderly (2, 14, 17). Of persons 65 years of age or older, admitted to the hospital during the winter with acute cardiopulmonary conditions or influenzae-like illness, 13% were caused by influenzae and 10% were caused by RSV (18). During RSV outbreaks in long term care facilities, rates of pneumonia ranged from 5% to 67% and death from 0% to 53% (17). Clinical manifestations of RSV infection in the elderly range from mild cold symptoms to acute respiratory distress and death (19). Distinguishing influenzae from RSV infection in the elderly is frequently not possible by clinical grounds alone (17). Of older patients with RSV infection requiring admission, 18% needed intensive care, 10% ventilatory support and 10% died (18). Besides supportive care, aerosolized ribavirin may be used to treat RSV pneumonia in the immune compromised and elderly. Other viruses that can cause severe pneumonia in the elderly but rarely result in death includes parainfluenza and corona virus (17).

Chronic Lymphocytic Leukemia

Ninety percent of all cases of CLL occur in persons over age 50; nearly 70 percent of patients are older than 60 years (20). Infections are the leading cause of death in patients with CLL. The five year risk of developing severe infections in 125 patients with CLL (mean age 65.6 years) was 26%, and 21 out of 71 deaths could be attributed to infectious causes (21). Molica S *et al.* (21) found severe infection occurred more frequently in patients with CLL who had advanced clinical stage of CLL, diffuse bone marrow histology and hypogammaglobulinemia.

Cryptococcus neoformins(22), *Histoplasma capsulatum* (23), *Coccidioides immitis* (24), and *Nocardia asteroides* (25) can cause a progressive pneumonia or disseminated disease in patients with CLL especially if they're receiving corticosteroids. *Aspergillus, M. tuberculosis, M. kansasii, M. avium*-intracellular can present in a similar fashion with a progressive pneumonia in the setting of corticosteroid therapy. In addition to the afore mentioned organisms, other unusual infections occurring in patients with CLL are frequently found in HIV infected individuals. A 78 year old man with CLL who was HIV negative developed disseminated angiomatous papules following a cat scratch consistent with bacillary angiomatosis caused by Bartonella henselae (26). Lesions resolved completely after treatment with erythromycin (26).

Infection and secondary primary malignant tumors were the most common complications and cause of death in 105 patients with B cell CLL followed for a median period of 5.5 years (27). *Streptococcus pneumoniae,*

S. aureus, S. haemolyticus, E. coli and varicella zoster virus accounted for most infections (27). The sites affected were the lungs, skin and urinary tract (27). Advancing disease increased the liability to major infection (27). Immunoglobulin deficiency is the factor that correlates best with the frequency, severity, and pattern of infection (27).

Another study of 59 patients with CLL found that the majority of patients with severe or multiple infections (13/18) had low levels of both total IgG and specific antibodies to pneumococcal capsular polysaccharide (28). Although less than half of the patients with hypogammaglobulinemia developed severe or multiple infections, low levels of pneumococcal antibodies were associated with the former and latter (28).

Of 146 patients with CLL in another series, 292 infections were recorded (29). The incidence of moderate to severe infections was 0.47 per patient year, with 42 patients dying of a severe infection (46% of all causes of death) (29). Patients with hypogammaglobulinemia and advanced disease stage were the most susceptible to death from infection and would be the most likely to benefit from IVIG prophylaxis (29). Patients with CLL and hypogammuglobuliremia, or a history of infection can be substantially protected from bacterial infection by every 3 week administration of immunoglobulin (30). After one year of therapy, 14 patients developed a bacterial infection versus 36 patients receiving placebo (30).

Intravenous immunoglobulin (IVIG) to provide protection for encapsulated bacterial infection such as pneumococcal pneumonia is frequently used for patients with CLL and multiple myeloma. Sklenar I *et al.* (31) have come up with recommendations on dosage and scheduling of IVIG in these patients. The dosage recommendation in CLL is .4g/kg every 3 weeks until week 12, followed by a maintenance dosage of .4 g/kg every 5 weeks (31). Because of a faster elimination rate of antibodies in multiple myeloma patients, the recommended loading dose is .8 g/kg, followed by .4g/kg every week as continuous treatment (31).

Fludarabine, an effective therapy for CLL, is also lymphotoxic especially for CD_4 lymphocytes (32). Fludarabine can produce neutropenia, with associated pneumonia and bacteremia, and opportunistic protozoal and mycobacterial infections have been described after therapy with this drug (33). Anaissie E *et al.* (34) found fludarabine and prednisone resulted in an increased incidence of listeriosis in patients with CLL. A dramatic reduction in CD_4 lymphocytes developed after fludarabine and prednisone treatment and coincided with the development of Listeriosis (34). Of 248 patients with CLL who received fludarabine and prednisone, 7 developed Listeriosis, whereas none of the 160 patients treated with fludarabine alone developed Listeriosis (34). Infections occurred regardless of whether patients were in remission, had active CLL, were neutropenic or hypogammaglobulinemic (34). Age appeared to play a role for developing Listeriosis, the median age for those infected was 70 years old, whereas the noninfected were 62 years old (34). Listeria infection manifested as bacteremia or meningitis. The major causes of meningitis in the aged are *S. pneumoniae*, enteric gram negative bacteria (GNB), *M. tuberculosis*, and *Listeria monocytogenes* (4). A brain abscess due to Listeria in a patient with CLL treated with fludarabine has also been reported (35). The authors propose that prednisone and fludarabine work synergistically to lower the threshold for listerial infection because high doses of prednisone alone did not increase the risk for Listeriosis. Patients with CLL who receive this combination therapy are advised to avoid foods which may contain large concentrations of Listeria, including unpasteurized milk, raw vegetables, and undercooked poultry or meat. The risk period of Listeriosis in patients with CLL treated with this combination could be as long as 2 years after completion of therapy even with a normal CD_4 lymphocyte count (36).

Non infectious causes of fever are not infrequent in patients with CLL and is probably due to the progression of the disease itself. A sudden development of fever, weight loss, increasing lymphadenopathy, hepatosplenomegaly, lymphopenia, or paraproteinemia should arouse suspicion of Richter's syndrome or other acute transformations which portend a poor prognosis (20).

Multiple Myeloma

Infection occurs most often during the first 2 months after diagnosis of multiple myeloma and accounts for 20–50% of all deaths (37). Recurrent infections are the presenting signs of myeloma in 25% of patients, and more than 75% of patients will develop a serious infection during the course of their illness (37). GNB have replaced *Streptococcus pneumoniae* as the most common cause of infection in myeloma patients. This change of spectrum of infection to favor GNB over pneumococcus may be due to more nosocomial infections, more aggressive chemotherapeutic regimens, longer periods of neutropenia, and greater use of pneumococcal vaccination (37). The occasional infections with fungi, herpes viruses, *M. tuberculosis* and *Pneumocystic carinii* most likely result from steroids and cytotoxic chemotherapy rather than from the myeloma itself (33,37,38).

Over a 13 year period, 141 patients with multiple myeloma were studied (39). Fifty-five percent developed an infectious complication, most commonly in the first month of diagnosis. During the study period, there was a significant rise in the overall incidence of infection especially those due to GNB. Risk factors for subsequent infection included renal insufficiency and anemia. Infection was associated with 275-fold increased risk of death, independent of other risk factors. Azotemia (BUN >35) is significantly related to infection with GNB, but not with *S. pneumoniae* or *H. influenzae* and is associated with a poor prognosis in multiple myeloma patients (38).

Of 75 bacterial infections in 57 patients with multiple myeloma, episodes of infection with *Streptococcus pneumoniae* and *Haemophilus influenzae* occurred at presentation, early in the disease, and in patients responding to chemotherapy (40). Episodes of infection

with GNB occurred in patients with active and advancing disease and in those responding to chemotherapy when neutropenic (40). Gram-negative bacilli (GNB) and *Staphylococcus aureus* caused 80% of infections seen after diagnosis and 92% of deaths from infection (40).

The high mortality associated with *S. aureus* infections in patients with myeloma was highlighted from a review of bacteremia in Denmark. Of 6,253 cases of *Staphylococcus aureus* bacteremia between 1975–1984, 479 occurred in patients with hematological malignancies and/or agranulocytosis (41). There was a lower incidence of endocarditis in cancer patients than in noncancer patients, 0.4 vs 4.7% respectively, probably due to a central line accounting for the focus of infection more often in the former (41). However, mortality was higher in patients with hematologic malignancy or agranulocytosis and *S. aureus* bacteremia than noncancer patients, 49%, 46% vs 33% respectively (41). The highest mortality was found in patients with multiple myeloma (71%) and the lowest in patients with ALL 28%, possibly related to older patients in the former (41).

The trend favoring GNB over pneumococcal infections in patients with myeloma held true in a study of male veterans. Thirty-three infectious episodes occurred in 60 patients (mean age of 63 years) with multiple myeloma over a 10 year period (42). Urinary tract infections caused by GNB (*Enterobacteriaceae* 31%, *Pseudomonas aeruginosa* 22%) were the most common, and most were due to bladder catheterization (42). Pneumococcal pneumonia occurred infrequently (2 cases) as did herpes zoster infection (2 cases) (42).

Another study found infectious complications developed in 71 of 126 (56.3%) of patients with multiple myeloma (43). Most infections manifested in the acute stages, the onset, relapse, and the terminal stage of myelomatosis, and during and after induction therapy. Old age, third clinical stage of disease, light chain myelomas, lambda light chain secretions, leukopenia, azotemia, polyclonal suppression of immunoglobulins and inadequate therapeutic response were statistically significant risk factors for an infectious complication (43). However, unlike prior studies, infections did not significantly impact survival in these patients.

When evaluating patients with multiple myeloma for infectious complications, the duration and stage of disease, prior and current therapy, and presence or absence of neutropenia should be taken into account when choosing empiric antibiotics, as the causative pathogens may vary with each factor (40). Hargreaves RM *et al* (44) investigated 102 patients with myeloma to assess whether immunological risk factors predisposing to serious infection could be identified. Low antipneumococcal and anti Escherichia coli titers correlated with risk of serious infection (44). The overall serious infection rate was 0.92 per patient year and was four times higher during periods of active disease (1.90) compared with plateau phase myeloma (0.49) (44). The majority of infections involved the respiratory tract. Several studies have found a subgroup of patients with myeloma with poor IgG responses to exogenous antigens, who are at increased risk of serious infection, can be identified and may benefit from replacement immunoglobulin therapy to reduce the risk of infection (44,45).

Because patients with plateau-phase myeloma have an increased risk of life-threatening bacterial infections and polyclonal humoral immune suppression, the value of IVIG prophylaxis was evaluated by Chapel HM *et al* (45). Monthly infusions of IVIG at 0.4g/kg or placebo was given to 82 patients with stable multiple myeloma. Sepsis or pneumonia occurred in 10 patients receiving placebo but in none receiving IVIG. Of 57 serious infectious complications, 38 occurred in 470 patient-months on placebo, compared with 19 in 449 patient-months on IVIG (45). Patients who had a maximum benefit from IVIG were identified by a poor pneumococcal IgG antibody response (less than 2-fold increase) (45).

In addition, IVIG had a statistically significant effect in protecting against recurrent infections in 60 patients who completed a year of therapy when compared to placebo (45). Although prophylactic IVIG is not routinely recommended in myeloma patients, a decreased incidence and severity of infections may be seen with its use (46, 47). No episodes of bacteremia or pneumonia occurred and less-serious infections and recurrent infections developed in patients treated with monthly IVIG (0.4 g/kg) than compared with placebo (47). Prophylactic penicillin may be useful in patients who are non responders or who cannot tolerate IVIG and who develop recurrent pneumococcal infections, but no published data supports this approach (37).

Myelodysplastic Syndromes

The myelodysplastic syndromes, occur predominantly in elderly patients and frequently lead to death from complications of cytopenias or transformation to leukemia. Response to chemotherapy is usually short-lived and infectious related deaths are very high. Lowenthal RM *et al* (48) gave Idarubicin to 14 patients with a median age of 74 years with an overall response rate of 14%. Three patients developed life-threatening infections and two died from cytopenias during therapy (48).

Oguma S *et al.* (49) assessed risk factors for infection in 430 patients with myelodysplastic syndromes (MDS). The frequency of infectious complications was highest just after diagnosis of MDS (4 per 1000 patient days) and declined rapidly within 4 years of diagnosis (.3 per 1000 patient days) (49). The most frequent infection was that of the respiratory tract followed by sepsis and fever of unknown origin (FUO) (49). Sepsis and FUO comprised the highest proportion of complications resulting in death (40%), followed by respiratory tract infections (39%) (49). *Staphylococcus sp.* were the most frequent pathogens isolated. Subtype, dependence on red blood cell transfusions, sex, and age, were risk factors for fatal infection (49).

Pomeroy C *et al.* (50) analyzed 86 patients with MDS to determine the incidence, characteristics, outcome and risk factors of infection. One infectious complication occurred per patient year of observation (50). Bacterial pneumonias and skin abscesses were the most common infections (50). Infection accounted for the majority of deaths (64%), and was more common than transformation to acute leukemia as a cause of death. Neutropenia and MDS subgroup were independent risk factors for infection (50).

Acute Myeloid Leukemia

The treatment of patients greater than 55 to 70 years of age with acute myeloid leukemia (AML) is associated with a treatment-related mortality of 25% (51). Those older than 50 with AML often do poorly compared to younger patients. They frequently die during induction therapy, usually as a result of infection during periods of prolonged neutropenia (52). Because elderly patients do not fare well during prolonged periods of neutropenia, chemotherapeutic regimens which are less myelosuppressive are often used. Low dose cytarabine was given to 44 patients (median age 72) with untreated AML for 42 days or less (53). Complete responses occurred in 10 patients (23%) but infection associated with granulocytopenia was the predominant complication (53).

Most elderly patients with AML should be considered for treatment with intensive chemotherapy (54). However, with intensive chemotherapy programs, the elderly have a greater risk of early death related to drug toxicity or infection (54). In several studies, more than half of patients over 60 years of age died from complications within 2 months, before receiving an adequate trial of antileukemic therapy (54). However, high-dose cytarabine, a mainstay for treatment of AML in young patients, is associated with significant neurotoxicity and infectious complications in the elderly and should not be routinely used in the latter population except in the context of controlled clinical trials (54).

Cytotoxic therapy-related epithelial damage in the gut due to high-dose cytarabine correlated with invasive fungal disease (55). Another potential infectious complication of high dose cytosine arabinoside is viridans streptococcal bacteremia complicated by ARDS, hypotension, and endocarditis (56,57). Multivariate analysis of predisposing factors showed that high doses of cytosine arabinoside, the presence of mucositis, and the absence of previous therapy with parenteral antibiotics were independent risk factors for the development of viridans streptococcal bacteremia (56).

In another study, 76 patients with newly diagnosed or relapsed AML developed streptococcal bacteremia (58). Pulmonary symptoms developed in 7 patients and death due to respiratory failure resulted in 5 of the 7 (58). The infections all occurred in the phase of maximum myelosuppression 1–3 weeks after the start of chemotherapy (58). Streptococcal bacteremia was not limited to patients treated with ARA-C but also occurred with the use of other regimens of intensive chemotherapy (58).

Lazarus HM *et al.* (52) concluded that high dose cytosine arabinoside and daunorubicin was effective antileukemic therapy but too toxic to recommend for most patients over 60 years of age with AML. Life threatening infection, the major toxicity or complication, consisted of 13 cases of pneumonia, bacteremia, or fungemia, and 5 resulted in death. Fever, infection, and low Karnofsky performance status at diagnosis predicted an unfavorable outcome with 6 of 7 patients with all three characteristics dying within 30 days after beginning antileukemic therapy. Another study found one half of 193 patients older than 50 years of age died during induction, and 63% of these deaths were due to infection (59). The degree of myelosuppression of the chemotherapeutic regimen may have been the major limiting toxicity. The mean time to achieve a neutrophil count in excess of 2000 per ml in this study was 27 days (range 23–37) after beginning either induction or consolidation therapy. Seven patients had antecedent myelodysplastic syndromes with impaired bone marrow reserve leading to greater potential for developing serious infection as the period of neutropenia or failure of BM recovery lengthens.

Although the best results for AML have been obtained with intensive consolidation chemotherapy, in the elderly this approach carries a higher risk of morbidity and mortality due to toxicity and infection (54). Most elderly patients cannot tolerate more that one to three courses of consolidation treatment (54). The intensity of these programs must often be reduced in elderly patients. Because of the intensity of cytoreductive therapy, patients over 50 years of age rarely survive bone marrow transplantation and have a higher incidence of graft-versus-host disease (54).

Infectious morbidity, myelosuppression profiles, and outcome of antileukemic therapy using standard cytarabine (ARA-C) plus duanorubicin ("7 + 3") remission-induction therapy and high dose ARA-C (HDARA-C) consolidation was studied in treated adult AML (60). For one, two, and three induction courses, the mean number of days the patients experienced severe neutropenia (<500 absolute neutrophil count ANC) were 22.5, 39.3 and 47.4 days respectively (60). The infection rates were 1.45, 2.45, and 3 infections per course respectively (60). The use of multiple induction courses had consequences of prolonged myelosuppression, increased blood product use, and incremental risks of infectious complications (60). HDARA-C was the most significant factor related to prolonged disease free survival and myelosuppression and infection risk were similar to those for the single 7+3 induction courses (60).

After induction chemotherapy with daunorubicin and cytarabine, 124 patients received GM-CSF or placebo if a day-10 bone marrow was aplastic without leukemia (51). Median times to neutrophil recovery was reduced with GCSF compared with placebo 13–14 days versus 17–21 days for an ANC >500/mL or 1,000/mL respectively (51). Similarly, infectious complications were significantly reduced on the GM-CSF arm (51). Of 30 patients over the age of 65 years with newly diagnosed or relapsed AML, GMCSF resulted in neutrophil recovery 6–9 days earlier than without this cytokine

and rapid clearance of infections in most patients (61). However, in another study, GCSF given before, during, and after treatment with fludarabine and cytarabine in elderly patients (median age 63 years) with newly diagnosed AML or MDS had no effect on complete response rates or infection rates (62). Cytokines and antimicrobial prophylaxis combined with an intensive chemotherapy regimen will allow more elderly patients to benefit from high dose antileukemic therapy (52). In one study, prophylactic penicillin G and ciprofloxacin given to patients receiving remission induction or intensive consolidation treatment for AML significantly reduced infectious morbidity and mortality due to streptococcal and gram-negative bacterial infection, respectively (63).

Febrile Neutropenia

Management of the febrile neutropenic patient is fairly standard with infectious complications similar across all age groups. One third of patients with absolute granulocyte counts less than $500/mL^3$ will develop fever or other clinical evidence of infection (64). A culture documented infection is never found in 40% of febrile neutropenic patients but clinical improvement frequently occurs after instituting broad spectrum antimicrobials (64). Early empiric therapy for febrile neutropenia with combination antipseudomonal antibiotics followed by an antistaphylococcal and streptococcal antibiotic and then an antifungal agent has become standard in cancer centers in the U.S. Neutropenic episodes (greater than 2 weeks) frequently requires antimicrobial modification to control for the development of resistant pathogens. Prolonged neutropenia (greater than 4 weeks) from failure to induce remission, consecutive chemotherapy cycles with a short pause and refractory bone marrow aplasia from chemotherapy or the disease itself, invariably results in breakthrough infection usually with resistant GNB and fungal pathogens. Antimicrobial modification beyond 4 weeks is based on suspected likely pathogens, prior antibiotic and antifungal therapy and toxicity of current therapy. The protocol for the management of febrile neutropenia at The H. Lee Moffitt Cancer Center is presented in Table 53.1.

The duration of granulocytopenia appears to be the most useful index for gauging the risk for infectious complications (65). Whereas less than 30% of patients with short term neutropenia (less than 1 week) develop fever or evidence of infection, 100% of patients with long term neutropenia (greater than 1 week) will do so (65). The longer the period of neutropenia, the more serious the infectious complications (65). For example, the risk of Aspergillus infection in patients with leukemia increases from 1% per day during the first several weeks of neutropenia to greater than 4% per day after 3 weeks (66). In addition to knowing the predominant pathogens for each week of neutropenia, the infectious diseases acquired during prior periods of neutropenia may be very crucial, with certain fungi and viruses. Aspergillus pneumonia and herpes simplex stomatitis has a recurrence rate with subsequent

Table 53.1   H. Lee Moffitt Cancer Center Protocol.

Empiric antibiotic therapy of febrile neutropenic patients

AGC < 1000/ml + temperature ≥ 101 F   Day 0
Complete evaluation + culture + no identifiable focus of infection
↓
Fortaz 2 gm IV q 8 h
+
Gentamycin 1.5 mg/kg IV q 8 h
↓

Specific Antibiotics	←	Pathogen Identified	←	→	Clinical Response	→	Continue Same Antibiotics

↓
No clinical response after 3 days and/or temperature _ 101 FDay 3
+
No identifiable focus of infection
↓
ADD Vancomycin 1 gm IV q 12 h

Specific Antibiotics	←	Pathogen Identified	←	→	Clinical Response	→	Continue Antibiotics

↓
No clinical response and/or temperature ≥ 101 FDay 5
+
No identifiable focus of infection after 5 days
↓
ADD Amphotericin B 0.5 mg/kg/d/IV
or
Fluconazole 400 mg IV qd
↓

Specific Antibiotics	←	Pathogen Identified	←	→	Clinical Response	→	Continue Antibiotics

↓
Change Fluconazole to   Day 10
Amphotericin B .5 mg/kg/d IV
↓

Specific Antibiotics	←	Pathogen Identified	←	→	Clinical Response	→	Continue Antibiotics

↓
Modify antibiotics and Amphotericin B dose based on cultures or suspected pathogens

1.   If abdominal pain suggestive of typhlitis or if oral ulcers suggestive of anaerobic infection, add:
Flagyl 500 mg IV q 6
or
Clindamycin 900 mg IV q 8

2.   If orolabial lesions suggestive of herpes simplex infection, add:
Acyclovir .5 mg/kg IV q 8

3.   If renal insufficiency with creatinine > 2.0, or rapidly increasing creatinine, or excessive fluid retention from renal insufficiency, then:
   A.   Change Amphotericin B to ABELCET 3.0–5.0 mg/kg/d
   B.   Change Aminoglycoside to Ofloxin

neutropenia of 50% and 40–80% respectively, unless prophylactic or early empiric therapy directed at each organism is initiated.

Inpatient management of neutropenia associated with therapy of hematologic malignancies is necessary because of transfusional, nutritional and antimicrobial requirements during this period. Because patients with cancer, neutropenia, and fever do not make up a homogenous group, Talcot JA et al. (64) developed a risk stratification system. Presenting clinical features were used to identify groups that could be managed with less medical supervision, paving the way for outpatient management. Patients with anticipated short-term neutropenia (less than 1 week) who generally have benign outcomes can be safely managed as outpatients.

Outpatient treatment for short term low risk febrile neutropenia can be successfully done with GCSF or GMCSF and a quinolone plus augmentin or clindamycin until resolution of neutropenia. Although advanced age may be a significant risk factor, many elderly patients can be treated as outpatients if they are functional, otherwise healthy and compliant with the recommended treatment protocol.

In general, therapy for older patients with malignancy is becoming more intensive. As oncologist push the limits of chemotherapy to improve disease-free survival in the older cancer patient, the use of cytokines and prophylactic and early empiric antimicrobial therapy with subsequent modification of the latter is crucial to reduce infectious related mortality.

References

1. Norman DC, Toledo SD. Infections in elderly persons. *Clinics Geriatr Medicine* 1992; **8**: 713–719.
2. Crossley KB, Peterson PK. Infections in the elderly. In *Principles and Practice of Infectious Diseases*, 4th edition, edited by GL Mandell, JE Bennett, R Dolin. New York: Churchill Livingstone, 2737–2742, 1995.
3. Gleckman RA, Hibert D. Afebrile bacteremia — A phenomenon in geriatric patients. *JAMA* 1982; **248**: 1478.
4. Crossley KB, Peterson PK. Infections in the elderly. *Clin Infect Dis* 1996; **22**: 209–215.
5. Esposito AL, Gleckman RA. Fever of unknown origin in the elderly. *J Am Geriatr Soc* 1979; **26**: 498.
6. Schwab R, Walters CA, Weksler ME. Host defense mechanisms and ageing. *Seminars Oncology* 1989; **16**: 20–27.
7. Ben-Yehuda A, Weksler ME. Host resistance and the immune system. *Clinics Geriatr Med* 1992; **8**: 701–711.
8. Charpentier B, Fournier C, Fries D, et al. Immunological studies in human ageing: I. In vitro function of T-cells and polymorphs. *J Clin Lab Immunol* 1981; **5**: 87.
9. Wayne SJ, Rhyme RL, Garry PJ, et al. Cell-mediated immunity as a predictor of morbidity and mortality in subjects over 60. *J Gerontol* 1990; **45**: M45.
10. Ershler WB. Introduction: Geriatric oncology comes of age. *Seminars Oncology* 1989; **16**: 1–2.
11. Marrie TJ. Epidemiology of community-acquired pneumonia in the elderly. *Semin Respir Infect* 1990; **5**: 260.
12. Rajul L, Khan F. Pneumonia in the elderly. *Geriatrics* 1988; **43**: 51
13. Valenti WM, Trudell RG, Bentley DW. Factors predisposing to oropharyngeal colonization with gram-negative bacilli in the aged. *NEJM* 1978; **298**: 1108.
14. Crossley KB, Thurn JR. Nursing home-acquired pneumonia. *Semin Respir Infect* 1989; **4**: 64–72.
15. Dutt AK, Stead WW. Tuberculosis. *Clin Geriatr Med* 1992; **8**: 761–75.
16. Holden M, Dubin MR, Diamond PH. Frequency of negative intermediate-strength tuberculin sensitivity in patients with active tuberculosis. *NEJM* 1971; **285**: 1506.
17. Falsey AR. Viral respiratory tract infections in elderly persons. *Infect Dis Clin Pract* 1996; **5**: 53–58.
18. Falsey AR, Cunningham CK, Barker WH, et al. Respiratory syncytial virus and influenza A in the hospitalized elderly. *J Infect Dis* 1995; **172**: 389–394.
19. Mathur U, Bentley DW, Hall CB. Concurrent respiratory syncytial virus and influenza infections in the institutionalized elderly and chronically ill. *Ann Intern Med* 1980; **93**: 49–52.
20. Johnson LE. Chronic lymphocytic leukemia. *Amer Fam Pract* 1988; **38**: 167–176.
21. Molica S, Levato D, Levato L. Infections in chronic lymphocytic leukemia. Analysis of incidence as a function of length of follow-up. *Haematologica* 1993; **78**: 374–377.
22. Whitley TH, Graybill JR, Alford RH. Pulmonary cryptococcosis in chronic lymphocytic leukemia. *South Med J* 1976; **69**: 33–36.
23. Kauffman CA, Israel KS, Smith JW, et al. Histoplasmosis in immunosuppressed patients. *Am J Med* 1978; **65**: 923–932.
24. Deresinski SC, Stevens DA. Coccidioidomycosis in compromised hosts: experience at Stanford University Hospital. *Medicine* 1975; **54**: 377–395.
25. Young LS, Armstrong D, Bleuint A, et al. Nocardia asteroides infection complicating neoplastic disease. *Am J Med* 1971; **50**: 356–367.
26. Torok L, Viragh SZ, Borka I, et al. Bacillary angiomatosis in a patient with lymphocytic leukaemia. *Brit J Dermatol* 1994; **130**: 665–668.
27. Robertson TI. Complications and causes of death in B cell chronic lymphocytic leukemia: A long term study of 105 patients. *Aust N Z J Med* 1990; **20**: 44–50.
28. Griffiths H, Lea J, Bunch C, et al. Predictors of infection in chronic lymphocytic leukaemia. *Clin Experiment Immunol* 1992; **89**: 374–377.
29. Itala M, Helenius H, Nikoskelainen J, et al. Infections and serum IGG levels I in patients with chronic lymphocytic leukemia. *Europ J Haematol* 1992; **48**: 266–270.
30. Cooperative group for the Study of Immunoglobulin in Chronic Lymphocytic Leukemia. Intravenous immunoglobulin for the prevention of infection in chronic lymphocytic leukemia. *NEJM* 1988; **319**: 902–907.
31. Sklenar I, Schiffman G, Jnsson V, et al. Effect of various doses of intravenous polyclonal IgG on in vivo levels of 12 pneumococcal antibodies in patients with chronic lymphocytic leukaemia and multiple myeloma. *Oncology* 1993; **50**: 466–477.
32. Boldt DH, Von Hoff DD, Kuhn JG, et al. Effects of human peripheral lymphocytes of in vivo administration of 9-beta-D-arabinofuranosyl-2 fluoroadenine-5 monophosphate (NSC 312887), a new purine antimetabolite. *Cancer Res* 1984; **44**: 461–466.
33. Scully RE, Mark EJ, McNeely WF, et al. Case records of the Massachusetts General Hospital. *NEJM* 1994; **330**: 557–564.
34. Anaissie E, Kontoyiannis DP, Kantarjian H, et al. Listeriosis in patients with chronic lymphocytic leukemia who were treated with fludarabine and prednisone. *Ann Int Med* 1992; **117**: 466–469.
35. Cleveland KO, Gelfand MS. Listerial brain abscess in a patient with chronic lymphocytic leukemia treated with fludarabine. *Clin Infect Dis* 1993; **17**: 816–817.
36. Girmenia C, Mauro FR, Rahimi S. Late Listeriosis after fludarabine plus prednisone treatment. *Brit J Haematol* 1994; **87**: 407–408.
37. Furman AC, Sepkowitz KA. Infections in patients with multiple myeloma. *Infect Med* 1995; **12**: 353,356,351–362.
38. Jacobson DR, Zolla-Pazner S. Immunosuppression and infection in multiple myeloma. *Seminars Oncol* 1986; **13**: 282–290.
39. Rayner HC, Haynes AP, Thompson JR, et al. Perspectives in multiple myeloma: survival, prognostic factors and disease complications in a single centre between 1975 and 1988. *Quart J Med* 1991; **79**: 517–525.

40. Savage DG, Lindenbaum J, Garrett TL. Biphasic pattern of bacterial infection in multiple myeloma. *Ann Intern Med* 1982; **96**: 47–50.

41. Espersen F, Frimodt-Milner N, Rosdahl VT, *et al. Staphylococcus aureus* bacteremia in patients with hematological malignancies and/or agranulocytosis. *Acta Medica Scand* 1987; **222**: 465–470.

42. Doughney KB, Williams DM, Penn RL. Multiple myeloma infectious complications. *South Med J* 1988; **81**: 855–858.

43. Goranov S. Clinical problems of infectious complications in patients with multiple myeloma. *Folica Medica* 1994; **36**: 41–46.

44. Hargreaves RM, Lea JR, Griffiths H, *et al.* Immunological factors and risk of infection in plateau phase myeloma. *J Clin Pathol* 1995; **48**: 260–266.

45. Chapel HM, Lee M, Hargreaves R, *et al.* Randomized trail of intravenous immunoglobulin as prophylaxis against infection in plateau-phase multiple myeloma. The UK Group for Immunoglobulin Replacement Therapy in Multiple Myeloma. *Lancet* 1994; **343**: 1059–1063.

46. Chapel HM, Lee M. The use of intravenous immune globulin in multiple myeloma. *Clin Exp Immunol* 1994; **97**: S2S24.

47. Chapel HM, Lee M, Hargreaves R, *et al.* Randomized trial of intravenous immunoglobulin as prophylaxis against infection in plateau-phase multiple myeloma. *Lancet* 1994; **343**: 1059–1063.

48. Lowenthal RM, Lambertenghi-Deliliers G. Oral idarubicin as treatment for advanced myelodysplastic syndrome. *Haematologica* 1991; **76**: 398–401.

49. Oguma S, Yoshida Y, Uchino H, *et al.* Infection in myelodysplastic syndromes before evolution into acute non-lymphoblastic leukemia. *Internat J Hematol* 1994; **60**: 129–136.

50. Pomeroy C, Oken MM, Rydell RE, *et al.* Infection in the myelodysplastic syndromes. *Am J Med* 1991; **90**: 338–344.

51. Rowe JM, Anderson JW, Mazza JJ, *et al.* A randomized placebo-controlled phase III study of granulocyte-macrophage colony-stimulating factor in adult patients (>55 to 70 years of age) with acute myelogenous leukemia: A study of the Eastern Cooperative Oncology Group (E1490). *Blood* 1995; **86**: 457–462.

52. Lazarus HM, Vogler WR, Burns P, *et al.* High-dose cytosine arabinoside and duanorubicin as primary therapy in elderly patients with acute myelogenous leukemia. *Cancer* 1989; **63**: 1055–1059.

53. Powell BL, Copizzi RL, Muss MB, *et al.* Low-dose ARA-C therapy for acute myelogenous leukemia in elderly patients. *Leukemia* 1989; **3**: 23–28.

54. Champlin RE, Gajewski JL, Golde DW. Treatment of acute myelogenous leukemia in the elderly. *Seminars Oncology* 1989; **16**: 51–56.

55. Bow EJ, Loewen R, Cheang MS, *et al.* Invasive fungal disease in adults undergoing remission-induction therapy for acute myeloid leukemia: the pathogenic role of the antileukemic regimen. *Clin Infect Dis* 1995; **21**: 361.

56. Boshud P-Y, Eggiman PH, Calandra TH, *et al.* Bacteremia due to viridans streptococcus in neutropenic patients with cancer: clinical spectrum and risk factors. *Clin Infect Dis* 1994; **18**: 25–31.

57. Tasaka T, Nagai M, Sasaki K, *et al.* Streptococcus mitis septicemia in leukemia patients; clinical features and outcome. *Internal Med* 1993; **32**: 221–223.

58. vander Lelie H, Vanketel RJ, von dem Borne AE, *et al.* Incidence and clinical epidemiology of streptococcal septicemia during treatment of acute myeloid leukemia. *Scan J Infect Dis* 1991; **23**: 163–168.

59. Estey EH, Keating MJ, McCredie KB, *et al.* Causes of remission induction failure in acute myelogenous leukemia. *Blood* 1982; **60**: 309–315.

60. Bow EJ, Kilpatrick MG, Scott BA, *et al.* Acute myebid leukemia in Manitoba. The consequences of standard "7+3" remission-induction therapy followed by high dose cytarabine post remission consolidation for myelosuppression, infectious morbidity, and outcome. *Cancer* 1994; **74**: 52–60.

61. Buchner T, Hiddemann W, Koenigsmann M, *et al.* Recombinant human granulocyte-macrophage colony-stimulating factor after chemotherapy in patients with acute myeloid leukemia at higher age or after relapse. *Blood* 1991; **78**: 1190–1197.

62. Estey E, Thall P, Andreeff M, *et al.* Use of granulocyte colony-stimulating factor before, during, and after fludarabine plus cytarabine induction therapy of newly diagnosed acute myelogenous leukemia or myelodysplastic syndromes: comparison with fludarabine plus cytarabine without granulocyte colony-stimulating factor. *J Clin Oncol* 1994; **12**: 671–678.

63. de Jong P, de Jong M, Kuijper E, *et al.* Evaluation of penicillin G in the prevention of Streptococcal septicaemia in patients with acute myeloid leukaemia undergoing cytotoxic chemotherapy. *Europ J Clin Microbiol Infect Dis* 1993; **12**: 750–755.

64. Talcott JA, Finberg R, Mayer RJ, *et al.* The medical course of cancer patients with fever and neutropenia. *Arch Intern Med* 1988; **148**: 2561–2568.

65. Lee JW, Pizzo PA. Management of the cancer patient with fever and prolonged neutropenia. *Hem Onc Clin North Amer* 1993; **7**: 937–960.

66. Gerson SL, Talbott GH, Hurwitz S, *et al.* Prolonged granulocytopenia: The major risk factor for invasive pulmonary aspergillosis in patients with acute leukemia. *Ann Intern Med* 1984; **100**: 345–351.

54. Principles of Cancer Nursing

Karen Smith Blesch

Introduction

Oncology nurses have recognized the elderly as a special population for cancer prevention, detection, treatment and rehabilitation for over a decade. This recognition was formalized in 1992 by the publication of the Oncology Nursing Society Position Paper on Cancer and Aging (1). The position paper contains ten statements which form a set of recommendations for nursing practice in geriatric oncology. The ten statements are summarized in Table 54.1, and provide a framework for considering nursing practice in this population. The purpose of this chapter is to discuss concepts of geriatric oncology nursing practice. For information about specific clinical problems the reader is referred to the appropriate chapter in this text.

Personal Biases Toward Aging

Although most nurses and health care professionals would be reluctant to consider themselves "ageist," a substantial literature exists which documents the importance and independence of advanced age as an

Table 54.1 Summary of position statements for oncology nursing practice in geriatric oncology.

- Recognize personal biases toward aging and the elderly
- Advocate cancer prevention and early detection activities
- Acknowledge interrelationships between cancer and aging
- Intervene to prevent or minimize age-specific sequelae of cancer and cancer treatment
- Integrate comprehensive geriatric assessment in nursing care
- Assess availability and capability of support networks
- Increase communication with colleagues and other providers regarding older cancer patients
- Consider age-related factors that affect learning and performance of self care activities related to cancer
- Maximize advocacy role in ethical decision-making regarding quality of life
- Recognize effects of healthcare policy on geriatric oncology nursing care

important and independent predictor of cancer diagnosis and treatment decisions (2–6). Berkman and colleagues have detailed myths and biases related to cancer and aging which, if held by elderly persons and their families, or the health professionals who care for them, may mitigate against optimal cancer care (6). These myths are listed in Table 54.2.

It is important for nurses and other providers to be aware of consciously and unconsciously held beliefs that may negatively affect the care they deliver. Many providers who identify themselves as specialists in gerontology and/or oncology will not identify with the beliefs listed in Table 54.2. Others will note that successful efforts to dispel these beliefs have been made by the geriatric oncology community. However, a substantial amount of cancer care is delivered to elderly patients by providers who do not identify themselves as specialists in either gerontology or oncology. This includes nurses practicing in home care, extended care facilities, hospital inpatient and outpatient areas, and ambulatory surgery centers, as well as many physicians. It is incumbent upon providers who do not hold these myths and biases to educate patients and providers who do, in the interest of optimizing cancer care to all.

Prevention and Early Detection

Despite the fact that people over the age of 65 are at highest risk of developing cancer, there is much to be understood regarding cancer prevention and early detection activities in this age group. Although primary prevention of cancer can be initiated in old age, it is complicated by the long induction period from carcinogen exposure to clinically apparent disease for many tumors (7). Primary prevention of cancer in old age is best accomplished by assuming risk reducing behaviors and avoidance of carcinogenic exposures at much younger ages.

Smoking cessation is recommended at all ages, not only to prevent lung cancer, but for its more immediate effect on reducing risks of heart and other lung diseases and has received a substantial amount of attention in older age groups (8–11). Colorectal cancer may be prevented by removal of benign, premalignant polyps, and certain skin cancers may be prevented by avoiding sun and other ultraviolet exposures at all ages (7). Primary chemoprevention of breast cancer with tamoxifen in older women is currently under investigation (12). Avoiding excessive dietary fat, salted and pickled foods, and increasing intake of fiber, antioxi-

Table 54.2 Myths and biases that may negatively affect cancer care in the elderly (from (6)).

Myths that affect early detection and diagnosis

- cancer is contagious
- cancer is caused by accidental injuries or carelessness
- cancer is caused by stress
- once you have cancer it is "too late"
- pain is an early symptom of cancer
- health symptoms are due to normal aging or other chronic diseases
- elderly patients are not good sources of information about their health
- cancer screening is not valuable in the elderly

Myths that affect cancer treatment

- cancer is inevitably accompanied by unrelieveable pain
- older people are less sensitive to pain
- opiate pain medications cause addiction, respiratory depression, mental distortion, and death
- cancer is incurable
- cancer treatment is worse than the disease
- radiation therapy is painful, dangerous, and a treatment of last resort
- chemotherapy is extremely hazardous and inevitably accompanied by severe side effects
- the severity of side effects is positively correlated with the effectiveness of chemotherapy
- elderly patients cannot tolerate aggressive cancer work-ups, surgery, or adjuvant therapy
- elderly patients are not suitable candidates for clinical trials

Myths and biases that affect cancer rehabilitation

- elderly people are too frail and sick
- elderly people cannot learn adaptive behaviors
- elderly people have too little survival time
- elderly people can't cope with knowledge that they have cancer

dants, and fruits and vegetables should be lifetime habits in order to obtain maximum cancer prevention benefits, however, it is believed that benefits from these habits accrue even when they are started later in life (13,14).

An important barrier to primary cancer prevention efforts in the elderly is the notion, discussed above, that by old age, carcinogenic exposures have already been accrued and that the benefits of adopting risk

reducing behaviors do not outweigh the difficulties involved in changing lifelong habits. This belief, alluded to in Table 54.2, is prevalent among both lay persons and their health providers. While it is never too late to adopt a healthier lifestyle, it is likely that primary prevention of cancer in old age begins in youth and continues throughout a lifetime.

Understanding that cancer development in old age is related to behaviors adopted early in life is critical to primary prevention of cancer in future generations of elderly people. While adoption of risk-reducing behaviors by those already in old age has some benefits, adoption of these behaviors early in life may have a large impact on primary cancer prevention in old age. Nurses play an important role in encouraging smoking cessation and discouraging any kind of tobacco use among younger people. They are also active in skin cancer prevention activities, promoting the use of sunscreen and protective clothing among younger populations. Nurses and practitioners in all practice settings, but particularly those who work with children and younger adults are likely to have the largest impact over the long run on primary cancer prevention efforts for the elderly.

Early detection of cancer in the elderly has been a focus of attention ever since a classic article by Holmes and Hearne (15) documented that many common cancers are diagnosed at a more advanced stage in older people than in younger people. Many of these age/stage at diagnosis relationships have not been consistently demonstrated (16,17). There are four potential reasons why age/stage at diagnosis relationships may exist: (1) differences in biological behavior and histologic subtypes of various tumors with age; (2) patient delay in obtaining medical care once symptoms are apparent; (3) physician delay in diagnosis; and (4) lack of cancer screening in asymptomatic individuals. Age differences in tumor biology and histologic subtypes have been widely investigated and well-documented (18). While hypotheses regarding patient delay once symptoms arise are popular, they have not been as well-supported (4,16,18,19). Physician related factors contributing to delay in diagnosis have been somewhat better supported (20), although not consistently.

A major cornerstone of theories regarding both patient and physician delay when cancer symptoms are present is the notion of "symptom confusion" in the elderly. This occurs when symptoms actually due to cancer are attributed to other processes common in the elderly (4), and is rooted in the myths about cancer symptoms and health information presented in Table 54.2. However, it is also important to remember that by the time cancer causes symptoms such as anorexia, weight loss, decrease in performance status, or even coughing or bleeding, it is likely to be at a more advanced stage than it would be if asymptomatic screening had been done.

There are many reasons why asymptomatic older people do not receive regular cancer screening tests. For some common cancer sites (e.g., lung, ovary, bladder) there are no reliable screens. For other sites (pros-

Table 54.3 Barriers to cancer screening in the elderly.

- physician or health provider did not recommend
- not aware of increased risk of disease in old age
- reimbursement issues
- inability to access facilities
- lack of knowledge about screening tests
- physical discomfort of exams
- focus of health/medical care does not include cancer screening
- not wanting to feel or appear weak or vulnerable
- lack of confidence in ability to do self-administered exams/tests
- not comfortable with self-examinations
- not aware of screening benefits
- lack of consensus in professional community regarding cancer screening

Table 54.4 Strategies nurses can implement to encourage asymptomatic cancer screening in the elderly.

- Make cancer screening educational materials available in all health and social settings frequented by senior citizens
- Be aware of the controversies and lack of consensus surrounding cancer screening
- Discuss the issues and concepts surrounding cancer screening in the elderly with colleagues and other health professionals
- Discuss or provide opportunities to learning about cancer screening to patients regardless of practice setting
- Discuss cancer screening with patients and physicians in all practice settings
- Establish mechanisms for promoting cancer screening activities among older patients in your work setting
- Identify barriers to cancer screening in your patient population
- Have a list available of nearby and accesible screening facilities
- Have simply written instructions for obtaining Medicare or other insurance reimbursement for screening activities available

tate, colorectal, breast, cervix) there are well-established screens available. Although the misconceptions about cancer causation and prognosis identified in Table 54.2 may contribute to lack of screening for screenable cancers there are multiple other reasons. Table 54.3 presents a synthesis of barriers to cancer screening activities in the elderly that have been identified and discussed by multiple authors (21–31).

Nurses have historically taken an active role in promoting and furthering the understanding of cancer screening activities at all ages . The barriers to cancer screening identified in Table 54.3 present multiple opportunities for nursing interventions in any setting. Table 54.4 identifies specific strategies nurses and others can use to enhance cancer screening efforts in the elderly.

Acknowledge Interrelationships between Cancer and Aging Processes

Old age carries with it multiple changes in physiologic functioning, functional status and overall physical health. Although these changes may not occur at the same rate nor with the same severity among individuals, it is important to be cognizant of the impact of physiologic age on the elderly patient with cancer. Cancer in the older person must be considered within the context of other health and physical deficits that may be occurring simultaneously. It is possible that cancer does not carry the same threats to survival, functional status and quality of life as other health problems the elderly person may be facing.

In a study of comorbidity and disability in the elderly, cancer had only a moderate impact on disability, behind cerebrovascular disease, hip fractures, visual impairment, osteoporosis, diabetes, ischemic heart disease, arthritis, and age itself (32). Cancer does not occur as frequently in older people as these more disa-

bling diseases (32,33). In a study of hope in the elderly, declining physical health and lower socioeconomic were perceived as threats to hope, but having cancer did not threaten hope (34).

In a series of studies of comorbidity, physical functioning and breast cancer, younger breast cancer patients experienced more difficulties with physical functioning than did older breast cancer patients, when compared to women their own age without breast cancer (35). The presence of comorbid conditions increases the risk of death from causes other than breast cancer in elderly women with breast cancer (36,37). It is not clear how comorbid conditions and functional status affect participation in breast cancer screening, although they do affect, at least in part, cancer treatment decisions and survival (38).

It is easy for oncology nurses to focus exclusively on the cancer problems a patient has, without considering them in the broader context of other, possibly more threatening health problems. In the elderly, nurses must be aware of the presence and potential impact of aging and comorbid conditions, understanding that these may pose more of the threat to the patient than cancer itself. A thorough assessment of the patient's other health problems and how the cancer problem relates to them is an important part of geriatric oncology nursing.

Intervene to Prevent or Minimize Age-Specific Sequelae of Cancer and Cancer Treatment

Nurses have a critical role in assessing and managing side and toxic effects of cancer treatment in hospital, outpatient, and home care settings. The role of advanced age in determining the severity of the effects of cancer and its treatment in any particular individual is not well-understood.

Certain anatomic and physiologic changes that accompany normal aging in the absence of specific illness may affect an elderly patient's response to cancer treatment (39). These include declines in hepatic and renal function, an increased ratio of fat to lean body mass, decreased amounts of body water, and reduced ability of protective mechanisms (skin, mucous membranes, hematopoietic system) to cope with insults.

Whether or not cancer treatment is attenuated in an elderly cancer patient, the nurse should be aware that side effects and toxicities may arise in different patterns than they usually do in younger patients. Side effects and toxicities may arise earlier or later than usual, with a greater or lesser degree of severity, or with different presenting symptoms (4).

What looks like chemotherapy toxicity in an older patient, may be some other health problem. This author recalls a 77 year old, otherwise healthy woman who was receiving cis-platinum as part of a chemotherapy and radiation therapy protocol for lung cancer. Shortly after the start of chemotherapy, she complained of unilateral hearing loss, and suggested to the nurse that she might have a cerumen impaction. Without checking her ears, the nurse oncologist and medical oncologist referred the patient to an audiologist, who could not examine her hearing because of impacted cerumen in the affected ear.

As people age, they grow more heterogeneous. The nurse caring for elderly patients with cancer must be fully aware of the potential impact of normal aging changes as well as co-morbid conditions on the effects of cancer and its treatment. Critical, individualized assessment at each visit is important. Paying attention to the patient's symptoms and his or her interpretation of them may help to distinguish cancer-related problems from other problems. Shedding preconceptions about what is "normal" or "expected" for an individual cancer patient is critical to individualizing patient care at any age, but is particularly important in old age.

Integrate Comprehensive Geriatric Assessment in Nursing Care

The term, "comprehensive geriatric assessment" refers to the objective measurement of an individual's physical, psychological, functional, social, economic, and environmental status. This differs from routine functional status assessments that are commonly used, such as the Karnofsky Performance Status Scale. Comprehensive geriatric assessment is much more detailed and specific, using formal instruments to assess the patient's ability to perform individual basic activities of daily living (bathing, grooming, dressing, toileting, ambulating, feeding) and instrumental activities of daily living (shopping, cooking, cleaning, transportation, handling finances, taking medication, using the telephone). Formal instruments may also be used to measure mental status (cognitive and affective), social

Table 54.5 Purposes of comprehensive geriatric assessment and how they apply to nursing assessment.

1. Assist with improved diagnostic accuracy
   - determine etiology of symptoms that arise while patient is undergoing cancer treatment (eg, disease progression vs treatment toxicity vs other organic or inorganic problems)
   - determine etiology of problems with functional and mental/emotional status

2. Selection of appropriate interventions
   - patient education for self-care versus teaching a caregiver
   - appropriate use of medications versus other interventions for pain and other symptoms
   - response to preventive self-care practices and anti-cancer therapies

3. Identification of the optimal environment for care
   - hospital-based discharge planning
   - solving problems that arise during home or ambulatory care

4. Prediction of outcomes
   - patient/family education re treatment, side effects, toxicities
   - aid in planning home or clinic visits
   - assessment of rehabilitation needs and goals

5. Monitoring of changes over time
   - assessment of progress toward goals
   - assessment of new problems that develop

6. Assessment of patient's ability to perform self-care
   - psychomotor skills necessary for self-administration of treatments involving high-level technology

support systems, and environmental conditions. Comprehensive geriatric assessment generally relies on direct observation of behaviors and activities rather than self reports, as patients tend to overestimate their functional abilities while family caregivers tend to underestimate them. Numerous formalized scales and instruments for use in conducting geriatric assessment have been developed, many of which can be found in (40).

Six purposes of the comprehensive geriatric assessment (41) and examples of how they apply to nursing assessments of elderly cancer patient are listed in Table 54.5. While it is not practical or necessary for the nurse to conduct a full formalized comprehensive geriatric assessment of every elderly cancer patient using formal tools, the oncology nurse should be alert to clues that a comprehensive assessment is needed. A full comprehensive geriatric assessment is most readily

Table 54.6 Elements of comprehensive geriatric assessment and how they can be incorporated into routine nursing assessment for geriatric oncology patients.

Reliance on direct observation rather than self-report

- Observe patient performing basic activities of daily living

- Observe patient performing instrumental activities of daily living (ambulatory; home care)

- Make home visit (or arrange home visit) to observe patient in home environment

- Observe patient or caregiver performing self-care tasks

Use of formalized instruments

- Structure nursing assessment forms to include cues for conducting elements of geriatric assessment

- Incorporate specific assessment questions in nursing assessment forms and reports

Include multiple aspects of patient's life in assessment

- Incorporate assessment of family structure, social networks, environment in addition to physical and mental status

Focus on individual elements of functional status

- Assess and report ability to bathe, feed self, ambulate, etc rather than reporting on "ADLs"

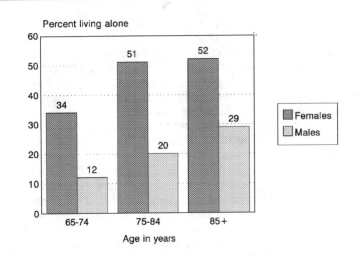

Figure 54.1 Percent of persons over age 65 living alone by age and sex, United States, 1987

accomplished by gerontologic consultation teams (42,43).

Nurses may integrate aspects of comprehensive geriatric assessment into their routine nursing assessments. Table 54.6 gives examples of how nurses in all practice settings can incorporate elements of comprehensive geriatric assessment into their practice.

Assess Availability and Capability of Support Networks

The importance of an elderly person's social support network is most often appreciated in the home care and ambulatory settings, where the meeting of most patient needs is left to the patient and his or her family and friends. The shift in cancer care settings from inpatient acute care to home and ambulatory care places unprecedented demands on support networks, not only for direct patient care, but also for other needs such as transportation, meals, and sensory stimulation. Nurses are frequently the first to identify weaknesses and strengths in a patient's support network and are often called upon to fill in the gaps.

Assessment of a patient's social support networks should not be incidental, and in many cases, should be a high priority. This is particularly true if a patient is being discharged from an inpatient setting to home or

outpatient care. The demands of cancer are superimposed on a support network that may already be wearing thin from the changes associated with normal aging and other chronic illnesses (44). Hermann and Carter (45) have noted that cancer patients are often discharged from the inpatient setting with "elaborate" home care regimens to follow and no supports for following through. This results in feelings of frustration on behalf of health care providers and feelings of alienation and powerlessness on behalf of patients and families.

Assessment of social support includes the quantity, nature, and quality of relationships and available supports, as well as cultural and ethnic considerations, and the patient's willingness to accept help (1). An important aspect of the social support network is the patient's living arrangement. Nearly one-third of all persons over the age of 65 live alone, and that proportion increases with age (Figure 54.1). Elderly persons who live alone often experience more health and socioeconomic problems and have fewer social supports than those who live with others. The typical elderly person who lives alone is a widowed female, over the age of 75 (46).

An illness such as cancer may force a change in living arrangements for an elderly person (47,48). An elderly person who has successfully lived alone may need to move in with a relative or other caregiver on at least a temporary basis. In other cases, some kind of long-term care facility may be needed. This disruption in living arrangements, coupled with the effects of a cancer diagnosis may create very high levels of stress for the patient and his or her support network. While patients living alone pose obvious demands on social support networks and systems, providers may be lulled into a false sense of security by patients who are living with a spouse or others. These living arrangements, whether or not they existed prior to the cancer diagnosis, may also be stressed by the new demands of the cancer diagnosis and its treatment. When the patient is living with others, particular attention should be given to the caregivers. It is not wise to assume that caregivers are capable of meeting the demands placed on them by the disease and it's treatment. These may include needs for personal care, nutrition, medication administration, monitoring and administration of intravenous medications, wound care and dressing changes, transportation, and pain management, among others. For example, a five week course of outpatient radiation therapy requires, at a minimum, 25 round trips to and from the radiation therapy facility, usually in the middle of the day, during the week, when job and other responsibilities are also making their demands.

When the caregiver is a spouse, sibling, or friend, the "hidden patient" syndrome must be considered. Is the caregiver elderly or chronically ill? The responsibilities of caring for the patient may quickly or suddenly exhaust the caregiver's supportive capacity, and may aggravate chronic illnesses such as heart disease that were previously under control.

Caregiver role strain is a second consideration. The change in established roles and interpersonal relationships that caregiving often demands (particularly of men, adult children, siblings, or others who are not used to assuming a caregiving role) may result in severe emotional strain for everyone involved. Another aspect of caregiver role strain involves the middle-aged daughters of elderly patients. In addition to assuming primary caregiving responsibilities for their sick, elderly parents (whether or not they are living with them), these women are also often responsible for their own younger families. These middle-aged children are often referred to as the "sandwich generation," and are likely to grow in numbers as lifespans increase and childbearing continues into middle age (1).

While the support needs of patients living alone with no one to rely on may be obvious, those of patients living with others or who have designated caregivers may be more complex, and less obvious, creating double jeopardy for all involved. Critical assessment, selection, preparation, and care of caregivers is a critical aspect of geriatric oncology that ultimately affects the success of cancer treatment.

Increase Communication with Colleagues and Other Providers Regarding Older Cancer Patients

Elderly patients with cancer are living longer with their disease than ever before, and are being treated in many different settings, for health problems both related and unrelated to their cancer. They are also receiving cancer care in many settings, at many stages of the disease, from diagnosis until death, particularly at home, from providers who may not be familiar with the body of knowledge surrounding cancer in the elderly.

Nurses are in an excellent position to inform other members of the health care team about the special

Table 54.7 Age-related considerations for cancer patient education.

- Functional illiteracy
- Neurosensory compromise — vision, hearing, touch
- Increased learning time
- Short-term memory loss
- Anxiety, stress over life changes
- Negative past experiences with cancer
- Age-appropriateness of teaching tools and methods
- Physical ability to perform necessary motor skills

needs and concerns of elderly patients with cancer. This can be done on an individual basis, when referring a patient from one setting to another (e.g., hospital to home care), or within disciplines (e.g., physical therapy or social work). Nurses can identify providers and members of disciplines who deal with large numbers of elderly cancer patients and make efforts to communicate with them about the needs of elderly cancer patients along the disease trajectory.

Consider Age-Related Factors that Affect Learning and Performance of Self-Care Activities Related to Cancer

Patient and family education are key components of cancer nursing care at all ages. Patient education occurs in cognitive, affective and psychomotor domains. With the increasing emphasis on ambulatory and home care, the learning and performance of self-care activities for cancer patients and their caregivers has assumed unprecedented importance.

In any age group, there are special considerations for patient/caregiver education, and the elderly are no exception. Table 54.7 lists considerations for patient education in this age group.

Functional illiteracy is an important consideration, since we place heavy reliance on booklets, pamphlets, written instructions and other teaching aids. Fully one-third of persons aged 65 and over in the United States have eight or fewer years of formal schooling (49), yet many patient education materials are written at a grades 9–12 reading level (50). A recent study (51) of literacy and the readability of 30 cancer patient education pamphlets found that most the materials were written at a grades 8–9 reading level. Of 63 veterans (aged 22–74) in the study, 27 percent read below a sixth grade level (below all 30 pamphlets tested) and 17 percent read between sixth and eighth grade levels (47 percent of the pamphlets). The formal education of many older persons ended long before current cancer treatment concepts, language, and technologies were developed. This may pose extra challenges when teaching or even talking to patients about their disease and treatment.

Neurosensory changes that accompany aging may affect visual acuity, hearing, and touch. Visual acuity is necessary for reading written instructional materials as well as medication labels and indicators on pumps and machines that may be used to deliver intravenous therapy at home. Heavy reliance on verbal instructions necessitates that patients be able to hear and process what is being said. Many people (of all ages) are reluctant to ask physicians and nurses to slow down or repeat themselves, and many physicians and nurses tend to only give instructions quickly and once.

In the absence of dementia, older people are capable of learning much new material, although the learning process may take longer, and short term memory loss may occur. Coupled with neurosensory declines, these aspects of teaching the elderly may make the patient education process more time-consuming and laborious than usual, tempting the nurse to direct instructions to the caregiver rather than the patient. This strategy often backfires as the patient senses that he or she is being overlooked and reduced to a passive role in this process.

Anxiety and emotional stress revolving around the cancer diagnosis and life changes it may entail (e.g., changing living arrangements), also interfere with effective learning. The patient may have had negative past experiences with cancer. Understanding the importance of these experiences and the impact they have on the patients' ability to understand and absorb new information related to cancer and its treatment is vital to effective patient education.

Many patient education materials are not geared specifically to the needs of elderly patients. Although written materials contain valuable information, print may be small, illustrations may not be clear enough, and information may be presented in a way that is difficult to understand. Audiovisual materials may be fast-paced, with excessive narration and high vocabulary levels (52–56).

Finally, activities such as wound care, management of feeding tubes, intravenous lines, injections, pumps, and solutions all require a certain amount of visual acuity and manual dexterity. Arthritic and sensory changes in fingers and hands many interfere with the patient's or elderly caregiver's ability to perform necessary tasks, and the tasks may need to be adapted to the patient's limitations or performed by someone else. Table 54.8 lists specific interventions for maximizing patient education in geriatric oncology.

The importance of effective patient education for optimizing cancer treatment and rehabilitation efforts in this age group cannot be overemphasized. Failure to adapt patient education efforts to the special needs of elderly cancer patients and their caregivers may hamper the achievement of treatment outcomes and possibly result in serious complications.

Maximize Advocacy Role in Ethical Decision-Making Regarding Quality of Life

Cancer care and treatment decisions become increasingly complex as a patient's age increases. Decisions

Table 54.8 Interventions for maximizing patient/ caregiver education efforts in geriatric oncology.

- Assess ability of patient/caregiver to read and comprehend written materials
- Assess ability to see and hear
- Give patient/caregiver permission to ask for repetitions, decrease or increase in speed of presentation
- Give patient/caregiver permission to admit that she/ he does not understand something
- Be sensitive to cues that patient/caregiver is not absorbing material (e g, cannot paraphrase what has just been taught)
- Allow extra time for patient education
- Give information in small amounts, with frequent repetitions and checks that patient is comprehending
- Have a detailed plan for patient education, specifying exactly what will be taught when
- Adapt instructional materials to patient needs, supplementing with customized materials such as signs, lists, etc
- Avoid directing conversation and education solely to the caregiver unless the patient is clearly uninterested or incapable
- Assess ability of patient/caregiver to perform motor tasks and adapt as possible
- Obtain feedback in all domains (cognitive, affective, psychomotor) after material has been taught in order to clarify what was learned and what still needs to be taught

regarding cancer prevention, screening, diagnosis, and treatment must be weighed in consideration of the patient's remaining life expectancy, other co-morbid conditions, functional status, mental status, psychosocial status, and ability to tolerate treatment. The role of patient advocate has long been considered an important role of the nurse (57–62) and is expected to increase in importance (63). It entails assisting patients and their families to explore their own values related to clinical options when faced with difficult decisions. In order to be an effective advocate the nurse must understand his or her own biases and values to ensure that they do not interfere with the patient's decision making (64–66).

Making the effort to ensure that a balance is reached between the elderly individual's acknowledged right to self-determination and his or her need or desire for surrogate decision-making is critical. Issues such as the patient's level of autonomy and the existence of or need for advance directives are best resolved before a critical health decision is necessary, and should be part of the initial nursing assessment.

Ensuring that the patient and/or his or her designated others have sufficient information to make decisions, and that they understand the information that has been given to them is another important aspect of patient advocacy. This can be difficult if healthcare team or family members are inclined (for any reason) to withhold various options from the decision-making process, or favor one option over another. Examples of decisions for which there are options include cancer treatment, pain management, setting of care, or disclosure of a diagnosis or prognosis.

Regardless of age or perceived frailty, patients must be included in decision-making activities (1). This can be difficult and time-consuming, particularly if the patient and family do not understand the issues surrounding a particular decision, if providers involved in the patient's care do not agree among themselves on the issues surrounding a decision, or if providers do not agree with family members.

Hundreds of decisions must be made in the course of cancer care, from prevention and screening to diagnosis, treatment and rehabilitation. The vast majority of these decisions do not assume crisis proportions, and many do not carry strong ethical concerns. However, all health care decision-making concerning cancer and the elderly should be driven by ethical considerations.

In 1991 the Oncology Nursing Society (ONS) convened an Ethics Task Force to address the oncology nurse's role in dealing with issues and decision making related to ethics. The full report of this task force was published in 1993 (67) and includes discussions of the moral context of oncology nursing, the role of professional associations in relation to ethics and society, ethical issues in oncology nursing practice, and the ethical context of healthcare reform. Priority ethical issues for oncology nurses were identified by the ONS Ethics Advisory Council, which grew out of the Ethics Task Force. They include topics surrounding: assisted suicide, end of life decisions, pain management, healthcare reform, access to healthcare, truth-telling and informed choice, scientific integrity, confidentiality, and advance directives (68). A professional code of ethics for oncology nurses was published in 1995 (69).

Recognize Effects of Healthcare Policy on Geriatric Oncology Nursing Care

Few topics have generated as much controversy and concern as healthcare policy in the late 20th century. Efforts to control healthcare costs have driven unprecedented changes in the healthcare system including shifts from acute inpatient to outpatient and home care, shortened inpatient stays, increasing use of unlicensed personnel to provide care, and attempts to predict and evaluate outcomes of care.

The effects of these changes on geriatric oncology patients, their families, and the nurses who care for them are many. Home and outpatient care rely heavily on informal caregivers and strong social support networks, not only for basic needs, but also for transportation to and from physician visits, monitoring of changes in patient condition, and management of symptoms and treatment. We have already seen that many elderly patients live alone, and many social support networks are insufficient to meet these demands.

Health care reimbursement places a high priority on treatment of disease and lower priority on prevention and maintenance of health and well-being (1). This results in inadequate coverage for long-term care, whether at home or in an institution. As long as the need for care by a registered nurse or other registered therapist at home, or institutional care for treatment and rehabilitation and progress toward outcomes can be documented, reimbursement is available for some care. However, when the patient has reached treatment goals, or fails to progress, reimbursement for care is often denied. The support network must then assume the burden of care which can be considerable, if the patient is physically or mentally incapacitated. Nurses are often placed in the position of deciding when care can no longer be reimbursed and a patient must either be transferred to another setting or discharged.

Although volunteer and private sector efforts to provide social supports to the elderly are laudable and meet many needs, most are inadequate to meet all the needs of their clients. The patient, family, nurse, social worker are often forced to piece together services (eg, meals on wheels, volunteer driver, volunteer housekeeper) in order to maintain the patient at home while treatment is in progress and after treatment stops in order to avoid costly and perhaps unnecessary institutionalization.

Health care policy and reimbursement also affect cancer treatment patterns (1). One form of treatment may be given over another because reimbursement is available. For example, injections and certain drugs may be paid for if administered by a nurse in a hospital outpatient setting, but not if self-administered by the patient at home. "Off-label" use of antineoplastic drugs (use of Food and Drug Administration (FDA)-approved agents for non-FDA approved indications or in nonapproved routes or dosages) may not be reimbursed, despite documented effectiveness. Health policy also dictates access to clinical trials, since many of the costs of clinical trial involvement may not be covered.

The effects of health care policy on the day to day practice of nurses who care for elderly cancer patients are ubiquitous. Because nurses are often employed by others rather than self-employed, they may not directly see the relationship between health policy and their practice. It is important for nurses to realize that nearly every aspect of their practice is dictated by health care reimbursement policy on either the local, state, or national level. Nurses need to be aware of the policies that affect their practice and the importance of involvement in the creation of health policy.

Conclusion

Geriatric oncology nursing practice encompasses a broad spectrum of activities and considerations. In order to optimize patient care the nurse must be aware of the multiple factors that affect the cancer experience in the elderly in general, and how they affect the individual patient. There is great heterogeneity among the elderly, and their responses to cancer and cancer treatment will be equally heterogeneous. As the population ages, it is important for health care providers to develop new paradigms about aging and health that may contradict long-held assumptions, and to have a voice in health policy decision-making, so that health policies and practices reflect the health needs of the population.

Acknowledgement

Supported in part by a grant from the National Institute on Aging, AG002310-03.

References

1. Boyle DM, Engelking C, Blesch KS, et al. ONS position paper on cancer and aging: The mandate for oncology nursing. Onc Nurs Forum 19: 913–933, 1992.

2. Walsh SJ, Begg CB, Carbone PB. Cancer chemotherapy in the elderly. Semin Oncol 16: 66–75, 1989.

3. Wetle T. Age as a risk factor for inadequate treatment. JAMA 258: 516, 1987.

4. Cohen HJ. Oncology and aging: General principles of cancer in the elderly. In Principles of Geriatric Medicine and Gerontology, 3rd edition, edited by WR Hazzard, et al. New York: McGraw-Hill, pp. 77–89, 1994.

5. McKenna R. Clinical aspects of cancer in the elderly: treatment decisions, treatment choices, and follow-up. Cancer 74 (suppl): 2107–2117, 1994.

6. Berkman B, Rohan B, Sampson S. Myths and biases related to cancer in the elderly. Cancer 74 (suppl): 2004–2008, 1994.

7. Patterson WB, Williams TF. Epilogue: future directions for cancer control in older persons. In Cancer in the Elderly, Approaches to Detection and Treatment, edited by R Yancik and JW Yates. New York: Springer, pp. 224–231, 1989.

8. Rimer BK, Orleans CT. Tailoring smoking cessation for older adults. Cancer 74 (suppl): 2051–2054, 1994.

9. Cummings KM. Involving older Americans in the war on tobacco: the American Stop Smoking Intervention Study for Cancer Prevention. Cancer 74 (suppl): 2062–2066, 1994.

10. Orleans TC, Jepson C, Resch N, et al. Quitting motives and barriers among older smokers: the 1986 Adult Use of Tobacco Survey Revisited. Cancer 74 (suppl): 2055 2061, 1994.

11. Bal DG, Lloyd J. Advocacy and government action for cancer prevention in older persons. Cancer 74 (suppl): 2067–2070, 1994.

12. Love RR. Prospects for antiestrogen chemoprevention of breast cancer. J Natl Cancer Inst 82: 18–21, 1990.

13. Merskens FL. Strategies for prevention of cancer in humans. Oncology 6 (suppl): 15, 1992.

14. Yates JW. Cancer prevention in older adults. In Geriatric Oncology, edited by L Balducci. Philadelphia: JB Lippincott, pp. 99–104, 1992.

15. Holmes FF, Hearne E. Cancer stage-to-age relationship: Implications for cancer screening in the elderly. J Am Geriatr Soc 29: 55–57, 1981.

16. Mor V. Malignant disease and the elderly. In Research and the Ageing Population, edited by D Evered, J Whelan. Chichester: Wiley (Ciba Foundation Symposium 134), p. 160, 1988.

17. Goodwin JS, et al. Stage at diagnosis varies with the age of the patient. J Am Geriatri Soc 43: 20–26, 1986.

18. Samet JM, et al. Delay in seeking care for cancer symptoms: a population-based study of elderly New Mexicans J Natl Cancer Inst 80: 432–438, 1988.

19. Prohaska TR, Funch D, Blesch KS. Age patterns in symptom perception and illness behavior among colorectal cancer patients. Behavior, Health and Aging 1: 27–39, 1990.

20. Robinson E, et al. Factors affeeting delay in diagnosis of breast cancer: Relationship of delay of disease. Isr J Med Sci 22: 333–338, 1986.

21. Rubenstein L. Strategies to overcome barriers to early detection of cancer among older adults. Cancer (suppl) 74: 2190–2193, 1994.

22. Blesch KS, Prohaska TR. Cervical cancer screening in older women: issues and interventions. Cancer Nursing 14: 141–147, 1991.

23. Maddox MA. The practice of breast self-examination among older women. Oncol Nurs Forum 18: 1367–1371, 1991.

24. Frank-Stromborg M. The role of the nurse in early detection of cancer. Oncol Nurs Forum 13 (3): 66–74, 1986.

25. Powe BD. Cancer fatalism among elderly Caucasians and African Americans. Oncol Nurs Forum 22: 1355–1359, 1995.

26. Burnett CB, Steakley CS, Tefft MC. Barriers to breast and cervical cancer screening in underserved women of the District of Columbia. Oncol Nurs Forum 22: 1551–1558, 1995.

27. Gelfand DE, et al. Digital rectal examinations and prostate cancer screening: attitudes of African-American men. Oncol Nurs Forum 22: 1253–1258.

28. Sensiba ME, Stewart DS. Relationship of perceived barriers to breast self-examination in women of varying ages and levels of education. Oncol Nurs Forum 22: 1265 1268.

29. Blalock SJ, et al. Participation in fecal occult blood screening: a critical review. Preventive Medicine 16 (1): 9–18.

30. Park SI, et al. Does use of the Colo-screen Self-Test improve patient compliance with fecal occult blood screening? Am J Gastroenterol 88: 1391–1394.

31. Mahon SM. The impact of mailing fecal occult blood test kits on return rate in a community cancer screening center. Oncol Nurs Forum 22: 1259–1263, 1995.

32. Verbrugge LM, Lepkowski JM, Imanaka Y. Comorbidity and its impact on disability. The Milbank Quarterly 67: 450–484, 1989.

33. Guralnik JM, et al. Aging in the eighties: the prevalence of comorbidity and its association with disability. Advance data from Vital and Health Statistics, no. 170. Hyattsville, MD: National Center for Health Statistics, 1989.

34. McGill JS, Paul PB. Functional status and hope in elderly people with and without cancer. Oncol Nurs Forum 20:

35. Satariano WA, et al. Difficulties in physical functioning reported by middle-aged and elderly women with breast cancer: a case-control comparison. J Gerontol 45: M3–M11, 1990.

36. Satariano WA, Ragland DR. The effect of comorbidity on 3-year survival of women with primary breast cancer. Ann Intern Med 120: 104–110, 1994.

37. Charlson ME, et al. A new method of classifying prognostic comorbidity in longitudinal studies: development and validation. J Chron Dis 40: 373–383, 1987.

38. Satariano WA. Comorbidity and functional status in older women with breast cancer: implications for screening, treatment, and prognosis. J Gerontol 47 (special issue): 24–31.

39. Blesch KS. The normal physiological changes of aging and their impact on the response to cancer treatment. Semin Oncol Nurs 4: 178–188, 1988.

40. Kane R, Kane R. Assessing the Elderly. Lexington, MA: Lexington Books, 1981.

41. Solomon D. NIH consensus Development conference statement: geriatric assessment methods for clinical decision making. J Am Geriatr Soc 36: 342–347, 1988.

42. Barker WH, et al. Geriatric consultation teams in acute-care hospitals. J Am Geriatr Soc 33: 422–428, 1985.

43. McVey LJ, et al. Effect of a geriatric consultation team on functional status of elderly hospitalized patients. Ann Intern Med 110: 79–84, 1989.

44. Engelking C. Comfort issues in geriatric oncology. Semin Oncol Nurs 4: 169–177, 1988.

45. Hermann JF, Carter J. The dimensions of oncology social work: intrapsychic, interpersonal, and environmental interactions. Semin Oncol 21: 712–717, 1994.

46. Kasper JD. Aging Alone. Profiles and Projections. A Report of the Commonwealth Fund Commission on Elderly People Living Alone. The Commonwealth Fund, 1988.

47. Prohaska T, et al. Functional status and living arrangements. In Health Data on Older Americans: United States, 1992, edited by JF Van Nostrand, et al. Vital Health Stat, Hyattsville MD: National Center for Health Statistics, pp. 23–40, 1993.

48. Miller B, *et al*. Changes in functional status and risk of institutionalization and death. In *Health Data on Older Americans: United States, 1992*, edited by JF Van Nostrand, *et al*. Vital Health Stat, Hyattsville MD: National Center for Health Statistics, pp. 41–76, 1993.

49. U.S. Bureau of the Census. *Statistical Abstract of the United States. 109th ed*. Washington, DC: 1989.

50. Meade CD, *et al*. Readability of American Cancer Society patient education literature. *Oncol Nurs Forum* 19: 61–55, 1992.

51. Cooley ME, *et al*. Patient literacy and the readability of written cancer educational materials. *Oncol Nurs Forum* 22: 1345–1351, 1995.

52. Welch-McCaffrey D. To teach or not to teach? Overcoming barriers to patient education in geriatric oncology. *Oncol Nurs Forum* 13 (4): 25–31, 1986.

53. Weinrich SP, Weinrich MC. Cancer knowledge among elderly individuals. *Cancer Nurs* 9: 301–307, 1986.

54. Rimer B, *et al*. Health education for older persons: lessons from research and program evaluations. *Adv Health Educ Promo* 1: 369–396, 1986.

55. Weinrich SP, Boyd M. Education in the elderly: adapting and evaluating teaching tools. *J Gerontol Nurs* 18 (1): 15–20, 1992.

56. Watson PM. Patient education: the adult with cancer. *Nurs Clin North Am* 17: 739–751, 1982.

57. American Nurses Association Committee on Ethical Standards. A suggested code. *Am J Nurs* 26: 599–601, 1926.

58. American Nurses Association. Standards and scope of gerontological nursing practice. Kansas City, MO: ANA, 1987.

59. American Nurses Association, Oncology Nursing Society. *Standards of Oncology Nursing Practice*. Kansas City: MO, ANA, 1987.

60. Oncology Nursing Society. *Scope of Oncology Nursing Practice*. Pittsburgh, PA: ONS, 1988.

61. Oncology Nursing Society. *Standards of Oncology Nursing Education*. Pittsburgh, PA: ONS, 1989.

62. Oncology Nursing Society. *Standards of Advanced Practice in Oncology Nursing*. Pittsburgh, PA: ONS, 1990.

63. National League for Nursing. *Nursing 2020: a study of future hospital-based nursing*. NLN Pub. No. 14:2217. New York: NLN, 1988.

64. Gadow S. An ethical case for patient self-determination. *Semin Oncol Nurs* 5: 99–101, 1989.

65. Donovan C. Toward a nursing ethics program in an acute care setting. *Top Clin Nurs* 5 (3): 55–62, 1983.

66. Welch-McCaffrey D. Ethical issues: advocacy responsibilities of nurses caring for the elderly cancer patient Arlington, VA: Proceedings of the Fifth National Conference on Cancer Nursing, 1987.

67. Carroll-Johnson RM (ed). Ethics and Oncology Nursing: Report of the Ethics Task Force. *Oncol Nurs Forum* (suppl) 20 (10): 1–56, 1993.

68. Ersek M, *et al*. Priority ethical issues in oncology nursing: current approaches and future directions. *Oncol Nurs Forum* 22: 803–808, 1995.

69. Scanlon E, Glover J. A professional code of ethics: providing a moral compass for turbulent times. *Oncol Nurs Forum* 22: 1515–1526 1995.

55. Cancer Pain in the Elderly

J.F. Cleary

Introduction

At some stage of their illness, almost all patients with cancer will need palliation of symptoms, either those caused by the disease itself or those related to treatment. Pain is one of these symptoms and its management has often been given little attention by health professionals. Although most pain from cancer can be adequately controlled with oral analgesics, a significant minority of cancer patients receive analgesics that are inadequate in type or potency to manage their pain. In a recent multi-center study of outpatients with metastatic cancer, 42% of those with pain did not receive the type of analgesics recommended by standard cancer pain management guidelines (1). In that study, patients aged greater than 70 were among specific populations at greater risk for inadequate analgesia. Poorly-controlled pain may have such catastrophic effects on the patient and his or her family that proper pain management must have the highest priority for those who routinely care for cancer patients. Special care must be exercised to see that older patients get pain relief. Severe pain may be a primary reason why both patients and their families stop cancer treatment, and is often given as a reason that patients and families entertain the idea of euthanasia. Improving the practice of anticipating, evaluating, and treating pain will benefit all cancer patients. Recognizing the specific barriers confronting our management of pain in the older patient will help assure adequate pain relief.

Prevalence, Severity and Risk of Pain

Although only 15% of patients with non metastatic disease had pain associated with their tumor at the time of diagnosis (2), pain is pervasive as disease progresses. With the diagnosis of metastatic disease, this increased to 74%. In a multi-centered study, 67% of outpatients who had metastatic disease had disease related pain or were taking analgesia on a daily basis (1). Thirty-six percent of the patients in this Eastern Cooperative Oncology Group Study had pain severe enough to compromise their daily function.

Etiology of Cancer Pain

The sensation of pain is generated either by stimulation of peripheral pain receptors or by damage to afferent nerve fibers. Peripheral pain receptors can be stimulated by pressure, compression, and traction as well as by disease-related chemical changes. Pain due to stimulation of pain receptors is called *nociceptive* pain. Damage to visceral, somatic, or autonomic nerve trunks produces *neurogenic* or *neuropathic* pain. Neuropathic pain is thought to be caused by spontaneous activity in nerves damaged by disease or treatment. Cancer patients often have both nociceptive and neuropathic pain simultaneously. In patients with advanced cancer, the majority have pain at multiple sites caused by multiple mechanisms.

Direct tumor involvement is the most common cause of pain, present in approximately two thirds of patients with pain from metastatic cancer. Tumor invasion of bone, common in breast and prostate cancer and with multiple myeloma accounts for pain in about 50% of these patients. The remaining 50% experience tumor-related pain that is due to nerve compression or infiltration, or involvement of the gastrointestinal tract or soft tissue. Up to 25% of patients may have pain related to their therapy (3). Persistent post-therapy pain, from long term effects of surgery, radiotherapy, and chemotherapy, accounts for up to 20% of those who report pain with metastatic cancer. The effect of aging on the side effects of chemotherapy has been documented. Begg and Carbone (4) assessed the toxicities of 25,000 patients treated on Eastern Cooperative Oncology Group studies and concluded in relation to hematological toxicity, that the elderly tolerate chemotherapy as well as younger patients. They showed a non statistically significant increase in the incidence of neurotoxicity in elderly patients who were treated for sarcoma. However they suggested that the elderly in general appear more susceptible to the neuropathy associated with cisplatin and the vinca alkaloids and recommended that these agents should be used sparingly in the elderly population.

A new complaint of pain in a patient with metastatic cancer should first be thought of as disease-related, but non-cancer causes may need to be considered and ruled out. The prevalence of co-morbidities that cause pain, such as osteoarthitis, is obviously much greater for an older population. Elderly persons experience more pain in general than the young. The prevalence of pain in those older than 60 is 250/1000, double that of those who are younger. The predominant cause of pain in the elderly is musculoskeletal, with 80% people over the age of 65 suffering from arthritis (5). 25–50% of community dwelling elderly suffer important pain problems (6) while up to 80% of patients living in nursing homes have pain (7). The older patient with cancer, is not only likely to experience pain in association with his/her cancer, but is more likely than a younger person

Table 55.1 Barriers to cancer pain relief.

Problems related to health care professionals

    Inadequate knowledge of pain management

    Poor assessment of pain

    Concern about regulation of controlled substances

    Fear of patient addiction

    Concern about side effects of analgesics

    Concern about patients becoming tolerant to analgesics

Problems related to patients

    Reluctance to report pain

    Concern about distracting physicians from treatment of underlying disease

    Fear that pain means disease is worse

    Concern about not being a "good" patient

    Reluctance to take pain medications

    Fear of addiction or of being thought of as an addict

    Worries about unmanageable side effects

    Concern about being tolerant to pain medications

Problems related to the health care system

    Low priority given to cancer pain treatment

    Inadequate reimbursement

    Appropriate treatment may not be reimbursed or may be too costly

    Restrictive regulation of controlled substances

    Problems of availability of treatment or access to it.

to have pain associated with other disease processes. However, it has been suggested that apart from pain associated with joints (arthritis), elderly patients have less pain than younger patients. and differences in the perception of pain in the elderly have been recorded. Despite these findings, biological aging appears to have no impact on the sensory or perceived unpleasantness of pain (8).

Barriers to Good Pain Management in Older Patients

There are many barriers to good cancer pain management and they have been detailed by the Agency for Health Care Policy and Research (AHCPR) Cancer Pain guidelines (9) (Table 55.1). These barriers may be related to health practitioners, to patients themselves or to the health care system of which they are part.

Doctors have acknowledged that they are not properly trained in pain assessment (10) and will often not raise the issue of pain unless it is volunteered by the patient. To provide adequate pain control, health professionals need to seek a patient's report of pain as the primary of assessment. Many cancer patients fear that reporting pain will distract their clinicians from their disease and its treatment and therefore do not report it (11). This may be of more importance in the elderly who often have multiple disease processes present. Poor or absent pain assessment has been identified as major reasons for poor cancer pain management.

Reimbursement issues are of significance in the management of cancer pain. A proper pain assessment, particularly for a patient with multiple pains, takes time and may be limited by the time a doctor can afford to spend with each patient. Proper pain assessment and management is poorly rewarded as it does take time. Cost can be a factor in relation to other issues including the availability of medications. Most cancer patients should be able to have their pain managed as an outpatient. However, many elderly patients in the United States are covered by Medicare which has not reimbursed the cost of outpatient oral analgesics even though it pays for the cost of inpatient medications. Patients themselves may not fill prescriptions for opioids despite the pain they may be experiencing because of the extra cost of these drugs to them. Proposed changes to health care in the United States may impact severely on funding to Medicare and consequently on cancer pain management in the elderly. Other health care organizations (HMOs, Insurance Companies) already vary greatly in what they provide for pain management but may become a driving force in "standard pain management", not necessarily through optimizing patient care but in optimizing profits.

What patients think about pain and its treatment can be very important in the provision of adequate pain management. Ward *et al.* (11) assessed pain severity and pain interference together with concerns about reporting pain and using pain medication in 270 cancer patients. The 8 specific issues addressed included fear of addiction, beliefs that 'good' patients do not complain about pain, and concerns about side effects. Some patients felt that doctors were not interested in their pain (37% of patients), many were concerned about addiction (55%) and most were anxious about constipation as a side effect of cancer pain management (85%). There were more concerns in those with less education, lower incomes, higher levels of pain and those who were under medicated. Of importance, older patients had *more concerns* in all areas.

Fear of addiction is a special concern for older patients and may also be a concern for their families and their health care providers. There is little rational evidence to support this concern. Of 12,000 patients prescribed opioids for medical purposes, less than one tenth of one percent (0.1%) became addicted to these medications (12). Confusion in the terminology associated with addiction and physical dependence is part of the problem. Physical dependence is a physiological phenomenon characterized by the development of an abstinence syndrome following abrupt discontinuation of therapy, substantial dose reduction or the administration of an antagonist drug (13). Physical dependence will develop in patients who are prescribed opioids for any length of time in a situation similar to that of any patient who has been prescribed corticosteroids over time. When an opioid is stopped suddenly, the patient experiences physiological withdrawal symptoms which may include fever, tachycardia and abdominal cramps. The occurrence of withdrawal symptoms has been used by many, including the authors of the Diagnostic and Statistical Manual, to establish the diagnosis of substance dependence. A more usable definition of addiction or psychological dependence allows the diagnosis to be made on the presence of three types of aberrant behavior. These are a) a patient's loss of control over drug use b) a patient's compulsive use of the drug and c) continued use of the drug despite evidence of harm to the patient (13). Care must be taken with the use of opioids in patients who are addicted to other drugs and guidelines have been established for their use (14). Confusion over drug seeking behavior in people with pain has resulted in the definition of the syndrome, pseudoaddiction. This syndrome refers to "drug seeking" behavior by patients in their search for adequate pain relief and is the direct result of inadequate pain management (15).

Assessment of Pain

Inadequate pain assessment and poor physician-patient communication about pain are major barriers to good pain care. Proper pain management requires a clear understanding of the characteristics of the pain and its physical basis. The changing expression of cancer pain demands *repeated assessment*, as new causes for pain can emerge rapidly. The essentials of cancer pain assessment are similar to those taught for disease assessment in the early years of professional education, principles used extensively for diagnostic purposes in patients with ischemic heart disease, appendicitis or renal colic to name a few examples. However as health care professionals, we rarely use these very same principles for the assessment of pain in patients with a diagnosis of cancer. The use of these principles can tell us so much about the pain and provide a guide to the best possible treatment options without the need to perform invasive tests. Pain assessment needs to occur repeatedly and at regular intervals throughout the treatment of a patient and most importantly with any new report of pain.

Components of Pain Assessment

It is essential to ask a patient about each component of their pain. It is possible from these individual components to identify pain syndromes, for instance based on the distribution of pain together with the character and radiation. However in seeking such patterns, a clinician must be careful to ensure that a total assessment is performed.

Intensity: How severe is your pain?

Physicians and nurses tend to underestimate pain intensity, especially when it is severe. Patients whose doctors underestimate their pain are at high risk for poor pain management and compromised function. Communication about pain is greatly aided by having the patient use a scale to report pain severity. A simple rating scale ranges from 0 to 10, with 0 being "no pain" and 10 being "pain as bad as you can imagine." Used properly, pain severity scales can be invaluable in titrating analgesics and in monitoring for increases in pain with progressive disease. Daut *et al.* (16) using a numeric rating index (0–10) to develop the Brief Pain Inventory (BPI) (Figure 55.1) a tool where patients self rate their pain (pain worst, pain average, pain least and pain now) along with a self assessment of the interference of pain with everyday functions such as activity, mood and relationships with others. The BPI has been validated for cancer patients in several languages (17) and has been used extensively in pain research. Based on continued work with this tool in cancer patients, Serlin *et al.* (18) have been able to define three levels of pain. Mild pain ("pain worst" score of 0–4) is often well tolerated with minimal impact on a patient's activities. At "pain worst" scores of 5–6, patients experience some disruption in these daily activities. However, there is a threshold beyond which pain is especially disruptive and is generally reached when the "pain worst" score is 7 or more on a 0–10 scale. At this level, pain becomes the primary focus of attention and prohibits most activity not directly related to pain. While it may not be possible to totally eliminate pain, reducing its severity to 4 or less ought to be a minimum standard of pain therapy.

Character: How would you describe your pain?

Verbal descriptors of pain used by the patient may help in establishing the etiology of pain. It is important that a physician be aware of the diversity of terms used by patients. Often a patient will deny that they have pain but that the "pulling" sensation that they are experiencing in their back would rate as a seven out of 10 on a 0–10 pain scale. A common descriptive term used by patients is that of an "ache." Other terms used include pressure, tightness, burning, tingling, numbness and electric shock like pain. A patient's description of a shooting pain down his/her arm would suggest that there is a neuropathic component of the pain.

Location: Where is your pain?

The discrimination between generalized versus localized pain is an important one in the consideration of both diagnoses and treatment options. It is equally important to remember that pain can be distributed over dermatomal patterns. This is as important in cancer related pain as it is when used in the diagnosis of appendicitis (periumbilical pain) or gall bladder disease (right shoulder tip pain). Patients may present with knee pain with no evidence of pathology in that joint. The pain may in fact be referred pain (not radiating) from L3 area in the spine or from disease associated with the hip. Localized pain may be best managed with systemic analgesic agents together with a localized therapy e.g. radiotherapy or nerve block. If adequate analgesia is obtained through such an intervention, the

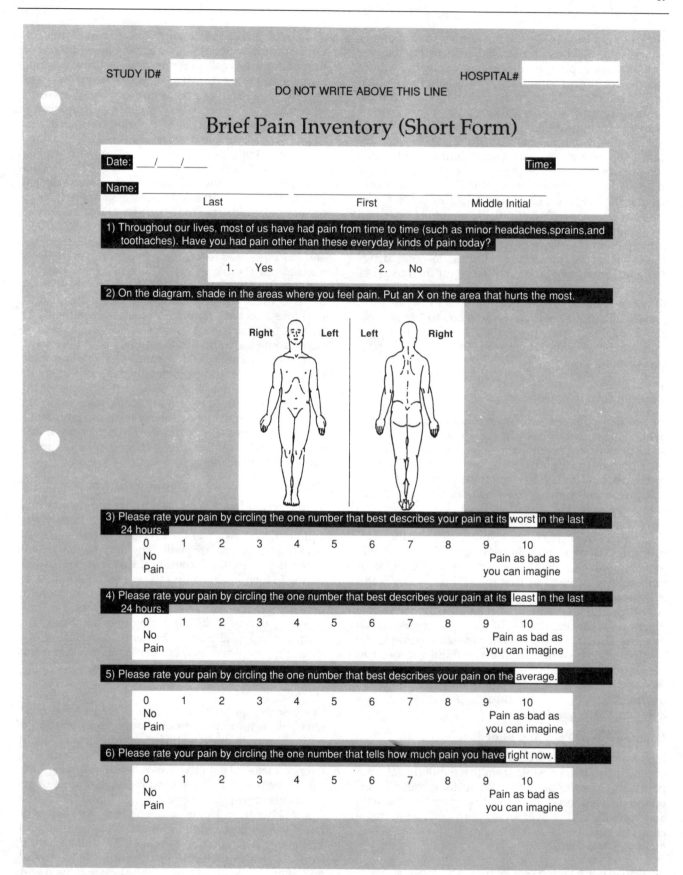

Figure 55.1

7) What treatments or medications are you receiving for your pain?

_____

8) In the last 24 hours, how much relief have pain treatments or medications provided? Please circle the one percentage that most shows how much relief you have received.

0%	10%	20%	30%	40%	50%	60%	70%	80%	90%	100%
No Relief										Complete Relief

9) Circle the one number that describes how, during the past 24 hours, pain has interfered with your:

A. General Activity

0	1	2	3	4	5	6	7	8	9	10
Does not interfere										Completely interferes

B. Mood

0	1	2	3	4	5	6	7	8	9	10
Does not interfere										Completely interferes

C. Walking ability

0	1	2	3	4	5	6	7	8	9	10
Does not interfere										Completely interferes

D. Normal work (includes both work outside the home and housework)

0	1	2	3	4	5	6	7	8	9	10
Does not interfere										Completely interferes

E. Relations with other people

0	1	2	3	4	5	6	7	8	9	10
Does not interfere										Completely interferes

F. Sleep

0	1	2	3	4	5	6	7	8	9	10
Does not interfere										Completely interferes

G. Enjoyment of life

0	1	2	3	4	5	6	7	8	9	10
Does not interfere										Completely interferes

Pain Research Group
Department of Neurology
University of Wisconsin-Madison

analgesic agent may consequently be diminished or stopped. Disseminated pain is usually best managed with analgesic agents but a particularly painful location in a patient with disseminated pain may need specific treatment, e.g. radiotherapy.

Radiation: Does your pain go anywhere else?

The radiation of a patient's pain can be a crucial factor in the diagnosis of a pain syndrome. The description of pain in the lower back radiating down both legs tells us much about the diagnosis especially when coupled with the verbal description of "shooting" or "like an electric shock" suggesting a neuropathic component.

Timing: When does your pain occur?

Pain may be breakthrough in nature, a term use to describe the transitory flare of pain in the setting of chronic pain managed by opioids. Portenoy and Hagen (19) defined this more specifically as a "transitory increase in pain to greater than moderate intensity (i.e., severe pain) which occurred on a baseline pain of moderate intensity or less (i.e. moderate or mild pain)." Such pain is also called incident pain when it occurs in association with a specific activity.

Correlated factors: What things make your pain better or worse?

Specifically defining these correlated factors can help greatly in establishing a diagnosis. Does coughing make low back pain worse and send it shooting down the back? Does straining make a headache worse? It is important to elicit the medications (not always analgesics) that a patient has been taking for the pain, together with the impact of these medications. This information helps in the assessment of pain severity and together with the use of equianalgesic dose tables will allow the adequate dose of other analgesic agents to be prescribed.

Implications of the pain: How does this pain effect your daily living?

Pain may limit a patient's activity which may already be dramatically affected by other cancer related symptoms. Therefore, it is imperative to document the effect of the pain on all patients' lives. This is more so in the elderly who, because of decreased reserves, may be more severely compromised by pain. When pain is of moderate or greater severity, we can assume that it has a negative impact on the patient's quality of life. That impact, including problems with sleep and depression, must be evaluated. The number of hours the patient is now sleeping compared with the last pain-free interval, difficulties with sleep onset, frequent interruptions of sleep, and/or early morning awakening suggest the need for appropriate pharmacological intervention. This may include the addition of a low-dose antidepressant at bedtime. Equally important is an assessment of how pain interferes with a patient's ability to interact with others. The Brief Pain Inventory, while used initially as a research tool, provides assessment of pain interference and has been found to be useful in clinical practice.

Significant depression should be treated through psychiatric or psychological consultation, especially if it persists in the face of adequate pain relief. Just as patients hesitate to report severe pain, they may hesitate to report depression. Having the patient report depression or tension on a scale of 0 to 10 may help overcome some of this reluctance. It is also known for physicians to misdiagnose true pain as depression or anxiety. Patients who are cognitively impaired, particularly those with agitation, may be extremely difficult to assess. In these patients, the differentiation between agitated delirium and pain may be extremely difficult. Patients in whom pain was well controlled before the development of delirium are unlikely to be agitated due to uncontrolled pain. Frequent discussions between various health care professionals and the patient's family are often required.

Meaning of the pain: What does this pain mean to you?

The implication of pain to a cancer patient is a very important part of the pain assessment. A patient's understanding of an initial minor increase in pain may dramatically influence his/hers perceived severity of the pain which could then result in the need to escalate the dose of an opioid. Does the pain mean the recurrence of a malignancy, that the patient thought had he he been "cured"? Is the worsening of a pain indicate that the patient's disease is progressing despite chemotherapy or is it related to the treatment? Will the pain mean more investigations, many of which are uncomfortable and painful? Considerations such as these may lead to the under reporting of pain in some patients while in others, will increase the anxiety associated with pain.

Further Assessment: Examination and Imaging

The physical examination should include a full disease assessment as well as a careful examination of the painful area or areas. This examination should be as least distressing for the patient as possible while respecting that analgesics may mask some of the signs necessary to fully make a diagnosis. Equally, the treatment of pain should not have to wait for the full diagnosis of a patient's disease. How often is a patient transferred to a radiology department with inadequate pain management, only to return with an inadequate procedure because of poor analgesia? Pain management should commence as soon as possible in the treatment of a cancer patient and should be based soundly on the suspected pathophysiology of the disease together with the pharmacology of the analgesic agents. The use of short acting opioids administered intravenously can provide this balance and ensure both patient and physician are comfortable.

The decision as to how extensively to investigate pain depends on a careful balance between what we know of the etiology of the pain in relation to the stage of the patient's disease and their associated prognosis. It may be that sudden severe back pain represents a collapsed vertebrae together with an impending spinal cord compression and that investigation with MRI needs to be performed to identify the lesion. A more gradual increase in pain in the same area may represent progressive bony disease that can be managed with an increase in analgesic agents without further investigation, although cord compression must always be a consideration. The absence of neurological signs does not exclude an impending spinal cord compression. A thorough understanding of the pathophysiology of the disease being assessed is imperative.

Bone metastases are a common cause of pain and lesions are often detected on plain X-ray. Pain in the limbs with weight bearing may indicate the possibility of an impending fracture, the occurrence of which may severely debilitate a patient and which may be prevented with orthopedic and radiotherapy intervention. However since painful metastases can occur without changes on plain x-ray, bone scans can be helpful in many disease situations; they are not helpful in multiple myeloma. CT or MRI scanning is useful in the evaluation of retroperitoneal, paravertebral, and pelvic areas as well as the base of the skull. Myelography may also be necessary in determining the cause of pain. Diagnostic nerve blocks can provide information concerning the pain pathway and can also determine the potential effectiveness of neuroablative procedures. It is important to remember that medical intervention is not always welcomed by patients. One of the fears that patients report is of pain associated with investigations and procedures. Patients may not report pain or they may underplay the severity pain of their pain for fear of being ordered yet another procedure or X-ray.

Pain Management

The principles of cancer pain management have been reviewed in a number of forums (3, 9, 20) that are widely available in paper and electronic forms* in English and other languages. In order in discuss the impact of aging on the management of cancer pain, it is necessary to review those principles here.

Pharmacological Management

The World Health Organization has recommended the use of the analgesic ladder for the treatment of cancer pain. With this comes the basic tenants for the management of cancer pain;

> by the ladder
> by mouth,
> by the clock
> and for the individual.

There has been some confusion concerning the best way to use the ladder. The WHO recommends that the treatment of cancer pain progress through the various steps of the ladder until relief from cancer pain is achieved (20). This has been tested and found to be a satisfactory means of providing pain relief (21).

However, patients' pain intensity ratings at the various steps were not reported nor was the duration of inadequate analgesia prior moving up the next step of the ladder. Zech *et al.* (22) reviewed their experience with pain relief in 2266 cancer patients, 74% of whom were on step II or III opioids at the time of admission to their pain service. While useful analgesia was obtained using the ladder (efficacy of pain relief was "good" in 76%), it is difficult to conclude from this study that all patients should be commenced at step 1 of the ladder. 25% of patients on Step 1 analgesics had pain intensity that was rated moderate to severe using a verbal rating scale, supporting concerns that by progressing through each step, many patients will be without pain relief for some time.

The recent AHCPR guidelines (9) for the management of cancer pain recommend use of the WHO ladder for cancer pain management but that patients be treated according to the severity of their pain. Mild pain can treated at step 1 with analgesics such as NSAIDs or acetaminophen. For moderate pain, opioids are commenced with either codeine, or low doses of oxycodone or morphine. Severe pain is treated at step 3 with full doses of opioids including morphine, oxycodone, hydromorphone or fentanyl. Consideration of the use of adjuvant medications is recommended in all cases and should include the use of NSAIDs together with opioids in the case of bony metastases. Adjuvant medications may result in a decrease in opioid dose with an associated decrease in side effects although this is still the subject of further study.

Physicians have a vast array of analgesic agents available for use with their patients. It is essential that physicians treating cancer pain understand the pharmacology of two to three drugs from each of the steps of the cancer pain ladder. The dose of pain medications are titrated upwardly until either a patient's desired pain relief or until *unmanageable* side effects are reached. In the case of NSAID's and acetaminophen, dose escalation will be limited by either side effects or the expectation of side effects. Opioids in their own right do not have a fixed ceiling in their dose, the highest dose being that which provides analgesia or results in *unmanageable* side effects. When opioids are combined with acetaminophen or aspirin such as in codeine/acetaminophen or oxycodone/acetaminophen formulations, the dose limiting component of these preparations is usually the total daily dose of acetaminophen or aspirin.

Analgesic agents are recommended to be taken on a regular around the clock basis, not on a "prn" or "as needed" basis. This relates to the need to maintain adequate levels of an opioid in the body and is more likely to maintain a patient in a pain free state (23). Rescue or "as needed" medications should be ordered for all patients and should be used for episodes of breakthrough pain and during periods of titration (either upward or downward titration) of analgesic agents. Current recommendations for rescue doses range from 5–15% of the daily dose (19) (or 10–30% of the 12 hourly dose).

---

* http://www.stat.washington.edu/TALARIA/TALARIA.html

The initial treatment and titration with opioids should take place with immediate release preparations of opioids (24). The prolonged absorption of a sustained release product may result in prolonged side effects in a patient who is receiving opioids for the first time. However a patient who is taking Percoset® is not opioid naive and can be changed to a sustained release product. 12 Percoset® tablets are the equivalent of 60 mg day of oral morphine. Oxycodone, the active ingredient in Percoset, is a drug that has an analgesic activity similar to morphine and which is now available as a sustained release product. The use of sustained release products has made twice a day dosing of analgesics a reality for cancer patients and once a day morphine products have been developed. There is however no measured difference in the side effects and analgesia between immediate release morphine administered every 4 hours and sustained release morphine administered twice a day (25). It is recommended that currently available sustained release opioids be administered twice a day and that the dose should be escalated if inadequate analgesia is obtained. Patients who are experiencing side effects from twice daily morphine, but in whom analgesia is not sustained for the full twelve hours, may benefit from 8 hourly dosing. Methadone, another oral opioid more commonly associated with drug withdrawal programs, is a cheap and effective alternative for the treatment of cancer pain. Methadone has a long half life and therefore dose escalation must proceed cautiously, especially in the elderly in order to the reduce the occurrence and severity of side effects.

Ideally pain medications should be given by mouth. However some patients cannot tolerate the oral route. In the study of Zech et al. (22), approximately 80% of the 2118 patients were managed with oral medications throughout their illness. This decreased to 50% of 864 patients being cared for in hospital at the time of death. Alternative methods of drug delivery therefore need to be considered in those in whom oral administration is not possible. Many people use the sublingual route feeling that this provides rapid analgesia. There is increasing evidence that the sublingual administration of morphine provides no benefit over oral administration. Peak plasma concentration of morphine occur later and at lower levels following sublingual administration than for oral administration (26). It may also be preferable to use morphine solutions rather than sublingual tablets which have a bitter taste. The rectal administration of opioids is not limited to drugs for which there is a suppository formulation; sustained release tablets administered rectally provide effective analgesia.

The transdermal delivery of opioids is currently limited to fentanyl. The rate of delivery of fentanyl (μg/hr) is dependent on the surface area of the patch applied, with rates ranging from 25 to 100 μg/hr. When administered transdermally, the drug accumulates in the subcutaneous fat. which results in sustained plasma concentrations. Current recommendations are that patients should be stabilized on oral opioids prior to starting transdermal fentanyl and that dose changes should not be made more frequently than every 72 hours (27). As always, patients need to be ordered a short acting opioid, such as immediate release morphine, for breakthrough pain; oral transmucosal fentanyl citrate, currently approved for preoperative sedation in children may be a useful rescue medication for cancer patients.

The parenteral administration of opioids may be necessary in those who cannot swallow, who have intractable side effects or in whom rectal delivery is not desirable. Subcutaneous infusions have been extensively used in Canada (28) and Australia but are not commonly used in the USA, possibly because many cancer patients have intravenous ports. The steady plasma concentrations of opioids, resulting from either intravenous or subcutaneous infusions, may result in a diminution of side effects and therefore an optimization of analgesia. Only a small percentage of cancer patients (2–5%) will require interventions or the direct delivery of opioids to the CNS (22). Patients with unmanageable side effects may benefit from epidural or intrathecal administration of opioids. Approximately one tenth of the intravenous dose of an opioid needs to be administered epidurally and one hundredth the dose administered intrathecally. These procedures are costly and need catheters and pumps to deliver drug. A patient should be expected to use such devices for more than 3 months and without complications in order to show any cost effectiveness.

The intramuscular injection of opioids is to be avoided. Apart from being painful for the patient, absorption following injection is erratic and in most cases results in an analgesic effect that parallels the oral administration of an equivalent dose of the same drug. One opioid commonly given by intramuscular injection is meperidine or pethidine (Demerol®). Meperidine is in fact a drug that has very few indications in the treatment of pain. Meperidine has short acting analgesic activity (one tenth that of morphine) and is mostly prescribed at subtherapeutic doses (50–75 mg 3 4qh IM). It is metabolized to normeperidine, a toxic metabolite that accumulates with repeated hallucinations. If used at all, meperidine should be used for no more than 48 hours and with a dose limitation of 600 mg/day. This dose limitation should be 450 mg/day in the presence of renal impairment which occurs more commonly in the elderly. Given these limitations, meperidine is not recommended for the routine treatment of pain.

A small minority of patients who have alcoholism or drug addiction may request analgesics for psychological effects. This is unlikely to occur in patients without a clear history of severe addictive behavior. Patients who are recovered alcoholics or drug abusers may be difficult to treat because of their resistance to taking analgesics. Although their care is more complex, patients with drug or alcohol addiction or a history of addiction, should never be denied appropriate pain medications. If drug addiction is suspected, the patient should be presented with these suspicions and agreement should be made about the use of opioids for the management of pain as opposed to the alteration of mood (14). The use of long-acting opioids or continuous infusions are preferable to short-acting opioids or patient-controlled analgesia. The writing of prescriptions by a single physician can simplify the negotiation process with such patients.

While opioids are the mainstay of cancer pain management, the use of adjunct therapy is recommended by both the WHO and AHCPR guidelines. Nonsteroidal anti-inflammatory drugs (NSAIDs) are particularly useful in the management of metastatic bone pain. While many prefer to use agents such as ibuprofen and naproxen, aspirin is equally effective in the management of bone pain. Steroids may be also useful in the management of bone pain but may cause unwanted side effects. Steroids are particularly useful in the management of painful liver metastases, where they act by reducing pressure on the liver capsule, the cause of hepatic pain. Anti-depressants such as amitriptyline and desimpramine are a useful adjunct for all cancer pain but particularly important for the treatment of neuropathic or nerve pain. Anti-epileptics such as carbamazepine have also been used as second line treatment for neuropathic pain. Gabapentin is a newer antiepileptic which has also been shown to be useful for neuropathic pain.

Nonpharmacological Management

One alternative, and often very effective, way of treating cancer associated pain is to treat the cancer itself. This is particularly true for those diseases that are responsive to chemotherapy or radiotherapy. However, it is imperative that a clinician carefully balances the potential benefit of anti cancer therapy in palliating symptoms with the expected toxicity of the treatment. Patients in whom anti cancer therapy is being administered for a palliative intention should have a symptom to be palliated. "Prophylactic" treatment of symptoms may often make further management of a symptom more difficult at a later date. Many of the diseases in which pain is a particular problem e.g., pancreatic cancer, are not responsive to chemotherapy agents.

Radiotherapy is a useful tool in the palliation of cancer associated pain. This is particularly true in the treatment of bone metastases but there is some discrepancy in the administration of radiotherapy for these lesions. In the United Kingdom, Canada and Australia, the common practice is to administer a single fraction of 6 Gy to painful bone metastases. This will provide good analgesia equivalent to that obtained with the administration of 20 Gy over 2 weeks (29). In some cases, lesions treated with a single fraction may need to be retreated earlier than those administered multiple fractions. Retreatment with single large fractions can have implications long term to the vasculature of the irradiated area but many patients do not live long enough for this to be an issue. It is important to balance the overall prognosis and the quality of life of the patient with the treatment administered. The maximum analgesic effect of radiotherapy may not occur for two to four weeks from administration of treatment. It is essential to provide adequate pharmacological management in the interim. With the onset of the antitumor effect of the radiotherapy and with it analgesia, these agents can be slowly decreased. Even in generalized pain, therapy such as hemibody radiation may provide adequate relief of pain.

Nerve blocks, either with chemicals or neuroablative methods may be useful in the pain management of some patients. A coeliac plexus block can be very useful in the treatment of pain associated with pancreatic cancer and may be best performed at the time of laparotomy. Diagnostic blocks with lidocaine are often performed before the instillation of a longer acting agent. In some cases, chordotomy (ablation of pain pathways in the spinal cord) may be useful for the management of pain. Bilateral cordotomies can be performed but will result in increased incidence of complications, particularly loss of bladder function (30). As with all procedures, it is imperative that staff are properly trained and maintain their proficiency in these procedures in order to minimize potential complications. Improvements in imaging techniques with CT Scans has improved the ability to perform many of these procedures.

Particular Issues of Pain Management in the Elderly

A number of issues are important in the management of cancer pain in the elderly. Despite concerns that these issues raise, the relief of cancer associated pain must remain a priority in the elderly. The repeated assessment of pain and consequent titration of opioids should proceed in the elderly until either adequate analgesia is reached or unmanageable side effects develop. Some refinement in the titration of opioids may be necessary in older patients.

Diferences in Analgesia in the Elderly

There is clear evidence of differences in the analgesic effect of opioids in older people when compared to a younger population. Bellville et al. (31) studied pain relief in 712 acute post operative patients administered 10mg of morphine or 20mg of pentazocine or both. They used a pain measurement tool developed by Houde and Beaver which assessed the mean Sum Pain Intensity Difference (SPID). The authors found that over the age of 40, age was the most important variable in predicting with degree of analgesia from morphine. Younger patients, who reported more pain initially, received less pain relief than older patients administered the same dose of opioids. Defining those older than 58 as elderly, the authors noted that was no change in sedation in "the elderly" and that the difference in analgesia was related to a difference in pain sensation with age and not to differences in the metabolism or disposition of the drug. Harkins and colleagues (8) have reviewed many studies and concluded that age does not impact on the sensory or perceived unpleasantness of pain in individuals.

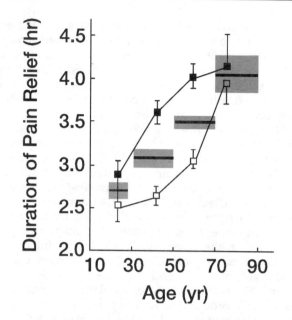

Figure 55.2 Duration of pain relief in relation to age after 8 mg (*lower curve*) and 16 mg (*upper curve*) morphine. The duration of pain relief is the hour after drug that the patient reports the last positive pain relief score. Each point represents mean duration of relief concurrent with the mean ages of four age groups. The *vertical bars* represent ±SEM. The *shaded areas* represent comparable data for the combined doses, extending horizontally to define the range of each age group (With permission ref 32).

A further explanation for the findings of Belville has been suggested by Kaiko *et al.* (1980). Using the same measurement tool, 947 post operative cancer patients were studied following the intramuscular administration of either 8 and 16 mg of morphine (32). Patients were analyzed according to four age divisions, 18–29, 30–49, 50–69, and 70–89 years. For both dose levels administered to the oldest group (70–89 years), analgesia was maintained for 1.5–2.5 times longer than the younger group (18–29 years) experienced for the administration of 16 mg of morphine. The authors suggested that this prolonged analgesia in the older group was probably related to functional changes in the hepatic and renal elimination of morphine. The same authors reviewed the situation with 714 chronic cancer pain sufferers (33) and again found a clear difference with total analgesic effect with age with the pain relief provided by 8mg of morphine in the elderly equal to the pain relief of 16 mg of morphine in the middle aged. The difference in pain relief observed between the extremes of adult age was twice that of the increase in relief provided by the doubling of the dose. On the basis of both studies, Kaiko and coworkers suggested that there was a difference in age related morphine pharmacokinetics and that this difference should be used to choose the initial dosing frequency rather than the initial dose.

Pharmacokinetics

The pharmacokinetics of morphine have been studied in relation to age. Analysis has been performed on the effect of age on the metabolism of 10 mg/70 kg of morphine administered intravenously to anesthetized humans (34). Patients aged 51–75 had almost twice the serum concentration of morphine than the younger group in the first 5 minutes following injection. However, there was no difference, in relation to age, in drug concentration from 10 to 240 minutes or in the half life of the drug. On the basis of these last two findings, the authors concluded that the metabolism of morphine did not appear to be age dependent. They did agree that early increased plasma concentrations of morphine may contribute to the increased analgesia seen with the elderly.

Owen *et al.* (35) found initial plasma concentrations of morphine to be higher in a group of older patients administered intravenous morphine and documented a more rapid β elimination phase for morphine. They also found both the clearance and the apparent volume of distribution of morphine to be less than in younger patients. They suggested that the dose of morphine should be reduced in relation to this decreased clearance (0.8 that of younger subjects). The effect of age on the bioavailability of morphine was compared in eight healthy young and nine healthy elderly who each received 10 mg of morphine sulfate as an intravenous injection, an oral suspension and as a slow release tablet (36). There was no difference in absorption in relation to age but the elderly group achieved a higher maximum plasma concentration and had a larger area under the concentration-time curve (AUC) than the younger group. The elderly also showed decreased clearance of morphine (35%) and the authors claimed that this reduction was of the similar scale to the decrease in liver size and blood flow in the elderly. The markedly increased AUC in the elderly was explained by decreased systemic drug clearance and reduced first pass hepatic extraction, both of which would result from decreased hepatic blood flow.

The effect of hepatic blood flow has been studied. Wynn *et al.* found a 28% fall in liver volume in those over 65 compared to those who were under 40 using an ultrasound technique (37). Liver size is important determinant of the elimination of capacity limited drugs. The authors also found a 35% reduction in blood flow in the same volunteers. As morphine is a highly extracted drug, one might expect to see the clearance of morphine decrease in patients in whom liver flow decreases. Therefore in the elderly, one would expect to see decreased clearance of morphine (38). But the question remains as to whether this accounts for the total change that we would see in the decreased clearance of morphine.

All of these studies considered the pharmacokinetics of morphine alone and did not address issues pertaining to its metabolites. Early studies must be viewed with caution as assays for morphine often did not have the ability to differentiate morphine from its glucuronides. Morphine-6-glucuronide which represents some 10% of the metabolism of morphine is an active analgesic agent with a potency 10 times that of morphine. 60% of morphine is metabolized to morphine-3-glucuronide (M-3-G), a compound with no analgesic properties but which may in fact be antagonistic to the analgesic actions of morphine (39) while contributing to its side effects. Given the potential role of these glucuronide metabolites, it is important to address the effect of age on glucuronidation. Herd *et al.* (40) found no correlation of age with the glucuronidation of acetaminophen. The authors used liver tissue obtained from patients aged 40–89 and studied in metabolic process *in vitro*. However, all were fit healthy patients and only 6 patients were older than 70 years. While the conclusions of this study are true, there is no data presented as to the effect of aging on glucuronidation in the aged. The same assessment can be made of other studies that have addressed the activity of hepatic microsomal monooxygenase function in relation to age. These enzymes are involved in the metabolism of opioids such as codeine, oxycodone and methadone. Major changes in mixed function oxidases (P450) with age have been documented in rats but are believed to be specific to loss of testosterone in males of the species. Similar findings have not been confirmed in primate studies and Schmucker *et al.* (41) found no correlation between enzyme activity and age in humans but again liver samples from only 7 patients above the age of 70 were included in the study. Given the variability of morphine metabolism between individuals, longitudinal studies of both the pharmacokinetics and pharmacodynamics of morphine and its metabolites are needed in populations of patients that include a significant proportion of elderly patients.

Polypharmacy and Toxicity

Polypharmacy can dramatically increase the risk of side effects and drug interactions in an individual. Many elderly patients have other illnesses and are already prescribed medications therefore increasing the risk of drug interactions. Aging itself may not be an independent variable in the development of adverse drug reactions. But 20–25% of patients over the age of 65 have been documented to be inappropriately using prescription drugs (42). Our priority in cancer patients should be the management of pain and the role of drug interactions in the development of side effects should be considered. It may be more sensible to cease an antihypertensive medication that is contributing to side effects than to decrease a dose of morphine that is ensuring adequate analgesia.

The use of non steroidal anti-inflammatory drugs (NSAIDs) must be cautious in elderly patients given the toxicity profile of these drugs especially in those with preexisting renal impairment. While we know that there is an age specific decline in renal function (43), each person should be assessed individually rather than assuming that all older persons have decreased renal function. Many practitioners are hesitant to prescribe NSAIDs in the elderly because of increased r isk of gastrointestinal hemorrhage. Careful analysis of the data on the use of NSAIDs would suggest that the elderly are not at increased risk of upper gastrointestinal hemorrhage (44). They are at increased risk of death if a hemorrhage does occur possibly due to a decreased ability to cope with the hemodynamic consequences of a major gastrointestinal bleed. The ability to cope with side effects is a factor that is important for many of the side effects encountered following the administration of other analgesic agents. Tricyclic antidepressants should be used with care in the elderly as the risk of postural hypotension may be greater due to disease or other medications that predispose them to this side effect. An low initial dose of tricyclic antidepressants is needed in most patients and in the elderly, escalation should proceed slowly and cautiously.

It is unknown whether the elderly have more side effects to opioids or whether they do not cope as well with side effects when they occur. Of the pharmacological factors related to drug delivery, namely absorption, distribution, metabolism and excretion, only absorption is not effected by aging. Although older patients show a decline in drug metabolism with aging, the age of the patient only accounted for 3% of this and much more of the decline was related to smoking (44). Many other issues influence the side effects of opioids in the elderly. The risk of respiratory depression from opioids is increased in patients with renal and liver impairment, conditions seen commonly in elderly patients with cancer. The effect of decreased metabolism or delayed excretion in the elderly is greater with drugs with longer half lives e.g. methadone, with which there may be an increase in the incidence of side effects. There are also concerns about the use of many generic drugs in the elderly patient given that bioequivalence studies performed for the registration of these products are usually performed in healthy young volunteers.

Conclusion

Cancer is a disease that is clearly associated with aging and pain is a symptom experienced by many cancer patients regardless of their disease stage. In order to ensure the proper management of cancer pain in older cancer patients, it is imperative that we understand more clearly those factors that effect pain relief. These include barriers to cancer pain relief as well as factors that effect both the pharmacodynamics and pharmacokinetics of analgesic agents in the elderly. The available evidence would suggest that the initial dose of opioids may need to be reduced slightly in the elderly and in some patients the dosing interval for opioids may be longer than in younger patients. While this may be an initial strategy, the management of pain in elderly cancer patients should proceed aggressively with more frequent reassessment of both analgesia and side effects than for a younger patient to ensure optimization of cancer pain relief.

References

1. Cleeland CS, Gonin R, Hatfield AK, Edmondson JH, Blum RH, Stewart JA, Pandya KJ. Pain and its treatment in outpatients with metastatic disease. *New Engl J Med* 1994; **330**: 592–6.
2. Daut RL, Cleeland CS. The prevalence and severity of pain in cancer. *Cancer* 1982; **50**: 1913–8.
3. Foley KM. The treatment of cancer pain. *New Engl J Med* 1985; **313**: 84–95.
4. Begg CB, Carbone PP. Clinical trials and drug toxicity in the elderly *Cancer*. 1982; **52**: 986–92.
5. Davis MA. Epidemiology of osteoarthritis. *Clin Geriatr Med* 1988; **4**: 241.
6. Cook J, Rideout E, Browne G. The prevalence of pain complaints in a general population. *Pain* 1984; **18**: 299.
7. Ferrell BA, Ferrell BR, Osterweil D. Pain in the nursing home. *J Amer Geriatr Soc* 1990; **38**: 409–14.
8. Harkins SW, Kwentus J, Price DD, Bonica J, Loeser JD, Chapman CR, Fordyce WE. *Pain and Suffering in the Elderly The Management of Pain*, (2nd Edition). Philadelphia: Lea and Febiger, 552–559, 1990.
9. Jacox A, Carr DB, Payne, R, *et al. Management of Cancer Pain: Clinical Practice Guideline No 9*. Rockville, Md: Agency for Health Care Policy and Research. US Dept of Health and Human Services, Public Health Service; March 1994, AHCPr Publication, 94–052.
10. Von Roenn JH, Cleeland CS, Gonin R, *et al.* Physician attitudes and practice in cancer pain management: A survey of the Eastern Cooperative Oncology Group *Ann Intern Med* **119 (2)**, 121–126.
11. Ward SE, Goldberg N, Miller-McCauley V, *et al.* Patient-related barriers to management of cancer pain. *Pain* 1993; **52**: 319–24.
12. Porter J, Jick H. Addiction is rare in patients treated with narcotics. *New Engl J Med* 1980; **302**: 123.
13. Portenoy, RK. Opioid therapy for chronic nonmalignant pain: current status. In *Progress in Pain Research and Management*, edited by HL Fields, JC Liebeskind, Vol 1. Seattle: IASP Press, pp. 247–287, 1994.
14. Reidenburg MM, Portenoy RK. The need to keep an open mind about the treatment of chronic nonmalignant pain *Clin Pharmacol Ther* 1994; **55**: 367–9.
15. Weissman DE, Haddox JD. Opioid pseudoaddiction — an iatrogenic syndrome *Pain* 1989; **36**: 363–6.
16. Daut RL, Cleeland CS, Flanery RC. Development of the Wisconsin Brief Pain Questionnaire to assess pain in cancer and other diseases. *Pain* 1983; **17**: 197–210.
17. Cleeland CS, Ryan KM. Pain assessment: global use of the Brief Pain Inventory. *Ann Acad Med* Singapore 1994; **23**: 129–38.
18. Serlin RC, Mendoza, TR, Nakamura Y, *et al.* When is pain mild, moderate or severe?: Grading pain severity by its interference with function. *Pain* 1995; **61**: 277–284.
19. Portenoy RK, Hagen NA. Breakthrough pain: definition and management. *Oncology* 1989; **3**: 25–9.
20. World Health Organization. *Cancer Pain Relief and Palliative Care: Report of a WHO Expert Committee*. Geneva, Switzerland: World Health Organization: 1990 Technical Report Series 804.
21. Ventafridda V, Oliveri E, Caraceni A, *et al.* A retrospective study on the use of oral morphine in cancer pain. *J Pain Sympt Manage* 1987; **2**: 77–81.
22. Zech DF, Grond S, Lynch J, *et al.* Validation of World Health Organization guidelines for cancer pain relief — a 10-year prospective study. *Pain* 1995; **63**: 65–76.
23. Lipman AG. Opioid analgesics in the management of cancer pain. *Amer J Hospice Care* 1989 **6**: 13–23.
24. Portenoy RK. Pain management in the older cancer patient. *Oncology* 1992; **6**: S86–98.
25. Walsh TD, MacDonald N, Bruera E, *et al.* A controlled study of sustained-release morphine sulfate tablets in chronic pain from advanced cancer. *Amer J Clin Oncol* 1992; **15**: 268–72.
26. Davis T, Miser AW, Loprinzi CL, *et al.* Comparative morphine pharmacokinetics following sublingual, intramuscular, and oral administration in patients with cancer. *Hospice J* 1993; **9**: 85–90.
27. Payne R, Chandler S, Einhaus M. Guidelines for the clinical use of transdermal fentanyl. *Anti-Cancer Drugs* 1995; **6 Suppl 3**: 50–3.
28. Macmillan K, Bruera E, Kuehn N, *et al.* A prospective comparison study between a butterfly needle and a Teflon cannula for subcutaneous narcotic administration. *J Pain Sympt Manage* 1994; **9**: 82–4.
29. Kilbride P. The role of radiotherapy in palliative care. *J Palliative Care* 1995; **11**: 19–26.
30. Stuart G, Cramond T. Role of percutaneous cervical cordotomy for pain of malignant origin. *Med J Australia* 1993; **158**: 667–670.
31. Bellville JW, Forrest WH, Miller E, Brown BW. Influence of age on pain relief from analgesics. *JAMA* 1971; **217**: 1835–1841.
32. Kaiko RF. Age and morphine analgesia in cancer patients with postoperative pain. *Clin Pharmacol Ther* 1980; **28**: 823–826.
33. Kaiko RF, Wallenstein SL, Rogers AG, Houde RW. Sources of variation in analgesic responses in cancer patients with chronic pain receiving morphine. *Pain* 1983; **15**: 191–200.
34. Berkowitz BA, Ngai SH, Yang JC, Hempstead BS, Spector S. The disposition of morphine in surgical patients. *Clin Pharmacol Ther* 1975; **17**: 629–635.
35. Owen JA, Sitar DS, Berger II, Brownell II, Duke PC, Mitenko PA. Age related morphine kinetics. *Clin Pharmacol Ther* 1993; **34**: 364–368.
36. Baillie SP, Bateman DN, Coates PE, Woodhouse KW. Age and the pharmacokinetics of morphine. *Age Ageing* 1989; **18**: 258–262.
37. Wynne, Cope LH, Mutch E. Liver Volume, blood flow and perfusion in ageing man-an explanation for altered drug metabolism in the elderly. *J Hepatol* 1987; **5**: 573.
38. Woodhouse KW, Wynne HA. Age-related changes in liver size and hepatic blood flow. The influence on Drug Metabolism in the Elderly. *Clin Pharmacokin* 1988; **15**: 287–294.
39. Watt J, Cramond T, Smith M. Morphine-6-glucuronide: analgesic effects antagonized by morphine-3-glucuronide. *Clin Exp Pharmacol Physiol* 1990; **S17**: 83.
40. Herd B, Wynne H, Wright P, James O, Woodhouse K. The effect of age on glucuronidation and sulphation of paracetamol by human liver fractions. *Brit J Clin Pharmacol* 1991; **32**: 768–770.
41. Schmucker DL, Woodhouse KW, Wang RK, *et al.* Effects of age and gender on *in vitro* properties of human liver microsomal monoxygenases. *Clin Pharmacol Ther* 1990; **48**: 365–74.
42. Willcox SM, Himmelstein DU, Woolhandler S. Inappropriate drug prescribing for the community-dwelling elderly *JAMA* 1994; **272**: 292–296.
43. Lindeman RD. Changes in renal function with aging. Implications for treatment *Drugs Aging* 1992; **2**: 423–431.
44. Gurwitz JH, Avorn J. The ambiguous reaction between aging and adverse drug reactions. *Ann Intern Med* 1991; **114**: 956–965.

56. Nutritional Therapy

N. Simon Tchekmedyian and David Heber

Introduction

There are several age-related variables that have a bearing on nutritional assessment and therapy. Aging is associated with decreasing bone mass and height. On average, there is a decrease of 2 inches between the 3rd and 6th decades of life (1). Between ages 60 and 80, the rate of decrease in stature has been estimated to be about 1/4 inch per year (2). Multiple myeloma, osteoporosis, or metastatic disease with vertebral compression fractures can cause a substantial decrease in height (several inches) over a short period of time.

Intra-abdominal fat increases with age (1). The centralization of body fat coupled with decreased height can mask severe progressive undernutrition in an older patient with cancer and weight loss. Aging is associated with a decrease in total body water, lean tissue, and skeletal muscle mass (1,3), and these changes make older patients more sensitive to acute reductions in calorie, protein, and water intake.

Aging is also associated with reduced activity levels and decreased total caloric intake. Progressive impairment in the sense of taste and smell can add to an underlying decrease in appetite. Furthermore, various degrees of impairment in digestive and absorptive functions are seen with aging. These include disordered esophageal motility, atrophic gastritis, hypochlorhydria, delayed gastric emptying, and decreased intestinal blood flow.

Elderly patients are at an increased risk for socioeconomic problems that can lead to isolation and difficulties with availability and preparation of meals. Older patients also have a higher prevalence of concomitant physical and psychological factors that range from difficulty chewing to depression. The latter is a common cause of undernutrition in older patients (4).

Problems and Questions

While undernutrition in older patients with cancer is a significant problem, there is a need for specific clinical parameters to grade the levels of undernutrition, study its prevalence, and guide effective therapy. Furthermore, once there is agreement on defined levels of undernutrition, it could be asked whether intervention is necessary and, if so, for what specific goals.

Clinical Nutritional Parameters

Weight Loss

Involuntary weight loss is a key indicator of undernutrition, and it is often a sign associated with a poorer prognosis and survival. The rate of weight loss is also important. It is accepted that an involuntary weight loss of ≥10% of the patient's usual body weight over a period of 6 months or less indicates undernutrition in patients with cancer (5).

One complicating factor in cancer patients is the development of edema or ascites; these should be kept in mind when interpreting weight data.

Current weight compared to the ideal body weight (IBW) and usual body weight (UBW)

Ideal body weight is the weight associated with optimal survivorship in populations studied by life insurance companies. A commonly used reference is the 1983 Metropolitan Life Insurance tables. With these tables, ideal weight range is calculated on the basis of height, body frame size, and sex, but no adjustments are made for age. Studies undertaken at the Gerontology Research Center (GRC), however, indicate that age significantly affects ideal body weight while sex differences are not significant (6). Table 56.1 shows a comparison of data from the two tables. The main finding is that for a given height older subjects have a higher ideal body weight than younger individuals. Importantly, both tables are based on the same data base, except that age is introduced as a variable only by the more recent GRC tables. Since cancer affects both the young and the aged, with the majority of patients being in the older age groups (7), it is more appropriate to utilize the age-adjusted tables to calculate ideal body weight range. Serious shortcomings still exist since there is no correction for disease-related changes in height, and no guidelines are provided in these tables for patients 70 years old or older.

Based on these ideal body weight ranges, we determine whether the patient is above, within, or below the ideal weight range. Thus, percent ideal weight (current weight compared to the expected or ideal body weight range) may help us determine the patient's nutritional status. An additional variable for consideration is usual or pre-illness weight. Therefore, both information on percent ideal weight and percent usual or pre-illness weight should be collected on all patients.

There are healthy individuals who are below their projected weight for many years. From a clinical standpoint, stable weight and an adequate diet often equate with good nutrition even if the individual is below the ideal body weight range.

Absence or Presence of Anorexia and/or Decreased Food Intake

Anorexia and decreased food intake have long been

Table 56.1 Comparison of the weight-for-height tables from actuarial data: non-age-corrected metropolitan life insurance company and age-specific gerontology research center recommendations.

Height (ft. and in.)	Metropolitan 1983 Weights* (25–59 yr.)		Gerontology Research Center* (Age-specific Weight Range for Men and Women)				
	Men	Women	20–29 yr.	30–39 yr.	40–49 yr.	50–59 yr.	60–69 yr.
4' 10"		100–131	84–111	92–119	99–127	107–135	115–142
4' 11"		101–134	87–115	95–123	103–131	111–139	119–147
5' 0"		103–137	90–119	98–127	106–135	114–143	123–152
5' 1"	123–145	105–140	93–123	101–131	110–140	118–148	127–157
5' 2"	125–148	108–144	96–127	105–136	113–144	122–153	131–163
5' 3"	127–151	111–148	99–131	108–140	117–149	126–158	135–168
5' 4"	129–155	114–152	102–135	112–145	121–154	130–163	140–173
5' 5"	131–159	117–156	106–140	115–149	125–159	134–168	144–179
5' 6"	133–163	120–160	109–144	119–154	129–164	138–174	148–184
5' 7"	135–167	123–164	112–148	122–159	133–169	143–179	153–190
5' 8"	137–171	126–167	116–153	126–163	137–174	147–184	158–196
5' 9"	139–175	129–170	119–157	130–168	141–179	151–190	162–201
5' 10"	141–179	132–173	122–162	134–173	145–184	156–195	167–107
5' 11"	144–183	135–176	126–167	137–178	149–190	160–201	172–213
6' 0"	147–187		129–171	141–183	153–195	165–207	177–219
6' 1"	150–192		133–176	145–188	157–200	169–213	182–225
6' 2"	153–197		137–181	149–194	162–206	174–219	187–232
6' 3"	157–202		141–186	153–199	166–212	179–225	192–238
6' 4"			144–191	157–205	171–218	184–231	197–244

*Values in this table are for height without shoes and weight without clothes.

Printed by permission from *Oncology* **6 (2)**:105–111, 1992

recognized as key causes of undernutrition in patients with malignancies (8,9). Anorexia is now a treatable symptom of cancer which, if left untreated, leads to significant patient discomfort in addition to malnutrition (10).

The clinician should inquire about the presence, duration, and severity of anorexia and decreased food intake. The impact of these and other nutrition-related complaints on the patient's overall well being and quality of life can be evaluated further with questionnaires. We currently are testing one such questionnaire as part of the FACT (Functional Assessment of Cancer Therapy), a quality of life scale developed by Dr. David Cella (11).

Anthropometric and Biochemical Measurements

Detailed anthropometric measurements (such as mid-arm circumference and triceps skin fold) have long been utilized to determine skeletal muscle mass and nutritional status (12). Although the value of these measurements can be limited if done in the hospital setting, serial measurements by the same professional in the outpatient clinic can help assess the patient's ongoing nutritional state. Problems with these measurements include inter-observer variability and interference by edema or patient positioning. The decision to do these measurements should often be individualized according to the acuity of the underlying process, the availability of trained personnel, and the goals of interventions. It should be noted that muscle wasting and loss of adipose tissue reserves seen on physical examination are important but late signs of undernutrition. Ideally, early diagnosis and intervention should be directed at avoiding this advanced stage of undernutrition or cachexia.

The role of laboratory parameters, such as albumin or prealbumin level, transferrin, or total lymphocyte count are less well defined in patients with cancer. These and other tests can be useful to assess protein depletion but are difficult to interpret in patients with advanced cancer who often have metastases to visceral sites with organ dysfunction as well as metabolic and immunologic derangements due to cancer therapy.

Routine chemistry panels include albumin levels which may be a useful indication of nutritional state. Albumin has a half-life in the circulation of about

3 weeks. Hypoalbuminemia may result from malnutrition, but is also associated with liver disease, disseminated malignancies, protein-losing enteropathy, nephrotic syndrome, and conditions leading to expanded plasma volume such as congestive heart failure.

Prealbumin has a half-life of just under 2 days and its level may increase with the use of steroid hormones and decrease in presence of liver disease, disseminated malignancies, nephrotic syndrome, inflammatory bowel disease, use of salicylates, or malnutrition (13,14).

Transferrin levels may be measured as transferrin antigen and are roughly similar to iron binding capacity. The half life of transferrin is about one week and it may increase with storage iron depletion or the use of hormonal agents, while it may decrease with infection, malignancy, inflammation, liver disease, nephrotic syndrome, or malnutrition (15). Absolute lymphocyte counts may be reduced by malnutrition as well as by a variety of other factors. More sophisticated tests of malnutrition (bioimpedance, total body K, basal metabolic rate [BMR] and others) belong to the realm of clinical research.

In many instances, a brief clinical nutritional assessment based on the degree of weight loss from usual or pre-illness weight, current weight as a percentage of usual and ideal body weight, and dietary history are sufficient to determine the clinical situation and consider potential interventions. We therefore reserve the use of anthropometric and laboratory evaluations to specific individual situations. Interpretations of these evaluations should be based on the clinical context.

Factors Affecting Food Intake

A number of associated conditions are prevalent in older patients with cancer and can affect their food intake and nutrition. Mucositis, as a side effect of chemotherapy, is more common in the elderly. Oral pain and dryness, poor dentition, periodontal disease, and ill fitting dentures are also common. Other problems requiring consideration are dysphagia, alteration in taste, fatigue, nausea, vomiting, and diarrhea or constipation. Pain and other symptoms such as dyspnea can also interfere with nutrition. Depression is a well known cause of weight loss in older patients, and depression can worsen due to the stress of coping with cancer. Feelings of isolation and actual social isolation are not uncommon, especially in those patients who do not have strong family support. Socioeconomic and living conditions must be taken into account because they may impact food availability and preparation. These may represent very serious problems for older patients with cancer and require a multidisciplinary effort for proper management.

Nutrition-Related Variables and Age

An understanding of the frequency and severity of malnutrition amongst cancer patients is necessary to better plan preventive, diagnostic, and therapeutic approaches including the allocation of a variety of resources. To this end and as part of a more comprehen-

Table 56.2 Patient characteristics in 644 consecutive cancer patients*.

Characteristics	
Age — Median (range) in years	66 (22–91)
	Percent of Patients
Age <65	45
Age ≥65	55
Sex	
Women	53
Men	47
Type of cancer	
Breast	16
Colon/Rectum	14
Leukemia/Lymphoma	13
Lung/Non-small Cell	14
Prostate	5
Stomach	4
Head/Neck Squamous	4
Ovary	3
Kidney/Urinary Bladder	3
Lung/Small Cell	2
All Others	22
Stage of Cancer	
Metastatic	52
Non-metastatic	48

* Seen at Pacific Shores Medical Group and St. Mary Medical Center, Long Beach, California

sive effort, we studied nutrition-related clinical variables in 644 consecutive oncology patients regardless of type, status, or stage of cancer. Patient characteristics are shown in Table 56.2. The majority were seen as outpatients. We divided patients by age (<65 vs ≥65), and we analyzed the entire group as well as the subset of patients who had metastatic disease (Table 56.3). Ideal body weight range was calculated using the Gerontology Research Center tables. The vast majority of the patients sustained the weight loss shown within a period of 6 months from cancer diagnosis.

The incidence of weight loss is very high in all patients, but particularly in those over the age of 65 (Table 56.3). Thus, 80% of all patients 65 or older with metastatic cancer had some degree of weight loss, 58% were underweight, 58% had decreased appetite, and 71% reported a decrease in food intake. Forty-three percent of patients 65 or older with metastatic disease had weight loss of 10% or more of their usual body

Table 56.3 Nutritional variables in 644 consecutive cancer patients*.

Variable	All Ages		<65 years old		≥65 years old	
	All Stages (N=644)	Patients with Metastases	All Stages (N=292)	Patients with Metastases (N=145)	All Stages (N=353	Patients with Metastases (N-192)
Weight Loss						
Any	74%	76%	68%	68%	80%	83%
Up to 5%	15%	15%	11%	10%	18%	18%
>5->10%	20%	22%	20%	18%	24%	21%
10–20%	27%	26%	24%	23%	28%	30%
>20%	15%	11%	13%	17%	10%	13%
None	24%	26%	33%	32%	20%	17%
Underweight	54%	49%	37%	45%	58%	61%
Normal Weight	33%	37%	44%	39%	32%	29%
Overweight	13%	14%	19%	17%	10%	10%
Decreased Appetite	59%	54%	49%	53%	58%	63%
Decreased Food Intake	67%	61%	58%	61%	63%	71%

*Seen at Pacific Shores Medical Group and St. Mary Medical Center, Long Beach, California

weight. As seen on Table 56.3, weight and other variables seemed more compromised in patients 65 and older. These data suggest that undernutrition at various stages is highly prevalent among oncology patients, particularly in the older population. Attention to the nutritional status of patients may afford the clinician opportunities for early diagnosis and intervention.

Mechanisms of Cachexia

The causes of cachexia in each individual patient appear to be multifactorial and complex (Figure 56.1). Certainly anorexia and decreased food intake are primarily involved in many cachexia patients. Increases in resting energy expenditure have been found only in a minority of patients (16). Disease- or therapy-induced nausea and vomiting, as well as gastrointestinal obstruction or dysfunction, may also play significant roles. Of great interest is the suspected role of cytokines (17,18). Thus, various peptides released by lymphocytes and monocytes, seemingly in response to the malignant process, can lead to profound derangements in multiple systems. As shown in Figure 56.1, interferon, tumor necrosis factor, and interleukin-1 can lead to anorexia and decreased food intake (19). Tumor necrosis factor may also lead to proteolysis and catabolism with lean tissue cell loss and compositional depletion. Several cytokines interfere with metabolic processes at the level of the hepatocyte, leading to increased gluconeogenesis and glucose turnover as well as to alterations in protein and lipid metabolism. These combined effects may lead, again, to proteolysis, lipolysis, and com-

positional depletion. In addition, inhibition of lipogenic enzymes of adipocytes by cytokines may enhance the depletion of energetic stores. The end result of these mechanisms is profound anorexia, decreased food intake, compositional depletion, cachexia, and eventually, death of the host from starvation.

As shown in Figure 56.1, some tumors can directly secrete mediators, e.g., bombesin, serotonin, and others, that cause paraneoplastic syndromes characterized in part by cachexia. However, these mediators seem to be produced by a minority of tumor types (18). A better understanding of the etiology of cachexia may help develop treatment strategies. Effective antitumor therapies may reverse all abnormalities, but are available only in a limited number of instances. An alternative approach includes pharmacologic interventions aimed to offset the mechanisms of cachexia (Figure 56.1).

When is Nutritional Intervention Needed?

The need for intervention in undernourished cancer patients needs to be based on several factors:

Nutritional Status

Clinical assessment of the nutritional status is an essential first step towards a management strategy. There are no defined rules to determine when to intervene. However, we feel that any weight loss that is progressive and associated with decreased appetite and food intake should immediately lead to further evaluation and patient education as well as close follow-up. The need for intervention is more urgent in patients who are underweight, but severe undernutrition demon-

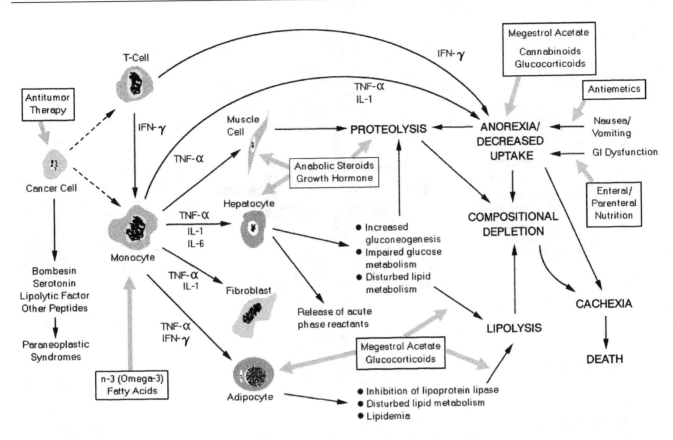

Figure 56.1 Mechanisms of Cachexia/Opportunities for Therapy.

strated by rapid weight loss can also affect patients who are "overweight."

Patient's Desires and Concerns

All clinical decisions need to be individualized and the patient's input is crucial. Palliative therapy should be focused on patient comfort. It is therefore important to understand whether anorexia and decreased food intake, as well as changes in body image associated with weight loss, are of major concern to the involved patient.

Overall Clinical Situation

Nothing can substitute for a comprehensive clinical assessment of a patient's condition. Therefore, the type of tumor, the outlook for potential treatments, the prognosis, the constellation of symptoms, and the therapeutic goals (palliative versus curative), need to be taken into account by the practitioner.

Quality of Life Aspects

Patients with advanced cancer depend on relief from uncomfortable symptoms in order to recover a basic sense of physical comfort and well-being. Thus, consistent and meticulous attention to the assessment and treatment of such common complaints as nausea, vomiting, pain, anorexia, dyspnea, constipation, and a variety of other disease and treatment-related problems is essential to the patient's quality of life (Figure 56.2).

Anorexia, because of its impact on food intake, can lead to depletion of energy stores as well as a catabolic state that eventually results in profound weakness. A meal is often a gratifying experience and an opportunity for the family to be together, and therefore anorexia has psychological as well as social implications.

Goals of Interventions

In the setting of palliative care, the goal of nutritional intervention is to stabilize or reverse the underlying progressive undernutrition. This may improve the patient's comfort, performance status, and quality of life. Early detection and treatment of anorexia and undernutrition can also help initiate steps to prevent cancer cachexia. In instances of treatable malignancies, (such as lymphoma and ovarian cancer), nutritional support can be an essential component of an overall aggressive strategy of antitumor therapy. Reversing or entirely preventing cachexia in patients with end-stage malignancies may be an unrealistic goal, but even in this setting the symptom of anorexia can often be palliated.

Nutrition Support and Tumor Biology

Protein-calorie deprivation can cause a reduction in spontaneous tumorigenesis, and a decline in the rate of establishment of transplanted tumors (20,22). In contrast, an increase in spontaneous tumor develop-

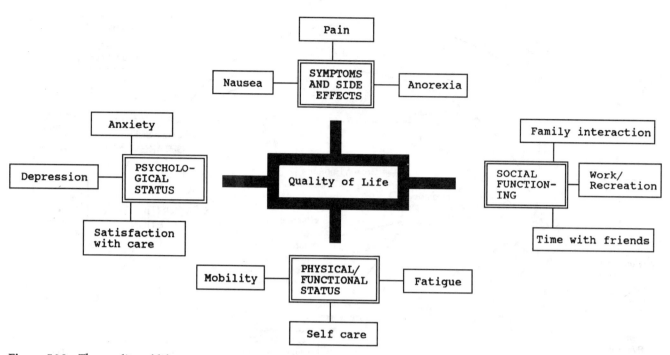

Figure 56.2 The quality of life construct.

ment in animal models has been associated with diets high in calories and fat (20,21). Animal studies have revealed an increase in tumor growth and metastases during periods of nutritional repletion (23,24). The animal model is generally different from the human model because of a much higher tumor/host weight ratio and a faster tumor doubling time (25). In cancer patients, there has been no clear effect of nutrition support on survival time. Whether tumor promotion by nutrition support has any significance at the clinical level remains unknown.

Interventions, Benefits, Risks, and Costs (see Table 56.4)

Counseling

The benefits of initial and follow-up evaluations and counseling by a registered dietitian, preferably in the context of a team approach, can be enormous, although difficult to quantify (26). The main benefits relate to patient satisfaction, nutrition improvement or maintenance, compliance with team or institutional management protocols and guidelines, and a judicious use of risky and expensive treatments. The costs of nutritional counseling are modest when compared to other interventions (Table 56.4).

Nutritional evaluation and counseling, usually undertaken by a registered dietitian, is a first and important step. Ideally, a dietitian should be an integral part of the cancer care team.

In addition to assessing the clinical nutritional parameters it is our practice to first determine, through the dietary history, whether the patient is consuming a "balanced diet." The dietitian obtains a 24–72 hour recall diet history either verbally or, preferably, recorded at home. This diet record is then examined to assess the adequacy of calories and protein utilizing food analysis tables as compared to estimated energy and protein needs. Usually a weight maintenance diet depends on the BEE (Basal Energy Expenditure) and is calculated based on the Harris-Benedict formula (27) which, on an average, results in a daily requirement of 20–25 kcal per kg of body weight. The minimum recommended protein need is at least .8 grams per kg/per day (28). These values need to be adjusted according to whether weight gain is desirable and to match the metabolic needs of the patient.

One goal of nutrition education and counseling is to have the patient increase consumption of nutrient-dense foods to correct nutritional imbalances and deficiencies in order to achieve and maintain a desirable weight. Nutrient-dense foods are those with a high content in calories, protein, fat, and vitamins relative to their volume. Liquid supplements are the most common types of nutritional supplements and are readily available for patient consumption. Patients may be anorectic due to illness or be affected by disabling factors such as difficulty chewing, inability to prepare foods for themselves, visual difficulties, decreased energy level or poor access to foods. Nutritional supplements may be homemade and are usually milk-based or commercially prepared and packaged. Although somewhat expensive, commercial supplements provide balanced, fortified (vitamin and mineral enriched) nutrition which require little or no preparation.

Food Supplements

Liquid concentrated food supplements provide high calorie and protein, low volume nutrients and are

Table 56. 4 Benefits, risks, and costs of nutrition interventions.

Intervention	Benefits	Risks	Average Monthly Cost in Dollars (Range)	Included Services and Products
1. Counseling	Patient satisfaction. Nutrition maintenance. Adherence to protocols.	None	125 (50–200) (Cost calculated based on prevailing hospital and office based dietitian compensation. Overhead not included).	1 initial and 2 follow-up visits by registered dietitian.
2. Food Supplements	Nutrition maintenance.	Limited risks: Diarrhea, nausea		
a. Home Made	Avoid or delay need for more expensive therapy.	a. Diarrhea with lactose intolerance.	a. 52 (34–59)	a. 3 eight oz servings = 750 kcal/day
b. Commercial		b. Patients may not like taste.	b. 132 (112–150) (Average retail prices in 5 grocery stores in Long Beach, California.)	b. 3 eight oz servings = 750–1080 kcal/day
3. Appetite Stimulants a. Megestrol Acetate Oral suspension.	a. Improved appetite, weight, well being, quality of life (see text).	a. Impotence, vaginal bleeding deep vein thrombosis.	a. 101 (73–165) 174 (146–213) 346 (290–426)	a. 200 mg/d, 1 month supply 400 mg/d, 1 month supply 800 mg/d, 1 month supply
b. Dronabinol	b. Improved appetite, no sigluficant weight change (see text).	b. Euphoria, somnolence, dizziness, confusion.	b. 119 (104–148) 230 (181–285)	b. 2.5 mg/d, 1 month supply 5 mg/d, 1 month supply
c. Prednisone	c. Short-term (4 weeks) appetite stimulation (see text).	c. Hypokalemia, muscle weakness, cushingoid features, hyperglycemia, immune suppression, others (see text).	c. 12 (11–14) (Average retail prices from 5 pharmacies in Long Beach, California.)	c. 40 mg/d, 1 month supply
4. Enteral Nutrition	Maintenance of nutrition via enteral route when oral route is not possible.	Requires nasogastric, gastrostomy, or jejunostomy tube placement. Aspiration, diarrhea, nausea, bloating, infection, bleeding.	990 (750–1,500) (Medicare allowable charges). See ref 39.	(See items in Table 56.4. Costs of tube placement and care of complications not included).
5. Home Parenteral Nutrition	Maintenance of nutrition when no other alternative is appropriate. No evidence of improved survival in end-stage cancer.	Catheter-related pneumothorax, sepsis, thrombosis, bleeding. Hepatic dysfunction, fluid and electrolyte imbalance.	8,400 (7,140–11,700) (Medicare allowable charges). See ref 39.	(See items in Table 56.4. Costs of indwelling venous devices and their placement as well as care of complications not included).

(Printed by permission from *Oncology* **9(11)**: 79–84, 1995), ref. 76.

reviewed elsewhere (26). Instant breakfast and milk provide an inexpensive and usually well-tolerated alternative. Commercial products may be more convenient and better tolerated in those patients with lactose intolerance. Dietitians will help patients select products on the basis of tolerance and palatability.

These products are particularly helpful when patients can not maintain an adequate intake through a regular diet but are able to swallow and have a relatively intact gastrointestinal tract.

Commercially prepared supplements are available in a variety of flavors (including unflavored) and in a variety of nutrient compositions. Most commercially prepared supplements are available in ready-to-drink eight ounce cans or boxes and are usually lactose free, which for the patients is often more acceptable due to the increased incidence of perceived milk intolerance in this population. When patients have difficulty consuming adequate volumes of enteral supplement, then a high caloric supplement containing 2 kcal/ml (e.g. Isocal HCN [Mead Johnson] or Magnacal [Sherwood Medical]) can be used. Homemade supplements can also be made with commercially available products comprising a dry milk base to which whole milk and flavoring is added for a nutrient-dense beverage. Commercially prepared powdered breakfast drinks (e.g. Ultra Slim-Fast, Instant Breakfasts) to which whole milk is added is an inexpensive effective supplement when lactose intolerance is not an issue. This supplement has similar vitamin, mineral, calorie, fat, carbohydrate and protein content as most commercially prepared supplements.

An eight ounce supplement varies in nutrient density from 240–480 kcals, 7–20 grams of protein, 5–19 grams of fat and 12–25 percent of the U.S. Recommended Dietary Allowances (U.S.R.D.A.) for vitamins and minerals.

A nutritional supplement is advisable for patients whose gastrointestinal (GI) tract is functional but who are unable to obtain adequate nutrition from a regular diet. The volume and choice of supplement is based on patients' individual nutrient needs and preferences, and GI tolerance. Supplements with fiber, generally soy or oat fiber, are available and may be beneficial to the patient who has diarrhea or constipation. Nutritional supplements are generally well accepted and may offer relief to a patient who has difficulties eating solid food. Tolerability can be enhanced by starting with small quantities and by diluting the supplement with water or ice to decrease osmolality. A patient will usually accept one to three, 8 ounce supplements per day, but there is great individual variability. Patients who have alterations in taste or nausea may tolerate an unflavored supplement better.

A common concern of patients and families is whether adding vitamins and other micronutrients to the patients' diet is beneficial. An analysis of the dietary record for the recommended number of servings from the Basic Four Food Groups (milk, meat and meat substitutes, vegetable and fruit, and grain) helps establish whether the minimum vitamin and mineral requirements are met. A computerized diet analysis program may help to quickly and accurately assess the nutrient content including vitamins and minerals. When intake is inadequate, we prescribe a daily multivitamin.

Patients should be provided with practical dietary advice about how to improve daily caloric intake, and the following are some simple tips to increase food intake:

- Avoid favorite foods after highly emetogenic chemotherapy to prevent the development of food aversions.

- Unless medically contraindicated patients should be encouraged to consume any foods regardless of them being labeled "non-nutritious" such as potato chips, nuts, or ice cream.
- Emphasize consumption of "nutrient dense" foods as part of main meals or snacks, i.e., peanut butter, cheese, whole milk, and yogurt.
- Avoid the "Why don't you eat?" complaint. The patient should not be psychologically punished by the cancer care team and/or the family for not eating but rather should be supported to overcome anorexia and other problems that lead to decreased food intake.
- Emphasize the pleasurable as well as social aspects of meals. Encourage patients to have their meals in a relaxed, friendly and familiar atmosphere.
- Moderate alcohol intake is usually compatible with treatments and should be allowed before meals unless contraindicated.
- Avoid odors that can cause nausea. A short walk outside while meals are being prepared is advisable.
- Encourage food supplements and snacks between meals without being concerned that they may affect intake at meal time.

Patients are often deeply interested in the topic of nutrition as an unproven treatment. However, many will not bring up this topic unless encouraged and listened to in a non-judgmental fashion. Open discussion and patient education may help prevent untoward effects of these diets and introduce nutrition-related issues into the mainstream of oncology care.

Hypercholesterolemia and hypertriglyceridemia are also common in older cancer patients, and it is often necessary to emphasize that an improvement in caloric intake is far more important than a low cholesterol diet when undernutrition is the main problem.

Appetite Stimulants

Anorexia and wasting have been a focus of research over the last decade, particularly in patients with cancer or AIDS. Therefore, references to results in both the AIDS and cancer fields are relevant here. Several drugs have been tested with the goal of stimulating the appetite of patients with AIDS or cancer and anorexia (29–31). Two drugs (megestrol acetate and dronabinol) have been recently approved by the Food and Drug Administration for use in patients with AIDS and weight loss. In addition, corticosteroids have been used in cancer patients with end-stage disease for short term (3–4 weeks) effects on appetite and well being. Anabolic steroids are also often utilized especially in AIDS patients, although data of their efficacy is lacking.

Megestrol acetate

This orally active progesterone hormone derivative was initially proposed as a treatment for cancer cachexia when it was recognized as a cause of marked weight gain in patients with breast cancer, when used at relatively large doses (32) Megestrol acetate is now available in the form of an oral suspension (40 mg/ml) and was recently approved for use in patients with AIDS-related weight loss. In these patients, two randomized placebo-controlled clinical trials indicate that megestrol acetate can stimulate appetite, food intake, and weight gain with associated patient-reported improvement in an overall sense of well being and quality of life parameters (33,34). Maximum weight change is seen in 2 to 6 weeks in about one fourth of patients, but it is not achieved until after 10 weeks of therapy in over a third of patients (30). The effects on appetite and weight are dose related and sustained so long as the medication is continued. Four previously published randomized double-blind, placebo-controlled trials in patients with advanced cancer, anorexia, and weight loss, demonstrated substantial appetite enhancement in patients receiving megestrol acetate (35–38).

The benefits of megestrol acetate are related mainly to a favorable symptomatic effect that results in improved appetite, food intake, sense of well being and quality of life parameters. This hormone derivative is well tolerated and side effects are infrequent and probably dose dependent. Side effects reported include impotence, vaginal spotting, and deep vein thrombosis. In the largest published AIDS trial, impotence was a reported side effect in 3% of placebo patients and in 4%, 6%, and 14% of megestrol acetate patients receiving 100 mg/day, 400 mg/day, and 800 mg/day respectively. Deep vein thrombosis was reported in one patient out of 232 receiving megestrol acetate. Although thrombotic complications have been infrequent, a trend for a dose related increase in thromboembolic events has been reported in cancer patients (39). The weight gain seen with megestrol acetate is due to increased body mass and is not due to edema (33,37). The charges according to drug dose are shown in Table 56.4. Although the recommended starting dose is 800 mg/day (20 ml PO Q am), appetite enhancement and weight gain is seen at lower doses as well.

Dronabinol

This marijuana derivative has been in use as an antiemetic and was recently tested in a randomized double-blind placebo-controlled trial in patients in AIDS-related anorexia and weight loss (40). Patients receiving dronabinol reported improved appetite and mood compared to placebo. There was no significant effect on body weight. Adverse events consisted of euphoria, somnolence, dizziness, and confusion. No randomized clinical trials have been so far reported in patients with cancer. Charges according to dosage are listed in Table 56.4.

Prednisone

This and other corticosteroids have been used by oncologists as appetite and mood enhancers in patients with end-stage disease and very poor short-term prognosis. Randomized trials in cancer patients have shown a short-lived (usually four weeks) period of appetite enhancement, without weight gain (41–44). Corticosteroids are generally contraindicated in patients with AIDS because of their immunosuppressive effects and

therefore have not been tried as appetite enhancers in this disease. Side effects of corticosteroids are frequent and can be serious. They include immune suppression, dysphoria, insomnia, hyperglycemia, muscle weakness, cushingoid features, edema, hypokalemia, and gastrointestinal intolerance. The cost of prednisone is low and is shown in Table 56.4; the cost of using this drug may be higher when one includes the need for monitoring glucose and potassium levels.

Other compounds

Other compounds such as cyproheptadine and hydrazine sulfate have been tried and shown to be ineffective in patients with cancer induced anorexia/cachexia (45–47). Anabolic steroids are indicated in males with hypogonadism. Definitive clinical studies of the effects of androgenic compounds in undernourished cancer patients are lacking. Androgens may cause hirsutism, cholestatic jaundice and other liver toxicities, and edema.

Enteral Nutrition

Enteral nutrition via nasogastric, gastrostomy or jejunostomy tube feedings is indicated generally in patients who are unable to swallow or who have obstructions or dysfunctions that prevent them from safely transferring liquid or solid food into the upper gastrointestinal tract. It is important that the decisions about tube feedings be made by the nutrition support team after proper evaluation and counseling of the patient. This will avoid initiating enteral nutrition in instances where a more conservative approach may be successful (48,49). Gastrostomy tube feedings have been reported to offer an advantage in terms of nutrition parameters, quality of life, and functional status in patients who are receiving combined modality treatments for head and neck cancer or upper gastrointestinal malignancies (50–52). Decisions in these patients need to be individualized however, because many patients will do well if instructed and helped from the onset of therapy by a skilled dietitian. If the reason for tube feedings is anorexia per se, without obstruction, strong consideration should be given first to counseling, food supplements, and appetite enhancers because they can be quite effective, less risky, and certainly much less expensive. The main serious risk of enteral feeding is aspiration, a complication more likely to occur where there is impaired gastric emptying, tube misplacement, or when the patient is fed in the supine position. Additional side effects include diarrhea or constipation, nausea, vomiting, abdominal cramps, bloating, and distention (49). The costs of home enteral feeding are presented in Tables 56.4 and 56.5. Cancer accounts for the majority of new cases of home enteral nutrition (Figure 56.3) (53), and it is estimated that the yearly cost for home enteral nutrition nationally is $357 million (53).

Parenteral Nutrition

Parenteral nutrition is indicated in patients who can not be fed via the gastrointestinal tract. Outside this indication, its use in the settings of advanced cancer or

Table 56.5 Medicare allowable charges for HPEN therapy.

	Parenteral (per day)	Tube Enteral (per day)
Nutrient solution		
Glucose	$158–$298	
Amino acids		$10–$35
Lipids	$30–$40	
Additives	$7	
Dressing kit	$7	$0.5–$2.0
Administration set	$22	$11
Pump loan (15 months only)	$12	$3.6
Mean (range)	$280($238–$390)	$33 ($25–$50)

HPEN = home parenteral and enteral nutrition

Adapted, with permission, from Howard *et al.* 53

AIDS is controversial. It has recently been reported that cancer patients, however, account for the majority of home parenteral nutrition cases in the U.S. (Figure 56.3) (53).

Ethical issues are important when consideration is given to nutritional support in end-stage cancer or AIDS. One must distinguish between hydration therapy which is obviously less expensive and total parenteral nutrition. The wishes of the patient and family as well as the clinical circumstances must be carefully balanced in order to make appropriate decisions. Parenteral nutrition is clearly not advisable as an adjunct to cancer therapy and should be used judiciously because of the limited benefits and high risks and expenses it imposes (54,55). It is in fact unclear whether any additional life or quality of life is gained with parenteral nutrition in patients with advanced cancer.

Parenteral nutrition is associated with serious risks, including complications of intravenous devise placement and maintenance (pneumothorax, venous thromboembolism, hemorrhage, exit site infection, bacteremia, and sepsis), and side effects of intravenous nutrition (electrolyte imbalance, hepatic dysfunction, fluid imbalance) (56). Parenteral nutrition requires close supervision, catheter care, frequent laboratory tests, and consequently multiple ongoing human resources are required including physician, pharmacist and nurse. The costs of home parenteral nutrition are shown in Tables 56.4 and 56.5. As shown in Figure 56.3, cancer accounts for the majority of new cases of home parenteral nutrition. It is estimated that the yearly cost of home parenteral nutrition is $780 million (53). The yearly cost for hospital parenteral nutrition has been estimated at $6 billion (57).

Method for Choosing Among Alternative Therapies

Figure 56.4 represents a method for choosing between alternative therapies directed to a common goal (i.e., improving health-related quality adjusted life years [HR-QALYs]). From a health-care stand point, an intervention may be indicated provided it improves the length of life and/or its quality. A therapy will be beneficial and acceptable if the combination of its effects on HR-QALYs warrants its use and supports the expense it requires (56). As a point of reference, a cost of $42,000 to $80,300 per life year has been quoted in patients receiving renal dialysis (57). When choosing between two or more alternative therapies, it is helpful

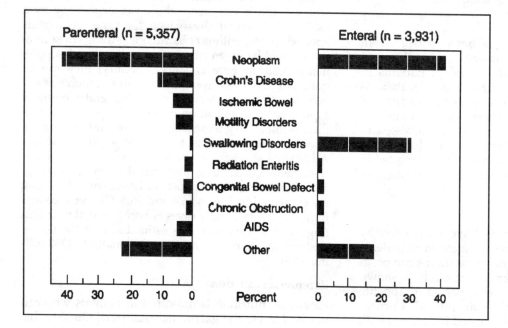

Figure 56.3 Home Parenteral and Enteral Nutrition — The distribution of diagnoses in new patients receiving home parenteral nutrition and home enteral nutrition reported to the North American home Parenteral and Enteral Nutrition (NAHPEN) Registry from 1985 to 1992. The values shown were percents of the total for each therapy category. Adapted, with permission, from Howard *et al.* (53)

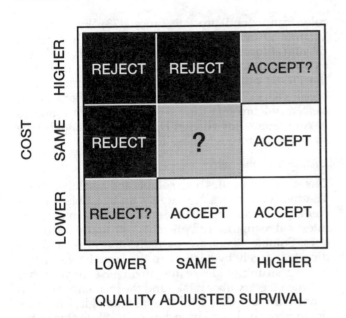

Figure 56.4 Health-Care Decision making – Weighing cost and quality-adjusted survival time in choosing between alternative therapies.

to determine which therapy offers the most favorable ratio of cost versus quality adjusted survival. The case of nutrition support in cancer offers an opportunity to apply this type of analysis. Since in most instances the length of survival is not affected, quality of life is the one dimension that determines the benefits obtained.

The conclusion to be drawn is that in order to make rational decisions, the effects of nutrition support interventions on quality of life must be measured and reported, and similarly, the cost of such interventions must be known. The clinician and patient may then choose from available nutrition support maneuvers by evaluating their effects on quality of life, and their costs.

Research Issues

Muscle Mass and Performance Status

Improved caloric intake may provide enough fuel to support increased function and the restoration of adipose tissue stores. Performance status and muscle mass also improve as a result of enhanced physical activity. It has been well demonstrated recently that even in institutionalized, frail, elderly patients (with an average age of 90), a relatively short-term (8 weeks) exercise program can markedly increase muscle strength and muscle size (35). It is therefore important that nutritional counseling as well as drug intervention are coupled with proper strategies to induce a better functional status. In patients with a relatively stable, chronic course, obtaining advice from the institution's rehabilitation and physical therapy programs can be rewarding. It has not been established whether patients with cancer are able to build muscle at times when cytokines

are actively affecting metabolism. During periods of remission such patients are clearly able to build muscle, but the variations with age and hormonal status have not been established. The best protocols for achieving these results and enhancing overall quality of life are clearly a research priority.

The Prevention of Cancer Recurrence or Progression

Epidemiologic and experimental findings imply both dietary patterns and specific nutrients in the pathogenesis of common neoplasms such as breast, colon, endometrial and prostate cancer. Moreover, nutrition may play a synergistic role together with smoking in lung and head and neck cancer. These tumors are particularly prevalent in the elderly. Lifestyle in general which includes diet, tobacco and alcohol use may account for up to 70% of avoidable cancer mortality in this country. The modification of these risk factors through intervention holds promise for reducing age-adjusted cancer incidence and mortality.

International comparisons across a wide range of dietary patterns in many countries indicate a strong correlation between dietary fat and cancers of the breast, colon, and prostate (58). Migration studies have also demonstrated a correlation of dietary fat intake with cancer (59,60). Controversy on the role of dietary fat in the causation of breast cancer has resulted from the demonstration of a correlation in some analytical epidemiology studies , but not in all studies (61). In particular the lack of any correlation in 89,538 nurses between fat consumption and breast cancer risk has been used to deny the existence of any association (62). Others (63) have argued that the range of dietary fat intakes was small by comparison to the international studies and may have been too small to demonstrate any correlation. In a subsequent epidemiologic study an association was demonstrated between intake of red meat and animal fat intake and the incidence of colon cancer among 88,751 nurses (64).

The primary mechanisms proposed for the effects of dietary fat on carcinogenesis is via tumor promotion, although some studies demonstrate an effect on initiation as well. Mechanisms may be direct or indirect. Mechanisms for direct effects include effects on cell membrane fluidity, prostaglandin metabolism, and formation of lipid peroxidation products. Polyunsaturated fats in particular are prone to formation of peroxidated products. The production of these metabolically active intermediates can be inhibited by antioxidants such as BHA, BHT, vitamins A, C, and E, selenium and carotenoids. Indirect effects of fat may be mediated via hormonal, paracrine, or immune mechanisms. Most studies of nutrition in colon cancer etiology have concentrated on biochemical processes, while most studies of breast cancer have concentrated on hormonal mechanisms.

Calories and obesity in carcinogenesis

Both animal studies and some population studies support a role for calories and obesity in cancers of the breast, colon, rectum, uterus and kidney (65). Calorie intake varies with activity level so that an active non-obese construction worker may take in 4500 kcal/day while an obese postmenopausal woman at increased risk for breast cancer might maintain her weight at a daily caloric intake of 1500 calories per day. Obesity defined as excess body fat results from increased intake of calories relative to energy expenditure and has been positively correlated with breast cancer in some studies (66,67), but not others (68,69). One case-control study supports this association (61).

Breast, ovarian and endometrial cancers are promoted by estrogens, and adipose tissue can convert androstenedione, an adrenal androgen to estrone. Estrone can subsequently be converted to estradiol. Thus, there are two sources of estrogens in women, the ovaries and the fat tissue conversion of adrenal hormones. After the menopause, the primary source is the fat tissue, so that obesity in postmenopausal women is correlated with increased breast cancer incidence. Other growth factors, such as insulin or IGF-1 may be produced in excess in obesity and promote carcinogenesis. Cell-cell interactions between stromal fibroblast/adipocytes and epithelial cells with developing tumors may be important in the process of carcinogenesis. Transplantable breast tumors grow well within fat pads, suggesting there may be trophic factors produced and released in a paracrine fashion by stromal cells in the breast and other endocrine organs.

Vitamin a, vitamin d, deltanoids and carotenoids

A prospective study of an elderly cohort in Massachusetts correlated a decreased incidence of all cancers with an increased intake of carotenoid-containing vegetables (70). A vitamin A index is used in studies to lump the dietary sources of preformed vitamin A (primarily retinyl esters) found in animal sources with different foods containing carotenoids, such as green and yellow leafy vegetables. A number of case-control studies demonstrate that lower intakes of these carotenoid-containing foods are associated with increased incidence of lung cancer in smokers (71,72). It is not clear from these studies which of the substances contained in fruits and vegetables are protective. Protective factors might include indoles, found in cruciferous vegetables, or vitamin C. While unmeasured substances may also prevent cancer, it is important to examine the overall effect of increased fruit and vegetable intake on total calories, dietary fat and obesity in order to control for other factors associated with the observed dietary patterns found to be protective. Vitamin A may directly prevent cancer by promoting normal epithelial cell differentiation. In addition, carotenoids and related substances serve as oxygen radical scavengers. Through this mechanism these substances may reduce the levels of active peroxidated intermediates within cells. Vitamin A, Vitamin C, and selenium may be part of a protective network called the antioxidant defense system by Ames.

There is epidemiologic support for the notion that exposure to sunlight via the production of vitamin D may provide some protection from development of colon cancer and prostate cancer (73). Furthermore, Vitamin D analogs which only minimally increase calcium absorption (called deltanoids) have been shown to lead to differentiation of cancerous cells including the HL-60 cell, acute promyelocytic leukemia cells, breast cancer, and prostate cancer cells. Both breast cancer and prostate cancer cells have been found to have receptors for vitamin D, and the deltanoids presumably act through these receptors (74).

Dietary fiber and cancer

Dietary fiber includes both soluble and insoluble fibers. The insoluble fibers are largely undigestible and include those bran products commonly used to promote intestinal regularity and prevent gastrointestinal disorders. Soluble fibers are partially digestible and are digested largely by bacteria in the large bowel. There is very strong evidence for an inverse relationship between dietary fiber intake and the incidence of colon cancer. In one review 33 of 42 epidemiological analyses demonstrated this relationship (75). While this is the most studied form of cancer with regard to dietary fiber intake there are potential mechanisms for effects on other commonly occurring cancers.

Mechanisms of action range from changes in stool transit time in the colon to the mutagenic actions of secondary bile acids and putative fecal mutagens. Fiber may also act to dilute bowel contents so that mutagenic substances are less likely to come into contact with the bowel mucosa.

Other specific nutrients

Vitamin C, Vitamin E, selenium, protein, pickled and smoked foods, food additives and alcohol have all been proposed to have a role in the nutritional etiology of cancer. While vitamin E, selenium, and vitamin C are all believed to acts as antioxidants, evidence for their preventive effects in cancer is still being collected. Pickled and smoked food have been found to contain carcinogens including nitrites. These latter foods are not thought to play a significant role in cancers in the U.S. but may be important in Asia. A number of fungi and molds have also been shown to contain carcinogens and mutagens. The ingestion of spoiled or moldy foods which contain aflatoxin and other toxins has been associated with the occurrence of hepatoma in many parts of the world. Aflatoxin forms a DNA adduct detectable in the urine. There is also evidence of an interaction between the genome of hepatitis B virus and aflatoxin in the pathogenesis of hepatoma.

Dietary recommendations and current clinical trials

Current dietary recommendations for primary prevention provided by the National Cancer Institute and the American Cancer Society include:

1. Eat at least five servings a day of fruits and vegetables.
2. Decrease total fat in the diet including both saturated and polyunsaturated fats.
3. Increase dietary fiber intake from cereals and grains.

4. Avoid excess calorie intake and attempt to achieve desirable body weight through exercise and a healthy diet.
5. Avoid excessive consumption of alcohol.
6. Avoid smoked, pickled, or poorly preserved foods.

A number of national multicenter clinical trials are currently examining diet and cancer prevention including: 1) Women's Intervention Nutrition Study (WINS) in which women with early stage breast cancer are placed on a 15% fat diet or control diet after primary treatment. Recurrence in the opposite breast is used as an outcome variable. There have been over 500 patients entered on this trial which has already established the feasibility of this diet intervention. 2) The Womens' Health Initiative (WHI): In this study of 148,000 postmenopausal women, all-cause mortality including breast and colon cancer will be examined. Women will receive either a 20% fat diet or a control diet. There will also be arms simultaneously receiving different postmenopausal hormone replacement (estrogen alone, estrogen plus progesterone, or placebo) and different calcium and vitamin D supplementation (supplements or placebo). This 3 by 2 by 2 design will follow women until the year 2005 and has the necessary statistical power to resolve whether a 20% low fat diet will be a useful preventive approach for breast cancer or colon cancer. 3) The Colonic Polyps Trial in which a combined low fat, high fiber diet is compared to a control diet for the prevention of polyp formation and colon cancer in this high risk group. The outcomes of these various trials will provide useful data for evaluating the potential of nutrition intervention in cancer. Nutrition may not only restore normal nutrition status in the malnourished cancer patient but also help to retard cancer progression in the future.

Conclusion

Changes associated with aging include decreasing height, muscle mass, total body water, and energy expenditure and increasing intra-abdominal adipose tissue. Variables that the clinician can assess to determine the nutritional status of cancer patients include percent and rate of weight loss from usual body weight, current weight compared to age-adjusted calculated ideal body weight (Table 56.1), and levels of appetite and food intake. Our studies show that eighty percent of patients with cancer who are over the age of 65 have had some degree of weight loss, and that more than half are underweight, have loss of appetite, or complain of a decrease in food intake (Table 56.3). The need for nutritional support depends on the clinical context as well as on patient preferences. The first step in management is nutritional evaluation, dietary counseling, and follow-up. Nutritional support is available in the form of homemade or commercial food supplements, enteral nutrition, and parenteral nutrition. In addition, medications can be used to improve appetite, food intake, and well being. Conservative cost estimates for these interventions range from $52 per month

for homemade supplements to $8,400 per month for home parenteral nutrition (Table 56.4). Clinicians must be familiar with the benefits, risks and costs of these therapies in order to suggest appropriate options.

Future research is focused on the nutritional modulation of the process of tumor progression following initial treatment. This work includes the use of low fat, high fiber diets, micronutrients and some phytochemicals found to have anti-tumor effects in experimental model systems. Ongoing clinical trials should provide new information on the use of nutritional interventions for the prevention of cancer recurrence and/or progression.

References

1. Kuczmarski RJ. Need for body composition information in elderly subjects. *Am J Clin Nutr* **50**: 1150–7, 1989.
2. Chumlea WC, Garry PJ, Hunt WC, Rhyne RL. Serial changes in stature and weight in a healthy elderly population. *Hum Biol* **60**: 918–25, 1988.
3. Morley J. Nutritional Status of the Elderly. *Am J Med* **81**: 679–695, 1986.
4. Silver AJ. Nutritional modulation of life span and gene expression. In *Nutrition in the Elderly*, edited by Morley JE, moderator, pp. 892–894. *Ann Intern Med* **109**: 890–904, 1988.
5. Blackburn G, Bistrian B, Maini B, *et al.* Nutritional and metabolic assessment of the hospitalized patient. *JPEN* **1**: 11–22, 1977.
6. Andres R, Elahi D, Tobin JD, *et al.* Impact of Age on Weight Goals. *Ann Intern Med* **103(6 pt 2)**: 1030–1033, 1985.
7. Boring C, Squires T, Tong T. Cancer Statistics, 1991. CA. *A Cancer Journal of Clinicians* **41(1)**: 19–36, 1991.
8. DeWys W. Management of cachexia. *Semin Oncol* **12**: 452–460, 1985.
9. Theologides A. Anorexia as a general effect of cancer. *Cancer* **43**: 2013–2019, 1979.
10. Tchekmedyian NS, Hickman M, Jessie Siau, *et al.* Treatment of Cancer Anorexia With Megestrol Acetate. Impact on Quality of Life. *Oncology* **4**: 185–192, 1990.
11. Cella DF, Bonomi AE. Measuring Quality of Life: 1995 Update. *Oncology* **9(11)**: 47–60, 1995.
12. Chumlea WC, Baumgartner RN. Status of anthropometry and body composition data in elderly subjects. *Am J Clin Nutr* **50**: 1158–66, 1989.
13. Henry JB. Clinical Chemistry. In *Clinical Diagnosis and Management by Laboratory Methods*, 18th ed. WB Saunders Co., pp. 316, 1991.
14. Sacher RA, McPherson RA, Campos JM. Tables 56.9–56.11. Serum Proteins of Diagnostic Significance. In *Widmann's Clinical Interpreter of Laboratory Tests*, 10th ed. FA Davis Company, pp. 352, 1991.
15. Brittenham GM. Disorders of Iron Metabolism. Iron Deficiency and Overload. In *Hematology. Basic Principles and Practice*, edited by Ronald Hoffman. Churchill Livingstone Inc., pp. 334, 1991.
16. Heber D, Byerley L, Tchekmedyian NS. Hormonal and Metabolic Abnormalities in the Malnourished Cancer Patient. Effects on Host-Tumor Interaction. *J Parenter Enter Nutr* **16**: 60S–64S, 1992.
17. Moldawer L, Rogy M, Lowry S. The Role of Cytokines in Cancer Cachexia. *J Parenter Enter Nutr* **16**: 43S–49S, 1992.
18. McNamara M, Alexander R, Norton J. Cytokines and Their Role in the Pathophysiology of Cancer Cachexia. *J Parenter Enter Nutr* **16**: 50S–55S, 1992.
19. Langstein HN, Norton JA. Mechanisms of Cancer Cachexia. *Hematol Oncol Clin North Am* **5**: 103–123, 1991.
20. Tennenbaum A, Silverstone H. Nutrition in relation to cancer. *Adv Cancer Res* **1**: 451–501, 1953.
21. Green JW, Benditt EO, Humphreys EM. The effect of protein depletion on the host response to transplantable rat tumor Walker 256. *Cancer Res* **10**: 769–774, 1950.

22. White FR, Belkin M. Source of tumor proteins. Effect of a low-nitrogen diet on the establishment and growth of a transplanted tumor. *JNCI* 5: 261–263, 1944.

23. Cameron IL, Ackley WJ, Rogers W. Responses of hepatoma-bearing rats to total parenteral hyperalimentation and to ad libitum feeding. *J Surg Res* 23: 189–195, 1977.

24. Ota DM, Copeland EM, Strobel HW, *et al*. The effect of protein nutrition on host and tumor metabolism. *J Surg Res* 22: 181–188, 1977.

25. Torosian M. Stimulation of Tumor Growth by Nutrition Support. *J Parenter Enter Nutr* 16: 72S-75S, 1992.

26. Bowman BB, Rosenberg IH. Digestive Function and Aging. In *Human Nutrition. Clinical Nutrition* 37C, 75–89, 1983.

27. Harris JA, Benedict FG. *Biometric studies of basal metabolism in man*. Publication no: 279. Carnegie Institute of Washington, 1919.

28. *Recommended Dietary Allowances*, 10 Edition. Subcommittee on the Tenth Edition of the RDAs. Food and Nutrition Board, Commission on Life Sciences, National Research Council, National Academy Press, Washington, D.C., 1989.

29. Von Roenn JH. *Pharmacologic interventions for HIV-related anorexia and cachexia. Oncology* 7(11): 95–99, 1993.

30. Tchekmedyian NS, Heber D. Cancer and AIDS cachexia. Mechanisms and approaches to therapy. *Oncology* 7(11): 55–59, 1993.

31. Loprinzi CL. Pharmacologic management of cancer anorexia/cachexia. *Oncology* 7(11): 101– 103, 1993.

32. Tchekmedyian NS, Tait N, Moody M, Aisner J. High-Dose Megestrol Acetate. A Possible Treatment for Cachexia. *JAMA* 257(9): 1195–1198, 1987.

33. Von Roenn JH, Armstrong D, Kotler DP, *et al*. Megestrol acetate in patients with AIDS- related cachexia. *Ann Intern Med* 121(6): 393–399, 1994.

34. Oster MH, Enders SR, Samuels S. Megestrol Acetate in Patients with AIDS and Cachexia. *Ann Intern Med* 121: 400–408, 1994.

35. Loprinzi CL, Ellison NM, Schaid DJ, *et al*. Controlled trial of megestrol acetate for the treatment of cancer anorexia and cachexia. *J Natl Cancer Inst* 82: 1127–1132, 1990.

36. Bruera E, Macmillan K, Kuehn N, *et al*. A controlled trial of megestrol acetate on appetite, caloric intake, nutritional status, and other symptoms in patients with advanced cancer. *Cancer* 66: 1279–1282, 1990.

37. Tchekmedyian NS, Hickman, Siau J, *et al*. Megestrol acetate in cancer anorexia and weight loss. *Cancer* 69(5): 1268–1274, 1992.

38. Feliu J, Gonzalez-Baron M, Berrocal A, *et al*. Treatment of cancer anorexia with megestrol acetate. Which is the optimal dose? *J Nat Cancer Inst* 83: 449, 1991.

39. Loprinzi CL, Michalak JC, Schaid DJ, *et al*. Phase III evaluation of four doses of megestrol acetate as therapy for patients with cancer anorexia and/or cachexia. *J Clin Oncol* 11: 762–767, 1993.

40. Beal JE, Olson R, Laubenstein L, *et al*. Dronabinol as a treatment for anorexia associated with weight loss in patients with AIDS. *Journal of Pain & Symptom Management* 10(2): 89–97, 1995.

41. Moertel CG, Schutt AJ, Reitemeier RJ, *et al*. Corticosteroid therapy of preterminal gastrointestinal cancer. *Cancer* 33: 1607–1609, 1974.

42. Wilcox J, Corr J, Shaw J, *et al*. Prednisolone as an appetite stimulant in patients with cancer. *British Medical Journal Clinical Research Ed*: 288(6410). 27, 1984.

43. Popiela T, Lucchi R, Giongo F. Methylprednisolone as palliative therapy for female terminal cancer patients. *Dur J Cancer Clin Oncol* 25: 1823–1829, 1989.

44. Bruera E, Roca E, Cedaro L, *et al*. Action or oral methylprednisolone in terminal cancer patients. A prospective randomized double-blind study. *Cancer Treat Rep* 69(7): 751–754, 1985.

45. Kardinal CG, Loprinzi CL, Schaid DJ, *et al*. A controlled trial of cyproheptadine in cancer patients with anorexia and/or cachexia. *Cancer* 65: 2657–2662, 1990.

46. Kosty M, Fleishman S, Herndon J, *et al*. Cisplatin, vinblastine and hydrazine sulfate (NSC #150014) in advanced non-small lung cancer (NSCLC). A randomized, placebo-controlled, double-blind phase III study. *Proc Am Soc Clin Oncol* 11: 294, 1992.

47. Loprinzi CL, Goldberg RG, Su JQ, *et al*. Randomized double-blind, placebo-controlled trial evaluating hydrazine sulfate (HS) in patients with newly diagnosed non-small lung cancer. *Proc Am Soc Clin Onc* 12: 337, 1993.

48. Bloch A. Nutritional Management of Patients with dysphagia. *Oncology* 7(11): 127–137, 1993.

49. Shike M. Enteral Feeding. In *Modern Nutrition in Health and Disease*, 8th Ed, edited by ME Shils, JA Olson, M Shike. PA: Lea & Febiger, pp. 1417–1429, 1994.

50. Daly JM, Weintraub FN, Shou J, *et al*. Enteral nutrition during multimodality therapy in upper gastrointestinal cancer patients. *Ann Surg* 221(4): 327–338, 1995.

51. Fietkau R, Iro H, Sailer D, *et al*. Percutaneous endoscopically guided gastrostomy in patients with head and neck cancer. *Recent Results in Cancer Research* 121: 269–282, 1991.

52. Koehler J, Buhl K. Percutaneous endoscopic gastrostomy for postoperative rehabilitation after maxillofacial tumor surgery. *International Journal of Oral & Maxillofacial Surgery* 20(1): 38–39, 1991.

53. Howard L, Ament M, Fleming CR, *et al*. Current use and clinical outcome of home parenteral and enteral nutrition therapies in the United States. *Gastroenterology* 109(2): 355–365, 1995.

54. American College of Physicians Position Paper. Parenteral nutrition in patients receiving cancer chemotherapy. *Ann Intern Med* 110(9): 734–736, 1989.

55. Klein S. Clinical efficacy of nutritional support in patients with cancer. *Oncology* 7(11): 87–92, 1993.

56. Shils M. Parenteral Nutrition, in Shils ME, Olson JA, Shike M (eds). *Modern Nutrition in Health and Disease*, 8th Ed, pp. 1430–1458. PA: Lea & Febiger, 1994.

57. Goel V. Economics of total parenteral nutrition. *Nutrition* 6(4): 332–335, 1990.

58. Wynder EL, McCoy GD, Reddy BS, Cohen L, Hill P, Spingarn NE, and Weisburger JH. Nutrition and metabolic epidemiology of cancers of the oral cavity, esophagus, colon, breast, prostate, and stomach. In *Nutrition and Cancer. Etiology and Treatment*, edited by GR Newell and NM Ellison. New York: Raven Press, 1981.

59. Gori GB. Dietary and nutritional implication in the multifactorial etiology of certain prevalent human cancers. *Cancer* 43: 2151–2161, 1979.

60. Kolonel LN, Hankin JH, Lee J, Chu SY, Nomura NMY, and Hinds MW. Nutrient intakes in relation to cancer incidence in Hawaii. *Br J Cancer* 44: 332–339, 1981.

61. Newman SC, Miller AB, Howe GR. A study of the effect of weight and dietary fat on breast cancer survival time. *Am J Epidemiol* 123(5): 767–74, May, 1986.

62. Willet WC, Stampfer MJ, Colditz GA, *et al*. Dietary fat and the risk of breast cancer. *New Engl J Med* 316: 22–28, 1987.

63. Prentice RL, Sheppard L. Dietary fat and cancer. consistency of the epidemiologic data, and disease prevention that may follow from a practical reduction in fat consumption. *Cancer Causes and Control* (Oxf.) 1: 81–97, 1990.

64. Willett WC, *et al*. Relation of meat, fat and fiber intake to the risk of colon cancer in women. *New Engl J Med* 323: 1664–1672, 1990.

65. Doll R, Peto R. *The causes of cancer*. New York: Oxford University Press, 1981.

66. Rohan TE, Bain CJ. Diet in the etiology of breast cancer. *Epidemiol Rev* 9: 120, 1987.

67. Howe GR, Hirohata T, Hislop G, *et al*. Dietary factors and risk of breast cancer: combined analysis of 12 case-control studies. *J Nat Canc Inst* 82: 561–569, 1990.

68. Jones, DY, Schatzkin A, Green SB, *et al* Dietary fat and breast cancer in the National Health and Nutrition Survey I. Epidemiologic follow-up study. *J Nat Canc Inst* 79: 465–71, 1987.

69. Buell P. Changing incidence of breast cancer in Japanese-American women. *J Nat Cancer Inst* 65: 1141, 1980.

70. Colditz GA, Branch LG, Lipnick RJ, Willett WC, Rosner B, Posner BM, and Hennekens CH. Increased green and yellow vegetable intake and lowered cancer deaths in an elderly population. *Am J Clin Nutr* 41: 32–36, 1985.

71. Potter JD, McMichael AJ. Diet and cancer of the colon and rectum: a case-control study. *J Natl Cancer Inst* 76: 557–69, 1986.

72. Lyon JL, Mahoney AW, West DW, *et al*. Energy intake: its relationship to colon cancer risk. *J Natl Cancer Inst* **78**: 853–61, 1987.

73. Graham S, Marshall J, Haughey B, *et al*. Dietary epidemiology of cancer of the colon in western New York. *Am J Epidemiol* **128**: 490–503, 1988.

74. Elstner E, Lee YY, Hachiya M, Pakkala S, Binderup L, Norman AW, Okamura WH, Koeffler HP: 1,25 dihydroxy-20-epi-vitamin D_3. An extraordinarily potent inhibitor of leukemic cell growth in vitro. *Blood* **84**: 1960–67, 1994.

75. Jain M, Cook GM, Davis FG, Grace MG, Howe GR, Miller AB. A case-control study of diet and colo-rectal cancer. *Int J Cancer* **26**: 757–68, 1980.

76. Tchekmedyian NS. Costs and Benefits of Nutrition Support in Cancer. *Oncology* **9(11)**: 79–84, 1995.

57. Oncological Rehabilitation

Dario Dini and Alberto Gozza

Introduction

The main goals of cancer research and cancer treatment are cure of cancer, and, when cure is not achievable, meaningful prolongation of patient survival. The cure rate has improved over the past decade for numerous adult malignancies, including some forms of acute leukemia, malignant lymphomas, breast cancer, germ cell tumors, epithelial carcinoma of the ovaries, cancer of the lung and of the large bowel. For many more malignancies the patient disease-free survival has been substantially prolonged by aggressive systemic therapy. In these cases, restoration and preservation of the functions, which may be impaired by cancer and by cancer treatment alike, allows the cancer patient to resume the activity of life prior to the diagnosis of cancer. Yet, in many cases, neither cure or disease-free survival can be obtained. In these cases, the practitioner can mainly offer comfort to the dying patient, by relieving the most vexing symptoms of the disease. Rehabilitative and supportive care frequently interface and thus are best discussed together.

Over the past two decades, impressive advances in supportive care and rehabilitation have improved the quality of life of most cancer patients. Better symptom control has allowed terminal patients to enjoy fully the limited time left to them. Effective rehabilitation has allowed patients who had undergone major surgery, or were debilitated by aggressive chemotherapy and radiotherapy, to resume their regular activities. A major tenet of the practice of oncology is that, whatever the prognosis, the quality of life of the cancer patient must be preserved with all available means. Based on these principles, the management of the cancer patient is becoming more and more a multidisciplinary endeavor, aimed to provide pain control, nutritional therapy, social support, emotional care, and functional rehabilitation, in addition to specific antineoplastic treatment.

Supportive care and rehabilitative interventions are particularly important for the older person with cancer. In frail patients, supportive care may also have a life-prolonging role.

The management of older cancer patients is becoming more and more common for two reasons. First, the prevalence of most malignancies increases with the age of the population and approximately 50% of cancers occur in patients over 65 (1). Second, older people are often affected by concomitant illnesses, functional restrictions, social isolation and economic limitations. Any treatment plans for older persons with cancer must take these issues into account (2).

The Meaning of Oncological Rehabilitation

The rehabilitation of the cancer patient must address physical and functional damages caused by either progression of cancer or by cancer treatments, and requires a highly individualized approach, accounting for variations in the course of the disease and in treatment plans. The rehabilitation of the aged is further complicated by age-related disabilities and comorbid conditions, whose effects may be overimposed to those of cancer and cancer treatment. The rehabilitation program cannot follow rigid guidelines, but need to be continuously molded to the evolving clinical picture (3).

The rehabilitation team members require a general knowledge of oncology, physiatrics and geriatrics; the qualities of sympathy and understanding are necessary to help both patients and their families. Whenever possible, patients must be helped and encouraged to resume their usual life-style and independence (4).

For the older patient, the possibility of recovery is contingent not only on resolution of cancer-related disabilities, but also on preexisting physical disabilities and on comorbidities (cardiovascular, pulmonary and renal insufficiency, diabetes, neurological and rheumatological diseases) and on the patient's ability to follow the treatment plan. These conditions compel us, when planning rehabilitation for an elderly patient, to evaluate the limitations on autonomy imposed by impaired physical function(s). Reversal of these impairments and restoration of some degree of autonomy are the first steps toward further rehabilitation. The improvement of physical function is essential to motivate the older person to achieve and to maintain independence, whenever possible.

Team of Cancer Rehabilitation

Cancer rehabilitation is a team effort. The importance of working as a team is illustrated in the following cases:

Case #1

In November 1992 we were asked to see a 75 year old man who had undergone surgery for rectal cancer 7 years before. He also had Parkinson's disease with continuous hand tremors, that worsened as he tried to perform purposeful movements, such as buttoning his clothes or cutting his food. Though his 71 year old wife helped him regularly with activities of daily living (ADL), he was embarrassed to let her manage his colostomy.

The patient changed colostomy appliances five times daily, because, he believed, he was unable to place them correctly, due to his tremor. He also reported irregular evacuation, which he ascribed to inappropriate diet. The examination showed maceration of the skin surrounding the colostomy, with infection and areas of necrosis. There was evidence of frequent fecal contact with the skin. Of interest, the diameter of the stoma was 3 cm and that of the bag hole 6.4 cm. Also, the patient had never been instructed in bowel irrigation.

After assessment, the stoma care nurse prescribed a suitable bag with adhesive and taught the patient to apply the bag by himself, despite his tremor. After a few days of training, the patient learned to use the appliance, which was effective in containing the effluences. Healing of the skin soon ensued.

In a second group of sessions, the patient was instructed in bowel irrigation, but due to tremors, showed extreme difficulty in following instructions. The intervention of the social worker removed the reluctance of the patient to allow the wife to participate in his care. In two days the wife became able to practice bowel irrigation and since then she practices it at home on alternate days. The primary care nurse reinforces the collaboration of the couple with regular home calls, during which both spouses are allowed to express feelings, concerns, and frustrations. This team effort led to perfectly healed skin and marked improvement in the quality of life of the patient and his family. The timely intervention of different team members was critical to the success of this case.

Case #2

In June, 1992, a 70 year old woman with locally advanced adenocarcinoma of the right breast and osteolytic metastases to the proximal third of the right femur received radiotherapy of the breast and the femur, in combination with polychemotherapy. That included intravenous epidoxorubicin (75 mg/m2). The drug was administered at home, into peripheral veins of the left arm, via a butterfly needle. During the fourth cycle of chemotherapy, in September 1992, the patient experienced a burning sensation on the back of the left hand, which lasted approximately 20 minutes. This was followed by intense local pain and erythema, two hours after the end of the infusion. At the emergency room the patient received s.c. prednisolone around the extravasation site.

Seven days later the patient was referred to our division, with severe local pain, and an extensively blistered area, which involved the dorsal surface of the ulnar half of the left forearm, wrist and hand. The overall area was 15x10 cm in diameter and was erythematous, edematous, and hot. Range of motion was maintained and pin-prick sensibility was intact. The patient was treated with topical applications of ice and 99.9% dimethyl sulfoxide (DMSO), hyaluronic acid dress and systemic antibiotics, and was instructed to repeat the same treatment at home three times daily.

Days later she developed a dry eschar on the forearm and a moist eschar on the hand, which were removed surgically. Postsurgical treatment consisted of saline irrigation and hyaluronic acid dressing. Treatment management suffered a setback as the patient was admitted to the hospital for a pathological fracture of the left femur, in another town on October, 1992, while on a family visit. When she returned to our observation in January 1993, she had a severe ulceration with exposure of the extensor tendons of the hand. A dermo-epidermic graft from the left inguinal area allowed adequate repair of the lesions of the forearm and the wrist. The ulceration of the hand was treated with soft laser therapy (He/Ne/Ir laser), and was completely healed after 30 applications lasting 30 minutes each. Physical therapy allowed resumption of full range of motion of the upper extremities.

It should be emphasized that the intervention of the social worker has been essential in coordinating the transportation of the patient to the treatment center by different family members and in supporting the patient through periodic bouts of depression, while the primary nurse supervised the appropriateness of the home care and provided proper education.

This case has multiple facets. First, and foremost, it illustrates the importance of a tightly coordinated team effort in the successful management of a potentially devastating situation. It also illustrates the importance of continuity of care in the treatment of serious soft tissue extravasation in older patients: the lack of patient contact during admission to a different institution delayed the healing of the lesion for several months. Last but not least, this case emphasizes the need for carefully planning of the logistical aspects of treatment of older individuals.

The team operating in an oncological rehabilitation department is composed of physicians expert in oncology, physiatrics and geriatrics, physiotherapists and occupational therapists, stoma care nurses, primary nurses and medical social workers (Table 57.1). The

Table 57.1 Members of the rehabilitation team and their respective functions.

Physician:	Diagnosis Medical treatment Prescription of physical and of instrumental therapy.
Physiotherapist:	Physical and instrumental therapy Application of prosthesis Patient and family education.
Stoma care specialist:	Stoma management Bowel irrigation Stoma appliances.
Primary nurse:	Management of medical treatment general assistance to patient and family.
Social worker:	Emotional support of patient and family management of social and financial issues.

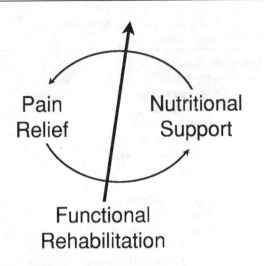

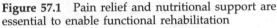

Figure 57.1   Pain relief and nutritional support are essential to enable functional rehabilitation

efforts of the rehabilitation team are coordinated with those of the nutrition and teams and with the practitioner providing primary oncological care. (Figure 57.1). Proper pain control and nutritional support are essential to successful rehabilitation as illustrated by the following case:

A 92 year old manager of a "prank shop" developed back pain and experienced a 20 lb weight loss over three months. When the diagnosis of adenocarcinoma of the pancreas was established, she asked that no attempt be made to prolong her life but she be allowed to die pain free and as functional and independent as she had been for the rest of her life. Pain management with sustained release morphine (30 mg po every 12 hours) caused severe nausea and vomiting and so did low dose radiation therapy to the pancreas. Over the following month the patient had lost 10 additional lbs, her albumin levels had dropped to 2.1 gm/dl and she had become wheel chair-bound.

Block of the retroperitoneal plexus with alcohol produced partial relief of pain with some improvement in function. The administration of intrathecal morphine at low daily doses produced complete relief of pain with insignificant nausea and vomiting. That allowed resumption of ambulation and food intake. The patient died two months later in her sleep and was still able to perform her ADLs up to the last day of her life. She was not taking any antinausea medications at the time of her death.

It is essential to enroll the support of family members, whenever possible, and to instruct them on rehabilitative interventions that may be carried out at home. Frequently, the intervention of family members is the most effective as it involves personal knowledge of the patient, lifelong trust, emotional support and encouragement.

The cooperation of various team members with the patient's primary caregiver guarantees the most suc-

cessful rehabilitative outcome (3). A common problem in dealing with the family of elderly cancer patients in need of home care is preexisting family dynamics. Underlying conflicts may be exacerbated by a serious disease in the family; different family members may use the patient to promote their different and sometimes antagonistic agendas. When such a dynamic is allowed to surface, the patient's care may be seriously compromised as the patient is caught in the middle of a battlefield. It is very important that the social worker of the rehabilitation team assess the family dynamics and promote the resolution of conflicts through meetings involving different family members. During these meetings, the proposal of a common goal targeted to the rehabilitation of the patient, and the definition of specific roles for each family member may promote harmony within a family, which could otherwise be torn apart. The identification of a primary caregiver, i.e. of a family member responsible for coordinating the efforts of all other members is the key to successful home care in both functional and dysfunctional families. The primary caregiver is generally an adult daughter of the patient, must have the trust of all family members. The dedication of this person to the patient and the absence of any plan of secondary gain must be clear to everybody and beyond suspicion. A person who has already proven him/herself a leader of the family in previous times of distress is the most natural choice for primary caregiver. The primary caregiver must be knowledgeable about the patient's daily progress, must establish realistic short term objectives of patient care, must control the performance of each family member and must prevent "role blurring" which may cause new conflicts between family members.

Cancer Related Damages

In oncological rehabilitation it is useful to classify organ damages leading to disabilities according to the main etiology (Table 57.2). Thus, we recognize *iatrogenic damages*, due to cancer treatment, *pathological damages*, due to the effects of cancer, and *immobility damages*, which are a consequence of prolonged bed rest and immobilization.

In the following discussion we will examine the pathogenesis and the management of each condition. In Table 57.3 we summarize principles, indications, advantages and disadvantages of common rehabilitative techniques.

Iatrogenic Damages

Surgery, radiotherapy and chemotherapy may cause numerous and frequent disabling effects. The organ damages may be permanent or temporary, depending on the seriousness and the duration of the injury. Some iatrogenic complications, such as lymphedema from lymph node dissection, radiation neuropathy, or anthracycline induced cardiomyopathy may become evident months or years after the treatment has been discontinued.

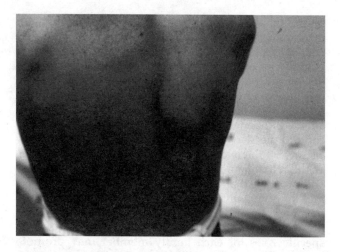

Figure 57.2 Winged scapula.

Surgery-Related Damages

Scar pathology

Adhesions and retractions are common after cervical, axillary or inguinal dissection. These complications may cause lymphatic stasis and lymphedema, paresthesias and weakness from nerve entrapment and may limit the range of motion of the limbs and neck.

The management of these conditions involves massage, lymphatic drainage, and vacuum therapy. Soft massage and vacuum therapy are useful to reduce the adhesion of the tissues, to prevent the formation of scar retraction, and to preserve the range of motion. Lymphatic drainage is important to minimize the lymph stasis around the scar which facilitates the scar formation.

Nerve injuries

The injury of a visceral nerve may lead to derangements in visceral function. In head and neck surgery, nerve injury may cause dysarthria, dysphagia and disturbances of mastication. In pelvic surgery, nerve injury may cause urinary and/or fecal incontinence and erectile dysfunction.

The surgical damage of a motor nerve causes paresis or palsy of a muscle or of a group of muscles. A typical example of this sort of complications is the winged scapula (Figure 57.2) due to injury of the thoracic long nerve, which may limit the abduction of the arm (5).

A frequent symptom of sensory nerve injury is neuropathic pain that presents the characteristics of deafferentation pain: shooting of electrical shock-like pain on a background of burning, constricting sensations. These symptoms are reported as dysesthesia and hyperesthesia and are accompanied by allodynia of significant degree on examination (6). Frequent clinical manifestations of nerve injury are postmastectomy, post-thoracotomy and stump pain. The treatment of motor disability involves physical therapy and facilitating techniques (Table 57.3), which exploit the neurogenic interactions of muscles within the same muscle

Table 57.2 Types of organ damage leading to disability in the older cancer patients.

A. Iatrogenic Damage
      Surgery-related
          Scar pathology
          Nerve injury
          Muscular injury
          Lymphedema
          Cutaneous stomas
          Amputations

      Radiotherapy-related
          Early complications
          Late Complications
             Contractures
             Pulmonary fibrosis
             Osteoporosis and fractures
             Myelitis
             Plexopathy and neuropathy
      Chemotherapy-related
          Central and peripheral neuropathies
          Extravasation of drugs

B. Pathological Damage
      Skeletal metastases
          Pain
          Pathologic fractures
      Central Nervous System Metastases
          Disturbances of Motility, Speech, Consciousness, Sensory, Sensations
          Vegetative Functions
      Peripheral Nervous System Metastases
          Muscular weakness
          Paresthesias
          Neuropathic pain
          Lymph node metastases
          Lymphedema

C. Immobility Damage
      Respiratory problems
      Deep vein thrombosis
      Pressure sores
      Muscle atrophy and contractures
      Bone loss.

district. For the success of these techniques it is important that some of the muscles of the district not be injured.

The treatment of neuropathic pain may benefit from transcutaneous electrical nerve stimulation (Table 57.3) (7,8), topical application of anesthetics or capsaicin (9,10), antidepressant and antiepileptic drugs and acupuncture (Figure 57.3). In older individuals, who are particularly sensitive to the side-effects of antidepressant medications, capsaicin may have a primary role. Capsaicin (Zostrix in USA), is the pungent principle of red pepper and similar plants and is supposed to in-

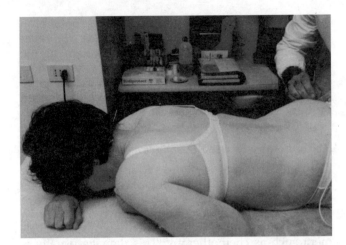

Figure 57.3 Acupuncture.

terrupt nociceptive transmission by depleting substance P from the ending of unmyelinated fiber. Capsaicin causes a burning sensation at the site of application, which may be prevented by lidocaine ointment, and is otherwise devoid of side-effects. In concentrations of 0.025% capsaicin may be applied 3–4 times daily for at least two months. Another advantage of capsaicin is low cost. In out patients we try capsaicin first, TENS and acupuncture thereafter, or a combination of these techniques prior to instituting treatment with amitriptyline, nortriptyline or carbamazepine.

Muscle injury

Muscle injury includes muscular retractions, a frequent finding during functional assessment for rehabilitative purposes. Muscle retractions are a result of soft tissue tumor surgery, and may be worsened by radiotherapy. Retractions may also be originated by a defense reflex (11) which makes the muscle shorter in response to the trauma of a surgical procedure; this outcome is a common complication of axillary dissection.

Physical therapy is the main form of prevention of muscle injury. Adjunctive therapy with ultrasound therapy or laser therapy (Figure 57.4) is indicated in the cases in which muscle retraction is likely or when the patient is unable or unwilling to cooperate with physical therapy. Adjuvant therapy with ultrasound or low level laser energy is particularly helpful in the case of older patients with preexisting cognitive or physical impairments that interfere with physical therapy. Adjunctive treatment may be continued until the maximal rehabilitative effects have been obtained. With the proper combinations of these techniques satisfactory results are obtained in the large majority of patients.

Lymphedema

Lymphedema is one of the most frequent issues in oncological rehabilitation. Commonly, lymphedema complicates radical lymph node dissection of important lymph nodal chains. Lymphedema is a common

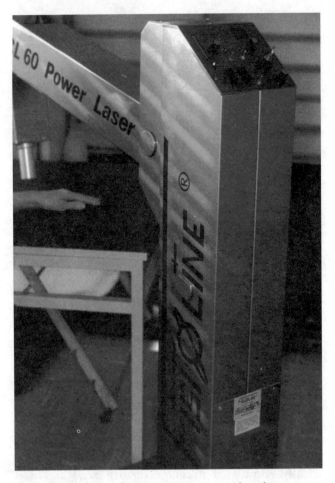

Figure 57.4 Laser therapy of cutaneous ulcer from extravasation of cancer chemotherapy.

complication of iliac or lumbar dissection. The occurrence of lymphedema is more unpredictable after axillary or femoral dissection. A number of external factors may increase the risk and worsen the severity of lymphedema. These include radiotherapy, infections (cellulitis and lymphangitis), venous obstruction, prolonged exposure to heat and excessive exercise of the limb, especially isometric exercise. These factors may aggravate preexisting problems of lymphatic drainage, by obliterating the remaining superficial lymphatic vessels of the skin and subcutaneous tissue.

Lymphedema may also signal recurrent disease (secondary lymphedema) and as such it pertains to pathological damages.

There is almost universal consensus that both iatrogenic and pathologic lymphedema may be controlled, but may not be completely reversed (12, 13, 14). Nevertheless, pressotherapy (Table 57.3), electrical drainage (Table 57.3) and compressive garments (elastic bandages or sleeves) effectively reduce the edema of the extremities. Recently, manual lymphodrainage has produced the best results in postsurgical edemas (15, 16, 17). Pharmacological therapy, including diuretics, vasoconstrictors and, occasionally, anticoagulants (18) has been effective in decreasing the sense of tension of

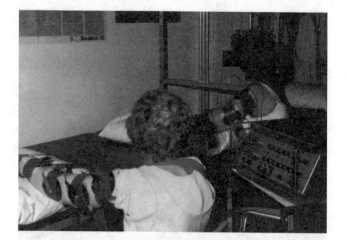

Figure 57.5 Electrically stimulated limb drainage.

the arm and in partially maintaining the result of compressive therapies.

The management of lymphedema varies with the seriousness and with the age of lymphedema. Manual lymphodrainage is the most effective treatment of lymphedema of recent onset and small volume. The first course of lymphodrainage consist of 15 sessions, the following courses are repeated every six months and consists of 10 sessions. Every session lasts approximately one hour and 15 minutes. Elastic bandages should be continuously worn. Pressotherapy and electrically stimulated drainage (Figure 57.5) are used mainly for inveterate lymphedema.

Cutaneous stomas

Cutaneous stomas are the end results of radical surgery involving larynx, bladder and rectum. Stomas affect both the physical and the emotional welfare of the patient. Often stomas may cause a chronic dependence of the patient on the care-giver and may result in strain within interpersonal relationships (19). For this reason, counseling should be seriously considered for all patients destined to wear a permanent colostomy and for their caregivers. A realistic outline of the function and of the possible complications of a stoma may defuse the anxiety related to the stoma. It may also be useful to allow the patient and his/her caregiver to express their feelings related to the new situation and to work out mutually satisfactory solutions. Detailed instructions on stoma management should be conveyed to patients and family members in order of avoiding common cutaneous complications, such as maceration and abrasion (20). Periodical bowel irrigation allows the bearers of a definitive colostomy for colorectal cancer to recover an intermittent intestinal function, to control fecal excretion and thus to maintain their quality of life (21, 22).

Limb amputations

Limb amputations may represent the end result of the management of melanomas or sarcomas of the

extremities. Limb amputation may have serious physical, social and emotional implications (3). The rehabilitative plan aims to rebuild the balance among the remaining muscle, to maintain strength, to promote circulation and to prepare the patient to use the prostheses (23). Pain and phantom sensations are managed by transelectrical cutaneous stimulation and medications (6).

Radiotherapy-Related Damages

The functional complications of radiotherapy may be divided into early and late complications (24). Acute radiation-induced injuries are related to the damage of surface epithelial cells and may delay the completion of treatment and the institution of other forms of treatment such as chemotherapy. This damage usually is reversed in a few weeks.

Early complications include: erythema, moist desquamation, ulceration. The treatment is based on topical application of substances that promote healing and prevent further lesions (25).

Late radiotherapy complications have more serious rehabilitative implications. Late complications occur months or years after completion of treatment and are due to a progressive compromise of the small blood vessels (endarteritis obliterans with chronic alteration of connective and nervous tissues). The most frequent conditions include: joint or muscle contractures, subcutaneous fibrosis, pulmonary fibrosis, spontaneous bone fractures, myelitis and brachial/lumbar plexopathies.

The seriousness of the clinical picture depends on the site of irradiation, on the dosage and on the time since completion of treatment (26). The management of late complications includes segmental physiotherapy for muscular lesions, pulmonary physiotherapy for lung lesions, and support devices able to stabilize fractures and to sustain paralyzed limbs. Neuropathic pain is a common sequela of peripheral nerve damage and is managed with transelectrical cutaneous stimulation, local application of anesthetics or capsaicin and antidepressants.

Outcomes from Chemotherapy

Chemotherapy is associated with numerous side effects: nausea and vomiting, hair loss, visceral dysfunctions, peripheral neuropathies and local tissue damage following drug extravasation. Of these complications, peripheral neuropathies and contractures from drug extravasation are susceptible to rehabilitative intervention.

Peripheral neuropathies are common consequences of treatment with cisplatin, vinca alkaloids, podophyllotoxins, and taxanes (27, 28). Impairment of sensations (paresthesias and numbness, sensory ataxia) may make the patient susceptible to skin injuries and Charcot's joints, while neuropathic pain and loss of tendons reflexes may hinder the patient's motility. Even if chemotherapy is discontinued as soon as the first neurophatic signs and symptoms become apparent, the neurophaty may continue to develop and spontaneous regression

Table 57.3 Common techniques of oncological rehabilitation.

Acupuncture (Figure 57.3): Mechanism of action unknown. **Indications:** Most forms of pain and fatigue. Advantages: Low cost, low time involved (1–2 weekly sessions of half hour each, for 2–3 months), low technology, does not require patient active participation. **Disadvantages:** Unpredictable effectiveness; needs specifically trained personnel.

Electrically stimulated lymphatic drainage (Figure 57.5): The lymphatic flow is stimulated by electric impulses starting from the most proximal portion of the limbs. **Indications:** lymphedema, both from obliteration of regional lymph nodes and from tumor recurrences. **Advantages:** can be used for tumor recurrences, does not require patients active participation, safe, inexpensive. **Disadvantages:** Time consuming (three yearly treatment, each involving 10 daily sessions lasting 60 minutes each); limited effectiveness

Edemacenthesis (Figure 57.6): Multiple punctures of the hardest part of the edematous limb with 25 gauge needles. After many punctures the limb is gently massaged to promote the outflow of third space fluid. Heparin (5000U) and normosaline (10 ml) are added to the dressing to prevent early coagulation of the drainage. Thorough disinfection of the limb before and after the procedure are mandatory. **Indications:** refractory edema. **Advantages:** effective, inexpensive. **Disadvantages:** Painful; high risk of infections. Should be reserved for few selected cases.

Facilitating techniques: Methods of muscular rehabilitation based on stimulation of peripheral receptors, both extero and proprioreceptors. As an example, the Kabat facilitating technique (7) is based on scheme of movement involving groups of muscles functionally connected. Exercises are performed along spiral and diagonal axes, starting from the greatest muscle elongation. Exercises against resistance exploit the phenomenon of "irradiation", i.e. the possibility of spreading the voluntary efforts of healthy muscles to weaker muscles belonging to the same muscular scheme. **Indications:** muscle weakness from peripheral or central nervous injury. **Advantages:** Low technology, low cost. **Disadvantages:** time consuming, require patient active participation, require normal joints, intact proprioception and intact posterior columns.

Lasertherapy (low level) (Figure 57.4): The mechanism of action involves increased intracellular concentration of ATP and stimulation of prostaglandin synthesis. **Indications:** Management of pain, fibrosis, soft tissue, ulcers from drug extravasation, wounds. **Advantages:** High effectiveness, safety, does not require patient active participation. **Disadvantages:** Time consuming, expensive, requires high technology and trained personnel.

Pressotherapy: Has been considered for many years the standard treatment of lymphedema. The mechanism of action consists in 'pressing" the third space fluid into the lymphatic and venous capillaries. A special form of pressotherapy, recently introduced, is the intermittent gradient therapy, which facilitates the proximal drainage of the lymphedema fluid. **Indications:** lymphedema of the extremities, from obliteration of regional lymph nodes due to surgery or irradiation. Not indicated for tumor recurrence. **Advantages:** effective and safe; may be used for home therapy. **Disadvantages:** costly, especially the intermittent gradient form; may require some degree of patient participation in case of home care.

Transcutaneous electrical nerve stimulation (TENS): This technique is based on the "Gate theory" of pain holding that counterstimulation of the nervous system may decrease the perception of pain. It requires a stimulator connected with electrodes applied to the skin. **Indications:** Most forms of localized pain, especially neuropathic pain manifested as hyperesthesia, dysesthesia and allodynia. **Advantages:** low cost, easy management, even for older patients. **Disadvantages:** Low effectiveness in severe pain.

Ultrasound therapy: Mechanism of action includes increased blood flow, increased extensibility of collagen, thermal effect, mast cell degranulation, increased intracellular Ca^{++} levels, increased fibroblast protein synthesis, increased vascular permeability, increases angiogenesis, and increased tensile strength of collagen. **Indications:** muscle retractions, joint contractures, delay healing of wounds and ulcers. **Advantages:** low cost, safety, does not require specialized training or active patient participation. **Disadvantage:** Time consuming; unpredictable results.

is slow and incomplete; similarly to other neurologic disorders, a rehabilitative management with electrical stimulation and physiotherapy is necessary in order to reduce consequences of peripheral nerve involvement.

Inadvertent extravasation of antitumor agents during intravenous administration is a potential complication of cancer chemotherapy; it can cause local tissue reactions ranging from minor erythema, acute pain and swelling in the area of vesicant infiltration, to severe necrosis (29, 30).

The list of vesicant drugs includes anthracyclines, alkylating agents, and plant alkaloids. The appropriate management of these iatrogenic accidents, including their prevention, as a part of supportive care in the elderly has been addressed by several experimental and clinical studies; they demonstrate the usefulness of a combined management: medical, surgical and rehabilitative, in the appropriate care of extravasation (30, 31). Topical dimethyl sulfoxide (DMSO) showed great effectiveness in preventing cutaneous ulcers while laser therapy may facilitate ulcer healing (32).

Pathological Damages

More demanding for the rehabilitation team is the management of elderly patients affected from disabling outcomes of cancer progression. Needless to say, in elderly cancer patients, the progression of disease can further deteriorate pre-existent pathological situations such as incontinence, restricted mobility, impaired cognition and communication. A multidisciplinary approach associating antineoplastic treatment with emotional support and appropriate therapy of specific dysfunctions is the clue to successful rehabilitation of elderly patients with advanced cancer.

Common problems include:

Bone metastases

Bone metastases are frequent and cause considerable suffering and disability. Skeletal involvement results from many types of tumors: breast, lung, kidney, prostate etc. It may also represent the site of primary bone lesion. Vertebral metastases may lead to vertebral collapse and spinal cord compression.

Long bones bearing lytic metastatic lesions are subjected to spontaneous fractures. In the elderly, the risk of vertebral collapse or weight-bearing long bone fracture is increased from coexistent osteoporosis.

Pain is almost universal in bone metastases and may further limit a patient's motility. Painful bony metastases likely enhance the dependence of elderly patients on the assistance of family members. The rehabilitative approach must be coordinated with other forms of treatment, such as surgery, radiotherapy, and chemotherapy. The initial rehabilitative step is aimed to reduce the risk of vertebral collapse and of bone fractures with orthotic devices which tend to reduce the load on the affected bone and permit a partial recovery of mobility (3). The pharmacological management of pain in the elderly must avoid dangerous complications of analgesic drugs such as non steroid anti-inflammatory drugs, corticosteroids and antidepressants. Bisphosphonates, however, seem to be well tolerated by the aged, but produce effective pain control in only 20–25% of cases (33). Bisphosphonates (sodium etidronate, clodronate, pamidronate) inhibit osteoclastic bone reabsorption and decrease both neoplastic and age-related bone loss. They seem to prevent fractures and to ameliorate bone pain, but clinical studies of these drugs are still ongoing. Persisting clinical problems include difference in activity between fist generation bisphosphonates and newer drugs (alendronate, tiludronate, risedronate), optimal duration of treatment; optimal dosage; long term risks and benefits. In general, corticosteroid and nonsteroidals are the first line management of bone pain from metastases, but in older patients the complications of these drugs may be substantial and bisphosphonates may be safer and more effectively used as front line treatment. The following case illustrates the effects of bisphosphonates in older persons with bone metastases:

An 85 year old woman with metastatic breast cancer to the bone since 1989 was seen by us in 1993. Her tumor had progressed with tamoxifen, aminogluthetimide, progestins and estrogen at high doses. She had pain in her left femur and a radiograph showed a 3 cm lytic lesion that was surgically stabilized with an intramedullary rod. She received several 6 week courses of navelbine IV at 20 mg/m2, but myelotoxicity caused delay of treatment in three occasions. Her Ca 15-3 increased in the meantime from 80ng/dl to 154 ng/dl, and her bone pain progressed. She refused further chemotherapy and we initiated treatment with pamidronate (Aredia) 60 mg IV over three hours every three weeks, and oral calcium. The patient experienced immediate relief of pain that has been maintained for four months.

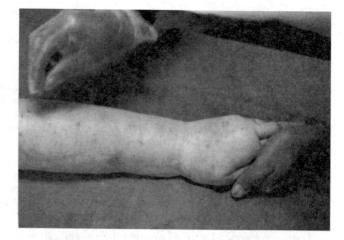

Figure 57.6 Edemacentesis.

Central and peripheral nervous system recurrences

The disabling effects of tumors on the nervous system vary in intensity from minimal to severe. The location and the extent of the lesion determine the functional effects.

Neoplastic involvement of the central nervous system may cause abnormality in the cognitive (language, cognition, memory and personality), the motorial and the sensory functions. Patients with lesions of the central nervous system are often dependent on caregivers (34, 35, 36).

The involvement of cranial nerves, as seen in recurrences of the head and neck cancer, and in neoplastic meningitis, may affect important visceral functions such as swallowing, respiration and speech (37, 38).

The rehabilitation program involves physiotherapy and is aimed at minimizing the patient's disability and allowing the patient to recover some degree of autonomy. One mainstay of recovery is maintenance of strength and function of non-paralyzed muscles. The patient is taught to use orthotic devices and to become self-supporting as much as possible. To assure the comfort of the patient at home in a familiar environment, it is important to enlist the cooperation of family members and to instruct all potential caregivers in the family in the use of orthotic devices.

Skin and lymphonodal recurrences

Skin and lymphonode recurrences generate similar clinical pictures. The most frequent symptoms are: pain which presents often the characteristics of deafferentation pain, decreased range of motion of certain muscular groups, and secondary lymphedema. This sort of lymphedema differs from that following surgery. Secondary lymphedema generally presents a rapid onset, with dramatic enlargement of the limb volume and hardening of soft tissues. There is often a widespread redness of the limb which presents some telangiectasias at its root due to venous compression. The treatment of secondary lymphedema is palliative and quite different from that of surgical lymphedema. Treatment involves edemacentesis (Figure 57.6; Table 57.3), low compression pressotherapy, electrical lymphatic drainage, pharmacological therapy with steroids, diuretics and anticoagulants, and active and passive limb mobilization. Generally, high compression pressotherapy and lymphodrainage have been considered contraindicated in secondary lymphedema due to the possibility of dislodgement and distant spreading of tumor cells. It should be underlined however, that this risk is more theoretical than real. Also, dealing with recurrent and generally widely metastatic cancer, further spreading may have only a limited impact on survival or quality of life. Though effective, edemacentesis should be limited to the most refractory and most discomforting forms of lymphedema. This technique is painful and may cause serious infections.

The most effective rehabilitation of secondary lymphedema is the effective antineoplastic treatment. Palliative measures, when successful, may improve the quality of life of patients with metastatic cancer.

Consequences of Immobility

Elderly patients with cancer often require prolonged bed rest. This may ensue prolonged and difficult surgical procedures, debilitation from cancer and from antineoplastic treatment. Aging processes, concomitant illnesses and functional restrictions are risk factors which cause common complications of immobility more frequently in older than in younger adults. Metabolic and physiological changes associated with bed rest may compromise the patient's medical and functional recovery (3).

The most important consequences of immobility are (39):

Respiratory problems

Respiratory complications are likely to develop after general anesthesia. The patient may present difficulties in breathing and coughing from retained secretions, reduced thoracic expansion and fear of pain. In elderly people, physiotherapy is performed both before and soon after surgery to prevent further complications such as atelectasis, postoperative pneumonia and aspiration pneumonia. Deep breathing exercises should be taught preoperatively to obtain the patient's utmost collaboration immediately after recovery from the anesthesia. After the operation the physiotherapist should teach the patient to cough effectively and with as little pain as possible in order to facilitate the removal of secretions.

Deep vein thrombosis

Advanced age and malignancies are both risk factors for deep vein thrombosis, which occurs more frequently in the lower extremities. Often pain and edema signal the presence of deep vein thrombosis, but a silent presentation of this complication is not uncommon.

Compression devices and physical therapy may prevent deep vein thrombosis in older patients bedridden for prolonged periods of time. Active exercises of the lower extremities and deep breathing exercises should be practiced several times daily both during the preoperative and the postoperative periods. Patients at high risk of deep vein thrombosis should also be treated with anticoagulants. If a deep vein thrombosis does develop, active exercises can usually be continued while the patient is receiving anticoagulant therapy. Elastic bandages may control swelling and aid venous return.

Pressure sores

Pressure sores can be superficial or deep. Superficial sores involve the skin and present a shallow, painful ulcer. Deep pressure sores involve the subcutaneous tissues. Malnutrition is a major risk factor both for pressure sores and for delayed wound healing.

The most common sites of pressure ulcers are the heels, malleoli, great trochanter, sacrum and elbows where the continued pressure induces the occlusion of blood vessels and deprives the tissues of nutrition. Other causes of pressure ulcers: ill fitting splints, friction from rough sheets, persistent soaking of the skin with urine, secondary to incontinence.

Prevention of pressure sores involves changing position every two hours. Sheepskins are often used under paralyzed or heavy patients to prevent friction. Air and water beds are very expensive devices, but are very effective in reducing the risk of pressure sores. They may be indicated for patients subjected to prolonged immobilization. Treatment of pressure ulcers involves debridement of the necrotic tissue, accurate cleansing, application of cicatrizing ointments and laser therapy.

Muscle atrophy

Prolonged bed rest leads to atrophy and hypotonia of muscles and the most remarkable effect of this is alteration in posture and difficulty in walking.

Muscle atrophy may be avoided with active movement either in the form of active exercises or as static (isometric) work.

Contractures

These complications are of special concern to the elderly as they cause serious limitation of range of motion and pain. They are caused by shortening of muscles, tendons and ligaments due to a prolonged bed rest resulting in a loss of joint motion. To prevent the contractures the patient should have stretching exercises once or twice daily. Other preventative modalities include ultrasound and laser therapy.

Bone loss

Osteoporosis from immobility is more common in older than in younger patients. Pathologic fractures may complicate osteoporosis. Frequent mobilization and oral biphosphonates are the mainstay treatment of this complication.

The most common cancer related lesions seen at our institutions in patients over 65 are summarized in Table 57.4.

Table 57.4 Iatrogenic lesions in 150 patients over 65 seen at our institution during 1994. Sum > 100% because several patients presented more than one lesion.

Muscle retractions:	55%
Nerve injuries:	40%
Pain:	35%
Abdominal stomas:	25%
Lymphedema:	18%
Scar pathology:	4%
Drug extravasation:	2%
Tissue fibrosis:	2%

Rehabilitative Assessment

A large body of literature deals with functional and quality of life assessment in disabled cancer patients. The various methods of assessment may differ in methodology according to pathology and patient characteristics. Irrespective of the method of assessment, maintenance of the patient's autonomy and preservation of meaningful social relationships are major rehabilitative goals for the elderly (40). Thus, it is important to define impairment, disability and handicap as a framework of reference to assess older individuals with cancer who present potentially disabling conditions (41).

1. Impairment: loss or abnormality of physiological or anatomical structure or function (e.g. restricted gait).
2. Disability: restriction or lack of ability to perform an activity (e.g. inability to write due to loss of hand movements or to dyslexia).
3. Handicap: disadvantage suffered by individuals as a result of ill-health due to inability to fulfil a role which is normal for someone of that age, sex and culture.

The concept of quality of life in rehabilitation is connected with the impairment of function, overall autonomy and social relationships. The definition of quality of life lacks full consensus and unambiguous methods of evaluation (42, 43, 44, 45). Nevertheless, there seems to be general agreement on some of the components of quality of life in persons with disease (health-related quality of life). These include: physical function, emotional or psychological function, social function and symptoms related to the disease or to its treatment.

The rehabilitative assessment of elderly cancer patients is a dynamic process which begins at diagnosis and continues throughout the course of the illness. Although the methods of assessment may vary with the condition of the patient and the course of the disease, the focus of the assessment is always the same: to measure the impact of an anatomical or functional impairment on the patient's overall well-being.

In the evaluation of elderly cancer patients we make a distinction between patients with metastatic cancer and those without metastases. This distinction stems from our experience. In general, full functional recovery may be obtained in the absence of metastases. In patients with metastatic cancer the chances of full functional recovery are poorer and the main goals of rehabilitation are to ameliorate functional impairment and to delay the development of new dysfunctions and disabilities.

We subscribe to the classification of rehabilitative outcome of elderly cancer patients proposed by Rustmeyer (46). This author envisioned three different situations:

1. Patients with favorable prognosis for whom we can predict a full recovery of the damage or an incomplete recovery, which is still adequate to preserve previous autonomy and social relationship (Complete recovery).
2. Patients who are still able to maintain some degree of autonomy and some meaningful social life, but at a poorer level than that preexisting the disabling event (Incomplete recovery).
3. Patients affected by serious and irreversible motor or functional impairments for whom treatment aims to prevent a further deterioration and to relieve the symptoms related to the disease (Palliative treatment).

The different stage of disease and the different functional impairment lead us to assume a distinct approach in assessing the quality of life of nonmetastatic and metastatic patients. In this assumption we agree with authors who sustain that quality of life can only be defined by the patients themselves in their current situation.

Young and Longmann (47) define quality of life as the degree of satisfaction with present life circumstances. For Gerson, quality of life is measured by the degree to which an individual succeeds in accomplishing his/her desires, despite the constraints imposed upon him/her by a hostile or indifferent nature, God or social order (48). Lewis emphasizes the psychological impact of disease on quality of life and measures quality of life from self-esteem, the presence of a purpose in life and the degree of anxiety (49).

Clearly, irrespective of the definition, cancer and cancer treatment have a substantial impact on the quality of life of each person (50).

Non Metastatic Patient Assessment

The rehabilitative assessment is performed about one month after hospital discharge or treatment completion, when the patient is aware of the treatment outcome and of the implications related to autonomy and social relationship. The first step is the assessment of voluntary motility of the muscle districts involved by surgery or radiotherapy. The oncological treatment can impair one or more of the following voluntary functions: swallowing, moving and speaking capabilities, urinary and fecal continence, motorial function of the face, of the spine and of the upper and lower extremities. The second and third steps evaluate how far the impairment of segmental voluntary motility affects overall autonomy (in feeding, in dressing, in providing for personal hygiene and in standing up/lying down), and social relationships (working occupation, leisure activities and use of means of transport).

Metastatic Patient Assessment

The rehabilitation team, when facing the elderly metastatic patients goes beyond the traditional concepts of physiatric evaluation and focuses on the influence of the progression of disease and of the treatment on quality of life. This includes physical, psychological and social dimensions, in addition to the symptoms related to cancer and cancer treatment.

An essential part of the examination involves activities of daily living (ADL), that pertain to functional autonomy, instrumental activities of daily living (IADL), that pertain to personal autonomy, and advanced activities of daily living (AADL) that pertain to enjoyment of one's life. It is extremely important to realize that some AADLs may be maintained and preserved even when ADLs and IADLs are lost. For example, we saw a mildly demented 72 year old man with metastatic transitional cell carcinoma of the bladder who needed assistance in grooming and feeding and was unable to manage his own affairs, but still enjoyed his morning golf game. Cytotoxic chemotherapy produced marked relief of bone pain from bone metastases and allowed him to play golf for six additional months after diagnosis of his disease.

The most frequent and disabling symptoms of metastatic cancer include: pain, asthenia, sleeping abnormalities, with reversal of daytime sleeping pattern, depression or anxiety. It is important to weigh the capacity of the family to support the needs of the patient in the home environment.

Conclusion

The rehabilitation of elderly cancer patients is a multidisciplinary endeavor which may involve strict coordination with the work of other treatment teams. In particular, control of disabling problems, such as pain and malnutrition, is the first step toward successful rehabilitation.

The support and the cooperation of the patient's family is essential to provide effective home care both in functional and dysfunctional families. The recognition of a primary care giver within the family, is critical to the success of the rehabilitative effort. Family education should be incorporated in all rehabilitative plans involving patients who may spend a substantial amount of time at home.

The focus of all rehabilitative efforts is improvement and preservation of the quality of life of the older cancer patient. This goal may be reached with different modalities in different sets. For patients with a substantial chance of cure or prolonged disease control, it is reasonable to attempt to restore the function preexisting the diagnosis of cancer. For patients with advanced and incurable malignancies the main objective is control of the discomfort from symptoms of cancer.

Age itself does not impair rehabilitative efforts. The treatment plans of older patients should be continuously reviewed in the light of the progression of cancer and of other coexisting conditions.

The rehabilitation of the older patient with cancer is an open area of continuous research to improve the present outcome.

Rehabilitation is probably the youngest field of oncology, borne from the continuous improvement of cancer treatment and the increasingly prolonged survival of cancer patients. The research in this field is still in the initial phases.

We would like to propose the following priority in research related to oncological rehabilitation of the older patient:

1. Uniform evaluation, definition, and quantification of rehabilitative outcome;
2. Correlation between rehabilitation and quality of life;
3. Social rehabilitation; and
4. Continuous exploration of new rehabilitative techniques, such as laser therapy, which appear very effective and require minimal active participation from the patient.

References

1. Fentiman IS, Tirelli U, Monfardini S, Scheneider M, Festen J, Cognetti F, Aapro MS. Cancer in the elderly: why so badly treated? *The Lancet* April 1990; **28**: 1020–1022.
2. Balducci L, Ades T, Carbone P, Friedman M, Fulmer T, Galakotos A, Yancik R. Issues in treatment. *Cancer* 1991; **68**: 2527–2529.
3. Gerber L, Levinson S, Hicks JE, Gallelli P, Whitehurst J, Scheib D, Sonies BC. Evaluation and management of disability: rehabilitation aspects of cancer. In *Cancer: Principles and Practice of Oncology (fourth edition)*, edited by VT DeVita, S Hellman, SA Rosemberg. Philadelphia: JB Lippincott, pp. 2538–2569, 1993.
4. Raven RW. *Rehabilitation and continuing care in cancer*. UICC, The Parthenon Publishing Group Limited. Carnforth, England: 1986.
5. Tish Knobf MK. Primary breast cancer: physical consequences and rehabilitation. *Sem Oncol Nurs* 1985; **1**: 214–224.
6. Foley KM. Pain assessment and cancer pain syndromes. In *Oxford Textbook of palliative medicine*, edited by D Doyle, GW Hanks, N MacDonald. Oxford: Oxford University Press, pp. 148–165, 1993.
7. Mannheimer JS, Lampe GN. *Clinical transcutaneous electrical nerve stimulation*, edited by FA Davis. Philadelphia, 1984.
8. Thompson JW, stimulation (TENS) Filshie J. Transcutaneous electrical nerve and acupuncture In *Oxford Textbook of palliative medicine*, edited by D Doyle, GW Hanks, N MacDonald. Oxford: Oxford University Press, pp. 229–244, 1993.
9. Dini D, Bertelli G, Gozza A, *et al*. Treatment of the post mastectomy pain syndrome with topical capsaicin. *Pain* 1993; **54**: 223–226.
10. Watson CP, Evans R. The post mastectomy pain syndrome and topical capsaicin: a randomized trial. *Pain* 1992; **51**: 375–379.
11. Sherrington CS. *The integrative action of the nervous system*, Second Edition. New York: Charles Scribner's Sons, 1906. New Haven: Yale University Press, 1947.

12. Foldi E, Foldi M, Clodius L. The lymphedema caos: a lancet. *Ann Plast Surg* 1988; **22**: 505–515.

13. Bertelli G, Venturini M, Forno G, *et al.* Conservative treatment of postmastectomy lymphedema: a controlled, randomized trial. *Ann Oncol* 1991; **2**: 575–578.

14. Gillham L. Lymphoedema and Physiotherapists: control not cure. *Physiotherapy* 1994; **80** (12): 835–843.

15. Zanolla R, Monzeglio C, Balzarini A, Martino G. Evaluation of the results of three different methods of postmastectomy lymphedema treatment. *J Surg Oncol* 1984; **26**: 210–213.

16. Swedborg I. Effects of treatment with an elastic sleeve and intermittent pneumatic compression in postmastectomy patients with lymphoedema of the arm. *Scand J of Rehab Med* 1984: **16**: 35–41.

17. Mirolo BR, Bunce IH, Chapman M, Olsen T, Eliadis P, Hennessy JM, Ward RD, Jones LC. Psychosocial benefits of postmastectomy lymphedema therapy. *Cancer* 1995 **18** (3): 197–205.

18. Casley-Smith JR, Morgan RG, Piller NB. Treatment of lymphedema of the arms and legs with 5,6-Benzo-alfa-Pyrone. *N Engl J Med* 1993; **329**: 1158–1163.

19. Costello AM. Supporting the patient with problems relating to body image. In *Proceedings of the National Conference on Cancer Nursing.* Chicago: American Cancer Society, 36–40, 1974.

20. Kunrtzman SH, Gardner B, Kellner WS. Rehabilitation of the Cancer Patient. *Am J Sura* 1988; **155**: 791–803.

21. Venturini M, Bertelli G, Forno G, Grandi G, Dini D. "Colostomy irrigation in the elderly." *Diseases of the colon-rectum* 1990; **33**(12): 1031–1033.

22. Dini D, Venturini M, Forno G, Bertelli G, Grandi G. Irrigation for colostomized patients: a rational approach. *International Journal of Colorectal Disease* 1991; **6**: 9–11.

23. Davis BC. Amputations. In *Cash's Textbook of Physiotherapy in Some Surgical conditions,* edited by PA Downie. London: Faber and Faber, pp. 133–160, 1979.

24. Bentzen SM, Overgaard M. Early and late normal tissue injury after postmastectomy radiotherapy. In *Recent Results in Cancer Research,* vol. 130.Berlin-Heidelberg: Springer-Verlag, 1993.

25. Dini D, Macchia R, Gozza A, Bertelli G, Forno G, Guenzi M, Bacigalupo A, Scolaro T, Vitale V. Management of acute radiodermatitis. *Canc Nurs* 1993; **16**(5): 366–370.

26. Dutreix J. Human skin: early and late reactions in relation to dose and its time distribution. *Br J Radiol* 1986; **59**(19): 23.

27. Kaplan RS, Wiernik PH. Neurotoxicity of antineoplastic drugs. *Semin Oncol* 1982, **9**: 103.

28. Hildebrand J. *Neurological adverse reactions to anticancer drugs.* European School of Oncology Monographs. Berlin: Springer Verlag, 1991.

29. Gallina EJ. Practical guide to chemotherapy administration for physicians and oncology nurses. In *Cancer: Principles and Practice of Oncology (fourth edition),* edited by VT DeVita, S Hellman, SA Rosemberg. Philadelphia: JB Lippincott, pp. 2570–2580, 1993.

30. Dorr RT. Antidotes to vesicant chemotherapy exstravasations. *Blood Rev* 1990; **4**: 41–60.

31. Bertelli G, Gozza A, Forno GB, Vidili MG, Silvestro S, Venturini M, Del Mastro L, Garrone O, Rosso R, Dini D. Topical dimethylsulfoxide (DMSO) for the prevention of soft tissue injury after extravasation of vesicant cytotoxic drugs: a prospective clinical study. *J Clin Oncol* 1995, in press.

32. Kitcher SS, Partridge CJ. A review of low level laser therapy. *Physiotherapy* 1991; **77**: 161–168.

33. Portenoy RK. Adjuvant analgesics in pain management. In *Oxford Textbook of palliative medicine,* edited by D Doyle, GW Hanks, N MacDonald. Oxford: Oxford University Press, 1993.

34. Zochodne DW, Cairncross JG. Metastasis to the central nervous system. *Cancer Growth Prog* 989; **8**: 32.

35. Black PM. Brain Tumors (I) *N Engl J Med* 1991; **324**: 1471–1476.

36. Black PM. Brain Tumors (II) *N Engl J Med* 1991; **324**: 1555–1564.

37. Dudgeon B, DeLisa L, Miller R. Head and neck cancer: a rehabilitative approach. *Am J Occup Ther* 1980; **34**: 243.

38. Mathog RH. Rehabilitation of head and neck cancer patients: consensus on recommendations from the International Conference on rehabilitation of the head and neck cancer patient. *Head Neck* 1991; Jan/Feb: 1–2.

39. Thompson KM. Complications following surgery. In *Cash's textbook of physiotherapy in some surgical conditions,* edited by PA Downie. London: Faber & Faber, 1979.

40. Simpson JM, Forster A. Assessing elderly people. Should we all use the same scales? *Physiotherapy* 1993; **79**(12): 836–842.

41. Ebrahim S. Measurement of impairment, disability and handicap. In *Measuring outcomes of medical care,* edited by A Hopkins and D Costain. Royal College of Physicians of London, 1990.

42. Forer S, Granger C, *et al. Functional Independence measure.* Buffalo, NY: The Buffalo General Hospital, State University of New York at Buffalo, 1987.

43. Donovan K, Sanson-Fisher RW, Redman S. Measuring quality of life in cancer patients. *J Clin Onc* 1989; **7**(7): 959–968.

44. Cella DF, Tulsky DS, Gray G, Sarafian B, *et al.* The functional assessment of cancer therapy scale: development and validation of the general measure. *J Clin Oncol* 1993; **11**(3): 570–579.

45. Linacre JM, Heinemann AW, Wright BD, Granger CV, Hamilton BB. The structure and stability of the functional independence measure. *Arch Phys Med Rehabil* 1994; **75**: 127–132.

46. Rustmeyer J. *Rehabilitation. Physical and clinical aspects.* In *Geriatrics,* edited by D Platt. Berlin: Springer-Verlag, 1993.

47. Young K, Longmann A. Quality of life and persons with melanoma: a pilot study. *Cancer Nurs* 1983; **6**: 219–225.

48. Gerson E. On the quality of life. *Am Soc Rev* 1976; **41**: 793–806.

49. Lewis F. experienced personal control and quality of life in late-stage cancer patients. *Nurs Res* 1982; **31**: 113–119.

50. Glaus A. Quality of life. A measure of the quality of nursing care. *Support Care Cancer* 1993; **1**: 119–123.

58. Assessing Needs and Providing Comfort to Geriatric Cancer Patients and Their Families

Stephanie B. Hoffman and Joan A. Balmes

Introduction

Comforting and communicating clearly and empathically with the cancer patient and family is a difficult undertaking. Moreover, interacting with the family of the geriatric cancer patient has special challenges. These challenges will be discussed below, along with a variety of communication techniques to build trust, compliance, and empathic interaction.

Geriatric patients may experience less psychosocial difficulties with their illness than younger cancer patients. This may in part be due to fewer obligations and responsibilities at that point in their lives. Also, elders sometimes make light of problems encountered as they grow older, while younger adults frequently emphasize the crises intruding upon their already stressful lives (1). Interactions with families of geriatric patients may sometimes be easier than dealings with the families of younger patients. The family of the older adult has probably coped with a number of health and role changes over the years, inoculating them to the rigors of the health care system and the increasing needs of their loved one. There are expectations that an older adult must indeed die of some disease, and cancer may be a less stressful diagnosis than that of a dementing illness. Caregiving responsibilities for cancer, though burdensome, are probably less than those of a dementia, which can last up to 20 years (2).

Too, the tragedy of a diagnosis of cancer is less traumatic in an older adult, who has lived a full life (3). And the slow progression of some geriatric cancers gives the patient and family time to adapt and to perhaps choose less invasive treatments. Older patients also are often very accepting of their time to die (4). They may in fact prefer death to limitations in functioning or fear of becoming a burden. Their refusal of aggressive interventions, however, can be troubling to younger generations, who may value them as the patriarch or matriarch of the family and not be able to handle their impending death so easily.

Impact of Cancer Stage on the Family

Cancer is a "disorder of change" (5). The progression of the disease causes the family system to go through a series of adaptive stages: acute, chronic, and resolution. In the acute stage, the initial disclosure of the illness is made, and the family must deal with the patient's pain and incapacitation. A support system to nurture the patient's emotional and physical needs is formed. The support system must include all members of the health profession, family, and friends. An older adult may have an attenuated support system, however, because of distance of family members, a past history of alienation, frailty of the spouse, death of friends, and discomfort with self-disclosure. Elderly patients going through crises can also become cognitively overwhelmed, resulting in a delirium. This can further scare and upset family members. The burden of support may rest on adult children if the patient is widowed or the spouse is sick or unable to provide physical care. The adult child may also feel uncomfortable with the necessity for role reversal, and the consequent role changes may impose stress on family functioning.

Those who should be providing support to the patient may need as much emotional support themselves. Spouses may feel alone and threatened in the situation, as more attention is usually given to the patient himself (6), even though both patient and caregiver usually devote the same amount of time to the treatment regimen. The caregiver frequently worries more about the prognosis of the patient than the patient does himself. This may be attributed to the fact that the caregiver is unable to understand how the patient is feeling physically, as the patient may try to conceal true feelings to shield his or her loved one from additional pain and worry. Patients may also be able to focus more on the day-to-day treatment regimens which consume so much of their time, while family members become distracted, looking more toward future complications (7).

As daily stress increases, the health of the primary caregiver is also a cause for concern. The caregiver must cope with the responsibilities of getting enough sleep and staying in good health in order to manage and provide the care the patient is relying upon her to provide. This can continue for extended periods of time as the disease slowly takes its toll (6). Regular medical check-ups for the caregiver are advisable during this difficult and often lengthy time period (7).

Spouses of cancer patients often suffer dispersed aches and physical exertion when the patient is discharged from hospital stays (8). A discharge may be riddled with mixed feelings of joy at having the loved person close again, along with feelings of skepticism over how well the present status will be managed within the home and whether his stay at home will last for a significant duration or soon result in an emergency visit to the doctor or hospital. Patients are frequently released on the basis of their desire to return home to their families, rather than solely on the basis of physical readiness. Although this keeps the choice of the patient paramount, it can contribute to much stress and guilt for the caregiver. Torn with fears and doubts, it may even result in confrontations between the physician and caregiver, in which the caregiver feels he must justify his concerns.

Family members and the patient himself pass through significant crises and emotional changes which have a marked impact on adjustment and acceptance for all that is to come. During these periods, the family may search for the meaning of this intrusion into their lives and how it can be managed now and in the future. This process of self-searching is accompanied by grief as the patient as well as family members acknowledge the emotional pain that they are presently feeling and the pain that may still lie ahead of them. Gone is the notion of being able to conquer all obstacles — the sense of immortality (9).

The chronic stage is a process of turmoil. The patient might return to the hospital periodically for treatment and may go through a period of remission. There is a sense of crisis orientation; families feel like they must always be in a state of emergency readiness. During times of patient decompensation, health professionals focus on patient survival, ignoring the information and participation needs of families (10). In some circumstances friends may even distance themselves socially from the patient in an effort to shield themselves from more pain later. This "anticipatory grief" is a coping mechanism of emotional detachment. When the patient is in remission and appears to no longer need treatment, emotional reattachments may occur (7).

A sense of helplessness pervades the family. As family members search for meaning and identity in their changing roles and lifestyles, there is an increase of stress for all involved. But finding a purpose to the crisis in their lives is essential for adaptation. In order to function adequately as a family unit, the family must develop a balance of facing new psychosocial challenges and conflicting demands on their time, while continuing to meet their already established obligations and routines. If a harmonious equilibrium is not achieved, the family will not be able to carry on (9). The demands of daily living can not succumb to the increasing impositions of a cancer diagnosis.

In the resolution stage, the patient is terminal. The family tries to come to terms with the impending loss. Family members can be in conflict, as some believe that all efforts should be made to save the patient, while others are in favor of only comfort care. Family members can form coalitions which include some members and exclude others. Guilt over an inadequate relationship with the parent can induce adult children to seek aggressive treatment, though this might not be in the best interest of the parent. While caregiving needs of a patient in the terminal stages increase dramatically, so do the tensions of the caregiver. As the patient is approaching the time of death, the caregiver is faced with the realization that the loss of their loved one is imminent (6).

Although it may appear much more comfortable to remain at home while receiving recuperative or palliative care, the burdens of home care can present complications which infringe upon the family's regular routines and heighten anxieties. Even maintaining activities of daily living, such as bathing and dressing, may necessitate calling upon outside services. If relatives and friends are not able to sufficiently care for the patient, treatment decisions may change, accompanied by a regression in the patient's physical and psychological state (1). To put the patient in hospice care can be emotionally wrenching, as it implies that there is no hope of recovery. However, hospice will be a source of caring support to the patient and family, and hospice will continue to provide support to the family after the death of the patient.

Emotional and Financial Costs to Families

Families must strive to resolve or reduce the effects of their problems instrumentally, while easing the pain caused by their current situation. The way in which the family members handle this stress is just as important as the frame of mind of the patient. There is great value to accepting the support of relatives and friends, in addition to utilizing community resources. How the family works together to cope can be linked to whether or not the situation develops into a crisis (11). The challenge of this critical situation provides the potential for the individuals to learn and gain by their endeavors (12).

Cancer presents an acute and chronic crisis because "the family's adjustment to cancer involves moving through . . . transitions in ways that facilitate the meaning of the experience, that maintain the family's ongoing functions, that respond to the illness-related demands, that maintain the self-esteem of the family members, and that foster new arrangements and relationships in the family that are responsive to the contingencies of the illness. Families experiencing cancer destructure and restructure themselves in response to the illness. Destructuring is the breakdown of operational and communication patterns that no longer adequately respond to the illness and to its contingencies. Restructuring is the creation of new forms of interpersonal exchange and operations that reflect the family's adjustment to its illness-related environment. When restructuring is successful, the family adapts to the illness-related demands and balances its commitments to both the diagnosed person and to the family's activities and functions" (9).

Many conflicts may surface for the partner of a cancer patient in their day-to-day living requirements. Along with the increased financial responsibilities incurred by the illness, there may also be the threat to job security for the partner as caregiver in addition to the patient. To analyze the expense of care within the home, caregivers' time and additional expenses incurred to manage the involvement should all be considered as part of the overall cost. "When family labor is included in the cost of calculations, average cancer home care costs for a 3-month period ($4,563) are not much lower than the costs of nursing home care. The substantial variation in home care costs appears to be unrelated to the type of cancer diagnosis, type of treatment, or time since diagnosis but seems to be driven by the functional status of the patient and the family living arrangements . . . Three important components of family costs often are neglected . . . (1) direct costs such as out-of-pocket cash expenditures for services not or only partially covered by third-party payers; (2) indirect costs in the form of foregone earnings opportunities resulting from the illness; and (3) indirect costs in the form of foregone household production and/or leisure time (13)."

There are the economic losses which may not even be recognized, such as the sacrifice of possible job promotions or salary increases due to limitations on income (sometimes for county or government-funded medical coverage) or from lack of commitment of time due to increasing needs at home. Additional expenses may be incurred; for example, more meals consumed outside the home because of lack of time or energy, housekeeping services, added fuel expenses for medical appointments or visits to the patient while in the hospital (13), and long-distance telephone calls to out-of-town relatives and friends.

It is becoming more and more common for families to act as the primary provider for the patient through all stages of treatment to the palliative phase approaching death. This may be the desired choice of some families or taken on due to financial necessity. Such care may involve many varied psychological as well as active responsibilities. While dispensing medications, keeping watch over physical complications leading to a medical emergency, and maintaining adequate exchange of communication with physicians, the caregiver is witnessing the decline of their loved one and making adjustments in their relationship. In a study of bereaved spouse caregivers, it was found that providing for the physical needs of the patient was the most demanding responsibility during the time care was given; but when looking back on that stressful period, the most arduous aspect of that time was steadily watching the family member slip farther away (14).

Assessing the Structure and Function of the Family

Although family assessment may seem far afield from the role of the oncologist, understanding the supportiveness of the family can give insight into the type and extent of treatment the geriatric patient can tolerate. A geriatric patient of Dr. Balducci's had alienated children living at a distance. He was not offered aggressive treatment for his small cell cancer of the lung, as there would be no support close at hand for transportation, comforting, or assistance with side effects.

Alternatively, in another case, a supportive family had a very different effect on treatment decisions. Here, the patient had mild dementia and transitional cell carcinoma of the bladder. However, he had a loving, younger wife and two caring daughters. One daughter was an intensive care nurse, quite concerned about treatment complications. The daughter sought a second opinion, and treatment was initiated. The patient experienced a complete remission of his disease for six months. Although the consultant recommended radiation therapy, the daughter turned it down. The daughters visited often, giving respite to the wife. The patient's disease recurred after six months, but no further treatment was given. The patient was able to engage in enjoyable activities, and eventually died as a result of renal failure due to urinary obstruction. Both wife and children were very satisfied with treatment and with the patient's quality of life. The case represents an example of how a supportive, loving family with a main decision-maker is able to help an older patient through a very toxic regimen with net positive results.

The family unit may well be the patient's most valuable resource as he passes through the stages of his disease. Outside counseling and support for the family can be beneficial only if the family is willing to receive it. At medical interventions, the family should be questioned concerning their own needs and views of the current situation to avoid any false assumptions. Although a family may be very receptive to the idea of providing care for the terminal patient, their ability to do so may be lacking (15). Also, role transitions may be a source of tension for all family members (12).

During the course of the illness, boundaries among the roles of the subsystems may become enmeshed or disengaged. In an enmeshed relationship, family members do not have distinct role expectations. All family members work together in demanding situations, regardless of their age or parental status. There is total family involvement and commitment. Family problems take priority over individual and external concerns. This type of familial relationship can lead to a lack of control over the dominating situation when concerns become too consuming. Physicians may not be able to discern which family member is the primary caregiver, as all are struggling and communicating their concerns. Conversely, in a disengaged relationship, family members act independently of each other with little interaction or family involvement. They are not in touch with each other's feelings, as they hold distinct roles and are reluctant to call upon one another for support. Due to their lack of communication, it is difficult to pull together during a crisis (12).

Communication is necessary between spouses during a terminal illness in order to maintain control of the relationship and cope effectively. Even if the two individuals hold differing viewpoints and goals, it is critical that they share information in an effort to support each other and cope effectively. Mutual respect and empathy are important. Health care personnel can also ease the couple through the transition. A family functions as a unit, with the feelings and reactions of one member influencing all the individuals and the way the family pulls together (6). Martocchio (10) suggests an assessment approach that includes the following questions:

(1) What is the family organization — what responsibilities does each family member have?
(2) What is considered a stressor to each family member?
(3) How has the family coped with change or crisis in the past?
(4) How many crises has the family recently experienced? Is this a time of stability or chaos?
(5) What are the available resources? Is the family aware of support groups?
(6) What kind of structure characterizes the family-egalitarian, accepting, cool, rigid?

Information gained from such questions can give the practitioner feedback about the extent of support the family can provide, the stress level of the family, who are the key decision makers, the information and participation needs of the family, the kinds of side effects the family can tolerate, initiation of conservative versus aggressive treatment approaches, and placement concerns.

When analyzing the pattern a family may take, it is helpful to observe family stage. As a family passes through the traditional patterns of development from a couple to the stages of childbirth, child rearing from early childhood through young adulthood, to eventual retirement, different roles and responsibilities are encountered, each with its individual needs and distinguishing conflicts if confronted with chronic illness. People are prone to the effects of stress particularly when adjusting to changing roles (12).

Ageism in the Medical Encounter

The first criterion for good doctor/patient interaction is genuine liking of the older age group. This liking cannot be forced or fabricated. However, much theorizing and some research documents the inadequate relationship between medical practitioners and elderly patients. In particular, the concept of "ageism" (16) has been postulated to interfere with such liking. Ageism, according to Butler (17) is "prejudice against the elderly as being unworthy of time and effort" (p. 99). This time unworthiness is actually reflected in current standards of practice — Radecki et al. (18) found that physicians spend significantly less time with their older patients. Green et al. (19) also researched the difference in medical encounters with young versus old patients. They found that physicians raised more psychosocial issues with their younger patients, even though older patients have far more concerns in this area. They also discovered that physicians provided better questioning, information, and support to younger patients, especially on patient-raised topics. Physicians were

rated by the younger patients as significantly more egalitarian, patient, interested, and respectful. The authors suggest that such findings corroborate the anecdotal evidence which abounds about physicians discounting elders' concerns (e.g., dizziness, falls, constipation, memory loss, depression) and their lack of attention to worrisome psychosocial issues.

"In the United States, the elderly comprise only 12% of the national census, yet they represent greater than 50% of all U.S. citizens who are diagnosed with cancer . . . To date, little attention has been given to the special needs of the elderly . . . The elderly cancer patient is often viewed as being a poor candidate for aggressive treatment, having a high-risk toxicity profile, lacking social support, and having a slim chance for both quality and long term survival (20)." Even nurses may demonstrate this prejudice in administering medications and in their care for the elderly patient.

Chronic illness frequently associated with aging sometimes influences cancer treatment regimens. Careful attention should be given to the proper administration of prescription and over-the counter medications to prevent overmedication and adverse drug reactions. With so many medications frequently prescribed for cancer patients, proper dosages need to be treated with even greater scrutiny for the elderly population. Typical traits of aging, such as confusion, lethargy, and depression, may actually be symptomatic of adverse side effects to medications (20). In an effort to advance the quality of care for the geriatric cancer patient, the medical profession should take a more realistic, accurate look at the effects of aging. Protocols for treatment should be founded on the principles of biological needs, unrelated to stereotypes of aging. "Cross-training and the integration of the science of gerontologic principles and findings in cancer care, . . . in addition to any action taken by oncology nurses to customize care, investigate corollaries of distress, and implementing innovative strategies are actions necessary to improve quality of life in the elderly who face cancer (20).

Coping with the losses incurred with cancer may be especially difficult for the elderly patient, who may be experiencing additional losses at this time of his life. With the emotional and physical burdens associated with sensory decline, decreased stamina, and possibly additional health complications, the patient may feel overwhelmed and unable to fight the stresses and regimens associated with cancer. He or she may have even lost close friends or a spouse to this disease (20). Such a patient is certainly in great need of a dedicated support system.

Communication Needs of Family Members of Cancer Patients

Family members of cancer patients have a variety of needs at different phases of the illness. However, Tringali (21) found that in all phases of the patient's illness, the top need was to have questions answered honestly. Information needs, rather than emotional or physical care needs, seemed to also have priority, e.g., to be informed of changes in the patient's condition, to know what treatment the patient is receiving, to know specific facts concerning the patient's prognosis. Information seeking, according to Weisman (22), is an important coping strategy in cancer and other illnesses. Physicians should hold family conferences to eliminate all ambiguity and to willingly answer any questions directly. Shields (23) suggests that the conspiracy of silence that has plagued the field of oncology for so long is at last ending, but families still engage in hovering, false reassurances, and role inflexibility. Because of their frailty or dependency, some older adults may be overprotected by children and thus not get their information needs met. Doctors too may be more comfortable in talking with adult children than with the older patient.

All family members should be able to take an active part in the patient's care if they express a need to do so. Even children or grandchildren may be shown ways to help, such as gathering needed supplies and providing comfort and companionship to the patient (15). Children can be a wonderful source of support to a dejected patient. They bring with them a spirit of vitality and seem able to make light of a solemn situation. Even in the most traumatic of times, children benefit from being kept informed and a part of family interaction. Nothing may be worse than the fears sometimes imagined by a child as a result of being shielded from the total picture. Children are resilient, as well as receptive, to what is happening around them. Being involved in the patient's care can be a form of therapy for loved ones.

The needs of the caregiver may change over the course of illness, with different aspects of the caregiving role contributing to more or less stress as the disease progresses. Health care personnel need to be open to these special needs and willing to confront the issues at hand in a supportive manner. Attention should always be given to the family's needs extending beyond the immediate concerns of the patient, as these matters may resurface as even more critical later (14). Depression may even be linked to a lack of social activity in the caregiver's life, rather than just to the patient's status *per se* (8).

Family members carry the additional psychological burden of coping with their own changing lifestyles while at the same time coping with the emotional responses of their loved one to the effects of the disease. There is a "loss of self" as they accept new responsibilities. Distress may be exhibited in any number of psychological reactions: anger, frustration, anxiety, depression, irritability, preoccupation, mood swings, denial, etc. Children may exhibit their frustration in temper tantrums, restless sleep, uncontrolled screaming or crying, or a return back to more dependency upon the other parent. How a person handles this stress is very individual. Cultural beliefs and moral values are enmeshed into the experience as he or she struggles to derive meaning and direction from the ordeal. Discretion should be observed in keeping a balance between denial of the impending situation and the surrender of hope (24).

Supportive Interventions

Physicians should keep families informed of available resources to draw upon for support during the difficult times. Many caregivers have later reported regrets about not taking advantage of support systems. Because the caregiver may be reluctant to seek help, the physician should emphasize how calling upon outside support is actually a constructive move in maintaining order in caregiving responsibilities (14).

Counseling can serve "as a dynamic process of problem solving directed at maintaining or improving quality of life (25)." Counseling can be beneficial from the time of diagnosis to the grieving period continuing after the patient's death. All stages of this illness are subject to heightened anxieties and unexpected pitfalls as the disease takes its unscrupulous route of remissions and reoccurrences.

Health professionals need to provide support to family members concerning three main issues in particular: 1) feelings of guilt about relinquishing caregiving responsibilities to professionals; 2) anticipating the patient's terminal status; and 3) acceptance of outside support to aid in the grieving process. Lack of acceptance of the illness as a terminal disease may be exhibited in repeated inquiries concerning the patient's prognosis (24).

A high level of anxiety in a patient himself frequently correlates with a high level of anxiety felt by the caregiver (8). Communication barriers may occur between the patient and his or her spouse due to fear of acknowledgment or wanting to shelter a loved one from increased psychological burden. With the emphasis on "positive thinking" popular in current literature, men often cope by fighting the threats of this disease with this concept. However, the female spouse may experience even more anxiety due to her husband's avoidance of talking together about their threatening issues. Likewise, significant concerns of the caregiver may not be voiced if they include resentment at how the disease has impacted her own lifestyle (6). These anxieties can then escalate. Outside support services can be extremely helpful for couples who are reluctant to talk about distressing concerns. The lines of communication between spouses are most effective when both share corresponding emotions (6).

Sexual problems may also be encountered. A spouse may feel vulnerable to the threat of impending death and may compensate by retreating from sexual activity. Also, the patient may feel too physically drained himself to be sexually active. The added separations of increased hospitalizations may further affect the situation. However, for some, there may be an increase in desire for sexual intimacy, and this physical bonding can be very beneficial to both partners.

Reasons to Enhance Communication Techniques

Why are communication skills so important to good diagnosis and treatment? For any practitioner who works with the geriatric patient and family, the quality of the interaction is very significant. High-quality communication with the geriatric patient can lead to a more thorough history, a more comfortable physical and mental status examination, and the development of trust between doctor and patient, which can increase compliance with treatment recommendations (17,26,27). Trust between the practitioner and the patient and family can create a climate for acceptance of the diagnosis, decreased doctor shopping, and a willingness to work on issues of patient compliance, comfort, and family support.

Doctor shopping comes from a disbelief in the diagnostic or treatment abilities of the physician, exacerbated by a lack of trust due to impaired communication, and by the physician's inability to break through the family's denial. The family who cannot trust their physician is also less likely to comply with difficult or complex treatment recommendations, or to take advice in seeking caregiving assistance. Thus, high-quality communication between the practitioner and the patient and family is critical.

The rationale for effective listening is based on the attaining of better, more complete information during diagnosis and greater patient cooperation during treatment. Although the busy practitioner may feel there is no need to patiently listen to a rambling, unclear client's recital of symptoms, problems, and concerns, active listening by the physician may help the patient express himself more clearly and concisely.

Active Listening

Active listening requires attention, concentration, and an open mind on the part of the practitioner. Active listening is both verbal and nonverbal. The nonverbal behaviors include a positive facial expression, head nods, a sitting posture close to the patient, gentle touch, and the use of the expression "Mmmm Hmmm." Verbal behaviors include asking open-ended questions (who, what, why, when, where, and how), repeating back key phrases for confirmation, and rephrasing. The outcomes of active listening are trust, cooperation, and patient compliance.

Trust

Active listening gains for the dyad a feeling of trust and comfort, a willingness to disclose embarrassing information, and confidence in each other. The patient who trusts the physician may more readily reveal symptoms that are crucial to the diagnosis. Patients with a life-threatening disease may be very sensitive to the nonverbal messages that others are conveying. The patient will quickly sense if a physician is hurried or impatient or uncaring. This may make the patient even more anxious, further eroding the opportunity for high-quality interaction.

The practitioner can determine how to build a trusting relationship with the particular family, in terms of explaining the disease and various treatment alternatives, gaining cooperation from key decision-makers, orienting the family to facility procedures and policies, providing written information about the members of the health care team, and giving family members a sense of control and hope.

Cooperation

Good communication during the physical examination or chemotherapy/radiation treatment can decrease patient discomfort. If the patient is anxious and upset, the slowness that normally accompanies aging may increase. This can infuriate the busy practitioner and create a cycle of anxiety, distrust, increased slowness, and acting out. A relaxed patient can more easily understand and cooperate with physician instructions. A pleasant, respectful, and empathic communication style will enhance the examination and treatment process.

Compliance

Good communication also improves patient compliance and facilitates patient education and counseling. However, physicians seriously underestimate the amount of time they spend in information giving. In fact, on the average, doctors spend only one minute out of 20 in providing information, although they overestimate this by a factor of nine (28). In a study by Cassileth *et al.* (29) of cancer patients, a majority of those over age 60 desired all information available and wanted maximum detail. Haug & Ory (26) suggest the following about compliance or its lack: "Communication skills of physicians have long been implicated in noncompliance or nonadherence to physician's instructions" (p. 26).

They, along with others, feel such a skill deficit is the most significant problem facing current medical practice (30). It is estimated that for those with chronic conditions, noncompliance occurs in about 50%, and can be as high as 92% for short-term medication recommendations (31). Haug and Ory suggest that a feeling of physician error, lack of understanding, lack of commitment, and forgetting account for these high rates of noncompliance (26). They recommend that better communication with both patient and family will lessen this significant problem.

The oncologist, however, may not want to take on the burden of having patients and families accept treatments solely to please the doctor. Lederberg *et al.* (32) suggest that there is tremendous stress generated in the field of oncology due to the uncertainty in treatment decisions, the difficult trade-offs in various interventions, patients' unrealistic expectations, the withholding or stopping of life support, and discussions with patient and family. It might be that the physician, as a form of self protection, purposefully turns away from close communication. However, the risks to the patient of poor communication seem to be greater than the risk to the oncologist of promoting a trusting, caring relationship (33).

Can Communication Skills be Effectively Learned?

The busy practitioner with little time for training might want to believe that communication effectiveness is an innate ability, with which one is either blessed or bypassed. Certainly, some physicians do seem to be nurturing and empathic by nature, women more so than men (34). Women physicians interrupt their patients far less than male physicians, for example.

As patients are turning into medical consumers, medical schools are adding psychosocial courses to their curricula, with a focus on interviewing and other communication skills (28). However, what about experienced physicians who have been in practice for many years? Can they benefit from communication skills training?

A study by Evans et al. (35) indicates that physicians can indeed learn emotional and cognitive communication techniques with very brief training, and that such knowledge impacts directly on patient satisfaction and anxiety. A random sample of doctors who had been in practice for an average of 16 years received two three hour seminars on communication plus a course booklet concerning "psychological variables in doctor-patient interactions; patient satisfaction; recall and understanding; patient compliance; and a range of suggested consulting techniques designed to increase satisfaction and understanding and reduce non-compliance" (p. 374). The treatment group did not have an opportunity to role-play or practice new skills, only to discuss them. A control group received no special training. Four hundred patients were tested four weeks following the training program. Patients from doctors in the training group were significantly more satisfied and less anxious than patients from doctors in the control group.

It is indeed surprising that such a brief training intervention could have produced such a significant change in patient satisfaction and attitude. It suggests that patients are so responsive to physician interaction style that even a small change can produce great appreciation for their efforts. The skills of showing empathy and respect in caring for patients, coupled with providing complete information of diagnosis and treatment using simple language and written information, are powerful indeed.

A Model for Communication Skill Development

Going beyond the simple training program of Evans et al (35), Hornsby and Payne (36) developed an extensive theory-based program involving a number of skills to enhance the patient-physician relationship. They use this model of skills training with family practice residents and faculty in 20 hours of instruction over a one-month period, with videotaping and feedback extending over a two-year period. These skills take into consideration the action oriented nature of physician interactions and move from the development of trust, through building a personal relationship, and ultimately to changed behaviors. The authors suggest that good communication skills are necessary in the following areas of practice: taking a patient history, performing the physical examination, prescribing, educating, and

counseling to ensure compliance. One aspect of communication skills that they emphasize is nonverbal communication — the use of gestures, posture, voice, tone, touch, and facial expression.

Practitioners must not only know how to use nonverbal techniques themselves, but they also must be able to assess nonverbal messages in their patients, such as the physical expression of pain. The skills model developed by Gazda, Walters, and Childers (37), which served as the basis for the training program, encompasses empathy, respect, warmth, concreteness, genuineness, self-disclosure, confrontation, immediacy, and behavior modification.

Empathy

Empathy is the ability to show understanding, to put oneself in the other person's shoes, and to identify feeling. The skill of identifying feelings is very helpful in making patients feel understood, as it takes the interaction beyond a superficial plane and makes possible a climate of closeness. Feeling identification is a no-lose skill, as the patient will almost always correct a wrongly identified feeling. If the physician says to a patient, "You seem to be somewhat anxious," and the patient is instead frustrated, he or she will invariably reply, "No, I'm frustrated at what is going on. As the physician uses this skill more frequently, observation of the nonverbal signals of different emotions will improve in accuracy. The use of this skill seems to say to the patient, "I'm not going to cast blame or defend myself; I'm going to try to understand where you are coming from."

Respect

The use of respect demonstrates that the physician values and believes in the patient and in his or her ability to follow through on an effective health care program. People want to be valued and respected, especially when they feel insecure and in situations of unequal power. Older patients do not feel respected in many medical encounters, and this feeling can lead them into a vicious cycle of dependency, poor self-esteem, and loss of independent functioning known as "the social breakdown syndrome" (38). Lack of respect is evidenced by arguing with the patient, making fun of his or her feelings, or saying those feelings are wrong. For example, "You shouldn't be upset by this" is a statement that shows a lack of respect for the natural emotions of an individual in an anxiety provoking situation. Lack of respect is also demonstrated when one forces opinions on the patient: "This is what you should do next." Rather, one should ask patients for their own ideas about how they might implement a treatment regimen: "How do you plan to go about losing the weight we discussed?"

Warmth

Warmth is the next skill in facilitating the physician-patient relationship. Caring naturally evolves from understanding and respecting the patient. Conveying warmth is usually done nonverbally through gentle touch, eye contact, and verbal/nonverbal congruence. For instance, saying "Nothing is wrong" to the patient while frowning over test results conveys an attitude of mistrust. With warmth, one conveys the sense of "I am concerned too." In fact, patients were more satisfied in encounters in which physicians showed tension and anxiety (39), perhaps because patients felt their physicians were revealing themselves to be human and caring, rather than distancing themselves with coldness or idle reassurances.

The warmth conveyed by gentle touch is also craved by most people. Older persons are the least touched patients in health care settings. They are also less touched by significant others, as these others die or move away. Thus, there is a tremendous need for touch in this age group, and a real thriving can come from a warm squeeze or hand clasp (40).

The three skills of empathy, respect, and warmth serve to encourage the patient to reveal his or her problems completely and build rapport between the physician and patient. Concreteness, genuineness, and self-disclosure develop the relationship further.

Concreteness

This skill helps the patient be specific about symptoms and experiences. The physician encourages the patient to discuss sensitive topics and, in turn, is willing to address such sensitive topics as cost, length of time needed for treatment, and the like. Instead of wondering about delicate matters, the patient and physician both can put energy into frank discussions that can clear the air. Also, it is far better to have the patient expect something to be tougher or more painful than it actually is than to feel betrayed by the casual statement, "Oh, this won't hurt a bit." Although the rationale of minimizing pain expectation is no doubt sound — to prevent anxiety that exacerbates pain — this belittling strategy can backfire.

Genuineness

Being yourself is what genuineness implies. For example, a physician who does not like a patient might say, "We're having a difficult time getting along here. Rather than conveying insincerity, this statement conveys a sense of honesty and integrity. A genuine physician offers compliments at times as well: "I'm impressed at your compliance efforts" or "You've come a long way in dealing with this issue." Genuineness also means being frank when the patient is ready for it: "You know, prostate cancer can mean loss in function in the future."

Self-Disclosure

Self-disclosure is the next skill that deepens a relationship. The physician confesses to problems or reactions similar to those of the patient. "I recently had to give up running because of a bad knee, so I know what you're going through." Physicians must not excessively disclose, as they are not their patients' parents. However, sharing some aspect of one's life with the patient says, "We're both human beings here, subject to losses

and pain and suffering. We share a common bond and want to comfort and motivate each other."

The next set of skills — confrontation, immediacy, and behavior modification — help the patient problem solve and ultimately change behavior. Only when trust and open communication are present can the physician successfully assist the patient in changing behavior.

Confrontation

With this skill, the practitioner points out the discrepancy between what the patient is saying and what the patient is doing. "You say you've given up smoking; yet you were smoking in the waiting room." Or, "You say you've been feeling alone and depressed; yet you haven't been attending your support group." These kinds of statements are potentially quite threatening, so they can only be made in an atmosphere of trust. Otherwise, the patient will contradict the physician, be offended, withdraw, resist, or even sever the relationship. In an atmosphere of trust, the patient may feel chagrin and no doubt reply, "You're right, doctor. I haven't been doing as well as I could. I was just afraid to tell you."

Immediacy

With the skill of immediacy, the physician comments on what is immediately happening between him or herself and the patient that might interfere with compliance or disclosure. "You say you're going to take the medication despite the side effects. But I sense you only want to please me and really aren't sure about this course of action. Am I reading you right?"

Behavior Modification

Behavior modification is the ultimate influence of human behavior, subsuming a host of skills including positive and negative reinforcement, modeling, shaping, prompting, and systematic desensitization. These skills require very specialized training for proper implementation.

Applications of the Communications Model

It is critically important that good communication skills be used by the entire health care staff, from the receptionist to insurance clerk, to ensure that the patient feels understood and respected. If the physician is rushed with the patient or the patient did not understand instructions, the patient may ask the nurse to explain further. If the nurse is similarly curt or brief, the patient may feel frustrated and be unable to comply with instructions. The American Association of Retired Persons (41) suggests that good communication should also be evident in telephone procedures, the appointment process, billing, and follow up, as well as during the history, examination, and education and counseling.

AARP's communication training manual for physicians emphasizes good nonverbal and verbal communication strategies. Nonverbal strategies include avoiding physical barriers, such as a desk between patient and physician, sitting during conversations to indicate the mutuality of power and a willingness not to rush off, using touch appropriately, and maintaining eye contact while avoiding doodling or fiddling. Environmental considerations, such as good lighting, a quiet room without interruptions, and the lack of prolonged waiting time, are also important. Some other authors suggest that additional subtle, yet powerful, techniques include displaying all diplomas prominently to inspire confidence and wearing traditional physician garb (42)

Verbal communication strategies according to AARP include asking the patient to write out symptoms and questions before a visit, using open-ended questions, asking patients what name they prefer to be called, avoiding medical jargon, speaking distinctly and slowly, stating expectations, summarizing information, giving patients written instructions and checklists, and providing positive feedback. AARP believes that good communication will reduce patient stress, improve self-esteem, increase patient compliance, keep patients loyal, increase office efficiency, and improve job satisfaction.

It is especially important in large, impersonal health care settings to provide the family and patient with a written list of their practitioners and phone numbers where they can be reached daily during an emergency.

Family Communication Issues

In one study, at least 20% of older patients who attended a general medical clinic were accompanied by a companion (15). It might be expected that family members would accompany an older patient to the oncologist in far greater numbers. Family members might attend initial medical encounters because their presence is comforting to the patient, they are needed for transportation, to provide medical or historical information, or they themselves are the impetus for the visit. However, the presence of another person at the medical encounter complicates the communication process. It creates a triad or even larger number of persons who can form coalitions with or against the physician to enhance or detract from his or her power and communication effectiveness.

According to Adelman et al (43), the companion at the medical encounter can take the role of advocate, antagonist, or passive party. These roles can be further subdivided. The most extreme type of advocate will be a patient activist. Other advocate roles include a patient extender who speaks for the patient who cannot talk coherently and a patient-physician mediator. The antagonist role can be subdivided into patient saboteur, who ignores or discounts the patient's agenda, and an opportunist, who brings his or her own agenda to the encounter. The opportunist takes over the encounter so that his or her own concerns and medical problems take precedence. The passive party may have been a driver for the patient or other neutral person and has no vested interest in the encounter.

Role of the Patient Activist

The patient activist might be expected to want to control the medical encounter for the patient's sake. The activist might question the practitioner's expertise of judgment, interrupt the physician frequently, challenge the diagnosis or prognosis, and demand alternative treatments. Although such tactics may embarrass the patient, the activist will persist with these issues. The practitioner must be extremely patient and tactful with the activist and be sure to communicate with the patient, as well as the companion. The physician should identify for the companion the underlying feelings of protectiveness and concern, but express the reality of the situation — that this is a difficult diagnosis to make and to hear.

Role of the Patient Extender

The patient extender's focus is on the patient, trying to represent the patient's concerns and explain the patient's perhaps unintelligible utterances. The extender is trying to be helpful in the encounter by assisting in the history-taking process and reinterpreting the physician's statements to the patient using language and gestures that the patient may understand. The physician can also be greatly helped by the extender to understand more fully the history of the disease and by having the extender ensure compliance with any treatment recommendations. The physician will be tempted to address remarks exclusively to the extender, but this should be avoided.

Role of the Patient-Physician Mediator

The patient-physician mediator will be active yet neutral during the encounter. The mediator is representing both physician and patient, explaining each to each other and working toward compromise if conflict exists.

Role of the Patient Saboteur

The patient saboteur may act in quite a charming manner, trying to set up a coalition with the physician against the patient. This alliance will serve the saboteur's needs while discounting those of the patient. Although the patient may be alarmed at his or her own symptoms, the saboteur will try to downplay them to the physician: "They're not that bad." The saboteur can complicate the diagnostic picture and must be handled carefully by the physician. The physician may need to bring in other family historians to corroborate or contradict the saboteur's statements.

Role of the Opportunist

The opportunist can create ethical conflicts for the practitioner (27). Just who is the identified patient? Whose needs should be served? Often, practitioners will ally themselves with the opportunist simply because the patient cannot easily communicate his or her needs and wishes. The opportunist might be histrionic in presenting the stressors of the caregiving situation and may create sympathy for the overwhelming problems faced every day.

Communication skills are challenged in situations that involve companions in the medical encounter. Certainly, the diagnosis and treatment of cancer patients and their families call for the greatest use of active listening, relationship-enhancing skills, behavior-change strategies, tact, and support.

Families that bring multiple roles to the medical encounter can cause the practitioner to feel he or she is doing family therapy, rather than diagnosis and treatment (44). However, the observation of family dynamics can shed light on the adequacy of the patient's caregiving situation. Dysfunctional family dynamics can create "excess disability" in the patient or even a clinical depression (45).

The maladjustment of one family member to the patient's condition can have an adverse affect on the whole family. Interpersonal conflicts of other members can hinder the daily management of treatments and how the patient adjusts to the disease himself. The unpredictability of this disease continues throughout its course. Families are continuously faced with the possibility of the inevitable finality while, at the same time, experiencing the ups and downs of remissions and recurrences without little time to adjust to the changes. To keep stability for this "emotional roller coaster" (15), it may be beneficial to anticipate an approaching fall and brace oneself for the ride that is to come.

Anticipating Future Needs

"Since 1991, the Patient Self-Determination Act (PSDA) has required most hospitals to inform patients, on admission of their right to have an advance directive (46)." It is especially important for the physician to be open and honest so the patient can make his or her own decisions to accept or decline life support systems in emergency situations. Without a clear and total picture of the true prognosis, the patient may not be able to make a valid judgment to do this. The immediate family can then be thrown into psychological turmoil when such a crisis arises in the absence of a living will. Without advance directives, a patient might be denied the opportunity to experience the type of dying process he would prefer. Relatives may become overwhelmed with feelings of guilt and confusion if a vital decision rests upon them. Nurses can facilitate the options available, as they may have an existing relationship with the patient and family as regular caregivers and liaisons. The establishment of a living will should be an integral part of care for a terminal patient (46).

A living will is a very personal, sensitive issue which calls upon individual morals and values. Quality of life and the quality for the lives of surrounding loved ones are factors which may influence life support decisions. As stated by one cancer patient: "I want to leave my children with memories of a father who gave them strength and a sense of security . . . If at all possible, I too want my death to be consistent with the life I have led . . . There is a time to fight death with every ounce of strength one has — and a time to let go . . . There is also the cost . . . I know my family would struggle to care for me at home and would feel guilty if they had to put me in a nursing home. Then they would be driven by love and a sense of obligation to visit my body — perhaps for years. I have seen what this can do to loved ones, and I know I do not want to put my family through that ordeal . . . If the time ever comes that I would desire assisted death, I will be powerless to act on my choice. I will need the understanding, love, and support of others to die with dignity. May God grant these others the courage to carry out this, my final wish (47)."

Comfort Measures vs. Aggressive Therapy in the Final Stages

As a patient nears the final stages of the disease, the family is faced with additional stressors and issues which may raise questions and conflict among its members. Basic physical needs, such as nutrition, hydration, and ventilation, can begin to surface as major concerns. At this point in the illness, the patient might become unresponsive to chemotherapy treatments, and the decision may lie with whether to continue with aggressive measures for life support or to principally aim to keep the patient as comfortable as possible.

For family members, witnessing a patient's refusal to eat or drink may signal impending death and create increased anxieties among the caregivers. Feelings of guilt and frustration come into play, as relatives feel compelled to encourage the loved one to maintain activities of daily living. However, clinicians recognize that this refusal is a natural step in the final stages of the disease and should be available to prepare and support the family members for this emotional disturbance (48).

Decreased appetite is usually not seen as a primary concern for the patient himself. Food aversions may be acquired for a number of reasons, such as the effects of chemotherapy treatment, tumor growth, and reactions to medications. For the caregiver, it can be very difficult to witness this gradual regression of a loved one. However, "the causes of malnutrition may be classified into three categories: (1) decreased intake, (2) increased caloric needs related to the malignancy, and (3) malabsorption . . . Cachexia, profound and progressive bodily wasting, and weight loss are significant problems for end-state cancer patients . . . .The tumor may be giving off chemicals that cause changes in the perception of taste, and the satiety or "fullness" center in the brain may also be affected by these chemicals. It is helpful to emphasize that this is a part of the disease and is something over which the patient and family have no control (48)."

Family members are usually inclined to promote caloric intake from feelings of guilt of not being more in control of the deteriorating situation, helplessness over not being able to care more actively for their loved one, and lack of knowledge of nutritional consequences in the final stages of cancer. "Despite the negative impact of malnutrition on survival, aggressive nutritional support, consisting of total parenteral nutrition (TPN) or enteral feedings, has not been successful in reversing the above-mentioned symptoms in most patients

... Patients being treated with TPN may have a shortened survival time because the enhanced nutrition may enhance tumor growth. Other studies indicate that artificially administered sustenance has no significant impact on tumor response to radiation or chemotherapy. Even when TPN has achieved weight maintenance, it has been through water and fat accumulation rather than improved protein status. Neither enteral or parenteral feedings have a place in the clinical management of patients with advanced cancer (48)." Recording the patient's caloric intake or keeping track of weight loss is usually not advisable or productive. Instead, it serves more purpose to make readily available the foods and liquids the patient desires (48). To entice appetite, serve food in smaller portions and prepare meals at the time of day the patient expresses an interest in eating. Aim to serve high-caloric foods (48), and add nutritional supplements as additional ingredients.

For the family member who was in charge of preparing meals, there may now be a void in her caregiving responsibilities which may be constructively filled. Guidance and support should be given to that person to help redirect her caregiving needs to other ways of providing pleasure to the patient, such as in companionship or tactile stimulation. The caregiver could read the daily news or sports page at bedside, revisit old memories with stories from their past, play relaxing music, or provide comfort in cool compresses to the forehead or light massage. By removing the emphasis of food persuasion, the patient will benefit in a more relaxed atmosphere and will feel more in control of his own needs (48).

Dehydration is also a normal aspect in the dying phase of this disease and should be approached with similar prudence. As with nutritional therapies, there are detriments as well as advantages with hydration therapy. Many factors may contribute to a patient becoming dehydrated, from fluid loss due to diarrhea and/or vomiting, to less obvious causes, such as obstructions and infections. A patient may even have difficulty staying awake long enough to drink adequate amounts of fluid. Every possible effort should be made to prevent dehydration whenever possible. Careful observation should be kept during nausea and diarrhea. It is important for clinicians to alert caregivers to signals that a problem may be imminent and ways to help manage the situation (48).

When making decisions whether or not to induce hydration therapy, the key concern should be whether or not it will provide more comfort to the patient. "Beneficial effects of dehydration include: decreased urine output resulting in less incontinence and less need for toileting; decreased production of gastric fluids resulting in less nausea and vomiting; decreased pulmonary secretions resulting in less need for suctioning; and diminished incidence of edema and ascites ... Not only is dehydration not a painful condition, but a state of dehydration before death may even cause the patient to perceive less pain (48)."

To arrive at an appropriate decision, health care professionals need to provide guidance to the family on the duties involved for home infusion. The willingness of the family, in addition to the patient's desires and possibility of recovery, should all be taken into consideration. If the family decides not introduce hydration therapy, palliative measures should definitely be explored. Use of simulated tears and ointments to lubricate, and spoon-feeding ice chips, may make the patient more comfortable. Once the patient is no longer able to sip through a straw, fluids may then be given through an oral syringe. Sedatives might also be considered to help control muscle spasms and keep the patient calm (48).

One point to keep in mind is that once therapy is begun, it can be very difficult emotionally to cease treatment. Families might view it as failure and then battle with depression. It may be advisable to put a time restriction on the trial of such therapy to avoid future guilt. Then they may feel, at least, that they gave therapy a chance to remedy the situation. Hospice counselors should emphasize that nutrition and hydration therapies should actually be thought of as medicinal treatments which serve no purpose in being continued if they are not alleviating the situation. Therapies may be reduced slowly rather than abruptly. However, a patient may continue from days to weeks without nutrition (48).

Making a Difference

Although practitioners might want to resist a change in their habitual behaviors, as change is stressful and uncomfortable, making even modest adjustments in communication style could produce a significantly more comforted patient population. For example, using some of the relationship-enhancing skills described above, as well as providing more complete information and written instructions for identifying practitioners and following a treatment regimen, could go a long way toward alleviating patient/family anxiety about the medical encounter and increasing compliance.

The abilities of the older patient may be decreased by sensory changes, depression, and other chronic diseases accompanying aging, in addition to cancer (49). These conditions can lessen the motivation and energy available for interaction and even the ability to hear and see the physician. Thus, the practitioner's task of communicating is even more difficult with frail older patients. The gratitude and appreciation of patients who recognize these efforts can be very fulfilling. Older patients can be delighted by a minimal increase in functional status or the slowing of deterioration, which can create a significant difference in their lives (50). Their families can also be comforted through honest, direct interaction with the oncologist and thus adapt better to caregiving demands and grief work.

Cancer is a degenerative disease which invades the lives of the entire family unit. The family is in a constant state of remaining on-call in a roller coaster situation of remissions and reoccurrences. Caregivers are no longer in a position to make even short-term plans. An unexpected trip to the hospital emergency room or a spiked fever can be a frequent occurrence when a cancer patient is undergoing a regulated course of chemotherapy treatments. Needs unique to each person in the family, in addition to the needs of the whole group, change with the unpredictability incurred in their lives (12). The physician and health care team can learn skills which provide comfort and reassurance through the various stages of the illness and its treatment regimens.

References

1. Mor V, Allen S, Malin M. the Psychological Impact of Cancer on Older Versus Younger Patients and their families. *Cancer Supplement* 1994; **74 (4)**.

2. Light E, Lebowitz BD. *Alzheimer's Disease Treatment and Family Stress. Directions for Research*. Rockville, MD: National Institute of Mental Health, 1989.

3. Cassileth BR Lusk, EJ, Strouse TB, *et al*. Psychosocial status in chronic illness. A comparative analysis of six diagnostic groups. *N Engl J Med* 1984; **311**: 506–511.

4. Kalish RA, Reynolds DK. *Death and Ethnicity. A Psychoculural Study*. Los Angeles, USC: Press 1976.

5. Rait D. A family-system approach to the patient with cancer. *Cancer Invest* 1989; **7**: 77–81.

6. Germino B, Fife B, Funk S. Cancer and the Partner Relationship. What is its Meaning? *Seminars in Oncology Nursing* 1995; **11 (1)**.

7. Davis-Ali S, Chesler M, Chesney B. Recognizing Cancer as a Family Disease. Worries and Support Reported by Patients and Spouses. *Social Work in Health Care* 1993; **19 (2)**.

8. Kaye J, Gracely E. Psychological Distress in Cancer Patients and Their Spouses. *Journal of Cancer Education* 1993, **8 (1)**.

9. Lewis F. Psychosocial Transitions and the Family's Work in adjusting to Cancer. *Seminars in Oncology Nursing* 1993; **9 (2)**.

10. Martocchio BC. Family coping. Helping families help themselves. *Semm Oncol Nurs* 1985; **1**: 92–297.

11. Musci E, Dodd M. Predicting Self-Care with Patients and Family Members' Affective States and Family Functioning. *Oncology Nursing Forum* 1990; **17(3)**.

12. Gray-Price H, Szczesny S. Crisis Intervention with Families of Cancer Patients. A Developmental Approach. *Topics in Clinical Nursing* 1985; **7(1)**.

13. Stommel M, Given C, Given B. The Cost of Cancer Home Care to Families. *Cancer* 1993; **71(5)**.

14. Stetz K, Hanson W. Alterations in Perceptions of Care giving Stetz K, Demands in Advanced Cancer During and After the Experience. *The Hospice Journal* 1992; **8 (3)**.

15. Jassak P. Families. An Essential Element in the Care of the Patient with Cancer. *Oncology Nursing Forum* 1992; **19 (6)**.

16. Greene MG, Adelman R, Charon R, Hoffman S. Ageism in the medical encounter. An exploratory study of the doctor-elderly patient relationship. *Lang Communication* 1986; **6**: 113.

17. Butler RN. The doctor and the aged patient. *Hosp Pract* 1978; **1**: 38. 99.

18. Radecki SW, *et al*. Do physicians spend less time with older patients? *J Am Geriatr Soc* 1988; **36**: 713.

19. Greene MG, Hofman S, Charon R, Adelman R. Psychosocial concerns in the medical encounter. *J Gerontol* 1987; **27**: 164.

20. Boyle D. Realities to Guide Novel and Necessary Nursing Care in Geriatric Oncology. *Nursing Care in Geriatric Oncology* 1994; **17 (2)**.

21. Tringali CA. The needs of family members of cancer patients. *Oncol Nurs Forum* 1988; **13**: 65–70.

22. Weisman A. *Coping with Cancer*. New York: McGraw-Hill Book Co, 1979.

23. Shields P. A supportive bridge between cancer patient, family and health care staff. *Nurs Forum* 1984; **21**: 31–36.

24. Hinds C. Suffering. A Relatively Unexplored Phenomenon Among Family Caregivers of Non-Institutionalized Patients with Cancer. *Journal of Advanced Nursing* 1992; **17 (8)**.

25. Reele B. Effect of Counseling on Quality of Life for Individuals with Cancer and Their Families. *Cancer Nursing* 1994; **17 (2)**.

26. Haug MR, Ory MG. Issues in elderly patient-provider interactions. *Res Aging* 1987; **9**: 3.

27. Iahnigen DW, Schrier RW. The doctor/patient relationship in geriatric care. *Clin Geriatr Med* 1986; **2**: 4567.

28. Waitzkin H. Doctor patient communication. Clinical implications of social scientific research. *JAMA* 1984; **252**: 2441.

29. Cassileth B, Zupkis R, Suttojn-Smith K, Marsh V. Information and participation preferences among cancer patients. *Ann intern Med* 1980; **94 (4)**: 832.

30. Eraker SA, Kirscht JP, Becker MH. Understanding and improving patient compliance. *Ann Intern Med* 1984; **100**: 258.

31. Becker MH. Patient adherence to prescribe therapies *Med Care* 1985; **23**: 539–555.

32. Lederberg MD, Holland JC, Massil MJ. Psychosocial aspects of patients with cancer. In *Cancer. Principles and Practice on Oncology*, 3rd ed, edited by VT DeVita, S Hellman, SA Rosenberg. Philadelphia: JB Lippincott Co, vol 2, pp. 2198–2205, 1989.

33. Wanzer SH, *et al*. The physician's responsibility toward hopelessly ill patients. *N Engl J Med* 1984; **310**: 955–959.

34. West C. When the doctor is a lady. In *Women, Health and Medicine*, edited by A Stromberg. Palo Alto, CA: Mayfield Publishers, 1984.

35. Evans BJ, *et al*. A communication skills programme for increasing patients' satisfaction with general practice consultation. *Br J Med Psychol* 1987; **60**: 373.

36. Hornsby JL, Payne FE. A model for communication skills development for family practice residents, *J Fam Pract* 1979; **8**: 71.

37. Gazda GM, Walters RP, Childers WC. *Human Relations Development — A Manual for Health Sciences*. Boston: Allyn and Bacon, 1975.

38. Kypers IA, Bengston VL. Competence and social breakdown. A social-psychological view of aging. *Human Dev* 1973; **16**: 37.

39. Carter WB, *et al*. Outcome-based doctor-patient interaction analysis. II. Identifying effective provider and patient behavior. *Med Care* 1982; **20**: 550.

40. Blondis MN, Jackson BE. *Nonverbal Communication with Patients. Back to the Human Touch*. New York: John Wiley, 1982.

41. American Association of Retired Person. *Older Patients and You*. Washington, DC: American Association of Retired Persons, 1987.

42. Dew PE, Wood SD, Trenter SW. Developing patient satisfaction. The physicians's role. *Group Pract J* **March/April**, p. 6, 1989.

43. Adelman RD, Greene MG, Charon R. The physician-elderly patient-companion triad in the medical encounter. The development of a consensual framework and research agenda. *Gerontologist* 1987; **27**: 729.

44. Hahn SR, Feiner JS, Bellin EH. The doctor-patient family relationship. A compensatory alliance. *An Intern Med* 1988; **109**: 884.

45. Kahn RI. Excess disabilities. In *Readings in Aging and Death*, edited by SH Zarit. New York: Harper and Row, 1977.

46. Neumark D. Providing Information About Advance Directives to Patients in Ambulatory Care and Their Families. *Nursing Forum* 1994; **21 (4)**.

47. Hensel W. A Piece of My Mind — My Living Will. *JAMA* 1996, **275 (8)**.

48. Holden C. Nutrition and Hydration in the Terminally Ill Cancer Patient. The Nurse's Role in Helping Patients and Families Cope. *Hospice Journal* 1993; **9** (2–3).

49. Root MJ. Communication barriers between older women and physicians. *Pub Health Rep Suppl* **July/Aug**, p. 152, 1987.

50. Libow LS. General concepts of geriatric medicine. In *The Core of Geriatric Medicine. A Guide for Students and Practitioners*, edited by LS Libow, FT Sherman. St. Louis: CV Mosby Co, 1981.

59. Family Caregiving Issues

William E. Haley, Laurie A. Ehrbar and Ronald S. Schonwetter

Introduction

Family caregiving for older adults is receiving increasing attention as an issue central to research, clinical care, and policy related to chronic illness (1). Caregiving research has grown dramatically due to several demographic changes (2). Increasing life expectancies, with a resulting higher prevalence of a number of chronic illnesses, have led to more older Americans unable to care for themselves. Furthermore, people tend to live longer with these chronic ailments due to medical advances and due to a steadily increasing life expectancy among those surviving to old age (3). Families commonly prefer to care for disabled relatives themselves, and older adults are usually highly motivated to remain in their homes even with illness and disability. There are additional pressures for families to provide caregiving due to the limits of community services, and the high financial burden associated with hospital and nursing home care. These changes have resulted in more families, particularly spouses and adult daughters, assuming the role of caregivers.

Home care may be seen as a way of reducing expenditures and humanizing the effects of chronic and terminal illness by allowing patients to remain at home; however, these benefits may come at a cost to the caregiver. Caregiving may lead to "hidden" costs of care that are borne by family members, such as negative effects on psychological, social, or physical health functioning (4,5). Since caregivers may experience adverse effects, attention to caregiving issues is important in understanding how this major, unpaid segment of our health care and long-term care system works and what we can do to minimize the burdens of caregiving.

While a variety of chronic conditions precipitate families into the caregiving role, the majority of research within this area has focused on caregivers of elderly patients with Alzheimer's disease (AD) and other forms of dementia (2,5–7). This is unfortunate because policy, practice, and research have neglected special caregiving issues associated with other illnesses. Cancer is highly prevalent and a leading cause of death in late life, with age emerging as a primary risk for the subsequent diagnosis of cancer (8) Compared to men and women in their mid-forties to mid-sixties, the incidence of cancer quadruples among elderly men and doubles among elderly women (8). By 2030, cancer prevalence is projected at over six million elderly adults (8). The rising rate of cancer among this increasing population will affect the number of families assuming responsibility for these family members. This trend is apparent in the growing number of articles concerning family caregiving issues; however, there has not been extensive, systematic research conducted on cancer caregivers (9).

Until recently, most psychosocial work in oncology focused on the patient, rather than the caregiver (10). Although some caregiving stressors may be similar between AD and cancer, there are likely to be several vastly different stressors that heighten the danger of overgeneralizing from one illness to another. In general, research suggests that dementia caregiving leads to greater ill effects for the caregiver (11,12), or equivalent effects (13,14). However, given the various forms of cancer, and the greatly differing issues faced by caregivers at varying stages of cancer, it would be premature to assume that cancer has a lesser impact on family members.

The present chapter will provide an overview of the field of caregiving research, emphasizing a stress process model as an organizing theme. General findings from the field of caregiving research will be presented, including available information on issues specific to caregiving for older cancer patients. A number of issues that have received considerable attention in the literature on caregiving, such as the stresses of caregiving, possible mediators within the stress process model, mental and physical health outcomes of caregiving, interventions for caregivers, and issues around bereavement will also be addressed, to provide direction for future work on cancer caregiving.

The Stress Process Model of Caregiving

Drawing from broader investigations in the field of stress and coping (15), family caregiving for chronically ill relatives has been viewed as an example of a major life stress which individuals adjust to with a variety of coping mechanisms. Stress process models of caregiving, widely applied to AD caregiving, typically focus on the specific stressors produced by the patient's illness, the caregiver's appraisals of these stressors, how the caregiver copes with these stressors, the extent and perceived quality of their social support system, and how the caregiver is affected by these stressors (2,6,7,16). Similar stress process models have been discussed in the context of cancer (17,18), but have been applied predominantly to the patient response to stress rather than the caregiver. Much of the current research on cancer caregiving has been atheoretical or focused on a specific aspect of the stress process, rather than utilizing a comprehensive stress process model. Fundamental to these stress process models is that there are marked individual differences in reactions to caregiving. Some caregivers react with depression, poor health, or feel substantial burden, while other families show little or no negative impact (and may even report benefits from caregiving).

Within a stress process model, common caregiving stressors include caring for the disabilities that accompany illness, or coordinating medical regimens. Objective measures of caregiving stressors' severity are commonly found to predict surprisingly little variance in caregiver well-being, suggesting that mediating variables deserve attention (4,6,7) Appraisals, another component of this model, include the caregiver's subjective perceptions of the patient's problems and the acceptability of recent changes in the caregiver's life due to the demands of caregiving (6,7,19,20). Another element of this model includes the coping responses of the caregiver. These can include such efforts as problem solving, emotional discharge, and seeking information (21). Social support is another widely studied potential mediator of caregiving stress, with the premise that a larger and more supportive social network would assist caregivers (22). Other potential mediators of stress have also been described, including financial resources, and the availability of formal and informal help.

Studies assessing the outcome of caregiving commonly include an assessment of the caregiver's well-being, including outcomes such as the caregiver's mental and physical health. More recent work on caregiving has also examined positive outcomes of caregiving, including improvement on measures of the caregiver's level of mastery, satisfaction, marital communication (23), and other perceived benefits of caregiving.

These factors within the stress process model will now be reviewed. When possible, we highlight knowledge about caregiving specific to cancer; when necessary, we emphasize research drawn from other areas and suggest future directions for research in cancer caregiving.

The Stressors

Primary stressors of caregiving include stressors that directly relate to caregiving tasks, such as assisting the patient with daily dependencies, managing the patient's symptoms including their treatment related side-effects, and handling the behavior problems or emotional reactions of the patient. As noted by Sales *et al.* (24), researchers studying cancer caregiving have used a variety of indices to estimate the severity of caregiving stressors, including stage of illness, prognosis, demands of caregiving, duration of illness, site of cancer, and patient distress (24). Greater caregiver distress has generally been found to be associated with more advanced cancer, higher caregiving demands, and elevated patient distress. However, few existing projects have included a number of desirable methodological features, such as a longitudinal follow-up of caregiving families through the progression of cancer symptoms and caregiving. Another limitation of this work is that

it is unclear what mechanisms might be involved with a given stressor, e.g. prognosis may be a marker for the caregiver having more caregiving tasks, versus an indication of anticipatory grieving.

One tactic used to study caregiving stressors includes identifying specific caregiving tasks or patient behaviors and then evaluating the prevalence of these demands. For example, having the caregivers report the number of activities the patient requires assistance with is one measure of primary stressors. Typically, these measures include the Activities of Daily Living (ADL), which include tasks such as dressing and bathing, and the Instrumental Activities of Daily Living (IADL), which include tasks such as shopping or meal preparation (25,26). Many studies that have examined the burdens cancer caregivers face combine patients with different cancer diagnoses, even though these self-care behaviors may vary greatly for patients with varying disease stages (i.e. metastasized cancer often entails more management due to the possibility of multiple organs being impaired). In Sales *et al.*'s review (24), the literature supports the notion that greater psychosocial problems, such as an increased sense of being overwhelmed, more impaired family relations, and greater mood disturbances, arise when cancer metastasizes.

A major primary stressor that has emerged in dementia caregiving is the patients' disruptive behavioral problems. In dementia caregiving, research has extensively described the prevalence of these primary stressors and there are well-validated measures of these dementia-specific primary caregiving stressors (27,28). Although behavioral problems were less common in one cancer caregiving project, these problems were described as the most difficult, upsetting, tiring, and hardest to manage among caregivers of terminally ill elderly patients (29). In general, this research suggests that severity of patient self-care impairments has relatively little direct relationship to caregiver well-being, but that patient behavioral problems are more likely to be related to caregiver depression and burden (4). Kurtz *et al.* (30) reported that cancer patient symptoms indirectly predict caregiving depression, mediated by patient depression, again suggesting that the provision of physical care is less important in predicting caregivers' distress than the potential "emotional contagion" (4) of assisting a distressed relative.

A few studies assessing the impact of cancer on caregivers have shown that certain stressor factors place caregivers at risk for adverse effects. For example, Jensen and Given (31) found that caregivers experience greater fatigue when their schedules become more burdened (the demands and expectations placed upon them have increased). Other researchers have also found that relatives of cancer patients have poorer psychological well-being (high anxiety levels, mood disturbance, and overall mental health) during palliative care than active treatment or follow-up periods (32,33). Palliative care is typically associated with impending bereavement, aimed at comforting the patient rather than battling the cancer.

Older cancer patients may have self-care impairments that increase the need for caregiving assistance, but they rarely display the disruptive behavioral problems that are seen in dementia patients unless additionally burdened with cognitive impairment or delirium. However, cancer caregivers face a number of other stressors which are extremely difficult, but have not been systematically characterized. Many of these occur because cancer patients may be undergoing aggressive treatment regimens aimed at either palliative care, cure, or the remission of cancer. For example, depending on the type of cancer, family caregivers may coordinate and witness complex medical regimens, such as chemotherapy, in an ambulatory or home setting. Family caregivers may also be responsible for escorting their loved one to radiation or chemotherapy sessions, and must assist the patient in coping with treatment-related side-effects, such as nausea and vomiting. Caregivers also face increasing stressors related to newer treatments such as infusion therapy in the home, given that they may face exposure to toxic drugs that represent a biological hazard (34). These diverse stressors need to be systematically studied in order to understand the role that primary stressors may have upon caregivers' mental and physical health outcomes.

Terminal care provides other unique stressors. Family caregivers must deal not only with special in-home care tasks, but also with managing the death of their relative, including such sensitive aspects as closing the eyes upon death or dealing with material expelled upon death (35). Most of the published reports that do examine possible stressors of cancer caregiving are descriptive and lack a measure that quantifies the broad range of caregiving stressors that are involved in cancer care. Existing research suggests that assisting with self-care tasks, managing patient symptoms (36) and the treatment regime (37), and witnessing the suffering of the relative with cancer (38) are major stressors identified by cancer caregivers. Future research that could better quantify common caregiving stressors faced by families of older cancer patients would be quite valuable in providing an objective measurement of the daily caregiving stressors faced by these families.

Finally, caregiving can also lead to secondary stressors such as role strain, strains on finances and employment, changes in family structure and other areas due to providing care to the patient, and intrapsychic strains, or changes in the caregiver's self-concept (2). These are "spillover" effects which can occur, but may not universally occur. Contextual stressors include the difficulties that the caregiver is exposed to in the environment, independent of caregiving. As Aneshendel et al. (39) note, the difficulties faced by caregivers do not occur in a vacuum. Existing reports support that finances, managing the household, alterations in roles, and employment changes (36,37) are secondary stressors identified as problems by cancer caregivers.

Appraisals of Stress

Appraisals of caregiving stress have generally been measured in two ways. First, caregivers may be asked to report on their subjective appraisals of specific caregiving tasks, such as managing incontinence or dressing the patient (40). Such ratings have been used in concert with scales assessing primary caregiving stressors, e.g. by asking caregivers to rate the subjective stressfulness of each caregiving problem. Such studies generally show that self-care problems are rated as mildly to moderately stressful by families, with incontinence emerging as the most distressing self-care impairment. Disruptive behavioral problems, which include agitation, wandering, and dangerous behaviors, are common in patients with cognitive impairments and are rated as highly stressful by families (40). Families also report that patient depression is highly stressful to the caregiver (27). In general, subjective appraisals of caregiving stressors have been found to be more predictive of caregiver burden and depression than objective severity of patient illness (41).

Another tactic to assess caregiver appraisal focuses on appraisal of the general circumstance of caregiving. Lawton and his colleagues (42) utilized measures of appraisal that included caregivers' sense of satisfaction from caregiving, perceived burden, caregiving mastery, and caregiving as an intrusion. These measures allow for the assessment of the caregiver's reaction to all caregiving stressors, rather than individual stressors.

There has been some effort to study cancer caregivers' appraisals of their general circumstances. Stetz (37), using a measure of caregivers' general appraisal of the demands of caregiving, found that female cancer caregivers appraised greater strain than did male caregivers. Oberst, Gass, and Ward (43) found that cancer caregivers appraised the challenges of caregiving (i.e., meeting responsibilities, managing problems, creating solutions), as the most stressful area of caregiving on the Appraisal of Caregiving Scale (ACS). Carey et al. (44) reported that a negative appraisal of the caregiving situation mediated the relationship between caregiver burden and patient dependency; however, most caregivers in their study appraised caregiving as challenging, benign, or beneficial rather than as negative.

Little is known about the role of appraising specific stressors in caregiving for older patients with cancer. While some primary stressors, including patient ADL and IADL impairment, and patient depression, are common to AD and cancer caregiving, the different problems specific to cancer deserve greater attention. As noted above, the development of measures of primary caregiving stressors in cancer is quite important, and these could include assessments of caregiver appraisals as well. For example, an instrument that could assess the prevalence and appraised stressfulness of cancer caregiving stressors would be valuable.

Social Support and Activity

Extensive literature has suggested that social supports are valuable in coping with a variety of life stresses (22). Research on AD caregiving has shown that being a caregiver does not diminish the objective size of the social support network, but significantly reduces caregivers' perceived satisfaction with their levels of social support (45,46). Caregiving in AD also leads to a clear reduction in social activities for the caregiver, including visiting others outside of the home, lowered church attendance, and decreased formal social activities (45,46). In turn, smaller numbers of social supports, lower satisfaction with support, and fewer social activities have been found to be predictive of greater caregiver depression (6,41). As caregiving continues over a long period of time, changes in social support may become persistent and resistant to recovery even when caregiving ends (47).

Research on cancer caregiving and social support has been surprisingly sparse (9). Most of the research has focused on examining the impact of cancer on the patient's supportive network, neglecting the caregiver's social support. The few studies available suggest that family caregivers of cancer patients experience a lack of perceived support from family members and the medical staff (34,38,48). Northouse (48) found an inverse relationship between spouses' of mastectomy patients scores on social support, measured with the researcher's Social Support Questionnaire (SSQ), and the spouses' level of adjustment scores, measured by the Psychosocial Adjustment to Illness Scale (PAIS) (49). Spouses with lower levels of social support had more difficulty adjusting than those husbands with a higher level of social support. A longitudinal study (50) found that low levels of perceived social support predicted poor functioning in the caregiver.

Disruption of daily routines and reduced socializing by cancer caregivers was examined in a recent project (51) This study suggested that over half of cancer caregivers report disruption of their daily routines, with older caregivers reporting significantly fewer disruptions. Over half of the caregivers also reported reduced socializing with neighbors, friends, and others due to the demands of caregiving.

There is an important need for future cancer caregiving research to better specify the consequences of caregiving on the various dimensions of social activity and social support. For example, size of the social network, subjective satisfaction with the network, engaging in visits with family and friends, and opportunities for more structured social activities may all be diminished by caregiving. Comparison with noncaregiving groups would also be advantageous in allowing for estimates of the impact of caregiving beyond changes due to other factors, such as aging. It is important to recognize that the patterns of social support established during caregiving may have important implications for subsequent adjustment of the caregiver during bereavement in the case of terminally ill patients (47).

Coping

In recognition that life stress does not simply act on passive individuals, stress researchers have characterized the coping responses used in a variety of life stresses. A general taxonomy of coping includes approach coping, or efforts to directly face the stress through such means as seeking out information or problem solving, versus avoidance coping, which includes efforts to ignore problems, or wishful thinking

(21). While avoidance coping may be effective in reducing distress in the short run, in general, research finds that caregivers who use approach coping more extensively have better psychological adjustment (15).

Coping responses of family caregivers of patients with cancer have been characterized in a number of studies (9), but these studies have been more focused on description of typical coping responses than on identifying which coping responses are more adaptive. For example, a study by Hull (52) described several coping mechanisms used by a small sample of caregivers that were followed longitudinally. These strategies included: avoidance, cognitive reformulation, acceptance, rationalization, social comparisons, and "windows of time," or breaks in caregiving duties. Recently, several studies have reported the benefits derived from the caregiver's level of optimism as a coping mechanism. More optimistic caregivers appear less depressed and appraise the caregiving situation as having less of an impact upon their health and schedule than caregivers who scored low on optimism (30). Given et al. (53) also reported that the caregiver's disposition of optimism predicted the caregiver's mental health status and their reactions to caregiving. In other words, optimism appears to play an important role in helping caregivers adapt to the stressors of caregiving and may play a valuable role in designing interventions (53).

Several studies have identified particular variables that are similar to some aspects of the coping construct; for example, studies have assessed the extent to which prognosis is openly discussed with the patient. Generally, families that communicate more openly with a terminal cancer patient tend to adjust better following bereavement (54,55). A study by Schumacher et al (56). reported that the caregiver's perceived efficacy of coping strategies mediated the relationship between depression and strain, providing support for the stress process model; however, these researchers acknowledge the limitations of having only one item assessing coping strategies. Future research needs to pay greater attention to assessing which caregivers' coping mechanisms are empirically associated with better caregiving adjustment.

Mental and Physical Health Outcomes

There is strong evidence that caregiving leads to an increased risk for depression, and conflicting evidence suggesting a risk to the physical health of the caregiver (4,5). Depression has been found to have a higher prevalence in AD caregivers than in noncaregivers or population norms across most studies (4,5).

Physical health measures have not yielded consistent results across studies. Several studies suggest that caregivers have poorer health than noncaregivers or normative data (45,57–59), but results have been inconsistent (4). The lack of consistent results in the area of physical health is likely due in part to the difficulty in accurately measuring health through questionnaires, and the diverse groups of caregivers often included in studies. Several projects that have focused on specific subgroups of caregivers (e.g. older spouses, employed daughters) have found higher ambulatory blood pressure during episodes of caregiving (60), or altered immune function in caregivers (58).

An important caveat is that most of this research has been applied to dementia patients. The few studies that have attempted to assess the mental and physical health impact of caregiving for relatives with cancer have not detected marked negative effects. For example, in Sales *et al.*'s (24) review, several researchers indicate that most family members do not develop clinically problematic levels of emotional distress when coping with the demands of cancer. However, there are some families that do have difficult handling the impact of cancer. Mor and his colleagues (51) reported rates of depression in cancer caregivers that are somewhat higher than population norms, but are lower than rates found in AD caregivers. However, another recent study (61) reported substantial levels of depression among cancer caregivers. Hinds (38) reported that the percentage of families that would benefit from supportive services was greater than 30%.

However, research is lacking that includes a comparison of cancer caregivers on a broad range of physical and mental health outcomes with appropriate noncaregiving comparison groups — which would allow for clearer assessment of the potential impact of the stress of caregiving on caregiver well-being. The rather mixed findings on depression in cancer caregivers suggests that certain subgroups of cancer caregivers need to be identified based on risk factors for depression. For example, cancer caregivers' depression has been shown to relate to patient depression, which is strongly predicted by their symptoms, and to a lesser extent, their immobility (30).

Some caregivers do report benefits from the caregiving experience. For example, one study of men who survived testicular cancer found that the men and their wives experienced improvements in a number of dimensions of marital outcomes, including increased intimacy, as a result of the experience of coping with cancer (23) Further attention to perceived benefits, such as satisfaction from caregiving, may be particularly important in understanding ethnic differences in response to caregiving. Several studies (42,46) have reported that African-American caregivers of patients with AD report lower levels of distress, and higher levels of satisfaction and mastery related to caregiving, than do white families. It is unknown whether such ethnic differences are also found in the context of cancer.

Interventions for Caregivers

Because of the widely documented impact of AD caregiving on family members' depression, a variety of psychosocial interventions have been developed to enhance caregiver adjustment (62). These interventions have included support groups, individual and family interventions, and respite care. Besides descriptive studies of these programs, a good deal of work has provided systematic evaluation of the efficacy of these interventions for AD caregivers on such variables as caregiver well-being, and delaying institutionalization of the patient (63).

Support groups, although widely available and commonly very well-received by participants, have been found to lead to relatively little objective improvement in caregiver mental health (63). Caregivers often report such benefits as gaining information, or satisfaction from knowing that others share their problems, but the typical formats of support groups are not focused or intensive enough to successfully combat caregiver depression. Recent research has shown that group interventions which are more focused on teaching caregivers specific skills, such as anger management or increasing life satisfaction, have a greater impact on caregiver well-being (64). Other studies have shown that intensive individualized caregiver interventions not only decrease caregiver depression, but can delay nursing home placement (65). Evaluations of respite care programs have generally found that caregivers are highly satisfied with these programs, but they do not appear to significantly delay institutionalization or decrease caregiver depression (66).

A variety of psychosocial interventions have been developed which are relevant for cancer caregivers. Most of these intervention programs primarily target and evaluate the impact upon the patient with cancer (9), whereas the caregiver benefits have often been thought of as secondary. In particular, support groups, which usually include both the patient and the family caregiver, are increasing in popularity. However, there are few studies available evaluating the impact of these support groups on the cancer caregiver. A number of other caregiver educational intervention programs have been widely disseminated, but they have not been systematically evaluated in terms of their impact on objective caregiver adjustment measures. One randomized study of counseling for spouse caregivers of patients with lung cancer found no evidence that counseling led to greater change than a control group, although most of the patients and significant others were adapting well, leaving little room for improvement on the measures used in this study (67). Another individualized intervention that introduced problem solving skills to aid cancer caregivers did not find greater improvement in the treatment group and the control group on a broad range of psychosocial measures. However, many of the caregivers in this project were found to have relatively low levels of caregiving activities, and the authors suggest that greater benefits of intervention were found among a highly distressed subsample of caregivers (61).

Bereavement Issues

Since caregiving is highly stressful, some have thought that the end of caregiving might afford family members some relief after what is often a lengthy and highly stressful process. However, the available research suggests that caregivers may experience long-term sequelae after long-standing efforts at caregiving. When caregiving ends with the death of a relative, another major life stress begins: bereavement. The bereavement process may be made more difficult by the depletion of the caregivers' resources, alterations in their social supports and activities, and the lingering reminders of caregiving and loss. In one unique longitudinal project, Bodnar and Kiecolt-Glaser (47) found that, even after four years after the death of a relative with dementia, caregivers as a group reported levels of depression as high as when they had active caregiving responsibilities. Of interest is that two factors were found to be particularly predictive of continued distress: low levels of social support and high levels of rumination (repetitive thinking) about the caregiving situation. In another project (68) it was found that family strain during caregiving predicted greater subsequent distress after the death of the patient.

Cancer caregiving may also lead to such troublesome problems for bereaved caregivers (69). It appears likely that caregivers who become socially isolated or depressed after lengthy caregiving duties may have similar problems in resolving their grief and resuming an active life. For example, Mullan (70) suggests that caregiving can lead to problems during subsequent bereavement when psychological or social resources, that could assist with adjustment to bereavement, became depleted through the process of caregiving. It is noteworthy that one recent report (71) found that depression among bereaved spouses commonly begins six months before the death of the spouse, which may be related to anticipatory grief or the strains of caregiving.

A number of interventions have been used to assist families with the grieving process, including support groups, and family support offered through hospice programs. While such interventions appear promising, future research needs to more rigorous in assessing the impact of interventions on the long-term outcome of bereavement. Clinical experience tends to support the value of hospice bereavement services (72), but these benefits have been difficult to document with objective evidence (73). Of particular interest in the current context is whether psychosocial intervention during caregiving might prevent complications in the bereavement process. Many hospice programs attend to such issues by beginning bereavement counseling before the patient's actual death (73). Several recently developed measures assessing quality of life for patients and caregivers in the hospice setting appear promising in evaluating these interventions for hospice families (74). The impact of such intervention needs further research.

Implications for Health Care Delivery

Geriatric medical care has been described as differing from the typical care of younger adults because of the common inclusion of a triad of doctor, patient, and caregiver (75). In efforts to focus on the care of older patients with cancer, it is important to realize that the family member is much more than the person who delivers the patient for treatment. With older adults, the family caregiver is often an essential informant about patient status, and necessary to the implementation of any treatment regimen. Attention to caregiver concerns and distress is thus essential to successful comprehensive care of these patients. The American Medical Association Council on Scientific Affairs has recently released a statement strongly urging the formation of partnerships between physicians and family caregivers in the care of older adults (76). While not specific to oncology, the paper outlines a number of specific ways that physicians and other health care providers can improve care for older adults by recognizing the family context of late-life disease. For example, families greatly appreciate such simple assistance as brochures and referrals to information services. Caregivers of older patients often need referrals to community agencies. Family caregivers also value some acknowledgment from health care providers of the valuable and often heroic efforts made in caregiving, and attention to the caregiver's distress. Other recommendations specific to the context of cancer caregiving are provided in another report (77). This ideal of viewing the family, rather than just the patient (or their disease) as the target of treatment is currently difficult to attain in many settings, but should be a primary goal in geriatric care.

Summary and Future Directions

Family caregivers provide largely hidden care that is essential to the well-being of cancer patients, sometimes at a significant personal cost. More research focusing on the problems of cancer caregivers, using stronger methodologies, is clearly needed, in order to better understand the needs and concerns of these family caregivers. Since this is a relatively recent area of exploration, most of the research that has been conducted on cancer caregiving for older patients is limited methodologically, in terms of small, convenience samples collected at one point in time, across various types of cancer, with a primary focus on terminal patients (78). One high priority for future research in this area should be identification of cancer caregivers who are at risk for depression, so that these families can be targeted for services. The literature reviewed above points to factors likely to place cancer caregivers at risk: a combination of high levels of caregiving stressors, coupled with poorer social supports and/or maladaptive appraisals and coping responses. In terms of intervention, systematic evaluation of the efficacy of caregiver interventions will be important in improving these services, and justifying their existence in a cost-drive system of care. Intervention studies should target cancer caregivers who show evidence of significant depression, or risk factors for depression; previous research has shown that many caregivers cope well without special intervention programs. Attention to family caregivers is important not only because of the potential human costs that caregivers experience, but also because unpaid family caregivers are an essential part of the health care system that is being strained by efforts to cut costs, often by increasing demands on family members. Better information on the costs of caregiving, and on factors that help caregivers adjust better to the potentially overwhelming task of caring for a loved one at home, is essential.

References

1. Kane RA, Penrod J. *Aging and Family Caregiving Policy*. Newbury Park: Sage, 1995.
2. Pearlin LI, Mullan JT, Semple SJ, Skaf MM. Caregiving and the stress process: An overview of concepts and their measures. *Gerontologist* 1990; **30**: 583–594.
3. U.S. Senate. *Aging America: Trends and Projections*. Department of Health and Human Services. DHHS publication No. (FCOA) 91-28001. Washington, D.C., 1991.
4. Schulz R, O'Brien AT, Bookwala J, Fleissner K. Psychiatric and physical morbidity effects of dementia caregiving: Prevalence, correlates, and causes. *Gerontologist* 1995; **35**: 771–791.
5. Schulz R, Visintainer P, Williamson GM. Psychiatric and physical morbidity effects of caregiving. *J Gerontol* 1990; **45**: 181–191.
6. Haley WE, Levine EG, Brown SL, Bartolucci AA. Stress, appraisal, coping, and social support as predictors of adaptational outcome among dementia caregivers. *Psychol Aging* 1987; **2**: 323–330.
7. Gatz M, Bengtson, VL, Blum MJ. Caregiving families. In *Handbook of the Psychology of Aging, Third Edition*, edited by JE Birren, KW Schaie. San Diego: Academic Press, pp. 404–426, 1990.
8. Schonwetter RS. Geriatric oncology. *Cancer Epidemiol Prev Screening* 1992; **19**: 451–463.
9. Clark JC, Gwin RR. Psychosocial responses of the family. In *Cancer Nursing: Principles and Practice*, edited by SL Groenwald, MH Frogge, M Goodman, CH Yarbro. Boston: Jones and Bartlett, pp. 468–483, 1993.
10. Cassileth BR, Chou JN. Psychosocial issues in the older patient with cancer. In *Geriatric Oncology*, edited by L Balducci, GH Lyman, WB Ershler. New York: J.B. Lippincott Co., pp. 311–319, 1992.
11. Clipp EC, George LK. Dementia and cancer: A comparison of spouse caregivers. *Gerontologist* 1993; **33**: 534–541.
12. Krizek-Karlin N, Bell PA. Self-efficacy, affect, and seeking support between caregivers of dementia and non-dementia patients. *J Women Aging* 1992; **4**: 59–78.
13. Rabins PV, Fitting MD, Eastham J, Fetting J. The emotional impact of caring for the chronically ill. *Psychosomatics* 1990; **31**: 331–336.
14. Stommel M, Wang S, Given CW, Given B. Confirmatory factor analysis (CFA) as a method to assess measurement equivalence. *Res Nurs Health* 1992; **15**: 399–405.
15. Lazarus RS, Folkman S. *Stress, Appraisal, and Coping*. New York: Springer, 1984.
16. Vitaliano PP, Russo J, Young HM, Teri L, Maiuro RD. Predictors of burden in spouse caregivers of individuals with Alzheimer's disease. *Psychol Aging* 1991; **6**: 392–402.
17. McGee RF. Overview: Psychosocial aspects of cancer. In *Cancer Nursing: Principles and Practice*, edited by SL Groenwald, MH Frogge, M Goodman, CH Yarbro. Boston: Jones and Bartlett, pp. 437–448, 1993.
18. Jacobsen PB, Holland JC. The stress of cancer: Psychological responses to diagnosis and treatment. In *Cancer and Stress: Psychological, Biological and Coping Studies*, edited by CL Cooper, M Watson. New York: John Wiley & Sons, pp. 147–169, 1991.
19. Zarit SH. Issues and directions in family intervention research. In *Alzheimer's Disease Treatment and Family Stress: Directions for Research*, edited by E Light, BD Lebowitz. National Institute of Mental Health. DHHS publication No. ADM 89-1569. Washington, D.C., 1989.
20. Niedereche G, Fruge E. Dementia and family dynamics: Clinical research issues. *J Geriatr Psychiatry* 1984; **17**: 21–56.
21. Moos RH, Cronkite R, Billings A, Finney J. *Health and Daily Living Form Manual*. Palto Alto: Social Ecology Laboratory, Stanford University and Department of Veteran's Affairs Medical Centers, 1984.
22. Sarason BR, Sarason IG, Pierce GR. *Social Support: An Interactional View*. New York: John Wiley & Sons, 1990.
23. Gritz ER, Wellish DK, Siau J, Wang HJ. Long-term effects of testicular cancer on marital relationships. *Psychosomatics* 1990; **31**: 301–312.
24. Sales E, Schulz R, Biegal D. Predictors of strain in families of cancer patients: A review of the literature. *J Psychosoc Oncol* 1992; **10**: 1–26.
25. Katz S, Ford AB, Moskowitz RW, Jackson BA, Jaffe MW. Studies of illness in the aged. The index of ADL: A standardized measure of biological and psychological function. *JAMA* 1963; **185**: 914–919.
26. Lawton M, Brody E. Assessment of older people: Self-maintaining and instrumental activities of daily living. *Gerontologist* 1969; **9**: 179–186.
27. Teri L, Truax P, Logsdon R, Uomoto J, Zant S, Vitaliano PP. Assessment of behavioral problems in dementia: The revised memory and behavior problems checklist. *Psychol Aging* 1992; **7**: 622–631.
28. O'Leary PA, Haley WE, Paul PB. Behavioral assessment in Alzheimer's Disease: Use of a 24-hour log. *Psychol Aging* 1993; **8**: 139–143.
29. Yang C, Kirschling JM. Exploration of factors related to direct care and outcomes of caregiving: Caregivers of terminally ill older persons. *Cancer Nurs* 1992; **15**: 173–181.
30. Kurtz ME, Kurtz JC, Given CW, Given B. Relationship of caregiver reactions and depression to cancer patients' symptoms, functional states and depression — a longitudinal view. *Soc Sci Med* 1995; **40**: 837–846.
31. Jensen S, Given BA. Fatigue affecting family caregivers of cancer patients. *Cancer Nurs* 1991; **14**: 181–187.
32. Cassileth B, Lusk E, Brown L, Cross P. Psychosocial status of cancer patients and next-of-kin: Normative data from POMS. *J Psychosoc Oncol* 1985; **3**: 99–105.
33. Cassileth BR, Lusk E, Strouse T, Miller D, Brown L, Cross P. A psychological analysis of cancer patients and their next-of-kin. *Cancer* 1985; **55**: 72–76.
34. McNally JC. Home care. In *Cancer Nursing: Principles and Practice*, edited by SL Groenwald, MH Frogge, M Goodman, CH Yarbro. Boston: Jones and Bartlett, pp. 1403–1431, 1993.
35. Hine V. Dying at home: Can families cope? *Omega* 1979–1980; **10**: 175–186.
36. Blank JJ, Longman, AJ, Atwood JR. Perceived home care needs of cancer patients and their caregivers. *Cancer Nurs* 1989; **12**: 78–84.
37. Stetz KM. Caregiving demands during advanced cancer. *Cancer Nurs* 1987; **10**: 260–268.
38. Hinds C. The needs of families who care for patients with cancer at home: Are we meeting them? *J Adv Nurs* 1985; **10**: 575–581.
39. Aneshendel CS, Pearlin LI, Mullan JT, Zarit SH, Whitlatch CJ. *Profiles in Caregiving: The Unexpected Career*. San Diego: Academic Press, 1995.
40. Haley WE, Brown SL, Levine EG. Family caregiver appraisals of patient behavioral disturbance in senile dementia. *Clin Gerontol* 1987; **6**: 25–34.
41. Haley WE, Roth DL, Coleton MI, Ford GR, West CAC, Collins RP, Isobe TL. Appraisal, coping, and social support as mediators of well-being in Black and White Alzheimer's family caregivers. *J Consult Clin Psychol* 1996; **64**: 121–129.
42. Lawton MP, Rajagopal D, Brody E, Kleban MH. The dynamics of caregiving for a demented elder among black and white families. *J Gerontol: Soc Sci* 1992; **47**: S156–S164.
43. Oberst MT, Gass KA, Ward SE. Caregiving demands and appraisal of stress among family caregivers. *Cancer Nurs* 1989; **12**: 209–215.
44. Carey PJ, Oberst MT, McCubbin MA, Hughes SH. Appraisal and caregiving burden in family members caring for patients receiving chemotherapy. *Oncol Nurs Forum* 1991; **18**: 1341–1348.

45. Haley WE, Levine EG, Brown SL, Berry JW, Hughes GH. Psychological, social, and health consequences of caring for a relative with senile dementia. *J Am Geriatr Soc* 1987; **35**: 405–411.

46. Haley WE, West CAC, Wadley VG, Ford GR, White FA, Barrett JJ, Harrell LE, Roth DL. Psychological, social, and health impact of caregiving: A comparison of Black and White dementia family caregivers and noncaregivers. *Psychol Aging* 1995; **10**: 540–552.

47. Bodnar JC, Kiecolt-Glaser JK. Caregiver depression after bereavement: Chronic stress isn't over when it's over. *Psychol Aging* 1994; **9**: 372–380.

48. Northouse LL. Social support in patients' and husbands' adjustment to breast cancer. *Nurs Res* 1988; **37**: 91–95.

49. Derogatis LR. *Psychosocial Adjustment to Illness Scale*. Baltimore: Clinical Psychometric Research, 1975.

50. Ell K, Michimoto R, Mantel J, et al. Longitudinal analysis of psychosocial adaptation among family members of patients with cancer. *J Psychosom Res* 1988; **32**: 429–438.

51. Mor V, Allen S, Malin M. The psychosocial impact of cancer on older versus younger patients and their families. *Cancer Suppl* 1994; **74**: 2118–2127.

52. Hull MM. Coping strategies of family caregivers in hospice home care. *Oncol Nurs Forum* 1992; **19**: 1179–1187.

53. Given CW, Stommel M, Given B, Osuch J, Kurtz ME, Kurtz JC. The influence of cancer patients' symptoms and functional states on patients' depression and family caregivers' reaction and depression. *Health Psychol*; **12**: 277–285.

54. Cohen P, Dizenhuz I, Winget C. Family adaptation to terminal illness and death of a parent. *Soc Casework* 1977; **58**: 223–228.

55. Northouse LL, Swain MA. Adjustment of patients and husbands to the initial impact of breast cancer. *Nurs Res* 1987; **36**: 221–225.

56. Schumacher KL, Dodd MJ, Paul SM. The stress process in family caregivers of persons receiving chemotherapy. *Res Nurs Health* 1993; **16**: 395–404.

57. Fuller-Jonap F, Haley WE. Mental and physical health of male caregivers of a spouse with Alzheimer's disease. *J Aging Health* 1995; **7**: 99–118.

58. Kiecolt-Glaser JK, Dura JR, Speicher CE, Trask OJ, Glaser R. Spousal caregivers of dementia victims: Longitudinal changes in immunity and health. *Psychosom Med* 1991; **53**: 345–362.

59. Pruchno RA, Potashnik SL. Caregiving spouses: Physical and mental health in perspective. *J Am Geriatr Soc* 1990; **45**: 697–705.

60. King AC, Oka RK, Young DR. Ambulatory blood pressure and heart rate responses to the stress of work and caregiving in older women. *J Gerontol* 1994; **49**: M239–M245.

61. Toseland RW, Blanchard CG, McCallion P. A problem solving intervention for caregivers of cancer patients. *Soc Sci Med* 1995; **40**: 517–528.

62. Zarit SH, Orr NK, Zarit JM. *The Hidden Victims of Alzheimer's Disease: Families Under Stress*. New York, New York University Press, 1985.

63. Knight BG, Lutzky SM, Macofsky-Urban F. A meta-analytic review of interventions for caregiver distress: Recommendations for future research. *Gerontologist* 1993; **33**: 240–248.

64. Gallagher-Thompson D, DeVries H. "Coping with Frustration" classes: Development and preliminary outcomes with women who care for relatives with dementia. *Gerontologist* 1994; **34**: 548–552.

65. Mittelman MS, Ferris SH, Steinberg G, Shulman E, Mackell JA, Ambinder A, Cohen J. An intervention that delays institutionalization of Alzheimer's disease patients: Treatment of spouse-caregivers. *Geronotologist* 1993; **33**: 730–740.

66. Lawton MP, Brody EM, Saperstein AR. *Respite for Caregivers of Alzheimer's Patients: Research and Practice*. New York: Springer, 1991.

67. Goldberg RJ, Wool MS. Psychotherapy for the spouses of lung cancer patients: Assessment of an intervention. *Psychother Psychosom* 1985; **43**: 141–150.

68. Bass DM, Bowman K. The transition from caregiving to bereavement: The relationship of care-related strain and adjustment to death. *Gerontologist* 1990; **30**: 35–42.

69. McHorney CA, Mor V. Predictors of bereavement depression and its health services consequences. *Medical Care* 1988; **26**: 882–893.

70. Mullan JT. The bereaved caregiver: A prospective study of changes in well-being. *Gerontologist* 1992; **32**: 673–683.

71. Lichtenstein P, Gatz M, Pedersen NL, Berg S, McClearn GE. A Cotwin-control study of response to widowhood. Presented at The Gerontological Society of America, Los Angeles, California, 1995.

72. Longman AJ. Effectiveness of a hospice community bereavement program. *Omega* 1993; **27**: 165–175.

73. Hayslip B Jr, Leon J. *Hospice Care*. Newbury Park: SAGE Publications, 1992.

74. McMillan SC, Mahon M. The impact of hospice services on the quality of life of primary caregivers. *Oncol Nurs Forum* 1994; **21**: 1189–1195.

75. Silliman RA. Caring for the frail older patient: The doctor-patient-family caregiver relationship. *J Gen Intern Med* 1989; **4**: 237–241.

76. Council on Scientific Affairs American Medical Association: Physicians and family caregivers: A model for partnership. *JAMA* 1993; **269**: 1282–1284.

77. Northouse LL, Peters-Golden H. Cancer and the family: Strategies to assist spouses. *Semin Oncol Nurs* 1993; **9**: 74–82.

78. Biegel DE, Sales E, Schulz R. *Family Caregiving in Chronic Illness*. Newbury Park: Sage, 1991.

60. The Case for a Geriatric Oncology Program in a Cancer Center

Janine Overcash

Introduction

The addition of a geriatric oncology program is a beneficial approach to the treatment of cancer in the older person. Cancer is predominately a disease of the old and the aged are quickly becoming the fastest growing cohort in the United States. Data suggest that 50% of all cancers are diagnosed in people 65 and older, and 60% of all cancer deaths occur in people over 65 (1). It is important to explore ways to improve the medical care offered to seniors and a geriatric oncology program is the most effective means to face this challenge. Given the diversity of the older population, a geriatric oncology program may help individualize treatment and research plans to recognize and account for changes that occur in aging (2). The purpose of this chapter is to point out reasons why this type of program is necessary, define the geriatric oncology program concept, identify disciplines included in the program and the roles they perform, the target population served, and some advantages and disadvantages of this type of service.

Definition of a Geriatric Oncology Program

A geriatric oncology program is a team of professionals that specialize in the care of the older person with cancer (Table 60.1). A program includes a variety of disciplines that contribute to a specific aspect of the assessment which result in interventions established in the plan of care. These professionals work together to assess the patient and family, develop a plan, and provide continued follow-up care even beyond anticipated therapy. The program is also useful in intervening with caregiving concerns, addressing patient and family needs that may be appropriate for referral to community resources and providing continued emotional support.

Much of the assessment provided by the geriatric program is coordinated through the use of a Comprehensive Geriatric Assessment (CGA) commonly used in geriatric medicine. The CGA will be discussed in further detail later in this chapter. After the assessment process has been completed, it is important for the team, or program members, to collaborate on the establishment of a treatment plan for the patient, family and/or the caregiver. A holistic approach is essential, because the treatment of the older person with cancer is influenced by comorbidities, functional status, financial issues, transportation problems and caregiving concerns as well as from the diagnosis and stage of cancer. It would be unwise to formulate an elaborate treatment plans for the patient if basic services such as transportation are not available. In a study looking at the functional status and social support networks of people over 65 with a diagnosis of cancer, it was concluded that poor functional status and diminished social support networks may explain why many older cancer patients do not receive adequate medical attention (3). The geriatric team is very effective in addressing these considerations and networking with various resources.

The following case presentations are situations in which a geriatric oncology program proved beneficial in the care of the older person with cancer. The Senior Adult Oncology Program mentioned in the presentation is a geriatric oncology program established at the H. Lee Moffitt Cancer Center and Research Institute in Tampa, Florida.

Mr. B. is a 83 year old gentleman with basal cell and squamous cell carcinoma of the skin, diagnosed in 1984. He had several lesions removed in 1984 and received no further treatment at that time. The patient presented to the Senior Adult Oncology Program with a 6 × 6 right mandibular mass that the patient states appeared in mid September over a very short period of time. The patient also presented with a 4cm bleeding ulceration to the right aspect of his forehead which he states has been draining for several months. Upon assessment by the Senior Adult Oncology Social Worker, it was revealed that patient lived alone, had limited income and no means of transportation. The patient had not received medical care for several years and stated that he was aware of his declining health and just expected to die in his home because he had no means of receiving medical attention. The patient was only able to receive medical attention, after a neighbor witnessed Mr. B's failing health and made the arrangements for an evaluation at the cancer center. A nutritional assessment by the program dietitian revealed a poor diet of conven-

Table 60.1 Program members.

- Medical Oncologist/Geriatrician
- Medical Oncology Fellow
- Geriatric Nurse Practitioner
- Primary Care Nurse
- Pharmacist
- Dietitian
- Social Worker

ience store food (the convenience store was the only store within walking distance) and a 23 lb weight loss over one year. The program pharmacist detected that the patient was not taking any of his medications for hypertension due to lack of transportation to the physician's office and poor financial situation. Physical examination revealed a frail 83 year old gentleman, with soiled clothes, unsteady gait and unable to perform his activities of daily living. After initial workup by the team, the patient was referred to the surgical service for removal of his mandibular tumor which was shown to be a malignant, squamous cell carcinoma and for surgical repair of the ulcer on his forehead. He was also scheduled to receive several courses of radiation therapy following surgery. Interventions established by the Program were to first address patient's lack of transportation and to arrange rides for his daily radiation therapy and follow up office visits. These arrangements were made through the American Cancer Societies' Angel Wings volunteer program as well as the county transportation service. Next, the social worker and the dietitian addressed the issue of malnutrition and arranged for meals to be delivered to patient's home daily at a minimal charge that was well within the patient's financial means. The social worker also helped the patient understand his Medicare benefits and is currently looking into Medicaid services. A home health nurse and aide were provided to perform daily dressing changes after surgery and to assist with activities of daily living. The pharmacist contacted the primary care physician regarding the medication situation and arrangements were made for an office visit to reassess this diagnosis of hypertension and subsequent treatment planning. The Senior Adult Oncology Program has assisted the patient in regaining his optimal level of functioning and therefore maintaining his independence. The patient was able to return home and maintain the lifestyle in which the patient is comfortable.

Another case in which a geriatric oncology program was helpful is the case of Mrs. O.

Mrs. O. is a 84 year old lady that presented to the Senior Adult Oncology Program for her six month follow up visit. In 1988, the patient underwent a right modified radical mastectomy and was shown to have infiltrating ductal carcinoma, with a 2 cm tumor and lymph nodes negative for malignancy. She was maintained on Tamoxifen and underwent radiation therapy following surgery. The patient continues on her Tamoxifen at this time, receives an annual mammogram, and regular follow up visits. Upon assessment by the social worker, the patient states that she is extremely anxious and has difficulty sleeping which is continuing to get worse. The patient states her primary care physician had just prescribed an antianxiety medication for complaints of nervousness and insomnia. Further investigation revealed that patient's husband of 54 years has recently undergone his ninth cardiac artery bypass and has been very ill. The patient has had to be her husband's caregiver as well as a cancer patient and she has no caregiver support. The patient does not drive and she relies on her husband for this service even with his current health situation. Upon review of the case, the team provided recommendations for caregiver support via a community volunteer agency which is able to provide support in the home for approximately 4 hours per day. Transportation was also arranged via a county transportation service so the patient could maintain her follow up visits to monitor her cancer diagnosis. The Program nurse practitioner instructed the patient as to sleep hygiene and nonmedical interventions that could be used to treat the insomnia. Contact was also made with the primary care physician's office, per patient permission, to discuss the support issues the patient and her husband are facing and to establish communication regarding patient's oncology history and treatment. Also in the discussion with the primary care physician's office, was the issue of discontinuing the antianxiety medication and establishing interventions to reduce patient's anxiety such as assistance with caregiving and transportation. The primary care physician agreed to discontinue the medication and to monitor patient's anxiety and complaints of insomnia as well as general health status. Transportation was provided to and from the cancer center so the patient could continue her regular follow up care. The Senior Adult Oncology Program will continue to follow the patient and her husband and will maintain communication with the primary care physician.

How did the geriatric oncology program make a difference in the care of these patients? First, in the case of Mr. B. several issues were uncovered that had an impact on the outcome of cancer therapy, such as transportation, untreated comorbidities, malnutrition, poor financial situation and lack of caregiver support. By performing a holistic assessment, interventions were implemented that made it possible for Mr. B. to receive cancer therapy and to preserve independence. The availability of the various disciplines and immediate treatment planning were beneficial in the cases of both Mr. B. and Mrs. O. in that interventions were established before the emergence of an acute situation such as an emergency hospitalization. In the case of Mrs. O., her cancer diagnosis was not her primary concern, and the source of her anxieties and insomnia were the result of a poor caregiver situation and the lack of adequate transportation services. Proactive interventions were established by the team before more costly and invasive considerations such as nursing home placement were implemented.

As one can see, a geriatric oncology program intervenes on issues other than the diagnosis of cancer. Both case presentations point out the many other challenges confronted by older people diagnosed with cancer. By focusing only on the malignancy, many of the challenges identified in the two case presentations would not have been addressed and an optimal situation for the treatment of cancer would not have been provided.

The purpose of a geriatric oncology program includes: a) to identify and treat the cancer, as well as comorbid conditions that may affect cancer therapy, b) to establish or maintain patient health while undergoing both cancer therapy and cancer follow up, c) to detect and treat any geriatric syndromes (malnutrition, polypharmacy, social isolation), d) to provide psychosocial support for both the patient/family and caregiver, e) to educate patient/families regarding issues related to the cancer diagnosis, f) to educate the community, and, g) to provide a medium of opportunity to enroll the older cancer patient in various clinical trials specifically for seniors.

The program aides not only the patient and families, but the community as well, to provide education and support to older people with and without a diagnosis of cancer. Community elders need to be served by education programs that provide information as to cancer screening recommendations, risk factors and some of the cancer warning signs of which to be aware. Guided tours of the local cancer center may help reduce fears and anxieties associated with a diagnosis of cancer. Cancer is a frightening experience, and hospitals can be intimidating for any patient, and even more so for many senior patients. A geriatric oncology program can help reduce these frightening experiences by making themselves accessible and acting as a resource to provide cancer information to the community.

Table 60.2 Reasons why older people require specialized care.

- Comorbid conditions
- Psychosocial Issues
- Conditions easily missed during routine examination

Rationale for Implementing a Geriatric Oncology Program

Many older adults suffer from more than one medical diagnosis. A diagnosis of cancer is many times just one of a long list of diagnoses that affect the health of an older person. The average number of diagnoses for a person over 70 is five and many older patients do not have an illness that follows a single disease medical model (4). The fact that many older people suffer from comorbid conditions and that the medical model of diagnosis and treatment is not always effective is a primary motivation for the utilization of a geriatric oncology program (Table 60.2).

Another significant rationale for such a program is the increased need for psychosocial support within the senior adult population. Many older patients have a variety of psychosocial issues such as the lack of a caregiver or support person to provide assistance during cancer therapy, poor socioeconomic situation and limited social networks. The social work component of a geriatric oncology program provides interventions for many of these situations encountered by older cancer patients, as well as continued support throughout the experience of cancer. Psychosocial interventions are a large part of what a geriatric program provides and commonly involve disciplines other than social work, all of which contribute to finding solutions for these diverse challenges.

Another goal of a geriatric oncology program is to discover conditions that may not be detected by a routine evaluation. This includes not only comorbid conditions but geriatric syndromes, such as incontinence, poor skin integrity, or confusion, that can be caused by many confounding factors. Polypharmacy, malnutrition and depression are problems commonly missed during routine examination, and these are important medical concerns that can account for many of the signs and symptoms of poor health. Below is a patient/family case that presented to the Senior Adult Oncology Program at the H. Lee Moffitt Cancer Center and Research Institute.

Mrs. C. is a 72 year old lady with a diagnosis of adenocarcinoma of unknown origin who presents to the outpatient clinic for a second opinion regarding further treatment options. She is currently undergoing treatment with chemotherapy by her local oncologist. Mrs. C. has been a very active member of her community until approximately three months ago when she began feeling fatigued. The fatigue correlated with the onset of the chemotherapy administration and no further attention was given to this symptom. Mrs. C. lives with her husband of 25 years and has two very supportive children who live locally and have daily interaction with the patient and her husband. Upon initial assessment Mrs. C. appears upbeat and optimistic regarding her cancer diagnosis and current treatment plan. History reveals no serious illness or surgery throughout her life. The patient is on no medication with the exception of her chemotherapy and an antiemetic when necessary. Physical examination is found to be negative. Upon examination by the Program social worker, the psychosocial history reveals that the patient is coping well with her disease and her family voiced admiration for "keeping such a positive attitude." The social worker, using a geriatric depression screening instrument with only the patient present in the room, reveals a score of 11/15 which does screen positive for depression. Mrs. C. confides with the social worker that she is feeling increasingly depressed each day and finds it more difficult to get out of bed. The patient also shared that she does not want her family aware of her depression, although requests treatment at this time. The patient's primary oncologist was notified of this diagnosis and social support was arranged in her area. The Senior Adult Oncology pharmacist and social worker, together with the Program physician and the local physician, prescribed Amitriptyline 25mg q hs. Mrs. C. will receive regular follow up care with her primary care physician.

This diagnosis may have been undetected, or even masked under the effects of chemotherapy unless the social worker was able to perform a thorough psychosocial assessment, including a screening assessment for depression. The important aspect of this case history is that the patient wanted to be treated for her depression, and wanted, or even needed, to maintain a positive attitude for her family throughout her disease process. Providing privacy for the patient by administering the assessment without the family present, the patient was able to ventilate her concerns and receive medications that may help her with her feelings. The social worker also suggested the patient share some of her feelings with her family and talk about some of the fears and concerns she and her loved ones are facing. Depressive symptoms are frequent and persistent in the geriatric population (5). In a study to determine whether old age is related to the under reporting of depressive symptoms, it was found that many older patients do not report depression (6). A geriatric oncology program looks specifically for these types of problems and provides the necessary interventions so that the older cancer patient can experience optimal health while undergoing cancer therapy.

Goals of a Geriatric Oncology Program

The scope of a geriatric program is multifaceted. In addition to providing individualized care to the older person with cancer the program also concerns itself with clinical research, prevention and screening, and education for the patient, family, health care staff and the community. The effectiveness and feasibility of screening asymptomatic seniors for breast, colorectal and cervical cancers; the removal of barriers to cancer prevention and care; and the study of cancer in the oldest old are of great interest to a geriatric oncology program (7). By pursuing these types of interests and formulating projects to further investigate these topics, better cancer care will be offered to many older people diagnosed with a malignancy. The mission of

Table 60.3 Roles of team members.

Medical Oncologist/Geriatrician is responsible for team interventions and recommendations. Develops treatment plans based on each discipline's assessment. Formulates research plans, assesses funding opportunities and conducts weekly team conferences.

Medical Oncology Fellow provides patient and family care. Conducts both clinical and basic research.

Nurse Practitioner coordinates and plans team activities. Provides patient care. Formulates research proposals, manages data for the program. Coordinates community education/marketing strategies and research projects.

Primary Care Nurse acts as case manager for patient/families within the Program. Provides education and patient support. Orchestrates clinic so that each discipline evaluates the appropriate patient. Acts to communicate medical information between team members.

Social Worker provides psychosocial assessment which includes coping, social networks, financial issues, emotional support, and caregiver support. Conducts depression and dementia assessment. Provides continued ongoing support. Networks with various community agencies.

Dietitian preforms a complete nutritional assessment. Provides diet education including vitamins and nutritional supplements.

Pharmacist evaluates medication that are both over-the-counter and legend drugs. Assesses for harmful drug interactions and provides education regarding these interactions. Communicates with primary care physician regarding possible discontinuation of medication.

a geriatric oncology program is to promote optimal cancer therapy outcomes and prolong the meaningful survival of older persons with cancer.

Developing an Interdisciplinary Geriatric Oncology Team

When deciding what disciplines should make up a geriatric program, it is important to think of the needs of older cancer patients. A registered dietitian, social worker, pharmacist, geriatric nurse practitioner, primary care nurse and a cancer specialist interested in geriatrics, are vital. Together they are able to identify and treat many of the health concerns and syndromes present in older patients. The program cancer specialist may include a medical oncologist, radiation oncologist, surgical oncologist or pain specialist. In the case of the Senior Adult Oncology Program at the H. Lee Moffitt Cancer Center and Research Institute, the only two full time physician members are medical oncologists. Although a geriatric oncology program is an expensive approach to care, the service provided to the patient and family is an important element in the treatment of cancer. Again, as mentioned earlier in the chapter, many of the signs and symptoms an older person experiences do not follow the clinical path of a presenting symptom which yields a diagnosis. Symptoms can be a wide array of possibilities when it comes to making a diagnosis and a complete interdisciplinary team can be pivotal in identifying and correctly treating the older cancer patient.

Geriatric teams need to be composed of team members that have some experience in assessing and treating older people with cancer. Many of the assessment instruments used in geriatrics (ADL, IADL, Mini-Mental State Examination) are specific to geriatrics and not commonly used with other age groups. Interviews with

older people tend to require more time and patience and very often older people require an intricate treatment plan because of complex physical and psychosocial problems. Team members must be aware of these facts and possess the patience and knowledge this process requires.

The Roles Performed by Each Member of a Geriatric Oncology Program

In order for all disciplines to fulfill their roles, collaboration by the entire team becomes extremely important. Program members perform discipline specific assessments, but together they are able to identify and analyze problems, formulate treatment plans and interventions, and monitor follow up care. To make it possible for team members to be effective in their roles, it is important to define the roles in the initial program development process (Table 60.3). When each team member is clear on what piece of the assessment in which they are responsible, the assessment process will run smoother.

For many teams however, roles are blurred and, for example, the primary care nurse may have to instruct the patient on indications of medication instead of the pharmacist. This blurring of roles is a common occurrence, which team members must understand and work together to attain the goals of the established treatment plan. Team members must learn about the roles of other disciplines and how they play a part in the total team function. "Professionals must solidify their own identity to deal with territorial overlap, stereotyping and inappropriate demands" (8). Professionals with no understanding of the models subscribed to by the other team members are more likely to make wrong assumptions about their colleagues' roles and the interventions they recommend. Professionals who function most efficiently and comfortably in team settings are those that respect and acknowledge model differences. Team members who possess a narrow range of flexibility toward other disciplines will be least effective in a team setting (9).

Who Should Be the Team Leader?

The program leader functions to coordinate the work of the team members and to facilitate their interactions. The leader must represent the continuously evolving consciousness of the team as it relates to new advances in cancer therapy and in the understanding of aging and oncological management. Promoting appropriate change in team roles and focuses, encountering budgetary considerations, and administrative concerns are also responsibilities of this position.

Several professionals from different disciplines may be successful team leaders. Whatever discipline or individual is identified for this responsibility, knowledge of current literature and geriatric training is essential. The organizational ability and the time required to fulfill the program obligations is extensive and requires a full time position.

Geriatric Medical Oncologist

The physician works with the team members to provide patient and family care, with attention to cancer care issues and general health issues. Other responsibilities include: formulation of research ideas, assessment of funding opportunities, leadership in weekly patient/family care conferences, implementation of clinical research, and the establishment of general operating plans to provide direction to the entire team.

Geriatric Nurse Practitioner

The role of the geriatric nurse practitioner (GNP) or geriatric nurse specialist (GNS) can be utilized to coordinate team operations. In a busy outpatient geriatric oncology clinic, extensive planning is required to establish a process so each team member can assess the targeted patient/family, communicate the results of the assessment and form a treatment plan. In the case of the Senior Adult Oncology Program at the H. Lee Moffitt Cancer Center and Research Institute, a GNP performs the history and physical, coordinates the CGA and is responsible for documenting the complete interdisciplinary plan in the permanent record. The nurse practitioner also coordinates and initiates many of the community education programs and develops marketing strategies appropriate for the designated target population. With emphasis on research in the area of geriatric oncology, the advanced practice nurse (GNP or CNS) is responsible to coordinate much of the clinical research aspects of the team. Formulation of research proposals, data management and data entry, or coordination of data entry, are well within the scope of this role.

Primary Care Nurse

The role of the primary care nurse (PCN) is that of case manager, and educator. Patient/families are instructed to call the PCN for any issues or concerns they may be experiencing or for diagnostic results. All lab values, diagnostic results and other patient information are directed to the primary care nurse and then are reported to the physician and the rest of the geriatric team. The PCN is responsible to teach the patient/families techniques such as how to care for an infusion port or the importance of reporting potentially harmful signs and symptoms such as a fever. The PCN builds a strong relationship with the patient/families and provides ongoing emotional support. This role is also effective in orchestrating the daily clinic operations and reporting accurate medical information to the program members. The PCN is also responsible for conducting a nursing assessment to obtain information regarding general health and effects of cancer therapy the patient may be experiencing as well as any acute health issues.

Social Worker

A psychosocial evaluation is a large part of a geriatric assessment. Many seniors experience complex psychosocial situations that involve alteration in coping, poor social networks, poor emotional support and financial concerns. These issues for many seniors can be a major hurdle in the treatment of cancer. The social worker is very effective in providing the necessary support and networking with various community agencies to assist in these matters. Screening for depression and dementia can also be included in the role of the social worker. Frequently, instruments such as the Geriatric Depression Scale (GDS) and the Mini-Mental State Examination (MMSE) are very helpful screening tools used to uncover a diagnosis of depression, or dementia possibly caused by medications that may have otherwise gone unnoticed and untreated. The social worker provides an invaluable service by allowing seniors to ventilate concerns and anxieties they may be experiencing due to the diagnosis of cancer.

Dietitian

A complete nutritional assessment, including lab studies and 24-hour dietary intake, can provide information helpful in the treatment of malnutrition. The prevalence of malnutrition in older persons is generally high. Malnutrition has been defined as a decrease in nutrient reserves and up to 15% of ambulatory seniors experience this condition (10). The dietitian educates patients and families to the dietary requirements necessary to sustain, increase or reduce current weight. Nutritional supplements are advised when necessary and ongoing nutritional follow up is continued throughout the cancer treatment process.

Pharmacist

The assessment of medication is an important part of the role performed by a pharmacist in a geriatric oncology service. Approximately 12% of Americans are over the age of 65, and yet this age group consumes 30% of all prescriptions and 40% of all over-the-counter medications (11). The older person usually has a number

Table 60.4

Inpatients that benefit from a CGA	Outpatients that benefit from a CGA.
Patients with potentially treatable problems that are medical, functional, or psychosocial and impair independent living. • confusion • polypharmacy • failure to thrive • abusive home situation	• decreased functional status • falls • confusion • incontinence • death of a spouse • polypharmacy • failure to thrive • use of in-home assistive services • use of adult day-care
Inpatients that do not benefit from a CGA	Outpatients that do not benefit from a CGA
• terminal illness (six months or less) • severe dementia patients without alternative to nursing home placement	• need for urgent hospitalization • absence of any significant functional impairment

of medications prescribed by several physicians, and prescription medication is only part of the problem, as over-the-counter medications and vitamins are also a concern. A complete review of medication, both prescription and over-the-counter agents, including vitamin supplements, is performed. If any changes are recommended, or if the patient has numerous medications, the primary care physician is contacted so a plan can be established. The pharmacist also educates the patient/family regarding medication schedules, interactions, and indications. Again, ongoing pharmacist support is continued throughout the cancer therapy.

Targeting a Population for the Geriatric Oncology Program

We have established that cancer is a disease whose risk increases with age. We also know that the older cancer patient requires a specialized approach to cancer therapy which includes the consideration of issues such as psychosocial concerns, functionality and comorbidities. Now, the question that should be addressed is which older patients would benefit from an interdisciplinary geriatric team? This portion of the chapter will discuss various factors to consider when including patients in a geriatric oncology program.

The CGA has been shown to be effective in both inpatient and outpatient settings. Table 60.4 describes criteria established by a committee composed of members of the American Geriatrics Society and was created for use in Medicare reimbursement issues (12) (Table 60.4).

It has been suggested that the patients in need of a CGA are the "frail elderly" (13). The frail elderly can be defined as older people who are; (a) entering a

nursing home, (b) have experienced repeated hospitalizations, (c) comorbid conditions, (d) functional dependencies, and (e) psychosocial problems. Older people that have been identified as having geriatric syndromes such as falls, polypharmacy, incontinence and malnutrition could also benefit from a CGA.

In the case of geriatric oncology, it is important to perform a CGA on all patients regardless of current health status. For the active, seemingly healthy senior adult, a CGA can detect potentially harmful conditions that may interfere with cancer therapy. A consistent characteristic of aging is a loss in functional reserve. Thus, conditions of stress such as a diagnosis of cancer or cancer therapy, may cause severe functional impairment and loss of independence even in healthy older patients. The CGA is a proactive approach which may prevent or minimize these considerations.

People over 70 represent a very diverse segment of the population and many are extremely active members of society. The Senior Adult Program at the H. Lee Moffitt Cancer Center and Research Institute includes patients that are over the age of 70 and have a diagnosis of cancer. Each patient is initially provided a CGA in addition to attention given the cancer related diagnosis. Follow up care that addresses the geriatric and the oncological aspect of treatment is provided by all team members. Some of the senior adult patients may not require all of the services offered by the program and in those cases, patients are seen regularly by the nurse practitioner and the physician for regular follow-up care and screening for potential problems. Many older people have experienced a diagnosis of cancer but maintain a very active, independent lifestyle. Others are not so fortunate and require total assistance. Each treatment plan takes into account the

Table 60.5 Benefits of a geriatric oncology program.

- Inclusion of older people in clinical trials.
- Comprehensive approach to cancer therapy.
- Reduced mortality.
- Reduced nursing home placement.
- Reduced medical costs.
- Caregiver support.
- Detection of cormorbid conditions

Table 60.6 Barriers to inclusion of older cancer patients in clinical trials.

- Patient/family reluctance
- Physician biased
- Cost
- Lack of information or understanding

variation in health and functional status that exists in the older population.

Benefits of an Interdisciplinary Geriatric Oncology Team

Research has shown that there are many benefits that result from the assessment and intervention of a geriatric team (Table 60.5). The benefits stem from the fact that many disciplines are involved with the patient and family, each performing a specific aspect of the assessment and working together to establish a comprehensive treatment plan. This portion of the chapter will discuss the benefits of instituting a geriatric oncology program.

Inclusion of Older People in Clinical Trials

Research into the widespread problem of the lack of participation among older cancer patients in clinical research is a major goal of a geriatric oncology program. Historically, older people have not been included in clinical trials, and most treatments have been shown to be effective only in younger populations. Clinical protocols especially designed for people over 65 are extremely limited and this information is vital in the treatment of cancer in older patients. A geriatric oncology program can be instrumental in developing clinical protocols and enrolling appropriate subjects to help understand adequate dosing of chemotherapeutic regimes in older patients. Enrolling subjects has always been a considerable challenge in a geriatric population for many reasons. One reason is simply a lack of understanding regarding the meaning of clinical research. Many older patients state they do not want to be "guinea pigs" for any new type of therapy. A geriatric oncology program can take the time to educate the patient and family about the protocol being considered and help dispel the fears and anxieties the family and patient may have.

Another hindrance to the inclusion of older people in clinical trials is physician bias. Many physicians do not prescribe chemotherapy to patients of advanced age and therefore enrollment in clinical trials is not presented as an option. Cost may be another factor that keeps older patients out of clinical trials. Often additional medications, frequent diagnostic tests and evaluations that are necessary for participation in many

protocols are not covered by Health Maintenance Organizations or private insurance and many seniors are then excluded. Education of the patient, family and health care professionals are very important to the enrollment of seniors in clinical protocols and therefore important to geriatric oncology.

Reduced Mortality

Much attention has been given to reduced mortality as a benefit of a comprehensive team approach to geriatrics. One study found that patients admitted to an inpatient geriatric evaluation unit had a lower mortality at one year when compared to patients not assigned to the unit (14). In addition to a lower mortality, the researchers found a reduction in nursing home placement, less inpatient hospital days, and less acute care readmissions. A study conducted to look at the effects of an inpatient geriatric consultation team in a nonacademic environment, found that at 6 months, 12 of the 58 (21%) patients in the control group and 3 out of 62 (6%) patients in the experimental group had died. At one year, 10% of the experimental and 20% of the control patients had died. The patients that underwent the geriatric service experienced a greater functional status and fewer hospital readmissions (15).

As shown in the above studies, specialized geriatric medical care can be an important factor in the treatment of the older adult. In a geriatric oncology setting, a thorough assessment to uncover untreated diagnosis and potential risks from falls or medication interactions may be instrumental in reducing mortality.

Reduced Nursing Home Stay

Nursing home placement is often an appropriate option for many frail elderly. Sometimes however, nursing home placement is premature or inappropriate and other options should be explored. In the case of an older person with cancer, nursing home placement is often a consideration. The number of nursing home admissions was reduced in patients undergoing CGA, which prevented inappropriate admissions, provided rehabilitation and explored other alternatives to long term care (16). For the cancer patient, nursing home placement can be particularly traumatic as it may be perceived that there is an implied anticipation of death from the malignancy. Given the limited life expectancy of the older patient many viable alternatives often exist to nursing home placement by providing support and education to caregivers in the home care setting.

Reduced Hospital Costs

By providing a CGA by an interdisciplinary team to identify and treat various conditions revealed in the assessment, medical costs have been reduced. Rubin looked at inpatients receiving care from a geriatric assessment team and determined they had less hospital charges (17). The patients receiving geriatric care had less total hospital charges and higher home health charges suggesting a shift to home care or outpatient services. Another study conducted to look at the team oriented approach to geriatric assessment versus a traditional approach, showed that patients receiving the team approach realized a 25% reduction in institutional costs (18).

Comprehensive Approach to Cancer Therapy

The many aspects of a comprehensive approach to the older cancer patient have already been identified and discussed thus far in this chapter. One issue that deserves further attention is that of the caregiver assessment. Caregivers have many needs and concerns that also require intervention and support from the team members. Caregivers undergoing a CGA were found to be more likely to report good general health than the caregivers not undergoing the same type of assessment (19). Brown, Potter and Foster performed a study to determine the relationship between caregiver burden and the use of long-term care services and found that caregiver burden is a factor in deciding what patients will request these services (20). In a study conducted to look at the outpatient CGA, it was found that family strain was significantly decreased in families that received outpatient care by a geriatric team (21).

Caregiver concerns are an important aspect to the health of the senior cancer patient. A geriatric oncology program understands this concern and routinely provides both assessment and interventions for the caregiver. In a symposium given at the Gerontological Society of America in 1995 on the topic of stress perceived by caregivers of both dementia patients and cancer patients, it was stated that caregiver stress contributed more to patient stress than did the patient's own physical health (22).

Disadvantages of an Interdisciplinary Team

As cost saving is an advantage of a geriatric oncology team, cost is also a disadvantage. The staff required to provide team services to a single patient/family is significant. The initial visit will usually require 2.5 to 3 hours to preform the necessary assessments and develop the treatment plan. The value however, is realized in the results of the assessment such as possible prevention of acute or urgent situations or frequent hospitalizations. The investment is the amount of time and costs required for the initial assessment and development of the comprehensive treatment plan (Table 60.7).

The duration of the initial assessment may also represent a burden for patient and the family. As previously stated, the CGA requires several hours to

Table 60.7   Disadvantages of a geriatric oncology program

- Expensive
- Longer clinic visits which can be harder on the patients
- Complex clinic coordination

complete and this may be very taxing for many patients. Should the length of time become a major issue, then the assessment may be either trimmed down or divided into different sessions.

Clinic coordination, especially in the ambulatory setting, and the amount of effort required to coordinate an intradisciplinary team may represent a burden even for seasoned managers. Extensive planning is required to formulate a schedule in which each team member is able to provide an initial assessment and generate a treatment plan. Without a formalized schedule and clinic plan, it would be very difficult for at least six team members to conduct their portion of the assessment in a timely manner as to not exhaust the patient and/or violate the amount of time allowed for each patient visit. Good clinic organization is critical to the productive abilities of a geriatric oncology program and proves to be one of the greatest challenges to the implementation of such a service. Team members must arrange their schedules to be present at each geriatric oncology clinic. It is imperative that team members are available to assess patients and offer recommendations at the time of initial evaluation.

Problems Encountered By A Geriatric Oncology Program

Aside from advantages and disadvantages of a geriatric oncology program there can also be problems. One ongoing problem is communication. With so many team members, each performing a different part of the assessment, collaboration must take place, and this is not always easy in a busy ambulatory setting. The following is a case presentation of an example of poor communication between members.

Mrs. M. was a 77 year old lady with a diagnosis of metastatic breast cancer that was diagnosed in 1988 and shortly thereafter underwent treatment with chemotherapy and radiation therapy. In late 1994, Mrs. M. developed melanoma on her skin overlying her right knee. This was excised, but in 1995 she developed recurrence to the left groin which was also excised in the hospital. In 1978, a stroke left Mrs. M. with right hemiparalysis and unable to speak in complete sentences, so she relied on her husband for total care. Mrs. M. was married to her husband for approximately 50 years and they had four children living in the area but did not have much contact with the children or grandchildren. Upon initial assessment by the Senior

Table 60.8   Problems faced by a geriatric oncology program

- Communication between team members.
- Role territorialization among members, which can stimulate discord.

Table 60.9 Communication sheet.

Pharmacist

Medication currently Motrin 200mg PRN, Digoxin 0.125mg QD for arrhythmia, Vitamin A, Vitamin C, OTC Benadryl for sinus pain PRN.

Dietitian

Weight 125lb, Height 5'3". Currently maintaining weight with nutritional intake. Ideal body weight is $12 \pm 10\%$. Usual weight 125lb. No difficulties at this time.

Social Worker

Patient lives with husband of 25 years. She is a retired nurse. Has two supportive children that live locally. States she maintains frequent social interactions and is coping with diagnosis well. Will continue to monitor. Scores on the GDS 0/15, MMSE 30/30.

Nurse Practitioner

History positive for arrhythmia and is currently under treatment by a cardiologist. No allergies no past surgeries. Physical negative. ADL/IADL is independent.

Physician

Treatment plan with Tamoxifen 10mg BID. Will recommendation annual mammogram. Plan to see patient in clinic in one month.

Adult Oncology Program, Mr. M. stated that Mrs. M. could not communicate and therefore he would have to answer the assessment questions on her behalf. Mrs. M. appeared very quite and withdrawn on the many interactions the team had with the couple. On several occasions Mr. M. would display anger and aggressive behavior toward team members individually, when confronted about this behavior, Mr. M. would become tearful and apologetic. After several weeks of this inconsistent behavior, the team began to communicate these inappropriate interactions to other members of the program and realized that as the patient began to gradually decompensate and grow closer to death, these behaviors exhibited by Mr. M. became more violent. Several days before death, the patient was admitted to the inpatient service for a diagnosis of pneumonia. A social worker, not knowing that Mr. M. had announced that the patient was unable to communicate, sensed something was bothering the patient and began to speak directly to Mrs. M. while Mr. M. was not present in the room. Upon further assessment, the patient indicated through consistent "yes" and "no" answers that something was harming her at home. A speech pathologist was able to help the social worker discover that Mr. M. had been the source of the patients harm and that she was afraid to return home with her husband. When Mr. M. was confronted about these allegations, he became extremely abusive, threatening the nursing staff and accusing the social worker of manipulating the patient into reporting the information. HRS then had to be notified and after an investigation, it was revealed that the children had been afraid of Mr. M. for many years and that he had been abusive to his entire family. It was also found that Mr. M. had murdered his father for abusing his mother many years ago. After these dramatic events took place and this story unfolded, Mrs. M. died quietly in her sleep in the presence of her children while in the hospital. A conference directly following Mrs. M's death, was called to process the unfortunate incidents that had taken place. After review, it was found that each team member was aware of Mr. M's aggressive, inappropriate behavior but did not communicate this information to each other. It was also assumed that the patient was unable to communicate, which was not the case. After this case, relevant information regarding caregivers is communicated and patients are psychosocially assessed without the presence of the caregiver.

This case shows the importance of complete communication between team members. This overall situation may not have been avoided if each team member

reported that Mr. M. had shown aggressive behavior or had acted inappropriately, but better communication may have prevented the situation to have become as acute. As a result of this case, it is now standard practice for the Senior Adult Oncology Program to perform a segment of the psychosocial assessment without the presence of the caregiver or family. Patients may be more likely to discuss matters that are of personal concern or issues they feel are likely to upset the family as a result of this privacy. Appropriate information concerning the family and caregivers should be detailed in the psychosocial report provided by the social worker to ensure adequate interventions are included in the treatment plan.

Communication difficulties can also become evident during the initial patient evaluation when each discipline is performing their part of the CGA. Interventions such as a communication sheet, which is a form used by all disciplines to record observations, assessments' results, diagnostic results, and recommendations. This equips the physician and the rest of the team, with a brief summary of relevant information on which to base the comprehensive treatment plan. The following figure provides an example of what information is included on the communication sheet (Table 60.9).

Another intervention to improve communication is a weekly team meeting. In this meeting, patients and families are presented to the entire program and decisions are formulated regarding further treatment options, referral to community services, psychosocial interventions and treatment outcomes. Each member will give report on their portion of the treatment plan and note where further additional follow up is necessary. Any problems that arise are also discussed so the team can work together to provide the best possible care for the patient and the family.

Table 60.10

Advantages.	Disadvantages	Problems
Enroll seniors in clinical trials	Expensive	Inadequate communication
Comprehensive approach to cancer therapy	Clinic visits are linger which can be harder on the patient and family	Role confusion among team members which may produce discord
Reduced nursing home placement	Complex clinic coordination	

Role territorialization is another problem for any intradisciplinary team. As mentioned earlier in this chapter, role blurring is a concept in which issues can be assessed and intervened upon by several team members that are within their scope of practice. For instance, the primary care nurse may be asked whether a particular type of nutritional supplement should be used. The nurse may feel comfortable in giving a recommendation without consulting the dietitian. This happens frequently in an interdisciplinary setting and it becomes a problem when a team member may feel his or her territory has been invaded. This territorialization may be avoided by educating the team members that blurring does, and will occur, and to the importance of communication between team members. When recommendations are provided by team members other than the discipline primarily responsible for the particular aspect of the care, report must then be communicated. This will diminish any confusion amongst team members about how and why various interventions were established.

Comprehensive Geriatric Assessment for Use in a Geriatric Oncology Program

Each geriatric setting can modify a CGA to fit the needs of the patient population. A geriatric oncology program uses the CGA as an instrument for the detection of geriatric concerns in addition to the specific assessments required of the cancer diagnosis. A CGA usually contains a thorough history and physical, functional assessment, depression and a cognition screening instrument. In the case of the oncology assessment, it can be expanded to include questionnaires regarding coping, quality of life, pain, social network or general emotional status. For clinicians, time is usually a consideration, especially in the ambulatory setting, so the instruments included in the CGA must be easily administered and require a short amount of time to complete. Many of the questionnaires can be mailed to the patients prior to the initial assessment and brought to the clinic for the initial evaluation .

The purpose of the CGA, as used by an intradisciplinary program, is to act as a tool to guide the holistic evaluation and bring together the many different aspects of this type of assessment. Components of the CGA can also function as a measure of treatment outcomes established by the program. An example is the following case history.

Mrs. B. is an 85 year old lady with a diagnosis of iron deficiency anemia. She presents to the Senior Adult Oncology Program for monitoring and treatment of this diagnosis and for a new onset of confusion. The patient had recently come to live with her granddaughter in Florida from Ohio where she has lived all of her life. A CGA revealed that patient required minimal assistance in performing her activities of daily living and moderate assistance performing instrumental activities of daily living. The depression screening instrument did not screen positive for depression, but the cognition instrument did indicate dementia with a score of 22/30. Upon assessment by the Senior Adult Oncology pharmacist, the patient was found to be taking 13 medications, many prescribed by various physicians while she lived in Ohio. After several return visits to the clinic and contact with the primary care physician in Ohio, 3/4 of the patient's medications were discontinued. During this time, Mrs. B. was slowly readjusting to her environment and life with her granddaughter and other family members, as her family states she continued to become less confused. Upon reassessment using the cognition screening instrument, the patient's score had greatly increased from, 22/30 to 27/30. Mrs. B's granddaughter reported that the patients is much more alert and oriented and able resume many of her normal activities. The Senior Adult Oncology Program continues to monitor the patient's anemia, psychosocial status, as well as her general health status.

In this case, Mrs B. most likely suffered from a disorientation caused by her relocation from Ohio, and the geriatric syndrome of polypharmacy. Mrs. B. was taking a great many medications, most of which she had collected over the years and neither she nor her family had any idea why these medications were continued. After gathering information from Mrs. B's primary care physician, and reviewing her medical history, many of the medications were discontinued and her dementia lessened considerably. The CGA coordinated the collection of this data from the patient, family and local physician so a treatment plan could be established. The cognitive screening instrument was used as an empiric indicator regarding the patient's improved mental status.

After the team retrieves all of this information, it is important for all the team members to agree on how to interpret the instruments. Each instrument has its own score and norms that warrant interpretation. The team then has to decide how to proceed after a patient or caregiver screens for cognition problems, decreased functional status, depression or one of the other psychosocial indicators. It is important to be clear on the parameters specific to each instrument and what further techniques or consultations could be utilized to further diagnose and treat any conditions that may be uncovered.

Example of a Geriatric Oncology Program

The Senior Adult Oncology Program (SAOP) at the H. Lee Moffitt Cancer Center and Research Institute began seeing patients in August of 1994. During the first year of operation 235 patients and families were offered a comprehensive approach to cancer treatment. Of those 235 patients, 109 had a diagnosis of breast cancer, 25 colon cancer, 22 prostate cancer, 22 lymphoma, 7 leukemia, 6 pancreatic cancer and the rest were cancers of unknown origin and various other malignancies. Approximately 50% continued with the SAOP for cancer treatment and follow up appointments, and the rest presented for second opinion consultation. Most of the patients included in the SAOP were found to be independent upon assessment of functional status using Katz ADL and Lawton IADL scales. As cancer therapy progressed, many patients required assistance with 2 or more activities of daily living. Using the GDS, 76% (99/130) scored <5, which does not indicate depression, however 18% (24/130) did screen positive for depression and required further evaluation. Using the Mini-Mental State Examination (MMSE) to screen for cognition problems, it was found that 73% (77/105), screened negative for dementia and that 27% (28/105) did show some dementia. Approximately half (60%) of the SAOP live with a spouse, 20% live with an adult child and 14% live alone. The average number of medications was 4.3 and 80% of the patients were prescribed more than 3 drugs. Approximately 35% of the patients suffered from some type of malnutrition.

The disciplines that make up the SAOP are a medical oncologist, who also functions as the team leader, a medical oncology receiving advanced training in geriatric oncology, with a special interest in geriatrics, a nurse practitioner, registered nurse, dietitian, pharmacist and a social worker. These disciplines work together to provide care to patients and families that are over the age of 70 and who have a diagnosis of cancer. Unlike many programs at the cancer center, the SAOP does not define a patient population according to disease site, but to age and functional status. Because of this selection criteria, the SAOP sees patients with many different types of malignancies and cancer issues.

Patients in need of an initial examination are scheduled for one day selected as the "new patient" day, and are routinely assessed by each discipline represented in the SAOP. Patients are contacted before their initial visit both by letter and by telephone to provide information as to what to expect during their visit, and what medical records are essential they obtain and bring with them. Treatment plans are established and many times initiated immediately prior to the initial visit for patients that plan to receive treatment with the SAOP. For patients presenting for a second opinion consultation, recommendations are provided and communication via telephone, and/or letter is directed to the primary care physician or local oncologist. All patients are encouraged to use the SAOP as a resource for any information regarding cancer, regardless of where they receive cancer treatment.

Aside from clinical duties, the SAOP is an active part of the community, providing educational programs to senior centers and organizations. Sensitivity training is an important part of the educational service, and is helpful to health care staff that care for the aged.

Many departments with the University of South Florida interact with the SAOP for purposes of research studies and for student internships. Students get a look at interdisciplinary team functioning, interviewing techniques, clinical skills and management responsibilities. Work is continuing with the Florida Mental Health Institute in the Department of Aging and Mental Services to study caregiver stress and interactions between caregivers, of dementia patients and cancer patients. The Department of Sociology is currently involved in writing personal narratives of patients and their caregivers about their experiences as a cancer patient and/or caregiver of a cancer patient to be used as training exercises for medical and nursing students and to offer patients and caregivers an insight into the lives of other people that have been affected by cancer. Frequently, the Department of Gerontology is consulted for projects concerning the older person with cancer. Projects regarding quality of life, pain assessment in the older population, and caregiver stress are currently being conducted and regular research meeting are held for the formulation of ideas that would improve the care of the older person with cancer.

Summary

Cancer is mainly a disease of the older person and it is therefore important to provide specialized care to this segment of the population. The diversity of the geriatric population mandates individualized treatment programs based on a intradisciplinary assessment of the patient. A geriatric oncology program consists of a team of disciplines that function together to provide a comprehensive approach to the geriatric oncology patient. This service can be provided as an inpatient or an outpatient service and include a physician, primary care nurse, nurse practitioner, dietitian, pharmacist and a social worker. The goals of the geriatric oncology program are to provide a holistic assessment, looking not only at the diagnosis of cancer, but at other health issues as well. Research regarding cancer therapies in the aged, prevention and screening, and community education are also goals of a geriatric oncology program in addition to improved outcomes of cancer and patient satisfaction.

A Geriatric Oncology Program is a team of professionals that specialize in the care of the older person with cancer. A program should include a medical oncologist, a primary nurse, a geriatric nurse practitioner, a social worker, a dietitian, and a pharmacist. These professionals work together, assessing, treating and monitoring patients and families throughout the cancer therapy process.

In general, the CGA was found beneficial mostly for the "frail" elderly. In the case of cancer patients, a comprehensive assessment may be beneficial to all patients over 70. Benefits derived from a geriatric program are reduced mortality, reduced nursing home stay, reduced medical costs, caregiver support, and detection of comorbid conditions.

Developing an interdisciplinary geriatric oncology program involves identifying disciplines that can contribute to the needs of the older person with cancer. Team members must be experienced with the assessment instruments commonly used in geriatrics and possess the patience and understanding this speciality requires. It is important to identify the roles of each discipline involved with a geriatric program. Each team members must understand that role blurring and flexibility are beneficial to the function of the team.

Conclusion

As the senior adult population increases, the need for health care designed for the older adult is necessary. Interdisciplinary geriatric oncology programs can provide a specialized aspect to cancer therapy in the effort to improve the meaningful survival of the older person with cancer. A geriatric oncology program requires commitment from both the facility and the individuals that make up the program. This type of commitment in the area of geriatric medicine will provide patients and families with excellent cancer care while answering some pressing research questions.

References

1. Yancik R, Ries L, Yales J. Breast cancer in aging women, population based study of contrasts in stage, surgery and survival. *Cancer* 1989; **63**: 976–981.
2. Balducci L. Perspectives on quality of life of older patients with cancer. *Drugs and Aging* 1994; **4(4)**: 313–324.
3. Goodwin JS, Hunt WC, Samet JM. A population-based study of functional status and social support networks of elderly patients newly diagnosed with cancer. *Archives of Internal Medicine* 1991; **151**: 366–370.
4. Fried LP, Storer DJ, King DE, Lodder F. Diagnosis of illness presentation in the elderly. *Journal of the American Geriatrics Society* 1991; **39(2)**: 117–123.
5. Callahan CM, Hui SL, Nieaber NA, Musick BS, Tierney WM. Longitudinal study of depression and health services use among elderly primary care patients. *Journal of the American Geriatrics Society* 1994; 42 (8): 833–838.
6. Lyness JM, Cox C, Curry J, Conwell, Y, King DA, Caine ED. Older age and the under reporting of depressive symptoms. *Journal of the American* 1995; *Geriatrics Society* **43(3)**: 216–221.
7. Balducci L, Cox CE, Greenburg H, Lyman GH, Miguel R, Karl R Fabri D. Management of cancer in the older person. *Cancer Control* 1994; **1 (2)**: 132–137.
8. Robertson D. The roles of health care teams in the care of the elderly. *Family Medicine* 1992; **24**: 136–141.
9. Qualls SH, Czirr R. Geriatric health teams: Classifying models of professional and team functioning. *Gerontologist* 1988; **28 (3)**: 372–376.
10. Beck JC. Geriatrics Review Syllabus. *A core Curriculum in Geriatric Medicine*. New York: American Geriatric Society, 1991.
11. Drake AC, Romano E. How to protect your older patient from the hazards of polypharmacy. *Nursing 95* 1995; **25 (6)**: 34–39.
12. Rubenstein LZ, Goodwin M, Hardley E, Patten SK, Rempusheski VF, Reuben D, Winagrad CH. Working group recommendations: Targeting criteria for geriatric evaluation and management research. *Journal of the American Geriatric Society* 1991; **39Supp**: 37S–41S.
13. Beghe' C, Robinson BE. Comprehensive geriatric assessment: Diagnostic, therapeutic and prognostic value. *Cancer Control* 1994; **1(2)** 121–125.
14. Rubenstein LZ, Josephson KR, Wieland GD, English PA, Sayre JA, Kane RL. Effectiveness of a geriatric evaluation unit. *The New England Journal of Medicine* 1984; **311 (26)**: 1664–1670.
15. Thomas DR, Brahan R, Haywood BP. Inpatient community-based geriatric assessment reduces subsequent mortality. *Journal of the American Geriatrics Society* 1993; **41**: 101–104.
16. Brumer CD, Kohm CA, Naglie G, Skekter-Wolfson L, Zorzitto ML, O'Rouke K, Kirkland JL. Do geriatric programs decrease long-term use of acute care beds? *Journal of the American Geriatric Society* 1995; **43**: 885–889
17. Rubin DC, Sizemore MT, Loftis PA, Adams-Huet B, Anderson. The effect of geriatric evaluation and management on Medicare reimbursement in a large public hospital: A randomized clinical trial. *Journal of the American Geriatric Society* 1992; **Q (10)**: 989–995.
18. Williams ME, Williams F, Zimer JG, Hall WJ, Podgorski CA. How does the team approach to outpatient geriatric evaluation compare with traditional care: A report of a randomized controlled trial. *Journal of the American Geriatric Society* 1987; **35 (12)**: 1071–1078.
19. Silliman RA, McGarvey ST, Raymond PM, Fretwell MD. The senior care study: Does inpatient interdisciplinary geriatric assessment help the family caregivers of acutely ill older patients? *Journal of the American Geriatrics Society* 1990; **38 (4)**: 461–466.
20. Brown LJ, Potter JF, Foster BG. Caregiver burden should be evaluated during geriatric assessment. *Journal of the American Geriatric Society* 1990; **38 (4)**: 455–460.
21. Silverman M, Musa D, Martin DC, Lave JR, Adams J, Ricci ME. Evaluation of outpatient geriatric assessment: A randomized multi-site trial. *Journal of the American Geriatrics Society* 1995; **43**: 733–740.
22. Parr J. In J Parr (chair), A new look a multidimensional assessment of older persons in medical settings: Different foci in different settings. Symposium conducted at the meeting of the American Gerontological Society of American. Los Angles, November 1995.

Index

360   PO# 163800 $180.99 US